Advances in Haptics

Edited by

Mehrdad Hosseini Zadeh

Advances in Haptics
Edited by Mehrdad Hosseini Zadeh

Republished by InTech
Janeza Trdine 9, 51000 Rijeka, Croatia

Additional hard copies can be obtained from orders@intechopen.com

Advances in Haptics,
Edited by Mehrdad Hosseini Zadeh
p. cm.
ISBN 978-953-307-093-3

For EU product safety concerns:
IN TECH d.o.o., Prolaz Marije Krucifikse Kozulić 3, 51000 Rijeka, Croatia,
info@intechopen.com or visit our website at intechopen.com.

Preface

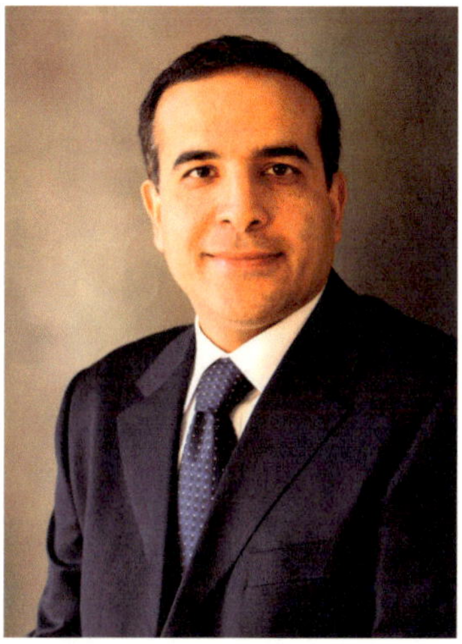

In everyday life, we use our senses to interact with the environment. We can see, touch, smell, hear and taste the external world surrounding us through interactions that usually occur with an initial contact between an organism and its environment.

Particularly, we have physical experiences such as texture, stiffness, and resistance to movement through our sense of touch. To experience these in virtual environments (VEs), computer interfaces are required to enable us to interact with virtual objects. Haptic technology enables computer users to touch and/or manipulate virtual or remote objects in virtual environments or tele-operation systems. If haptic cues (e.g., touch sensations) are displayed in addition to visual and auditory cues, these VEs are called haptic-enabled virtual environments.

Haptic interfaces are divided into two main categories: force feedback and tactile. Force feedback interfaces are used to explore and modify remote/virtual objects in three physical dimensions in applications including computer-aided design, computer-assisted surgery, and computer-aided assembly. Tactile interfaces deal with surface properties such as roughness, smoothness, and temperature.

Haptic research is intrinsically multi-disciplinary, incorporating computer science/engineering, control, robotics, psychophysics, and human motor control. By extending the scope of research in haptics, advances can be achieved in existing applications such as computer-aided design (CAD), tele-surgery, rehabilitation, scientific visualization, robot-assisted surgery, authentication, and graphical user interfaces (GUI), to name a few.

Advances in Haptics presents a number of recent contributions to the field of haptics. Authors from around the world present the results of their research on various issues in the field of haptics. The contributions are organized in five sections:

Section I deals with the design, control, and analysis of haptic interfaces. Issues such as stability and achievable performance of haptic interfaces are addressed. Stability is one of the main issues in the control of haptic interfaces. Instability might cause an undesirable feeling to the user and unrealistic interaction with the virtual environment. Stability and achievable performance of a haptic system are among the fundamental indices for evaluation of a high-precision stable haptic rendering.

In Section II, several important issues are addressed in the haptic rendering of haptic-enabled VEs. The contributed chapters in this section deal with the development and enhancement of algorithms and software associated with generating, transmitting, and rendering the feel of virtual objects.

Section III covers several human factors studies that investigate the effects of various factors on user perception and performance in various applications of haptics. Haptic applications require interactions between humans and computers. Due to the complexity and variability of the user's physical motion, it is difficult to generate a precise mathematical description of human motor control behavior. In addition, to ensure that VEs are compatible with users, VE designers need knowledge about human perception to obtain an understanding of design constraints influenced by sensory perception. Thus, human factors studies are required to recognize the limitations and capabilities of the user.

Section IV presents topics focusing on various aspects of the haptic interaction between humans and computers. An understanding of the nature of user-computer interaction is essential for the design of haptic interfaces. Several interaction issues are investigated to ensure the effectiveness of haptic interfaces. The results of these studies can improve the design of usable and effective haptic interfaces.

Finally, Section V presents recent selected applications in the field of haptics.

Mehrdad Hosseini Zadeh, Ph.D
Grand Blanc, Michigan
April 2010

Contents

Preface V

I. Haptic Interfaces: Design, Control, and Analysis

1. Novel Actuation Methods for High Force Haptics 001
Stephen P. Buerger and Neville Hogan

2. Using Magnetic Levitation for Haptic Interaction 031
Peter Berkelman and Michael Dzadovsky

3. Solving the Correspondence Problem in Haptic/Multisensory Interface Design 047
Charles Spence, Mary K. Ngo, Ju-Hwan Lee and Hong Tan

4. Cartesian Control of a Cable-Driven Haptic Mechanism 075
Martin J.D. Otis, Vincent Duchaine, Greg Billette, Simon Perreault, Clément Gosselin and Denis Laurendeau

5. Stability Boundary and Transparency for Haptic Rendering 103
Iñaki Díaz, Jorge Juan Gil and Thomas Hulin

6. Implementation of a Wireless Haptic Controller for Humanoid Robot Walking 127
Eun-Su Kim, Man-Seok Kim, Johwan Kim, Sang Woo Kim and Jong-Wook Kim

7. Head-Tracking Haptic Computer Interface for the Blind 143
Simon Meers and KorenWard

8. Passivity-based Analysis and Design of Multi-contact Haptic Systems via LMIs 155
Gianni Bianchini, Marcello Orlandesi and Domenico Prattichizzo

9. Analysis and Experimental Study of a 4-DOF Haptic Device 171
Ma and Payandeh

10. A Haptically Enhanced Operational Concept for a Hydraulic Excavator 199
Henning Hayn and Dieter Schwarzmann

11. Five Fingers Haptic Interface Robot HIRO: Design, Rendering, and Applications 221
Osama Halabi and Haruhisa Kawasaki

12. Optimal Design of Haptic Interfaces 241
Volkan Patoglu and Aykut Cihan Satici

13. Transparent and Shaped Stiffness Reflection for Telesurgery 259
BertWillaert, Pauwel Goethals, Dominiek Reynaerts, Hendrik Van Brussel and Emmanuel B. Vander Poorten

14. Mechanism Design of Haptic Devices 283
Han Sung Kim

II. Computer Haptics and Haptic Rendering

15. Haptic-Based 3D Carving Simulator 299
Gabriel Telles O'Neill, Won-Sook Lee and Jeff William

16. Manipulation of Dynamically Deformable Object using Impulse-Based Approach 315
Kazuyoshi Tagawa, Koichi Hirota and Michitaka Hirose

17. Haptic Interaction with Complex Models Based on Precomputations 333
Igor Peterlík and Luděk Matyska and Jiří Filipovič

18. A Haptic Modeling System 357
Jeha Ryu and Hyungon Kim

19. Haptic Data Transmission based on the Prediction and Compression 375
Yonghee You and Mee Young Sung

III. Human Factors

20. Digitizing literacy: reflections on the haptics of writing 385
Anne Mangen and Jean-Luc Velay

21. Kinesthetic Illusion of Being Pulled Sensation Enables Haptic Navigation for Broad Social Applications 403
Tomohiro Amemiya, Hideyuki Ando and Taro Maeda

22. Perceptual Issues Improve Haptic Systems Performance 415
Marco Vicentini and Debora Botturi

23. Temporal perception of visual-haptic events in multimodal telepresence system 437
Zhuanghua Shi, Heng Zou and Hermann J. Müller

24. On the Influence of Hand Dynamics on Motion Planning of Reaching Movements in Haptic Environments 451
Igor Goncharenko, Mikhail Svinin, Shigeyuki Hosoe and Sven Forstmann

25. Haptic touch and hand ability 463
Miriam Ittyerah

26. Force Scaling as a Function of Object Mass when Lifting with Peripheral Fatigue 481
James C. Larmer, Camille Williams and Heather Carnahan

27. Neuromuscular Analysis as a Guideline in designing Shared Control 499
Abbink D.A. and Mulder M.

28. Factors Affecting the Perception-Based Compression of Haptic Data 517
Mehrdad Hosseini Zadeh, David Wang and Eric Kubica

IV. Haptic Interaction

29. Real-Time Support of Haptic Interaction by Means of Sampling-Based Path Planning 543
Michael Strolz and Martin Buss

30. Sensory Properties in Fusion of Visual/Haptic Stimuli Using Mixed Reality 565
Itaru Kitahara, Morio Nakahara and Yuichi Ohta

31. Expanding the Scope of Instant Messaging with Bidirectional Haptic Communication 583
Youngjae Kim and Minsoo Hahn

32. Realistic Haptics Interaction in Complex Virtual Environments 603
Hanqiu SUN and Hui CHEN

V. Selected Haptic Applications

33. Mapping Workspaces to Virtual Space in Work Using Heterogeneous Haptic Interface Devices 621
Ayano Tatematsu and Yutaka Ishibashi

34. Collaborative Tele-Haptic Application and Its Experiments 637
Qonita M. Shahab, Maria N. Mayangsari and Yong-Moo Kwon

35. Using Haptic Technology to Improve Non-Contact Handling: the "Haptic Tweezer" Concept 649
Ewoud vanWest, Akio Yamamoto and Toshiro Higuchi

36. Haptics and the Biometric Authentication Challenge 675
Andrea Kanneh and Ziad Sakr

37. Haptic virtual reality assembly – Moving towards Real Engineering Applications 693
T. Lim, J.M. Ritchie, R. Sung, Z. Kosmadoudi, Y. Liu and A.G. Thin

1

Novel Actuation Methods for High Force Haptics

Stephen P. Buerger and Neville Hogan
Massachusetts Institute of Technology
United States of America

1. Introduction

Most haptic devices are intended primarily, if not exclusively, to exchange information with a human operator, and often replace or augment traditional computer displays with backdrivable, force-producing tactile interfaces. This includes popular commercial devices such as the PHANTOM (Massie & Salisbury, 1994) that are typically limited to at most several Newtons of endpoint force capacity, just enough to display simple virtual environments to the operator. Less conventional wearable haptic devices operate differently, but similarly have a low force capacity sufficient only to convey information (e.g. see devices described in (Biggs & Srinivasan, 2002)). By contrast, a class of applications that we refer to as *high force haptics* requires devices that exchange significant forces (and sometimes power) with an operator, often up to and exceeding the force to move limbs or even large fractions of body weight. While achieving high forces, these devices must also present low mechanical endpoint impedance to the operator (i.e. be backdrivable or feel "gentle") in order to avoid injury and, frequently, to exchange information with the operator by representing virtual environments. We propose the following working definition:

> *High force haptic device:* A mechanical device for physical interaction with humans in one or more degrees of freedom that can actively produce controlled force and motion comparable to the capability of the limbs it interacts with and can be back-driven over the same motion range by forces much less than the capacity of the same limbs.

This definition is not intended to be rigid or comprehensive but to provide a framework to elucidate the challenges of developing devices with high force capacity and low mechanical endpoint impedance capable of rendering virtual environments. "Force" and "motion" are considered here to be generalized quantities that include force and position as well as their derivatives or integrals, which are often important. For instance, velocity is important to accommodate typical limb motion, and the rate of change of force is important to display impact-like experiences. This applies to controlled outputs from the devices as well as to backdriving. "Comparable to" means exceeding X% of (force and motion capabilities of relevant limbs), where X is as close to 100 as practical—often tens to hundreds of Newtons or more. "Much less than" means less than Y%, where Y << X; in fact the ratio X/Y is a key measure of high force haptic performance, and maximizing this ratio is the central challenge.

The application of robots to provide sensory-motor physiotherapy is a flagship application of high force haptics, and provides an instructive example of the engineering challenges unique to this emerging area. The ultimate goal is to promote, enhance and accelerate recovery after any injury that affects motor behavior. Common examples include stroke (cerebral vascular accident) (Volpe et al., 2009) and cerebral palsy (Krebs et al., 2009). Scientific and clinical evidence has shown that movement of the affected limbs is a key element of the recovery process. The compromised ability to move that immediately follows injury such as stroke may lead to permanent motor disability if left unaddressed, even though the peripheral neural, muscular and skeletal system is intact, a phenomenon that has been termed "learned non-use" (Taub and Uswatte, 2006; Wolf et al., 2006). In the case of cerebral palsy, unaddressed motor deficits also interfere with a child's development, leading to severe, permanent motor disability. In contrast, studies (Nudo, 2007) have shown that activity-dependent neural plasticity can offset these degenerative trends and, in some cases, even reverse them.

The process of recovery resembles motor learning (Hogan et al., 2006) though there are notable differences, such as abnormal muscle tone or spasticity, that do not occur in motor learning. Providing a high "dosage" or "intensity" of movement experience (many repetitions) is one of the ways robotic tools may augment conventional physiotherapy. However, repetition alone is not enough: voluntary participation is essential (Volpe et al., 2004). To ensure voluntary participation, the machine must assist only as needed. Even more important, the machine must not suppress any productive movements a patient can make. It must "get out of the way" of appropriate movements while gently resisting inappropriate movements; *guidance* is more important than *assistance* (Krebs et al., 2003). The requirement to provide permissive guidance—encouraging "good" movements while discouraging "bad" movements—is perhaps the most important distinction between therapeutic robotics and assistive technologies such as amputation prostheses, powered orthoses, etc. The latter compensate for a motor deficit; the former attempt to ameliorate it.

This may account for the contrasting results to date with upper-extremity and lower-extremity robotic therapy. Robotic treatment of upper-extremity stroke-related motor disorders has consistently succeeded, typically providing more than twice the benefit of conventional therapy alone (Kwakkel et al., 2007; Prange et al., 2006). It has even proven beneficial for stroke survivors in the "chronic phase", many years after injury, when all recovery had apparently ceased. In contrast, clinical studies to date have shown that robotic treatment of lower-extremity motor disorders is about half as effective as conventional approaches (Hidler et al., 2009; Hornby et al., 2008). This may be due, in part, to the relatively smaller number of clinical studies but it may also be due to the fact that early lower-extremity therapy robots were designed to impose motion rather than provide guidance (Neckel et al., 2008; Israel et al., 2006). More recent designs for locomotor therapy have begun to address the formidable challenge of providing highly "back-drivable" (low impedance) interaction (Roy et al., 2009; Veneman et al., 2007) while supporting substantial fractions of body weight (Roberts, 2004).

Additional examples of high force haptic applications include human-assistive and exoskeletal devices (Guizzo & Goldstein, 2005, Kazerooni & Guo, 1993), physically cooperative man-machine systems (Peshkin et al., 2001) and similar applications. Like these other high force haptic devices, successful therapy robots must simultaneously embody a formidable set of capabilities, usually including all of the following:

1) The capacity to deliver large forces, sufficient to move human limbs actively against strong muscular effort by the subject (e.g. due to abnormal tone), and in some cases (e.g. balance & locomotion) to support substantial fractions of body weight
2) The ability to represent controlled, virtual environments (e.g. virtual walls or springs), in order to provide physical guidance, assistance (but only as needed), protection from force spikes, resistance (e.g. for strength training), and to communicate information
3) The ability to be backdriven, to avoid inhibiting a patient or operator's attempts to move or observe the outcomes of these efforts
4) Large workspaces, up to a cubic meter or more, to accommodate the range of motion of human limbs
5) A number and arrangement of degrees of freedom compatible with large and small scale human movement
6) Guaranteed stability and safety while exchanging significant force and power with non-expert, impaired and unpredictable human subjects

In contrast, most existing haptic and robotic systems embody some subset of this list of features, but not all. More specifically, most existing robotic devices have either low force capacity with low mechanical impedance or high force capacity with high intrinsic impedance. Achieving this full set of features is a formidable engineering challenge that is limited by existing actuator and control technologies.

In this chapter we provide an overview of the tools available to address the high force haptic challenge by summarizing and critiquing available techniques, discussing several advanced approaches that show promise, and presenting a novel actuator architecture that may provide a superior solution for certain high force haptic applications. In the next section performance and stability considerations for high force haptic systems are summarized. Section 3 discusses the utility of available actuator and interaction control technologies for high force haptics. Section 4 introduces a novel hybrid actuator architecture that circumvents the fundamental limitations plaguing actuators for high force haptics. Analysis and experimental validation of a simple example are included. Concluding remarks are provided in Section 5. The prior and novel work presented here provides the foundation of a nascent toolkit of methods to design and build effective high force haptic machines.

2. Performance and Stability of High Force Haptic Systems

Haptic systems consist of a union between an engineered mechanical system (a haptic device) and a human operator. While haptic devices and robots both include actuators, sensors, control software, and mechanisms designed to achieve particular kinematics, haptics differ from most common robots because the physical coupling to an unknown and unpredictable human subject has a strong influence, by design, on the system's behavior. From a control standpoint, this significantly influences how both performance and stability are understood. For a traditional motion-controlled robotic system, performance is measured by the system's ability to track trajectories or move to locations in space. Stability is determined by the robot and its controller, possibly with consideration of static payloads.

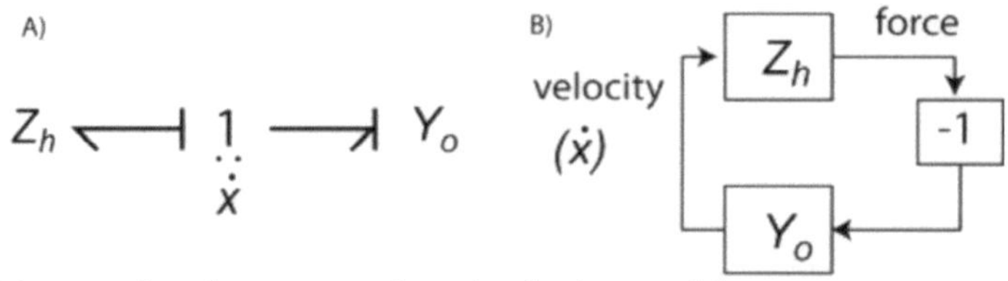

Fig. 1. Physical interaction between a haptic device and human operator, represented by port functions. A) Bond graph representation. B) Block diagram representation.

For haptic devices, the considerations are quite different. Rather than control motion, haptic devices are intended to represent virtual objects, meaning that they must convincingly transition between apparent free motion and apparent contact with objects with specified physical properties. Performance is best understood as the quality of the virtual environment, or the "feel" presented to the operator by the haptic device. Furthermore, the operator is a dynamic system that is physically coupled to the haptic device. A critical distinction between typical robots and haptic devices is as follows: In robotic systems, performance and stability are both properties of the robot. In haptic systems, including high force haptic systems, performance is solely a property of the haptic device, while stability depends on *both* the human operator and the haptic device. This indicates that traditional methods of analyzing the performance and stability of robotic systems are not ideally suited to analyzing high force haptic systems.

A proven method for analyzing physically coupled systems uses *port functions* to model energy flow between systems at physical points of interaction, or *power ports* (Hogan & Buerger, 2005). Port functions define the behavior of each system in terms of the relationship between conjugate "effort" and "flow" power variables, depending on causality. Impedance (Z) provides the effort output in response to a flow input, while admittance (Y) is the inverse. In the mechanical domain, force (or torque) is the effort variable while velocity (or angular velocity) is the flow variable. Figure 1 shows two interacting systems: a haptic system represented by its impedance (Z_h) and a human operator represented by its admittance (Y_o). In this representation, the direction of power flow is purely a matter of convention; it is depicted as positive into each system. No assumption is required regarding the magnitude of either the impedance or admittance port functions.

The performance of the haptic device can be derived from its port impedance, which can be loosely thought of as dynamic stiffness, can be linear or nonlinear, and includes stiffness, inertia, friction and other dynamic behaviors, e.g. modes of vibration. Specifically, the intended feel at the interface can be represented by some virtual environment, which can be quantified by some impedance function, which may be linear or nonlinear and may vary in space and time. Performance can then be quantified by measuring the difference between the target impedance (or the target virtual environment) and that achieved in hardware. Phenomena that may detract from this performance can include unwanted inertia, compliance, or friction as well as unhelpful or distracting vibrations. This is consistent with the definitions of "fidelity" found in the haptics literature. A related performance metric, "transparency," generally refers to only the quality of the haptic hardware and its ability to minimize or disguise parasitic dynamics that are not part of the software-generated virtual environment (Carignan & Cleary, 2000). Specific high force haptic applications may benefit from differing performance metrics based on the port impedance. For instance, when port impedance is linear or can be approximated as such, performance can be defined as a cost function C that consists of a frequency-weighted integral of the difference between the magnitudes of the actual (Z) and target (Z_{targ}) impedance functions (normalized to 1 Ns/m to make the argument of the log dimensionless), yielding a single number to minimize:

$$C = \int_{\omega_0}^{\omega_1} W(\omega) \Big| \log\left|Z(j\omega)\right| - \log\left|Z_{targ}(j\omega)\right| \Big| d\omega \qquad (1)$$

The weighting function W can be used to emphasize general frequency regions of interest or particular features such as precise resonances, and ω can be replaced with its log to achieve logarithmic frequency weighting. In other cases more insight may be gained by quantifying performance in terms of intuitively familiar physical quantities such as the apparent inertia, Coulomb friction, etc. Metrics may be more complex when the port impedance is nonlinear, and performance can also be measured in the time domain, based on the desired and actual response to particular excitation at the port. Regardless of the specific metric used, we contend that performance of a high force haptic system derives from the port behavior as quantified by the mechanical impedance.

In contrast, the stability of an interactive system like that shown in figure 1 depends on the dynamic properties of both coupled ports. If both port functions are linear, the characteristic polynomial of the system in Fig. 1B is

$$1+Z_h Y_o. \qquad (2)$$

The stability of the coupled system, termed *coupled stability* (Colgate & Hogan, 1988), is determined by the real part of the roots of this quantity. Clearly, the dynamics of the human operator contribute fundamentally to total system stability. This fact, taken with the previous paragraph, highlights an important distinction between physically interactive systems and servo controlled systems. In linear servo controlled systems, the same characteristic equation determines closed-loop stability and influences performance (in terms of frequency response, time response, etc.) In linear interactive systems, performance is dictated by the port function of the haptic system alone (Z_h) while stability is determined by equation 2, which includes properties of the operator as well (Buerger & Hogan, 2007).

Because the dynamic properties of the operator cannot be controlled by the haptic system designer, guaranteeing coupled stability poses a challenge. One valuable concept for understanding coupled system stability is *passivity*. A power port with a passive port function cannot release more energy than has been put into it. For the linear time-invariant case, a system defined by the linear 1-port impedance function $Z_p(s)$ is passive iff:

1. $Z_p(s)$ has no poles in the right half plane
2. Any imaginary poles of $Z_p(s)$ are simple, and have positive real residues
3. $Re(Z_p(j\omega)) \geq 0$ (3)

Such a port function has phase between -90° and +90° for all frequencies. Colgate showed that when two passive port functions are coupled together as in Fig. 1, the total open-loop phase must be between -180° and +180° at all frequencies, and the Nyquist stability criterion cannot be violated, so the coupled pair is guaranteed to be stable (Colgate & Hogan, 1988).

This is consistent with the energy properties of passive ports. If two passive ports are coupled, neither can generate energy indefinitely, and therefore stability is guaranteed. Because it is energy based, this extraordinarily powerful result works for linear and nonlinear systems (for nonlinear extensions, see e.g. (Wyatt et al., 1981)), and applies (perhaps with fine tuning) to all physical domains. To the extent that humans can be assumed to act as passive mechanical systems at their ports of interaction, passivity provides a powerful stability metric for high force haptics. While this has not been conclusively proven, given the complexities of the neuromuscular system, available empirical results and theory strongly suggest that this is indeed the case (Hogan, 1989). Unfortunately, making high force haptic systems passive can often limit performance. Certain simple control laws can preserve passivity, but given the limitations of available actuator hardware, these simple controllers often can not achieve adequate performance at the haptic system port. These challenges are reviewed in the next section.

3. Actuator and Control Technology for High Force Haptic Systems

Ideal high force haptic systems would achieve high forces while representing port impedance ranging from near zero to near infinite stiffness, friction and inertia, while guaranteeing passivity and coupled stability. Actuators for these idealized systems would require similar properties, plus some additional properties (e.g. low mass), depending on the system configuration. In this section we assess the value of various technologies in approaching this ideal, first by seeking a purely physical solution in the form of actuators effective at human scales (tens to hundreds of N, cm to m motions, frequencies less than 10 Hz), then by exploring the benefits of available advanced control methods.

3.1 Classical Actuator Technologies for High Force Haptics

Electromagnetic actuators can represent desired forces with extremely high fidelity when used in direct drive configurations. Friction can be extraordinarily low, especially at the low frequencies typical of interaction with humans (at higher frequencies eddy current or IR losses create drag). With the low intrinsic impedance of these actuators, simple and robust control algorithms, discussed below, may be used to provide a stiff interface and to preserve passivity. The main drawback is limited force density (Hollerbach et al., 1992), meaning that high forces lead to large, heavy actuators. Electromagnetic actuators are easy to use, and in many cases systems can be successfully designed to meet certain limited requirements in spite of force density limitations. An example is the MIT-MANUS robot for upper-limb physical therapy, which uses direct-drive rotary motors with a two-DOF (degree of freedom) planar closed-chain configuration that allows both actuators to remain stationary (Krebs et al., 2004). Other devices are effective due to very small translational workspaces (Berkelman et al., 1996). The force density limitation is far more difficult to overcome for open-chain serial systems. If the actuator for DOF #1 is carried by DOF #2, as is common for serial robot arms, then the mass of the actuator not only increases the force required for the DOF #2 actuator, but also adds to the endpoint inertia of that DOF. This problem emerges for most non-planar mechanisms, and is therefore very common. As forces increase, carrying the full weight of direct drive actuators rapidly becomes prohibitive. When rotary motors cannot be used, large motions pose an additional problem, as the high mass per unit force increases nearly linearly with range of motion.

An obvious way to improve the force density of electromagnetic or other actuators is to add gearing. This approach makes carrying actuators in a serial mechanism feasible and is used extensively in robots. Unfortunately a gear train compromises endpoint impedance, increasing the actuator's apparent inertia and friction due to eddy current or IR losses, as observed at the endpoint, by the square of the gear ratio. Coulomb friction and stiction in the actuator are amplified linearly by the gear ratio. Furthermore, the gear train adds its own friction, inertia and backlash. As a result, even when transmissions are designed explicitly to minimize friction, high impedance is difficult to escape (Buerger et al., 2001). While some applications are amenable to modest gear ratios (typically less than about 5:1), larger gear ratios rapidly lead to unacceptable levels of reflected inertia and friction. The failure of gearing to solve the underlying force density problem in high force haptics distinguishes this problem from most robotics, where gearing is generally very successful.

The most significant problem with using direct-drive electromagnetic actuators for high force haptics is the need to carry their substantial mass when complex or serial mechanisms are used. Mechanical transmissions such as cables, belts, tapes and rods offer a potential opportunity to keep the actuators stationary or nearly stationary, in some robot configurations, while transmitting their force, motion and impedance properties to the interaction port. Cable transmissions, in particular, have been elegantly and cleverly designed to achieve reasonable force and impedance capabilities in high-DOF serial arms, e.g. the WAM arm (Townsend & Guertin, 1999). The complexity of the mechanisms that enable the WAM underscore the fact that routing of mechanical transmission members can be extremely challenging. When actuators for multiple DOFs of a serial mechanism are mounted at the base, the transmission elements for one or more DOFs must pass through or around other joint(s). This presents an extreme packaging challenge as the number of DOFs grows, and this challenge is compounded by the fact that fixed separation must generally be maintained between transmission nodes (e.g. between pulleys in a cable system). Cables, belts and transmission tapes must be held in tension, requiring tight, deterministic coupling between the actuators and the intermediate and terminal joints that they actuate, even as the intermediate joints are independently actuated. These flexible members also tend to introduce problematic dynamic resonances (a "guitar-string" effect) and can severely limit bandwidth. Transmission rods can be made more rigid, but present an even more difficult plumbing challenge, as the gears that mate adjacent rods must be kept in tightly controlled contact. In certain configurations, mechanical transmissions can offer an acceptable high force haptic solution, and thus represent an important tool. However, for other applications their limitations are insurmountable, and other options must be sought.

Appealingly, hydraulic actuators can achieve force densities at least an order of magnitude better than ungeared electromagnetic motors (Hollerbach et al., 1992). Because the working fluid is nominally incompressible, hydraulics can achieve very high stiffness relative to humans. Pressure sources and valves can be located remotely, with force and motion coupled to the interaction port through flexible tubing, which can be routed with greater flexibility than mechanical transmission elements. In spite of these apparent advantages hydraulics have been little-used for haptic interfaces (with some exceptions, e.g. see (Kazerooni & Guo, 1993, Lee & Ryu, 2008)). This is because the operation of conventional servovalves causes hydraulic actuators to have high intrinsic impedance, and in fact generally to be non-backdrivable. Hydraulic actuators rely on nonzero valve impedance to

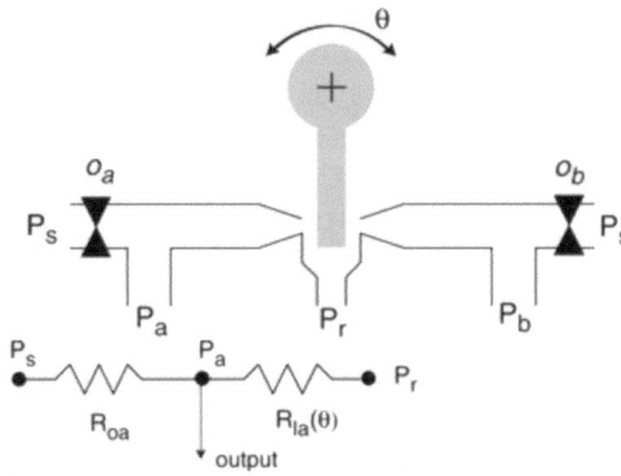

Fig. 2. Schematic of flapper servovalve, with resistor model of left half.

regulate output, placing a lower limit on the output impedance. The fundamental nature of this limit can be demonstrated by considering a typical pressure control valve design.

A servohydraulic system includes a high-pressure energy source, usually controlled to produce nominally constant pressure P_s, and a servovalve connected to a control system that meters the flow (or pressure, depending on the valve design and control structure) to the actuator, where energy is converted to mechanical energy. The servovalve determines the mechanical characteristics of the output, including force or motion as well as the mechanical impedance. A common valve architecture for pressure regulation is the flapper valve, shown schematically in Fig. 2 (jet-pipes offer a different configuration subject to largely similar tradeoffs). The flapper configuration is used, for example, as the first stage of the Moog Series 15 pressure control valves (www.moog.com). The output of this valve is the differential pressure (P_a-P_b). Two streams of fluid from the high-pressure source P_s push in opposite directions against the flapper, which is attached to the rotor. Both fluid streams then drip to the return at pressure P_r. The flapper rotates to partially restrict one side and raise the fluid pressure in that branch. For the change in fluid resistance at the flapper to have an impact on P_a and P_b, each side of the valve must be separated from P_s by an orifice (o_a and o_b). Unfortunately, any fluid supplied to the load must pass through one of these orifices, increasing the impedance and degrading the valve's quality as a pressure source.

This can be seen if the left half of the valve is modeled as a pair of fluid resistors, as shown below the schematic. The input orifice is modeled as the resistor R_{oa}, and the flapper opening is modeled as the resistor $R_{la}(\theta)$, which creates a pressure drop between P_a and the return pressure P_r and depends on the rotor angular position θ. If $R_{oa}=0$, then the output pressure $P_a= P_s$, and the actuated flapper has no effect on output. If a single fixed rotor position $\theta=\theta_o$ is considered, $R_{la}=R_{la}(\theta_o)$. Deriving the output impedance $Z_a = P_a / Q_a$, where Q_a is the volumetric output flow rate, produces:

$$Z_a = \frac{R_{oa} R_{la}}{R_{oa} + R_{la}} \tag{4}$$

A pure pressure source would have $Z_a=0$. If R_{oa} is too small, then changes in $R_{la}(\theta)$ have little effect on the output pressure P_a, and the valve will not function. Z_a can be made small by minimizing R_{la}. However, the total valve output impedance is:

$$Z = Z_a + Z_b \tag{5}$$

where Z_b is the port impedance for the other side of the valve, and has the same form as Eq. (4). But $R_{lb}(\theta)$ increases when $R_{la}(\theta)$ decreases, so the only way for the total output impedance to be low is for both flapper resistances to be low. This would allow substantial leakage through the flapper and would significantly reduce the output pressure. To achieve high output pressure requires amplification in a second stage (as in the Moog series 15 valve). The problems with this amplifier are twofold: first, even if it operates perfectly, it amplifies the impedance of the first stage at the endpoint by acting as a gear mechanism (hydraulic gearing is analogous to mechanical gearing); and second, it introduces more small orifices through which the fluid must flow. Enlarging the orifices in both valve stages simply produces a leaky valve, increasing power consumption and reducing efficiency. Thus without pressure feedback, the only way to avoid high impedance is with substantial leakage flow, which increases compressor size. Given the stringent impedance requirements of high force haptics, the leaky valve approach is generally impractical. High impedance in the valve is directly related to the ability generate output pressure, and cannot be eliminated. Furthermore, sliding cylinder seals represent another source of unwanted friction that can be challenging to avoid, particularly if operating at high pressures. Narrow pressure lines also contribute viscous damping and inertia. Another disadvantage of hydraulics is that at high pressures, safety risks can arise if lines rupture; however, the modest forces (by hydraulic standards) required for human interaction mitigate this hazard. Finally, the compressors needed for servohydraulic systems are usually heavy and noisy and therefore problematic for close proximity to human subjects. In section 4 of this chapter, we argue that in spite of these limitations, the force density advantage of hydraulics warrants further consideration in different configurations for high force haptics, and we present an architecture that circumvents the high-impedance servovalve challenge.

Pneumatic actuators are also capable of high force densities (Hollerbach et al., 1992) and provide behaviors unique among actuator technologies. While regulators that control gas pressure rely on flow restriction, much like hydraulic servovalves, low impedance is readily achieved due to the compressibility of the working fluid. Indeed gas compressibility presents one avenue to modulate the endpoint impedance, by directly manipulating the properties of the enclosed volume of gas in the actuator. However, representing high stiffness requires high pressure, and transitioning from low to high stiffness (e.g. to represent a virtual wall) requires rapid pressure changes. This can be understood by considering the simple example of a closed cylinder in compression due to force from a piston with cross-sectional area A, shown in Fig. 3. For simplicity isothermal conditions are assumed. Adiabatic conditions yield similar conclusions. Behavior at the port of interaction with the operator is characterized by the applied force F and displacement x. The gas in the cylinder is at the absolute pressure P, and the specific gas constant R and temperature T are fixed, while the volume V varies with x. P_{amb} denotes ambient pressure. A mass m of an ideal gas with molar mass M, is contained in the cylinder. The ideal gas law for this volume is:

$$PV = \frac{m}{M} RT \tag{6}$$

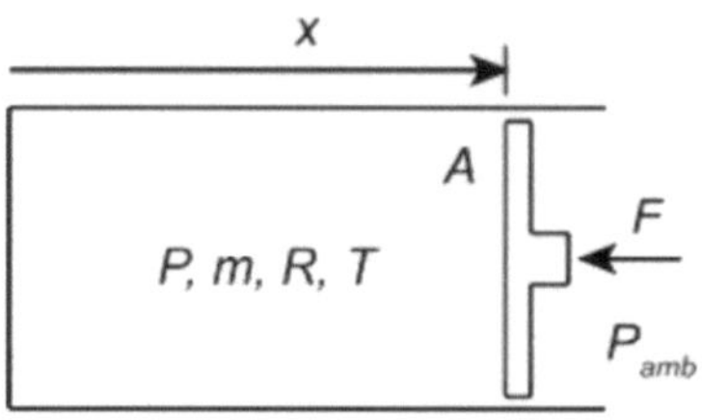

Fig. 3. Schematic of an ideal gas under isothermal compression in a piston-cylinder.

Pressure consists of ambient plus that due to the applied force:

$$P = \frac{F}{A} + P_{amb} \tag{7}$$

Substituting $V=Ax$ and eq. (7) into eq. (6) and rearranging produces:

$$F = \frac{RT}{M}\frac{m}{x} - P_{amb}A \tag{8}$$

Differentiating produces the stiffness:

$$\frac{dF}{dx} = -\frac{RT}{M}\frac{m}{x^2} \tag{9}$$

For fixed (or nearly fixed) x, for example when traversing a virtual wall, stiffness is proportional to the enclosed mass. To simulate a virtual wall with stiffness 100 times greater inside the wall than out purely by manipulating the properties of the enclosed fluid requires increasing the enclosed mass by a factor of 100 within the period of simulated contact with the wall. From eq. (6), this means that the pressure also must increase 100-fold. (For a real implementation, something must also offset the force due to increased pressure, usually a pressure against the other face of the piston). Thus discrete virtual environment features such as virtual walls are extremely difficult and inefficient to implement in this way. Another problem shown by eq. (9) is that stiffness is highly nonlinear in x, meaning the pressure must also be varied to maintain linear stiffness, if that is desired. An alternative approach would be to always operate at high pressures, keeping the transmission stiff, and modulating impedance at the valve source. Unfortunately this presents the same high intrinsic impedance challenge described in detail above for hydraulics. Pneumatic actuators are notoriously difficult to control, and the additional challenges of high force haptics exacerbate the problems. The fluid dynamics of pneumatic actuators are also forbidding for implementing closed-loop control using a regulator to respond to measured endpoint forces. Venting can be used to eliminate resistance from the gas, but this can be quite inefficient. Finally, compressed gas stores orders of magnitude more energy than liquids at the same pressures, and this can raise potential safety concerns. In spite of their challenges, pneumatic actuators have been proposed for certain haptic and high force haptic applications where their intrinsic compliance can be beneficial, including exoskeletal devices (Tressler et al., 2002) and other devices employing pneumatic muscles (Tondu & Lopez, 2000).

3.2 Interaction Control

Physical interaction requires control strategies that differ significantly from the more common position or velocity servo problems. Because of the unique characteristics of physical interaction described above, the prevailing approach is explicitly to regulate dynamic behavior at the port(s) of interaction, e.g. by using *impedance control* (Hogan, 1985). The most straightforward embodiment of this theory, termed simple impedance control, uses motion feedback with torque- or force-producing actuators to implement virtual dynamics on low-impedance hardware. Proportional position feedback produces virtual stiffness, and proportional velocity feedback (or derivative position feedback) produces virtual viscous damping. If implemented ideally with positive gains and co-located sensors and actuators, the result is passive port impedance (Hogan & Buerger, 2005). This approach is powerful, robust and easily implemented, and has been applied successfully (Krebs et al., 2004). Its major limitation is the need for low-impedance hardware. Simple impedance control can do nothing to counteract inertia and friction in the physical system. Thus while simple impedance control can effectively stabilize interaction by guaranteeing passivity, it can do little to address the limitations of actuator technology discussed in the previous section, providing significant motivation for the alternative techniques discussed here.

A class of control methods has been developed that uses measured forces (torques) at the port of interaction to close a feedback loop and expand the range of apparent dynamics that can be presented. This approach has the potential to mask the physical properties of the hardware, presenting a desired dynamic response at the port of interaction that closely tracks target dynamics derived independent of the physical hardware. For instance, the apparent inertia and friction can be reduced below the physical values by using the actuators to drive the device in the direction of applied force. When the target impedance is zero, this is termed force control. Unfortunately this approach seriously threatens coupled stability; in fact passivity is lost whenever the apparent inertia is reduced by more than a factor of two below the physical inertia (Colgate & Hogan, 1988, Newman, 1992). Natural admittance control exploits the fact that loss of passivity derives from reducing the apparent inertia, rather than the friction. This method provides a means of theoretically ensuring passivity while aggressively reducing the apparent friction well below the physical level by keeping the inertia at a level that ensures passivity (Newman, 1992). This approach can dramatically improve feel by virtually eliminating static friction, but cannot mitigate high levels of physical inertia, which are particularly common in geared actuator systems.

An alternative approach recognizes that passivity, though sufficient to stabilize interaction with human subjects, is not necessary. Passivity ensures stability when coupled to a wide range of environments including large inertial loads, kinematic constraints, highly nonlinear frictional contact, etc. On the other hand, the dynamic characteristics of human limbs are considerably more limited, even as they vary in time, configuration and across subjects. Port stability can be posited as a robust stability problem with conservative bounding values used for operator dynamic properties, and robust control methods can be used to shape the dynamics of the force feedback control loop to maximize performance (by minimizing impedance error) while guaranteeing coupled stability (Buerger & Hogan, 2007).

3.3 Advanced actuators

In spite of significant progress in advanced interaction control, achieving all six required characteristics of high force haptic devices listed in section 1 remains a persistent challenge, particularly for complex and high-DOF devices. Several recent advances in actuator development offer promising future alternatives for the high force haptic designer's toolbox.

Goldfarb has described monopropellant-powered actuators that chemically generate gas to produce pressure, and force output (Goldfarb et al., 2003). This approach dramatically improves energy density and eliminates the need for a compressor. However, force and impedance properties—and limitations—appear to be fundamentally similar to those of compressed-air systems. In particular, rapid changes of stiffness (to simulate contacting a surface) require high mass flow rates. Dramatic thermal changes would also impact endpoint impedance. In the authors' opinion, this approach seems quite promising, though as yet unproven for high force haptics.

Series elastic actuators, which include compliant members placed between high-impedance source actuators and the environment and use force feedback control, can achieve high force-density and low impedance (Pratt & Williamson, 1995). The elastic element provides several advantages for certain applications, but does not guarantee passivity, and a careful tuning process is generally required to achieve stability. This is problematic when interacting with variable, unpredictable humans. An alternative design method that includes carefully controlled physical damping in conjunction with natural admittance control can theoretically guarantee passivity (Dohring & Newman, 2002). Generally, the more aggressive the reduction of apparent impedance from the physical actuator level, the softer the compliant element must be. This limits the utility of this approach by limiting achievable stiffness. Still, carefully designed series dynamics are an important tool.

Research into electroactive and dielectric polymers has shown potential for high achievable stresses. These muscle-like materials could one day produce effective high force haptic actuators, but have not yet been shown to scale up to the forces needed (Bar-Cohen, 2004).

To the best of our knowledge, no existing actuator technology or control strategy provides a comprehensive solution for high force haptics. Additional tools are needed to improve the tradeoffs between force capacity, DOFs, workspace size, interface fidelity, and coupled stability. An alternative way of evaluating the potential of major human-scale actuator technologies is by available stress, which is strongly related to force density. The force output of electromagnetic actuators is limited by the shear stress in the air gap between moving and stationary components, which is typically tens of pounds per square inch (psi). Pneumatic actuators can achieve hundreds of psi but rapidly introduce hazards as pressure is elevated, due to high levels of stored energy. By contrast, hydraulic actuators routinely achieve thousands of psi (McBean & Breazeal, 2004). This fundamental promise warrants a second look at hydraulics to see if the underlying high impedance of servovalves can be avoided, and if the tradeoffs between the six criteria listed in section 1 can be improved.

4. Hybrid hydraulic actuators for high force haptics

Among actuator technologies available at the human scale, hydraulic actuators are alone in offering high force density, high stiffness, and flexible connectivity between power sources and the interaction port. Their main drawback is high impedance, which derives primarily from servovalves, and because of this they have been little-used for haptic interfaces. By contrast, electromagnetic actuators are widely used for haptics due to their favorable force and impedance behavior, but suffer from dramatically inferior force density. A hydraulic actuator capable of controlling pressure with low impedance rather than a high impedance servovalve would be a powerful development. We have investigated a hybrid architecture for actuators that exploits the benefits of both hydraulic and electromagnetic actuation while circumventing the weaknesses of each. In this design, sketched in Fig. 4, a hydraulic element is used purely as a transmission, while a remotely-located source actuator provides force and motion, and dictates the representation of the virtual environment. The hydraulic transmission is stiff in the direction of actuation but is embodied in flexible tubing, such that motion of the interaction port is decoupled from motion of the source actuator, and the source actuator may remain stationary. Critically, this architecture obviates the need for a hydraulic servovalve, eliminating the main cause of high impedance. The hydraulic transmission is analogous to a mechanical transmission but, unlike cables, tapes or rods, does not require a deterministic coupling between source and interaction port locations. This architecture also enables the use of effective source actuators, particularly direct-drive electromagnetic actuators, that can provide favorable force, motion and impedance properties. The source actuator can have large mass, because it need not move.

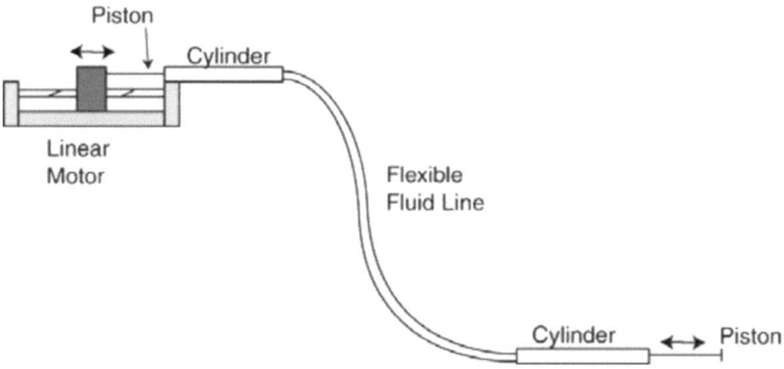

Fig. 4. Schematic of linear actuation scheme with fluid transmission.

While this proposed architecture can dramatically reduce endpoint mass, in its simplest form it actually increases the total system mass when compared to using only direct drive electromagnetic actuators. (The hydraulic transmission would be unnecessary if the actuator was connected directly to the endpoint.) Total mass is critically important for some applications (e.g. fully mobile exoskeletons), and this approach may not be suitable for those. However, in many cases the *placement* of mass is of equal or greater importance than total mass. Therapeutic robots, for instance, may tolerate being tethered to a stationary or independently mobile collection of heavy components, e.g. for power (Roberts, 2004). On the other hand, the absence of a compressor may lead to a lower system mass than a pure hydraulic system. This passive hydraulic architecture decouples a portion of the drivetrain from the mobile interaction port and conducts energy to it in hydraulic, not electrical, form.

4.1 Design Model and Tradeoffs

Figure 4 shows a schematic of one embodiment of this architecture that uses a linear electromagnetic motor as a source actuator and a passive hydraulic system as a power transmission. The hydraulic system consists of a piston/cylinder on each end for conversion between mechanical and fluid power, and a flexible hose connecting the two. One piston connects to the source motor, and the other acts as an actuator. Unlike servovalve-controlled hydraulics, the mechanical piston-cylinders, each of which acts as both an energy and signal source for the hydraulics, and the tubing that joins them need not include small orifices to regulate pressure, and can be designed to have relatively low intrinsic impedance.

If the source actuator is capable of providing the desired force and impedance, then an ideal transmission is mechanically *transparent*. In this context, transparency (previously used to describe an objective for bilateral teleoperation systems (Lawrence, 1993)) means that the force, motion, and energy exchanged between a load and the transmission is equal to that exchanged between the transmission and the source actuator. The goal is to transport actuator behavior to a remote endpoint package that weighs less than the source. Figure 5 depicts a generic transmission architecture. If the transmission is perfectly transparent, the motion trajectories of ports 1 and 2 are identical for all time, the force exchanged at port 2 equals that exchanged at port 1, and the impedance at the interface to the environment exactly equals the actuator impedance. That is, a perfectly transparent transmission is lossless and has the following properties:

$$\begin{aligned} x_2(t) &= x_1(t) \\ F_2(t) &= F_1(t) \\ Z_p &= Z_r \end{aligned} \tag{10}$$

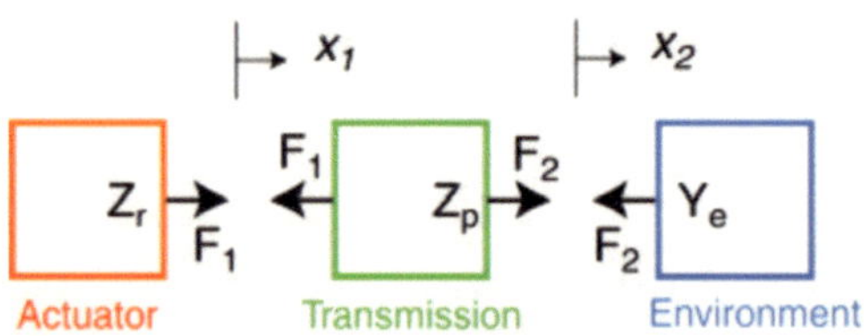

Fig. 5. Schematic depiction of a transmission between a source actuator and environment.

Any practical transmission will drain some energy and will therefore not be perfectly transparent. Furthermore any real physical system has nonzero inertial and compliant dynamics. To approach ideal behavior, the transmission should be designed to minimize inertia, compliance, and friction (although transmission dynamics may be used to advantageously shape the port impedance; see 4.3). While transparency is an important performance objective, an effective transmission must also be *flexible*. A perfectly flexible transmission would allow infinite separation (in all spatial degrees of freedom) of the endpoint package from the source actuator with zero reaction forces (torques). A practical transmission must provide sufficient freedom of motion from the source to cover the robot's workspace. Forces and torques required to bend and twist the fluid line should be minimized. The requirements of flexibility and transparency are often in conflict, as detailed below. Whether a transmission is intended to be transparent or to shape impedance, its design specifications focus on how it impacts endpoint impedance. This distinguishes high-force haptic applications from conventional servo problems. Below we provide a model that enables the prediction of the transmission's transparency and its impact on endpoint impedance. First several issues must be addressed to ensure that useful actuators capable of bilateral power transmission can be configured and controlled to operate as intended.

From Figure 4 it is straightforward to envision the hydraulic components transmitting force, motion and power in compression. However most high force haptic systems must sometimes actuate bilaterally (pulling as well as pushing). If tensile forces are applied to a closed liquid volume, its pressure drops below ambient and the fluid evaporates locally (cavitates). If the seals are imperfect, air leaks in. Two simple options enable bilateral actuation: a bias pressure that exceeds the pressure needed to transmit tensile forces can be introduced, or actuator pairs can be used together. The latter is depicted in Figure 6, wherein the two actuation paths exist within the same two cylinders, joined by two separate fluid lines, one for "tension" and the other for "compression." This configuration introduces several difficulties, including additional weight and complexity as well as additional seals. Seals where the pistons exit the cylinders are particularly problematic, as any liquid that leaks there leaves the constant-volume system and must be replaced.

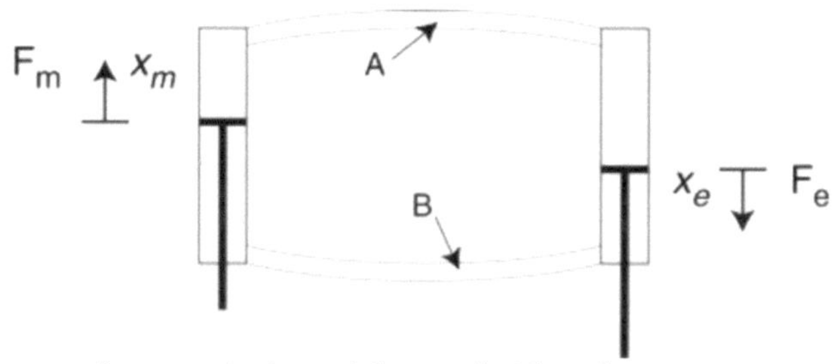

Fig. 6. Bilaterally actuated transmission with two fluid paths.

A simpler method of tensile force transmission that uses a single fluid path requires mechanically creating a bias pressure such that the fluid pressure is elevated above ambient without force applied by the actuator or environment. This can be accomplished by applying a constant compressive force to each piston. When the system is at rest, the forces on each side cancel, but the fluid in the chamber is at an elevated pressure. Tensile forces reduce the pressure, but if the force does not exceed the bias force level, the fluid pressure remains above ambient and cavitation and gas leakage into the system are avoided. This approach requires additional hardware to create the applied load, and increases the operating fluid pressure, but requires only two moving seals rather than four.

Using this mechanical bias force approach, the transmission can be modeled for design purposes as the simple straight-pipe system shown in Fig. 7. This model, used as the design basis for determining transmission impedance, includes each of the piston-cylinders (with diameters D_1 and D_2 and length L_1) and approximates the flexible line that connects them as a straight, smooth and rigid cylindrical pipe (with diameter D and length L). The forces applied to the two pistons are F_1 and F_2, and the piston velocities are v_1 and v_2. The bulk fluid velocity in the line is v. The transition from piston diameter to hose diameter must also be considered. This simplified model can be used to predict losses due to friction, the weight of the fluid in the system, and the inertia due to fluid acceleration. Calculations based on this particular model are summarized below to illustrate the relationship between transmission geometry and system performance. From Fig. 7 it is evident that this hydraulic transmission can also provide an intrinsic gear reduction for force (or motion) amplification or reduction, without adding mechanical parts that might contribute backlash or friction. In this case, the gear ratio is equal to the ratio of the piston areas.

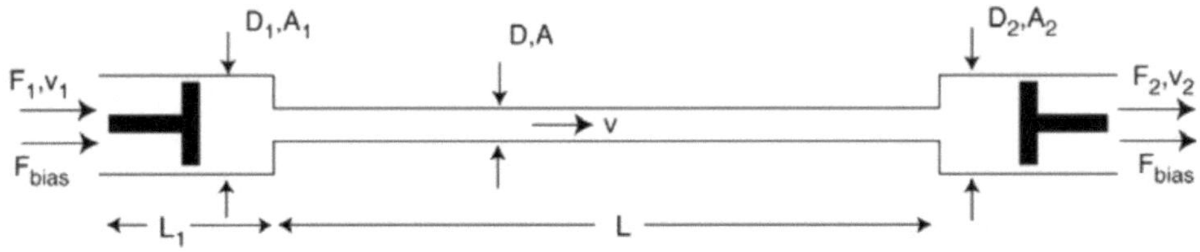

Fig. 7. Straight-pipe, dual piston model for a linear passive hydraulic transmission.

To be viable, the proposed actuator architecture must be amenable to control. By introducing a significant separation between the source actuator and the endpoint where behavior is controlled, with accompanying transmission dynamics, the structure of the system poses a potential challenge for effective and highly stable control. Because stability and passivity are paramount, one way to represent target impedance is to feed back motion only at the source actuator, closing a simple impedance control loop around only the well-characterized electromagnetic source actuator, yielding a robustly stable implementation. This arrangement depends on the transmission to reliably (and nearly transparently) transmit impedance between the source actuator and operator, but without using a sensor at the interaction port, it may be vulnerable to small and accumulating position errors. Fortunately, although humans excel at gathering information from physical contact, they are not generally sensitive to small changes in position. Provided that physical contact is represented as intended, small positioning errors can be tolerated with very little consequence, especially if the device is used in conjunction with a visual display. Compared to alternative transmission implementations (e.g. cable drives), a hydraulic transmission may provide superior damping of resonant transmission line modes via the intrinsic viscous behavior of the working fluid, and in fact the dynamics of the transmission may be intentionally sculpted to improve both interaction stability and performance via *impedance shaping*, as discussed briefly below.

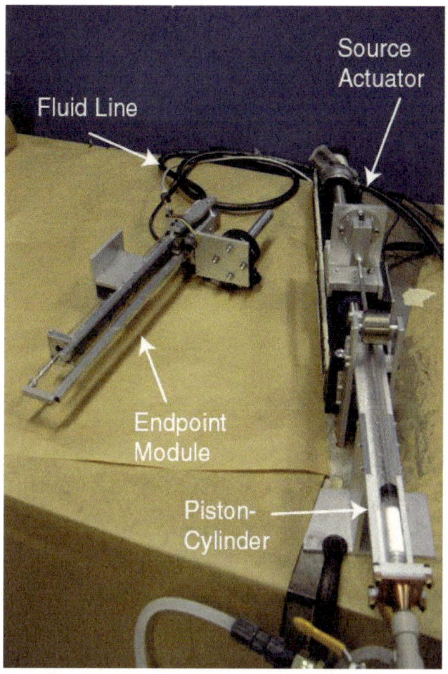

Fig. 8. Prototype passive hydraulic transmission system with linear source actuator.

To illustrate the key design issues for this architecture, a representative design problem is presented by applying the model in Fig. 7 to the specifications for an actuator for an upper-limb physical therapy robot device. This is intended as an out-of-plane "anti-gravity" addition to the planar MIT-MANUS robot, and has previously been addressed with two designs, one using a rotary electric motor and a low-friction roller screw and the other a direct-drive linear electromagnetic motor (Buerger et al., 2001, Krebs et al., 2004). The stringent and challenging target specifications for this application include a range of motion of 0.4 m, a force capacity of at least 65 N, a mass of less than 2 kg at the endpoint, a separation of at least 3 m between the stationary source actuator and the mobile endpoint, achievable stiffness of at least 2 kN/m, and minimal endpoint impedance including inertia less than 2 kg, Coulomb friction less than 2 N, and linear damping coefficient of no more than 10 Ns/m. Both previous designs violated the mass specification by nearly a factor of four. In this section the design model is developed to predict frictional and inertial dynamics of the transmission, and compliance is discussed. A prototype actuator (Fig. 8) was fabricated and its measured properties are discussed in the next section.

Damping: A major advantage of this configuration is its ability to avoid or minimize the viscous losses that arise in conventional hydraulics from forcing large volumes of fluid through small control orifices. Nevertheless, the long, narrow transmission line contributes some damping due to viscous drag. Assuming the fluid in Fig. 7 is incompressible, steady flow between any two points in the pipe is governed by the following expression, derived from the energy equation:

$$\left(\frac{P_1}{\rho}+\alpha_1\frac{v_1^2}{2}+gz_1\right)-\left(\frac{P_2}{\rho}+\alpha_2\frac{v_2^2}{2}+gz_2\right)=h_{lt} \tag{11}$$

P_1 and P_2 are the pressures at each point in the pipe. ρ is the fluid density, α_1 and α_2 are kinetic energy coefficients related to the flow profile, z_1 and z_2 represent elevation, and g is the acceleration due to gravity. h_{lt} is the total head loss, representing the energy (per unit mass) lost between the two points. Selecting the two pistons as points 1 and 2, with equal cross-sectional areas, bulk velocities, and flow profiles, with no net change in elevation and a force F_1 applied to piston 1 but no force applied to piston 2, eq. (11) reduces to:

$$F_1 = A_1 \rho h_{lt} \tag{12}$$

which also uses the relationship:

$$P_1 = \frac{F_1}{A_1} \tag{13}$$

The head loss h_{lt} results from major losses due to the main fluid line body in addition to minor losses due to the changes in pipe area. The prototype was designed with tapered cylinder ends to restrict the minor losses to less than 5% of the major losses, so only the major losses need be considered. Major loss can be computed for laminar and turbulent flow with separate calculations, where turbulence depends on the piston velocities. For laminar flow (with Reynolds number less than 2300), the effective damping seen at the piston is linear with velocity and with the fluid viscosity μ, and is governed by the expression:

$$F_1 = 8\pi\mu L \left(\frac{D_1}{D}\right)^4 v_1 \tag{14}$$

The major damping at the piston is proportional to the *fourth power* of the ratio of piston diameter to pipe diameter (or the square of the area ratio A_1/A). In other words, decreasing the pipe diameter increases damping dramatically in the laminar region. The same can be said of the turbulent region, where the Blasius equation can be used to predict losses when the Reynolds numbers exceeds 4000. The resulting expression is:

$$F_1 = \frac{\pi}{8} 0.3164 \mu^{0.25} \rho^{0.75} L \frac{D_1^{5.5}}{D^{4.75}} v_1^{1.75} \tag{15}$$

Turbulent damping is nonlinear in velocity, and even more highly dependent on the piston and line diameters.

Given the specification of a 3 m flexible line for the representative prototype, a design figure depicting the predicted friction versus velocity for several different hose diameters is shown in Fig. 9. A specification of a maximum of 10 Ns/m damping is also shown. Because the overwhelming majority of human patient subjects never exceed 0.4 m/s hand speed in the course of therapy, a hose with an inner diameter of 5/16" (0.79 cm) was selected for the prototype as it satisfies the design requirement for all relevant speeds. This hose has an outer diameter of approximately ½" (1.27 cm), and is comparable in size and flexibility to the electrical power cables that drive the source motor.

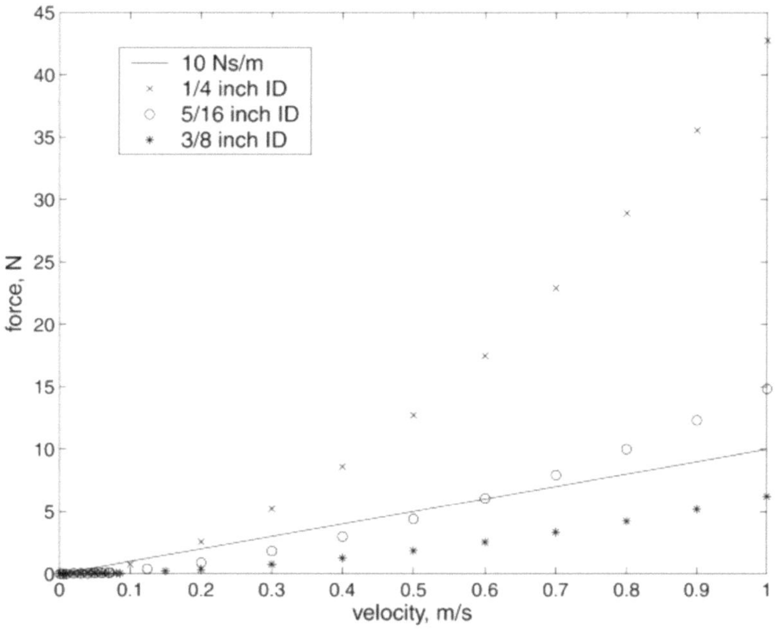

Fig. 9. Predicted fluid friction versus piston velocity, several hose diameters.

Inertia: The apparent endpoint inertia of the fluid transmission is another important factor that can be predicted from the Fig. 7 design model. Assuming incompressibility, the apparent mass m_{eq} at piston 1 can be determined from the total kinetic energy of the fluid:

$$m_{eq}\frac{v_1^2}{2} = m_{cyl}\frac{v_1^2}{2} + m_{line}\frac{v^2}{2} \tag{16}$$

m_{cyl} is the mass of the fluid in the two cylinders, while m_{line} is the mass of the fluid in the hose. Computation of m_{cyl} and m_{line} is straightforward from the density and system geometry but to determine m_{eq} the following relationship must be used:

$$v = \frac{A_1}{A}v_1 \tag{17}$$

The resulting equivalent inertia is:

$$m_{eq} = \rho L_1 \pi \frac{D_1^2}{4} + \rho L \pi \frac{D_1^4}{4D^2} \tag{18}$$

When the fluid line is long or narrow, the second term dominates. Decreasing the piston diameter D_1 decreases the system inertia but decreasing the line diameter D increases the inertia dramatically despite the fact that a smaller volume of fluid is used. This is because the fluid in the smaller line must accelerate much more rapidly, more than compensating for the fact that there is less of it.

Compliance: Assuming that the working fluid is incompressible and that air can be effectively eliminated from the transmission system, compliance can still result from the radial flexibility of the hose. Flexibility of the hose in bending is a direct performance requirement, and it is nearly impossible to create a tube that is very flexible in bending but very stiff radially. Designs that use radial reinforcements (for example braided fibers) to maximize the anisotropy of the hose are reasonably effective, but some radial compliance is unavoidable. This results in a fluid volume that expands as the pressure increases, changing the relative position of the two pistons. To maximize transparency, compliance should be minimized. Although hose anisotropy makes it difficult to predict compliance exactly, geometric effects can be inferred from the mechanics of pressure vessels. Compliance can be decreased by increasing hose thickness, reducing hose length, or reducing the internal hose diameter.

The simple calculations described above elucidate the geometric tradeoffs in the hydraulic transmission architecture. Because this application uses hydraulics differently from prior work, this model facilitates scaled designs for various applications and requirements. Transparency requires low friction, compliance, and inertia. From eqs. (14), (15) and (18), short and wide (large diameter) lines provide low friction and inertia. However, flexibility requires long and bendable (preferably small diameter) lines. Minimizing compliance requires using lines that are either materially rigid or thick-walled (and therefore unlikely to bend easily), or small in diameter and short. Design of line materials and geometry must include consideration of each of these requirements and the tradeoffs between them. Impedance can also be changed by altering the piston/cylinder geometry. Reducing the piston diameter can significantly reduce damping and inertia, as shown by Eqs. (14), (15) and (18), or permits smaller hose diameters for the same impedance properties, reducing compliance and improving flexibility. However, by Eq. (13) this increases the operating pressure, which has at least two negative consequences: greater part strength is required, and leakage is likely to increase, often requiring seals with greater friction. Thus changes in piston diameter can trade leakage and seal friction against reflected fluid friction and inertia.

Changes to system geometry improve certain aspects of performance at the expense of others. For any specific application the performance properties must be traded off against one another to find a suitable solution. Several rules of thumb should guide design:

1) To minimize reflected inertia, fluid friction, *and* compliance, the hydraulic line(s) should be made as large and radially rigid as possible.
2) Problem constraints should be used to determine how large, how heavy, and how rigid the line can be. These properties (related to flexibility) are traded against the endpoint impedance (transparency).
3) Decreasing the piston diameter decreases the reflected impedance but increases the operating pressure, and therefore the leakage rate and/or seal friction.

4.2 Proof of concept prototype and characterization

A prototype for the anti-gravity upper-limb application, shown in Fig. 8, was constructed to prove the concept of hybrid hydraulic actuation and to test the design model. A cogless tubular linear motor from Copley™, used previously as a version of the anti-gravity robot system, was selected as a source actuator for the system. A wound steel constant-force spring was used at each cylinder to apply the bias force. Springs are an advantageous means

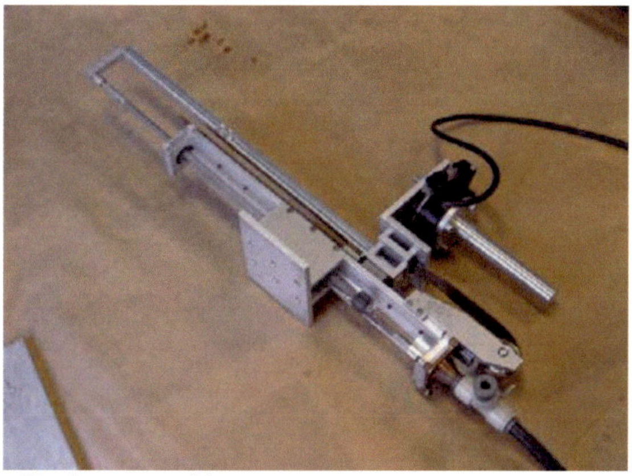

Fig. 10. Outer piston/cylinder assembly.

of applying a bias force because they contribute minimal inertia and friction. In choosing a working fluid for this application, fluid dynamics including the viscosity, density, and compressibility are especially important because they contribute to the endpoint impedance and haptic feel. Other factors (e.g. lubricity) that are important for other hydraulic applications are not important here because of the mechanical simplicity of the design. Water is cheap and available in abundance, and has minimal viscosity and compressibility with modest density. Water also poses minimal environmental threats (provided that it be separated from electrical and electronic equipment), and was therefore selected. The fittings that connect the flexible fluid line to solid structures are a critical component for design of a system with no small orifices. The analysis in 3.1 shows that losses from small orifices in servovalves lead to high endpoint impedance; the same can be said of orifices in a transmission line. Typical pipe and tube fittings generally obstruct the interior passages, greatly reducing diameter (and increasing damping) in a local area. In servo systems this effect is usually insignificant because the losses in the servovalve are so great as to dwarf fitting losses. For this application, however, an unobstructed fluid path is critical, and small orifices must be aggressively eliminated. Quick-release hose fittings that grip only the outside of the hose and leave the inside unobstructed were chosen for this prototype. To use such fittings, only hoses with relatively rigid walls are acceptable. A fuel hose meeting the SAE30R3 specification was selected. Perhaps the most challenging practical issue in hydraulic transmission design is the selection of moving seals with sufficiently low friction. In general, sliding seals require increased friction to reduce leakage. Because of the extreme low-friction needs of high-force haptic devices, static and Coulomb friction must especially be minimized. A wide array of seal types were considered, including elastomeric sliding seals, rolling diaphragm seals, bellows designs, and non-contacting seals. While rolling diaphragm seals show great promise, they generally provide a small ratio of travel to diameter. Non-contacting Airpot™ piston-cylinders were selected to minimize friction. This technology uses a precision ground sintered graphite piston that is diametrically matched to a high-precision glass tube to clearances that are generally between .0001" and .001". There is no physical seal, and the piston is designed to ride on a cushion of fluid between its outer edge and the cylinder's inner edge. This design minimizes friction but, because there is clearance between piston and cylinder, inevitably permits some leakage. Some amount of leakage of the working fluid across a low-friction seal is inescapable. When fluid leaks, the

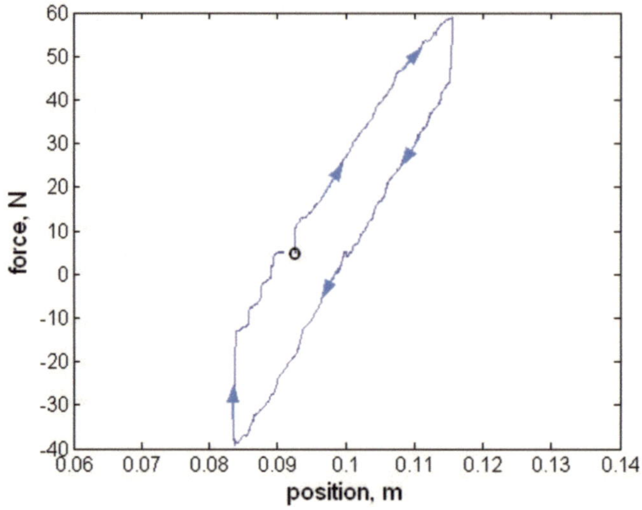

Fig. 11. Endpoint force versus position with virtual spring imposed, actuated by hand. The circle marks the start of the test and the arrows indicate the time course.

bias pressure prevents the replacement of the fluid with air. Instead the fluid volume is reduced. This is a positive feature of this bias pressure method; leakage produces a drift in endpoint position, but no significant change in dynamic transmission properties. To permit long-term operation, the leaked fluid must be replaced. For the prototype, a pump was used to replace leaked fluid. Because the pump is a high-impedance flow source, its supply rate is unaffected by changes in the transmission pressure, and it has a negligible impact on the system dynamics. Figure 10 shows the outer cylinder assembly.

Static and dynamic characterization tests were conducted to evaluate the prototype performance and validity of the design model. The force capacity, transmission stiffness, friction, inertia, weight and bandwidth were analyzed. The results are summarized and compared to the specification and the same quantities for a module based on the source actuator alone (Krebs et al., 2004) in Table 1.

	Specification	**Linear Motor**	**Passive Hydraulic Transmission**
Force capacity (N)	65	70	70
Endpoint weight (kg)	2	8.1	2.4
Core component weight (kg)	-	2.7	0.6
Endpoint inertia (kg)	2	2.7	4.5
Coulomb friction (N)	2	3.5	8
Stiffness (kN/m)	2	10	3.7

Table 1. Performance comparison of specifications, linear motor, and hydraulic transmission system for vertical therapy robot module. Improvement in weight is highlighted.

To determine the force capacity in tension and compression a high stiffness was commanded with the source actuator and a force was applied (and measured) at the endpoint until saturation was reached. The transmission supported over 50 N in tension (exceeding the bias spring force) and almost 70 N in compression (meeting the saturation level of the source motor). The endpoint stiffness at DC is a series combination of the effective transmission stiffness and the source actuator stiffness. The source actuator controller was calibrated to achieve target endpoint stiffness using proportional motion feedback (simple impedance control). To determine the transmission stiffness, a virtual spring was imposed at the source actuator and the transmission endpoint force and position were measured as the endpoint was actuated slowly and steadily by hand. An example of the resulting data is shown in Fig. 11. The endpoint stiffness was determined from the slope of a linear fit to this data. The test was repeated at several different stiffnesses and the results were averaged, producing a measured transmission stiffness of 4020 N/m. When coupled to the source motor with maximum stiffness of 50,000 N/m, the resulting system can achieve stiffness up to 3700 N/m. This exceeds the specification by 85% and signals that radial hose flexibility does not prevent the creation of desired haptic sensations.

The endpoint friction profile was determined by measuring the force required to backdrive the system at constant speeds with a separate servo system. This test revealed approximately 8 N of Coulomb friction at the endpoint, in addition to viscous damping around 15 Ns/m. Coulomb friction appears as the separation between the upper and lower parts of the trace in Fig. 11. Approximately 3.5 N of Coulomb friction results from the source actuator, and the rest is mostly due to the bearings on the outer assembly. Significantly, a test on only the two pistons and the fluid, decoupled from mechanical bearings on each end, revealed less than 0.5 N friction from these critical parts. Viscous damping is approximately twice the estimate from the model. This results from viscous drag at the source motor as well as the fact that the transmission is not an ideal straight pipe, as modeled, and indicates a need for further model development to capture additional damping.

The model predicts over 2.5 kg of apparent fluid inertia, plus the inertia of the linear motor forcer and the moving hardware (handle, bearing carriage, sensors, etc.) in the endpoint package, totaling 4.9 kg. This significantly exceeds the 2 kg specification, because the design of this prototype erred on the side of making the hose extremely flexible yet radially stiff, and therefore very small. The most straightforward way to reduce inertia is by changing the hose geometry, as described in the previous section. A segmented line could help to balance hose flexibility and endpoint inertia. To measure the inertia, the source actuator was used to create a virtual spring. The transmission endpoint was displaced and released, creating an initial condition response. The transient of this response was fit with a second order initial condition response using the known endpoint stiffness. Inertia measured in several trials averaged to 4.5 kg. This is slightly less than the prediction because the inertia is actually partially distributed across a compliant part of the system (the transmission), while the model assumes a lumped mass with compliance originating only from the source actuator.

The weight of the endpoint package, including all parts of the assembly downstream of, but not including, the fluid line was 2.43 kg. Perhaps more importantly, the total weight of the (non-structural) components required to produce force (the cylinder, piston, piston rod assembly, fluid, and constant force spring assembly) was less than 630 g. By contrast, the weight of the linear motor magnet rod and forcer (for the same amount of travel) is over 2.7

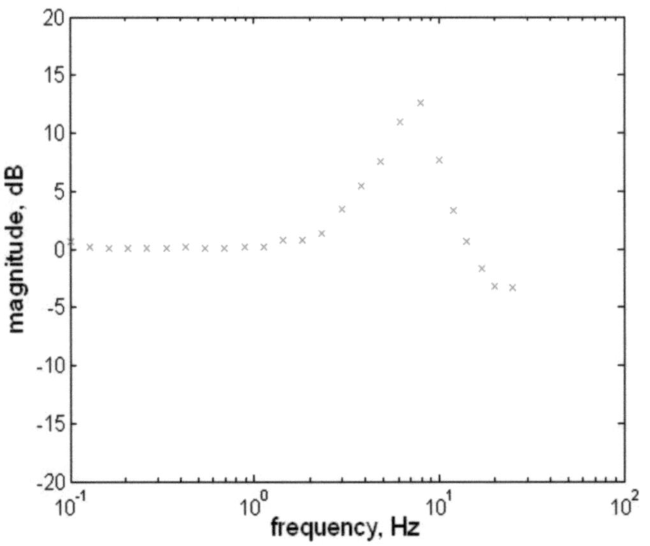

Fig. 12. Force magnitude output/input ratio versus frequency.

kg. The weight of the core technology to produce force, excluding bearings and structure, is reduced by approximately 77%—more than a factor of four. Additional weight reduction is achieved because the structure need not support such heavy core components.

Although not a direct performance requirement for this application, bandwidth was also measured by fixing the endpoint and commanding a sinusoidal force profile at various frequencies, with a magnitude of 12 N (approximately 20% of the peak force specification). A resulting plot of magnitude versus frequency is shown in Fig. 12. The system has a resonant peak around 8 Hz with a damping ratio between 0.1 and 0.2, and an open-loop bandwidth of approximately 20 Hz. The system geometry could easily be altered to increase viscous drag and reduce the resonant spike (e.g. by using more constrictive fittings) should this be desired. The bandwidth is more than adequate for human arm movement.

A critical assessment of the model's accuracy in predicting prototype impedance reveals moderate errors in the prediction of inertia, due to the assumption of lumped inertia in spite of the nonzero compliance, and somewhat larger errors in the prediction of damping, stemming primarily from the fact that damping is highly sensitive to tubing surface conditions, coiling, and interface losses. In general, over long stretches of tubing as implemented here, the primary goal is to keep friction below some level, rather than precisely achieve a specific value, so the simplified model suffices for this purpose. Prototype testing, along with the insights provided by the model, underscores the fact that seals are the core technology that determines performance. Smaller piston diameters can dramatically reduce apparent inertia and damping, but require higher pressures. At higher pressures, leakage increases unless seals are made tighter, which usually requires greater friction. It is clear from this work that improved seal technology that can better contain the fluid with minimal friction would substantially improve the capabilities of this technology.

4.3 Compliant Impedance Shaping

As discussed above, viscoelastic dynamics placed in series between a high-impedance actuator utilizing force feedback and the environment (termed series elasticity, mechanical

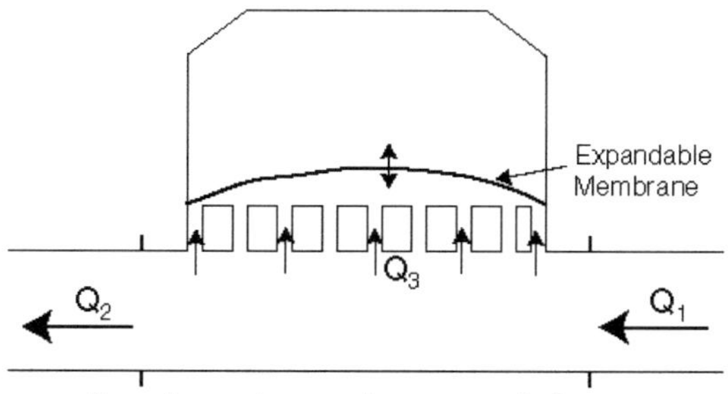

Fig. 13. Schematic of a cross-flow impedance shaper module.

filtering, or impedance shaping) can help to stabilize contact (Pratt & Williamson, 1995, Dohring & Newman, 2002). A passive hydraulic transmission can implement selected dynamic characteristics and is situated to place these dynamics in series, providing another potentially valuable aspect of this architecture. In the prototype described above, the source actuator friction and inertia contribute significantly to the endpoint impedance (half the friction and 1/3 the inertia), suggesting that it may be useful to use force feedback control around the actuator to reduce its apparent impedance, with series dynamics to improve coupled stability. An *impedance shaper* can be introduced to the transmission system to physically shape the dynamic characteristics of the actuator system as desired. A compliant impedance shaper (with compliance greater than that of the tubing alone) must introduce an alternative flow path so that the movement of each piston is not constrained absolutely by the movement of the other. A schematic depiction is shown in Fig. 13, where Q_1 and Q_2 represent the volumetric flow from each of the two pistons. Q_3 is the flow into or out of the impedance shaper. To make an impedance shaper with positive stiffness, there must be a means of expanding the volume in response to increases in fluid pressure (such as a flexible membrane). To endow the impedance shaper with dissipative behavior it suffices to regulate the geometry of the passages into and out of the stiffness chamber. In such simple and compact geometry, it is likely that damping can be more closely controlled and shaped than in the lengthy, flexible transmission line prototype. This architecture is dynamically analogous to a parallel spring and damper in series between the source actuator and the environment, as called for by Dohring and Newman (Dohring & Newman, 2002).

This simple impedance shaper can also introduce controlled inertia. The passageways can be designed to provide inertial forces that are proportional to the acceleration of the flow Q_3, the relative flow between Q_1 and Q_2, rather than the acceleration of either piston. The damping and inertia can be regulated independently either by varying both the diameter and length of the passageways, or by introducing obstructions of negligible length (e.g. small holes) that increase damping but not inertia. More complex dynamics can be designed using simple fluid circuits if advantageous. The passive hydraulic transmission provides a platform where desired dynamics can be implemented and adjusted with simple, lightweight physical structures. Aside from moving seals, hydraulic system dynamics are generally devoid of backlash, discontinuous nonlinear friction, and other "hard" nonlinearities, and physical laws that govern behavior are well understood. The benefits of impedance shaping can be added to remote power transmission and intrinsic gearing in an integrated package to improve high-force, low-impedance robot actuation capabilities.

5. Conclusions

This chapter presented and defined high force haptic systems, and articulated the specific constraints that make the selection of actuators for this application difficult. To provide context, the pioneering high force haptics application of therapeutic robotics, and the obstacles to continued advancement of the field, were discussed. We continue to develop therapeutic robots for human movement from lower body (including partial weight support) to fine finger motions, and the actuation problem is the core engineering challenge for almost all of the designs. Major actuation and control technologies suitable for human-scale interaction were explored and evaluated for their fitness for high force haptics. As existing technology does not meet all of the needs of this field, we described our development and proof-of-concept of a hybrid hydraulic actuation scheme. This approach exploits the high force density of hydraulic systems without producing inevitably high endpoint impedance. Though analogous to mechanical transmissions, the hydraulic approach enables a dramatically more flexible coupling between source actuators and interaction ports. The simplicity of this design architecture, and the relatively straightforward and validated impact of geometric design parameters, makes it amenable to scaling for use as modular actuators in robots of all shapes and sizes. With this architecture, a single integrated physical system, the passive hydraulic transmission, can provide remote power transmission (directly reducing endpoint actuator weight), intrinsic gear reduction (permitting variation in actuator sizing) and impedance shaping (stabilizing contact while more aggressive force feedback is used). The structure of hybrid hydraulic actuators may also permit operation in environments that are hostile to other actuator types, including near or inside medical neuroimaging equipment for use in concert with, for instance, functional magnetic resonance imaging (fMRI). Together with existing actuator and interaction control technology, as well as developing new capabilities for advanced interactive actuators, the hybrid hydraulic actuation approach contributes to a diverse and expanding suite of tools for addressing the high force haptics challenge. As a one-size-fits-all solution to this formidable challenge seems unlikely to emerge, the growing community of high force haptics researchers should consider each of these possible solutions for their applications and select those best suited to their needs.

Acknowledgements

Support: NDSEG Fellowship, NIH HD37397, Burke Medical Research Institute, New York State C019772.

6. References

Bar-Cohen, Y. (Ed.) (2004). *Electroactive Polymer (EAP) Actuators as Artificial Muscles: Reality, Potential, and Challenges.* SPIE Press, Bellingham, WA.

Berkelman, P., Butler, Z. & Hollis, R. (1996). Design of a Hemispherical Magnetic Levitation Haptic Interface Device. *Proc. ASME Int Mech Eng Cong Expo,* Vol. 58, pp. 483-488.

Biggs, S. & Srinivasan, M. (2002). Haptic Interfaces, In: *Handbood of Virtual Environments*, Stanney, K. (Ed.), pp. 93-115, Lawrence Erlbaum Associates, Inc., New Jersey.

Buerger, S. & Hogan, N. (2007). Complementary Stability and Loop-Shaping for Improved Human-Robot Interaction. *IEEE Trans Rob Autom*, Vol. 23, pp. 232-244.

Buerger, S., Krebs, H. & Hogan, N. (2001). Characterization and Control of a Screw-Driven Robot for Neurorehabilitation. *Proc. IEEE CCA / ISIC.*

Carignan, C. & Cleary, K. (2000). Closed-Loop Force Control for Haptic Simulation of Virtual Environments. *Haptics-e*, Vol. 1, No. 2, pp. 1-14.

Colgate, J. & Hogan, N. (1988). Robust Control of Dynamically Interacting Systems. *Int J Contr*, Vol. 48, pp. 65-88.

Dohring, M. & Newman, W. (2002). Admittance Enhancement in Force Feedback of Dynamic Systems, *Proc. IEEE ICRA*, pp.638-643.

Goldfarb, M., Barth, E., Gogola, M. & Wehrmeyer, J. (2003). Design and Energetic Characterization of a Liquid-Propellant-Powered Actuator for Self-Powered Robots. *IEEE / ASME Trans Mechatronics*, Vol. 8, pp. 254-262.

Guizzo, E. & Goldstein, H. (2005). The Rise of the Body Bots. *IEEE Spectrum*, Vol. 42, pp. 50-56.

Hidler, J., Nichols, D., Pelliccio, M., Brady, K., Campbell, D. D., Kahn, J. H., and Hornby, T. G. (2009). Multicenter Randomized Clinical Trial Evaluating the Effectiveness of the Lokomat in Subacute Stroke. *Neurorehabilitation and Neural Repair* Vol. 23, pp. 5-13.

Hogan, N. & Buerger, S. (2005). Impedance and Interaction Control, In: *Robotics and Automation Handbook*, Kurfess, T. (Ed.), ch. 19, CRC Press, New York.

Hogan, N. (1985). Impedance Control: An Approach to Manipulation. *ASME J Dyn Sys Meas Contr*, Vol. 107, pp. 1-24.

Hogan, N. (1989). Controlling Impedance at the Man/Machine Interface, *Proc. IEEE ICRA*, pp. 1626-1631.

Hogan, N., Krebs, H. I., Rohrer, B., Palazzolo, J. J., Dipietro, L., Fasoli, S. E., Stein, J., Hughes, R., Frontera, W. R., Lynch, D., and Volpe, B. T. (2006). Motions or muscles? Some behavioral factors underlying robotic assistance of motor recovery *Journal Of Rehabilitation Research And Development* Vol. 43, pp. 605-618.

Hollerbach, J., Hunter, I. & Ballantyne, J. (1992). A Comparative Analysis of Actuator Technologies for Robotics, In: *The Robotics Review 2*, Khatib., O. (Ed.), pp. 299-342, MIT Press, Cambridge, MA.

Hornby, T. G., Campbell, D. D., Kahn, J. H., Demott, T., Moore, J. L., and Roth, H. R. (2008). Enhanced Gait-Related Improvements After Therapist- Versus Robotic-Assisted Locomotor Training in Subjects With Chronic Stroke: A Randomized Controlled Study. *Stroke* Vol. 39, pp. 1786-1792.

Israel, J. F., Campbell, D. D., Kahn, J. H., and Hornby, T. G. (2006). Metabolic Costs and Muscle Activity Patterns During Robotic- and Therapist-Assisted Treadmill Walking in Individuals with Incomplete Spinal Cord Injury. *Physical Therapy* Vol 86, pp. 1466.

Kazerooni, H. & Guo, J. (1993). Human Extenders. *ASME J Dyn Sys Meas Contr*, Vol. 115, pp. 281-290.

Krebs, H. I., Ladenheim, B., Hippolyte, C., Monterroso, L., and Mast, J. (2009). Robot-assisted task-specific training in cerebral palsy. *Developmental Medicine and Child Neurology* Vol. 51, pp. 140-145.

Krebs, H. I., Palazzolo, J. J., Dipietro, L., Volpe, B. T., and Hogan, N. (2003). Rehabilitation robotics: Performance-based progressive robot-assisted therapy. *Autonomous Robots* Vol. 15, pp. 7-20.

Krebs, H., Ferraro, M., Buerger, S., Newbery, M., Makiyama, A., Sandmann, M., Lynch, D., Volpe, B. & Hogan, N. (2004). Rehabilitation Robotics: Pilot Trial of a Spatial Extension for MIT-MANUS. *J NeuroEng Rehab.* Vol 1, p. 5.

Kwakkel, G., Kollen, B. J., and Krebs, H. I. (2007). Effects of Robot-assisted therapy on upper limb recovery after stroke: A Systematic Review. *Neurorehabilitation and Neural Repair.*

Lawrence, D. (1993). Stability and Transparency in Bilateral Teleoperation. *IEEE Trans Rob Autom,* Vol. 9, pp. 624-637.

Lee, Y. & Ryu, D. (2008). Wearable Haptic Glove Using Micro Hydraulic System for Control of Construction Robot System with VR Environment. *Proc. IEEE Int Conf on Multisensor Fusion and Integration for Intelligent Systems,* pp. 638-643.

Massie, T. & Salisbury, K. (1994). The PHANTOM Haptic Interface: A Device for Probing Virtual Objects. *Proc. ASME Winter Annual Meeting, Symposium on Haptic Interfaces for Virtual Environment and Teleoperator Systems.*

McBean, J. & Breazeal, C. (2004). Voice Coil Actuators for Human_Robot Interaction. *Proc. IEEE/RSJ Int Conf on Intel Rob Sys,* pp. 852-858.

Neckel, N. D., Blonien, N., Nichols, D., and Hidler, J. (2008). Abnormal joint torque patterns exhibited by chronic stroke subjects while walking with a prescribed physiological gait pattern. *Journal of NeuroEngineering and Rehabilitation* Vol. 5, pp. 1-13.

Newman, W.S. (1992). Stability and Performance Limits of Interaction Controllers. *ASME J Dyn Sys Meas Contr,* Vol. 114, pp. 563-570.

Nudo, R. J. (2007). Postinfarct Cortical Plasticity and Behavioral Recovery. *Stroke* Vol. 38, pp. 840-845.

Peshkin, M., Colgate, J., Wannasuphoprasit, W., Moore, C., Gillespie, R. & Akella, P. (2001). Cobot Architecture. *IEEE Trans Rob Autom,* Vol. 17, pp. 377-390.

Prange, G. B., Jannink, M. J. A., Groothuis-Oudshoorn, C. G. M., Hermens, H. J., and Ijzerman, M. J. (2006). Systematic review of the effect of robot-aided therapy on recovery of the hemiparetic arm after stroke. *Journal of Rehabilitation Research and Development* Vol. 43, pp. 171-184.

Pratt, G. & Williamson, M. (1995). Series Elastic Actuators. *Proc. IEEE/RSJ Int Conf on Human Robot Interaction and Cooperative Robots,* pp. 399-406.

Roberts, M. H. (2004). "A Robot for Gait Rehabilitation." Massachusetts Institute of Technology.

Roy, A., Krebs, H. I., Williams, D. J., Bever, C. T., Forrester, L. W., Macko, R. M., and Hogan, N. (2009). Robot-Aided Neurorehabilitation: A Novel Robot for Ankle Rehabilitation. *IEEE Transactions on Robotics* Vol. 25, pp. 569-582.

Taub, E., and Uswatte, G. (2006). Constraint-Induced Movement therapy: Answers and questions after two decades of research. *NeuroRehabilitation* Vol. 21, pp. 93-95.

Tondu, B. & Lopez, P. (2000). Modeling and Control of McKibben Artificial Muscle Robot Actuators. *IEEE Contr Sys Magazine,* Vol. 20, Issue 2, pp. 15-38.

Townsend, W. & Guertin, J. (1999). Teleoperator Slave - WAM Design Methodology. *Ind Robot,* Vol. 26, p. 167.

Tressler, J., Clement, T., Kazerooni, H. & Lim, A. (2002). Dynamic Behavior of Pneumatic Systems for Lower Extremity Extenders. *Proc IEEE ICRA,* pp. 3248-3253.

Veneman, J. F., Kruidhof, R., Hekman, E. E. G., Ekkelenkamp, R., Asseldonk, E. H. F. V., and Kooij, H. v. d. (2007). Design and Evaluation of the LOPES Exoskeleton Robot for Interactive Gait Rehabilitation. *IEEE Transactions on Neural Systems and Rehabilitation Engineering* Vol. 15, pp. 379-386.

Volpe, B. T., Ferraro, M., Lynch, D., Christos, P., Krol, J., Trudell, C., Krebs, H. I., and Hogan, N. (2004). Robotics and Other Devices in the Treatment of Patients Recovering Stroke. *Current Atherosclerosis Reports* Vol. 6, pp. 314-319.

Volpe, B. T., Huerta, P. T., Zipse, J. L., Rykman, A., Edwards, D., Dipietro, L., Hogan, N., and Krebs, H. I. (2009). Robotic Devices as Therapeutic and Diagnostic Tools for Stroke Recovery. *Archives Of Neurology* Vol. 66, pp. 1086-1090.

Wolf, S. L., Winstein, C. J., Miller, J. P., Taub, E., Uswatte, G., Morris, D., Giuliani, C., Light, K. E., and Nichols-Larsen, D. (2006). Effect of Constraint-Induced Movement Therapy on Upper Extremity Function 3 to 9 Months After Stroke: The EXCITE Randomized Clinical Trial. *Journal of the American Medical Association* Vol. 296, pp. 2095-2104.

Wyatt, J., Chua, L., Gannett, J., Goknar, I. & Green, D. (1981). Energy Concepts in the State-Space Theory of Nonlinear n-ports: Part I – Passivity. *IEEE Trans Circ Sys*, Vol. 23, pp. 48-61.

2

Using Magnetic Levitation for Haptic Interaction

Peter Berkelman and Michael Dzadovsky
University of Hawaii-Manoa
USA

1. Introduction

Magnetic levitation as a means of motion and force/torque control can provide many advantages for high-fidelity haptic interaction, as compared to motorized linkage and cable actuation. Impedance-based haptic interface devices function both as force display devices, generating forces and/or torques to be felt by the user, and as input devices, sensing the motions imparted by the user to the device. The realism of the haptic interaction is related to the performance of these two functions, which can be quantitatively measured by their position and force accuracy and response times.

Magnetic levitation devices have been able to provide very high force & position control bandwidths, resolution, and impedance ranges for haptic interaction through a grasped tool handle. Only one moving part is required to provide precise, responsive, 6 degree-of-freedom frictionless motion with force and torque feedback to interact with a simulated or remote environment. With no friction from contacts with actuation or sensing mechanisms, magnetic levitation devices are ideally backdriveable and dynamic nonlinearities such as cogging and backlash are eliminated.

The small motion ranges of current tabletop magnetic levitation devices in translation and rotation have been a severe limitation on the size and type of interactive environments and tasks, however. Small motion ranges of magnetic levitation devices are due to a combination of narrow magnetic field gaps and linearized magnetic actuation models which are only valid in a neighborhood of a given setpoint. As a result, magnetic levitation haptic interfaces which have been previously developed focus on fingertip-scale motions, and provide variable indexing, rate control, and scaling methods through software to simulate interaction with larger environments.

The mass and rotational inertia perceived by the user as the haptic interface device is manipulated affects the realism of haptic interaction, as well as the position control bandwidths of the device. The transparency of haptic interaction is improved when the encountered mass and inertia are minimized.

We have developed two different magnetic levitation devices which provide unprecedented ranges of motion in both translation and rotation to a levitated handle to be used for tool-based haptic interaction. The first device levitates a handle attached to a thin spherical shell of flat coils suspended in permanent magnet fields using Lorentz forces. A novel coil type and magnet configuration provides double the translation and triple the rotation ranges of previous Lorentz levitation haptic devices.

The second device uses a planar array of cylindrical coils to levitate a platform of one or more magnets. By using redundant control methods and an experimentally measured high resolution model of the forces and torques generated on the levitated magnets from each coil, the translation range of the magnet in horizontal directions and its rotation in all directions can be extended indefinitely. These new devices permit fuller wrist and forearm motions of the user for haptic interaction rather than the fingertips-only motions provided by previous magnetic levitation haptic interface devices. Design, analysis, and control methods are presented with measured haptic performance characteristics and haptic interaction task results from both devices.

The following section surveys current technology background in magnetic levitation and grasped haptic interaction devices actuated by motorized linkages and/or cables. Section 3 describes early Loretz force magnetic levitation devices developed for haptic interaction by Hollis, Salcudean, and Berkelman. Sections 4 and 5 describe our current development of a Lorentz force magnetic levitation haptic interface device with a new magnet and coil configuration to increase its translation and rotation ranges and a levitation system using an array of cylindrical coils to levitate one or more disk magnets, followed by a future work and conclusion section.

2. Research Background

2.1 Magnetic Levitation Systems

Magnetic levitation systems can provide advantages for applications in manipulation (Oh et al., 1993; Khamesee & Shameli, 2005) fine positioning (Kim & Trumper, 1998; Kim et al., 2004), and haptic interaction (Hollis & Salcudean, 1993; Berkelman & Hollis, 2000). Surveys of magnetic levitation technology for rail transportation are given in (Lee et al., 2006) and for magnetic bearings in (Schweitzer et al., 1994). Other existing systems (Wang & Busch-Vishniac, 1994; Lai et al., 2007; Robertson et al., 2005; Zhang & Menq, 2007) also typically have ranges of motion which are limited however to a small fraction of the dimensions of the levitated body in most or all directions, and to rotation angles of less than 20 degrees.

High frequency feedback control is necessary to stabilize magnetic levitation. Non-contact position sensing for feedback control of magnetic levitation can be provided by optical methods using LED markers and position sensing photodiodes, Hall effect magnetic sensing (Gohin et al., 2007), or by laser interferometry which can provide submicrometer precision position sensing.

Lorentz force levitation was initially developed for compliant assembly robotic wrists (Hollis and Salcudean, 1993). Hollis and Salcudean pioneered the use of Lorentz force actuation from currents in flat racetrack-shaped coils suspended between horseshoe-shaped magnet assemblies, producing forces independent of coil positions provided that magnetic fields are constant.

A large range of motion levitation system for small magnets using multiple permanent magnets, pole pieces, and actuation coils to control magnetic fields is described in (Khamesee & Shameli, 2005). A gripper has been added to this system for magnetic levitation micromanipulation (Craig & Khamesee, 2007), however the spatial rotation of the magnet is uncontrolled.

Spherical motors (Yan et al., 2006; Chirikjian & Stein, 1999) have been developed to control spatial orientation of a rigid body using magnets and coils, yet these are supported by bearings and not levitated or controlled in position. A dipole model for simplified magnetic field torque computations in spherical motor is presented in (Lee et al., 2009).

The previous work most closely related to our current research on levitation of cylindrical magnets using a coil array was by (Groom & Britcher, 1992), who carried out extensive analysis of electromagnetic actuation, rigid body dynamics, and feedback control methods for levitation with large rotations. Owing to limitations in position and orientation sensing, implementation was limited to small motions however. Baheti and Koumboulis (Baheti, 1984; Koumboulis & Skarpetis, 1996) have also carried out related work on magnetic suspension and balance systems for models in wind tunnels.

2.2 High-Fidelity Haptic Interface Devices

Haptic interface devices are typically actuated by DC motors through linkages and low-friction drivetrains such as belts and cables. As the motors produce torque directly, it is straightforward to generate haptic forces to the user given the kinematics of the linkage. High fidelity haptic interaction with position control bandwidths greater than 100 Hz may be realized by designing the linkage to be as stiff and lightweight as possible, with minimal joint friction and backlash. Parallel linkage designs can be made particularly stiff and lightweight, although joint friction may be more significant. Many of these devices provide 3 DOF force feedback only, as this is sufficent for haptic interaction at a single "fingertip" point and a 6 DOF mechanism must add complexity, mass, and friction which reduce its dynamic performance.

The most widely used haptic interface devices are the *Phantom* devices from Sensable Technologies Inc (Massie & Salisbury, 1994). In these devices the user grasps a pen which is mounted on a gimbal to a counterweighted, cable-driven parallelogram linkage. 3 DOF force feedback and and 6 DOF force and torque feedback models of various sizes and configurations are available. The *Delta* haptic device (Grange et al., 2001) is based on 3 parallel link sets and has similar properties, and is also commercially available in 3 and 6 DOF feedback versions.

The *Pantograph* (Hayward et al., 1994) design maximizes the control bandwith obtainable from a 2 DOF planar parallelogram linkage. The *Freedom* 6/7 (Hayward, 1995) devices provide 6 and 7 DOF with an attached gripper using a complex linkage with cable drives.

3. Racetrack Coil Lorentz Force Magnetic Levitation Haptic Interfaces

3.1 IBM Magic Wrist

The *Magic Wrist* was adapted for haptic interaction by fixing it to a stationary base rather than a robotic arm (Berkelman et al., 1995), as shown in Figure 1. This device provided high control bandwidths, position resolution, and stiff haptic contacts, but its motion range is limited to less than 10 mm and 10 degrees rotation. The levitated coils in this device are embedded in a hexagonal box.

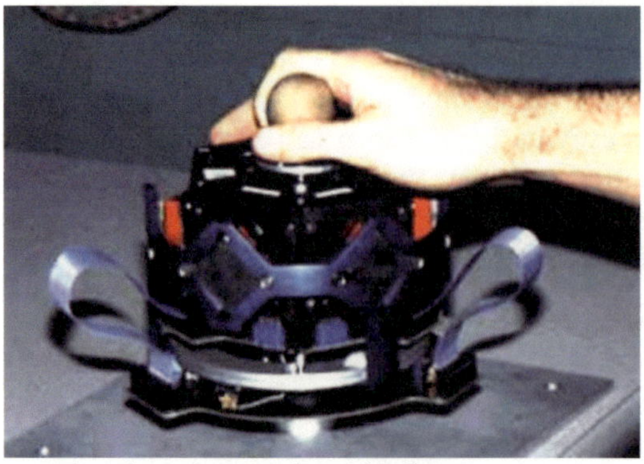

Fig. 1. IBM Magic Wrist used as haptic interface device

3.2 UBC Teleoperation Master and Powermouse

The *Teloperation Master* developed at the University of British Columbia (Salcudean et al., 1995) has a similar size and motion range as the Magic Wrist, yet has a novel magnet and coil configuration. Its structure, with the grasped cover removed, is shown in Figure 2(a). The *Powermouse* (Salcudean & Parker, 1997) is a smaller desktop device, with reduced mass and a small motion range adaped for fingertip interaction. Its levitation coils are arranged on the faces of a cube embedded inside the housing of the device shown in Figure 2(b).

3.3 CMU / Butterfly Haptics Maglev Haptic Interface

Another Lorentz force magnetic levitation haptic interface device was developed at Carnegie Mellon by Berkelman and Hollis (Berkelman & Hollis, 2000) , with the coil and magnet configuration and position sensing system modified to provide a large increase in the ranges of motion in both translation, at 25 mm, and rotation at 15 degrees. The main factor in the motion range increase was to embed large actuator coils tightly together in a thin hemispherical shell, with the interaction handle mounted at the center. The top of the device and its use with a graphically displayed environment on a PC are shown in Figure 3.

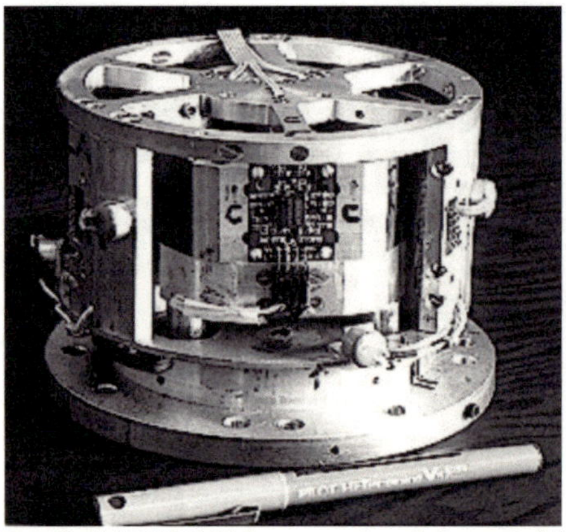

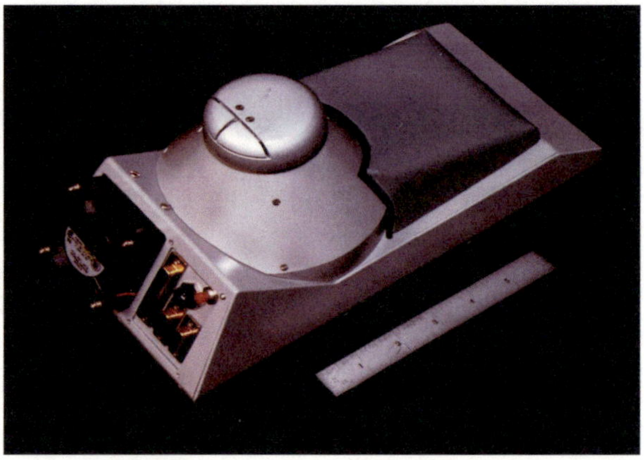

Fig. 2. (a) UBC Teleoperation Master, (b) UBC Powermouse

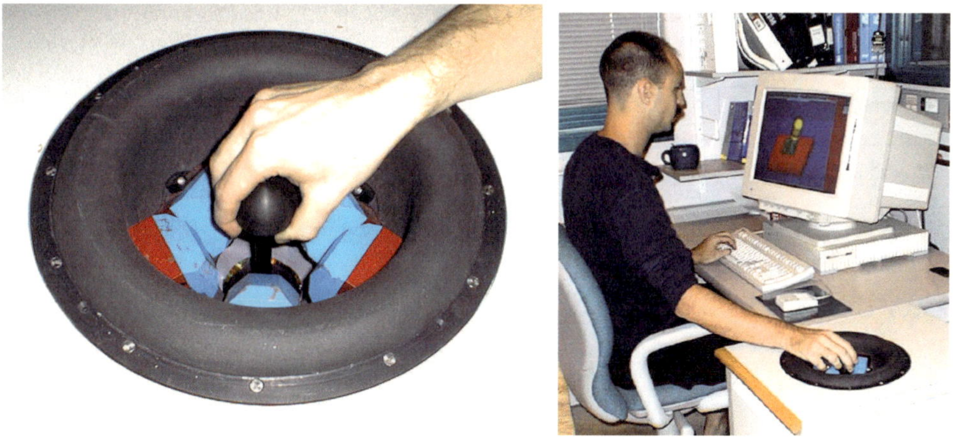

Fig. 3. Carnegie Mellon University Prototype (a) Levitated Handle Grasped by User, (b) Interaction with Simulated Environment

A commercial successor to this design, with improved position sensing feedback, a lighter, stiffer levitated hemisphere shell, and with a software programming interface, is currently produced by Butterfly Haptics LLC. At least 10 devices are in use in several different research labs composing a maglev haptic consortium.

4. Double Coil Layer Lorentz Magnetic Levitation Design

4.1 Design

Our first extended range magnetic levitation design is a Lorentz levitation device with coils on a spherical shell and a user handle mounted at the center of the shell, as in the Carnegie Mellon Lorentz devices. This device uses a novel coil shape, magnet configuration, and arranges the coils in two layers so that the magnetic field gap widths can be doubled at approximately the same field intensity as before and the coil areas can be increased many times more on a shell of approximately the same radius, resulting in a doubling of the translation range and a tripling of the rotation range in all directions. The basic design is described in more detail in (Berkelman, 2007) and shown in Figure 4. Instead of using racetrack-shaped coils in which the coil windings follow oval paths, a new coil shape shown in Figure 5(a) is used in which the windings follow straight paths across the centers of the coils, and curved return paths around the periphery of the round coils. This allows the coils to be arranged in two layers as in Figure 5(b), with the straight wires across the centers of the coils orthogonal to one another. In this arrangement, the areas of the coils can be increased considerably without increasing the radius of the spherical shell, and each pair of layered coils requires only two magnets to generate their shared magnetic field. Large, curved iron pole pieces pass above and around the levitated coil assemblies to form a magnetic flux path from one magnet to the other on the opposite sides of each gap. The centers of the coil pairs are arranged at 0, 120, and 240 degrees around the circumference at an angle of 35 degrees below the horizontal plane, on a spherical surface with a 125 mm radius, and each coil spans a solid angle of 90 degrees. The effective solid angle of each coil is reduced to approximately 70 degrees due to the width of the magnets and the return paths of the wires around the edges of the coils and the magnet gaps are 53 mm, so that the device can provide a motion range of 50 mm in translation and approximately 60 degrees in rotation in all directions.

As the translation range is approximately double and the rotation range is triple that of previous levitated haptic interaction devices, the workspace volume is actually increased by a factor of 8 and the rotation space by a factor of 27. The increased motion range

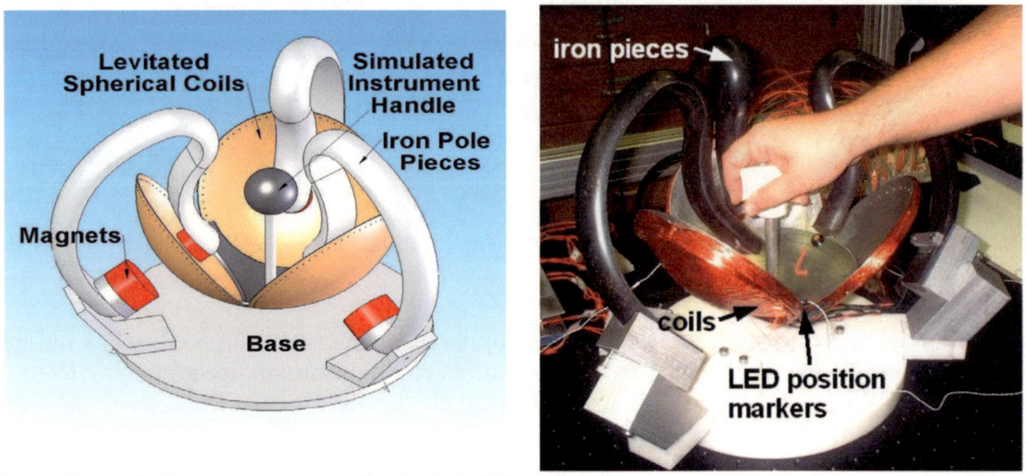

Fig. 4. Extended motion range spherical shell Lorentz force magnetic levitation device (a) Design, (b) device as fabricated

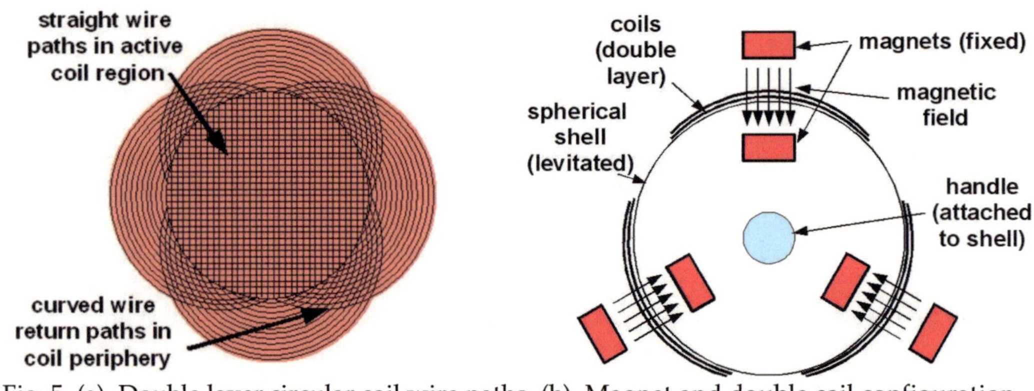

Fig. 5. (a) Double layer circular coil wire paths, (b) Magnet and double coil configuration

of the new device is not merely an incremental improvement, but enables a qualitatively much greater variety of interactive tasks to be simulated as the increased range is comparable to the full range of human wrist movement, whereas previous haptic levitation devices could accommodate fingertip motions only. For example, common manual manipulation tasks such as turning doorknobs, keys, and hexagonal nuts and screwheads can be realistically haptically simulated with the new device, and 60 degrees of rotation and 50 mm of translation is sufficient to simulate many tasks in minimally invasive surgery (Rosen et al., 2002).

The force generated by each coil can be modelled as a single force vector at the center of each coil, and one coil in each pair generates vertical and the other generates horizontal forces. The magnitude of the force generated by each coil is approximately 3.0 Newtons/Amp. With the coil center locations at:

$$r_{1,2} = 0.125\begin{bmatrix} \cos(35) \\ 0 \\ -\sin(35) \end{bmatrix}, \quad r_{3,4} = 0.125\begin{bmatrix} \cos(120)\ \cos(35) \\ \sin(120)\ \sin(35) \\ -\sin\ (35) \end{bmatrix}, \quad r_{5,6} = 0.125\begin{bmatrix} \cos(240)\ \cos(35) \\ \sin(240)\ \cos(35) \\ -\sin\ (35) \end{bmatrix} \tag{1}$$

in m, and the forces generated by each coil at:

$$\begin{gathered} f_1 = 3.0\begin{bmatrix} \sin(35) \\ 0 \\ \cos(35) \end{bmatrix} i_1, \quad f_2 = 3.0\begin{bmatrix} 0 \\ 1 \\ 0 \end{bmatrix} i_2, \quad f_3 = 3.0\begin{bmatrix} \cos(120)\ \ \sin(35) \\ \sin(120)\ \ \sin(35) \\ \cos(35) \end{bmatrix} i_3, \\ f_4 = 3.0\begin{bmatrix} -\sin(20) \\ \cos(35) \\ 0 \end{bmatrix} i_4, \quad f_5 = 3.0\begin{bmatrix} \cos(240)\ \ \sin(35) \\ \sin(240)\ \ \sin(35) \\ \cos(35) \end{bmatrix} i_5, \quad f_6 = 3.0\begin{bmatrix} -\sin(240) \\ \cos(240) \\ 0 \end{bmatrix} i_6, \end{gathered} \tag{2}$$

in Newtons, with angles in degrees, then the current to force and torque vector transformation matrix can be given as:

$$\begin{bmatrix} f_x \\ f_y \\ f_z \\ \tau_x \\ \tau_y \\ \tau_z \end{bmatrix} = \begin{bmatrix} f_1 & f_2 & \cdots \\ r_1 \times f_1 & r_2 \times f_2 & \cdots \end{bmatrix} \begin{bmatrix} i_1 \\ i_2 \\ i_3 \\ i_4 \\ i_5 \\ i_6 \end{bmatrix} \tag{3}$$

to relate currents in A to forces in N and torques in N-m. When the sphere radius and the force magnitudes are normalized to 1 to compensate for differences in force and torque units, the condition number of the transformation matrix is 3.7, indicating that the matrix is invertable and forces and torques can be efficiently generated in all directions without requiring excessively larger coil currents for some directions.

4.2 Analysis and Fabrication

Electromagnetic finite element analysis was performed to find magnet shapes and dimensions to concentrate and maximize magnetic fields necessary for levitation. This analysis indicated that the minimum field strength in between magnets is approximately 0.25 T, which is expected from experience (Berkelman & Hollis, 2000) to be sufficient for levitation and high-fidelity haptic interaction. The mass of the fabricated levitated body is 1200 g; by fabricating new coils using aluminum wire and using a more lightweight support structure we aim to reduce the levitated mass to 500 g or less. In Figure 4(b), the iron pole pieces on two of the magnet assemblies have been rotated about the magnet axes by approximately 30 degrees to provide more ergonomic access for the user to more easily grasp the levitated handle without affecting the magnetic fields or the range of motion of the device.

4.3 Experimental Results

A sample large scale vertical step input motion trajectory for the free-floating levitated coils in the vertical direction is shown in Figure 5. The control gains used were as follows:

	translation	rotation
Kp	2.0 N/mm	0.0875 N-m/degree
Kd	0.01 N-sec/mm	0.00035 N-m-sec/degree

As these are very preliminary results, it is expected that more careful modeling, calibration, and signal processing will result in considerable increases of the maximum stable gains and a more damped response.

Regarding the positioning accuracy of the levitated bowl and the stiffness of the coil structure, it is notable that any flexion of the coils from high actuation forces would not affect the position accuracy of the manipulation handle, as the position sensing feedback is from LED markers close to the center of the structure, which is reinforced with an additional layer of aluminum and a collar around the base of the handle. Furthermore, for haptic interaction applications, absolute position accuracy of the device is not as critical as the incremental position and force accuracy and control bandwidths to the perceived fidelity of the haptic interaction.

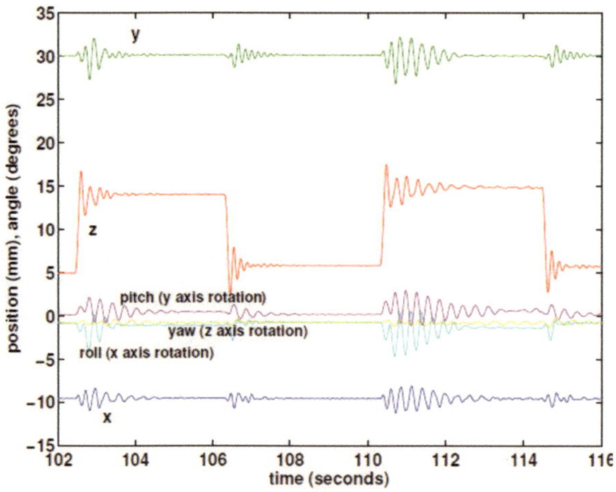

Fig. 6. Vertical step response results for new Lorentz levitation device

5. Magnet Levitation by Planar Array of Cylindrical Coils

5.1 Design

A redundant actuation method was used to levitate a single magnet by combining actuation forces and torques from more than 5 coils at a time. The potential advantages of redundant actuation compared to selections of coil subsets at each magnet position are that the maximum required coil currents for levitation may be reduced by distributing the generation of lifting forces over more coils, and discontinuous force disturbances due to measurement and position errors as coil currents are abruptly switched on and off during motion trajectories can be avoided. Sixteen coils of 25 mm diameter, 30 mm height, and 1000 windings are currently used, providing a motion range of approximately 100x80x30 mm with potentially unlimited tilt range. Rotation about the axis of a single disk magnet cannot be controlled due to its radial symmetry, so single magnet platform levitation leaves this yaw angle uncontrolled. The array levitation control methods, design, and initial results are described in further detail in (Berkelman & Dzadovsky, 2008). The levitated mass is approximately 125 g.

5.2 Control

To determine the model of force and torque generation between a single magnet and coil, an experimental setup of motion stages and a force sensor was used as in Figure 7(a). Although it is possible to obtain a force and torque generation model either analytically (as described in [5]) or from electromagnetic finite element analysis, in this case it is simpler and faster to obtain the model experimentally, and furthermore the effects of variations in the magnet material and its magnetization are accounted for directly.

The 6 force and torque elements generated between the magnet and coil were recorded at 1 mm intervals of vertical and radial separation and 30 degree angular intervals, resulting in the force and torque data partially shown in shown in Figure 7(b). The forces and torques generated by each coil were found to be independent and proportional to each coil current to a very close approximation, allowing the current to force and torque transformation to be represented in linear matrix form at any magnet position and orientation. This data was used to calculate the current to force and torque transformation for single magnet levitation. Defining the angle from each coil center i to the magnet center in the horizontal plane as ψ_i, the transformation from currents to forces and torques is as follows:

$$\begin{bmatrix} f_x \\ f_y \\ f_z \\ \tau_x \\ \tau_y \\ \tau_z \end{bmatrix} = \begin{bmatrix} \cos(\psi_1)f_x(r_1,z,\phi,\theta_i)-\sin(\psi_1)f_y(r_1,z,\phi,\theta_i) & \cdots \\ \sin(\psi_1)f_x(r_1,z,\phi,\theta_i)+\cos(\psi_1)f_y(r_1,z,\phi,\theta_i) & \cdots \\ f_x(r_1,z,\phi,\theta_i) & \cdots \\ \cos(\psi_1)f_x(r_1,z,\phi,\theta_i)-\sin(\psi_1)f_y(r_1,z,\phi,\theta_i) & \cdots \\ \sin(\psi_1)f_x(r_1,z,\phi,\theta_i)+\cos(\psi_1)f_y(r_1,z,\phi,\theta_i) & \cdots \\ f_x(r_1,z,\phi,\theta_i) & \cdots \end{bmatrix} \begin{bmatrix} i_1 \\ i_2 \\ \cdots \end{bmatrix} \tag{4}$$

where z is the levitation height of the magnet center above the coil plane, and r_i is the horizontal distance from the center of the coil i to the center of the magnet. Since the coil forces

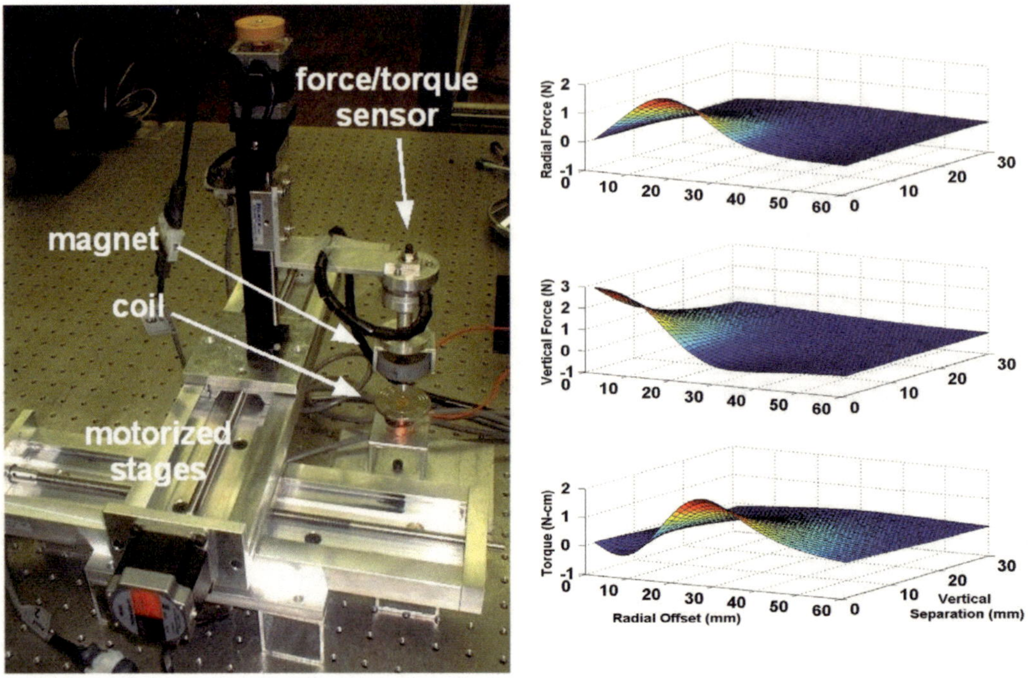

Fig. 7. (a) Motion stage and force/torque measurement setup, (b) Radial force, vertical force, and torque generated on magnet by coil with 1.0 Ampere current

and torques are measured at discrete values of θ, cubic interpolation is used to estimate the values of the continuous functions.

For 6 degree of freedom controlled levitation of platforms with multiple disk magnets, additional terms must be added due to the **r**×**f** torques from magnet forces **f** generated at a distance **r** from the center of mass of the levitated platform; it is these transformation terms which enable generation of τ_z torques to control the yaw angle.

As forces and torques are both produced in 3 dimensions, and there are 16 coils in the current setup, each resulting transformation matrix is 6x16 elements. This rectangular matrix is kinematically redundant, as the number of actuators is greater than the DOF to be controlled. For redundant systems in general, the Moore-Penrose pseudoinverse $\mathbf{A}^{+}$ of $\mathbf{A}$ (Moore, 1920; Penrose, 1955) can be used to calculate actuation currents $\mathbf{I} = \mathbf{A}^{+}\mathbf{F}$ with the lowest sum of squared currents for levitation control, adapting control methods developed for redundant actuation velocity control and execution of subspace tasks as described in (Nenchev, 1992; Baillieul, 1987). In our system however, the pseudoinverse of the transformation matrix cannot be directly inverted to produce the coil currents to produce a desired set of forces and torques, as no combination of coil currents can produce any torque on the magnet about its principal axis. For 5 DOF levitation control at arbitrary orientations, the torque vectors in the transformation matrices can rotated so that one of the torque directions is aligned with the magnet axis, and the row corresponding to these torques is reduced to approximately zero. This row can then be eliminated from the transformation matrix, and the pseudoinverse of the resulting reduced 5x16 transform matrix can then be used to calculate coil currents to generate two torques perpendicular to the axis of the magnet to control its orientation while leaving the rotation of the magnet about its principal axis uncontrolled.

The force/torque to current transforms are precalculated to the closest 1.0 mm in translation and 30 degrees in orientation, and stored in a lookup table for use during realtime control. Linear interpolation of the measured force and torque data described previously is used online for control, as the distance and angle from each coil to the magnet are not restricted to 1 mm and 30 degree intervals. Numerical computation software was used for the calculation of the force/torque to current transformation lookup tables.

Condition numbers of the transformation matrix across the motion plane are shown for a horizontal magnet orientation in Figure 8(a) and a vertical orientation in Figure 8(b) at a 25 mm levitation height. The locations of the 16 coil centers are indicated by asterisks '*', these are arranged in a hexagonal configuration with a spacing of 35 mm. The transformation condition numbers are greatest directly above the coil centers because the horizontal force and torque torque generation capabilites of the coil underneath are zero although the vertical force generation efficiencies are maximized at these locations.

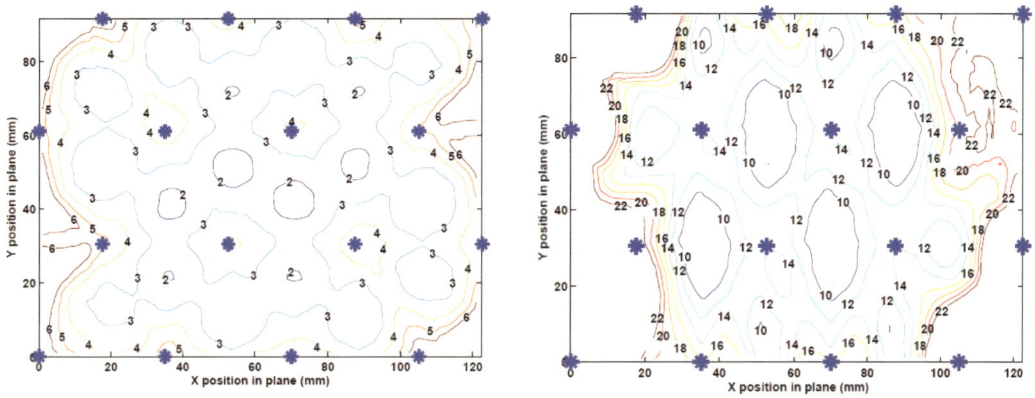

Fig. 8. Coil current to force/torque vector transformation matrix condition numbers, (a) Horizontal orientation, (b) vertical orientation

5.3 Results and Discussion

Using the system and methods described, we have realized stable levitation with 5 DOF control of a single disk magnet, as shown in Figure 9(a), and 6 DOF control of a magnet pair shown in Figure 9(b). A single levitated magnet may be embedded in a computer mouse shell for user interaction, as shown in Figure 10(a), and a single magnet may be levitated in any orientation by fixing 12 position markers to the levitated body oriented on the faces of a dodecahedron, so that at least 3 markers are visible to the position sensor at all times, as shown in Figure 10(b).

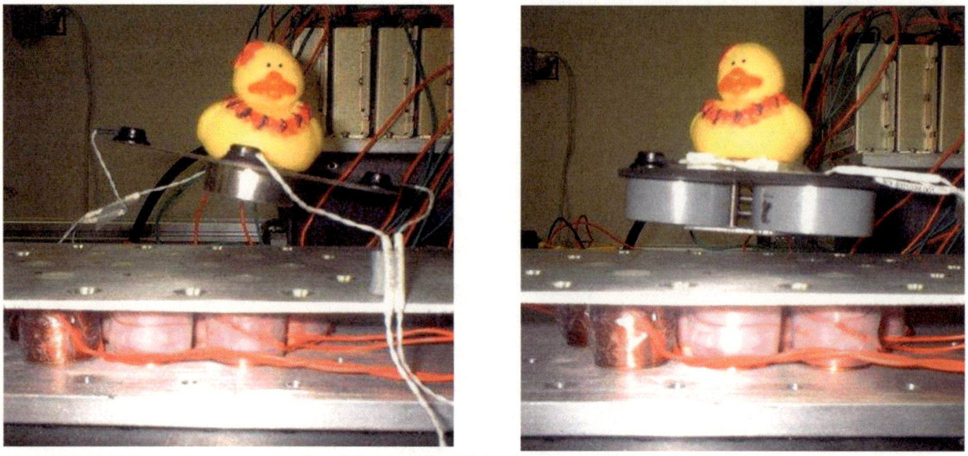

Fig. 9. (a) 5 DOF motion control with single disk magnet, (b) 6 DOF motion control

Large scale motion trajectories from a single free-floating levitated magnet are shown in Figure 11. The control gains used were as follows:

	translation	rotation
Kp	0.2 N/mm	5.25 N-mm/degree
Kd	0.002 N-sec/mm	0.0525 N-mm-sec/degree

The position control bandwidths of the system are limited by the maximum stable proportional gain, or stiffness of the controller, this gain is limited in turn by the resolution and noise level of the position sensor and the update rate of the controller. Initial levitation of two magnet platforms has also been demonstrated for 6 degree-of-freedom levitation control including yaw rotations.

6. Future Work and Conclusions

The planar array levitation system has greater potential for further expansion of its motion range in horizontal directions and rotations in all directions, but it is less efficient than the Lorentz levitation device, which can generate higher forces and torques without overheating. Each of the two systems will be interfaced to publically available haptic interaction software such as *Chai3d* and *H3D* to evaluate user perception and task performance using the devices.

Further development to be undertaken for each system includes modeling of the magnetic field variations in the Lorentz force device for better control performance, and modeling of magnetic actuation at any rotation angle for the planar system. Coils with iron cores will be used for more efficient actuation.

The two described magnetic levitation systems each provide greater motion ranges than any other previous magnetic levitation device for haptic interaction. The magnetic levitation systems and methods described are part of a larger research effort to investigate and develop magnetic levitation for high-fidelity haptic interaction.

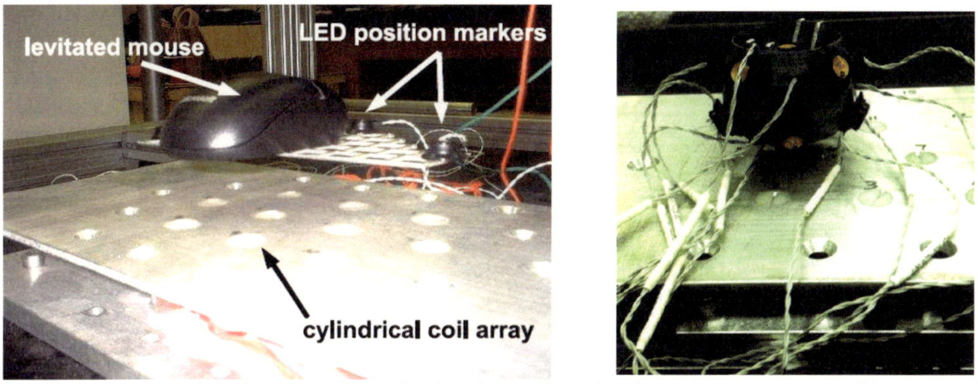

Fig. 10. (a) Levitated mouse with embedded magnet for haptic interaction, (b) 12 marker levitated body for levitation at any orientation

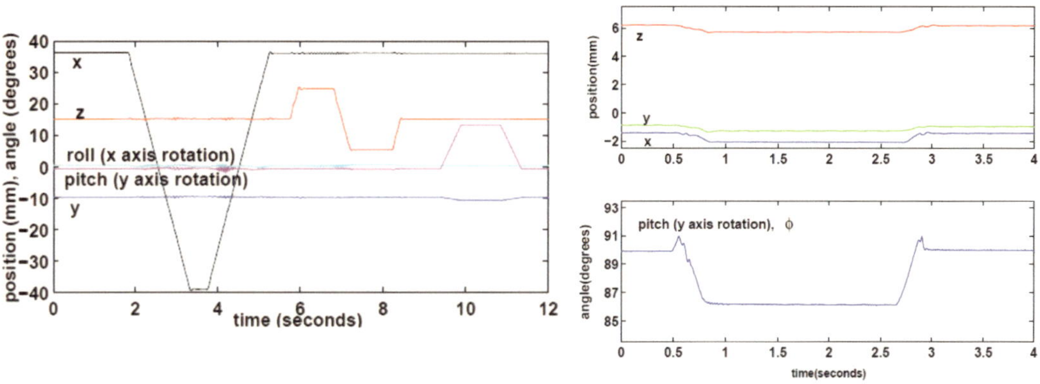

Fig. 11. (a) Motion trajectory for magnet in horizontal orientation, (b) vertical orientation

7. References

R. Baheti, "Multivariable frequency domain controller for magnetic suspension and balance systems," *IEEE Transactions on Automatic Control*, vol. 29, no. 8, pp. 725-728, 1984.

J. Baillieul, "A constraint oriented approach to inverse problems for kinematically redundant manipulators," *IEEE International Conference on Robotics and Automation*, Raleigh, March 1987, pp. 1827-1833.

P. J. Berkelman, R. L. Hollis, and S. E. Salculdean, "Interacting with Virtual Environments using a Magnetic Levitation Haptic Interface", Int'l Conf. on Intelligent Robots and Systems, Pittsburgh, August 1995.

P. J. Berkelman and R. L. Hollis, "Lorentz magnetic levitation for haptic interaction: Device design, function, and integration with simulated environments", *International Journal of Robotics Research*, 9(7):644-667, 2000.

P. J. Berkelman, "A novel coil configuration to extend the motion range of lorentz force magnetic levitation devices for haptic interaction", *IEEE/RSJ International Conference on Intelligent Robots and Systems*, San Diego, October 2007.

P. J. Berkelman and M. Dzadovsky, "Magnet levitation and trajectory following motion control using a planar array of cylindrical coils", *ASME Dynamic Systems and Control Conference*, Ann Arbor, October 2008.

G. S. Chirikjian and D. Stein, "Kinematic design and commutation of a spherical stepper motor", *IEEE/ASME Transactions on Mechatronics*, 4(4):342–353, December 1999.

D. G. Craig and M. B. Khamesee, "Motion control of a large gap magnetic suspension system for microrobotic manipulation," *Journal of Physics D: Applied Physics*, vol. 40, no. 11, pp. 3277-3285, 2007.

S. Grange and F. Conti, P. Rouiller, P. Helmer, and C. Baur, "Overview of the Delta Haptic Device", Eurohaptics, Birmingham UK, 2001.

A. Gohin, J. Simeray, W. X. Bing, and L. L. Qing, "Levitation device," *U. S. Patent No. 20,070,170,798*, July 2007.

N. J. Groom and C. P. Britcher, "A description of a laboratory model magnetic suspension test fixture with large angular capability", *IEEE Conference on Control Applications,,* Dayton, September 1992, pp 454–459.

V. Hayward, J. Choksi, G. Lanvin, and C. Ramstein, "Design and multi-objective optimization of a linkage for a haptic interface", ARK'94, 4th Int'l Workshop on Advances in Robot Kinematics, Ljubliana, June 1994.

V. Hayward, "Toward a Seven Axis Haptic Device", Int'l Conf. on Intelligent Robots and Systems, Pittsburgh, August 1995, pp. 113-139.

R. L. Hollis, S. Salcudean, and A. P. Allan, "A six degree-of-freedom magnetically levitated variable compliance fine motion wrist: design, modeling, and control", *IEEE Transactions on Robotics and Automation*, 7(3):320–332, June 1991.

R. L. Hollis and S. E. Salcudean, "Lorentz levitation technology: a new approach to fine motion robotics, teleoperation, haptic interfaces, and vibration isolation", *Proc. 6th Int'l Symposium on Robotics Research*, Hidden Valley, PA, October 1993.

W.-J. Kim and D. Trumper, "High-precision magnetic levitation stage for photolithography," *Precision Engineering*, vol. 22, pp. 66–77, 1998.

W.-J. Kim, N. Bhat, and T. Hu, "Integrated multidimensional positioner for precision manufacturing," *Proceedings of the Institution of Mechanical Engineers Part B: Journal of Engineering Manufacturing*, vol. 218, pp. 431–442, 2004

M. B. Khamesee and E. Shameli, "Regulation technique for a large gap magnetic field for 3d non-contact manipulation", *Mechatronics*, 15:1073–1087, 2005.

F. N. Koumboulis and M. G. Skarpetis, "Static controllers for magnetic suspension and balance systems," *IEE Proceedings–Control Theory and Applications*, vol. 143, no. 4, pp. 338–348, 1996.

Y.-C. Lai, Y.-L. Lee, and J.-Y. Yen, "Design and servo control of a single-deck planar maglev stage", *IEEE Transactions on Magnetics*, 43(6):2600–2602, June 2007.

H.-W. Lee, K.-C. Kim, and J. Lee, "Review of maglev train technologies," *IEEE Transactions on Magnetics*, vol. 42, no. 7, pp. 1917–1925, July 2006.

T. Massie and K. Salisbury, "The PHANToM Haptic Interface: A Device for Probing Virtual Objects", Symposium on Haptic Interfaces for Virtual Environment and Teleoperator Systems, Chicago, November, 1994.

E. H. Moore, "On the reciprocal of the general algebraic matrix", *Bulletin of the American Mathematical Society*, 26:394–395, 1920.

D. N. Nenchev, "Restricted jacobian matrices of redundant manipulators in constrained motion tasks," *International Journal of Robotics Research*, vol. 11, no. 6, pp. 584–597, 1992.

S.-R. Oh, R. L. Hollis, and S. E. Salcudean, "Precision assembly with a magnetically levitated wrist," in *IEEE Int'l Conf. on Robotics and Automation*, Atlanta, May 1993, pp. 127–134.

R. Penrose. "A generalized inverse for matrices", *Proceedings of the Cambridge Philosophical Society*, 51:406–413, 1955.

W. Robertson, B. Cazzolato, and A. Zander, "A multipole array magnetic spring," *IEEE Transactions on Magnetics*, vol. 41, no. 10, pp. 3826–3828, October 2005.

J. Rosen, J. D. Brown, L. Chang, M. Barreca, M. Sinanan, and B. Hannaford, "The blue DRAGON - a system for measuring the kinematics and the dynamics of minimally invasive surgical tools in vivo", *IEEE International Conference on Robotics and Automation*, Washington DC, May 2002.

S. Salcudean, N.M. Wong and R.L. Hollis, "Design and control of a force-reflecting teleoperation system with magnetically levitated master and wrist", IEEE Transactions on Robotics and Automation", 11:2, December 1995, pp. 844-858.

S. Salcudean and N. Parker, "6-dof desk-top voice-coil joystick", *International Mechanical Engineering Congress and Exposition*, Dallas, November 1997.

G. Schweitzer, H. Bleuler, and A. Traxler, *Active Magnetic Bearings - Basics, Properties, and Applications*. Zurich: Hochschulverlag AG, 1994.

I.-Y. Wang and I. Busch-Vishniac, "A new repulsive magnetic levitation approach using permanent magnets and air-core electromagnets," *IEEE Transactions on Magnetics*, vol. 30, no. 4, pp. 1422–1432, 1994.

L. Yan, I.-M. Chen, C. K. Lim, G. Yang, W. Lin, and K.-M. Lee, "Torque modeling of spherical actuators with double-layer poles", *IEEE/RSJ International Conference on Intelligent Robots and Systems*, Beijing, October 2006, pp. 5447–5452.

H. Zhang and C.-H. Menq, "Six-axis magnetic levitation and motion control," *IEEE Transactions on Robotics*, vol. 23, no. 2, pp. 196–205, April 2007.

3

Solving the Correspondence Problem in Haptic/Multisensory Interface Design

Charles Spence[1], Mary K. Ngo[1], Ju-Hwan Lee[1] and Hong Tan[2]
University of Oxford[1] & Purdue University[2]
Oxford, UK[1] & Indiana, USA[2]

1. Introduction

There has been a recent resurgence of interest in the use of haptic displays to augment human performance, and to provide an additional means of information transfer to interface operators whose visual and/or auditory modalities may be otherwise informationally-overloaded (e.g., Gallace et al., 2007; Kaczmarek & Bach-y-Rita, 1995; Spence & Ho, 2008a; Yannier et al., 2008; Zlotnik, 1988). Over the last few years, researchers have investigated the use of tactile interfaces to provide assistance in a wide variety of settings including everything from vibrating belts to provide navigation support (Nagel et al., 2005) through to wrist watches that allow the user to tell the time by the pattern of vibration that they feel on their wrist (Töyssy et al., 2008). However, the more extravagant predictions made by early researchers regarding the potential uses of vibrotactile interfaces – that people would soon be monitoring the latest stock market figures via vibrating waist displays (see Geldard, 1974; Hennessy, 1966), and/or watching television using nothing more than a 20 by 20 array of vibrators on the back of their chairs (the so-called "tactile television"; Collins, 1970) – have, as yet, proved to be too far-fetched (even allowing for extensive practice to familiarize themselves with the devices concerned).

The problem with the implementation of these predictions was that early researchers typically failed to account for the fundamental human limits on the processing of tactile information through artificial displays (e.g., see Gallace et al., 2007; Spence & Driver, 1997b, for reviews). Here, it is critical to note that humans are severely limited in their capacity to process information, and, if anything, the limits on the processing of tactile information seem to be far more restrictive than for visual or auditory modalities (see Spence & Gallace, 2007; Spence & Ho, 2008a). What is more, many vibrotactile interfaces were originally tested in the laboratory under conditions of unimodal sensory stimulation. In real-life environments, however, multiple senses are likely to be stimulated at the same time, and visual stimuli seem to have priority access to our attentional resources (Posner et al., 1976; Spence et al., 2001). Nevertheless, one area where there has been a lot of interest (and promise shown) in the last few years relates to the use of non-visual cues to facilitate people's visual search performance. It is on this aspect of tactile and multisensory displays that this chapter will focus.

It is our belief, given the known limitations on the processing of tactile information, that the primary role of tactile information displays in the coming years will be in terms of providing relatively simple information to interface operators in order not to overload their limited capacity for tactile information processing under conditions of concurrent multisensory stimulation (Spence & Ho, 2008a; see also Cao et al., 2007). However, it is important to note that we do not wish to imply by this that the haptic sense is necessarily fundamentally inferior to vision or hearing in terms of its ability to transmit information to an interface operator. In fact, it is often taken for granted (and hence under-appreciated) that the haptic sense is actually capable of processing vast amounts of information in our daily lives. This may be partly due to the fact that few of us encounter people who are haptically-challenged or are aware of the devastating effects caused by the loss of tactile/kinesthetic sensation. The story of Ian Waterman, an Englishman who lost his haptic sense from the neck down, provides a rare glimpse into the crucial role tactile/kinesthetic information plays in our daily tasks, such as helping us to maintain our posture, walk, and even button-up our shirt in the morning (see Cole, 1995).

Before we proceed, it is also worth pointing out that most tactile displays stimulate only a small part of the haptic sense. The term haptics is used here to refer to both tactile and kinesthetic sensing, as well as manual manipulation (Loomis & Lederman, 1986). The majority of tactile displays that have been developed for user interfaces only provide passive vibrotactile stimulation, and their bandwidth and spatial density (when an array of tactors are used) do not yet fully match the sensory capabilities of humans (e.g., Verrillo & Gescheider, 1992). Force-feedback devices constitute a type of kinesthetic display, but they are typically not portable and hence their usage is limited in applications such as collision avoidance systems and facilitating visual search in dynamic environments. It is therefore not too surprising that the success of tactile displays has, to date, been so limited, since we have yet to tap into the full potential of the haptic sense. It is important to note, however, that there are many 'small' mouse-like devices which provide force-feedback (Akamatsu & MacKenzie, 1995, 1996) or stylus pen type devices (Forlines & Balakrishnan, 2008) that have now been shown to be effective in daily computing situations (Viau et al., 2005). Therefore, size may not turn out to be as big a problem as previously thought when considering the use of kinesthetic feedback.

The deaf and deaf-and-blind community have long used methods such as fingerspelling and Tadoma (see Tan & Pentland, 2001, for a review) in order to communicate: With the Tadoma method (see Reed et al., 1985), deaf and blind individuals place their hand on a speaker's face with their thumb resting vertically on the center of the speaker's lips, and the fingers spread across the speaker's cheek and neck. Tadoma users are able to pick-up the naturalistic mouth opening, airflow, muscle tension and laryngeal vibration information through the hand. Tadoma users can achieve rates of information transfer of up to 12 bits/s (see Reed & Durlach, 1998), which is about half of the rate exhibited by able-bodied individuals when monitoring audiovisual speech.

The success of 'natural' tactile communication methods, such as Tadoma, provides living proof that haptics, when properly engaged, has the potential to provide an effective communication channel with a surprisingly high rate of information transmission. That said, it is also important to note that there are tremendous individual differences with regard to the limits of tactile information transfer (see Craig, 1977). For instance, two of the many thousands of sighted participants tested by Craig over the years were found to be able to read at a phenomenal rate of 70-100 words per minute (approximately 9-13 bits/s) through their fingertips using the vibrotactile patterns generated by the Optacon (Bliss et al., 1970); That is, at rates two to three times those seen in blind participants with an equivalent amount of practice. More impressive still was the fact that Craig's 'extraordinary observers', as he called them, were able to read at a higher rate through their fingertip than through an equivalent visual display! Thus, we would argue that while it is still important for tactile interface designers to consider the limits of human tactile processing, the opportunities for innovative tactile interfaces to provide useful information to interface operators in the coming years ought to be stressed. Some possibilities here for the increased use of tactile interfaces include the provision of alert and interrupt signals (Calhoun et al., 2003; Hameed et al., 2009), directional or waypoint navigation signals (e.g., Bosman et al., 2003; Ho & Spence, 2007; Jones et al., 2006; Nagel et al., 2005; Van Erp, 2005; Van Erp et al., 2004, 2005; Van Erp & Van Veen, 2004; Van Veen et al., 2004), orientation signals (e.g., for astronauts working in microgravity or deep-sea divers; Van Erp & Van Veen, 2006), signals to improve situational awareness (e.g., Raj et al., 2000) and/or spatial warning signals (e.g., Ho et al., 2006; Ho & Spence, 2008; Van Erp et al., 2007).

Compared to 'natural' tactile communication methods, most artificial tactile displays developed for tactile aids and human-computer interactions have yet to demonstrate information rates beyond 6-7 bits/s (see Reed & Durlach, 1998). In the future, this may be remedied by expanding haptic displays so that they can stimulate both the tactile and kinesthetic senses (e.g., Reed et al., 2003; Tan et al., 1999, submitted). It could also be argued that we have yet to learn how to communicate through the skin as effectively as we might using display technology and coding schemes that go beyond simply mimicking vision (the retina; see the next section) or hearing (the cochlea). Learning more about the perceptual grouping of tactile information, such as through the study of tactile Gestalts, will likely help here (see Gallace & Spence, submitted). However, when thinking about the presentation of tactile patterns to the skin of an interface operator, it is important to highlight an often under-appreciated problem relating to the question of what perspective we view stimuli/patterns that are 'drawn'/presented on the skin.

2. From what perspective do we view tactile stimuli presented on the skin?

It is interesting to note here that the issue of where to present vibrotactile information on an interface operator's body is becoming more and more important now that researchers are increasingly looking at the possibility of presenting letters and other meaningful, spatially-distributed patterns of vibrotactile stimulation using vibrotactile chairs, corsets etc. (Auvray & Spence, 2009; Jones et al., 2006; Jones & Sarter, 2008; Loomis, 1974; Tan et al., 2003; Yanagida et al., 2004). For example, Yanagida et al. reported up to 87% successful letter recognition in some cases using a 3 x 3 array of vibrators on the back of a chair. Note that the vibrators were activated sequentially, and in the same sequence (as if someone were tracing the letter on the chair's, or person's, back).

Given that nearly 50% of our skin surface is found on the torso, the back clearly offers great opportunities for the tactile presentation of information. One well-known psychological illusion that is relevant to the discussion here occurs when an ambiguous letter (such as a 'b', 'd', 'p', 'q') is drawn on a person's forehead (e.g., Krech & Crutchfeld, 1958, p. 205; Natsoulas, 1966; Natsoulas & Dubanoski, 1964). If the person on whom the letter is drawn is asked to identify the letter, they will often describe the mirror image of the letter that was actually drawn – e.g., frequently saying 'b' if a 'd' was drawn, etc. (see Kikuchi et al., 1979). Krech and Crutchfield (1958) found that about 75% of people take an internal perspective (i.e., as if looking out from an imagined perspective in the middle of the body; the so-called 'egocentre'; note that it is this perspective that leads to the mirror-reversals), while the remaining 25% took the external perspective (as if standing outside themselves), when a character was drawn on their forehead. A similar confusion has also been shown to occur for letters drawn (or presented) on the stomach. By contrast, the majority of people tend to report letters (or other symbols) that are drawn on the back of their head (or on their back) correctly. Such results have been taken to show that when trying to interpret the pattern of stimulation on their backs, people are likely to take an 'external' perspective (see Figure 1). In fact, it has been argued that we normally take this external perspective (as if standing behind ourselves) when trying to interpret patterns drawn on the body. This may perhaps help to explain why it is so easy to achieve 'out-of-body'experiences in precisely this situation (i.e., when it appears that we are standing outside and behind ourselves; see Aspell et al., 2009; Ehrsson, 2007; Lenggenhager et al., 2007).

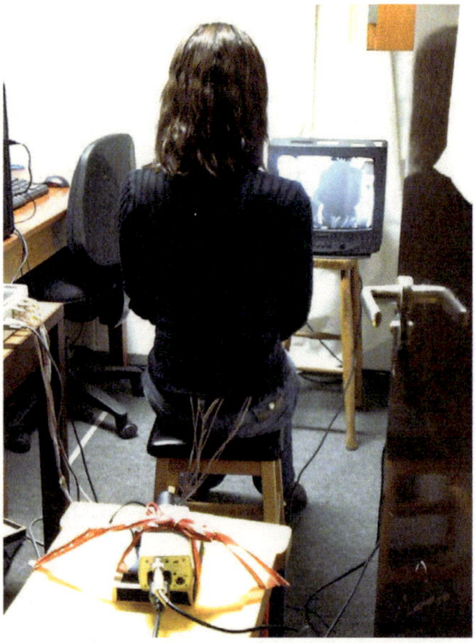

Fig. 1. When trying to interpret the pattern of tactile stimulation presented on our back, people can either take an 'internal', or an 'external', perspective (e.g., see Corcoran, 1977). Research has shown that people normally take an external perspective (Auvray & Spence, 2009); That is, they interpret the pattern of tactile stimulation as if standing outside and behind themselves (i.e., adopting the perspective shown in the figure).

Taken as a whole, the experimental literature that has investigated the viewpoint from which people interpret letters/symbols drawn on the skin suggests that presenting meaningful stimulus patterns to an interface operators' back may be easier than presenting the same stimuli to their stomach. It is certainly likely to result in a more consistent pattern of responding from interface operators. Back displays also have the advantage of keeping an interface operator's hands free. Pattern recognition also appears to be superior on the back than on the forearm (Jones et al., 2006). Furthermore, presenting tactile stimuli to stationary parts of the body (such as the back) also avoids the change numbness/blindness that can be experienced when tactile stimuli are presented to moving limbs (see Gallace et al., 2009).

3. The crossmodal correspondence problem in multisensory interface design

In recent years, there has been a rapid growth of research investigating the effectiveness of tactile cues in directing an interface operator's visual attention in a particular direction. Often the effectiveness of these tactile cues has been measured against the effectiveness of auditory cues (since both are non-visual). In this chapter, the focus will be on the vibrotactile (auditory and audiotactile) cuing of visual search in cluttered visual displays. Given that tactile cues will nearly always be presented in different spatial locations from the visual displays that they are designed to inform an interface operator about, this raises the correspondence problem (e.g., Fujisaki & Nishida, 2007; Marr, 1982).

In its traditional form, the correspondence problem referred to the difficult situation faced by the brain when it has to 'decide' which stimulus in one eye should be matched with which stimulus in the other eye (especially with stimulus displays such as random dot stereograms; e.g., Julesz, 1971; Marr, 1982). However, while it was originally framed as a purely unimodal visual problem, researchers have recently come to realize that (in complex real-world scenes) the brain also faces a crossmodal version of the correspondence problem (see Fujisaki & Nishida, 2007): How, for example, in a cluttered everyday, multisensory scene, does the brain know which visual, auditory, and tactile stimuli to bind into unified multisensory perceptual events and which to keep separate? A large body of basic psychological research has shown that spatiotemporal synchrony, semantic and synaesthetic congruency, and the 'unity effect' all play a role here in helping the brain decide which sensory stimuli should be bound, and which should be kept separate (Parise & Spence, 2009; see Spence, 2007, for a review).

Taking things one stage further, it can certainly be argued that the typical interface operator has a very similar (if not even more challenging) problem to solve. How does s/he know which location in the visual field s/he is being directed to look at on perceiving a completely-unrelated tactile stimulus that is presented on some part of their anatomy (often their back)? Clearly, while temporal synchrony can sometimes help here (but note that cues will sometimes need to be presented in advance of, or after, the relevant visual event; see below), precise spatial coincidence cannot. How then does an interface operator know which location in a distal visual display is being referred to by tactile stimuli on their body (e.g., back)? Is there a natural, dare we say 'intuitive' (Ho et al., 2007b; Van Erp, 2005), correspondence that interface designers can capitalize upon? If, as the literature briefly reviewed in the preceding section suggests, people take the perspective of standing behind themselves, looking forward as if 'seeing' their back from behind, then one might imagine that a tactile stimulus presented to the left side, say, of the participant's back, if projected forward, would lead the participant to attend to the left side of the visual display. We will move now to a review of the evidence on the tactile cuing of visual search.

4. Facilitating visual search using non-visual and multisensory cues

Van der Burg et al. (2009) recently investigated whether vibrotactile cues could be used to facilitate participants' visual search performance in cluttered displays. The visual search displays in their study consisted of 24, 36, or 48 line segments oriented at $\pm 22.5^{\circ}$ that regularly, but unpredictably, changed colour during the course of each trial (see Figure 2). The participants had to discriminate the orientation (horizontal vs. vertical) of the visual target that was presented somewhere in the display on each and every trial. The vibrotactile cue was presented from a mobile phone vibrator attached to the back of the participant's left hand. It should be pointed out that this non-visual cue was entirely spatially non-predictive with regard to the likely location of the visual target in the display, but that its onset was temporally synchronized with the colour change of the visual target.

Van der Burg et al.'s (2009) results showed that the vibrotactile cue had a dramatic effect on the efficiency of participants' visual search performance: Search slopes dropped from 91 ms/item in the baseline no-cue condition to just 26 ms/item when the vibrotactile cue was presented: For the largest set size, the benefit resulting from vibrotactile cuing equated to a mean reduction in search latencies of more than 1,300 ms (or 30%). While error rates increased as the set size increased, there were no differences as a function of whether the cue was present or absent (thus arguing against a speed-accuracy trade-off account of this RT benefit; see Spence & Driver, 1997a). Interestingly, the benefits of vibrotactile cuing on participants' visual search performance were of an equivalent magnitude to those that had been reported in an earlier study in which a spatially non-predictive auditory cue had been presented over headphones instead. In that study, the search slope was 31 ms/item when an auditory cue was present, as compared to 147 ms/item in the no-cue condition (see Van der Burg et al., 2008, Experiment 1).

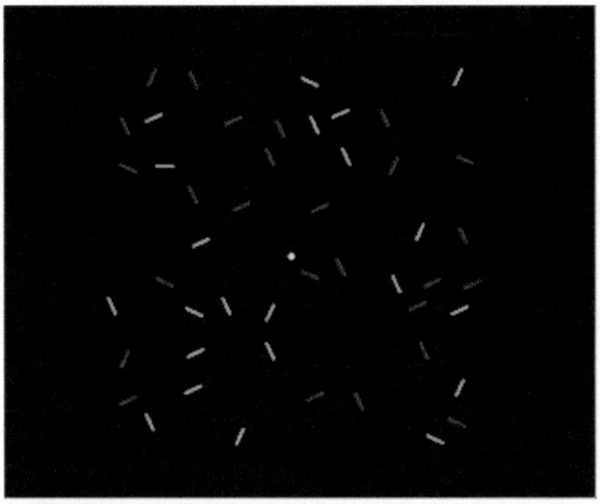

Fig. 2. An example of the kind of visual search display (with a set size of 48) used in Van der Burg et al.'s (2008, 2009) recent studies. The target was a horizontal or vertical line segment presented amongst tilted distractors. In this display, the horizontal target is located in the top left quadrant.

Ngo and Spence (in press, submitted) have recently extended Van der Burg et al.'s (2008, 2009) research findings: In their first experiment, they demonstrated that vibrotactile cues presented to both sides of the participant's waist (rather than to the participant's left hand as in Van der Burg et al.'s, 2008, study) led to an equivalent visual search benefit as compared to when an auditory cue was presented over a pair of loudspeakers, one placed to either side of the computer monitor on which the visual search displays were presented (rather than over headphones as in Van der Burg et al.'s, 2008, study). In a second experiment, Ngo and Spence (submitted) went on to show that bimodal audiotactile cues resulted in visual search performance that was no better than that seen when the unimodal (either tactile or auditory) cues were presented (see Figure 3).

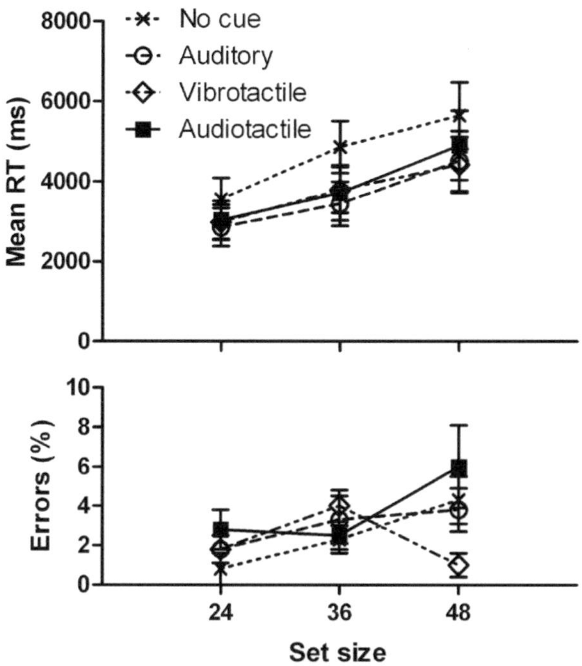

Fig. 3. Mean RT (in ms) and percentages of errors for the no cue, auditory, vibrotactile, and audiotactile conditions in Ngo and Spence's (submitted, Experiment 2) recent visual search study. Error bars represent the standard errors of the means.

In a subsequent experiment, Ngo and Spence (submitted) went on to investigate whether making the cue (either tactile or auditory) spatially informative with respect to the likely side of the target would lead to any additional performance advantage. In this study, the cue correctly predicted the side of the target on 80% of the trials and was invalid on the remaining 20% of trials. Under such conditions, participants' visual search performance was improved still further as compared to the spatially-uninformative central cuing condition (see Figure 4). It is, though, unclear whether this performance benefit should be attributed to the overt or covert orienting of participants' spatial attention to the side of the cue (see Spence & Driver, 1994, 2004). However, given the relatively long mean visual search latencies (> 3,000 ms), it would seem likely that the participants in Ngo and Spence's experiment would have moved their eyes around the visual display during the interval between its onset and the moment when they actually initiated their manual discrimination response (see Henderson, 2003; Henderson & Hollingworth, 1998; Tan et al., 2009; Van der Burg et al., 2008).

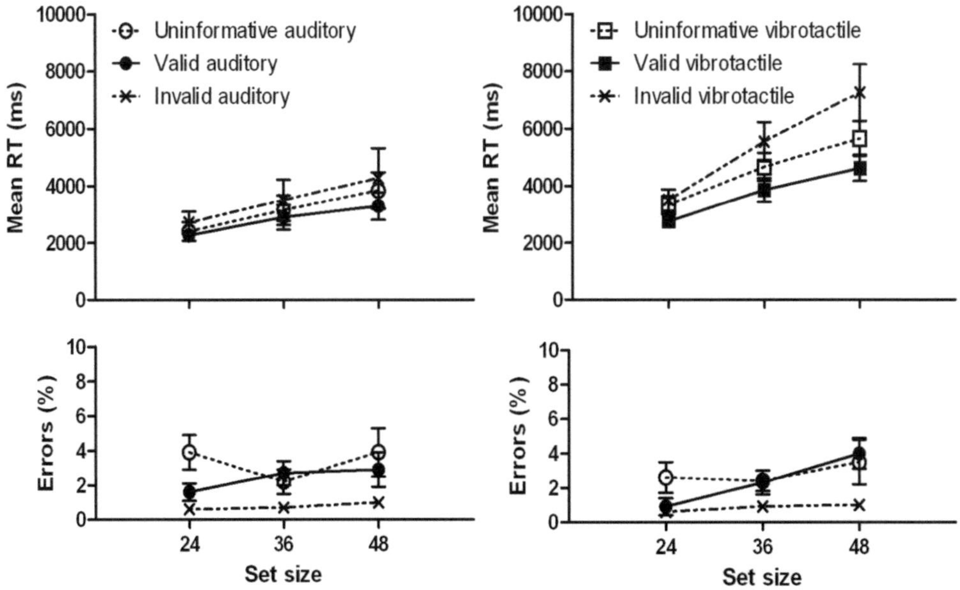

Fig. 4. Mean RT (in ms) and percentages of errors for the spatially uninformative, spatially valid, and spatially invalid auditory and vibrotactile cue conditions in Ngo and Spence's (submitted, Experiment 3) recent visual search study. Error bars represent the standard errors of the means.

Here, for the first time in the task popularized by Van der Burg et al. (2008, 2009), auditory cues were found to result in significantly faster overall visual search latencies than vibrotactile cues (there had been no difference in any of the previous studies using this paradigm). The visual search slopes were also shallower following auditory than following vibrotactile cuing. Why should this be so? Well, it may be that when a non-visual cue provides spatial information to a participant (or interface operator), it is more advantageous if the cue is presented from the same functional region of space as the target stimulus that the cue is informing the interface operator about (see Ho & Spence, 2008; Previc, 2000; Spence & Ho, 2008b, on this point).

5. Interim Summary

To summarize, Van der Burg et al.'s (2008, 2009) recent research has shown that spatially uninformative auditory and vibrotactile cues can be used to facilitate participants' visual search performance in cluttered visual displays. Ngo and Spence (in press, submitted) have extended these findings by showing that the performance benefits occur even when the auditory and vibrotactile cues are presented from different locations (in space and/or on a participant's body), and that bimodal audiotactile cues are no more effective than unimodal cues in facilitating participants' visual search performance. Ngo and Spence have also demonstrated that performance can be facilitated even further simply by making the cue spatially informative with regard to the likely side on which the target is presented. One obvious follow-up question to emerge from this line of research concerns whether operator performance could be facilitated still further simply by making the non-visual (i.e., tactile, or for that matter auditory, or audiotactile) cue even more informative with regards to the likely location of the visual target. While, as yet, no one has addressed this question using Van der Burg et al.'s specific 'pip and pop' or 'poke and pop' visual search tasks, other researchers have shown that visual search and change detection performance can benefit from the cuing of as many as three or four locations on a person's back.

6. From left/right cuing to quadrant cuing and beyond

Lindeman et al. (2003) highlighted a facilitatory effect of vibrotactile spatial cuing on participants' visual search performance using three possible cue locations on the left, middle, and right of a participant's back (presented using a chair-back mounted vibrotactile display). The participants in their study had to search a display of 24 random letters in order to find a target letter (that was specified at the bottom of the screen; see Figure 5). Participants responded by using the mouse to click on one of the letters in the display. The vibrotactile cues in this study were 100% valid with regard to the panel (left, middle, or right) in which the visual target would be found. Under such conditions, vibrotactile cuing led to a 12% reduction in search latencies as compared to a no-cue baseline condition. Interestingly, however, Lindeman et al. also reported that visually cuing the relevant section of the visual display (see the right panel of Figure 5) led to a much larger (30%) reduction in target detection latencies. Once again, bimodal visuotactile cuing was shown to result in performance that was no better than that seen following the most effective of the unimodal cues (cf. Ngo & Spence, submitted).

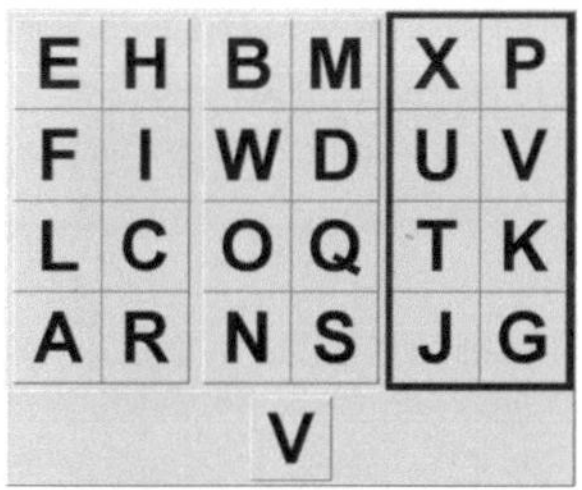

Fig. 5. Example of a visual search display used in Lindeman et al.'s (2003) visual search study. The search display is made up of three panels of 8 letters. A visual cue is shown highlighting the right panel. The target letter is indicated on the bottom of the screen.

It is, however, important to note here that it is unclear whether the reduced efficacy of vibrotactile (relative to visual) cuing reported by Lindeman et al. (2003) simply reflected uncertainty on the part of their participants with regard to the location of the vibrotactile cues on their back (since no measure of localization accuracy was provided in this study). Alternatively, however, this difference may also reflect the fact that, in this particular experimental setting, vibrotactile cues were simply not as effective as visual cues in facilitating participants' visual search performance. It is interesting to note at this point that simultaneous visual cuing (the presentation of a visual halo around the display coinciding with the visual target colour change) was found to be singularly ineffective in facilitating

participants' visual search performance in a visual search study conducted by Van der Burg et al. (2008; Experiment 2b). This difference in results suggests that different mechanisms may have been facilitating participants' performance in these two (at least superficially similar) experiments (see below for further discussion of this point).
Moving one stage further, Hong Tan and her colleagues at Purdue have conducted a number of studies over the last decade investigating whether the vibrotactile cuing of one quadrant of a person's back can facilitate their change detection performance in a version of the flicker paradigm (see Jones et al., 2008; Mohd Rosli et al., submitted; Tan et al., 2001, 2003, 2009; Young et al., 2003). In the flicker paradigm, two similar visual scenes/displays are presented in rapid alternation (e.g., Rensink, 2000). In Tan et al.'s studies, the visual displays typically consisted of a random array of horizontal and vertical line segments (see Figure 6). The two displays presented in each trial differed only in terms of the orientation of one of the elements (alternating between horizontal and vertical in successive screen displays). A 120-ms blank scene was inserted between the presentation of each of the two displays in order to mask any transient local motion cues associated with the changing orientation of the target. Previous research has shown that people need focal attention in order to detect the change in such situations. On each trial, a 250-300 Hz vibrotactile cue was presented 200 ms before the onset of the visual displays (the vibrotactile cue was presented for 60 ms, and was followed by a 140 ms empty interval), from one of the 4 corners of a 2-by-2 square array of tactors mounted on the back of the participant's chair (with a centre-to-centre spacing of approximately 16 cm). Importantly, Tan et al. confirmed that all of their participants could identify the quadrant from which each vibrotactile stimulus had been presented without error (on 60 trials) at the start of their experimental session. Upon detecting the changing item in the visual display, the participants had to click on a mouse button; They then had to move the cursor across the screen using the mouse and click again in order to identify the target item.

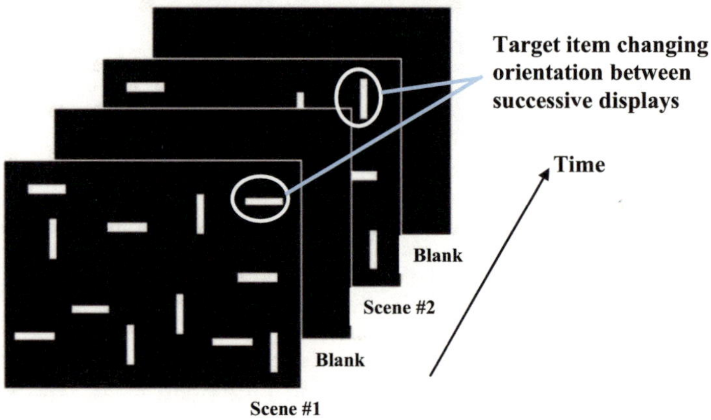

Fig. 6. Example of the flicker paradigm used in Tan et al.'s (2009) study.

Tan et al. (2009) varied the validity of the vibrotactile cue in different experiments. Often, the visual target would be presented in the screen quadrant indicated by the vibrotactile cue on 50% of the trials, while it was presented from one of the three other, uncued, quadrants on the remaining 50% of the trials (constituting valid and invalid trials, respectively; see Tan et al., 2003). The results of experiments using such spatially-informative vibrotactile pre-cues revealed that participants were able to respond significantly more rapidly, and no less accurately, to visual targets presented in the cued quadrant than to targets presented in one of the uncued quadrants. So, for example, the participants in one study responded 41% more rapidly on the validly-cued trials than in no cue baseline trials, and 19% more slowly than in the no cue conditions when the cue was spatially invalid (i.e., when the cue indicated that the target would be presented in one quadrant, whereas, in reality, it was actually presented from one of the other three quadrants; cf. Ngo & Spence, submitted, Experiment 3). Another interesting result to emerge from Tan et al.'s (2009; Mohd Rosli et al., submitted) research was that RTs increased as the location of the target moved further away from the centre of the cued quadrant (toward the periphery). This latter result would appear to suggest that participants' attention was initially focused on the centre of the cued screen quadrant before moving outward (or becoming more diffuse).

Recently, Tan et al. (2009; Jones et al., 2008) have started to monitor their participants' eye movements (using an eye tracker) in order to assess how the presentation of vibrotactile cues on a participant's back influences the overt orienting of their spatial attention around the visual search display situated in front of them. Under conditions where the vibrotactile cue validity was high (75% valid), Jones et al. reported that their participants' predominantly directed their saccades to the cued quadrant initially. (As in their previous research, RTs to detect the target were significantly faster as compared to those seen in a no-cue baseline condition.) Interestingly, however, when the vibrotactile cue was made completely non-predictive with regard to the quadrant in which the visual target was likely to occur (i.e., when the target was just as likely to appear in each of the four screen quadrants, regardless of the quadrant in which the vibrotactile cue had been presented), and when the participants were instructed to ignore the vibrotactile cues, then no significant differences were observed in the pattern of overt orienting from that seen in the no-cue condition. Under such conditions, the participants tended to direct their eyes to the top-left quadrant of the display first. Tan et al.'s results therefore suggest that non-predictive vibrotactile cues presented to a person's back can (under the appropriate conditions) be completely ignored. This result contrasts markedly with the results of other laboratory research highlighting the fact that people are unable to ignore vibrotactile cues presented to their fingertips (at least when the visual targets are presented from close by; i.e., from the same functional region of space; see Gray et al., 2009; Kennett et al., 2001, 2002; Spence et al., 1998).

One obvious question to emerge from this transition from 2, to 3, to 4 vibrotactile cue locations concerns just how many different spatial locations could potentially be cued on a person's back in the tactile interfaces of the future. Lindeman and Yanagida (2003) have already shown, for example, that participants can identify the source of a 1 s, 91 Hz, vibration using a 3-by-3 array of 9 tactors mounted on the back of a chair (with a minimum 6 cm spacing between adjacent tactors; and, importantly, no practice) at a level exceeding 80% correct. Unfortunately, however, no one has yet (at least as far as we are aware) investigated whether using a 3-by-3 matrix of vibrotactile cues would give rise to a performance benefit in a visual search or change detection task that was any larger than that already demonstrated by Tan et al. (2009) in their quadrant cuing studies. This certainly represents an important area for future study given that, at some point, increasing the specificity of spatial vibrotactile cuing will no longer lead to any further enhancement of visual search performance. Why? Well, because of the well-known limits of discriminating vibrotactile stimulation for touch displays on the back will have been reached (e.g., Weinstein, 1968; Wilska, 1954). Note also that there are systematic biases in tactile localization that need to be taken into account when presenting a large number of vibrotactile stimuli to a person's back/torso (e.g., see Cholewiak et al., 2004; Cholewiak & Collins, 2000; Van Erp, 2005). The influence of these biases on perceived vibrotactile localization is likely to become all the more pronounced as the density of cue locations (e.g., on the back) increases.

7. The importance of spatially co-localizing cue and target events

Ngo and Spence (submitted) have also investigated whether the reduced benefits of vibrotactile as opposed to auditory spatial cuing reported in one of their studies (Experiment 3), that was described earlier, may have resulted from the fact that vibrotactile cues have, of necessity, to be presented to an operator's body surface (Gregory, 1967). By contrast, the auditory cues used in their study were presented from close to the visual target display instead (i.e., from the same functional region of space as the target event; see Previc, 2000). In order to assess the potential importance of relative cue position on the facilitation of participants' visual search performance by non-visual cues, Ngo and Spence went on, in a final experiment, to compare their participants' performance under conditions in which the auditory cues were either presented from close to the visual display (i.e., from external loudspeakers situated to either side of the visual display) or via headphones (i.e., from close to the participant but further from the visual display, as in Van der Burg et al.'s, 2008, study). In separate blocks of experimental trials, the cue was either spatially nonpredictive (i.e., 50% valid) or 80% predictive with regard to the likely side of the visual display in which the target was presented. Note that exactly the same spatial information was provided in both cases (i.e., no matter whether the cue sound was presented over headphones or from the external loudspeakers). Ngo and Spence nevertheless still found that their participants were able to discriminate the orientation of the visual targets significantly (34%) more rapidly when the auditory cues were presented from close to the visual display than when they were presented from close to the participant (i.e., over headphones; see Figure 7). These results therefore suggest that, wherever possible, spatially co-localizing the non-visual cue (or warning) signal with the target visual event/display may be advantageous, especially when the cue provides spatial information to an interface operator.

Speaking more generally, we believe that Ngo and Spence's (submitted) results support the view that vibrotactile cues may, if anything, be inherently somewhat less effective in facilitating an interface operator's performance than auditory cues given that they have to be presented from the participants' body, which in many situations may be far away from the relevant visual event or display (see Spence & Ho, 2008b, for a review). By contrast, it is typically much easier to present auditory cues from close to the location of the relevant visual display (see Perrott et al., 1990, 1991, 1996). In fact, recent work by Ho and her colleagues (Ho et al., 2006) has come to a similar conclusion on the basis of their research investigating the effectiveness of vibrotactile versus auditory warning signals in alerting car drivers to the likely location of a potential danger on the road either in front or behind them. The possibility that the region of space in which non-visual cues are presented should play such an important role in determining their effectiveness, and the fact that the cue should, whenever possible, be presented from close to the relevant visual display (though see Ho & Spence, in press, for an exception) raise a number of interesting, but as yet unanswered, questions for future research. This research will likely have important implications for the future design of non-visual interfaces/warning signals.

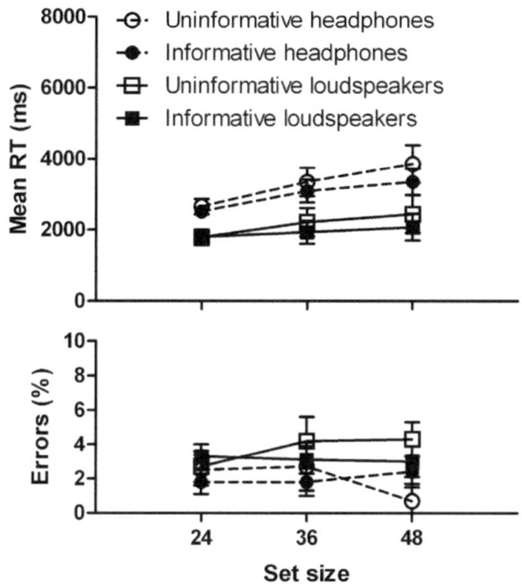

Fig. 7. Mean RT (in ms) and percentages of errors for the spatially uninformative and spatially valid (or informative) auditory cue conditions presented via headphones versus external loudspeakers (placed by the visual search display) in Ngo and Spence's (submitted, Experiment 4) recent visual search study. Error bars represent the standard errors of the means.

Given that the wrists/hands are increasingly being targeted as a potential site for vibrotactile stimulation in tactile/haptic interface design (e.g., Bosman et al., 2003; Chen et al., 2008; Hameed et al., 2009; Sklar & Sarter, 1999; Van der Burg et al., 2009), one interesting question for future research will be to determine whether the tactile enhancement of visual search performance would be modulated by the position of a person's hands relative to the visual display about which the vibrotactile cue was meant to provide information. If, for example, a vibrotactile stimulator were to be attached to either hand, and the side on which a vibration was presented were to indicate the likely side on which the visual target would appear (e.g., as in Ngo & Spence's, submitted, studies), then one might ask whether the benefit of vibrotactile cuing on participants' visual search performance would be any larger were the hands to be placed by the side of the visual display say, rather than down (away from the display) in the participant's lap (see Abrams et al., 2008; Hari & Jousmäki, 1996; Reed et al., 2005). At present, we simply do not know the answer to this question. Though should such a result be obtained, it would certainly have important implications for anyone thinking of presenting tactile cues to a car driver, say (since the cues could, in principle, either be presented by means of the vibration of the steering wheel when driving or by vibrating the sides of the driver's seat instead; Ho & Spence, 2008; Spence & Ho, 2008a).

Presenting non-visual spatial cues from the same location as the visual display that they are designed to refer to provides one obvious solution to the crossmodal correspondence problem in interface design (that was outlined earlier; see Section 3). However, it is important to note that in many real-world display settings, this may only be possible for auditory, but not necessarily for vibrotactile warning signals. What is more, in certain environments, it may simply not be possible to co-localize auditory cues with the relevant visual events either (see Fitch et al., 2007; Ho et al., 2009; Perrott et al., 1996). So, for example, Fitch and his colleagues recently reported that participants found it easier to localize vibrotactile than auditory cues in a vehicular setting. The participants in their study had to indicate which direction was indicated by the activation of one of an array of eight chair vibrators or eight loudspeaker cones. The participants in Fitch et al.'s study were significantly better at localizing the direction indicated by the vibrotactile cue (86% correct) than indicating the direction indicated by the auditory cue (32%). When presented with an audiotactile cue, the participants correctly localized the direction indicated by the cue on 81% of the trials (i.e., once again, multisensory cuing was no better than the best of the unimodal cues; Lindeman et al., 2003; Ngo & Spence, submitted).

Of course, the crossmodal correspondence problem could be solved when presenting vibrotactile cues if some way could be found to have people attribute a distal event to the source of stimulation on their body surface. However, to date, all attempts to achieve distal attribution using vibrotactile stimulation have failed (see Epstein et al., 1986). It should also be noted here that the crossmodal correspondence problem can be solved for auditory cues that are presented more-or-less simultaneously with a salient visual event by utilizing the so-called 'ventriloquism effect' (see Spence & Driver, 2000). The ventriloquism effect refers to the automatic visual capture of perceived auditory localization that occurs when a salient visual stimulus is presented at more-or-less the same time as a sound (see Slutzky & Recanzone, 2001). The harder it is to localize a sound, the larger the visual biasing of the perceived auditory localization is likely to be. The ventriloquism effect is larger for synaesthetically congruent pairs of auditory and visual events than for synaesthetically incongruent pairs. So, for example, Parise and Spence (2009) recently reported significantly larger spatial (and temporal) ventriloquism effects when large visual stimuli were paired with low frequency tones, and small visual stimuli with high frequency tones, than when large visual stimuli were paired with high tones or when small stimuli were paired with low tones. While tactile stimuli can also be ventriloquized toward stimuli presented in a different location in another sensory modality (see Caclin et al., 2002), it seems unlikely that tactile stimuli could ever be ventriloquized away from the body itself (i.e., and to the visual display/event to which they refer). Hence, the ventriloquism of relatively unlocalizable warning signals may only be of benefit for auditory cue (or accessory) stimuli.

8. What mechanism(s) underlie facilitation of visual performance by non-visual cues?

While the various studies reported in this chapter clearly demonstrate that various non-visual cues, be they tactile, auditory, or audiotactile, can be used to facilitate a person's ability to detect/identify visual targets in complex visual displays, the mechanism(s) underlying these effects have not, as yet, been fully worked out. Whenever a spatial cue provides information regarding the likely location of the target then any facilitation of participants' performance may be attributable, at least in part, to the endogenous (i.e., voluntary) orienting of their spatial attention to the location (side or quadrant) indicated by the cue (see Driver & Spence, 2004, for a review). Additionally, however, when the cue provides information about the likely identity of the target (or when the cue provides location information and the participant is required to make some sort of target localization response) then facilitatory effects may also reflect the direct priming of the participant's response by the cue (see Ho et al., 2006; Spence & Driver, 1994, 1997a).

The presentation of a non-visual cue (or accessory stimulus) may also bias participants' responses in detection tasks, simply by making them somewhat more likely to say that a target was present, regardless of whether or not it was actually in the display (see Odgaard et al., 2003; Stein et al., 1996). When a cue is presented at the same time, or slightly ahead, of the relevant visual event/display then it may also facilitate participants' performance by means of a non-spatial alerting effect (e.g., Posner, 1978; Spence & Driver, 1997a). Alerting effects have been characterized as a general speeding-up of a participant's responses, often together with a concomitant reduction in the accuracy of those responses (i.e., alerting can be thought of as equating to a lowering of the participant's criterion for initiating a response). Researchers in this area have managed to rule out alerting as the primary cause of the visual search benefits that they have observed by showing that certain cue-related effects only occur when the non-visual cue is synchronized with the visual target, and not when it is presented shortly before the visual target (e.g., see Van der Burg et al., 2008, Experiment 3; Vroomen & de Gelder, 2000, Experiment 2). This latter pattern of results is more consistent with some form of multisensory integration effect (as these tend to be maximal when events are presented simultaneously in different modalities; see Spence et al., 2004; Stein & Meredith, 1993; Stein & Stanford, 2008; Vroomen & de Gelder, 2000).

Finally, it is also possible that when spatial cues are presented (as in the studies of Lindeman et al., 2003; Ngo & Spence, submitted; Perrott et al., 1990, 1991, 1996; Tan et al., 2009) they may facilitate participants' performance by exogenously drawing their spatial attention toward the location of that cue (e.g., Dufour, 1999; Gray et al., 2009; Kennett et al., 2001, 2002; Spence et al., 1998). Researchers have shown previously that auditory or tactile cues briefly facilitate a participant's ability to detect and/or discriminate visual (and, for that matter, auditory and tactile) targets presented from more or less the same spatial location, even when they are non-predictive with regards to the likely location of the target. These benefits last for about 200-300 ms from the onset of the cue, and appear to be maximal at cue-leading asynchronies of 100-200 ms (see Spence et al., 2004). Neuroimaging studies have now revealed that the presentation of a vibrotactile cue on the same (rather than opposite) side as a visual target can lead to enhanced activation in early visual cortical areas, such as the lingual gyrus (e.g., see Macaluso et al., 2000), presumably via back-projections from multisensory parietal areas (Driver & Noesselt, 2008).

While it is easy to see that vibrotactile cues presented to the wrists/hands might lead to an exogenous shift of a participant's visual attention to the region of space around their hand/arm (Spence et al., 2004), it is less clear that vibrotactile cues presented to an interface operator's back would necessarily also lead to an exogenous shift of their spatial attention to a particular location in frontal visual space (i.e., where the visual display/event is often likely to be located). However, the large spatial separation between the vibrotactile cue presented to a participant's back and the visual event in frontal space (that it is designed to inform the interface operator about) also makes explanations for the facilitatory effects of spatial cues in terms of multisensory integration (see Stein & Meredith, 1993; Stein & Stanford, 2008) seem unlikely. One caveat that should, however, be noted at this point is that the rules of crossmodal attention and multisensory integration operating in the unseen part of space behind our heads (and, presumably also our backs) may be fundamentally different from the better-studied interactions that have been observed and documented in frontal (visual) space (see Ho & Spence, in press; Spence & Ho, 2008b). More research is needed on this topic.

What would be helpful here would be to conduct spatially-informative counter-cuing experiments (e.g., Chica et al., 2007), since that would really help researchers get a handle on the automatic nature of such exogenous crossmodal spatial cuing effects (see Tan et al., 2009). It has been reported previously that counter-cuing (i.e., when a cue on one side informs the participant about the likely localization of the target on the opposite side) can lead to very short-lasting exogenous cuing effects at the cued location (typically lasting for no more than 50 ms), followed by a later, longer-lasting endogenous cuing benefit at the likely target location (i.e., on the opposite side of the cue; see Chica et al., 2007; Driver & Spence, 2004). Results such as these have been taken to suggest that the cue automatically captures participants' attention spatially, prior to their being able to endogenously re-direct their attention on the basis of the informational content carried by the cue. Such a result, should it be found with vibrotactile cuing on a participant's back prior to the discrimination of a visual target in frontal space, would therefore suggest that under the appropriate conditions back cues can indeed exogenously direct a person's visual spatial attention in frontal space. Such an effect, should it be observed, might reflect some sort of mental set effect (i.e., showing that people can remap, or align, 'back' space to 'frontal' space under the appropriate conditions). However, if this crossmodal cuing effect were not to be observed (see Tan et al., 2009), it might then lead one to suggest that the mapping between an interface operator's back and the visual display in front of them is actually fairly arbitrary in nature. As such, it would imply that there might not be any special correspondence between locations on an interface operator's back and locations in frontal space. Given the importance of such an observation for our understanding of the facilitation of visual search using non-visual cues, this clearly reflects another important topic for future research.

It is at this point that one starts wondering whether the benefits from non-visual (especially vibrotactile) spatial cuing may result solely from the informational content provided by the cue. If this were to be the case, then the possibility emerges that perhaps the same information could be transmitted to an interface operator using a particular rhythm of tactile pulses delivered via a single vibrator attached to their wrist/back etc. (e.g., Brown et al., 2006; Frings & Spence, submitted; Peddamatham et al., 2008; Töyssy et al., 2008), rather than using a spatially-distributed, and potentially ambiguous (see Yana et al., 2008), vibrotactile display. At the very least, it is certainly worth pausing to consider whether the only benefit of spatial cuing relative to, say rhythmical, tactile cuing is the speed with which different cues can be differentiated in the former case (cf. Frings & Spence, submitted). However, even if such exogenous crossmodal cuing effects were not to be observed in a counter-cuing experiment, it could nevertheless still be argued that the spatial content of a vibrotactile cue on an interface operator's back might be capable of priming the appropriate orienting response (e.g., Gregory, 1967; Proctor et al., 2005). That is, there might still be some kind of 'natural' or intuitive mapping between back and frontal space which makes it easier to interpret the directional spatial cue, even if it does not lead to exogenous spatial attentional orienting: After all, just think how natural it feels to turn one's head in the appropriate direction when someone unexpectedly taps the back of one's shoulder.

9. Conclusions, caveats, and directions for future research

The research that has been reviewed in this chapter demonstrates that the presentation of non-visual cues (be they tactile, auditory, or audiotactile) can have a profoundly beneficial effect on participants' performance on a variety of different visual tasks, as evidenced by the findings from a number of visual search and change detection tasks (e.g., see Jones et al., 2008; Lindeman et al., 2003; Ngo & Spence, in press, submitted; Perrott et al., 1990, 1991, 1996; Tan et al., 2003, 2009; Van der Burg et al., 2008, 2009). It is interesting to note that non-visual warning signals, at least in certain circumstances, seem to provide benefits that visual cues simply cannot offer (Santangelo & Spence, 2008; Van der Burg et al., 2008; Experiment 2b; though see also Lindeman et al., 2003).

There is an important open question here as to whether, and under exactly what conditions, bimodal (i.e., multisensory) cues will facilitate performance more than unimodal cues. Bimodal cues appear to outperform unimodal cues under certain conditions (Ho et al., 2007a; Spence & Santangelo, 2009), but not others (e.g., Fitch et al., 2007; Lee & Spence, 2009; Ngo & Spence, submitted; Lindeman et al., 2003). One intriguing recent result that has now been demonstrated in a number of different experimental settings is that multisensory cues appear to capture people's spatial attention more effectively than unimodal cues when they are otherwise distracted (e.g., when performing another task), that is, under conditions of high perceptual (or cognitive) load (see Spence & Santangelo, 2009, for a recent review). Taken together, the most parsimonious conclusion to draw at the present time regarding the benefits of bimodal (or multisensory) over unimodal spatial cuing (i.e., attentional capture) is that it depends on the particular task conditions in which the cue is presented. Following on from this conclusion, researchers will, in the future, certainly need to demonstrate whether unimodal (as compared to bimodal) non-visual warning signals still retain their effectiveness (e.g., in visual search or change detection tasks) under conditions where the operator is overloaded, say answering a mobile phone while driving when the tactile warning signal comes in (e.g., Lee et al., 2009; Santangelo & Spence, 2008; Scott & Gray, 2008; Spence & Santangelo, 2009).

There are, however, also a number of potential caveats in terms of anyone thinking of applying these findings regarding the facilitation of visual search using non-visual cues to real-world settings. Perhaps the most important of which relates to the fact that in the majority (possibly all) of the studies reviewed here, the participants were instructed to fixate on a central fixation point at the start of each and every trial (i.e., prior to the presentation of the non-visual cue). This point is absolutely crucial because in any real-world setting it is unlikely that an interface operator would necessarily have their eyes and head nicely aligned in this way when the tactile, auditory, or audiotactile warning signal is presented. In fact, in many settings, the cue will be presented precisely because an interface operator's attention has been distracted off to the side (e.g., see Ho & Spence, in press). This means that there is an unresolved research question to be addressed here about the efficiency of non-visual cuing under conditions of unconstrained head/eye movements. The problem relates to the fact that the perceived location from which an auditory or tactile event is perceived to have been presented has been shown to change as a function of any change in their eye and/or head position (see Harrar & Harris, in press; Ho & Spence, 2007; Lewald & Ehrenstein, 1996a, b; Macaluso et al., 2002; Weerts & Thurlow, 1971). Now, it may be that these overt-orienting induced shifts are small enough not to deleteriously influence an interface operator's performance when using 2, 3, 4, and possibly even 9 vibrotactile cue locations (see Natsoulas & Dubanoski, 1964). However, at some point, the benefits of increased cue resolution will be offset by the mislocalization errors that are induced by any changes in head/eye position (see also Spence et al., 2004, on this point).

A second caveat that has to be noted here is that the actual tasks, paradigms, and visual displays used in the research that has been reviewed here have all been lifted straight from the psychologists' laboratory. That is, they are, in some important regards, very artificial (e.g., when in everyday life does one need to search for a horizontal or vertical line from amongst a large number of tilted distractors?). What we need to do now that we have demonstrated the efficacy of auditory, vibrotactile, and audiotactile cuing in facilitating people's ability to search amongst letters and line-segments in a laboratory setting, is to test the benefits using more realistic and dynamic displays, such as those found in air-traffic control settings (see Figure 8). We also need to bare in mind the fact that there is already evidence that certain of the cuing (accessory stimulus) benefits that have been reported to date may be specific to the particular tasks under investigation (e.g., compare Lindeman et al., 2003, and Van der Burg et al., 2008, as discussed above). On the other hand, though, there has also been a lot of exciting progress being made recently in applying the constraints on crossmodal attention that have been discovered in the laboratory to real-world interface settings (e.g., Ferris et al., 2006; Ferris & Sarter, 2008; Sarter, 2000, 2007; Spence & Ho, 2008b).

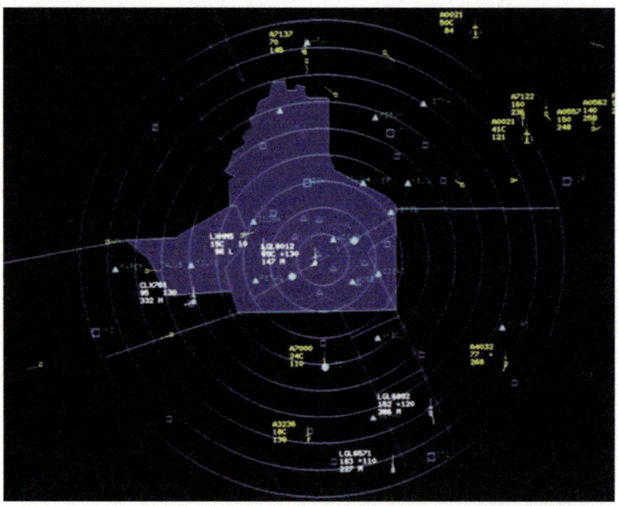

Fig. 8. An example of a complex visual display used by an air traffic controller containing data tags for different aircraft. Researchers will need to start demonstrating the benefits of using non-visual cues with such 'real-world' displays in the coming years.

Another important question for future research in this area concerns the determination of what constitutes the optimal asynchrony (if any) between non-visual cues, and the displays/events that they are designed to inform the interface operator about. To date, researchers have either looked at the synchronous presentation of the cue and target event (e.g., Ngo & Spence, submitted; Van der Burg et al., 2008, 2009), or else at conditions in which the cue has been presented prior to the onset of the target event (Tan et al., 2009; Van der Burg et al., 2008). While many researchers have been concerned about the effects of any perceived asynchrony on their participants' performance (Lindeman et al., 2003; Van der Burg et al., 2009), the only study that we are aware of that has conducted a full time-course analysis in order to determine the optimal cue-target stimulus onset asynchrony (SOA) was reported by Van der Burg et al. (2008, Experiment 3). They tested auditory cue-visual target (i.e., colour change) asynchronies from cue-leading asynchronies of 150 ms through to target-leading asynchronies of 100 ms. Their results showed that cue-target asynchronies from ±100 ms gave rise to significant cuing benefits, but intriguingly the benefits were maximal when the target actually preceded the cue by 25-50 ms (see Figure 9).

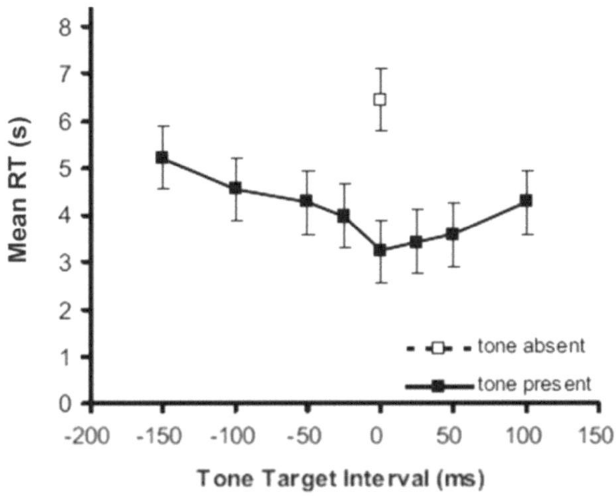

Fig. 9. Mean RT in the presence versus absence of an auditory tone presented at various tone-target intervals in Van der Burg et al.'s (2008, Experiment 3) recent visual search study. Error bars represent the standard errors of the means.

It is important to note that even when a non-visual cue stimulus is programmed to be delivered at the same time as a visual target stimulus, asynchronies can be induced either because of physical differences in equipment lags or because of biophysical differences in sensory transduction latencies (e.g., see Harrar & Harris, 2005; Shi et al., submitted; Spence et al., 2003; Spence & Squire, 2003). Note also that in certain situations the non-visual warning signal will, of necessity, have to be presented with some slight delay with respect to the external events that they are designed to inform the operator about (think, for example, about vehicle collision avoidance warning signals; see Ho & Spence, 2008; see also Chan & Chan, 2006). Researchers will therefore need to start focusing more of their research efforts on assessing the effectiveness of warning signals that are presented after the onset/occurrence of the event of interest. Furthermore, once we know more about the mechanism(s) underlying these crossmodal facilitatory effects on visual task performance in cluttered scenes (see above) we may want to try and utilize specific asynchronies in order to maximize attentional cuing and/or multisensory integration effects (see Spence et al., 2004;

Shore et al., 2006). That said, the evidence that we have reviewed in this chapter has hopefully highlighted the potential use that non-visual (in particular, vibrotactile, auditory, and audiotactile) cues (and accessory stimuli) may have in facilitating overloaded interface operators' visual search through complex and dynamic information displays in the coming years.

10. References

Abrams, R., Davoli, F., Du, C., Knapp, W., & Paull, D. (2008). Altered vision near the hands. *Cognition*, 107, 1035-1047.

Akamatsu, M., MacKenzie, I. S., & Hasbroucq, T. (1995). A comparison of tactile, auditory, and visual feedback in a pointing task using a mouse-type device. *Ergonomics*, 38, 816-827.

Akamatsu, M., & MacKenzie, I. S. (1996). Movement characteristics using a mouse with tactile and force feedback. *International Journal Human-Computer Studies*, 45, 483-493.

Aspell, J. E., Leggenhager, B., & Blanke, O. (2009). Keeping in touch with one's self: Multisensory mechanisms of self-consciousness. *PLoS ONE*, 4: e6488.

Auvray, M., & Spence, C. (2009). What perspective do people take when interpreting tactile letters presented on their bodies? Poster presented at the *10th International Multisensory Research Forum*. New York, NY, June 29-July 2.

Bliss, J. C., Katcher, M. H., Rogers, C. H., & Shepard, R. P. (1970). Optical-to-tactile image conversion for the blind. *IEEE Transactions on Man-Machine Systems*, 11, 58-65.

Bosman, S., Groenendaal, B., Findlater, J. W., Visser, T., De Graaf, M., & Markopoulos, P. (2003). GentleGuide: An exploration of haptic output for indoors pedestrian guidance. In *Proceedings of the Mobile HCI*, Udine, Italy.

Brown, L. M., Brewster, S. A., & Purchase, H. C. (2006). Multidimensional tactons for non-visual information presentation in mobile devices. *Proceedings of the Eighth Conference on Human-computer Interaction with Mobile Devices and Services*, 231-238.

Caclin, A., Soto-Faraco, S., Kingstone, A., & Spence, C. (2002). Tactile 'capture' of audition. *Perception & Psychophysics*, 64, 616-630.

Calhoun, G., Draper, M., Ruff, H., Fontejon, J., & Guilfoos, B. (2003). Evaluation of tactile alerts for control station operation. In *Proceedings of the Human Factors and Ergonomics Society 47th Annual Meeting* (pp. 2118-2122). Human Factors and Ergonomics Society, Santa Monica, CA.

Cao, C. G., Zhou, M., Jones, D. B., & Schwaitzberg, S. D. (2007). Can surgeons think and operate with haptics at the same time? *Journal of Gastrointestinal Surgery*, 11, 1564-1569.

Chan, A. H. S., & Chan, K. W. L. (2006). Synchronous and asynchronous presentations of auditory and visual signals: Implications for control console design. *Applied Ergonomics*, 37, 131-140.

Chen, H.-Y., Santos, J., Graves, M., Kim, K., & Tan, H. Z. (2008). Tactor localization at the wrist. *Proceedings of the EuroHaptics 2008 Conference* (pp. 209-218). Madrid, Spain, June 10-13.

Chica, A., Sanabria, D., Lupiáñez, J., & Spence, C. (2007). Comparing intramodal and crossmodal cuing in the endogenous orienting of spatial attention. *Experimental Brain Research*, 179, 353-364, 531.

Cholewiak, R. W., Brill, J. C., & Schwab, A. (2004). Vibrotactile localization on the abdomen: Effects of place and space. *Perception & Psychophysics*, 66, 970-987.

Cholewiak, R. W., & Collins, A. A. (2000). The generation of vibrotactile patterns on a linear array: Influences of body site, time, and presentation mode. *Perception & Psychophysics*, 62, 1220-1235.

Cole, J. (1995). *Pride and a daily marathon*. Cambridge, MA: MIT Press.

Collins, C. C. (1970). Tactile television–mechanical and electrical image projection. *IEEE Transactions on Man Machine Systems*, MMS-11, 65-71.

Corcoran, D. W. J. (1977). The phenomena of the disembodied eye or is it a matter of personal geography? *Perception*, 6, 247-253.

Craig, J. C. (1977). Vibrotactile pattern perception: Extraordinary observers. *Science*, 196, 450-452.

Driver, J., & Noesselt, T. (2008). Multisensory interplay reveals crossmodal influences on 'sensory-specific' brain regions, neural responses, and judgments. *Neuron*, 57, 11-23.

Driver, J., & Spence, C. (2004). Crossmodal spatial attention: Evidence from human performance. In C. Spence & J. Driver (Eds.), *Crossmodal space and crossmodal attention* (pp. 179-220). Oxford, UK: Oxford University Press.

Dufour, A. (1999). Importance of attentional mechanisms in audiovisual links. *Experimental Brain Research*, 126, 215-222.

Ehrsson, H. H. (2007). The experimental induction of out-of-body experiences. *Science*, 317, 1048.

Epstein, W., Hughes, B., Schneider, S., & Bach-y-Rita, P. (1986). Is there anything out there? A study of distal attribution in response to vibrotactile stimulation. *Perception*, 15, 275-284.

Ferris, T., Penfold, R., Hameed, S., & Sarter, N. (2006). The implications of crossmodal links in attention for the design of multimodal interfaces: A driving simulation study. *Proceedings of the Human Factors and Ergonomics Society 50th Annual Meeting*, 406-409.

Ferris, T. K., & Sarter, N. B. (2008). Cross-modal links among vision, audition, and touch in complex environments. *Human Factors*, 50, 17-26.

Fitch, G. M., Kiefer, R. J., Hankey, J. M., & Kleiner, B. M. (2007). Toward developing an approach for alerting drivers to the direction of a crash threat. *Human Factors*, 49, 710-720.

Forlines, C., & Balakrishnan, R. (2008). Evaluating tactile feedback and direct vs. indirect stylus input in pointing and crossing selection tasks. *Proceedings of the Twenty-Sixth Annual SIGCHI Conference on Human Factors in Computing Systems Table of Contents (CHI2008)* (pp. 1563-1572). Florence, Italy.

Frings, C., & Spence, C. (submitted). Seeing, hearing, and feeling the rhythm. *Attention, Perception, & Psychophysics*.

Fujisaki, W., & Nishida, S. (2007). Feature-based processing of audio-visual synchrony perception revealed by random pulse trains. *Vision Research*, 47, 1075-1093.

Gallace, A., & Spence, C. (submitted). To what extent do Gestalt grouping principles influence tactile perception? *Psychological Bulletin*.

Gallace, A., Tan, H. Z., & Spence, C. (2007). The body surface as a communication system: The state of the art after 50 years. *Presence: Teleoperators and Virtual Environments*, 16, 655-676.

Gallace, A., Zeeden, S., Röder, B., & Spence, C. (2009). Lost in the move? Secondary task performance impairs detection of tactile change on the body surface. *Consciousness & Cognition.*

Geldard, F. A. (Ed.). (1974). *Cutaneous communication systems and devices.* Austin, TX: Psychonomic Society.

Gray, R., Mohebbi, R., & Tan, H. Z. (2009). The spatial resolution of crossmodal attention: Implications for the design of multimodal interfaces. *ACM Transactions on Applied Perception*, 6, 1-14.

Gregory, R. L. (1967). Origin of eyes and brains. *Nature*, 213, 369-372.

Hameed, S., Ferris. T., Jayaraman, S., & Sarter, N. (2009). Using informative peripheral visual and tactile cues to support task and interruption management. *Human Factors*, 51, 126-135.

Hari, R., & Jousmäki, V. (1996). Preference of personal to extrapersonal space in a visuomotor task. *Journal of Cognitive Neuroscience*, 8, 305-307.

Harrar, V., & Harris, L. (2005). Simultaneity constancy: Detecting events with touch and vision. *Experimental Brain Research*, 166, 465-473.

Harrar, V., & Harris, L. R. (in press). Eye position affects the perceived locations of touches. *Experimental Brain Research.*

Henderson, J. M. (2003). Human gaze control during real-world scene perception. *Trends in Cognitive Sciences*, 7, 498-504.

Henderson, J. M., & Hollingworth, A. (1998). Eye movements during scene viewing: An overview. In G. Underwood (Ed.), *Eye guidance in reading and scene perception* (pp. 269-293). Oxford: Elsevier.

Hennessy, J. R. (1966). Cutaneous sensitivity communications. *Human Factors*, 8, 463-469.

Ho, C., Reed, N. J., & Spence, C. (2006). Assessing the effectiveness of "intuitive" vibrotactile warning signals in preventing front-to-rear-end collisions in a driving simulator. *Accident Analysis & Prevention*, 38, 989-997.

Ho, C., Reed, N., & Spence, C. (2007a). Multisensory in-car warning signals for collision avoidance. *Human Factors*, 49, 1107-1114.

Ho, C., Reed, N., & Spence, C. (2007b). 'Intuitive' vibrotactile collision warnings for drivers. In D. de Waard, G. R. J. Hockey, P. Nickel, & K. A. Brookhuis (Eds.), *Human factors issues in complex system performance* (pp. 169-176). Maastricht, Netherlands: Shaker Publishing.

Ho, C., Santangelo, V., & Spence, C. (2009). Multisensory warning signals: When spatial correspondence matters. *Experimental Brain Research*, 195, 261-272.

Ho, C., & Spence, C. (2007). Head orientation biases tactile localization. *Brain Research*, 1144C, 136-141.

Ho, C., & Spence, C. (2008). *The multisensory driver: Implications for ergonomic car interface design.* Aldershot: Ashgate Publishing.

Ho, C., & Spence, C. (in press). Using peripersonal warning signals to re-orient a driver's gaze. *Human Factors.*

Ho, C., Tan, H. Z., & Spence, C. (2006). The differential effect of vibrotactile and auditory cues on visual spatial attention. *Ergonomics*, 49, 724-738.

Jones, C. M., Gray, R., Spence, C., & Tan, H. Z. (2008). Directing visual attention with spatially informative and noninformative tactile cues. *Experimental Brain Research*, 186, 659-669.

Jones, L., & Sarter, N. (2008). Tactile displays: Guidance for their design and application. *Human Factors*, 50, 90-111.

Jones, L. A., Lockyer, B., & Piateski, E. (2006). Tactile display and vibrotactile pattern recognition on the torso. *Advanced Robotics*, 20, 1359-1374.

Julesz, B. (1971). *Foundations of cyclopean perception*. Chicago: University of Chicago Press.

Kaczmarek, K. A., & Bach-y-Rita, P. (1995). Tactile displays. In W. Barfield & T. A. Furness (Eds.), *Virtual environments and advanced interface design* (pp. 349-414). New York, NY: Oxford University Press.

Kennett, S., Eimer, M., Spence, C., & Driver, J. (2001). Tactile-visual links in exogenous spatial attention under different postures: Convergent evidence from psychophysics and ERPs. *Journal of Cognitive Neuroscience*, 13, 462-478.

Kennett, S., Spence, C., & Driver, J. (2002). Visuo-tactile links in covert exogenous spatial attention remap across changes in unseen hand posture. *Perception & Psychophysics*, 64, 1083-1094.

Kikuchi, T., Yamashita, Y., Sagawa, K., & Wake, T. (1979). An analysis of tactile letter confusions. *Perception & Psychophysics*, 26, 295-301.

Krech, D., & Crutchfield, R. S. (1958). *Elements of psychology*. New York: A. A. Knopf.

Lee, J.-H., & Spence, C. (2008). Assessing the benefits of multimodal feedback on dual-task performance under demanding conditions. *Proceedings of the 22nd British HCI Group Annual Conference on HCI2008* (pp. 185-192). Liverpool: UK.

Lee, J.-H., & Spence, C. (2009). Feeling what you hear: Task-irrelevant sounds modulate tactile perception delivered via a touch screen. *Journal on Multimodal User Interfaces*, DOI 10.1007/s12193-009-0014-8.

Lee, Y.-C., Lee, J. D., & Boyle, L. N. (2009). The interaction of cognitive load and attention-directing cues in driving. *Human Factors*, 51, 271-280.

Lenggenhager, B., Tadi, T., Metzinger, T., & Blanke, O. (2007). Video ergo sum: Manipulating bodily self-consciousness. *Science*, 317, 1096-1099.

Lewald, J., & Ehrenstein, W. H. (1996a). Auditory-visual shift in localization depending on gaze direction. *Neuroreport*, 7, 1929-1932.

Lewald, J., & Ehrenstein, W. H. (1996b). The effect of eye position on auditory lateralization. *Experimental Brain Research*, 108, 473-485.

Lindeman, R. W., & Yanagida, Y. (2003). Empirical studies for effective near-field haptics in virtual environments. *Proceedings of IEEE Virtual Reality 2003*, 287-288.

Lindeman, R. W., Yanagida, Y., Sibert, J. L., & Lavine, R. (2003). Effective vibrotactile cueing in a visual search task. *Proceedings of the Ninth IFIP TC13 International Conference on Human-Computer Interaction (INTERACT 2003)*, (pp. 89-98). Zuerich, Switzerland, Sept. 1-5.

Loomis, J. (1974). Tactile letter recognition under different modes of stimulus presentation. *Perception & Psychophysics*, 16, 401-408.

Loomis, J. M., & Lederman, S. J. (1986). Tactual perception. In K. R. Boff, L. Kaufman & J. P. Thomas (Eds.), *Handbook of perception and human performance: Cognitive processes and performance* (Vol. 2, pp. 31-41). New York: Wiley.

Macaluso, E., Frith, C., & Driver, J. (2000). Modulation of human visual cortex by crossmodal spatial attention. *Science*, 289, 1206-1208.

Macaluso, E., Frith, C. D., & Driver, J. (2002). Crossmodal spatial influences of touch on extrastriate visual areas take current gaze direction into account. *Neuron*, 34, 647-658.

Marr, D. (1982). *Vision: A computational investigation into the human representation and processing of visual information*. New York: W. H. Freeman and Company.

Mohd Rosli, R., Jones, C. M., Tan, H. Z., Proctor, R. W., & Gray, R. (submitted). The crossmodal spotlight of visual attention for proximal-distal tactile cueing. *ACM Transactions on Applied Perception*.

Nagel, S. K., Carl, C., Kringe, T., Märtin, R., & König, P. (2005). Beyond sensory substitution-learning the sixth sense. *Journal of Neural Engineering*, 2, R13-R26.

Natsoulas, T. (1966). Locus and orientation of the perceiver (ego) under variable, constant, and no perspective instructions. *Journal of Personality and Social Psychology*, 3, 190-196.

Natsoulas, T., & Dubanoski, R. A. (1964). Inferring the locus and orientation of the perceiver from responses to stimulation of the skin. *American Journal of Psychology*, 77, 281-285.

Ngo, M. K., & Spence, C. (in press). Comparing the effectiveness of auditory and tactile cues in facilitating visual search performance. *Lecture Notes in Computer Science (LNCS)*.

Ngo, M. K., & Spence, C. (submitted). Evaluating the effectiveness of temporally synchronous and spatially informative cues in visual search. *Attention, Perception, & Psychophysics*.

Odgaard, E. C., Arieh, Y., & Marks, L. E. (2003). Cross-modal enhancement of perceived brightness: Sensory interaction versus response bias. *Perception & Psychophysics*, 65, 123-132.

Parise, C., & Spence, C. (2009). 'When birds of a feather flock together': Synesthetic correspondences modulate audiovisual integration in non-synesthetes. *PLoS ONE*, 4: e5664.

Peddamatham, P., Peine, W., & Tan, H. Z. (2008). Assessment of vibrotactile feedback in a needle-insertion task using a surgical robot. *Proceedings of the Symposium on Haptic Interfaces for Virtual Environment and Teleoperator Systems* (pp. 93-99). Reno, NV, Mar. 13-14.

Perrott, D. R., Cisneros, J., McKinley, R. L., & D'Angelo, W. (1996). Aurally aided visual search under virtual and free-field listening conditions. *Human Factors*, 38, 702-715.

Perrott, D. R., Saberi, K., Brown, K., & Strybel, T. Z. (1990). Auditory psychomotor coordination and visual search performance. *Perception & Psychophysics*, 48, 214-226.

Perrott, D. R., Sadralodabai, T., Saberi, K., & Strybel, T. Z. (1991). Aurally aided visual search in the central visual field: Effects of visual load and visual enhancement of the target. *Human Factors*, 33, 389-400.

Posner, M. I. (1978). *Chronometric explorations of mind*. Hillsdale, NJ: Erlbaum.

Posner, M. I., Nissen, M. J., & Klein, R. M. (1976). Visual dominance: An information-processing account of its origins and significance. *Psychological Review*, 83, 157-171.

Previc, F. H. (2000). Neuropsychological guidelines for aircraft control stations. *IEEE Engineering in Medicine and Biology Magazine*, 19, 81-88.

Proctor, R. W., Tan, H. Z., Vu, K.-P. L., Gray, R., & Spence, C. (2005). Implications of compatibility and cuing effects for multimodal interfaces. *Proceedings of HCI International 2005*, 11, Paper No. 2733.

Raj, A. K., Kass, S. J., & Perry, J. F. (2000). Vibrotactile displays for improving spatial awareness. *Proceedings of the IEA 2000/HFES 2000 Congress*, 1-181 - 1-184.

Reed, C. M., Delhorne, L. A., Brughera, A., Durlach, N. I., Tan, H. Z., & Wong, A. (2003). Information-transfer rates for sequences of multidimensional tactual signals. In *Proceedings of the 7th International Sensory Aids Conference*, Portland, ME, USA, May 8, 2003.

Reed, C. M. & Durlach, N. I. (1998). Note on information transfer rates in human communication. *Presence: Teleoperators & Virtual Environments*, 7, 509-518.

Reed, C. M., Rabinowitz, W. M., Durlach, N. I., Braida, L. D., Conway-Fithian, S., & Schultz, M. C. (1985). Research on the Tadoma method of speech communication. *Journal of the Acoustical Society of America*, 77, 247-257.

Rensink, R. A. (2000). Visual search for change: A probe into the nature of attentional processing. *Visual Cognition*, 7, 345-376.

Santangelo, V., & Spence, C. (2008). Is the exogenous orienting of spatial attention truly automatic? Evidence from unimodal and multisensory studies. *Consciousness and Cognition*, 17, 989-1015.

Sarter, N. B. (2000). The need for multisensory interfaces in support of effective attention allocation in highly dynamic event-driven domains: The case of cockpit automation. *International Journal of Aviation Psychology*, 10, 231-245.

Sarter, N. B. (2007). Multiple-resource theory as a basis for multimodal interface design: Success stories, qualifications, and research needs. In A. F. Kramer, D. A. Wiegmann, & A. Kirlik (Eds.), *Attention: From theory to practice* (pp. 187-195). Oxford: Oxford University Press.

Scott, J. J., & Gray, R. (2008). A comparison of tactile, visual, and auditory warnings for rear-end collision prevention in simulated driving. *Human Factors*, 50, 264-275.

Shi, Z., Zou, H., Rank, M., Chen, L., Hirche, S., & Müller, H. (submitted). Effects of packet loss and latency on temporal discrimination of visual-haptic events. *ACM Transactions on Haptics*.

Shore, D. I., Barnes, M. E., & Spence, C. (2006). The temporal evolution of the crossmodal congruency effect. *Neuroscience Letters*, 392, 96-100.

Sklar, A. E., & Sarter, N. B. (1999). Good vibrations: Tactile feedback in support of attention allocation and human-automation coordination in event-driven domains. *Human Factors*, 41, 543-552.

Slutzky, D. A., & Recanzone, G. H. (2001). Temporal and spatial dependency of the ventriloquism effect. *Neuroreport*, 12, 7-10.

Spence, C. (2007). Audiovisual multisensory integration. *Acoustical Science & Technology*, 28, 61-70.

Spence, C., Baddeley, R., Zampini, M., James, R., & Shore, D. I. (2003). Crossmodal temporal order judgments: When two locations are better than one. *Perception & Psychophysics*, 65, 318-328.

Spence, C. J., & Driver, J. (1994). Covert spatial orienting in audition: Exogenous and endogenous mechanisms facilitate sound localization. *Journal of Experimental Psychology: Human Perception and Performance*, 20, 555-574.

Spence, C., & Driver, J. (1997a). Audiovisual links in exogenous covert spatial orienting. *Perception & Psychophysics*, 59, 1-22.

Spence, C., & Driver, J. (1997b). Cross-modal links in attention between audition, vision, and touch: Implications for interface design. *International Journal of Cognitive Ergonomics*, 1, 351-373.

Spence, C., & Driver, J. (2000). Attracting attention to the illusory location of a sound: Reflexive crossmodal orienting and ventriloquism. *Neuroreport*, 11, 2057-2061.

Spence, C., & Driver, J. (Eds.). (2004). *Crossmodal space and crossmodal attention*. Oxford, UK: Oxford University Press.

Spence, C., & Ho, C. (2008a). Tactile and multisensory spatial warning signals for drivers. *IEEE Transactions on Haptics*, 1, 121-129.

Spence, C., & Ho, C. (2008b). Multisensory warning signals for event perception and safe driving. *Theoretical Issues in Ergonomics Science*, 9, 523-554.

Spence, C., McDonald, J., & Driver, J. (2004). Exogenous spatial cuing studies of human crossmodal attention and multisensory integration. In C. Spence & J. Driver (Eds.), *Crossmodal space and crossmodal attention* (pp. 277-320). Oxford, UK: Oxford University Press.

Spence, C., Nicholls, M. E. R., Gillespie, N., & Driver, J. (1998). Cross-modal links in exogenous covert spatial orienting between touch, audition, and vision. *Perception & Psychophysics*, 60, 544-557.

Spence, C., & Santangelo, V. (2009). Capturing spatial attention with multisensory cues. *Hearing Research*. http://dx.doi.org/10.1016/j.heares.2009.04.015.

Spence, C., Shore, D. I., & Klein, R. M. (2001). Multisensory prior entry. *Journal of Experimental Psychology: General*, 130, 799-832.

Spence, C., & Squire, S. B. (2003). Multisensory integration: Maintaining the perception of synchrony. *Current Biology*, 13, R519-R521.

Stein, B. E., London, N., Wilkinson, L. K., & Price, D. P. (1996). Enhancement of perceived visual intensity by auditory stimuli: A psychophysical analysis. *Journal of Cognitive Neuroscience*, 8, 497-506.

Stein, B. E., & Meredith, M. A. (1993). *The merging of the senses*. Cambridge, MA: MIT Press.

Stein, B. E., & Stanford, T. R. (2008). Multisensory integration: Current issues from the perspective of the single neuron. *Nature Reviews Neuroscience*, 9, 255-267.

Tan, H. Z., Durlach, N. I., Reed, C. M., & Rabinowitz, W. M. (1999). Information transmission with a multifinger tactual display. *Perception & Psychophysics*, 61, 993-1008.

Tan, H. Z., Gray, R., Spence, C., Jones, C. M., & Rosli, R. M. (2009). The haptic cuing of visual spatial attention: Evidence of a spotlight effect. In B. E. Rogowitz & T. N. Pappas (Eds.), *Proceedings of SPIE-IS&T Electronic Imaging, Human Vision and Electronic Imaging XIV* (12 pp.). San Jose, CA, Jan. 18-22.

Tan, H. Z., Gray, R., Young, J. J., & Irawan, P. (2001). Haptic cuing of a visual change-detection task: Implications for multimodal interfaces. In M. J. Smith, G. Salvendy, D. Harris, & R. J. Koubek (Eds.), *Usability evaluation and interface design: Cognitive engineering, intelligent agents and virtual reality. Proceedings of the 9th International Conference on Human-Computer Interaction* (Vol. 1; pp. 678-682). Mahwah, NJ: Erlbaum.

Tan, H. Z., Gray, R., Young, J. J., & Traylor, R. (2003). A haptic back display for attentional and directional cueing. *Haptics-e: The Electronic Journal of Haptics Research*, 3 (1), June 11, 2003.

Tan, H. Z. & Pentland, A. (2001). Tactual displays for sensory substitution and wearable computers. In W. Barfield & T. Caudell (Eds.), *Fundamentals of wearable computers and augmented reality* (pp. 579-598). Mahwah, NJ: Lawrence Erlbaum Associates.

Tan, H. Z., Reed, C. M., & Durlach, N. I. (submitted). Optimum information-transfer rates for communication through haptic and other sensory modalities. *IEEE Transactions on Haptics*.

Töyssy, S., Raisamo, J., & Raisamo, R. (2008). Telling time by vibration. In M. Ferre (Ed.), *EuroHaptics 2008*, LNCS 5024, 924-929. Berlin: Springer-Verlag.

Van der Burg, E., Olivers, C. N. L., Bronkhorst, A. W., & Theeuwes, J. (2008). Non-spatial auditory signals improve spatial visual search. *Journal of Experimental Psychology: Human Perception and Performance*, 34, 1053-1065.

Van der Burg, E., Olivers, C. N. L., Bronkhorst, A. W., & Theeuwes, J. (2009). Poke and pop: Tactile-visual synchrony increases visual saliency. *Neuroscience Letters*, 450, 60-64.

Van Erp, J. B. F. (2005). Presenting directions with a vibrotactile torso display. *Ergonomics*, 48, 302-313.

Van Erp, J. B. F., Eriksson, L., Levin, B., Carlander, O., Veltman, J. E., & Vos, W. K. (2007). Tactile cueing effects on performance in simulated aerial combat with high acceleration. *Aviation, Space and Environmental Medicine*, 78, 1128-1134.

Van Erp, J. B. F., Jansen, C., Dobbins, T., & van Veen, H. A. H. C. (2004). Vibrotactile waypoint navigation at sea and in the air: Two case studies. *Proceedings of EuroHaptics 2004* (pp. 166-173). Munich, Germany, June 5-7.

Van Erp, J. B. F., & Van Veen, H. A. H. C. (2004). Vibrotactile in-vehicle navigation system. *Transportation Research Part F*, 7, 247-256.

Van Erp, J. B. F., & Van Veen, H. A. H. C. (2006). Touch down: The effect of artificial touch cues on orientation in microgravity. *Neuroscience Letters*, 404, 78-82.

Van Erp, J. B. F., Van Veen, H. A. H. C., Jansen, C., & Dobbins, T. (2005). Waypoint navigation with a vibrotactile waist belt. *ACM Transactions on Applied Perception*, 2, 106-117.

Van Veen, H.-J., Spapé, M, & van Erp, J. B. F. (2004). Waypoint navigation on land: Different ways of coding distance to the next waypoint. *Proceedings of EuroHaptics 2004* (pp. 160-165). Munich, Germany, June 5-7.

Verrillo, R. T., & Gescheider, G. A. (1992). Perception via the sense of touch. In I. R. Summers (Ed.), *Tactile aids for the hearing impaired* (pp. 1-36). London: Whurr Publishers.

Viau, A., Najm, M., Chapman, C. E., & Levin, M. F. (2005). Effect of tactile feedback on movement speed and precision during work-related tasks using a computer mouse. *Human Factors*, 47, 816-826.

Vroomen, J., & de Gelder, B. (2000). Sound enhances visual perception: Cross-modal effects of auditory organization on vision. *Journal of Experimental Psychology: Human Perception and Performance*, 26, 1583-1590.

Weerts, T. C., Thurlow, W. R. (1971). The effects of eye position and expectation in sound localization. *Perception & Psychophysics*, 9, 35-39.

Weinstein, S. (1968). Intensive and extensive aspects of tactile sensitivity as a function of body part, sex, and laterality. In D. R. Kenshalo (Ed.), *The skin senses* (pp. 195-222). Springfield, Ill: Thomas.

Wilska, A. (1954). On the vibrational sensitivity in different regions of the body surface. *Acta Physiologica Scandinavica*, 31, 285-289.

Yanagida, Y., Kakita, M., Lindeman, R. W., Kume, Y., & Tetsutani, N. (2004). Vibrotactile letter reading using a low-resolution tactor array. In *Proceedings of the 12th International Symposium on Haptic Interfaces for Virtual Environment and Teleoperator Systems* (pp. 400-406). Chicago, IL.

Yannier, N., Basdogan, C., Tasiran, S., & Sen, O. L. (2008). Using haptics to convey cause-and-effect relations in climate visualization. *IEEE Transactions on Haptics*, 1, 130-141.
Young, J. J., Tan, H. Z., & Gray, R. (2003). Validity of haptic cues and its effect on priming visual spatial attention. *Proceedings of the 11th International Symposium on Haptic Interfaces for Virtual Environment and Teleoperator Systems* (pp. 166-170). Los Angeles, CA: IEEE Computer Society, March 22-23.
Zlotnik, M. A. (1988). Applying electro-tactile display technology to fighter aircraft - Flying with feeling again. *Proceedings of the IEEE 1988 National Aerospace and Electronics Conference NAECON 1988*, 191-197.

4

Cartesian Control of a Cable-Driven Haptic Mechanism

Martin J.D. Otis, Vincent Duchaine, Greg Billette,
Simon Perreault, Clément Gosselin and Denis Laurendeau,
Laval University
Canada

1. Introduction

Haptic devices operated through a communication network require a trade-off between the stability of the interaction and the quality of the haptic display. A haptic device must be designed to provide the best haptic display in order to reproduce the tactile sensation of virtual objects, rigid or soft, while ensuring a stable operation to guarantee user safety. The challenges are greater when considering a locomotion interface where a walker can produce large wrenches. A Cable-Driven Locomotion Interface, used as a peripheral in a virtual environment, is designed to address some of the aforementioned issues, since the use of cables as a mechanical transmission is known to provide many advantages such as low inertia, which is helpful in attaining high speeds and high accelerations, and the potential lengths of the cables can allow for large workspaces. Using this mechanism, a walker could navigate in a virtual environment with the aid of two haptic platforms (one for each foot) which can be regarded as two independent parallel robots constrained to six degrees of freedom and sharing a common workspace.

The architecture of the framework is composed of two components: the *virtual environment manager* and the *controller manager*. The former contains the definition of the environment in which the user navigates, as expressed by a graphic rendering engine and a communication interface. The second component computes and controls the wrenches from two physical models to accurately simulate soft and rigid virtual objects. The challenge of high impact dynamics is addressed with the help of specialized reels that is also introduced as a potential solution to the issue. The aim of these new reels is to reproduce the vibrations that would normally be encountered during such an impact.

From kinematic-static duality principle, the total wrench applied on a platform is distributed optimally in each cable tension by an optimal tension distribution algorithm thereby allowing the haptic simulation of virtual objects using hybrid admittance/impedance control with multi-contact interactions. In the context of human-robot cooperation, some practical aspects of the software design for achieving a safe control (for avoiding accidents and injuries) with a safety management plan are presented. Finally, some stability issues are also developed specifically for the cable-driven parallel mechanism.

1.1 Review

The Cable-Driven Locomotion Interface (CDLI) design presented here is based on the concept of programmable platforms with permanent foot contacts, such as Gait Master (Iwata et al., 2001), (Onuki et al., 2007) and K-Walker or the Virtual Walking Machine in (Yoon et al., 2004). CDLI employs two independent cable-driven haptic platforms constrained in six degrees of freedom (Perreault & Gosselin, 2008). Each platform is attached to a foot of the walker. Its control system and its geometry are designed so as to support a wide range of walking patterns including left/right turns and going up/down slopes or stairs that are either rigid or soft virtual surfaces or objects. In the following paragraphs, a control algorithm made specifically for cable-driven platforms is presented to address the issue of the interactions between the virtual foot models linked to the platforms and any virtual object such as but not limited to uneven terrain.

Several concepts of locomotion interfaces have been developed in order to provide a better feeling of immersion in a virtual environment and for automated walking rehabilitation. For instance, the Rehabilitation Robot LOKOMAT (Bernhardt et al., 2005) uses a hybrid force-position control method for which the force component adjusts the movement of an actuated leg orthosis so as to influence the LOKOMAT's motion and to automate user gait-pattern therapy. Such a control method is implemented in the context of the Patient-Driven Motion Reinforcement paradigm. HapticWalker is a programmable robotic footplate device that allows arbitrary foot movements during user gait training via specialized motion generation algorithms (Schmidt et al., 2005). However these control strategies are not well adapted to a CDLI as well as haptic rendering of contacts with any virtual objects or uneven terrains. In fact, a CDLI shows substantial advantages over conventional locomotion interfaces and has the potential to achieve better performances than other devices. For instance, the haptic foot platform in a CDLI can reach higher accelerations and can move in a larger workspace. Some designs involving cable-driven mechanisms were devised as the primary haptic display in a virtual environment. For instance, cable-driven devices have proven their efficiency as haptic interfaces in virtual sport training such as a tennis force display (Kawamura et al., 1995) and a catch playing simulator (Morizono et al., 1997).

In this chapter, it is shown that a hybrid admittance/impedance strategy for controlling the CDLI combines the benefits of both control classes and exploits the contact points geometry and the physical properties (stiffness, friction, etc.) of the virtual surface colliding with the virtual foot model. Within the CDLI control algorithm, the measured action wrenches imposed by the walker's feet move the platforms while a virtual reaction wrench moves the walker in the virtual environment in the event that a contact is detected between a virtual object and the virtual foot model. The software also exploits the Newton Game Dynamics™ engine, labeled *"Newton engine"* in the following, for simulating rigid body interactions.

The second section of this chapter presents the software architecture for controlling the haptic foot platform. The third and the fourth sections covers the development of the control strategy for multiple-contact points geometry that is used for performing hybrid-controlled interactions in a CDLI. The fifth one presents a custom physics engine developed under QNX OS for force rendering on a haptic foot platform so as to manage soft object interactions. This physics engine includes a Force Optimization Problem (FOP) to distribute the wrench at each contact point uniformly and optimally. This custom engine is designed to overcome some drawbacks of the Newton engine, such as transient force computation and object penetration that occurs when a contact is detected between the virtual foot model and a compliant surface. Finally, the last section of the chapter presents simulations of the control strategy with the physics engines in normal gait walking conditions.

1.2 The geometry of the CDLI

As shown in figure 1, the geometry of the CDLI is optimized to cover the largest workspace possible in a limited volume (i.e. the overall dimension of the complete CDLI) so as to avoid cable interferences and to minimize human-cable interferences while the user is walking (Perreault & Gosselin, 2008). It must be noted that due to the unilaterality of the actuation principle, a cable-driven parallel platform needs at least seven cables in order to control a six DOF platform. Since each platform has six DOF so as to emulate human gait (Yoon & Ryu, 2006) and all cable attachment points are chosen so as to reach an optimal workspace, each haptic foot platform is actuated by eight cables.

The dimensions of the workspace along the X, Y and Z axis are respectively 2 metres, 0.6 metre and 1 metre, all within the overall dimensions of the complete CDLI whose size is approximately 6.0 metres by 3.5 metres by 3.0 metres. These dimensions allow users to perform a wide range of walking patterns.

The model of the virtual foot in the virtual environment, shown in figure 2, is mathematically related to the haptic foot platform by a translation vector and a rotation matrix between their respective reference frames.

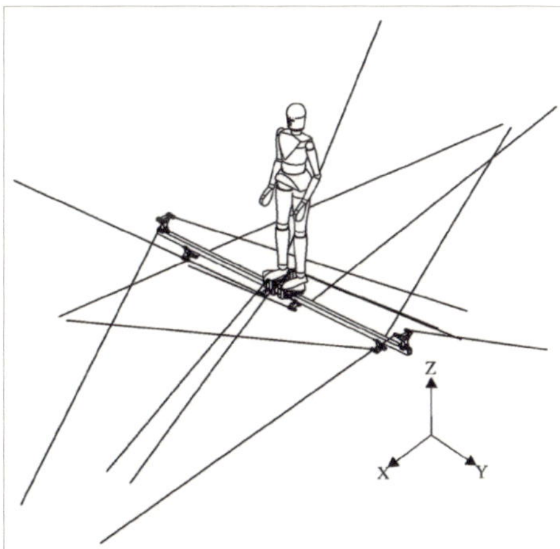

Fig. 1. CAD model of the complete CDLI taken from (Perreault & Gosselin, 2008)

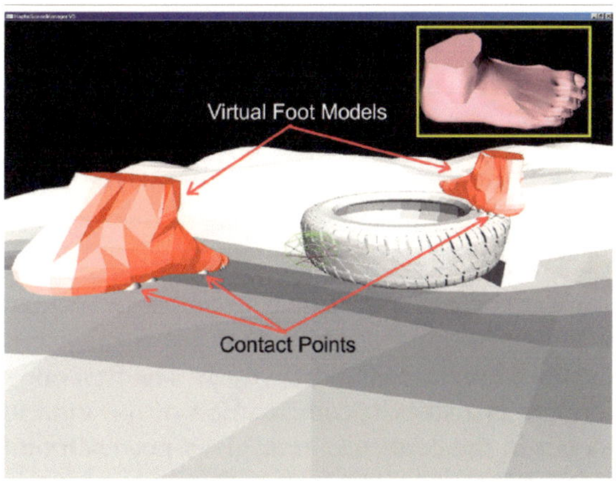

Fig. 2. Virtual foot models in contact with virtual objects

1.3 Control Classes for Haptic Rendering

Two control classes are generally employed for haptic rendering on the platforms: an impedance control class and an admittance control class similar to those described in (Carignan & Cleary, 2000). Since both control classes use pose and wrench inputs, they are instead defined by the output or the feedback loop. The properties of each approach are compared in table 1. The Cobotic Hand Controller (Faulring et al., 2007) and the HapticMaster (van der Linde & Lammertse, 2003) are both mechanisms that use admittance control. On the other hand, the Excalibur (Adams et al., 2000) and the Phantom (McJunkin & al., 2005) haptic devices have been designed as impedance displays that use impedance control.

Indeed, two virtual object models could be defined: an admittance model and an impedance model. Using linear circuit theory (quadripole or two-ports models), there are four possible topologies described by the immitance matrices: the impedance matrix, the admittance matrix, the hybrid matrix and the alternate hybrid matrix that the controller could manage as described in (Adams & Hannaford, 1999).

The hybrid control strategy combining these two control classes (interacting with the both virtual object models) ensure that free movements and contact with a rigid virtual object are rendered realistically by the platforms. Section 4 describes a method for selecting the appropriate control class using both the geometry of the contact points and the virtual object properties.

Impedance-controlled system (impedance control with force feedback)	Admittance-controlled system (admittance control with position/velocity feedback)
Controls the wrench applied by the haptic foot platform	Controls the pose or velocity of the haptic device
Is subject to instabilities when the user releases the device	Is subject to instabilities when the stiffness of the user's legs increases
Can simulate highly compliant virtual objects	Can simulate an unyielding virtual object

Table 1. Comparison of the control classes

1.4 Stability issues

The capability for a human to stabilize an unstable system or even to destabilize a stable system is a recurrent problem in the haptic interface control. Two methods are developed in the literature for stability analysis. The first one is based on human and environment models (on-line or real-time computation of the muscle stiffness) in order to adjust an admittance model in the controller that gives pose setpoints computed from the user applied wrench measured at the end effector. This method consists in adjusting the control law for ensuring stability of the system (Tsumugiwa et al., 2002). The analysis of the stability could then be performed with different strategies such as Routh-Hurwitz, root-locus, Nyquist, Lyapunov or μ-analysis among others. In the other case, the second method does not use any model. This method analyses the transfer of energy inside the system like in (Hannaford & Ryu, 2002). On the other hand, there exist numerous stabilizing techniques such as those exploited in adaptive or robust control.

A stable haptic system dissipates more energy than the overall control system produces. However, this diminishes the realism of the haptic display as the dissipated energy

increases. It is therefore a trade-off between performance and transparency. In cable tension control applications the dissipated energy should be compensated for so as to lead the system toward an unstable regime. The stabilizing method uses a virtual damping parameter in order to dissipate accumulated energy with a passivity observer (PO) and a passivity controller (PC). This method was used also for compensating the delay on the network.
Friction hysteresis in reel increases vibrations in the cables when the reel's mechanical parts stick and slip. Furthermore, rigid contacts between the virtual object and the foot produce discontinuities in cable tensions that have a tendency to create or emphasize cable vibrations. Finally, the stiffness of the reel and of the mechanical structure should be at least larger than the one of the virtual object so that mechanical deformation cannot generate more instability. From this analysis, which excludes the electronic hardware, six types of instability inside a hybrid control architecture for a Cable-Driven Mechanism can be considered:

1. Cable vibration and tension discontinuities;
2. Mechanical design (stiffness of the overall mechanical structure including motorized reel, friction hysteresis, actuator dynamic, encoder resolution, etc.);
3. Hybrid control architecture with uncertainty (Cheah et al., 2003) and with flexible joint (Goldsmith et al., 1999);
4. Contacts with a stiff virtual object with one or more contact points (Lu & Song, 2008);
5. Interaction between a human and a mechanism (Duchaine & Gosselin, 2009) and
6. Time delay (latency) over the network (Changhyun et al., 2008).

2. Software Architecture for Control

The hardware architecture is composed of two components: a soft real-time module implemented on a standard PC running Windows which manages the virtual environment with a graphic rendering engine, and a hard real-time module implemented on a standard PC running QNX whose primary tasks is to control and drive the cable-driven platforms and a server that ensures intercommunication and synchronization between different walkers. The software architecture is designed to exploit the above hardware and is thus composed of the two components shown in figure 3: the *Virtual Environment Manager* and the *Controller Manager* which are described in the next sections.

2.1 Virtual Environment Manager

The *Virtual Environment Manager* (VEM) is responsible for handling haptic objects (virtual foot model and virtual object), a physics engine, and a virtual user (an avatar) whose feet are shown to be moving in a virtual environment. The avatar therefore mimics the movements of the user so that he or she can observe his actions in the virtual environment. The *virtual user* defines the characteristics of the walker who can observe the virtual environment in coherence with his feet. For the *physics engine*, Newton Game Dynamics™ is used as a slave engine while the master physics engine is implemented on a second PC using QNX OS in the *controller manager* as described in section 2.2. The communication between both physics engines is ensured by a *client communication interface* and a *server communication interface*.

The *Haptic Scene Manager* (HSM) is the main interface with which the virtual environment is built and configured. The HSM is responsible for configuring the Newton engine according to the simulation requirements.

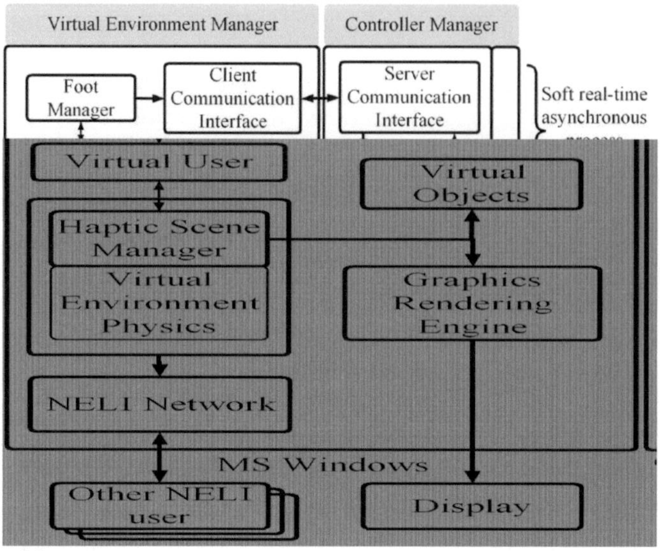

Fig. 3. Software architecture

It is also responsible for the creation, set up, and destruction of virtual objects having a haptic presence in the environment. Besides the HSM, the haptic module uses two other managers for the hands (*hand manager*) and feet (*foot manager* that define the avatar). The *foot manager*, which is connected to the *virtual user*, communicates with the *controller manager* using a TCP/IP connection. Over this communication link, the Newton engine provides the contact points between each virtual foot model and the virtual object to the *controller manager* and also provides the normal/tangent vectors to these contact points as well as the penetration into the virtual object. Conversely, the *controller manager* responds to these inputs by providing the *foot manager* with the pose and the speed of the haptic foot platform resulting from the contact, as well as the total wrench computed by the custom physics engine which then moves the virtual foot model and the virtual object in the scene.
The communication link between the VEM and the *controller manager* must support a minimum transmission rate of approximately 100 Hz in order to transfer a burst of 512 bytes with a maximum latency of one millisecond. Although there are hardware solutions satisfying these requirements, the main issue still remains the latency of the asynchronous process which is only executed whenever possible. Some solutions for resolving communication bandwidth limitations are given in (Sakr et al., 2009), where a prediction approach is exploited with the knowledge of human haptic perception (Just Noticeable Differences of Weber's law). The definition of a deadband is used for data reduction. This deadband consists of velocity and pose threshold values where there are no significant new informations. In the proposed system described in this chapter, the quantity of data transmitted over the network is based on the selection of meaningful contact points from those evaluated by the Newton engine. In fact, only three points are required by the *controller manager* to define the control class that will be applied in the appropriated DOF.

2.2 Controller Manager

The *controller manager* runs two processes: a hard real-time periodic process (labeled *control algorithm process*) responsible for the hybrid control algorithm, and a soft real-time asynchronous process that manages the virtual environment updates between the *foot manager* and the control algorithm process. The periodic process can be pre-empted any time by the asynchronous process. The rate of the periodic process for controlling the actuators and the sampling rate achieved for wrench sensing are both set at a multiple of the analog input signal number and has a minimal rate of 500 Hz, and in the best case, 1 kHz.

The *virtual torquer* in tandem with the control algorithm process runs the master physics engine (labeled *Haptic Display Rendering* (HDR) in figure 4) as well as a washout filter that maintains the walker at the centre of the workspace using a variable impedance model and position feedback as described in (Yoon & Ryu, 2006) and (Yoon. & Ryu, 2009).

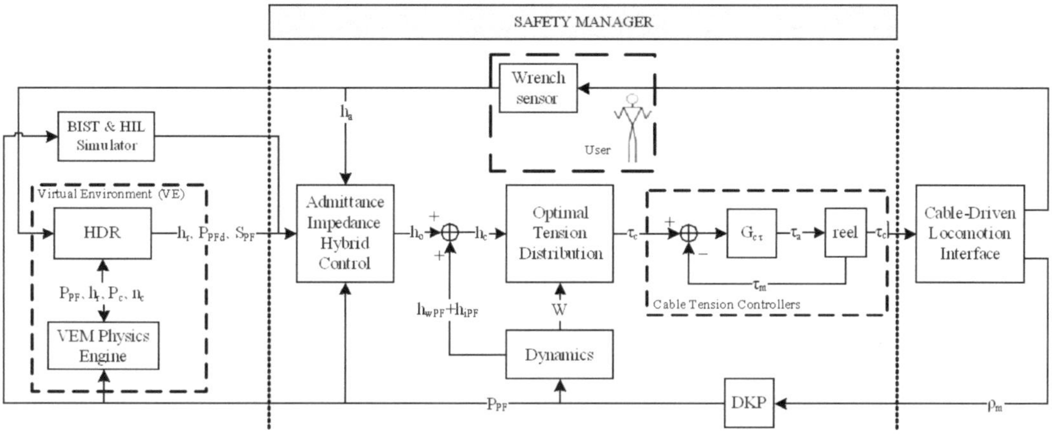

Fig. 4. Simplified control algorithm process with interactions of both physics engines

The control algorithm process, detailed in figure 4, accepts one input (the output of a 6 DOF wrench sensor) and produces two outputs (cable tensions $\boldsymbol{\tau}_c$ and platform poses $\mathbf{P}_{PF} \in \mathbb{R}^6$). The appropriate reaction wrench $\mathbf{h}_r \in \mathbb{R}^6$ is computed from the interaction between both physics engines. These engines also determine whether the degrees of freedom for each platform should be controlled in impedance or in admittance. Depending on the selected control class, the 6 DOF wrench sensor can produce, an action wrench $\mathbf{h}_a \in \mathbb{R}^6$ which moves each platform using a hybrid control scheme.

The total wrench $\mathbf{h}_c \in \mathbb{R}^6$ applied at the centre of mass of the platform is balanced with positive cable tensions using an Optimal Tension Distribution (OTD) algorithm as described in (Fang et al., 2004). The result being a set of equilibrium tension values $\boldsymbol{\tau}_c$, called the *setpoint*, that the cable tension controllers then attempt to follow. The pose of each platform is computed with the Direct Kinematic Problem (DKP) algorithm using the lengths of the cables ρ_m as input.

Since a virtual object can be rigid or soft, two physics engines are implemented to ensure a general approach that allows the physical reactions between the platforms and virtual objects to be adjusted. The HDR decides which reaction wrench computed by both engines must be transferred to the hybrid control. This choice depends both on the properties of the virtual object and on the contact points geometry. The contact point detection and the associated normal vector at the interface between a virtual object and a virtual foot model is evaluated by the Newton engine and dynamic proxy objects. The HDR exploits these values to compute its own reaction wrench $\mathbf{h}_r$ and for selecting which control class to use in order to get the best haptic rendering.

2.3 Cartesian Compensations

Mechanism transparency is crucial when a walker has to use a mechanical device inside a virtual environment. Indeed, in the virtual world, the user must be able to forget the fact that he is attached and that he is using a real device. Only the simulated physics (such as friction between foot and virtual object) inside the virtual environment must be reproduced under the user's foot. In order for this to happen, it is very important to know the exact behaviour of the mechanism at any time. This is made possible by knowing the dynamics of the device.
In a locomotion interface, the inertia and weight of platforms and sensors must be compensated for in order to increase the realism of the haptic display to the user. Therefore, $\mathbf{h}_c$ not only includes the variable load $\mathbf{h}_a$ applied by a walker's foot on the platform and the set of wrenches $\mathbf{h}_r$ computed from the interaction between walker's feet and its virtual environment, but also the effect of the weight $\mathbf{h}_{wPF} \in \mathbb{R}^6$ and inertia $\mathbf{h}_{iPF} \in \mathbb{R}^6$ of the platform and wrench sensors. For impedance control with force feedback, an additional $\mathbf{h}_r$ is added for haptic rendering of virtual contact between the platform and the virtual object.

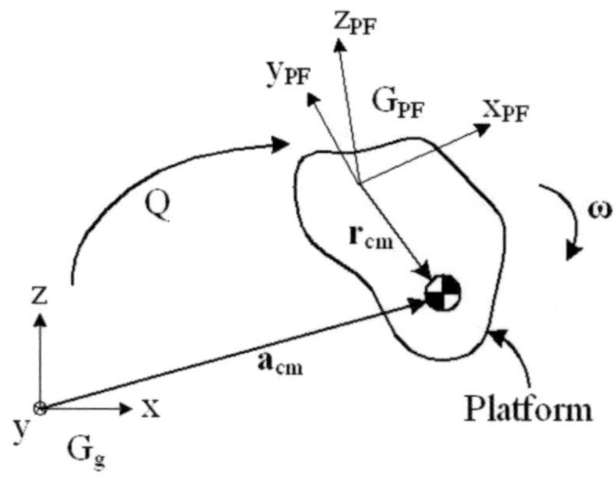

Fig. 5. Reference frame of the platform

The compensation for the mechanism inertia and weight (platforms and sensors altogether) is computed by dynamic wrenches $\mathbf{h}_{iPF}$ and $\mathbf{h}_{wPF}$ respectively. Since there are two working frames, the inertial frame G_g and the moving frame attached to the end-effector G_{PF} (as described in figure 5), and no deformation is permitted to the platform, $\mathbf{h}_{iPF}$ can be defined as follows:

$$\mathbf{h}_{iPF} = -\begin{bmatrix} m\mathbf{a}_{cm} \\ \mathbf{Q}[\mathbf{I}_{cm}]\mathbf{Q}^T\dot{\boldsymbol{\omega}} + \boldsymbol{\omega} \times \mathbf{Q}[\mathbf{I}_{cm}]\mathbf{Q}^T\boldsymbol{\omega} \end{bmatrix}, \qquad (1)$$
$$\mathbf{a}_{cm} = \mathbf{a} + \dot{\boldsymbol{\omega}} \times \mathbf{Q}\mathbf{r}_{cm} + \boldsymbol{\omega} \times (\boldsymbol{\omega} \times \mathbf{Q}\mathbf{r}_{cm}),$$

where the scalar noted m represents the mass of the platform, the vector noted $\mathbf{a}_{cm}$ represents the acceleration vector of the centre of mass of the platform in the inertial frame (i.e. the global reference frame), $\mathbf{I}_{cm} \in \mathbb{R}^{6\times 6}$ is the inertia matrix of the platform to its centre of mass and defined in the mobile frame G_{PF} (this matrix is constant since the mobile frame is fixed to the platform), $\boldsymbol{\omega}$ is the angular velocity vector of the moving frame G_{PF} compared to the inertial frame G_g, and $\mathbf{r}_{cm}$ is the vector connecting the origin of the moving frame to the centre of mass of the platform in G_{PF}.
The value of $\mathbf{h}_{iPF}$ is negative since it removes the inertia of the moving mechanism. Also the evaluation of $\mathbf{a}_{cm}$ with a low level of noise could be difficult with a low resolution of quadrature encoder inside the reel. This value should be evaluated with a six axis accelerometer/gyroscope module installed near the centre of mass. For the system presented in this chapter, it is not recommended to evaluate $\mathbf{a}_{cm}$ with the wrench sensor since the wrench sensor is used in the hybrid control.
Finally, to complete the part of dynamic relations related to the platform of the mechanism, it is needed to describe the wrench of the weight of the platform $\mathbf{h}_{wPF}$. Thus, this relation is defined as follows:

$$\mathbf{h}_{wPF} = \begin{bmatrix} m\mathbf{g} \\ \mathbf{Q}\mathbf{r}_{cm} \times m\mathbf{g} \end{bmatrix}, \tag{2}$$

where the vector $\mathbf{g}$ is the gravitational acceleration vector. As for the inertia of the motors and reels, they are accounted for by the cable tension controllers which also consider the effects of friction at low speed in order to accelerate the responses of their respective control loop.

2.4 Optimal Tension Distribution

Since each platform is driven by n-6 redundant cables, it is important that the tension be distributed among them according to kinematic and dynamic conditions so as to minimize the actuation power over all actuators (Hassan & Khajepour, 2008). It is desired to maintain the tension in the cables above a minimum threshold value $\boldsymbol{\tau}_{min}$ to limit cable sagging. Such a threshold must be greater than the minimal tension set by the precision of the acquisition system combined with a performance criterion obtained from cable behaviour (Otis et al., 2009a). Actuators (i.e. reel, motor and cable) are also limited by a maximum torque $\boldsymbol{\tau}_{max}$ which helps to avoid control problems. Hence, the following force distribution method is proposed to avoid cable sagging as well as excessive mechanical deformation of the CDLI:

$$\begin{cases} \text{minimize} & \frac{1}{2}\boldsymbol{\tau}^T\mathbf{G}\boldsymbol{\tau} \\ \text{under} & \left| \begin{array}{l} \mathbf{W}\boldsymbol{\tau} = \mathbf{h}_c \text{ , with} \\ \tau_{max} \geq \tau_i \geq \tau_{min} \\ \text{if interference, } \tau_{max} = \tau_{min} \end{array} \right. \end{cases} \tag{3}$$

$$
\begin{array}{rcl}
\mathbf{G} & = & \text{diag}(g_i) \\
\mathbf{h}_c & = & \mathbf{h}_{wPF} + \mathbf{h}_{iPF} + \mathbf{h}_o \\
\boldsymbol{\tau} & = & \left[\begin{array}{cccc} \tau_1 & \tau_2 & \dots & \tau_n \end{array} \right]^T \\
i & = & 1,\ 2,\ \dots,\ n \text{ cables,}
\end{array} \tag{4}
$$

where $\mathbf{h}_c$ represents the forces and torques that are applied on a single platform (i.e. the wrench applied by the cables on that platform), τ_i is the tension vector of the *i*th (of n) cable, **W** is the pose-dependent wrench matrix computed by the platform Jacobian matrix that links Cartesian to articular velocities, **G** is a weighting matrix with its diagonal elements such that $g_i = 1$ for all *i*, where the mathematical derivation of (3) is presented in (Barrette & Gosselin, 2005) and an application is described in (Perreault & Gosselin, 2008).

2.5 Human safety and security management plan

In the context of a human and a mechanism interacting within the same workspace, safety for human user is one of the utmost importance issues to be considered for avoiding accidents and injuries. The overall control algorithm process has a safety manager with an error handler that was designed with the help of a risk study. Each component of the software must have self-testing capabilities (or BIST for Build-In Self Test) for a general system test planning for the purpose of quality assurance (QA) and safety management. A Hardware-in-the-loop (HIL) simulator could be implemented as a way for running some parts of the BIST and partially control the platform. Documentations can be found in the IEEE 829 Standard for Software Test Documentation, CSA Z432-04 and ISO 14121. For Cable-Driven Mechanism applied to haptic applications, a minimum of four safety issues must be considered and documented:

1. Sensors reliability or fault tolerant (cable cut or failure by fatigue);
2. Mechanical interference like cable interference and platform interference with other parts of the mechanism or the user (Otis et al., 2009a);
3. Workspace limitations when the platform is going outside of its workspace;
4. Human and robot interaction like :
   - The mechanical device that safely disconnects the user from the mechanism when the mechanism is out of control (Lauzier & Gosselin, 2009) and,
   - The safety tether which maintains the equilibrium of the user when walking, falling or when the mechanism is out of control (Ottaviano et al., 2008), (Grow & Hollerbach, 2006).

Other safety aspects of the system must also be guaranteed. For example, the system must manage any sensor destruction and limits on control values (cable length, maximal and minimal cable tension, maximal current send to the motor, maximum wrench generated from the physics engine, etc.). Finally, a watchdog timer is included to ensure that the control algorithm process is executed within the prescribed period of the periodic process within an error of 5%. This watchdog and the timing period are set using a hardware interrupt implemented on a data acquisition board that is independent from the software to avoid control failure and to ensure hard real-time response. For computing derivative and for reducing noise on this value, the algorithm should consider the time shift generated by the latency (the 5% error on the prescribed period) of the OS context switching (or other process running).

3. Admittance/Impedance/Inertial-Wrench Hybrid Control

Hybrid control is a general approach that exhibits the combined advantages of impedance, admittance, and inertial-wrench control (or more precisely a null wrench control). The structure of the admittance/impedance hybrid control for one platform is shown in figure 4 and is detailed in figure 6. Two identical control structures are implemented, one per platform. The selection of the control class for each DOF of the platform is achieved by the $\mathbf{\Pi} \in \mathbb{R}^{6\times 6}$ matrix. The state of the $\mathbf{\Pi}$ matrix depends on the orientation of contact points geometry and the orientations of the platform.
When the reaction force $\mathbf{h}_r$ is null and the impedance control class is selected by the $\mathbf{\Pi}$ matrix, one simply chooses a null force control scheme with an open gain loop G_{ch}=K. Otherwise, impedance or admittance control is applied on the desired DOF for each platform. Admittance control could be performed by velocity or position feedback which could produce different experimental results, as described in (Duchaine & Gosselin, 2007). The desired platform positions $\mathbf{P}_{PFd}$ (or the desired velocities) are defined by the contact points given by the Newton engine. As the strategy used by the Newton engine, a wrench $\mathbf{h}_p$ must be added to the admittance control to avoid any large penetration inside a virtual object when a collision detection may have been missed because the refresh rate is not performed in time. This strategy also avoids the computation of a new set of contact points as the foot enters the object. In the Newton engine, the wrench $\mathbf{h}_p$ is computed with an impedance model of the object and must be controlled in the physics engine since the command is a null penetration for a rigid contact. From figure 6, the wrench $\mathbf{T}^{-I}{}_{cm}\mathbf{h}_o$ to be computed by the hybrid controller is defined by equations (5) to (8) :

$$\begin{aligned} \mathrm{T}^{-I}{}_{cm}\mathrm{h}_o &= \mathbf{\Pi}(G_{cp}(\mathrm{P}_{PFd} - \mathrm{P}_{PF}) + \mathrm{h}_p) + \\ &(\mathbf{I} - \mathbf{\Pi})(G_{ch}(\mathbf{h}_r - \mathbf{h}_a) + \mathbf{h}_r) - \mathbf{K}_h\mathbf{h}_a \text{ with,} \end{aligned} \quad (5)$$

$$\mathbf{\Pi} = \mathbf{Q}_o\mathbf{Q}_g\mathbf{S}_c\mathbf{Q}_g^T\mathbf{Q}_o^T, \quad (6)$$

$$\mathbf{Q}_o = \begin{bmatrix} \mathbf{Q} & \mathbf{0}_{3\times3} \\ \mathbf{0}_{3\times3} & \mathbf{Q} \end{bmatrix}, \quad (7)$$

$$\mathbf{Q}_g = \begin{bmatrix} \mathbf{Q}_c & \mathbf{0}_{3\times3} \\ \mathbf{0}_{3\times3} & \mathbf{Q}_c \end{bmatrix}, \quad (8)$$

where $\mathbf{G}_{cp}$ is a standard filter that controls the desired position $\mathbf{P}_{PFd}$ (or the desired velocity) of the platform ($\mathbf{P}_{PF}$ is the measured position), $\mathbf{Q}_c \in \mathbb{R}^{3\times3}$ is the rotation matrix between the contact points reference frame G_c and the platform reference frame G_{PF}. $\mathbf{Q} \in \mathbb{R}^{3\times3}$ is the rotation matrix between reference frame G_{PF} and its global counterpart G_g, which is computed by the DKP with the cable lengths ρ_m. $\mathbf{G}_{ch}$ is the wrench controller which should be set high enough (bounded by the appropriate stability criteria) to reduce the errors caused by the dynamics and friction of the cable-driven platform and of the motorized reels. A transfer matrix $\mathbf{T}_{cm}$ is used for computing the output wrench at the centre of mass of the platform since all haptic wrenches are under the foot and the OTD uses the centre of mass as its reference. Also, to prevent the platform form sticking to the contact point (i.e. when the hybrid control is oscillating between admittance and impedance), the action wrench $\mathbf{h}_a$ is added to the output of the hybrid controller with a gain $\mathbf{K}_h$. This gain and the two Cartesian controllers must consider the geometry of the mechanism and stability margins. In a Cable-Driven Mechanism, an anisotropy geometry could be designed and the control would need more energy in some DOF than other for obtaining the same transparency. Note that the initial conditions of the integrators and the filters inside both $\mathbf{G}_{ch}$ and $\mathbf{G}_{cp}$ must be adjusted for avoiding bouncing and instability. Furthermore, in some circumstances, kinematics and dynamics uncertainties must be considered in a hybrid control as described in (Cheah et al., 2003).

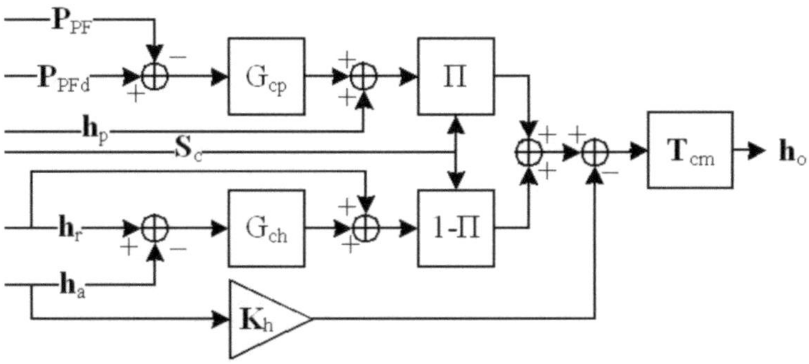

Fig. 6. Admittance/Impedance/Null Force Hybrid Control

The selection between control classes is achieved by the diagonal selection matrix $\mathbf{S}_c \in \mathbb{R}^{6\times 6}$ (1 or 0 on the diagonal and other values are set to 0) and is evaluated in the contact point reference frame G_c. The values on the diagonal of matrix $\mathbf{S}_c$ depend on friction, contact points geometry, and calibration based on experiments. A second selection matrix, $\mathbf{\Pi}_o$, defined in equation (9), is used to compute the force at each contact point by selecting the DOF under constraint using the *Force Optimization Problem* (FOP) algorithm defined in section 5.2:

$$\mathbf{\Pi}_o = \mathbf{Q}_o \mathbf{Q}_g \mathbf{S}_o \mathbf{Q}_g^T \mathbf{Q}_o^T \tag{9}$$

Thus, a 0 on the diagonal of matrix $\mathbf{S}_o \in \mathbb{R}^{6\times 6}$ allows a null force control by providing a corresponding null component for the wrench in contact points reference frame G_c. These two selection matrices ($\mathbf{S}_c$ and $\mathbf{S}_o$) are thereby quite similar in function, albeit not identical.

4. Definition of the multi-contact points geometry

Since the control strategy exploits two physics engines (Newton engine and HDR), each engine can control a given platform's DOF either in admittance or in impedance simultaneously. The virtual object properties and the contact points geometry are the criteria that determine the appropriate control class using the selection matrix $\mathbf{\Pi}$ that satisfies the following properties:

1. For a collision between a virtual foot model and a rigid virtual object for which a friction model is implemented, the selection could be based on the geometry described by the contact points between the virtual object and the virtual foot model;
2. To simulate friction, impedance control with force feedback could be chosen because there is a tangent force at the contact point reacting to an applied force from the user;
3. For compliant virtual objects, impedance control could be chosen and
4. Movement in free space could be simulated by a null force control, a special case of impedance control when some components of $\mathbf{h}_r$ are equal to 0.

The favoured method used for selecting a given control class is a multi-contact points strategy (shown in figure 7) that emphasizes control advantages relating to the simulation of rigid virtual objects which includes a friction model. Contact points are computed as the minimum set of points that completely define the boundary of the intersection between a virtual foot model and a given virtual object. They are represented in the Newton engine in conjunction with a corresponding set of normal vectors. For a haptic foot platform, a set of points whose relative distances are within ten millimetres can be viewed by the control algorithm as a single point.

The multi-contat points strategy used in this case involves the direction of the user-applied wrench for each foot: if a component of the measured wrench $\mathbf{h}_a$ is in the same direction as a normal vector describing contact points geometry, which means that the user pushes on the virtual object, this direction (or DOF) is then constrained by admittance control for rigid virtual objects; otherwise either null force control is selected to simulate free movement (i.e. the contact point is eliminated) or impedance control is employed to simulate friction. In the case of a soft virtual object, impedance control is selected in the direction normal to the contact points geometry. In figure 7, the normal vector describing contact points geometry is along the z_c axis.

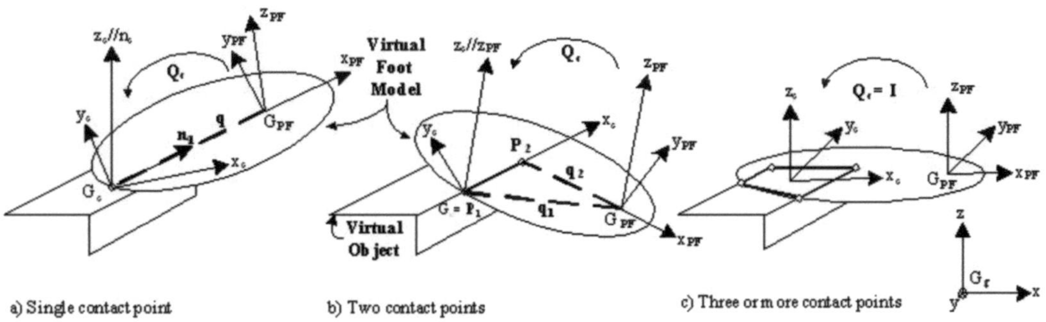

Fig. 7. Contact points description for the three cases

The theory, in the following, applies only for contacts with relatively low deformation. When the deformation is non-linear, alternative methods must be used. In the particular case of a linear deformation, there are three possibilities for which the constraints must be evaluated: the case of a single contact point (section 4.1), two contact points (section 4.2), and three or more contact points (section 4.3) when the wrench $\mathbf{h}_a$ is in the same direction as the normal vector describing contact points geometry.

4.1 Single contact point

The presence of a single contact point is a special case where the contact detection algorithm of the physics engine only finds points that are all situated within a minimal distance, and thus do not generate enough supporting action to some DOFs of the platform that would otherwise have been constrained. This case therefore only constrains the platform in the direction of the normal vector $\mathbf{n}_c$ defined by the tangent plane of the virtual object's surface at the contact point, assuming that friction vectors lie in this plane; the other directions are left unconstrained, i.e. free to move around, as shown in figure 7a). Thus, $\mathbf{S}_c[2][2]$ is set to one and all other values are set to zero, since the z_c axis is set in the normal direction of the contact point.

It must be noted that the determination of rotation matrix $\mathbf{Q}_c$ is difficult because only one z_c axis is defined. An alternative way to compute the force in the contact points reference frame G_c is to first compute $\mathbf{n}_c$, $\mathbf{h}_a$ and $\mathbf{q}$ in the global reference frame G_g, and then find the projection of $\mathbf{h}_a$ according to (10) instead of using the regular FOP (there is no force optimization on one contact point and $\mathbf{Q}_c$ is unknown):

$$\begin{aligned} \text{if}(\mathbf{q}^T\mathbf{h}_a[0:2] \geq 0) \ \Rightarrow \mathbf{\Gamma}_a &= \mathbf{n}_q(\mathbf{n}_q^T\mathbf{h}_a[0:2]) + \\ &\quad \text{skew}(\mathbf{q})^{-I}\mathbf{h}_a[3:5] \end{aligned} \tag{10}$$

$$\begin{aligned} \text{else } \mathbf{\Gamma}_a &= \mathbf{0}_{3\times 1} \text{ , with} \\ \mathbf{n}_q &= \mathbf{q}/\|\mathbf{q}\|. \end{aligned} \tag{11}$$

where [0:2] and [3:5] are operators that select the force and the torque vectors respectively and the *skew()* operator gives a square skew-symmetric matrix.

4.2 Two contact points

In the case of two contact points, the platform has only one free DOF left, as shown in figure 7b). The rotation around the x_c axis is constrained in impedance (null force control) while the other DOF can be controlled in admittance for a rigid virtual object. Rotation matrix $\mathbf{Q}_c$ is computed with the z_c axis parallel to z_{PF} and the x_c axis in the direction of the line linking the two contact points. This rotation matrix is thus defined by (12):

$$\mathbf{Q}_c = \begin{bmatrix} \cos\phi & \sin\phi & 0 \\ -\sin\phi & \cos\phi & 0 \\ 0 & 0 & 1 \end{bmatrix} \text{, with} \tag{12}$$

$$\text{if}(P_{2x} - P_{1x} \neq 0) \;\Rightarrow \phi = \arctan \frac{P_{2y} - P_{1y}}{P_{2x} - P_{1x}}, \tag{13}$$

$$\text{else } \phi = \pi/2 \; . \tag{14}$$

The diagonal of the selection matrix $\mathbf{S}_c$ is set so that only linear movements along the x_c and y_c axis with rotations around z_c can be controlled in impedance so as to allow friction forces to be applied, and such that linear movement along the z_c axis and rotation around the y_c axis are constrained in admittance for a rigid virtual object. Only the component representing rotations around the x_c axis in $\mathbf{S}_o$ is set to zero while all other values on the diagonal are set to one in order to select null force control.

4.3 Three or more contact points

This situation is simple because all haptic foot platform DOFs are constrained when some components of $\mathbf{h}_a$ push on the virtual object. Thus, rotation matrix $\mathbf{Q}_c$ and selection matrix $\mathbf{S}_o$ become identity matrices (figure 7c)) and the components of the diagonal of $\mathbf{S}_c$ are set to one except for the components representing linear movement along x_c and y_c axis that are set to zero so as to allow friction effects using impedance control.

5. Haptic Display Rendering (HDR)

To simulate soft objects, the collision detection algorithm from the Newton Game Dynamics™ engine is employed in conjunction with a custom physics engine, labeled HDR, based on the H3D API architecture and some algorithms in ODE (Open Dynamic Engine) optimized for the multi-contact points approach. This section describes the HDR in detail so as to be compatible with cable-driven locomotion interface applications and with the desired hybrid control scheme including wrench sensors designed to obtain the best possible haptic display.

The HDR developed in this paper is based on (Boyd & Wegbreit, 2007) simulation systems combined with (Ruspini & Khatib, 2000) definition of contact space. The solution to the force optimization problem, presented in section 5.2, which is computationally intensive, was proposed in (Baraff, 1994), (Cheng & Orin, 1990) and (Boyd & Wegbreit, 2007). The approach presented in this section assumes that an object is linearly deformable with respect to an impedance model as described in (Ramanathan & Metaxas, 2000) that include a static or dynamic proxy (Mitra & Niemeyer, 2005) and a friction cone law. Force display rendering can be done by other known engines like Chai3d[1]. As a secondary engine, Newton Game Dynamics, embedded in the virtual environment manager, has been chosen among others to provide force feedback of rigid body and collision detection algorithm.

[1]http://www.chai3d.org/

5.1 Computation of the Reaction Wrench

The computation of the reaction wrench $\mathbf{h}_r$ employs the action wrench $\mathbf{h}_a$ measured with the 6DOF force/torque sensors placed under the foot in the platform coordinates at origin position G_{PF}. Note that $\mathbf{h}_a$ is defined as the wrench applied by the walker on a haptic foot platform as described in figure 8 and $\mathbf{h}_r$ results from the impedance model of a virtual object and the friction model computed by equation (15):

$$\mathbf{h_r} = \begin{bmatrix} \sum\limits_{i=0}^{m-1} \mathbf{Q}_c \mathbf{\Gamma}_{r_i} \\ \sum\limits_{i=0}^{m-1} (\mathbf{q}_i \times (\mathbf{Q}_c \mathbf{\Gamma}_{r_i})) \end{bmatrix}, \tag{15}$$

where $\mathbf{\Gamma}_{ri} \in \mathbb{R}^3$ is the reaction force at the *ith* contact point $\mathbf{q}_i \in \mathbb{R}^3$. Although the presented algorithms can take into account an arbitrary number of contact points *m*, the demonstration and results uses only four points, for visual representation, around each rectangular prism that serves as a foot bounding box.

During a collision, each contact point must satisfy four constraints, which are defined similarly to what is presented in (Baraff, 1994):

1. $\mathbf{\Gamma}_{ri}$ can allow penetration between a virtual foot model and a virtual object;
2. $\mathbf{\Gamma}_{ri}$ can push but not pull (there is no glue on the virtual object);
3. $\mathbf{\Gamma}_{ri}$ occurs only at contact points defined on a virtual foot model bounding box, and
4. there is no torque on any point $\mathbf{q}_i$; the reaction torque applied on the virtual foot model is computed by $\mathbf{q}_i \, \mathrm{x} \mathbf{\Gamma}_{ri}$ as in equation (15).

The reaction forces $\mathbf{\Gamma}_{ri}$ (equation (16)) are composed of the friction forces $\mathbf{\Gamma}_{fi}$ described by the Coulomb law model (equation (19) under constraints (18)), the impedance models $\mathbf{\Gamma}_{Ii}$ (equation (17)), and a given forces $\mathbf{\Gamma}_{Mi}$ whose purpose are to ensure the conservation of linear momentum with a desired restitution coefficient (not presented in this paper):

$$\mathbf{\Gamma}_{r_i} = \mathbf{\Gamma}_{I_i} + \mathbf{\Gamma}_{f_i} + \mathbf{\Gamma}_{M_i} \text{ with,} \tag{16}$$

$$\mathbf{\Gamma}_{I_i} = \mathbf{A}_i \ddot{\mathbf{b}}_i + \mathbf{B}_i \dot{\mathbf{b}}_i + \mathbf{K}_i \mathbf{b}_i, \tag{17}$$

$$\text{if } (\mu_c \mathbf{n}_{ci}^T \mathbf{\Gamma}_{a_i} \leq \|(\mathbf{I} - \mathbf{n}_{ci}\mathbf{n}_{ci}^T)\mathbf{\Gamma}_{a_i}\|) \Rightarrow \tag{18}$$

$$\begin{aligned} \mathbf{\Gamma}_{f_i} &= (-\mu_c \mathbf{n}_{ci}^T \mathbf{\Gamma}_{ai})\mathbf{t}_{ci} \\ \text{else } \mathbf{\Gamma}_{f_i} &= -(\mathbf{I} - \mathbf{n}_{ci}\mathbf{n}_{ci}^T)\mathbf{\Gamma}_{a_i}, \end{aligned} \tag{19}$$

where $\mathbf{A}_i$, $\mathbf{B}_i$ and $\mathbf{K}_i$ are respectively the inertia matrices, the damping matrices and the spring matrices for given penetrations $\mathbf{b}_i$ of a virtual foot model inside a virtual object as shown in figure 9, for small displacements and for linear elasticities, since the contact model assumes the absence of coupling between each contact point. μ_c is the dynamic friction coefficient, while $\mathbf{n}_{ci}$ and $\mathbf{t}_{ci}$ are the normal and tangential vectors at the interface of a contact point between the virtual foot model and a colliding virtual object computed by the Newton engine and dynamic proxy objects.

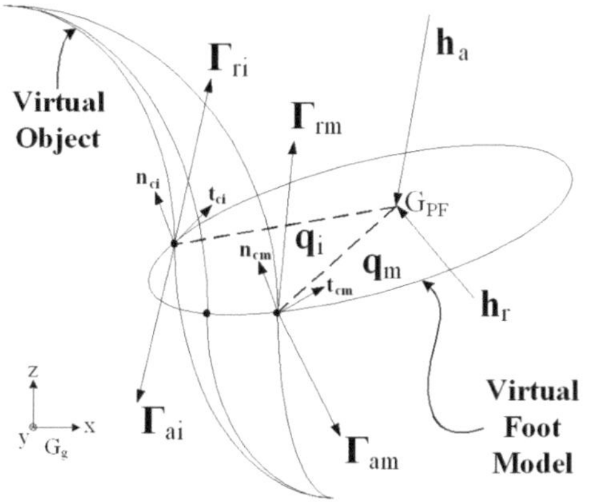

Fig. 8. Collision model with action and reaction wrenches

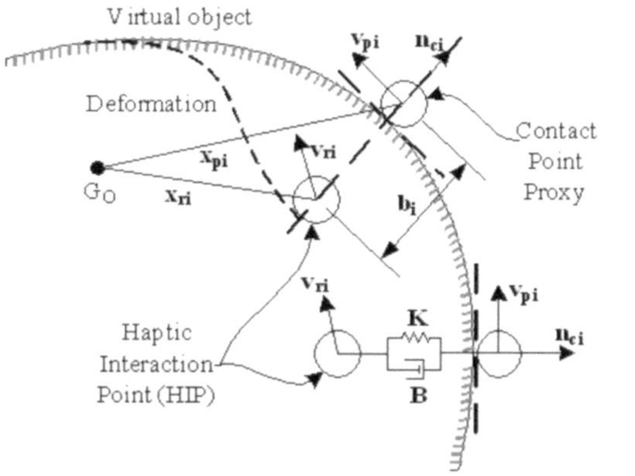

Fig. 9. Contact point proxy for each contact points with the respective penetration

5.2 Force Optimization Problem (FOP)

This section presents the methodology for computing the action forces $\mathbf{\Gamma}_{ai}$ at each contact point under friction cone constraints using the force optimization problem (FOP). The action wrench is measured in the platform reference frame at the location of the 6DOF sensor (G_{PF}). It must then be transferred to each contact point of the foot bounding box in order to obtain the desired virtual representation of the user-applied force. Because no model that calls for a specific force distribution under the foot is used, the action wrench is simply distributed uniformly and optimally, as described in (Duriez, et al. 2006). It is worth noting that this distribution should be evaluated by a walkway sensor array as specified in (Reilly, et al. 1991), but such a sensor has not yet been implemented in this work.

The FOP involves two constraints: the equilibrium constraint and the friction cone constraint, similar to (Melder & Harwin, 2004). The former constraint type is defined by a set of m linear equations (20), with contact matrices $\mathbf{R} \in \mathbb{R}^{6\times 3m}$ being defined by equations (21) and (22), where $\mathbf{\Gamma}_{ai} \in \mathbb{R}^3$ is the ith optimal force used to construct vector $\mathbf{\Gamma}_a = [\mathbf{\Gamma}_{a0} \ldots \mathbf{\Gamma}_{a(m-1)}]$:

$$\mathbf{\Pi}_o \mathbf{h}_a = \mathbf{\Pi}_o \mathbf{R} \mathbf{\Gamma}_a \text{ with,} \tag{20}$$

$$\mathbf{R} = [\mathbf{R}_0 \ldots \mathbf{R}_{m-1}], \tag{21}$$

$$\mathbf{R}_i = \begin{bmatrix} \mathbf{Q_c} \\ \mathbf{q}_i \times \mathbf{Q_c} \end{bmatrix}. \tag{22}$$

Friction cone constraints are used to define the friction force threshold values at which the virtual foot model transitions between slipping and sticking on an object surface occur. The FOP then attempts to compute the optimal forces when the virtual foot model sticks to the object, and assumes slipping motion when no solution can be found. Hence, the formulation of the FOP can be implemented using quadratic programming with non-linear constraints as represented by equation (23) for any $m \in \mathrm{N}^{+}$:

$$\begin{cases} \text{minimize} & \frac{1}{2}\mathbf{\Gamma}_a^T \mathbf{H} \mathbf{\Gamma}_a \\ \text{under} & \left| \begin{array}{l} \mathbf{\Pi}_o \mathbf{h}_a = \mathbf{\Pi}_o \mathbf{R} \mathbf{\Gamma}_a \\ \frac{-\mathbf{\Gamma}_{a_i}^T \mathbf{n}_{ci}}{\|\mathbf{\Gamma}_{a_i}\|} \geq \cos\alpha_i \\ \text{If no solution, try with} \\ \mu_c \mathbf{n}_{ci}^T \mathbf{\Gamma}_{a_i} \leq \|(\mathbf{I} - \mathbf{n}_{ci}\mathbf{n}_{ci}^T)\mathbf{\Gamma}_{a_i}\| \end{array} \right. \\ i = 0 \ldots m-1 \\ \tan\alpha_i = \mu_s \\ H = \mathrm{diag}(h_i), \end{cases} \tag{23}$$

where **H** is a weighting matrix with $h_i = 1$ which could represent the force distribution under the foot (unused for this work) and μ_s is the static friction coefficient.

5.3. Results for the FOP

This section presents results obtained from the HDR algorithm and its hybrid control strategy. For demonstration purposes, only the four points at the four vertices of the rectangular prism representing a virtual foot model bounding box are used. Note that the number of contact points has to be chosen so as to account for the maximum allowed communication bandwidth between the VEM and the *controller manager*. Figures 10 and 11 show the actual scaled version of the CDLI with a Kondo KHR-1HV.

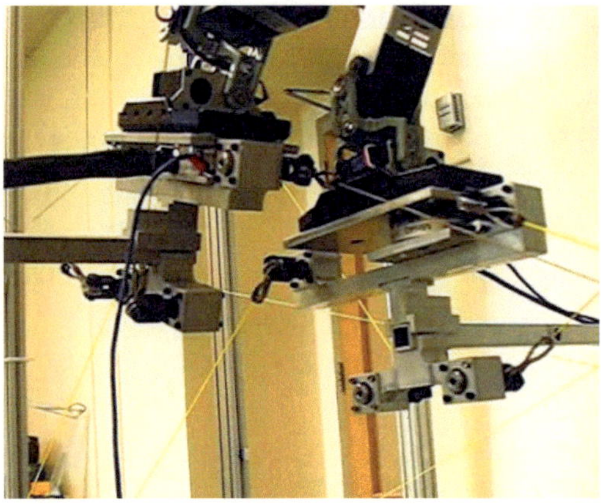

Fig. 10. Feet of the Kondo KHR-1HV on the scaled version of the CDLI

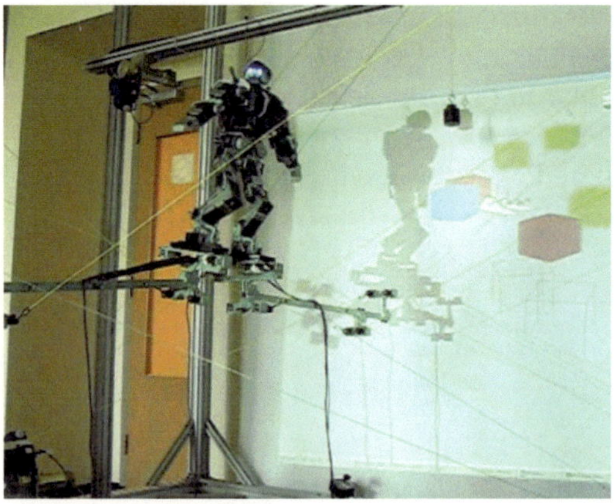

Fig. 11. Full view of the scaled version of the CDLI showing the platforms, the cables and the Virtual Reality screen displaying the scene

The simulation parameters are derived from a straight normal walking trajectory described in (McFadyen & Prince, 2002) with its corresponding wrench data defined over six DOFs for a walker mass of about 67 kg. The data consists of force and torque measurements that are collected at a sampling rate of 100 Hz, when the user walks on a rigid floor during a single gait cycle, as seen in figure 10.

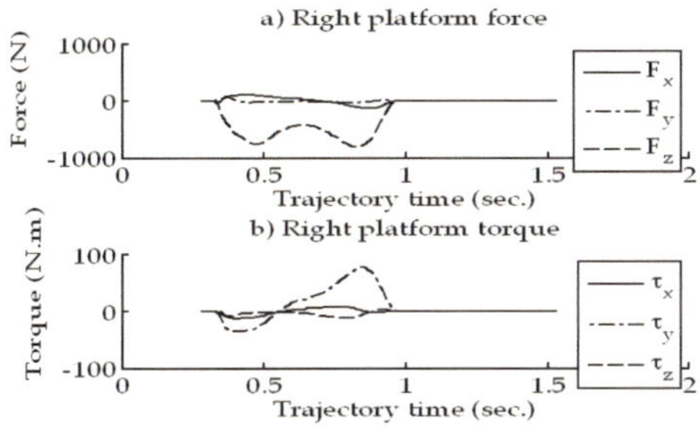

Fig. 12. Cartesian reaction wrench applied on the right haptic foot platform

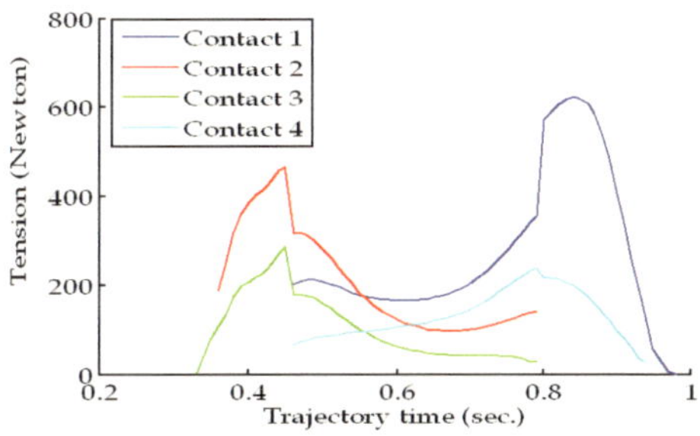

Fig. 13. Normalizes sum of reaction forces $\|\mathbf{\Gamma}_{ri}\|$ at each contact point

The forces generated at each contact point result from the contact points geometry under the virtual foot model and the action wrench, which partly explains why increasing the number of contact points enhances some contact force discontinuities that occasionally occur for a given wrench. Note that this type of discontinuity is expected since the system being optimized in the equation (20) changes its configuration. Figure 13 shows these discontinuities for a right foot trajectory that is subject to (16). Attempts to eliminate these discontinuities *a posteriori* is cumbersome and quite useless since they will be reduced and/or eliminated as the virtual foot model increases in complexity, thereby resulting in a contact distribution that better represents reality.

However, discontinuities in wrench $\mathbf{h}_o$ are still prohibited as they can potentially generate cable tension discontinuities when using the Optimal Tension Distribution (OTD) algorithm in conjunction with the cable tension controllers. When such discontinuities occur, the cable tension controllers cannot follow the computed cable tensions, and the resulting wrench applied on the haptic foot platform can then become unbalanced. Other stability problems are presented in (Joly & Micaelli, 1998).

Note that the presence of only four contact points per virtual foot model is advantageous for visual representation of force distributions, as shown in figure 16, which represents the frames of the video sequence extracted from the HDR and FOP algorithms over one walking gait cycle.

While a reaction force is applied to a haptic foot platform during impedance or admittance control, the action wrench $\mathbf{h}_a$ measured under the foot is employed by the FOP algorithm to compute friction forces at each contact point. The conditions represented by the friction cone are plotted in figure 14, and imply that some contact points slip on the virtual object when the tension forces go below $\cos(\alpha_i)$, thus indicating that a friction force, shown in figure 15, must be added as a reaction force at these points.

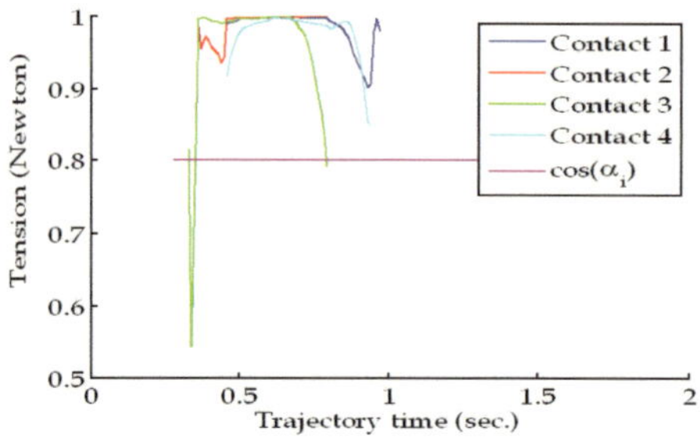

Fig. 14. Friction cone condition

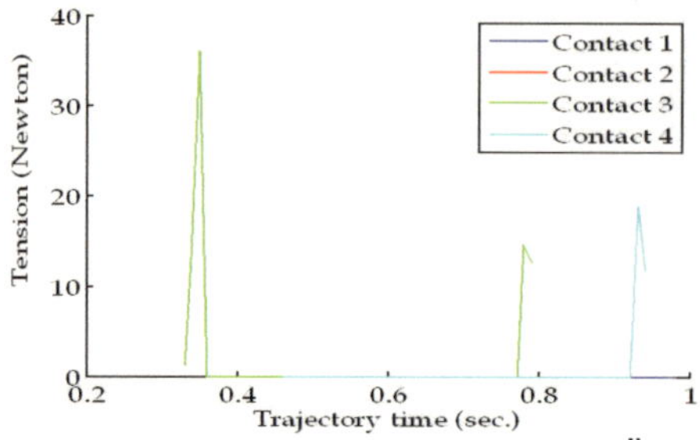

Fig. 15. Norm of the friction force $\|\mathbf{\Gamma}_{fi}\|$ as a part of reaction force

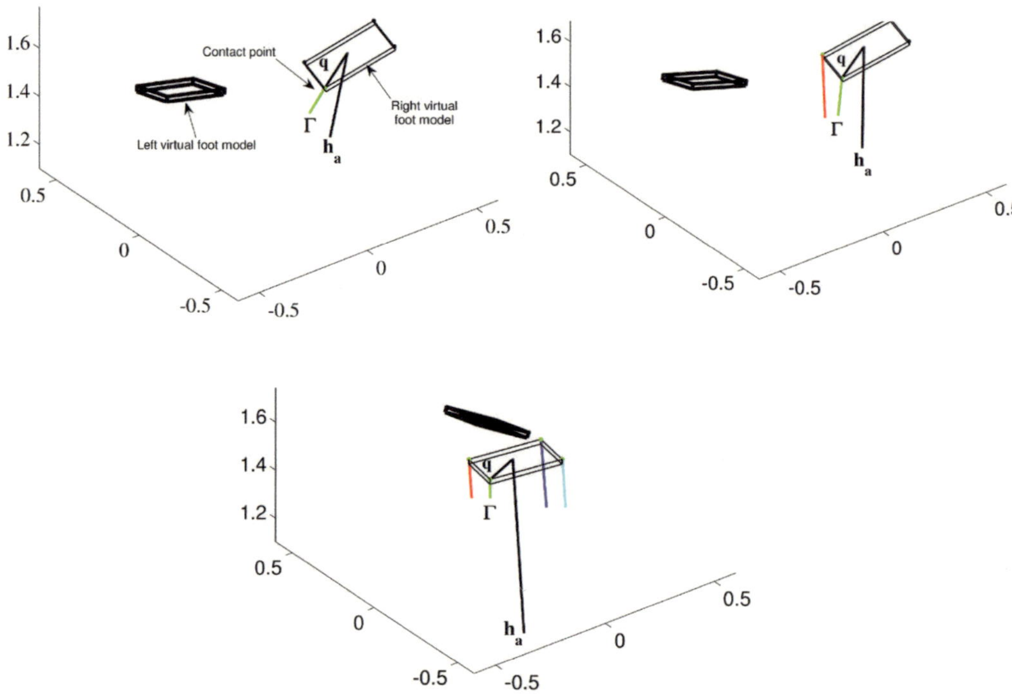

Fig. 16. Sequence of the walking simulation with four contact points

6. High dynamic impacts

The CDLI and the FOP presented in the preceding section were developed to render a haptic force feedback that was meant to stimulate the human kinesthetic sense. This sense is what gives humans the perception of force in their muscles. It is of course highly solicited during normal human gait, namely because of the reaction force that the ground inflicts on the foot which is also felt throughout the leg. There is however another sense that is neglected by this mechanism as well as by many other haptic mechanisms. This other sense is called the tactile sense and it is caused by tiny mechanoreceptors situated in glabrous skin. Some of these receptors are specialized in measuring the strength of deformation of the skin and others are specialized in measuring the changes in deformation of the skin. With this sense, a person is therefore able to feel a material's texture by pressing his or her skin on it's surface and is also able to determine an object's hardness and rigidity upon making contact. The former sensation is not within the scope of the present research and will therefore not be discussed any further. The latter sensation is the one that is most important to this research and it is caused by the transient vibration patterns that occur during a contact (more so during an impact) that are perceivable by these mechanoreceptors within human skin. Since different materials produce different vibration patterns, a person is therefore able differentiate between various materials (Westling and Johanson, 1987). If this sensation could be implemented in the CDLI, a walker could potentially be able to know which material constitutes the virtual floor on which he or she is walking.

The motorized reels presented in (Otis et al. 2009b) that are used in the CDLI were designed mainly to stimulate the human kinesthetic sense. In other words, they were designed to produce a wrench upon the user. These reels, shown in figure 17, are equipped with a transmission and for that reason they are also equipped with a cable tension sensor. In this way, tension control can be achieved via a closed-loop control method.

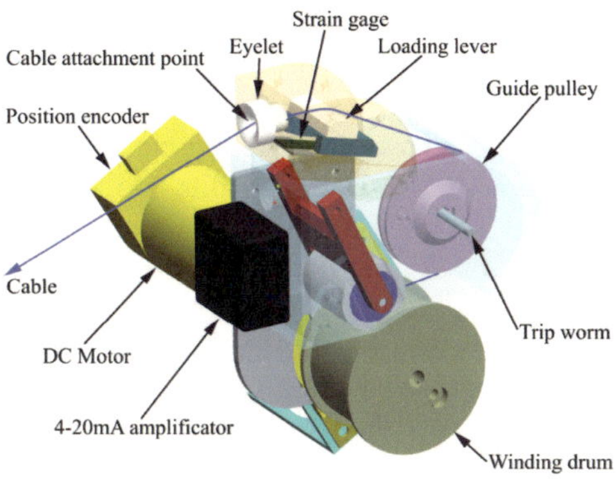

Fig. 17. First reel design

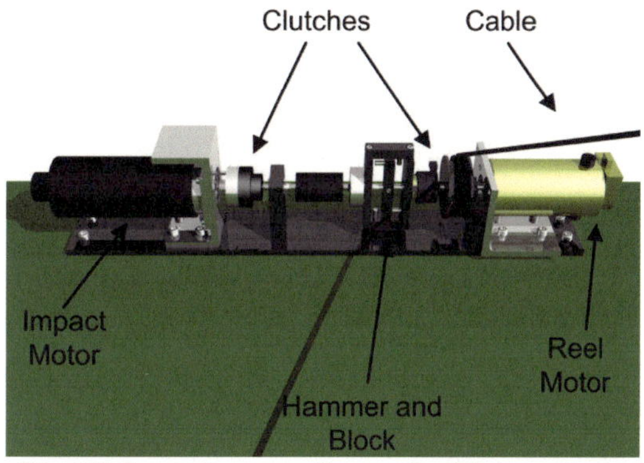

Fig. 18. Impact generating reel with two motors

A potential substitute for the previously mentioned reel is shown in figure 18. It was presented for the first time in (Billette and Gosselin, 2009) as a means of producing rigid contacts in simulations such as sword fighting simulations. It was designed to not only be able to stimulate the user's kinesthetic sense but also his tactile sense. To accomplish the latter with conventional reels would be quite hard given the fact that in order to stimulate the mechanoreceptors, they would need to create vibrations with frequencies much higher than 100 Hz. Evidently, if someone were to try and obtain such vibration frequencies with a standard electrical motor and reel he would be faced with the following conundrum: If he minimizes the mechanism's inertia enough to be able to reach these frequencies, the mechanism will not be strong enough to produce the required torque. The prototype in figure 18 addresses this issue by completely rethinking the contact strategy. Instead of trying to simulate impacts, this reel simply produces them by colliding two metal parts.

It takes just one quick look at the prototype reel to see that there is nothing standard about it. The most important parts are the hammer and the block. These are the actual metal parts that will collide during a contact. Since the block is attached permanently to the reel, it allows the transient vibrations to travel across the cable to the end-effector and the user. The other elements worth noticing are the fact that there are actually two motors instead of one and there are also two clutches added to the system. On the right side, there is the reel motor whose function is to keep tension in the cable at all times. The motor on the left side, called the impact motor, is the motor that will provide the energy for the impacts. The purpose of the two clutches is to control the angular spacing between the hammer and the block. Whenever the mechanism is in "no-contact" mode, the clutches make the two metal parts move together. The hammer is kept at a ready position in a similar manner with which the hammer of a firearm is cocked when ready to fire. In this mode, the impact motor is kept separated from the rest of the reel and the hammer and block assembly turns with the reel motor. When a contact (or impact) is ordered and generated, the clutches change states and this enables the impact motor to grab a hold of the hammer which then becomes free to move with respect to the block. The impact motor moves the hammer with an angular velocity that corresponds to the velocity of the virtual object and the block's movement corresponds to the velocity of the end-effector held by the user. The two metal parts will then collide and generate the required vibrations.

The challenge with the impact generation strategy described above comes from the fact that the vibrations must travel across all of the cables. Parallel cable driven mechanisms have typically small rigidity compared to solid member parallel mechanisms and it is therefore safe to assume that these vibrations will be dampened and that the highest vibrations frequencies generated at the reel may not travel across the cables. However, preliminary tests have shown that although the transient vibration patterns do not resemble those that would have occurred if the end-effector were to strike a real steel object, they do however show a close resemblance to the patterns of a material that can be considered as moderately rigid and hard (delrin). Applied to the CDLI, these reels could potentially give the walker an improved walking sensation by providing a punctuality to the reaction forces that he feels upon setting his foot on the virtual ground. Also, such reaction forces could also increase the haptic rendering for other activities such as striking a movable virtual object with a foot.

7. Conclusion

The haptic mechanism exploits software and hardware architectures that were specifically designed for managing a Cable-Driven Locomotion Interface driven by a haptic rendering engine for real-time applications. The architecture includes hybrid impedance, admittance and inertial-wrench control classes and two physics engines that permits the best haptic display for soft and rigid virtual objects. These components are implemented and generalized following an open-architecture paradigm in order to render a haptic display, and for facilitating physical model implementation.

The core of the control class selection mechanism is a selection matrix that depends on both the contact points geometry and the virtual object physical properties. Such a mechanism selects a particular control scheme for each haptic foot platform DOF, depending on the type of collision and friction conditions. The Force Optimization Problem then only needs to be solved over this spatial geometry, and is constrained by a friction cone which can be computed using non-linear quadratic programming algorithms. However, not only a standard reel design but also the cable-driven mechanism can not support high impact dynamics. Further investigation is needed for controlling vibrations that could occur between two rigid contacts.

8. Future work

The current model for the simulation of soft virtual objects is still under development. The coupling between each contact point is currently being neglected, and equation (12) is only valid for small penetrations and for linear elasticity tensors. It is possible to extend the friction model with more complex algorithms in order to consider nonlinearities like Signorini's law implemented in (Duriez et al., 2006). Haptic synthesis of interaction with novel materials (e.g., soil, sand, water, stone) with non-linear deformation and multimodal (audio and haptic) rendering will need to be developed for increasing realism. Such synthesis needs novel sensor network design for distributed interactive floor surfaces.
Concerning the locomotion interface, a washout filter with force feedback that uses an impedance model will be implemented to continuously drive the user toward the centre of the workspace. As for the haptic display accuracy, it can be increased by analyzing the real force distribution under a human foot.

Acknowledgment

The authors would like to thank CIRRIS (*Centre interdisciplinaire de recherche en réadaptation et intégration sociale*) and Dr. Bradford McFadyen for the gait trajectory data used in the simulation. The authors would also like to acknowledge the financial support of the Natural Sciences and Engineering Research Council (NSERC) through their strategic program.

9. References

Adams, R.J. & Hannaford, B. (1999). Stable haptic interaction with virtual environments. *IEEE Transactions on Robotics and Automation*, Vol. 15, No. 3, June 1999, pp. 465 - 74, ISSN 1042-296X.

Adams, R.J.; Klowden, D. & Hannaford, B. (2000). Stable haptic interaction using the Excalibur force display, *Proceedings of IEEE International Conference on Robotics and Automation*, pp. 770-775, ISBN-10: 0 78035 886 4, San Francisco, CA, USA, April 24-28, 2000, IEEE Robotics and Automation Society, Piscataway, NJ, USA

Baraff., D. (1994). Fast contact force computation for nonpenetrating rigid bodies, *Proceedings of Conference on Computer graphics and interactive techniques (SIGGRAPH)*, pp. 23 - 34, ISBN-10: 0 89791 667 0, Orlando, FL, USA, July 1994, ACM Press, New York, NY, USA

Barrette, G. & Gosselin, C. (2005) Determination of the dynamic workspace of cable-driven planar parallel mechanisms. *Journal of Mechanical Design, Transactions of the ASME*, Vol. 127, No. 2, March 2005, pp. 242 - 248, ISSN 0738-0666.

Bernhardt, M.; Frey, M.; Colombo, G. & Riener, R. (2005). Hybrid force-position control yields cooperative behaviour of the rehabilitation robot lokomat, *Proceedings of IEEE International Conference on Rehabilitation Robotics*, pp. 536 - 539, ISBN-10: 0780390032, Chicago, IL, USA, June-July 2005, IEEE Computer Society, Piscataway, NJ, USA.

Billette, G. & Gosselin, C. (2009). Producing Rigid Contacts in Cable-Driven Haptic Interfaces Using Impact Generating Reels, *Proceedings of International Conference on Robotics and Automation*, pp. 307-312, ISBN-13 9781424427888 , 2009, Kobe, Japan, IEEE, Piscataway, NJ, USA.

Boyd, S. & Wegbreit, B. (2007). Fast computation of optimal contact forces. *IEEE Transactions on Robotics*, Vol. 23, No. 6, December 2007, pp. 1117 – 1132, ISSN 1552-3098.

Carignan, C.; & Cleary, K. (2000). Closed-loop force control for haptic simulation of virtual environments. *Haptics-e*, Vol. 1, No. 2, February 2000, pp. 1 – 14.

Changhyun Cho; Jae-Bok Song & Munsang Kim (2008). Stable haptic display of slowly updated virtual environment with multirate wave transform. *IEEE/ASME Transactions on Mechatronics*, Vol. 13, No. 5, pp. 566 – 575, ISSN 1083-4435.

Cheah, C.C.; Kawamura, S. & Arimoto, S. (2003). Stability of hybrid position and force control for robotic manipulator with kinematics and dynamics uncertainties. *Automatica*, Vol. 39, No. 5, May 2003, pp. 847-855, ISSN 0005-1098.

Cheng, F.-T. & Orin, D. E. (1990). Efficient algorithm for optimal force distribution - the compact-dual lp method. *IEEE Transactions on Robotics and Automation*, Vol. 6, No. 2, April 1990, pp. 178 – 187, ISSN: 1042-296X.

Duchaine, V. & Gosselin, C. (2007). General model of human-robot cooperation using a novel velocity based variable impedance control, *Proceedings of EuroHaptics Conference and Symposium on Haptic Interfaces for Virtual Environment and Teleoperator Systems*, pp. 446–451, ISBN-10 0769527388, Tsukaba, Japan, March 2007, IEEE Computer Society, Los Alamitos, CA, USA.

Duchaine, V. & Gosselin, C. (2009). Safe, Stable and Intuitive Control for Physical Human-Robot Interaction, *Proceedings of International Conference on Robotics and Automation*, pp. 3383-3388, ISBN-13 9781424427888, Kobe, Japan, May 12-17, 2009, IEEE, Piscataway, NJ, USA.

Duriez, C.; Dubois, F.; Kheddar, A. & Andriot, C. (2006). Realistic haptic rendering of interacting deformable objects in virtual environments. *IEEE Transactions on Visualization and Computer Graphics*, Vol. 12, No. 1, January 2006 , pp. 36 – 47, ISSN 1077-2626.

Faulring, E.L.; Lynch, K.M.; Colgate, J.E. & Peshkin, M.A. (2007). Haptic display of constrained dynamic systems via admittance displays. *IEEE Transactions on Robotics*, Vol. 23, No. 1, February 2007, pp. 101-111, ISSN 1552-3098.

Fang , S.; Franitza D.; Torlo M.; Bekes, F. & Hiller, M. (2004). Motion control of a tendon-based parallel manipulator using optimal tension distribution. *IEEE/ASME Transactions on Mechatronics*, Vol. 9, No. 3, September 2004, pp. 561– 568, ISSN 1083-4435.

Goldsmith, P.B.; Francis, B.A.; Goldenberg, A.A. (1999). Stability of hybrid position/force control applied to manipulators with flexible joints. *International Journal of Robotics & Automation*, Vol. 14, No. 4, 1999, pp. 146-160, ISSN 0826-8185.

Grow, David I. & Hollerback, John M. (2006). Harness design and coupling stiffness for two-axis torso haptics, *International Conference on IEEE Virtual Reality*, pp. 83-87, ISBN 1424402263, Alexandria, VA, United states, 25-26 March 2006, Piscataway, NJ, USA.

Hannaford, B. & Ryu, J.-H. (2002). Time-domain passivity control of haptic interfaces. *IEEE Transactions on Robotics and Automation*, Vol. 18, No 1, February 2002, pp. 1-10, ISSN 1042-296X.

Hassan, M. & Khajepour, A. (2007). Optimization of actuator forces in cable-based parallel manipulators using convex analysis. *IEEE Transactions on Robotics*, Vol. 24, No. 3, June 2008, pp. 736 - 740, ISSN 15523098

Iwata, H.; Yano, H. & Nakaizumi, F. (2001). Gait master: a versatile locomotion interface for uneven virtual terrain, *Proceedings of IEEE Virtual Reality*, pp. 131 - 137, ISBN-10 0769509487, Yokohama, Japan, March 2001, IEEE Computer Society, Los Alamitos, CA, USA.

Joly, L. & Micaelli, A. (1998). Hybrid position/force control, velocity projection, and passivity, *Proceedings of Symposium on Robot Control (SYROCO)*, Vol. 1, pp. 325 - 331, ISBN-10 0080430260, Nantes, France, September 1997, Elsevier, Kidlington, UK.

Kawamura, S.; Ida, M; Wada, T. & Wu, J.-L. (1995). Development of a virtual sports machine using a wire drive system-a trial of virtual tennis, *Proceedings of IEEE/RSJ International Conference on Intelligent Robots and Systems, Human Robot Interaction and Cooperative Robots*, Vol. 1, pp. 111 - 116, Pittsburgh, PA, USA, August 1995, IEEE Computer Society, Los Alamitos, CA, USA.

Lauzier, N.; Gosselin, C. (2009). 2 DOF Cartesian Force Limiting Device for Safe Physical Human-Robot Interaction, *Proceedings of International Conference on Robotics and Automation*, pp. 253-258, ISBN-13 9781424427888, Kobe, Japon, 12-17 May 2009, IEEE, Piscataway, NJ, USA.

Lu , X.; Song, A. (2008). Stable haptic rendering with detailed energy-compensating control. Computers & Graphics, Vol. 32, No. 5, October 2008, pp. 561-567, ISSN 0097-8493.

McFadyen, B. J. & Prince, F. (2002). Avoidance and accomodation of surface height changes by healty, community-dwelling, young, and elderly men. *Journal of Gerontology: Biological sciences*, Vol. 57A, No. 4, April 2002, pp. B166–B174, ISSN 1079-5006.

McJunkin, S.T.; O'Malley, M.K. & Speich, J.E. (2005). Transparency of a Phantom premium haptic interface for active and passive human interaction, *Proceedings of the American Control Conference*, pp. 3060 - 3065, ISBN-10 0 7803 9098 9, Portland, OR, USA, 8-10 June, 2005, IEEE, Piscataway, NJ, USA.

Melder, N. & Harwin, W. (2004). Extending the friction cone algorithm for arbitrary polygon based haptic objects, *Proceedings of International Symposium on Haptic Interfaces for Virtual Environment and Teleoperator Systems (HAPTICS)*, pp. 234 - 241, ISBN-10 0769521126, Chicago, IL, United States, March 2004, IEEE Computer Society, Los Alamitos, CA, USA.

Mitra, P. & Niemeyer, G. (2005). Dynamic proxy objects in haptic simulations, *Proceedings of Conference on Robotics, Automation and Mechatronics*, Vol. 2, pp. 1054 - 1059, ISBN-10 0780386450, Singapore, IEEE, Piscataway, NJ, USA.

Morizono, T.; Kurahashi, K. & Kawamura, S. (1997). Realization of a virtual sports training system with parallel wire mechanism, *Proceedings of IEEE International Conference on Robotics and Automation*, Vol. 4, pp. 3025 - 3030, ISBN-10 0780336127, Albuquerque, NM, USA, April 1997, IEEE Robotic and Automation Society, New York, NY, USA.

Onuki, K.; Yano, H.; Saitou, H. & Iwata, H. (2007). Gait rehabilitation with a movable locomotion interface. *Transactions of the Society of Instrument and Control Engineers*, Vol. 43, No. 3, 2007, pp. 189 - 196, ISSN 0453-4654.

Otis, M. J.-D.; Perreault, S.; Nguyen-Dang, T.-L.; Lambert, P.; Gouttefarde, M.; Laurendeau, D.; Gosselin, C. (2009a). Determination and Management of Cable Interferences Between Two 6-DOF Foot Platforms in a Cable-Driven Locomotion Interface. *IEEE Transactions on Systems, Man and Cybernetics, Part A: Systems and Humans*, Vol. 39, No. 3, May 2009, pp. 528-544, ISSN 1083-4427.

Otis, M. J.-D.; Nguyen-Dang, T.-L.; Laliberte, Thierry; Ouellet, Denis; Laurendeau, D.; Gosselin, C. (2009b). Cable Tension Control and Analysis of Reel Transparency for 6-DOF Haptic Foot Platform on a Cable-Driven Locomotion Interface. *International Journal of Electrical, Computer, and Systems Engineering*, Vol. 3, No. 1, May 2009, pp. 16-29, ISSN 2070-3813.

Ottaviano, E.; Castelli, G.; Cannella, G. (2008). A cable-based system for aiding elderly people in sit-to-stand transfer. *Mechanics Based Design of Structures and Machines*, Vol. 36, No. 4, October 2008, pp. 310 - 329, ISSN 1539-7734.

Perreault, S. & Gosselin, C. (2008). Cable-driven parallel mechanisms: application to a locomotion interface. *Journal of Mechanical Design, Transactions of the ASME*, Vol. 130, No. 10, October 2008, pp. 102301-1-8, ISSN 0738-0666.

Ramanathan, R. & Metaxas, D. (2000). Dynamic deformable models for enhanced haptic rendering in virtual environments, *Proceedings of Virtual Reality Annual International Symposium*, pp. 31 - 35, ISBN-10 0769504787, New Brunswick, NJ, USA, March 2000, IEEE Computer Society, Los Alamitos, CA, USA.

Reilly, R., Amirinia, M. & Soames, R. (1991). A two-dimensional imaging walkway for gait analysis, *Proceedings of Computer-Based Medical Systems Symposium*, pp. 145 - 52, ISBN-10 0818621648, Baltimore, MD, USA, May 1991, IEEE Computer Society, Los Alamitos, CA, USA.

Ruspini, D. & Khatib, O. (2000). A framework for multi-contact multi-body dynamic simulation and haptic display, *Proceedings of International Conference on Intelligent Robots and Systems*, Vol. 2, pp. 1322 - 1327, ISBN-10 0780363485, Takamatsu, Japon, November 2000, IEEE, Piscataway, NJ, USA.

Sakr, N.; Jilin, Z.; Georganas, N.D; Jiying Z. & Petriu, E.M. (2009). Robust perception-based data reduction and transmission in telehaptic systems, *Proceedings of World Haptics Conference*, pp. 214-219, ISBN-13 9781424438587, Salt Lake City, UT, USA, March 2009, IEEE, Piscataway, NJ, USA.

Schmidt, H.; Hesse, S. & Bernhardt, R. (2005). Hapticwalker - a novel haptic foot device. *ACM Transaction on Applied Perception*, Vol. 2, No. 2., April 2005, pp. 166 - 180, ISSN 1544-3558.

SenseGraphics. H3D Open Source Haptics. http://www.h3dapi.org/.

Smith, R. ODE, Open Dynamics Engine. http://www.ode.org/.

Tsumugiwa, T.; Yokogawa, R. & Hara, K. (2002). Variable impedance control with virtual stiffness for human-robot cooperative peg-in-hole task, *Proceedings of IEEE International Conference on Intelligent Robots and Systems*, Vol. 2, pp. 1075 - 1081, ISBN-10 0780373987, Lausanne, Switzerland, September 2002, IEEE Robotics & Automation Society, Piscataway, NJ, USA.

van der Linde, R.Q. & Lammertse, P. (2003). HapticMaster - a generic force controlled robot for human interaction. *Industrial Robot*, Vol. 30, No. 6, 2003, pp. 515-524, ISSN 0143-991X

Westling, G. & Johansson, R. S. (1987). Responses in glabrous skin mechanoreceptors during precision grip in humans. *Experimental Brain Research,* Vol. 66, No. 1, 1987, pp. 128-140, ISSN 0014-4819.

Yoon, J. & Ryu, J. (2004). Continuous walking over various terrains - a walking control algorithm for a 12-dof locomotion interface, *Proceedings of International Conference Knowledge-Based Intelligent Information and Engineering Systems,* Vol. 1, pp. 210 - 217, ISBN-10 3540233180, Wellington, New Zealand, September 2004, Springer-Verlag, Berlin, Germany.

Yoon, J. & Ryu, J. (2006). A novel locomotion interface with two 6-dof parallel manipulators that allows human walking on various virtual terrains. *International Journal of Robotics Research,* Vol. 25, No. 7, July 2006, pp. 689 - 708, ISSN 02783649.

Yoon, J. & Ryu, J. (2009). A Planar Symmetric Walking Cancellation Algorithm for a Foot–Platform Locomotion Interface. *International Journal of Robotics Research, in press,* 19 May 2009, pp. 1 - 21.

Stability Boundary and Transparency for Haptic Rendering

Iñaki Díaz and Jorge Juan Gil
CEIT and TECNUN, University of Navarra
Spain

Thomas Hulin
Institute of Robotics and Mechatronics, German Aerospace Center (DLR)
Germany

1. Introduction

Over the past years haptic interfaces have been successfully integrated into a wide range of fields such as engineering (Borro et al., 2004) or surgery (Basdogan et al., 2004). Haptic devices allow users to interact with a certain environment, either remote or virtual, by the sense of touch. In these applications—unlike in conventional robotic systems—the user shares workspace with the device. Therefore, an unstable behaviour can damage the device, or even worse, harm the operator. Thus, stability must be guaranteed to ensure user safety and achieve high haptic performance. Unfortunately, preserving haptic stability usually implies reducing the range of dynamic impedances achievable by the system. Hence, rigid virtual objects cannot be perceived as stiff as real ones, and the overall haptic performance and transparency perception are considerably degraded.

Developing stable controllers able to exhibit a wide dynamic range of impedances is a persistent challenge in the field of haptics. This chapter describes main research carried out by the authors on stability issues for haptic rendering, as well as on the development of transparent haptic controllers.

In a haptic system, the stability boundary for haptic rendering depends on many factors, such as inherent interface dynamics, motor saturation, sensor resolution or time delay. Section 2 introduces the state-of-the-art on stability studies showing the influence of many of these phenomena. Beyond related work, Section 3 analyses the influence of viscous damping and delay on the stability boundary for haptic rendering. Although the shape of the stability boundaries found is quite complex, a linear condition which summarises the relation between virtual stiffness, viscous damping and delay is proposed.

Section 4 analyses the influence of the first vibration mode of the system on the stability boundary. The majority of haptic models used to analyse stability do not consider the existence of internal vibration modes. However, it will be shown that for certain interfaces vibration modes must be taken into account to correctly obtain the range of impedances achievable by the system.

Ensuring stability is of major concern in haptic interaction; however, preserving stability does not imply improving haptic transparency. A transparent haptic interface should be able to emulate any environment, from free-space to infinitely stiff obstacles without perceiving the dynamics of the haptic device. The stability boundary for haptic rendering is known to be independent of the mass of the device; yet, high inertia of haptic interfaces degrades both system usability and transparency. To cover this issue, Section 5 shows control algorithms that improve transparency on high-inertia haptic interfaces without compromising overall system stability. Finally, conclusions and future directions are drawn in Section 5.

2. Related Work

The authors of (Minsky et al., 1990) were the first to study the stability of haptic systems. They used the continuous model of a 1 DOF (degree-of-freedom) haptic device colliding against a virtual wall shown in Fig. 1. The interface has a mass m and a physical damping b. The user exerts a force F_u causing the displacement X_h of the device. An elastic model with stiffness K is used to compute the interaction force of the virtual environment.

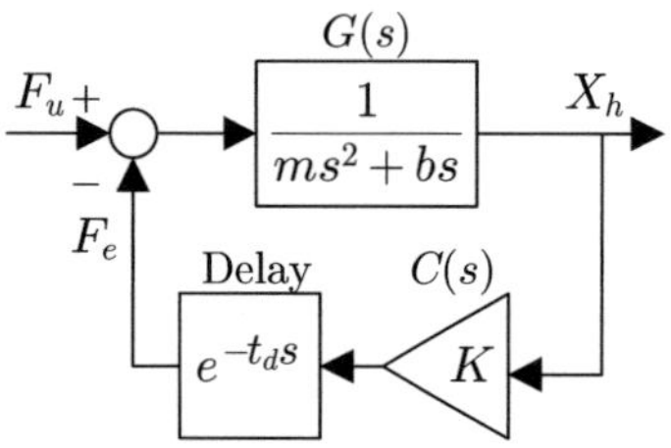

Fig. 1. Continuous haptic model.

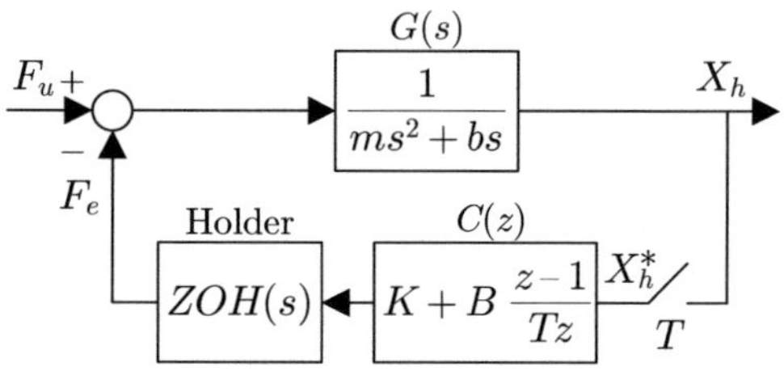

Fig. 2. Discrete haptic model.

In their study, system instabilities were attributed to the time delay introduced by the holder. To analyse its effect, but maintaining the continuous model, they included a time delay of one sampling period T to the actuation of the virtual environment. In this model, if the function of the delay is approximated by a second-order Taylor series expansion, it can be demonstrated that the system is stable if it satisfies the following condition:

$$b > KT \tag{1}$$

After this result, Minsky demonstrates experimentally that introducing in the model the user's mass m_h, damping b_h and stiffness k_h parameters, as well as a virtual damping B, the stability condition that must be guaranteed is:

$$B + b + b_h > \frac{(K + k_h)T}{2} \tag{2}$$

In this expression, the proportional factor $\frac{1}{2}$ is found from experimental results on the real system, but with no theoretical foundation. Later works (Brown & Colgate, 1994) show experimental results that obtain the stability boundary for haptic rendering as a function of many parameters of the device. Those results match the work carried out by Minsky.

From the control point of view, a haptic system is a sampled-data controlled mechatronic device. Unlike previous works, (Gil et al., 2004) analyse theoretically stability over a discrete haptic system (Fig. 2). $ZOH(s)$ represents the zero-order holder and the backwards difference is used to estimate velocity. The authors obtain the same stability condition (2) found by

previous works. Results of their work also show that this approximation is only valid for low values of virtual damping B. However, in most cases it is sufficient since common actuators used in haptic devices do not allow implementing large values of K and B.
The haptic models presented until now have not taken into account many parameters, such as user dynamics, friction, sensor quantization or time delays, that may have influence on stability. Regarding the user, (Gil et al., 2004), (Hulin, Preusche & Hirzinger, 2008) and (Diolaiti et al., 2006) show that the user only contributes positively to stability. Therefore, a haptic model without the user can be considered as the "worst-case scenario".
Fig. 3 shows the model of a haptic device colliding against a virtual wall with time delay t_d. This time delay can be the sum of several effects: computations, communications, etc. The model has also Coulomb friction c, and considers position sensor resolution q.

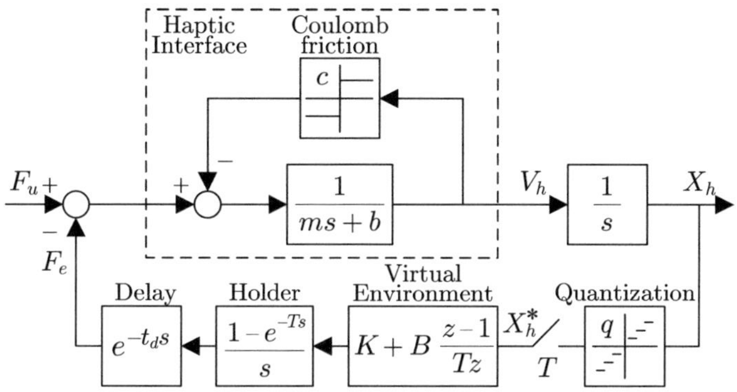

Fig. 3. Model of a haptic system with non-linear effects.

In (Diolaiti et al., 2006) and (Abbott & Okamura, 2005), it was found that Coulomb friction can dissipate the energy introduced by the quantization. Therefore, in some way both factors cancel each other and could be not considered for the stability analysis. Regarding the influence of the time delay, it will be covered in the following section.
Another way to guarantee the stability of the system is ensuring its passivity (Adams & Hannaford, 1999). The passivity condition for the system without time delay proposed by (Colgate & Schenkel, 1997) is

$$b > \frac{KT}{2} + B. \tag{3}$$

Notice that in (3) the virtual damping term does not contribute to obtain larger values of stiffness as in (2), but the opposite. Therefore, the passivity condition is considered a more restrictive condition than stability.
In later works, (Hannaford & Ryu, 2002) and (Ryu et al., 2005) have managed to adjust the passivity region using the "passivity controller". It consist of a variable virtual damping that dissipates the energy generated by the haptic interface. However, the model is still conservative compared to stability conditions.

3. Obtaining the Stability Boundary for Haptic Rendering

This section analyses the influence of viscous damping and delay on the stability boundary for haptic rendering. Assuming that Coulomb friction can dissipate the amount of energy introduced by quantization, and that the user only contributes positively to make the system more stable, Fig. 4 shows a simplified haptic model that can be considered as the "worst-case scenario".

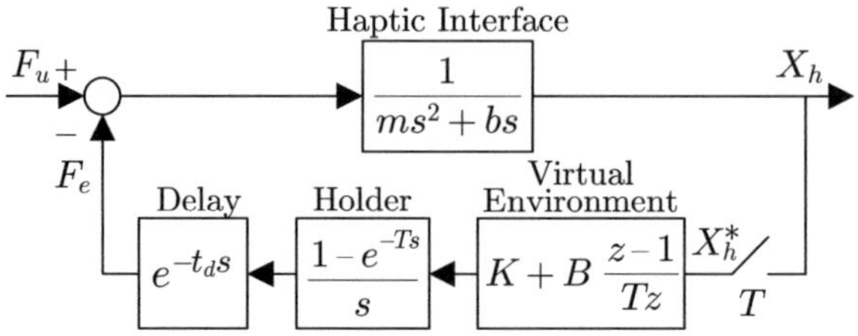

Fig. 4. Linear simplified model of a haptic system.

Following (Hulin et al., 2006), the dimensionless parameters that will be used in this section are shown in Table 1. Although some authors (Diolaiti et al., 2006) have used the virtual stiffness to normalise the parameters, here it will be used the mass (or the inertia for rotary joints), because this way the values of the device do not change with the contact force law.

Parameter	Variable	Dimensionless variable
Sampling period	T	-
Mass	m	-
Physical damping	b	$\delta = \frac{bT}{m}$
Virtual stiffness	K	$\alpha = \frac{KT^2}{m}$
Virtual damping	B	$\beta = \frac{BT}{m}$
Delay	t_d	$d = \frac{t_d}{T}$

Table 1. Dimensionless parameters.

Both real and dimensionless parameters can theoretically take any value ($m > 0, b > 0, T > 0$ and $t_d \geq 0$). However, typical sampling rates in haptics are quite fast ($\geq$ 1 kHz) and the relation between the physical damping and the mass cannot be supposed to be arbitrarily large. For example, some experimentally acquired values given in (Diolaiti et al., 2006) show that $\frac{b}{m} \ll 1\ \text{s}^{-1}$ for all investigated haptic devices. Therefore, the dimensionless physical damping δ is quite small in haptic systems. In this study it will be supposed that $\delta < 10^{-3}$. Classical control tools have been applied to the linear system in order to obtain the stability conditions. In (Gil et al., 2004), it was stated that, with no delay, $d = 0$, the stability condition of the linear system (using the dimensionless parameters of Table 1) is

$$\alpha < \delta(\delta + \beta) \frac{(1-\epsilon)(\beta\epsilon + \beta\delta\epsilon - \beta + \delta^2)}{(1-\epsilon-\delta\epsilon)(\beta\epsilon + \beta\delta - \beta + \delta^2)}, \tag{4}$$

where ϵ is a dimensionless number,

$$\epsilon = e^{-\frac{bT}{m}} = e^{-\delta}. \tag{5}$$

Stability condition (4) is consistent with (Gillespie & Cutkosky, 1996). Substituting ϵ by its Taylor approximation,

$$\epsilon = 1 - \delta + \frac{1}{2}\delta^2 - \frac{1}{6}\delta^3 + O(\delta^4), \tag{6}$$

makes it possible to linearise (4) around the origin and to obtain the following more compact stability condition:

$$\alpha < 2(\delta + \beta). \tag{7}$$

The fact that the dimensionless physical damping δ is a very small number enforces the validity of this approximation. Further experimental studies confirm the result that increasing both the physical viscous damping—i.e. electrically (Mehling et al., 2005), (Tognetti & Book, 2006) or magnetically (Gosline et al., 2006)—and the virtual damping (Colgate & Brown, 1994), (Janabi-Sharifi et al., 2000) allows for larger stable stiffness coefficients.
If the system contains a delay of one sampling period, $d = 1$, the stability condition that has been proposed in (Bonneton & Hayward, 1994) using the Padé approximation is

$$\alpha < \frac{2}{3}(\delta + \beta). \tag{8}$$

3.1 Stability Condition

In this section, a stability condition for the linear system including the effect of both delay and virtual damping is proposed. This stability condition may be seen as generalisation of previous conditions (7) and (8) for any delay, consistent with the study of the non-linear system (Diolaiti et al., 2006) but including the effect of the virtual damping β:

$$\alpha < \frac{2}{1+2d}(\delta + \beta). \tag{9}$$

Using the physical values of the parameters the proposed stability condition is

$$K < \frac{b+B}{\frac{T}{2} + t_d}, \tag{10}$$

and taking into account that the effect of the sampling and hold in the control loop can be approximated by a delay of half the sampling period $\frac{T}{2}$, the stability condition proposed (10) can be interpreted with the following statement:

$$\text{Critical stiffness} = \frac{\sum \text{Damping}}{\sum \text{Delay}}. \tag{11}$$

The critical stiffness of a haptic system is equal to the overall damping of the mentioned system divided by the total delay of the loop. Therefore, a double viscous damping in the system—physical plus virtual—will allow for a double stiffness; while a double delay in the haptic loop—no matter its nature—will half the maximum stable stiffness.
The validity of this formula will be checked by two different ways: 1) solving numerically the characteristic equation and performing a graphical approach, 2) with experimental results. The reader is addressed to (Gil, Sánchez, Hulin, Preusche & Hirzinger, 2009) for a complete theoretical analysis.

3.2 Graphical Analysis

The methodology followed in (Gil et al., 2004) can be used to receive the analytical stability condition from the characteristic equation of the system. In the Z-domain, this equation consists of a polynomial if the delay t_d is a multiple of the sampling period T (then d takes natural values):

$$\delta^2(z-\epsilon)(z-1)z^{d+1} - (1-\epsilon-\delta)(\alpha+\beta)z^2 \\ + [(1-\epsilon-\delta\epsilon)(\alpha+\beta) + (1-\epsilon-\delta)\beta]\,z \\ -(1-\epsilon-\delta\epsilon)\beta = 0. \qquad (12)$$

The validity of (9) is checked using the graphs of the stability boundaries. Two different ways have been used to obtain and depict the critical stiffness of the linear system with delay. The first one follows (Gil et al., 2004) and directly obtains the critical stiffness for different values of the virtual damping evaluating

$$\alpha < \mathrm{Gm}\left[\frac{1}{\frac{z^d(z-1)(z-\epsilon)\delta^2}{(\epsilon-1+\delta)z+1-\epsilon-\delta\epsilon}+\beta\frac{z-1}{z}}\right], \qquad (13)$$

where Gm[.] means gain margin of the Z-transfer function. The second method, used in (Hulin et al., 2006) and (Salcudean & Vlaar, 1997), numerically solves the poles of the characteristic equation (12) and finds the stiffness coefficients which place all the poles just within the unit circle. Although both methods obtain the same results, the gain margin can be computed easily in Matlab® if the delay is a multiple of the sampling period T, while the other method allows for introducing fractional numbers for the delay. Fig. 5 shows the stability boundaries for different delays d, setting $\delta < 10^{-3}$.

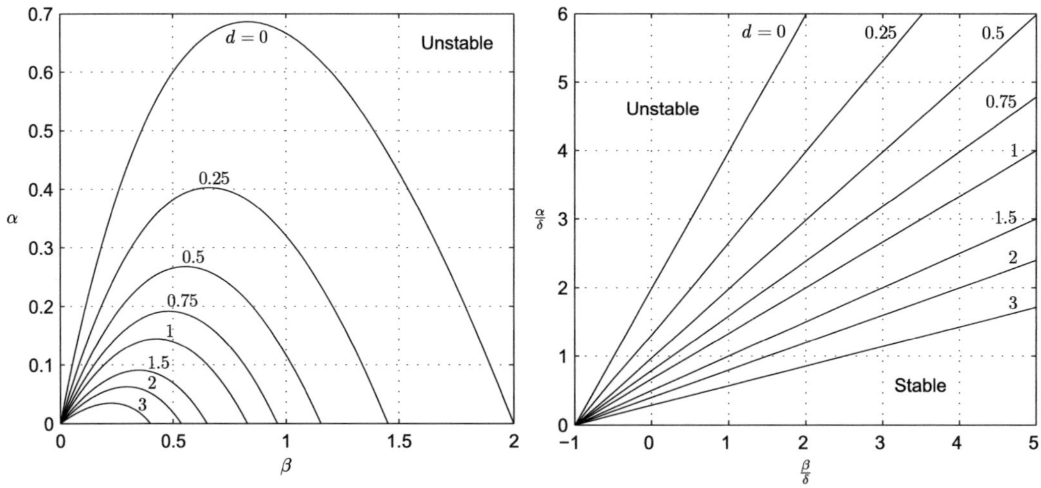

Fig. 5. Stability boundaries for small dimensionless physical damping ($\delta < 10^{-3}$) and delays $d = [0, 0.25, 0.5, 0.75, 1, 1.5, 2, 3]$ (left) and zoom near the point of origin (right).

The shown boundaries in Fig. 5 (right) fit perfectly the linearised stability condition (9). The initial slope of the stability boundaries becomes smaller with the delay. Therefore, the critical stiffness without virtual damping $\beta = 0$ decreases also with the delay. This means that, using the physical parameters, the critical stiffness depends on both the physical damping and the delay.

3.3 Experimental Results

Two different haptic interfaces have been used to perform experiments: the DLR Light-Weight Robot III (Hirzinger et al., 2002) and the LHIfAM (Savall et al., 2004). A bilateral virtual wall consisting of a virtual spring and damper was implemented using one joint of each interface. Limit-stable parameter values were obtained when sustained oscillations were observed increasing the stiffness. No user was involved in the experiments.

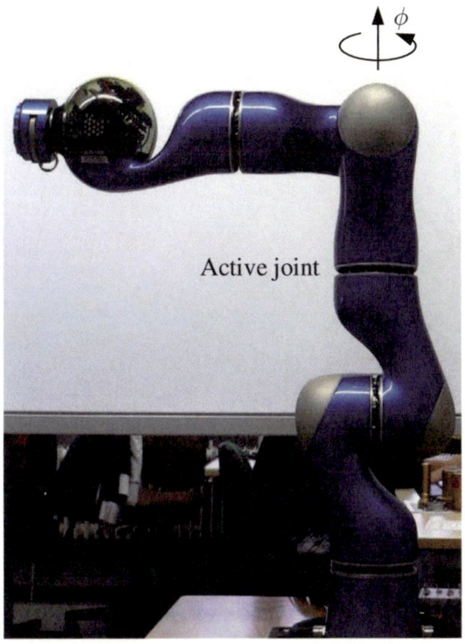

Fig. 6. Third generation of the DLR Light-Weight Robot arm.

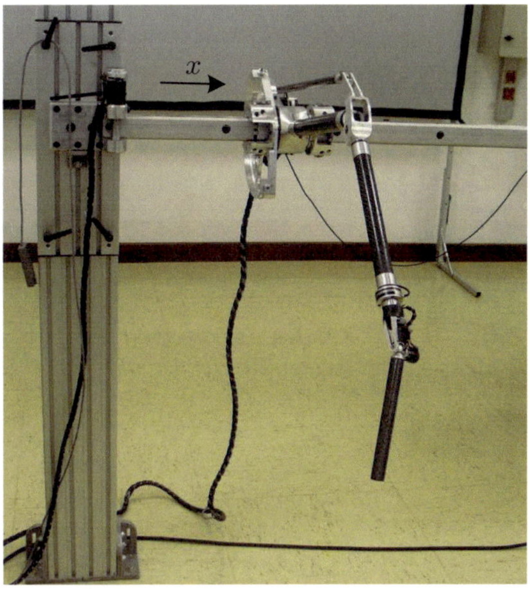

Fig. 7. LHIfAM haptic interface.

3.3.1 DLR Light-Weight Robot

The DLR Light-Weight Robot III (Fig. 6) is a 7 DOF robot arm with carbon fiber grid structure links. Though it weighs only 14 kg, it is able to handle payloads of 14 kg throughout the whole dynamic range. The electronics, including the power converters, is integrated into the robot arm. Every joint has an internal controller which compensates gravity and Coulomb friction. Since high-resolution position sensors are used to measure link orientation (quantization $q \approx$ 20"), non-linear effects can be neglected.

The virtual wall was implemented in the third axis of the robot, indicated by the rotating angle ϕ in Fig. 6. The environment was implemented using a computer connected to the robot via Ethernet. The sampling rate was 1 kHz and the overall loop contained a delay of 5 ms. Fig. 8 shows the experimental results, introducing several fixed values for the virtual damping. A set of experiments was performed with only the system delay of 5 ms, while additional delays were artificially introduced into the loop to obtain an overall delay of 6 and 10 ms. The theoretical behaviour is depicted with dashed lines. The experimental stability boundaries fit the linear condition remarkably well.

A significantly long delay was also introduced into the system in order to obtain a curved stability boundary. Fig. 9 shows the experimental stability boundary for an overall delay of 55 ms. The beginning of the stability boundary for a delay of 10 ms is also shown in the same figure. The theoretical stability curve has been computed using the device's inertia in the configuration selected for the experiments: 0.8 kg·m^2.

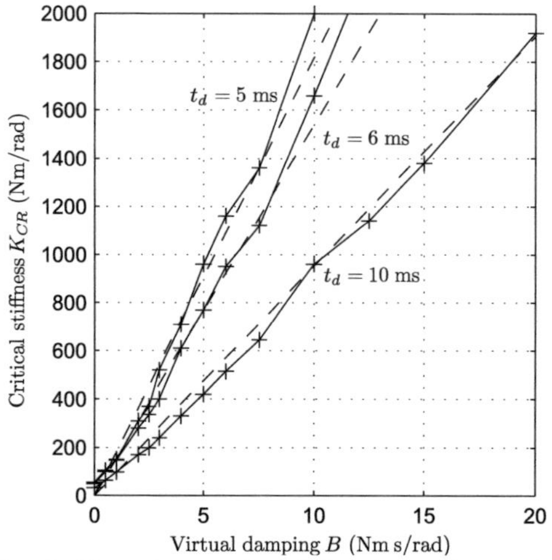

Fig. 8. Experimental stability boundaries for a delay t_d of 5, 6 and 10 ms (pluses and solid) and theoretical boundaries (dashed).

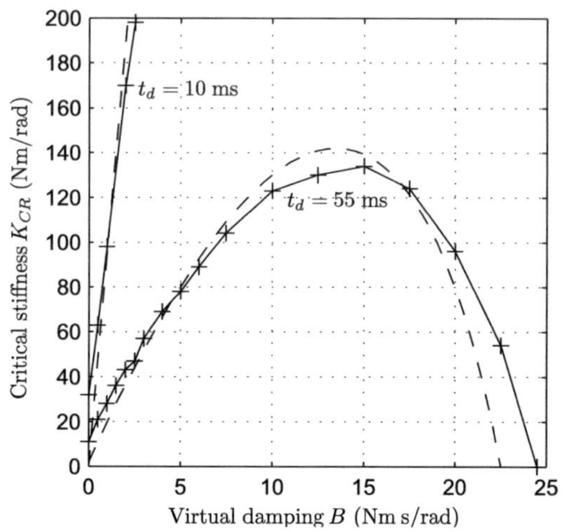

Fig. 9. Experimental stability boundaries for a delay t_d of 10 and 55 ms (pluses and solid) and theoretical boundaries (dashed).

3.3.2 LHIfAM

The LHIfAM (Fig. 7) is a haptic interface with a large workspace developed at CEIT. The mechanism consists of a counterbalanced parallelogram moving on a linear guide 1.5 m in length. The virtual wall was implemented in the direction of the translational movement of the guide (x axis in Fig. 7). In this direction, both the inertia of the device and the sensor resolution are quite high: 5.4 kg and quantization $q \approx 3.14$ μm, respectively. The Coulomb friction is compensated by the controller.

The controller can acquire the information from the sensor, compute the force of the virtual wall and command the motor within the same sampling period, that is, theoretically without delay in the loop. Therefore, significant stiffness coefficients can be implemented with stable behaviour. However, the motor is saturated with few millimeters of penetration in the virtual wall. In order not to saturate the actuator in the overall critical oscillation, artificial delays of 3, 6 and 12 ms have been introduced into the control loop.

Fig. 10 shows the experimental stability boundaries. It can be seen that experimental results match the stability condition proposed in (10). The theoretical stability boundaries have been computed using a physical damping of 4.6 Ns/m. Although the physical damping is quite high, since the sampling period was 1 ms, the dimensionless damping of the LHIfAM in the direction of x was $\delta = 0.85 \times 10^{-3}$ and therefore still within the $\delta < 10^{-3}$ range.

3.4 Valid Range of the Linear Condition

The shape of the stability boundary can be divided into two different parts. The first one follows the linear condition (10) for relatively small values of virtual damping (Fig. 8). The second one is a curve (Fig. 9) which can be obtained graphically or experimentally.

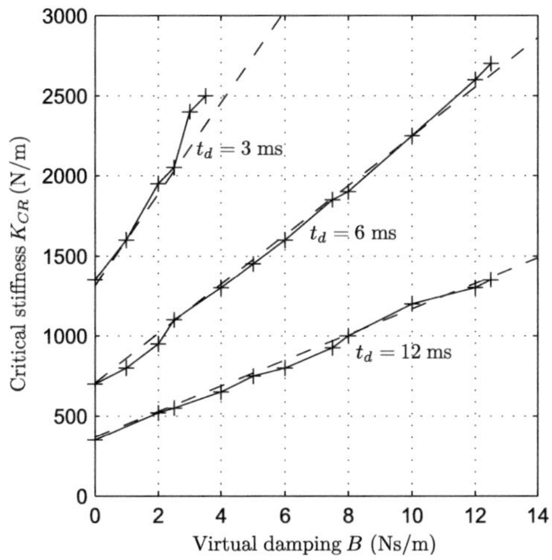

Fig. 10. Experimental stability boundaries for the LHIfAM and a delay t_d of 3, 6 and 12 ms (pluses and solid) and theoretical stability boundaries for a physical damping b of 4.6 Ns/m (dashed) and same delays.

Regarding the delay, several factors, such as computation of the collision detection algorithms for complex virtual environments, digital to analog conversion, and amplifier dynamics, introduce a certain delay in the haptic system that is usually equal to or less than one sampling period. Therefore the linear condition is appropriate for haptic devices. In other kinds of systems, which usually involve longer delays, the linear stability condition should no be used. For example, it is quite common to suppose a delay equal to hundreds of milliseconds in teleoperated systems.

4. Beyond Rigid Haptic Models: Influence of Internal Vibration Modes on Stability

The mathematical model used to analyse stability in previous section does not take into account the existence of internal vibration modes. This section presents a theoretical approach that studies the influence of internal vibration modes on the stability of haptic rendering (Díaz & Gil, 2008). In particular, it addresses the influence of the first resonant mode of cable transmission used in haptic devices. This type of mechanical transmission is widely used in haptic devices because it offers a number of advantages such as low friction, no backlash and low weight (Townsend, 1988).

4.1 Model Description

Fig. 11(a) illustrates the simplified model of a haptic device used in previous section to analyse the stability of haptic systems. It has a mass m and a viscous damping b, and the model assumes that the mechanical device is perfectly rigid. Although the force exerted by the motor F_r and the net force exerted by the user F_u are introduced in different places, a single transfer function is defined for this model, which is

$$G(s) = \frac{X}{F_r + F_u} = \frac{1}{ms^2 + bs}. \tag{14}$$

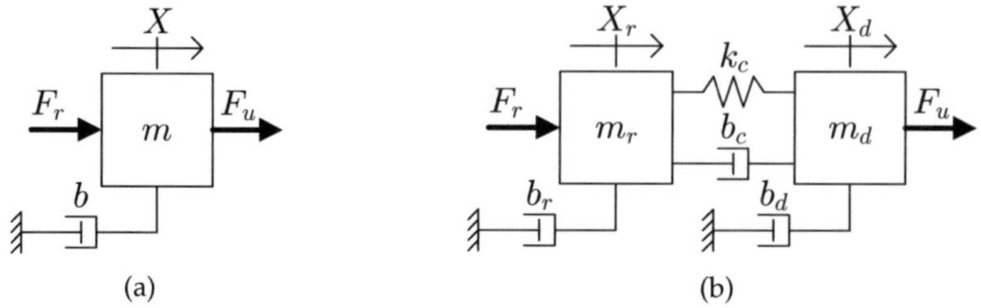

Fig. 11. Mechanical schematic of a perfectly rigid haptic device (a), and a haptic device with a single vibration mode (b).

Fig. 11(b) shows a haptic system with a single vibration mode. In this model, the device is divided into two masses connected by a link: mass m_r, pushed by the force of the motor, and mass m_d, pushed by the user. The dynamic properties of the link are characterised by a spring and a damper (k_c and b_c). This model is a two-input/two-output system, and the relationship between output positions and input forces is

$$\mathbf{x} = \begin{bmatrix} X_d \\ X_r \end{bmatrix} = \begin{bmatrix} G_d(s) & G_c(s) \\ G_c(s) & G_r(s) \end{bmatrix} \begin{bmatrix} F_u \\ F_r \end{bmatrix} = \frac{1}{p(s)} \begin{bmatrix} p_r(s) & k_c + b_c s \\ k_c + b_c s & p_d(s) \end{bmatrix} \begin{bmatrix} F_u \\ F_r \end{bmatrix} = \mathbf{Gf}, \tag{15}$$

where,

$$p_r(s) = m_r s^2 + (b_r + b_c)s + k_c, \tag{16}$$

$$p_d(s) = m_d s^2 + (b_d + b_c)s + k_c, \tag{17}$$

$$p(s) = p_r(s) p_d(s) - (k_c + b_c s)^2. \tag{18}$$

Introducing an impedance interaction with the virtual environment, the device can be analysed as a single-input/single-output system, as illustrated in Fig. 12. $C(z)$ is the force model of the virtual contact (which usually includes a spring and a damper), $H(s)$ is the zero-order-holder, T is the sampling period, and t_d represents the delay in the loop. The sampled position of the motor is given by

$$X_r^* = \frac{Z[G_c(s)F_h(s)]}{1 + C(z)Z[H(s)G_r(s)e^{-t_d s}]}. \tag{19}$$

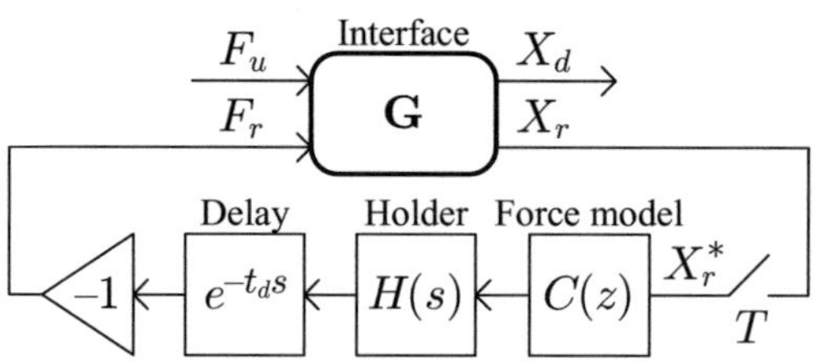

Fig. 12. Haptic system with impedance interaction.

If the force model only has a virtual spring with stiffness K, stability of the system depends on the following characteristic equation:

$$1 + KZ[H(s)G_r(s)e^{-t_d s}] = 0, \tag{20}$$

and the critical stiffness is

$$K_{CR} = \mathrm{Gm}\{Z[H(s)G_r(s)e^{-t_d s}]\}, \tag{21}$$

where Gm{.} means gain margin of the transfer function within brackets. From (21), it follows that $G_r(s)$ is the relevant transfer function for the stability of the system.

4.2 Model Parameters Identification

The physical parameters for $G_r(s)$ have been experimentally identified for two haptic interfaces, PHANToM 1.0 and LHIfAM. Since these interfaces are significantly different in terms of workspace and overall physical properties, the influence of the vibration modes may differ from one to another. Both devices are controlled by a dSPACE DS1104 board that reads encoder information, processes the control loop and outputs torque commands to the motor at 1 kHz.

A system identification method based on frequency response has been used to determine $G_r(s)$. This strategy has already been successfully used to develop a model of a cable transmission (Kuchenbecker & Niemeyer, 2005). The method yields an empirical transfer function estimate (ETFE), or experimental Bode plot (Ljung, 1999), by taking the ratio of the discrete Fourier transform (DFT) of the system's output response signal to the DFT of the input signal applied. A white noise signal is commonly used as input signal (Weir et al., 2008). Model parameters are identified by fitting the ETFE to the theoretical transfer function with six independent variables by performing an automatic iterative curve fitting using least-squares method.

The first rotating axis of a PHANToM 1.0 haptic interface has been used for the experiments (angle ϕ in Fig. 13). Only the motor that actuates this axis is active. A white noise torque signal is applied and the output rotation is measured. The experiment is performed without any user grasping the handle of the device.

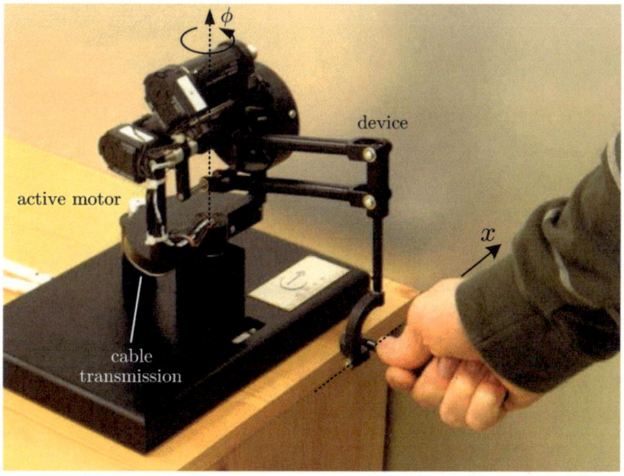

Fig. 13. PHANToM 1.0 haptic interface.

The frequency response of the system is presented in Fig. 14. It can be seen that the first vibration mode of the interface takes place at 62.5 Hz, which may correspond to the one detected in (Çavuşoğlu et al., 2002) at 60 Hz. The parameters obtained for $G_r(s)$ are presented in Table 2. These parameters have been identified with respect to the ϕ-axis.

Parameter	Variable	PHANToM	LHIfAM
Device mass	m	1.05 gm^2	5.4 kg
Device damping	b	0.0085 Nms/rad	3.5 Ns/m
Motor mass	m_r	0.895 gm^2	0.3 kg
Motor damping	b_r	0.0085 Nms/rad	0.1 Ns/m
Cable damping	b_c	0.0057 Nms/rad	15 Ns/m
Cable stiffness	k_c	18.13 Nm/rad	79.5 kN/m
Body mass	m_d	0.155 gm^2	5.10 kg
Body damping	b_d	0 Nms/rad	3.4 Ns/m

Table 2. Physical parameters of the PHANToM and the LHIfAM.

The equivalent translational parameters at the tip of the handle[1] (along the x-axis in Fig. 13) can be calculated by dividing the rotational parameters by $(12\ \text{cm})^2$. The linear inertia results as $m = 72.92$ g, which is consistent with the manufacturer specifications: $m < 75$ g; and the linear damping as $b = 0.59$ Ns/m.

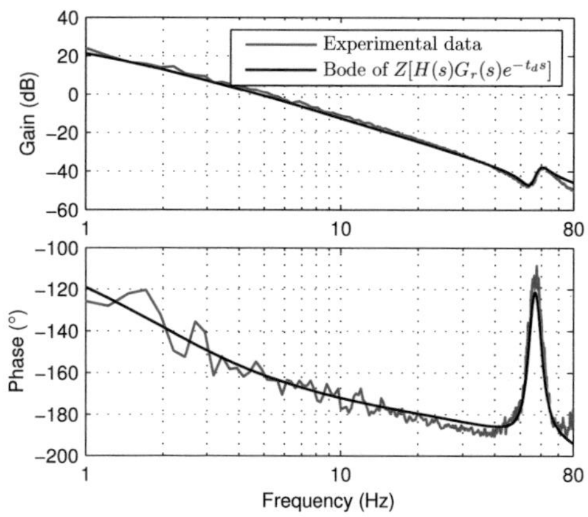

Fig. 14. Experimental (blue line) and theoretical (black line) Bode diagrams for the PHANToM.

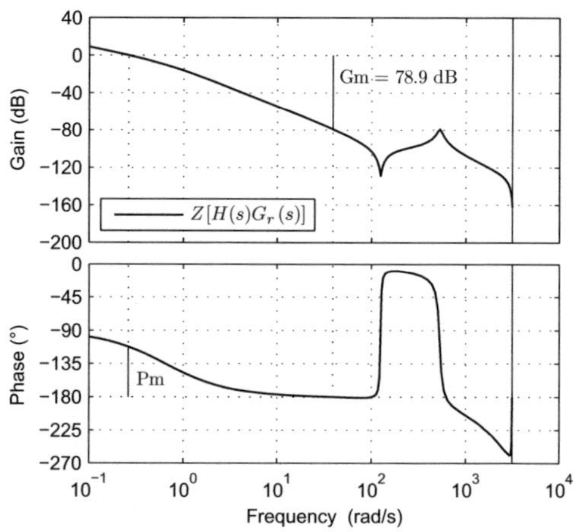

Fig. 15. Bode diagram and margins of $Z[H(s)G_r(s)]$ calculated for the LHIfAM.

Regarding the LHIfAM haptic interface, its translational movement along the guide has been used as a second testbed (Fig. 7). The cable transmission is driven by a commercial Maxon RE40 DC motor. Table 2 summarises the physical parameters obtained, and Fig. 15 shows the shape of $G_r(s)$ and the gain margin of the system.

4.3 Influence of the Vibration Mode

With the physical parameters obtained for both devices, $G_r(s)$ is known and the critical stiffness can be found by evaluating (21). If we compare those results with the linear condition (10) obtained in Section 3, the influence of the vibration mode on the critical stiffness, if any, can be found. Table 3 shows these theoretical gain margins for both devices.

[1] Placing the tip of the handle at the middle of the workspace is approximately at 12 cm from the joint axis.

Device	Model	Gm (dB)
PHANToM	Rigid	24.6
	Non rigid	22.41
LHIfAM	Rigid	76.9
	Non rigid	78.9

Table 3. Gain margins of PHANToM and LHIfAM.

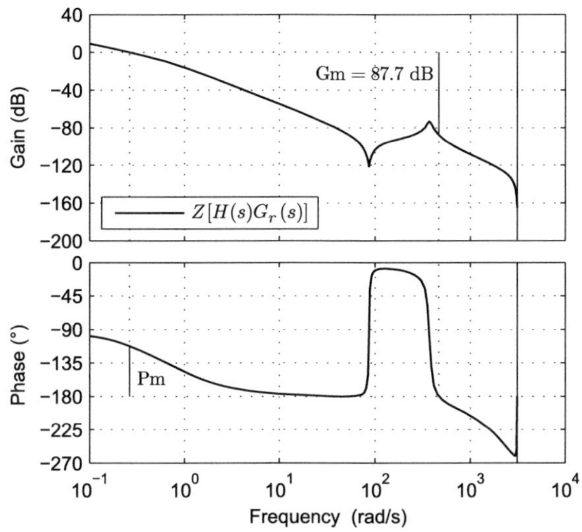

Fig. 16. Bode diagram and margins of $Z[H(s)G_r(s)]$ calculated for the LHIfAM after reducing cable pretension.

Gain margins obtained with the rigid haptic model are very similar to those obtained with a haptic model that takes into account the first vibration mode of the device. Therefore, it seems that the vibration mode does not affect stability. However, analysing Fig. 15, it can be seen that for the LHIfAM the resonant peak of the vibration mode could easily have imposed the stability margin. Therefore, further studies have been carried out on the LHIfAM to analyse the possible influence of the vibration mode. For that purpose, the initial pretension of the LHIfAM's cable transmission has been decreased. This affects directly the cable's dynamic parameters, thus the vibration mode. New parameters are: $k_c = 38$ kN/m and $b_c = 11$ Ns/m. Fig. 16 shows the Bode diagram of $Z[H(s)G_r(s)]$ for the new cable transmission setup. In this case, the first resonant mode of the cable does impose the gain margin of the system. Notice that the new gain margin is larger than the one of the original system, but placed at a higher frequency. Although it may not seem evident in Fig. 16, there is only one phase crossover frequency at 411.23 rad/s in the Bode diagram.

A possible criterion to estimate whether the resonant peak influences on the critical stiffness is to measure the distance Q from the resonant peak to 0 dB. This distance is approximately

$$Q \approx m_r z_n \omega_n, \tag{22}$$

where,

$$z_n = \frac{b_r + b_c}{m_r} + \frac{b_d + b_c}{m_d} - \frac{b_r + b_d}{m_r + m_d}, \tag{23}$$

$$w_n = \sqrt{\frac{k_c(m_r + m_d)}{m_d m_r}}. \tag{24}$$

Distance Q should be compared with the critical stiffness obtained using the criterion presented in (10), which gives a gain margin similar to the one shown in Fig. 15. If Q is similar or larger than that value, then the vibration mode should be taken into account in the stability analysis. Using the parameters of the LHIfAM, Q is approximately 78.16 dB (with original cable setup).

4.4 Experimental Results

Theoretical results of the influence of the vibration mode on the gain margin of the LHIfAM have been validated experimentally. Experiments have been performed after reducing cable pretension, therefore the gain margin obtained should be placed on the resonant peak of the vibration mode.

An interesting approach is to experimentally seek out—by tuning a controllable parameter in the same system—several critical stiffness values K_{CR}: some that are influenced by the resonant frequency and others that are not. This can be achieved by introducing an elastic force model with different time delays t_d:

$$C(z) = Kz^{-\frac{t_d}{T}}. \tag{25}$$

This way, the characteristic equation becomes

$$1 + Kz^{-\frac{t_d}{T}} Z[H(s)G_r(s)] = 0, \tag{26}$$

and the critical stiffness is

$$K_{CR} = \text{Gm}\{z^{-\frac{t_d}{T}} Z[H(s)G_r(s)]\} = \text{Gm}\{Z[H(s)G_r(s)e^{-t_d s}]\}. \tag{27}$$

Without any delay in the system, the gain margin should be imposed by the resonant peak of the vibration mode. Introducing certain time delay within the loop the gain margin should move to the linear region of the Bode where the slope is -40 dB/decade (as it is schematically shown in Fig. 17).

The critical virtual stiffness of the device has been calculated by means of the relay experiment described in (Barbé et al., 2006; Gil et al., 2004; Åström & Hägglund, 1995), with and without time delay. In this experiment a relay feedback—an on-off controller—makes the system oscillate around a reference position. In steady state, the input force is a square wave, the output position is similar to a sinusoidal wave, both in counterphase. These two signals in opposite phase are shown in Fig. 18.

It can be demonstrated (Åström & Hägglund, 1995) that the ultimate frequency is the oscillation frequency of both signals, and the critical gain is the quotient of the amplitudes of the first harmonic of the square wave and the output position. Since we are relating force exerted on the interface and position, this critical gain is precisely the maximum achievable virtual stiffness for stability.

Nine trials with varying delays in the input force (from 0 to 8 ms) were performed. Each one of these trials was repeated four times in order to have consistent data for further analysis. In each experiment, input-output data values were measured for more than 15 seconds (in steady state). Oscillation frequencies were found by determining the maximum peak of the average power spectral density of both signals. Gain margins were obtained by evaluating

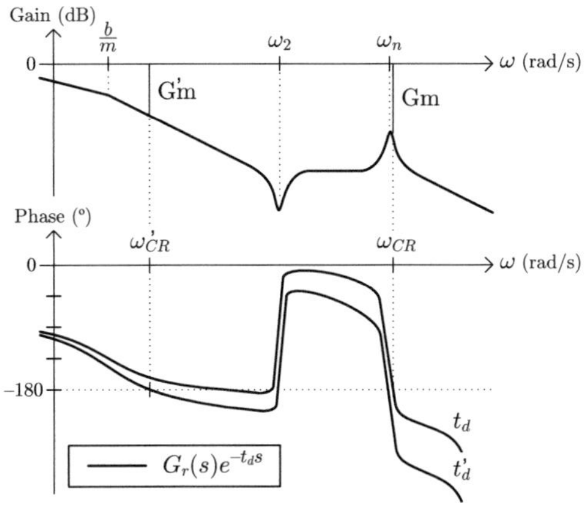

Fig. 17. Scheme of the Bode diagram of $G_r(s)e^{-t_d s}$ for two different time delays ($t_d < t'_d$).

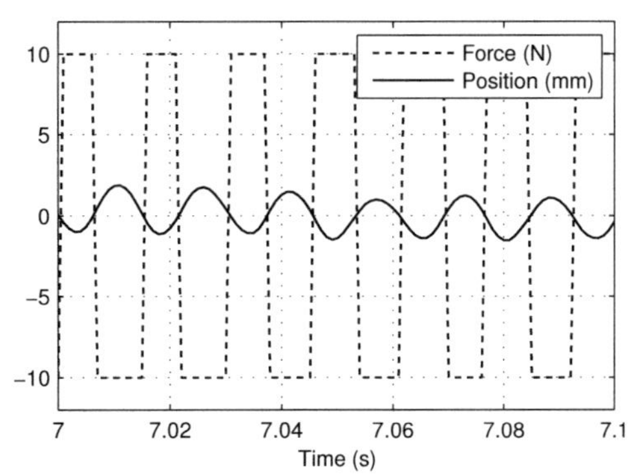

Fig. 18. Force input and position output of a relay experiment for time delay $t_d = 0$.

t_d (ms)	ω_{CR} (Hz)	Gm (dB)	t_d (ms)	ω_{CR} (Hz)	Gm (dB)	t_d (ms)	ω_{CR} (Hz)	Gm (dB)
0	64.9414	80.3149	3	4.3945	73.5975	6	3.1738	66.8281
0	64.4531	79.9414	3	4.3945	73.8443	6	3.1738	66.7219
1	60.0586	76.2336	4	4.3945	73.5919	7	2.6855	64.1268
1	59.0820	75.3235	4	4.3945	73.6444	7	2.8076	64.6013
2	4.8828	76.1063	5	4.5166	73.9604	8	2.3193	61.3209
2	4.8828	76.4240	5	4.3945	73.3171	8	2.3193	61.4755

Table 4. Critical oscillations of the LHIfAM.

the estimated empirical transfer function at that frequency. Table 4 presents these oscillation frequencies and gain margins.

Fig. 19 shows that results of Table 4 and the Bode diagram of $Z[H(s)G_r(s)]$ calculated for the LHIfAM match properly. Notice that the resonant peak of the vibration mode determines the stability of the system only for short delays.

Critical gain margins shown in Table 4 for the undelayed system should be similar to the gain margin obtained theoretically in Fig. 16. However, they differ more than 7 dB. A possible reason could be that most practical systems experience some amplifier and computational delay in addition to the effective delay of the zero-order holder (Diolaiti et al., 2006). This inherit delay has been estimated using the Bode diagram of Fig. 16, and is approximately 250 μs.

To sum up, the analysis carried out on this section shows that the first resonant mode of the haptic device can affect the stability boundary for haptic interfaces in certain cases. Therefore, the designer of haptic controllers should be aware of this phenomena to correctly display the maximum stiffness without compromising system stability.

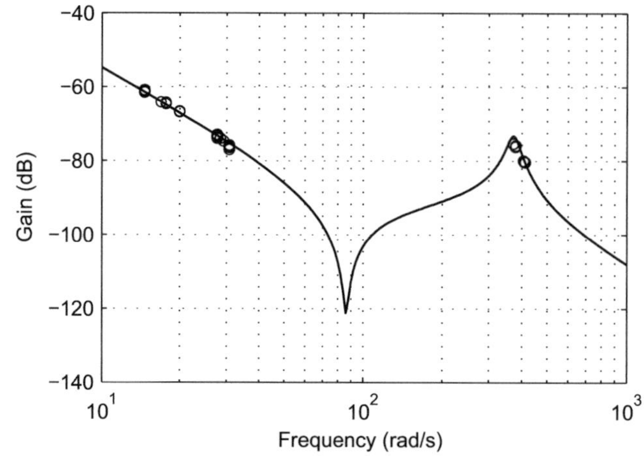

Fig. 19. Experimental gain margins obtained for several time delays by the relay experiment (circles), and the Bode diagram of $Z[H(s)G_r(s)]$ calculated for the LHIfAM (line).

5. Improving Transparency for Haptic Rendering

The need to decrease the inertia of an impedance haptic interface arises when a mechanism with large workspace is used. This occurs with the LHIfAM haptic device, which was designed to perform accessibility and maintenance analyses by using virtual reality techniques (Borro et al., 2004). One important objective of the mechanical design was to incorporate a large workspace while maintaining low inertia—one of the most important goals needed to achieve the required transparency in haptic systems. The first condition was met by using a linear guide (Savall et al., 2008). However, the main challenge in obtaining a large workspace using a translational joints is the high level of inertia sensed by the user. If no additional actions are taken, the operator tires quickly; therefore a strategy to decrease this inertia is needed.

A simple strategy used to decrease the perceived inertia is to measure the force exerted by the operator and exert an additional force in the same direction of the user. This type of feed-forward force loop, described in (Carignan & Cleary, 2000) and (Frisoli et al., 2004), has been successfully used in (Bernstein et al., 2005) to reduce the friction of the Haptic Interface at The University of Colorado. In (Ueberle & Buss, 2002), this strategy was used to compensate gravity and reduce the friction of the prototype of ViSHaRD6. It has also been used in (Hashtrudi-Zaad & Salcudean, 1999) for a teleoperation system. In (Hulin, Sagardia, Artigas, Schätzle, Kremer & Preusche, 2008), different feed-forward gains for the translational and rotational DOF are applied on the DLR Light-Weight Robot as haptic device.

To decrease the inertia of the haptic interface, the force exerted by the operator is measured and amplified to help in the movement of the device (Fig. 20). The operator's force F_u is measured and amplified K_f times. Notice that F_h is the real force that the operator exerts, but owing to the dynamics of operator's arm, $Z_h(s)$, a reaction force is subtracted from this force. It is demonstrated (28) that the operator feels no modification of his/her own impedance, while both the perceived inertia and damping of the haptic interface are decreased by $1 + K_f$.

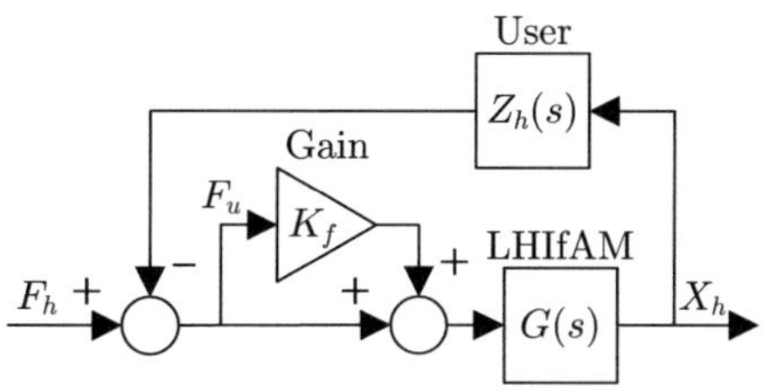

Fig. 20. Continuous model of the system in free movement.

The higher the gain K_f, the lower interface impedance is felt.

$$\frac{X_h(s)}{F_h(s)} = \frac{1}{\frac{m}{1+K_f}s^2 + \frac{b}{1+K_f}s + Z_h(s)} \tag{28}$$

A number of experiments have been performed demonstrating how this strategy significantly decreases the inertia felt. User's force F_h and position X_h have been measured in free movement with the motors turned off, and setting K_f equal to 2. Since inertia relates force with acceleration, abrupt forces and sudden accelerations have been exerted at several frequencies to obtain useful information in the Bode diagrams. The diagrams in Fig. 21 were obtained by using Matlab command *tfe* to the measured forces and displacements. This command computes the transfer function by averaging estimations for several time windows.

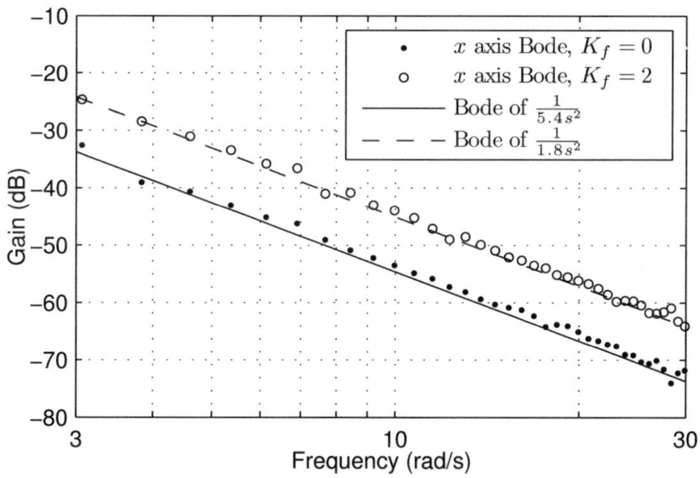

Fig. 21. Experimental gain Bode diagram of $\frac{X_h(s)}{F_h(s)}$ with $K_f = 0$ (dots) and $K_f = 2$ (circles); and theoretical gain Bode diagram of a mass of 5.4 kg (solid) and 1.8 kg (dashed).

As it could be expected, the gain Bode diagram of $\frac{X_h(s)}{F_h(s)}$ increases approximately 9.54 dB and the inertia felt is three times smaller. It can be also seen that, although it is not noticeable by the user, the force sensor introduces noise in the system. Its effect and other factors compromising the stability of the system will be studied in the following sections. The reader can found further details in (Gil, Rubio & Savall, 2009).

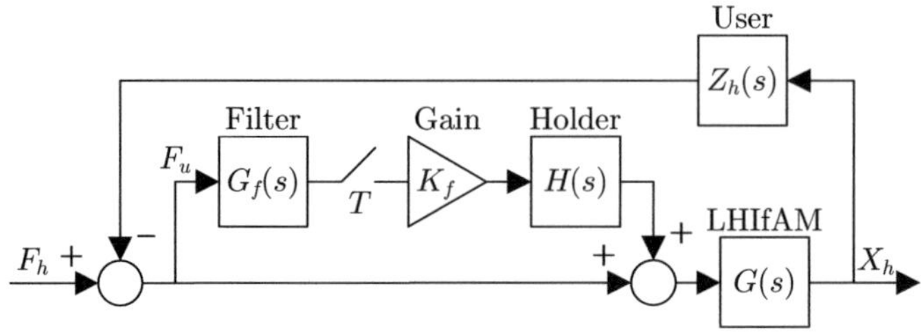

Fig. 22. Sampled model of the system in free movement.

5.1 Discrete Time Model

The sampling process limits the stability of the force gain K_f. A more rigorous model of the system, Fig. 22, is used to analyse stability and pinpoint the maximum allowable value of the force gain—and hence the maximum perceived decrease in inertia. This model introduces the sampling of the force signal, with a sampling period T, a previous anti-aliasing filter $G_f(s)$, and a zero-order holder $H(s)$. The characteristic equation of this model is

$$1 + K_f Z\left[H(s)\frac{G(s)Z_h(s)}{1+G(s)Z_h(s)}G_f(s)\right] = 1 + K_f G_1(z) = 0. \tag{29}$$

To obtain reasonable values for K_f, a realistic human model is needed. The one proposed by (Yokokohji & Yoshikawa, 1994) will be used in this case, because in this model the operator grasps the device in a similar manner. The dynamics of the operator (30) is represented as a spring-damper-mass system where m_h, b_h and k_h denote mass, viscous and stiffness coefficients of the operator respectively. Regarding the filter, the force sensor used in the LHIfAM (SI-40-2 Mini40, ATI Industrial Automation), incorporates a first order low-pass filter at 200 Hz (31). The control board of the system (dSPACE DS1104) runs at 1 kHz.

$$Z_h(s) = m_h s^2 + b_h s + k_h = 2s^2 + 2s + 10 \tag{30}$$

$$G_f(s) = \frac{1}{1+T_f s} = \frac{1}{1+0.005s} \tag{31}$$

Using these expressions, the critical force gain for the LHIfAM is

$$K_{fCR} = \mathrm{Gm}\{G_1(z)\} = 37.12. \tag{32}$$

This means that the inertia could be theoretically reduced from 5.4 kg up to 0.14 kg. However, phase crossover frequency coincides with the Nyquist frequency (see Fig. 23). At this frequency, as shown in previous section, vibration modes of the interface—which were not modelled in $G(s)$—play an important role in stability.

Possible time delays in the feedforward loop will reduce the critical force gain value because phase crossover will take place at a lower frequency. In case of relatively large delays, the worst value of the critical force gain is approximately

$$K^W_{fCR} = 1 + \frac{m}{m_h}, \tag{33}$$

where "W" denotes "worst case". This worst value has been defined within the wide range of frequencies in which the influence of inertia is dominant and the gain diagram is nearly constant (see Fig. 23). According to (33), several statements hold true:

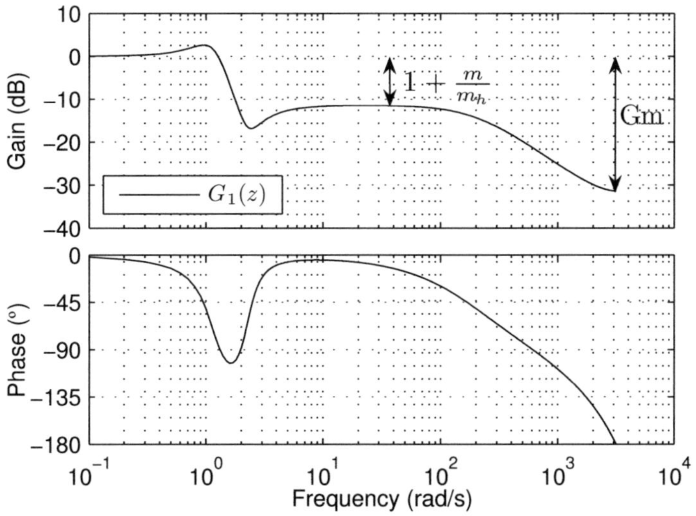

Fig. 23. Bode diagram of $G_1(z)$ using the estimated transfer function of the LHIfAM, the antialiasing filter (31) and the human model proposed by (Yokokohji & Yoshikawa, 1994). The gain is $1 + \frac{m}{m_h}$ (in dB) for a wide range of frequencies.

- The larger the human mass m_h which is involved in the system, the lower the critical force gain K_{fCR} will be. This equivalent human mass will be similar to the mass of the finger, the hand or the arm, depending on how the operator grasps the interface.
- Even in the worst-case scenario—assigning an infinite mass to the operator or a very low mass to the device—the force gain K_f can be set to one, and hence, the inertia can be halved.

The first statement is consistent with a common empirical observation, (Carignan & Cleary, 2000), (Gillespie & Cutkosky, 1996): the haptic system can be either stable or unstable, depending on how the user grasps the interface.

5.2 Inclusion of Digital Filtering

According to (Carignan & Cleary, 2000) and (Eppinger & Seering, 1987), since the force sensor of the LHIfAM is placed at the end-effector, the unmodelled modes of the mechanism introduce appreciable high-frequency noise in its measurements. Therefore, the inclusion of a digital filter in the force feedforward loop is required. Fig. 24 shows the block diagram with the digital filter, whose transfer function is $D(z)$.
The new theoretical critical force gain of the system,

$$K_{fCR} = \text{Gm}\{D(z)G_1(z)\}, \tag{34}$$

can be higher than (33). However, the phase crossover frequency will be placed at a higher frequency, where unmodelled dynamics introduces new poles and zeros that may drive the system into instability. Therefore, a more complete model of the system $G(s)$ including these vibration modes should be used in (34).
Nevertheless, it is not necessary to find a complex model of the system to tune the cut-off frequency of the digital filter. There are two boundaries for this frequency: a lower boundary

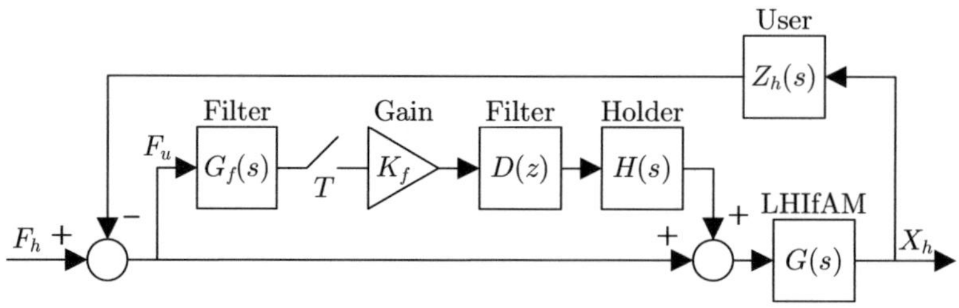

Fig. 24. Final force feedforward strategy with digital filter.

imposed by the bandwidth of human force and an upper one derived by the first vibration mode of the mechanism. Regarding the lower boundary, since the power spectrum of the human hand achieves about 10 Hz (Lawrence et al., 1996), the cut-off frequency should be above this value. Otherwise, the operator feels that the system is unable to track her/his "force commands". On the other hand, the first vibration mode of the interface mechanism should be considered as the upper boundary. Previous section has shown that a significant resonant peak appears around 82 Hz in the LHIfAM (Fig. 15). These facts motivate the inclusion of a second-order Butterworth digital filter at 30 Hz for this interface. And the final force gain K_f implemented in the system is equal to 5. With this value the apparent inertia of the device in the x direction is 0.9 kg, which matches the inertia in the other translational directions so the inertia tensor becomes almost spherical for this gain. In Fig. 25, the frequency response along the controlled x axis is compared with the y axis.

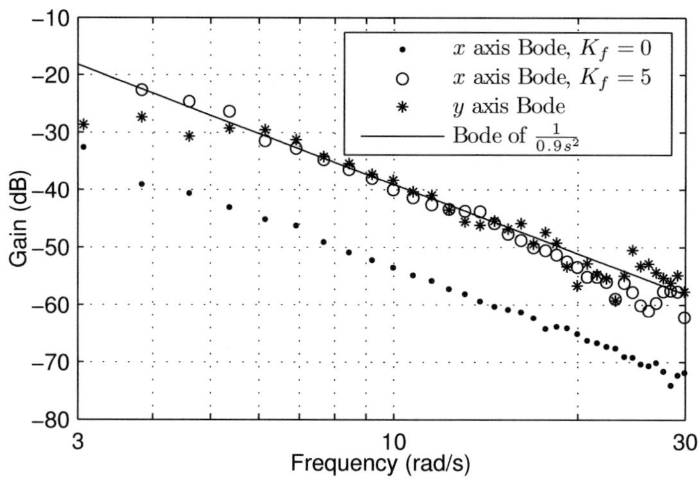

Fig. 25. Experimental gain Bode diagrams of the LHIfAM along y axis (stars), and along x axis with $K_f = 0$ (dots) and $K_f = 5$ (circles).

6. Conclusion and Future Directions

This chapter has started by analysing the influence of viscous damping and delay on the stability of haptic systems. Although analytical expressions of the stability boundaries are quite complex, a linear condition relating stiffness, damping and time delay has been proposed and validated with experiments.

Since the analyses presented in this chapter assume the linearity of the system, its results can only be taken as an approximation if non-linear phenomena (e.g. Coulomb friction and sensor resolution) are not negligible. Another limit is the required low bandwidth of the system compared to the sampling rate, which may be violated, e.g. if the haptic device collides with a real environment.

Beyond the rigid haptic model, the influence of internal vibration modes on the stability has also been studied. Haptic models commonly used to analyse stability rarely take into account this phenomenon. This work shows that the resonant mode of cable transmissions used in haptic interfaces can affect the stability boundary for haptic rendering. A criterion that estimates when this fact occurs is presented, and experiments have been carried out to support the theoretical conclusions.

Finally, a force feedforward scheme has been proposed to decrease the perceived inertia of a haptic device, thereby improving system transparency. The force feedforward strategy has been successfully applied to the LHIfAM haptic device, showing its direct applicability to a real device and its effectiveness in making LHIfAM's inertia tensor almost spherical.

In terms of future research, the investigation of nonlinear effects on stability is necessary to be carried out. Also the robustness against uncertainties of physical parameters and external disturbances has to be examined.

The authors hope that the research included in this chapter will provide a better understanding of the many phenomena that challenge the development of haptic controllers able to display a wide dynamic range of impedances while preserving stability and transparency, and thereby improve the performance of present and future designs.

7. References

Abbott, J. J. & Okamura, A. M. (2005). Effects of position quantization and sampling rate on virtual-wall passivity, *IEEE Trans. Robot.* **21**(5): 952–964.

Adams, R. J. & Hannaford, B. (1999). Stable haptic interaction with virtual environments, *IEEE Trans. Robotic. Autom.* **15**(3): 465–474.

Barbé, L., Bayle, B. & de Mathelin, M. (2006). Towards the autotuning of force-feedback teleoperators, *8th Int. IFAC Symposium on Robot Control*, Bologna, Italy.

Basdogan, C., De, S., Kim, J., Muniyandi, M., Kim, H. & Srinivasan, M. A. (2004). Haptics in minimally invasive surgical simulation and training, *IEEE Comput. Graph. Appl.* **24**(2): 56–64.

Bernstein, N. L., Lawrence, D. A. & Pao, L. Y. (2005). Friction modeling and compensation for haptic interfaces, *WorldHaptics Conf.*, Pisa, Italy, pp. 290–295.

Bonneton, B. & Hayward, V. (1994). Implementation of a virtual wall, *Technical report*, McGill University.

Borro, D., Savall, J., Amundarain, A., Gil, J. J., García-Alonso, A. & Matey, L. (2004). A large haptic device for aircraft engine maintainability, *IEEE Comput. Graph. Appl.* **24**(6): 70–74.

Brown, J. M. & Colgate, J. E. (1994). Physics-based approach to haptic display, *ISMRC Topical Workshop on Virtual Reality*, Los Alamitos, CA, USA, pp. 101–106.

Carignan, C. R. & Cleary, K. R. (2000). Closed-loop force control for haptic simulation of virtual environments, *Haptics-e* **1**(2).

Çavuşoğlu, M. C., Feygin, D. & Frank, T. (2002). A critical study of the mechanical and electrical properties of the phantom haptic interface and improvements for high-performance control, *Presence: Teleoperators and Virtual Environments* **11**(6): 555–568.

Colgate, J. E. & Brown, J. M. (1994). Factors affecting the z-width of a haptic display, *IEEE Int. Conf. Robot. Autom.*, Vol. 4, San Diego, CA, USA, pp. 3205–3210.

Colgate, J. E. & Schenkel, G. (1997). Passivity of a class of sampled-data systems: Application to haptic interfaces, *J. Robot. Syst.* **14**(1): 37–47.

Díaz, I. n. & Gil, J. J. (2008). Influence of internal vibration modes on the stability of haptic rendering, *IEEE Int. Conf. Robot. Autom.*, Pasadena, CA, USA, pp. 2884–2889.

Diolaiti, N., Niemeyer, G., Barbagli, F. & Salisbury, J. K. (2006). Stability of haptic rendering: Discretization, quantization, time-delay and coulomb effects, *IEEE Trans. Robot.* **22**(2): 256–268.

Eppinger, S. D. & Seering, W. P. (1987). Understanding bandwidth limitations in robot force control, *IEEE Int. Conf. Robot. Autom.*, Vol. 2, Raleigh, NC, USA, pp. 904–909.

Frisoli, A., Sotgiu, E., Avizzano, C. A., Checcacci, D. & Bergamasco, M. (2004). Force-based impedance control of a haptic master system for teleoperation, *Sensor Review* **24**(1): 42–50.

Gil, J. J., Avello, A., Rubio, A. & Flórez, J. (2004). Stability analysis of a 1 dof haptic interface using the routh-hurwitz criterion, *IEEE Tran. Contr. Syst. Technol.* **12**(4): 583–588.

Gil, J. J., Rubio, A. & Savall, J. (2009). Decreasing the apparent inertia of an impedance haptic device by using force feedforward, *IEEE Tran. Contr. Syst. Technol.* **17**(4): 833–838.

Gil, J. J., Sánchez, E., Hulin, T., Preusche, C. & Hirzinger, G. (2009). Stability boundary for haptic rendering: Influence of damping and delay, *J. Comput. Inf. Sci. Eng.* **9**(1): 011005.

Gillespie, R. B. & Cutkosky, M. R. (1996). Stable user-specific haptic rendering of the virtual wall, *ASME Int. Mechanical Engineering Congress and Exposition*, Vol. 58, Atlanta, GA, USA, pp. 397–406.

Gosline, A. H., Campion, G. & Hayward, V. (2006). On the use of eddy current brakes as tunable, fast turn-on viscous dampers for haptic rendering, *Eurohaptics Conf.*, Paris, France.

Hannaford, B. & Ryu, J.-H. (2002). Time domain passivity control of haptic interfaces, *IEEE Trans. Robot. Autom.* **18**(1): 1–10.

Hashtrudi-Zaad, K. & Salcudean, S. E. (1999). On the use of local force feedback for transparent teleoperation, *IEEE Int. Conf. Robot. Autom.*, Detroit, MI, USA, pp. 1863–1869.

Hirzinger, G., Sporer, N., Albu-Schäffer, A., Hähnle, M., Krenn, R., Pascucci, A. & Schedl, M. (2002). DLR's torque-controlled light weight robot III - are we reaching the technological limits now?, *IEEE Int. Conf. Robot. Autom.*, Washington D.C., USA, pp. 1710–1716.

Hulin, T., Preusche, C. & Hirzinger, G. (2006). Stability boundary for haptic rendering: Influence of physical damping, *IEEE Int. Conf. Intell. Robot. Syst.*, Beijing, China, pp. 1570–1575.

Hulin, T., Preusche, C. & Hirzinger, G. (2008). Stability boundary for haptic rendering: Influence of human operator, *IEEE Int. Conf. Intell. Robot. Syst.*, Nice, France, pp. 3483–3488.

Hulin, T., Sagardia, M., Artigas, J., Schätzle, S., Kremer, P. & Preusche, C. (2008). Human-scale bimanual haptic interface, *Enactive Conf. 2008*, Pisa, Italy, pp. 28–33.

Janabi-Sharifi, F., Hayward, V. & Chen, C. (2000). Discrete-time adaptive windowing for velocity estimation, *IEEE Tran. Contr. Syst. Technol.*, Vol. 8, pp. 1003–1009.

Kuchenbecker, K. J. & Niemeyer, G. (2005). Modeling induced master motion in force-reflecting teleoperation, *IEEE Int. Conf. Robot. Autom.*, Barcelona, Spain, pp. 350–355.
Lawrence, D. A., Pao, L. Y., Salada, M. A. & Dougherty, A. M. (1996). Quantitative experimental analysis of transparency and stability in haptic interfaces, *ASME Int. Mechanical Engineering Congress and Exposition*, Vol. 58, Atlanta, GA, USA, pp. 441–449.
Ljung, L. (1999). *System Identification: Theory for the User*, Prentice Hall.
Mehling, J. S., Colgate, J. E. & Peshkin, M. A. (2005). Increasing the impedance range of a haptic display by adding electrical damping, *First WorldHaptics Conf.*, Pisa, Italy, pp. 257–262.
Minsky, M., Ouh-young, M., Steele, O., Brooks Jr., F. & Behensky, M. (1990). Feeling and seeing: Issues in force display, *Comput. Graph.* **24**(2): 235–243.
Åström, K. J. & Hägglund, T. (1995). *PID Controllers: Theory, Design, and Tuning*, Instrument Society of America, North Carolina.
Ryu, J.-H., Preusche, C., Hannaford, B. & Hirzinger, G. (2005). Time domain passivity control with reference energy following, *IEEE Tran. Contr. Syst. Technol.* **13**(5): 737–742.
Salcudean, S. E. & Vlaar, T. D. (1997). On the emulation of stiff walls and static friction with a magnetically levitated input/output device, *Journal of Dynamics, Measurement and Control* **119**: 127–132.
Savall, J., Borro, D., Amundarain, A., Martin, J., Gil, J. J. & Matey, L. (2004). LHIfAM - Large Haptic Interface for Aeronautics Maintainability, *IEEE Int. Conf. Robot. Autom.*, Video Proceedings, New Orleans, LA, USA.
Savall, J., Martín, J. & Avello, A. (2008). High performance linear cable transmission, *Journal of Mechanical Design* **130**(6).
Tognetti, L. J. & Book, W. J. (2006). Effects of increased device dissipation on haptic two-port network performance, *IEEE Int. Conf. Robot. Autom.*, Orlando, FL, USA, pp. 3304–3311.
Townsend, W. T. (1988). *The Effect of Transmission Design on Force-controlled Manipulator Performance*, Ph.d. thesis, MIT Artificial Intelligence Laboratory.
Ueberle, M. & Buss, M. (2002). Design, control, and evaluation of a new 6 dof haptic device, *IEEE Int. Conf. Intell. Robot. Syst.*, Lausanne, Switzerland, pp. 2949–2954.
Weir, D. W., Colgate, J. E. & Peshkin, M. A. (2008). Measuring and increasing z-width with active electrical damping, *Int. Symp. on Haptic Interfaces*, Reno, NV, USA, pp. 169–175.
Yokokohji, Y. & Yoshikawa, T. (1994). Bilateral control of master-slave manipulators for ideal kinesthetic coupling. formulation and experiment, *IEEE Trans. Robot. Autom.* **10**(5): 605–620.

6

Implementation of a Wireless Haptic Controller for Humanoid Robot Walking

Eun-Su Kim, Man-Seok Kim, Johwan Kim,
Sang Woo Kim* and Jong-Wook Kim
*Dong-A University, *Pohang University of Science and Technology*
Korea

1. Introduction

Humanoid robots are the most proper type of robots for providing humans with various intelligent services, since it has a human-like body structure and high mobility. Despite this prosperity, operation of the humanoid robot requires complicated techniques for performing biped walking and various motions. Thus, the technical advancement concerning humanoid motion is somewhat sluggish.

For attracting more engineering interest to humanoids, it is necessary that one should be able to manipulate a humanoid with such easiness as driving an remote control(RC) car by a wireless controller. In doing so, they will watch the motion and learn intrinsic principles naturally. Actually, however, only a few well-trained experts can deal with a humanoid robot of their own assembling as often seen in robot shows. This limitation may be due to the lack of unified and systemized principles on kinematics, dynamics, and trajectory generation for a humanoid.

For biped walking, modeling of the humanoid for deriving kinematics and dynamics is to be constructed first. Humanoid modeling can be roughly classified into two categories; the inverted pendulum model (Park et al., 1998; Kajita et al., 2001; Kajita et al., 2003) and the joint-link model (Huang et al., 2001; Lim et al., 2002; Jeon et al., 2004; Park et al., 2006). The former approach is such that a humanoid is simplified as an inverted pendulum which connects the supporting foot and the center of mass (CoM) of the whole body. Owing to the limited knowledge in dynamics, this approach considerably relies on feedback control in walking. On the contrary, the latter approach requires the precise knowledge of robot specification concerning each link including mass, moment of inertia, and the position of CoM. This complexity in modeling, however, leads to an inevitable intricateness of deriving dynamics.

We have been building the humanoid walking technologies by constructing the unique three-dimensional model, deriving its dynamics, generating motor trajectories that satisfy both stability and performance in biped walking and upstairs walking since 2007 (Kim & Kim, 2007; Kim et al., 2008a; Kim et al., 2009a; Kim et al. 2009b). All the computer simulations were validated through implementation of walking with a small humanoid robot.

Based on the experience, we newly propose in this paper a wireless humanoid walking controller considered as a simple human-robot-interface. The target users of the controller are children and above, and thus it should be easy to command. The controller is equipped with a joy stick for changing walking direction and speed, function buttons for stop and start of walking or any other motions, and a haptic motor for delivering the current walking status to the user.

The proposed humanoid controller will arouse the popular interest on humanoids, and the related principles will bring about an improvement in the current walking techniques. The proposed controller can be applied to the remote medical robot, the exploration robot, the home security robot, and so on.

2. Humanoid Model

This section describes the kinematics of a humanoid robot in consideration of variable-speed biped walking and direction turning. Humans can walk, run, and twist by rotating joints whose axes are placed normal in three orthogonal planes; the sagittal, coronal, and transverse planes. These planes are determined from viewing angles to an object human. In the sagittal plane, a human walks forward or backward, while he or she moves laterally by rotating joints in the coronal plane. It is apparent that the joints locating in the transverse plane have to be rotated for turning the body.

Figure 1 illustrates the present humanoid model described in the three planes. There are three types of angles in the model; θ, ϕ, and ψ. The sagittal angles $\theta_i, i = 1,\cdots,6$ are the joint angles that make a robot proceed forward or backward. As shown in Figure 1(a), the joint angles $\theta_1, \theta_2,$ and θ_3 are associated with the supporting leg and an upper body, while $\theta_4, \theta_5,$ and θ_6 are assigned to move a swaying leg.

Treating the motor angles is more straightforward and simpler than using the sagittal angles. These motor angles are shown in Figure 1(a) as $\theta_i^j, i = an, kn, th,\ j = l, r,$ where the subscripts *an*, *kn*, and *th* represent ankle, knee, and thigh, and the superscripts *l* and *r* stand for left and right, respectively. Every sagittal joint motor has its own motor angle that has a one-to-one relationship with the six sagittal angles (Kim & Kim, 2007).

The coronal angle ϕ plays the role of translating the upper body to the left or right for stabilizing the robot at the single support phase. Figure 1(b) shows that there are four joints, i.e. two ankle joints and two hip joints, in the coronal plane. These joints, however, consistently revolve with one degree-of-freedom (DOF) to maintain the posture in which the upper body and the two feet are always made vertical to the ground in the coronal view.

The transversal joints with revolute angles $\psi_i, i = l, r$ actuate to twist the upper body and lifted leg around each axis and thus change the current walking direction. The left transverse joint (ψ_l) undertakes a right-hand turning by its first revolving in left leg supporting and by its second doing in right leg supporting. On the contrary, the right transverse joint (ψ_r) has to be rotated for turning to the left.

The present modeling approach is based on the projection technique onto the sagittal and coronal planes, and axis rotation for the transverse plane. While a humanoid is walking in three dimensions, the six links of the lower body seem to be simultaneously contracted from

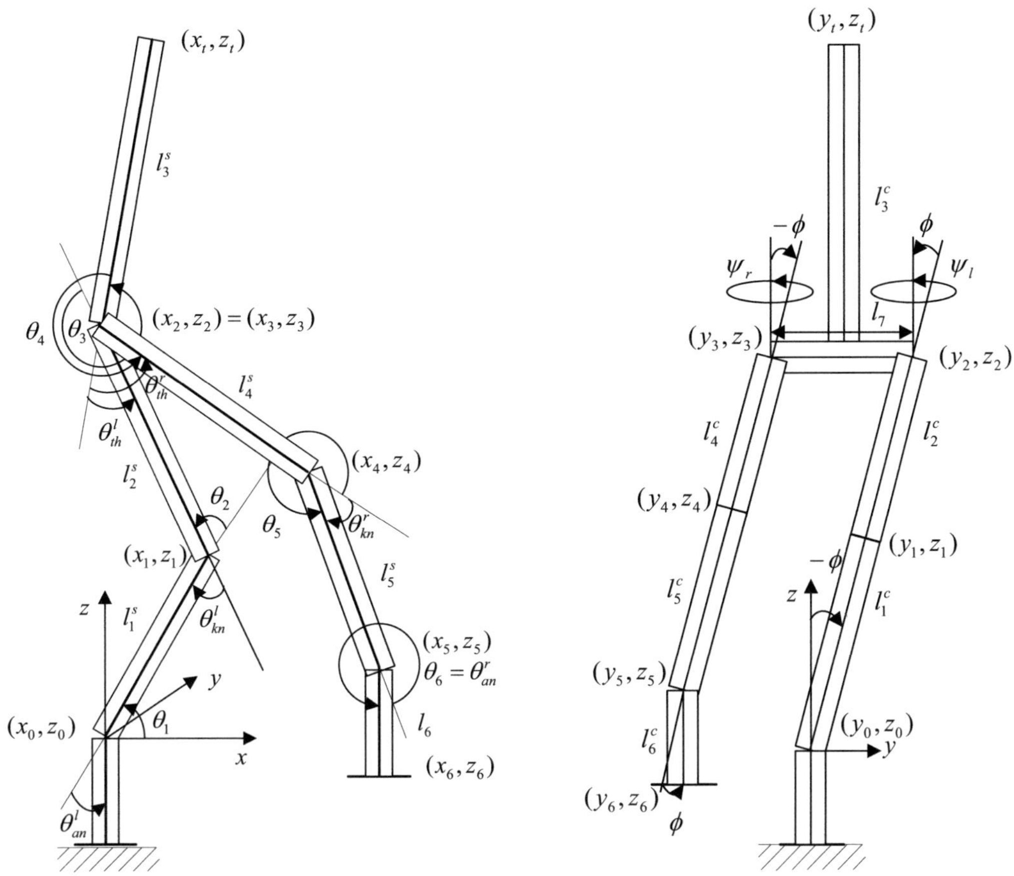

(a) sagittal plane (side view) (b) coronal plane (front view)

Fig. 1. Stick diagrams of a biped robot seen from the side and the front.

the viewpoint of the sagittal and coronal planes.
The projected links viewed from the sagittal plane are written as

$$l_1^s(t) = l_1 \cos\phi(t),\ l_2^s = l_2 \cos\phi(t), l_3^s = l_3, l_4^s = l_4 \cos\phi(t), l_5^s = l_5 \cos\phi(t), l_6^s = l_6 \quad (1)$$

where the superscript s denotes the sagittal plane. In the same manner, the links projected onto the coronal plane are described as

$$\begin{aligned}
&l_1^c(t) = l_1 \sin(\theta_1(t)), l_2^c(t) = \sin(\theta_1(t) + \theta_2(t)), l_3^c = l_3 \sin(\theta_1(t) + \theta_2(t) + \theta_3(t)),\\
&l_4^c(t) = l_4 \sin(\theta_1(t) + \theta_2(t) + \theta_3(t) + \theta_4(t)),\\
&l_5^c(t) = l_5 \sin(\theta_1(t) + \theta_2(t) + \theta_3(t) + \theta_4(t) + \theta_5(t)),\\
&l_6^c(t) = l_6 \sin(\theta_1(t) + \theta_2(t) + \theta_3(t) + \theta_4(t) + \theta_5(t) + \theta_6(t)),
\end{aligned} \quad (2)$$

where the superscript *c* denotes the coronal plane. It should be noted from Eqs. (1) and (2) that the projected links are time varying quantities.
Using the projected links, coordinates of the six joints in left leg supporting are simply derived as direct kinematics from their structural relationship like the following:

$$\begin{aligned}
&x_1 = x_0 + l_1^s C_1,\quad y_1 = y_0 - l_1^c S_\phi,\quad z_1 = z_0 + l_1^s S_1,\\
&x_2 = x_1 + l_2^s C_{12},\quad y_2 = y_1 - l_2^c S_\phi,\quad z_2 = z_1 + l_2^s S_{12},\\
&x_3 = x_2,\quad y_3 = y_2 - l_7,\quad z_3 = z_2,\\
&x_4 = x_3 + l_4^s C_{1234},\quad y_4 = y_3 - l_4^c S_\phi,\quad z_4 = z_3 + l_4^s S_{1234},\\
&x_5 = x_4 + l_5^s C_{12345},\quad y_5 = y_4 - l_5^c S_\phi,\quad z_5 = z_4 + l_5^s S_{12345},\\
&x_6 = x_5 + l_6^s C_{123456},\quad y_6 = y_5,\quad z_6 = z_5 + l_6^s S_{123456}
\end{aligned} \tag{3}$$

where $C_{12\cdots j}$, $S_{12\cdots j}$, and S_ϕ represent $\cos(\theta_1+\theta_2+\cdots+\theta_j)$, $\sin(\theta_1+\theta_2+\cdots+\theta_j)$, and $\sin(\phi)$, respectively. In the case of supporting with the right leg, only y_3 is changed in Eq. (3) as $y_3 = y_2 + l_7$.
For turning in walking or standing, the kinematics in Eq. (3) should be extended to describe turning to an arbitrary angle. For example, let the robot turn to the right by rotating the hip joint of the left leg. At this time, the first rotation resulting from actuation of ψ_l leads to the circular motion of all the joints except those installed in the supporting left leg. Since the coordinate of the left transverse joint is (x_2, y_2, z_2) as shown in Figure 1(b), the resultant coordinates of the *k*-th joint $(x_k^t, y_k^t, z_k^t), k = 3,\cdots,6$ are derived by using the following rotation matrix:

$$\begin{bmatrix} x_k^t \\ y_k^t \\ z_k^t \end{bmatrix} = \begin{bmatrix} \cos\psi_l & -\sin\psi_l & 0 \\ \sin\psi_l & \cos\psi_l & 0 \\ 0 & 0 & 0 \end{bmatrix} \begin{bmatrix} x_k - x_2 \\ y_k - y_2 \\ z_k - z_2 \end{bmatrix} + \begin{bmatrix} x_2 \\ y_2 \\ z_2 \end{bmatrix},\quad k = 3,\cdots,6 \tag{4}$$

where the superscript *t* implies that joint coordinates are rotated on the transverse plane. Owing to the consistency in coronal angles, the pelvis link l_7 is parallel to the ground, and thus the *z*-coordinates remain the same as shown in Eq. (4).
Using Eqs. (3) and (4), the *x*- and *y*-coordinates of the six joints after the rotation are rewritten as follows:

$$
\begin{aligned}
&x_1^t = x_1,\ y_1^t = y_1,\ z_1^t = z_1,\\
&x_2^t = x_2,\ y_2^t = y_2,\ z_2^t = z_2,\\
&x_3^t = x_2^t + l_7 S_{\psi_l},\ y_3^t = y_2^t - l_7 C_{\psi_l},\ z_3^t = z_3,\\
&x_4^t = x_3^t + C_{\psi_l} l_4^s C_{1234} + S_{\psi_l} l_4^s S_\phi,\ y_4^t = y_3^t + S_{\psi_l} l_4^s C_{1234} - C_{\psi_l} l_4^s S_\phi,\ z_4^t = z_4,\\
&x_5^t = x_4^t + C_{\psi_l} l_5^s C_{12345} + S_{\psi_l} l_5^s S_\phi,\ y_5^t = y_4^t + S_{\psi_l} l_5^s C_{12345} - C_{\psi_l} l_5^s S_\phi,\ z_5^t = z_5,\\
&x_6^t = x_5^t + C_{\psi_l} l_6^s C_{123456},\ y_6^t = y_5^t + S_{\psi_l} l_6^s C_{123456},\ z_6^t = z_6.
\end{aligned} \tag{5}
$$

When $\psi_r = 0$, the joint coordinates in Eq. (5) become identical with those in Eq. (3).
For completion of turning to the right, direction of the left foot that was supporting should also be aligned with that of the right foot. Therefore, the second rotation in ψ_l is also to be carried while the right leg supports the upper body at this time. Thus the origin of the coordinate frames (x_0, y_0, z_0) is assigned to the ankle joint of the right leg, and the left transverse joint has the coordinate (x_3, y_3, z_3). In this case, the rotation matrix written in Eq. (4) is changed like the following:

$$
\begin{bmatrix} x_k^t \\ y_k^t \\ z_k^t \end{bmatrix} = \begin{bmatrix} \cos\psi_l & -\sin\psi_l & 0 \\ \sin\psi_l & \cos\psi_l & 0 \\ 0 & 0 & 0 \end{bmatrix} \begin{bmatrix} x_k - x_3 \\ y_k - y_3 \\ z_k - z_3 \end{bmatrix} + \begin{bmatrix} x_3 \\ y_3 \\ z_3 \end{bmatrix},\quad k = 4,5,6. \tag{6}
$$

Then the rotated coordinates are approximated as

$$
\begin{aligned}
&x_1^t = x_1,\ y_1^t = y_1,\ z_1^t = z_1,\\
&x_2^t = x_2,\ y_2^t = y_2,\ z_2^t = z_2,\\
&x_3^t = x_3,\ y_3^t = y_3,\ z_3^t = z_3,\\
&x_4^t = x_3^t + C_{\psi_l} l_4^s C_{1234} + S_{\psi_l} l_4^s S_\phi,\ y_4^t = y_3^t + S_{\psi_l} l_4^s C_{1234} - C_{\psi_l} l_4^s S_\phi,\ z_4^t = z_4,\\
&x_5^t = x_4^t + C_{\psi_l} l_5^s C_{12345} + S_{\psi_l} l_5^s S_\phi,\ y_5^t = y_4^t + S_{\psi_l} l_5^s C_{12345} - C_{\psi_l} l_5^s S_\phi,\ z_5^t = z_5,\\
&x_6^t = x_5^t + C_{\psi_l} l_6^s C_{123456},\ y_6^t = y_5^t + S_{\psi_l} l_6^s C_{123456},\ z_6^t = z_6.
\end{aligned} \tag{7}
$$

3. Zero Moment Point (ZMP)

For stable biped walking, all the joints in a lower body have to revolve maintaining ZMP at each time in the convex hull of all contact points between the feet and the ground. ZMP is the point about which the sum of all the moments of active forces equals zero, whose *x*- and *y*-coordinates are defined as (Huang et al., 2001)

$$x_{ZMP} = \frac{\sum_{i=1}^{6} m_i (\ddot{z}_{im} + g) x_{im} - \sum_{i=1}^{6} m_i \ddot{x}_{im} z_{im}}{\sum_{i=1}^{6} m_i (\ddot{z}_{im} + g)}, \tag{8}$$

$$y_{ZMP} = \frac{\sum_{i=1}^{6} m_i (\ddot{z}_{im} + g) y_{im} - \sum_{i=1}^{6} m_i \ddot{y}_{im} z_{im}}{\sum_{i=1}^{6} m_i (\ddot{z}_{im} + g)}, \tag{9}$$

where g is the acceleration due to gravity, x_{im}, y_{im} and z_{im} denote the x-, y-, and z-coordinates of the CoM point in the ith link.

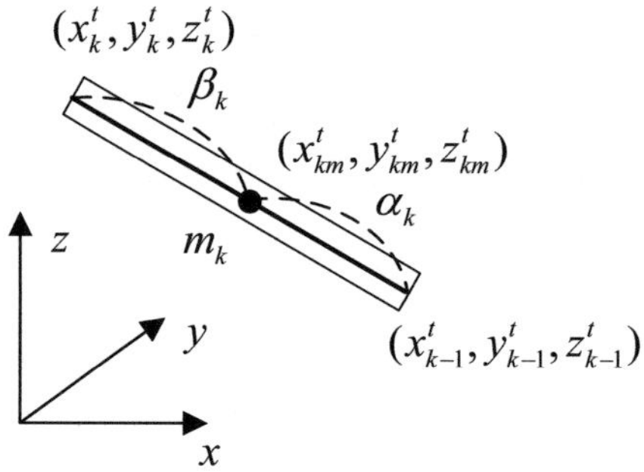

Fig. 2. Center of mass point of the kth link as an interpolated point with ratios of α_k and β_k

Considering that every link CoM point is rigidly fixed between its two end joints, only second-derivative expression of joint coordinates need to be derived. Using interpolation with two ratios as shown in Figure 2, the CoM point of the kth link connected between the (k-1)th and kth joints is expressed as

$$\left(x_{km}, y_{km}, z_{km}\right) = \left(\frac{\alpha_k x_k + \beta_k x_{k-1}}{\alpha_k + \beta_k}, \frac{\alpha_k y_k + \beta_k y_{k-1}}{\alpha_k + \beta_k}, \frac{\alpha_k z_k + \beta_k z_{k-1}}{\alpha_k + \beta_k} \right), \quad k = 1, \cdots, 6, \tag{10}$$

where α_k and β_k represent the CoM point division ratios of the kth link. Then the second derivatives of link CoM points required for computing Eqs. (8) and (9) are directly computed as

$$\left(\ddot{x}_{km}, \ddot{y}_{km}, \ddot{z}_{km}\right) = \left(\frac{\alpha_k \ddot{x}_k + \beta_k \ddot{x}_{k-1}}{\alpha_k + \beta_k}, \frac{\alpha_k \ddot{y}_k + \beta_k \ddot{y}_{k-1}}{\alpha_k + \beta_k}, \frac{\alpha_k \ddot{z}_k + \beta_k \ddot{z}_{k-1}}{\alpha_k + \beta_k} \right), \quad k = 1, \cdots, 6. \tag{11}$$

Therefore, computation of ZMP requires second-derivatives of all the joint coordinates that vary during walking.
In our recent work (Kim et al., 2009b), second-derivatives of the six joint coordinates in the lower body under actuation of the three-type joints have been derived like the following:

$$\begin{aligned}
&\ddot{x}_1 = l_1 A_{CC}(\phi,\theta_1),\quad \ddot{y}_1 = -l_1 A_{SS}(\phi,\theta_1),\quad \ddot{z}_1 = l_1 A_{CS}(\phi,\theta_1),\\
&\ddot{x}_2 = \ddot{x}_1 + l_2 A_{CC}(\phi,\theta_{12}), \ddot{y}_2 = \ddot{y}_1 - l_2 A_{SS}(\phi,\theta_{12}), \ddot{z}_2 = \ddot{z}_1 + l_2 A_{CS}(\phi,\theta_{12}),\\
&\ddot{x}_3 = \ddot{x}_2 + l_7\left(-S_\psi \dot{\psi}^2 + C_\psi \ddot{\psi}\right),\ \ddot{y}_3 = \ddot{y}_2 + l_7\left(C_\psi \dot{\psi}^2 + S_\psi \ddot{\psi}\right),\ \ddot{z}_3 = \ddot{z}_2,\\
&\ddot{x}_4 = \ddot{x}_3 + l_4 A_{CCC}(\phi,\theta_{1234},\psi) + l_4 A_{SSS}(\phi,\theta_{1234},\psi),\\
&\ddot{y}_4 = \ddot{y}_3 + l_4 A_{CCS}(\phi,\theta_{1234},\psi) - l_4 A_{SSC}(\phi,\theta_{1234},\psi),\ \ddot{z}_4 = \ddot{z}_3 + l_4 A_{CS}(\phi,\theta_{1234}),\\
&\ddot{x}_5 = \ddot{x}_4 + l_5 A_{CCC}(\phi,\theta_{12345},\psi) + l_5 A_{SSS}(\phi,\theta_{12345},\psi),\\
&\ddot{y}_5 = \ddot{y}_4 + l_5 A_{CCS}(\phi,\theta_{12345},\psi) - l_5 A_{SSC}(\phi,\theta_{12345},\psi),\ \ddot{z}_5 = \ddot{z}_4 + l_5 A_{CS}(\phi,\theta_{12345}),\\
&\ddot{x}_6 = \ddot{x}_5 + l_6 A_{CC}(\theta_{123456},\psi),\ \ddot{y}_6 = \ddot{y}_5 + l_6 A_{CS}(\theta_{123456},\psi),\\
&\ddot{z}_6 = \ddot{z}_5 + l_6\left(-S_{123456}\dot{\theta}^2_{123456} + C_{123456}\ddot{\theta}_{123456}\right),
\end{aligned} \tag{12}$$

where the functions have the following definitions

$$\begin{aligned}
A_{CCC}(\alpha,\beta,\gamma) &= \frac{d^2}{dt^2}\left(\cos\alpha(t)\cos\beta(t)\cos\gamma(t)\right),\\
A_{CCS}(\alpha,\beta,\gamma) &= \frac{d^2}{dt^2}\left(\cos\alpha(t)\cos\beta(t)\sin\gamma(t)\right),\\
A_{CSS}(\alpha,\beta,\gamma) &= \frac{d^2}{dt^2}\left(\cos\alpha(t)\sin\beta(t)\sin\gamma(t)\right),\\
A_{SSS}(\alpha,\beta,\gamma) &= \frac{d^2}{dt^2}\left(\sin\alpha(t)\sin\beta(t)\sin\gamma(t)\right),\\
A_{CC}(\alpha,\beta) &= \frac{d^2}{dt^2}\left(\cos\alpha(t)\cos\beta(t)\right),\\
A_{CS}(\alpha,\beta) &= \frac{d^2}{dt^2}\left(\cos\alpha(t)\sin\beta(t)\right),\\
A_{SS}(\alpha,\beta) &= \frac{d^2}{dt^2}\left(\sin\alpha(t)\sin\beta(t)\right).
\end{aligned}$$

Insertion of Eq. (12) into Eq. (11) and then Eqs. (8) and (9) enables one to directly compute ZMP.

4. Generation of Optimal Trajectories

In our previous works (Kim & Kim, 2007), the biped robot was modeled in two planes, and dynamics was derived based on it for calculating total energy consumed. For generation of six joint trajectories, the blending polynomial that is a connection of several cubic polynomials (Spong et al., 2006) is used with the optimization method named univariate dynamic encoding algorithm for searches (uDEAS) (Kim et al., 2008b). This method minimized the cost function composed of the sum of total energy consumed by six joint motors and of the penalty function representing the satisfaction of essential requirements such that the swaying foot should land on the desired position, the tip of swaying foot should be always higher than the ground, all the joint motors should rotate within their rotation angle limits, and ZMP should be located inside the convex hull of supporting foot area as much as possible while walking. This work updates the previous ones by recalculating kinematics suited to the three-dimensional model and by elaborating the cost function for walking with variable speed.

Specifically in fast walking, touching the ground of the swaying foot before normal landing gives more impact to the body than in slow walking. Thus, the swaying foot needs be sufficiently high, which can be implemented by adding a related term in the cost function like the following:

$$J = \gamma_1 \int_0^T E(t)dt + P, \tag{13}$$

$$E(t) = \frac{1}{2}\left(m_1(v_1(t))^2 + m_2(v_2(t))^2 + \cdots + m_6(v_6(t))^2\right) + \frac{1}{2}\omega^T I \omega,$$

$$P = \gamma_2\left(\frac{|x_6(T) - S|}{S} + \frac{|z_6(T)|}{h_f}\right) + \gamma_3(\text{violation of limit angle}) + \gamma_4(\text{violation of nontouching ground})$$

$$+ \gamma_5(\text{violation of ZMP}) + \gamma_6(\text{violation of maximum height}),$$

where $\gamma_i, i = 1,\cdots,6$ are the penalty weights chosen to keep from violating each constraint, m_i is the mass of the *i*-th link, v_i is the velocity of the CoM point in the *i*-th link, ω is the angular velocity vector, I is the inertia tensor, S is the stride length, h_f is the maximum height of the swaying foot, and T is the stride cycle. The walking speed can be adjusted by varying T in the optimization stage.

5. Controller Hardware and Experiment

5.1 Humanoid Control System

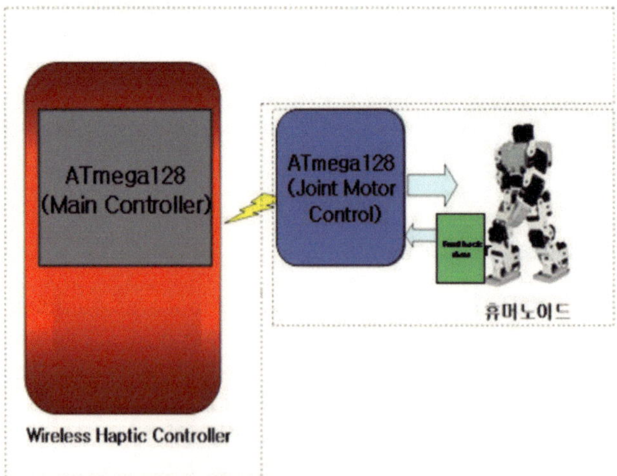

Fig. 3. Hardware structure of the humanoid walking control system.

Figure 3 shows a hardware structure of the proposed humanoid walking control system composed of two parts; a wireless haptic controller (WHC) part and a humanoid controller part.
WHC is executed by an Atmega128 board, where optimal trajectories of joint motors for each walking command are downloaded. Upon command, the motor trajectory data are transmitted to the humanoid controller, and the response data on walking status are feedback from the humanoid controller to WHC by Bluetooth communication.
The humanoid controller is executed by an ATmega128 board. This controller sends the optimal trajectory data received from WHC to each joint motor of the humanoid robot at sampled time.
The specification of the WHC is written in Table 1.

MCU	Atmega128
Memory	256Kbit (32Kbyte) SRAM
Network	Bluetooth Network (RS-232)
Haptic Module	Vibration Motor X 2
Controller	Direction Switch, Joystick, Button

Table 1. Specification of WHC board

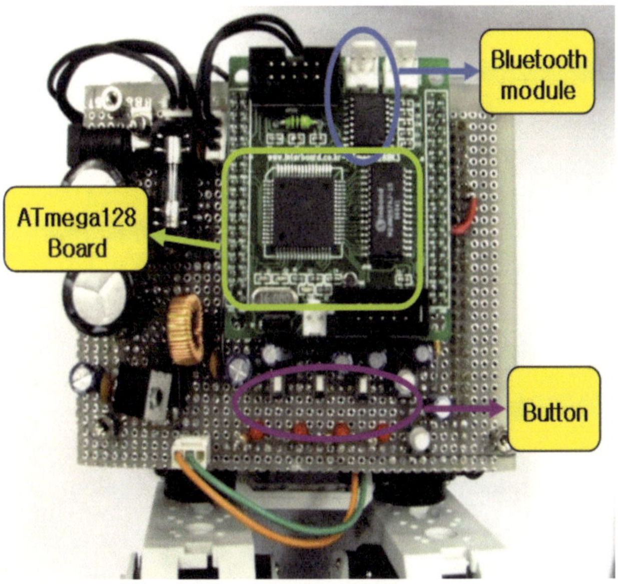

Fig. 4. Exterior of the humanoid control system

Figure 4 shows the manufactured humanoid control system which is composed of the following:

- Main processor is the ATmega128 processor.
- An attached Bluetooth module communicates with the robot in real-time.
- Upon user's command, the information on the corresponding optimal joint motor trajectories downloaded in WHC is transferred to the ATmega128 board.

- One can order the humanoid to walk or turn by using direction switches and a joystick, and command buttons.
- An haptic actuator delivers walking status to the user by vibrating its motor.

5.2 Haptic Controller

Figure 5 illustrates components in the proposed WHC. Detailed explanation is given below:

- Direction switches make the user select one of basic walking types; forward, left, right, and backward walking.
- Buttons are associated with the basic robot motions such as initial standing, starting to move, and waiting the next command.
- A joystick plays a role to modify walking direction and speed by user's will. For instance, a strong upward strike of it will command the robot to walk forward fast.
- A vibration motor makes the user feel the current robot status in motion.

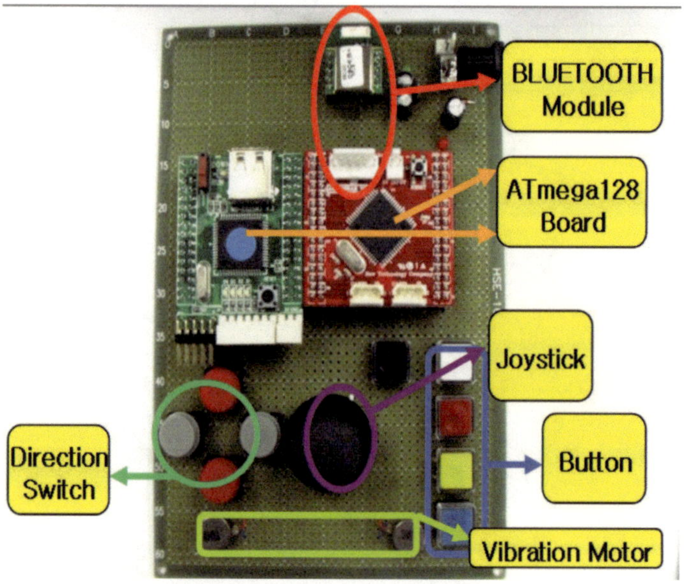

Fig. 5. Manipulation components in the wireless haptic controller

5.3 Simulation and Experiment

We employ uDEAS as a basic optimization method for attaining thirteen optimal parameters of blending polynomials that describe the joint trajectories. The stride length is fixed as $S = 0.1m$ and the stride cycle T is changed from 2 to 4 seconds for simulation of various-speed walking. As T increases, walking speed decreases, and vice versa.

Figure 6 illustrates the simulation result of biped walking for three representative walking cycles. As shown in Figure 6, uDEAS successfully finds out optimal parameters for the given T. Thus, a real-time adjustment of walking speed can be realized by subdividing T, searching for optimal parameters for each T in off-line, saving all the sets of optimal parameters into memory of WHC, and then generating motor trajectories for a requested T.

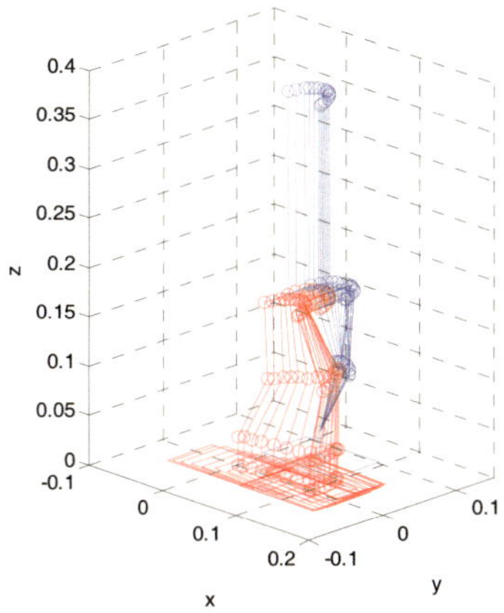

(a) fast walking (T = 2 sec)

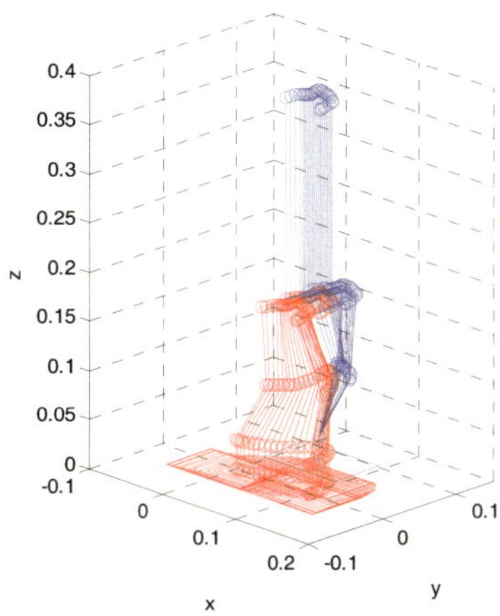

(b) mid-speed walking (T = 3 sec)

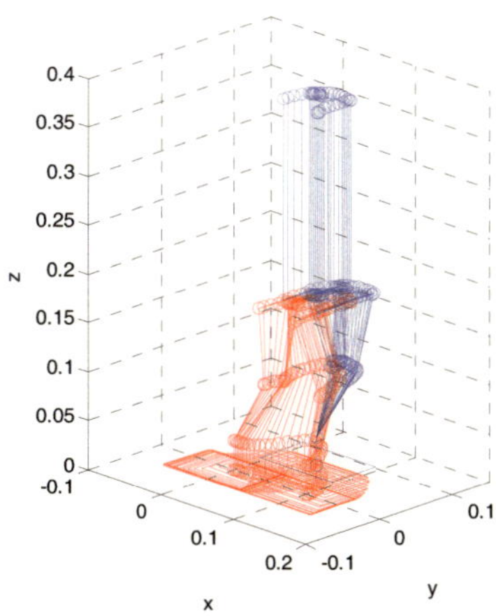

(c) slow walking (T = 4 sec)

Fig. 6. Simulation of variable-speed biped walking.

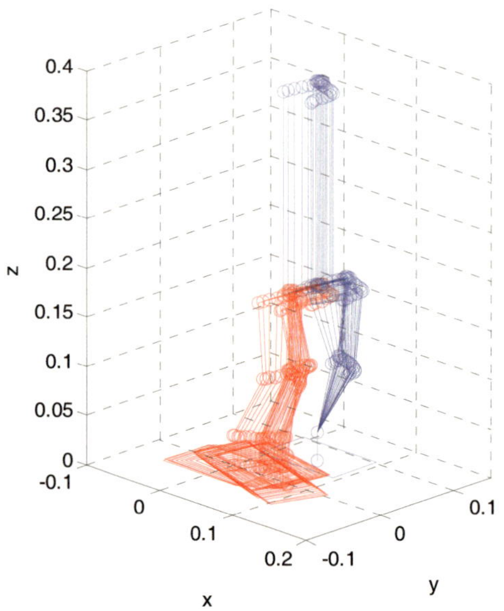

Fig. 7. Simulation of turning to the right with 20 degrees.

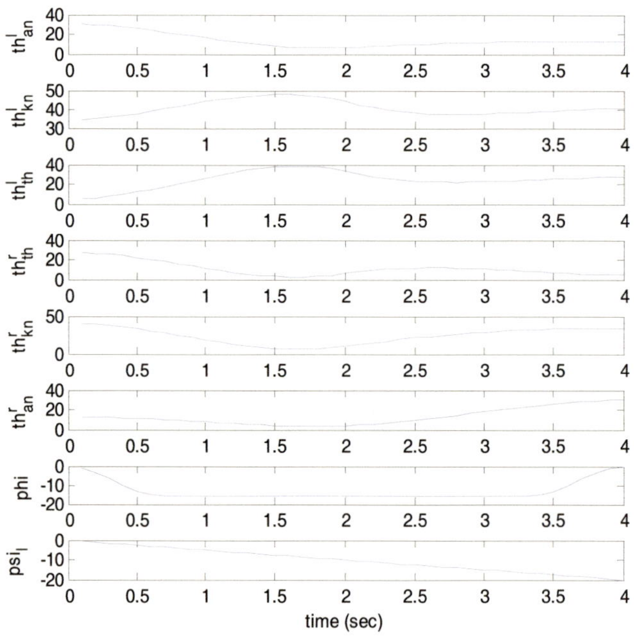

Fig. 8. Joint trajectories for biped turning to the right.

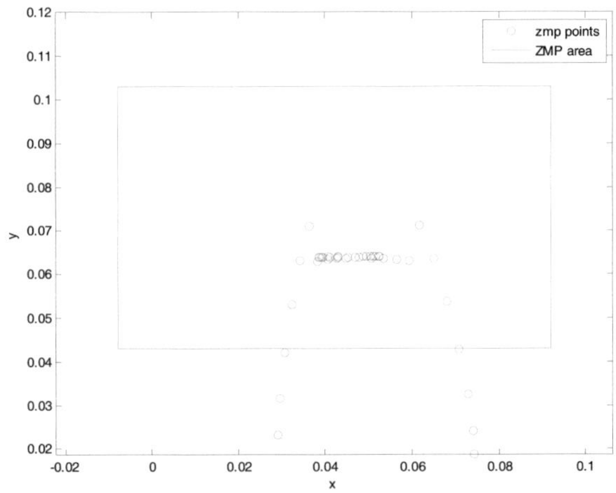

Fig. 9. Trajectories of ZMP during turning in walking.

Figure 7 shows simulation of bide turning to the right with 20 degrees during 4 seconds. All the joint trajectories involved in turning simulation are shown in Figure 8. The first seven motor angles are optimized by uDEAS for energy-minimal walking and the last angle ψ_l is newly added with a linear change from 0 to -20°. This simple trajectory is expected to affect dynamics minimally, and the ZMP's computed by Eqs. (8) and (9) stay inside the stable area, i.e. sole of the supporting foot, sufficiently long time as shown in Figure 9.
Figure 10 shows a snapshot of walking operation with WHC and a humanoid kit. Although the present feasibility of wireless humanoid control is limited to walking forward and turning in standing only, a wide variety of motion will be realized with high reliability in the near future.

6. Conclusion

This paper provides an innovative work concerning the principle and controller implementation on humanoid walking. A new humanoid model is described in three orthogonal planes, and kinematics equations are established based on the phenomena of projection and rotation. The feasibility of the proposed model is validated through the simulation result of variable-speed walking optimized by uDEAS with mere change in the stride cycle. Moreover, we newly succeeded in simulation of direction turning during walking with the aid of mathematical description of three-dimensional kinematics. In addition, the present work includes implementation of a wireless humanoid controller for the purpose of education and entertainment. This is in no doubt possible by virtue of new technologies to date. Our future research will be focused on wireless humanoid control for general human motions.

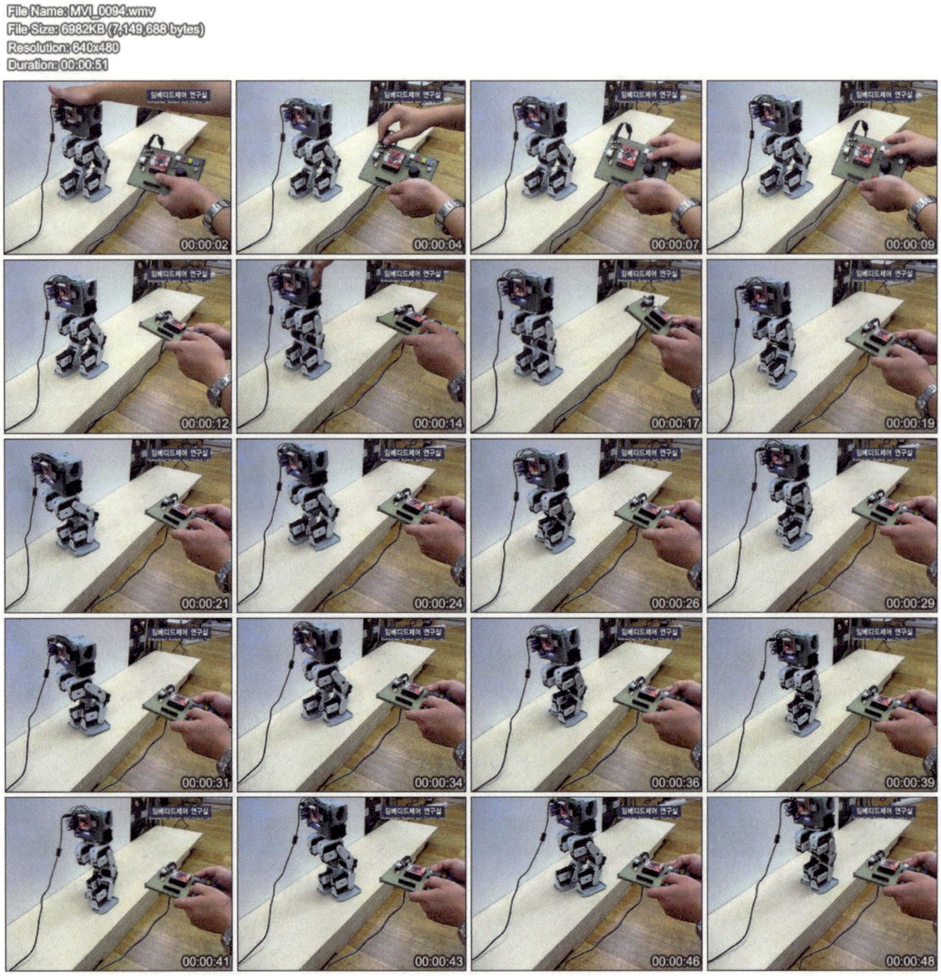

Fig. 10. Walking operation with WHC and a humanoid robot

Acknowledgement

This research was supported by Basic Science Research Program through the National Research Foundation of Korea (**NRF**) funded by the Ministry of Education, Science and Technology (2009-0073527).

7. References

Huang, Q.; Yokoi, K.; Kajita, S.; Kaneko, K.; Arai, H.; Koyachi, N. & Tanie, K. (2001). Planning walking patterns for a biped robot, *IEEE Trans. Robotics and Automation*, Vol. 17, No. 3, pp. 280-289

Jeon, K. S.; Kwon, O. & Park, J. H. (2004). Optimal trajectory generation for a biped robot walking a staircase based on genetic algorithm, *Int. Conf. on Intelligent Robots and Systems*, pp. 2837-2842, Sept. 2004, IEEE, Sendai, Japan

Kajita, S.; Kanehiro, F.; Kaneko, K.; Fujiwara, K.; Harada, K.; Yokoi, K. & Hirukawa, H. (2003). Biped walking pattern generation by using preview control of zero-moment point, *Int. Conf. on Robotics and Automation*, pp. 1620-1626, Sept. 2003, IEEE, Taipei , Taiwan

Kajita, S.; Kanehiro, F.; Kaneko, K.; Yokoi, K. & Hirukawa, H. (2001). The 3D linear inverted pendulum mode: a simple modeling for a biped walking pattern generation, *Int. Conf. on Intelligent Robots and Systems*, pp. 239-246, Oct. 2001, IEEE/RSJ, Maui, Hawaii

Kim, T. & Kim, J.-W. (2007). Planning walking patterns of a biped robot with uDEAS optimization, *Proceeding of International Conference on Control, Automation, and Systems*, pp. 2693-2698, Oct. 2007, ICROS, Seoul, Korea

Kim, E.; Kim, T. & Kim, J.-W. (2008a). Optimal trajectory generation for walking up a staircase of a biped robot using genetic algorithm (GA), *Proceeding of 39th International Symposium on Robotics*, pp. 713-717, Oct. 2008, Seoul, Korea

Kim, J. -W.; Kim, T.; Park, Y. & Kim, S. W. (2008b). On load motor parameter identification using dynamic encoding algorithm for searches (uDEAS), *IEEE Trans. on Energy Conversion*, Vol. 23, No. 3, pp. 804-813

Kim, E.; Kim, J. -H & Kim, J.-W. (2009a). Generation of optimal trajectory for ascending and descending a stair of a humanoid based on uDEAS, *Proceeding of International Conference on Fuzzy Systems (Fuzz-IEEE 2009)*, pp. 660-665, Aug. 2009, Jeju, Korea

Kim, E.; Kim, T. & Kim, J.-W. (2009b). Three-dimensional modelling of a humanoid in three planes and a motion scheme of biped turning in standing, IET Control Theory Appl., Vol. 3, No. 9, pp. 1155-1166

Lim, H.; Kaneshima, Y. & Takanishi, A. (2002). Online walking pattern generation for biped humanoid robot with trunk, *Int. Conf. on Robotics and Automation*, pp. 3111-3116, May 2002, IEEE, Washington, DC

Spong, M. W.; Hutchinson, S. & Vidyasagar, M. (2006). *Robot Modeling and Control*, John Wiley & Sons Inc.

Park, I. -W.; Kim, J. -Y.; Lee, J. & Oh, J. -H. (2006). Online free walking trajectory generation for biped humanoid robot KHR-3 (HUBO), *Int. Conf. on Robotics and Automation*, pp. 1231-1236, May 2006, Orlando, Florida

Park, J. H. & Kim, K. D. (1998). Biped robot walking using gravity-compensated inverted pendulum mode and computed torque control, *Int. Conf. on Robotics and Automation*, pp. 3528-3533, May 1998, Leuven, Belgium

7

Head-Tracking Haptic Computer Interface for the Blind

Simon Meers and Koren Ward
University of Wollongong
Australia

1. Introduction

In today's heavily technology-dependent society, blind and visually impaired people are becoming increasingly disadvantaged in terms of access to media, information, electronic commerce, communications and social networks. Not only are computers becoming more widely used in general, but their dependence on visual output is increasing, extending the technology further out of reach for those without sight. For example, blindness was less of an obstacle for programmers when command-line interfaces were more commonplace, but with the introduction of Graphical User Interfaces (GUIs) for both development and final applications, many blind programmers were made redundant (Alexander, 1998; Siegfried et al., 2004). Not only are images, video and animation heavily entrenched in today's interfaces, but the visual layout of the interfaces themselves hold important information which is inaccessible to sightless users with existing accessibility technology.

Screen reader applications, such as JAWS (Freedom Scientific, 2009b) and Window-Eyes (GW Micro, 2009), are widely used by the visually impaired for reading screen content and interpreting GUIs (Freitas & Kouroupetroglou, 2008). Although they allow the user to access the computer via control key commands and by listening to synthetic speech they can be slow and difficult for inexperienced users to learn. For example, JAWS has over 400 control key sequences to remember for controlling of the screen reader alone (Freedom Scientific, 2009a). Furthermore, a large amount of layout and format information is lost in the conversion from what is effectively a two-dimensional graphical interface into a linear sequence of spoken words.

Various interfaces have been devised which utilise force-feedback devices such as the PHANTOM (Massie & Salisbury, 1994), or (electro-)tactile displays (e.g. Ikei et al., 1997; Kaczmarek et al., 1991; Kawai & Tomita, 1996; Maucher et al., 2001) for haptic perception of three-dimensional models or simple two-dimensional images. Researchers such as Sjöström (2001) have demonstrated success with enabling blind users to interact with certain custom-built interfaces, but not typical GUIs.

Vibro-tactile devices such as the tactile mouse (Immersion Corporation, 2009; Hughes & Forrest, 1996; Gouzman & Karasin, 2004) are designed to provide characteristic tactile feedback based on the type of element at the mouse pointer location. Although a tactile mouse can give a blind user some sense of the spatial layout of screen elements, the inability of blind users to perceive exactly where the mouse pointer is located makes this form of interface ineffective for locating and manipulating screen elements.

Refreshable Braille displays have significantly higher communication resolution, and present information in a manner which is more intuitive for blind users, including the ability to represent text directly. Several projects have been undertaken to represent graphical interfaces using such displays. For example, HyperBraille (Kieninger, 1996) maps HyperText Markup Language (HTML) pages into Braille "pull down menu" interfaces. Recently, Rotard et al. (2008) have developed a web browser extension which utilises a larger pin-based tactile display with the ability to render simple images using edge-detection, as well as Braille representations of textual content. Such systems provide advantages beyond simple screen readers, but are still very limited in terms of speed of perception, layout retention and navigability.
To address these shortcomings we have been devising various interfaces for the visually impaired which involve head-pose tracking and haptic feedback. Our system utilises a head-pose tracking system for manipulating the mouse pointer with the user's 'gaze' which allows the user's hands to be free for typing and tactile perception.
This is implemented by mapping the graphical interface onto a large 'virtual screen' and projecting the 'gaze' point of the user onto the virtual screen. The element(s) at the 'focal' position are interpreted via tactile or voice feedback to the user. Consequently, by gazing over the virtual screen, the user can quickly acquire a mental map of the screen's layout and the location of screen elements (see Figure 1). By gazing momentarily at a single element, additional details can be communicated using synthetic speech output via the speakers or Braille text via a Braille display.

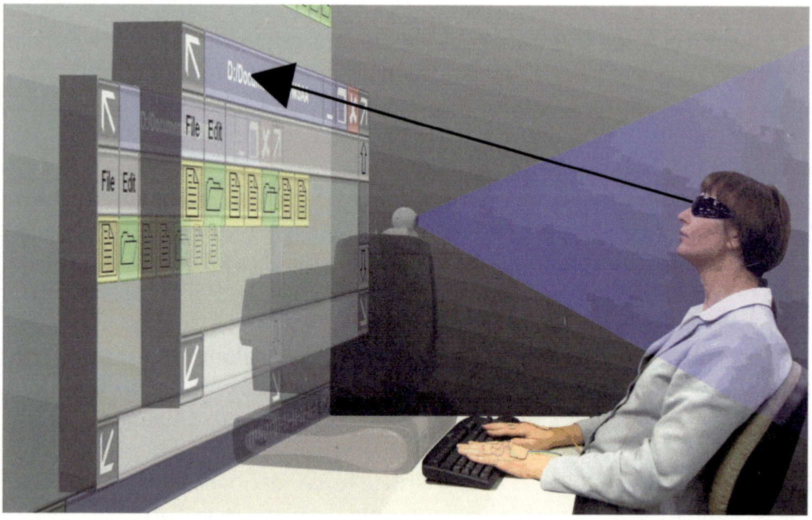

Fig. 1. Visual representation of the gaze-tracking "virtual screen" concept

We have experimented with a number of methods of mapping various graphical interfaces to blind gaze tracking virtual screens as well as a number of different haptic feedback devices. Details of these mapping techniques and haptic feedback devices are provided in the following sections.

2. Background

This project stems from our development of the Electro-Neural Vision System (ENVS) (Meers & Ward, 2004) – a device which allows its wearer to perceive the three-dimensional profile of their surrounding environment via Transcutaneous Electro-Neural Stimulation (TENS) and therefore navigate without sight or other aids. It utilises a head-mounted range-sensing device such as stereo cameras or an array of infrared sensors, pointed in the direction of the wearer's 'gaze'. The acquired depth map is divided into sample regions, each of which is mapped to a corresponding finger which receives electro-tactile stimulation of intensity proportional to the distance measured in that region. The frequency of the signal was used for encoding additional information such as colour (Meers & Ward, 2005b) or GPS landmark information (Meers & Ward, 2005a). Our experiments showed that this form of perception made it possible for unsighted users to navigate known environments by perceiving objects and identifying landmarks based on their size and colour. Similarly, unknown outdoor environments could be navigated by perceiving landmarks via GPS rather than their size and colour. Figure 2 shows the ENVS in use.

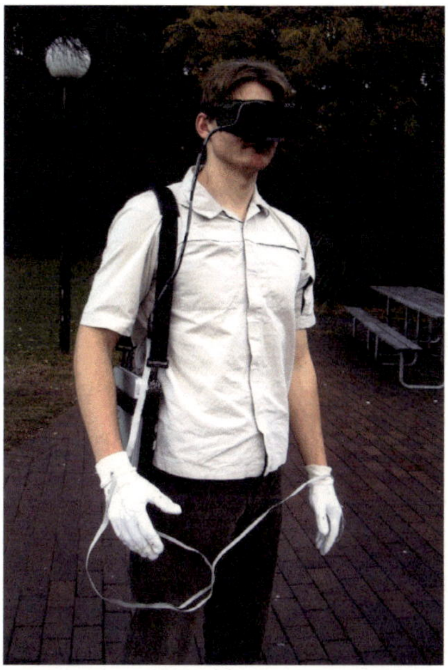

Fig. 2. Electro-Neural Vision System Prototype

Our ENVS experiments inspired us to implement a similar form of perception for interpreting the content of the computer screen. In this case, a large *virtual screen* was located in front of the user and a head-pose tracking system was used to track the 'gaze' position of the user on the virtual screen. To determine what is located at the gaze position on the virtual screen, pre-coded haptic feedback signals are delivered to the fingers via electro-tactile electrodes, a haptic keyboard or a refreshable Braille display. The following sections provide details of the head-pose tracking systems and haptic feedback devices deployed on our interface.

3. Gaze-Tracking Haptic Interface

The primary goal of our gaze-tracking haptic interface is to maintain the spatial layout of the interface so that the user can perceive and interact with it in two-dimensions as it was intended, rather than enforcing linearisation, with the loss of spatial and format data, as is the case with screen readers. In order to maintain spatial awareness, the user must be able to control the "region of interest" and understand its location within the interface as a whole. Given that we wanted to keep the hands free for typing and perception, the use of the head as a pointing device was an obvious choice – a natural and intuitive pan/tilt input device which is easy to control and track for the user (unlike mouse devices).

3.1 Head-pose tracking

While there are quite a number of head-pose tracking systems commercially available, we found that they were all either too cumbersome, computationally expensive or inaccurate for our requirements. Consequently, we developed our initial prototype using our own custom-developed head-pose tracker (Meers et al., 2006) which utilised a simple USB web camera and a pair of spectacles with three infrared LEDs to simplify the tracking process. This proved to be robust and accurate to within $0.5°$.

To avoid the need for the user to wear special gaze-tracking spectacles, we developed a head-pose tracking system based on a time-of-flight camera (Meers & Ward, 2008). This not only made our interface less cumbersome to set up, but also provided the advantage of in-built face recognition (Meers & Ward, 2009) for loading user preferences, etc.

3.2 The Virtual Screen

Once the user's head-pose is determined, a vector is projected through space to determine the gaze position on the virtual screen. The main problem is in deciding what comprises a screen element, how screen elements can be interpreted quickly and the manner by which the user's gaze passes from one screen element to another. We have tested two approaches to solving these problems as explained in the following sections

3.2.1 Gridded Desktop Interface

Our initial experiments involved the simulation of a typical "desktop" interface, comprising a grid of file/directory/application icons at the "desktop" level, with cascading resizable windows able to "float" over the desktop (see Figure 3). The level of the window being perceived (from frontmost window to desktop-level) was mapped to the intensity of haptic feedback provided to the corresponding finger, so that "depth" could be conveyed in a similar fashion to the ENVS. The frequency of haptic feedback was used to convey the *type* of element being perceived (file/folder/application/control/empty cell). Figure 4 illustrates the mapping between adjacent grid cells and the user's fingers. The index fingers were used to perceive the element at the gaze point, while adjacent fingers were optionally mapped to neighbouring elements to provide a form of peripheral perception. This was found to enable the user to quickly acquire a mental map of the desktop layout and content. By gazing momentarily at an individual element, the user could acquire additional details such as the file name, control type, etc. via synthetic speech output or Braille text on a Braille display.

A problem discovered early in experimentation with this interface was the confusion caused when the user's gaze meandered back and forth across cell boundaries, as shown in Figure 5. To overcome this problem, a subtle auditory cue was provided when the gaze crossed boundaries to make the user aware of the grid positioning, which also helped to distinguish con-

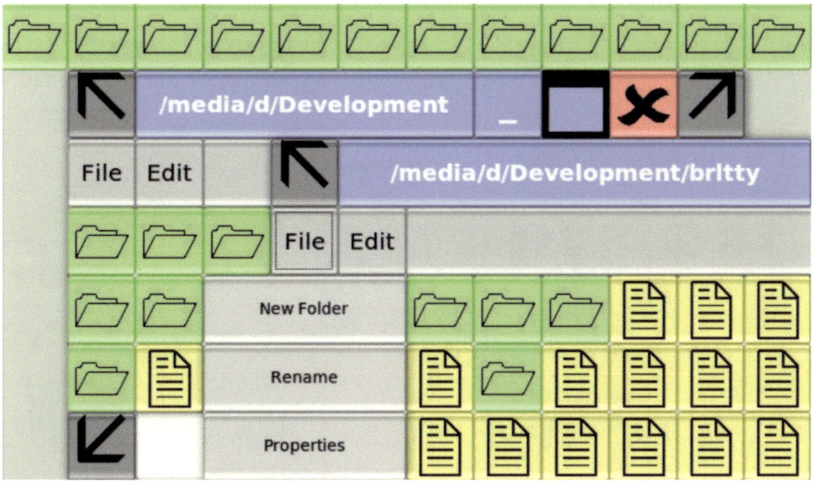

Fig. 3. Experimental desktop grid interface

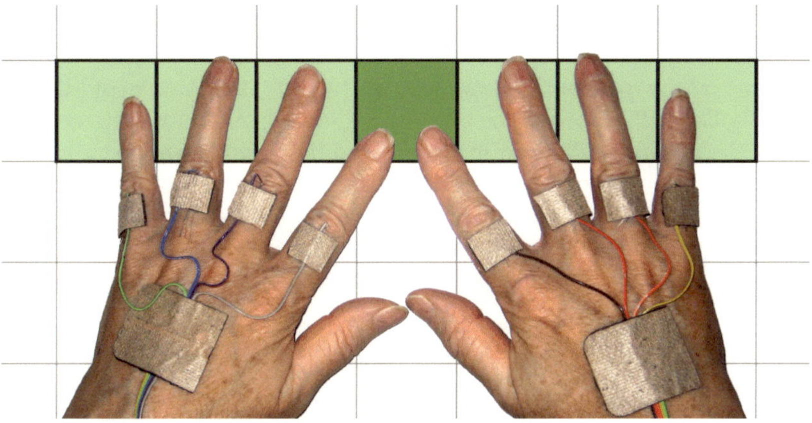

Fig. 4. Mapping of fingers to grid cells

tiguous sections of homogeneous elements. In addition, a stabilisation algorithm was implemented to minimise the number of incidental cell changes as shown in Figure 5.

3.2.2 Zoomable Web Browser Interface

With the ever-increasing popularity and use of the World Wide Web, a web-browser interface is arguably more important to a blind user than a desktop or file management system. Our attempts to map web pages into grids similar to our desktop interface proved difficult due to the more free-form nature of interface layouts used. Small items such as radio buttons were forced to occupy an entire cell, and we began to lose the spatial information we were striving to preserve. We therefore opted to discard the grid altogether, and use the native borders of the HTML elements.

Web pages can contain such a wealth of tightly-packed elements, however, that it can take a long time to scan them all and find what you are looking for. To alleviate this problem,

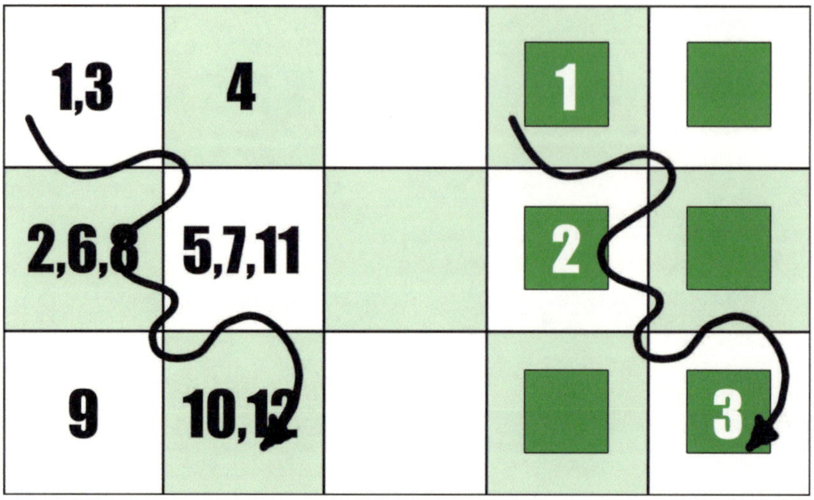

Fig. 5. Gaze travel cell-visiting sequence unstabilised (left) and with stabilisation applied (right)

we took advantage of the natural Document Object Model (DOM) element hierarchy inherent in HTML and "collapsed" appropriate container elements to reduce the complexity of the page. For example, a page containing three bulleted lists containing text and links, and two tables of data might easily contain hundreds of elements. If instead of rendering all of these individually we simply collapse them into the three tables and two lists, the user can much more quickly perceive the layout, and then opt to "zoom" into whichever list or table interests them to perceive the contained elements (see Figures 6(a) and 6(b) for another example).

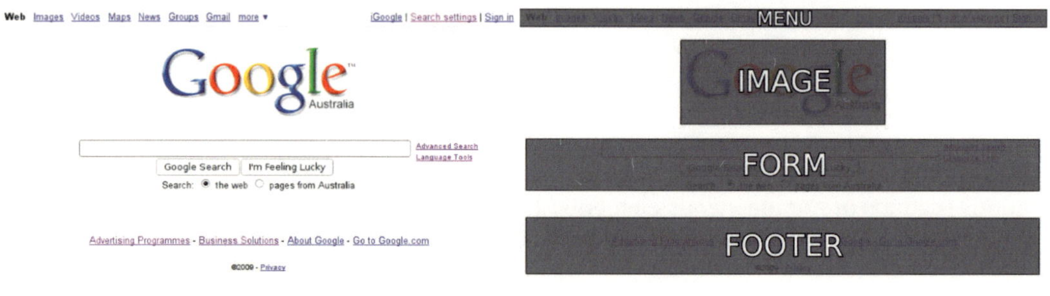

(a) Raw page (b) Collapsed page

Fig. 6. Example of collapsing a web page for faster perception

Our experimental interface has been developed as an extension for the Mozilla Firefox web browser (Mozilla Foundation, 2009), and uses the BRLTTY (Mielke, 2009) for Braille communication and Orca (GNOME Project, The, 2009) for speech synthesis. It uses JavaScript to analyse the page structure and coordinate gaze-interaction in real-time. Communication with the Braille display (including input polling) is performed via a separate Java application.

3.3 Haptic Output

We have experimented with a number of modes of haptic output during our experimentation, including glove-based electro-tactile stimulation, vibro-tactile actuators, wireless TENS patches and refreshable Braille displays. The following sections discuss the merits of each system.

3.3.1 Electro-Tactile Stimulation

Our initial prototype utilised a simple wired TENS interface as shown in Figure 7. The wires connected the electrodes to our custom-built TENS control unit (not shown). Each electrode delivers a TENS pulse-train of the specified frequency and amplitude (depending on what is being perceived in that region). The voltage and intensity can be varied for each electrode and for each different user. This is necessary given that each user's preferences vary greatly and the sensitivity of different fingers also varies for each individual. This interface proved effective in our experiments and allowed the user's fingers to be free to use the keyboard. However, being physically connected to the TENS unit proved inconvenient for general use.

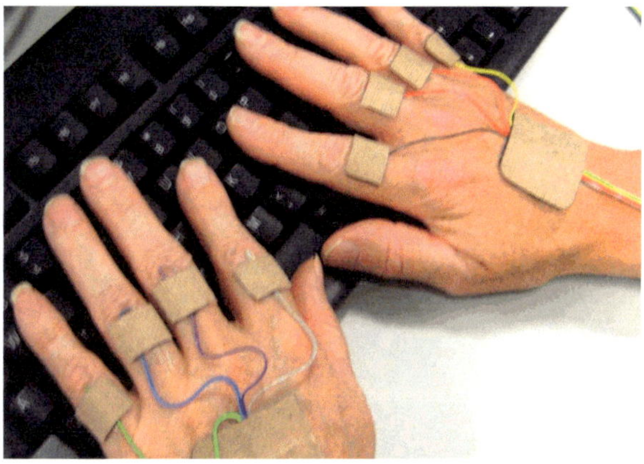

Fig. 7. Wired TENS system

To eliminate this constraint, we developed wireless TENS patches which communicate with the system via radio transmission. This not only allows the user to walk away from the system without having to detach electrodes, but also enables the electrodes to be placed anywhere on the body such as the arms or torso. A prototype wireless TENS patch can be seen in Figure 8.

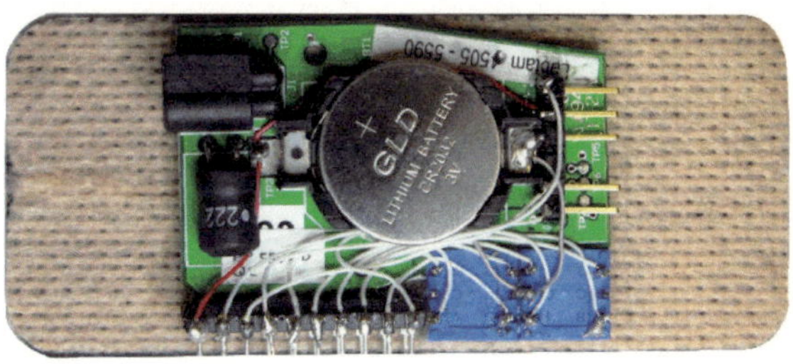

Fig. 8. Wireless TENS Patch

3.3.2 Vibro-Tactile Interface

Although the TENS interface is completely painless, it still requires wireless TENS electrodes to be placed on the skin in a number of places which can be inconvenient. To overcome this problem and trial another mode of haptic communication, we developed a vibro-tactile keyboard interface, as illustrated in Figure 9. This device integrated vibro-tactile actuators, constructed from speakers, which could produce vibration output of the frequency and amplitude specified by the system, analogous to the TENS pulse-train output.

This system has clear advantages over the TENS interface: 1) the user is not "attached" to the interface and can move around as they please, and 2) no TENS electrodes need to be worn and vibro-tactile stimulation is generally more palatable than electro-tactile stimulation despite having a lower bandwidth. Whilst we found this interface capable of delivering a wide range of sensations, the range and differentiability of TENS output was superior. Furthermore, the TENS interface allowed the users to simultaneously perceive and use the keyboard, whilst the vibro-tactile keyboard required movement of the fingers between the actuators and the keys.

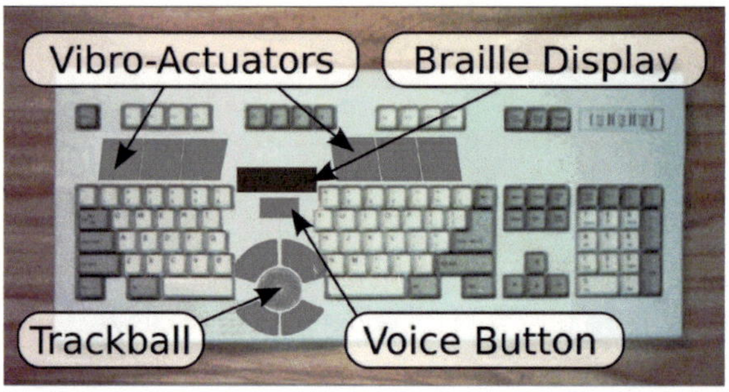

Fig. 9. Vibro-Tactile Keyboard

3.3.3 Refreshable Braille Display

We have also experimented with the use of refreshable Braille displays for haptic perception. Our experimentation revolved mainly around a Papenmeier BRAILLEX EL 40s (Papenmeier, 2009) as seen in Figure 10. It consists of 40 8-dot Braille cells, each with an input button above, a scroll button at either end of the cell array, and an "easy access bar" (joystick-style bar) across the front of the device. We found this device to be quite versatile, and capable of varying the "refresh-rate" up to 25Hz.

A refreshable Braille display can be used in a similar fashion to the TENS and electro-tactile output arrays for providing perception of adjacent elements. Each Braille cell has a theoretical output resolution of 256 differentiable pin combinations. Given that the average user's finger width occupies two to three Braille cells, multiple adjacent cells can be combined to further increase the per-finger resolution.

Whilst a blind user's highly tuned haptic senses may be able to differentiate so many different dot-combinations, sighted researchers have significant difficulty doing so without extensive training. For our preliminary experimentation we have therefore adopted simple "glyphs" for fast and intuitive perception. Figure 11 shows some example glyphs representing HTML elements for web page perception.

A further advantage of using a Braille display is the ability to display element details using traditional Braille text. Suitably trained users are able to quickly read Braille text rather than listening to synthetic speech output. Our experiments have shown that using half the display

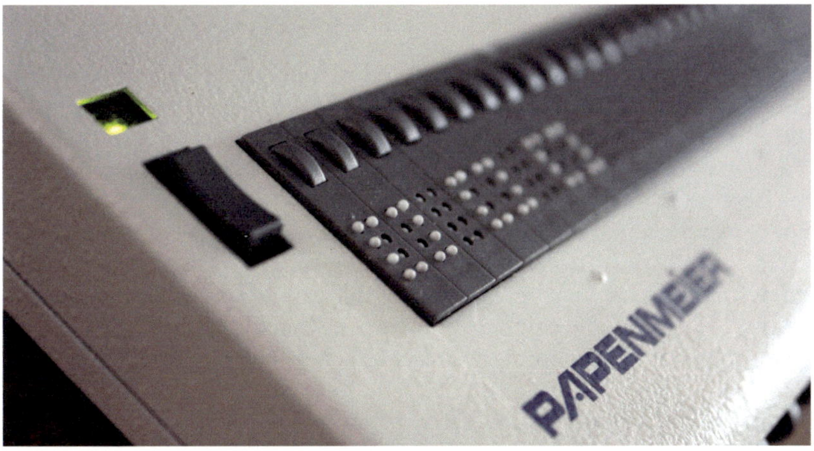

Fig. 10. Papenmeier BRAILLEX EL 40s Refreshable Braille Display

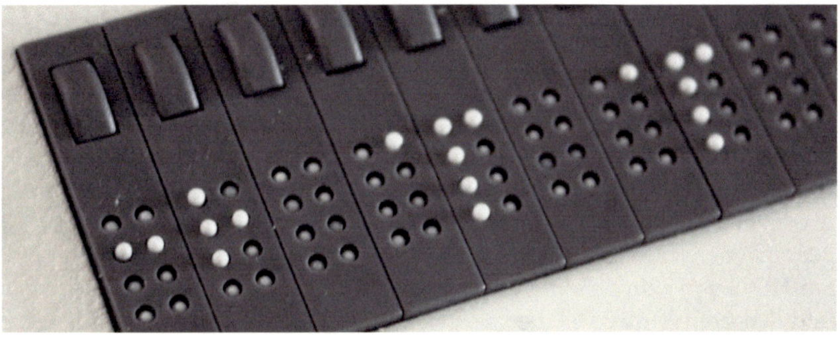

Fig. 11. Example glyphs – link, text, text

for element-type perception using glyphs and the other half for instantaneous reading of further details of the central element using Braille text is an effective method of quickly scanning web pages and other interfaces.

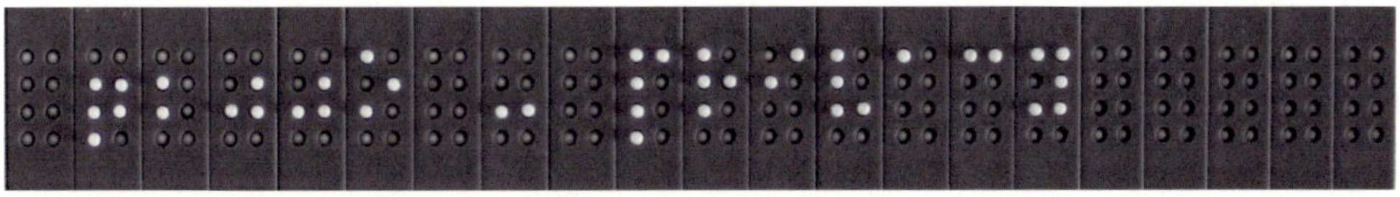

Fig. 12. Braille Text displaying details of central element

The Papenmeier "easy access bar" has also proven to be a valuable asset for interface navigation. In our prototype browser, vertical motions allow the user to quickly "zoom" in or out of element groups (as described in Section 3.2.2), and horizontal motions allow the display to toggle between "perception mode" and "reading" mode once a element of significance has been discovered.

4. Results

Through this work we have devised and tested a number of human computer interface paradigms capable of enabling the two-dimensional screen interface to be perceived without use of the eyes. These systems involve head-pose tracking for obtaining the gaze position on a virtual screen and various methods of receiving haptic feedback for interpreting screen content at the gaze position.

Our preliminary experimental results have shown that using the head as an interface pointing device is an effective means of selecting screen regions for interpretation and for manipulating screen objects without use of the eyes. When combined with haptic feedback, a blind user is able to perceive the location and approximate dimensions of the virtual screen as well as the approximate locations of objects located on the screen after briefly browsing over the screen area.

The use of haptic signal intensity to perceive window edges and their layer is also possible to a limited extent with the TENS interface. After continued use, users were able to perceive objects on the screen without any use of the eyes, differentiate between files, folders and controls based on their frequency, locate specific items, drag and drop items into open windows. Experienced users were also able to operate pull-down menus and move and resize windows without sight.

The interpretation of screen objects involves devising varying haptic feedback signals for identifying different screen objects. Learning to identify various screen elements based on their haptic feedback proved time consuming on all haptic feedback devices. However, this learning procedure can be facilitated by providing speech or Braille output to identify elements when they are 'gazed' at for a brief period.

As far as screen element interpretation was concerned, haptic feedback via the Braille display surpassed the TENS and vibro-tactile interfaces. This was mainly because the pictorial nature of glyphs used is more intuitive to the inexperienced users. It is also possible to encode more differentiable elements by using two Braille cells per finger.

Preliminary experiments with our haptic web browser also demonstrated promising results. For example, experienced users were given the task of using a search engine to find the answer to a question without sight. They showed that they were able to locate the input form element with ease and enter the search string. They were also able to locate the search results, browse over them and navigate to web pages by clicking on links at the gaze position. They were also able to describe the layout of unfamiliar web pages according to where images, text, links, etc were located.

5. Conclusion

This work presents a novel haptic head-pose tracking computer interface that enables the two-dimensional screen interface to be perceived and accessed without any use of the eyes. Three haptic output paradigms were tested, namely: TENS, vibro-tactile and a refreshable Braille display. All three haptic feedback methods proved effective to varying degrees. The Braille interface provided greater versatility in terms of rapid identification of screen objects. The TENS system provided improved perception of depth (for determining window layers). The vibro-tactile keyboard proved convenient but with limited resolution. Our preliminary experimental results have demonstrated that considerable screen-based interactivity is able to be performed with haptic gaze-tracking systems including point-and-click and drag-and-drop manipulation of screen objects. The use of varying haptic feedback can also allow screen objects at the gaze position to be identified and interpreted. Furthermore, our preliminary experimental results with our haptic web browser demonstrate that this means of interactivity holds potential for improved human computer interactivity for the blind.

6. References

Alexander, S. (1998). Blind Programmers Facing Windows, *Computer World* . Reprinted on-line by CNN: `http://www.cnn.com/TECH/computing/9811/06/blindprog.idg/`.

Freedom Scientific (2009a). JAWS keystrokes.
URL: *http://www.freedomscientific.com/training/training-JAWS-keystrokes.htm*

Freedom Scientific (2009b). Job Access With Speech (JAWS).
URL: *http://www.freedomscientific.com/fs_products/software_jaws.asp*

Freitas, D. & Kouroupetroglou, G. (2008). Speech technologies for blind and low vision persons, *Technology and Disability* **20**(2): 135–156.
URL: *http://iospress.metapress.com/content/a4665u784r582844*

GNOME Project, The (2009). Orca.
URL: *http://live.gnome.org/Orca*

Gouzman, R. & Karasin, I. (2004). Tactile interface system for electronic data display system. US Patent 6,762,749.

GW Micro (2009). Window-Eyes.
URL: *http://www.gwmicro.com/*

Hughes, R. G. & Forrest, A. R. (1996). Perceptualisation using a tactile mouse, *Visualization '96. Proceedings.*, pp. 181–188.

Ikei, Y., Wakamatsu, K. & Fukuda, S. (1997). Texture display for tactile sensation, *Advances in human factors/ergonomics* pp. 961–964.

Immersion Corporation (2009). iFeel Mouse.
URL: *http://www.immersion.com/*

Kaczmarek, K. A., Webster, J. G., Bach-y Rita, P. & Tompkins, W. J. (1991). Electrotactile and vibrotactile displays for sensory substitution systems, *Biomedical Engineering, IEEE Transactions on* **38**(1): 1–16.

Kawai, Y. & Tomita, F. (1996). Interactive tactile display system: a support system for the visually disabled to recognize 3d objects, *Assets '96: Proceedings of the second annual ACM conference on Assistive technologies*, ACM, New York, NY, USA, pp. 45–50.

Kieninger, T. (1996). The "growing up" of hyperbraille—an office workspace for blind people, *UIST '96: Proceedings of the 9th annual ACM symposium on User interface software and technology*, ACM, New York, NY, USA, pp. 67–73.

Massie, T. H. & Salisbury, J. K. (1994). The PHANTOM haptic interface: A device for probing virtual objects, *Proceedings of the ASME Winter Annual Meeting, Symposium on Haptic Interfaces for Virtual Environment and Teleoperator Systems*, Vol. 55, pp. 295–300.

Maucher, T., Meier, K. & Schemmel, J. (2001). An interactive tactile graphics display, *Signal Processing and its Applications, Sixth International, Symposium on. 2001*, Vol. 1, pp. 190–193 vol.1.

Meers, S. & Ward, K. (2004). A vision system for providing 3d perception of the environment via transcutaneous electro-neural stimulation, *Information Visualisation, 2004. IV 2004. Proceedings. Eighth International Conference on*, pp. 546–552.

Meers, S. & Ward, K. (2005a). A substitute vision system for providing 3d perception and gps navigation via electro-tactile stimulation, *Proceedings of the International Conference on Sensing Technology*.

Meers, S. & Ward, K. (2005b). A vision system for providing the blind with 3d colour perception of the environment, *Proceedings of the Asia-Pacific Workshop on Visual Information Processing*.

Meers, S. & Ward, K. (2008). Head-pose tracking with a time-of-flight camera, *Australasian Conference on Robotics & Automation*.

Meers, S. & Ward, K. (2009). Face recognition using a time-of-flight camera, *Proceedings of the 6th International Conference Computer Graphics, Imaging and Visualization*.

Meers, S., Ward, K. & Piper, I. (2006). Simple, robust and accurate head-pose tracking with a single camera, *The Thirteenth Annual Conference on Mechatronics and Machine Vision in Practice*.

Mielke, D. (2009). BRLTTY.
URL: `http://mielke.cc/brltty/`

Mozilla Foundation (2009). Mozilla Firefox.
URL: `http://www.mozilla.com/firefox/`

Papenmeier (2009). BRAILLEX EL 40s.
URL: `http://www.papenmeier.de/rehatechnik/en/produkte/braillex_el40s.html`

Rotard, M., Taras, C. & Ertl, T. (2008). Tactile web browsing for blind people, *Multimedia Tools and Applications* **37**(1): 53–69.

Siegfried, R. M., Diakoniarakis, D. & Obianyo-Agu, U. (2004). Teaching the Blind to Program Visually, *Proceedings of ISECON 2004*.

Sjöström, C. (2001). Designing haptic computer interfaces for blind people, *Proceedings of ISSPA 2001*, pp. 1–4.

8

Passivity-based Analysis and Design of Multi-contact Haptic Systems via LMIs

Gianni Bianchini, Marcello Orlandesi and Domenico Prattichizzo
Dipartimento di Ingegneria dell'Informazione, Università di Siena
Italy

1. Introduction

Stability is a key feature in haptic interaction with virtual environments, since unwanted oscillations can impair realism and, most importantly, may be potentially harmful for the human operator. The issue of stability in this context has been addressed by several authors since the early 90's (Minsky et al. (1990)) and involves quite a few aspects, since the systems at hand are complex and some of their components, namely the human operators, are difficult to model. Stability has been considered from multiple viewpoints, and passivity has often been exploited in this context, since it provides a powerful tool for analyzing etherogeneous interconnected systems (Lozano et al. (2000)). The fundamental paper Colgate & Schenkel (1997) and more recent works such as Stramigioli et al. (2005) provide different approaches to the characterization of passivity in sampled-data systems and in particular in haptics. In Miller (2000); Miller et al. (1999; 2000; 2004) a discrete-time passivity framework is proposed to deal with stability analysis and controller (virtual coupling) design also in the presence of non-passive virtual environments, and in particular Miller et al. (2000) addresses the presence of nonlinearities. In Naghshtabrizi & Hespanha (2006), an H_∞-type approach to the design of virtual couplings ensuring passivity and transparency is proposed. Most of the above contributions are mainly focused on the case of a single human operator interacting with a one-degree of freedom virtual environment, although also multivariable systems can be addressed to some extent.

In this chapter, we deal specifically with stability analysis and controller design for haptic systems involving several devices and human operators that interact with a common virtual environment through multiple points of contact. Multi-contact interaction is an important issue in virtual reality and haptics (Barbagli et al. (2005a)). Researchers from the computer haptics community, the branch of the haptic science closer to traditional robotics (Salisbury et al. (2004)), have investigated several aspects in this scenario such as friction modeling (Barbagli et al. (2004); Melder & Harwin (2003)) and interaction with deformable objects (Barbagli et al. (2005b)), but mostly neglected stability issues.

Our approach is related to the framework of Miller (2000); Miller et al. (1999; 2000; 2004) but exploits some features that are peculiar to multi-contact systems. Indeed, in a multi-contact scenario, several structural constraints arise due to the number, type and (physical or virtual) location of the devices that are coupled through the virtual environment. Moreover, virtual coupling implementation may be subject to structure constraints as well. As a matter of fact, it is often the case that the device and virtual coupling must be lumped together. More importantly, multi-contact systems may be physically distributed, and therefore the virtual coupling may share only limited information with the devices and virtual environment due to decentralization and limited communication requirements.

The contribution of this chapter is here summarized. First, we formalize the stability problem in a multi-user multi-contact setting. Then, we introduce a sufficient stability condition for the multidimensional haptic loop in the form of a single LMI problem. Moreover, we provide the parameterization of a class of stabilizing controllers satisfying structural constraints in terms of the solution of a sequence of LMI problems. This parameterization foreshadows the possibility of addressing several interesting performance problems in a computationally efficient way. Finally, the problem of optimizing controller transparency (in an H_∞ sense) within the proposed stabilizing controller class is considered.
The rest of the chapter is organized as follows. In Section 2 we report some preliminary and specific results on passivity-based analysis of multi-dimensional haptic systems; in Section 3 we derive the sought LMI stability condition, while in Section 4 we address controller parameterization. In Section 5 we formulate the controller transparency problem using the given parameterization. Finally, section 6 reports two illustrative application examples, and conclusions are drawn in Section 7.

Notation
For a square matrix X, $X > 0$ ($X < 0$) denotes positive (negative) definiteness, X^T denotes transpose and $\|X\|$ denotes some matrix norm of X. I_m is the $m \times m$ identity matrix. $X = \text{blockdiag}(X_1, \ldots, X_N)$ denotes a block-diagonal matrix with diagonal blocks $X_1, \ldots, X_N$. With $\mathcal{BD}(m; m_1, \ldots, m_N)$ we denote the set of $m \times m$ block-diagonal matrices whose N blocks have dimensions $m_1 \times m_1, \ldots, m_N \times m_N$, with $\sum_{i=1}^{N} m_i = m$. The latter notation is also used without ambiguity for block-diagonal transfer matrices of $m-$input, $m-$output linear systems and for generic $m-$input, $m-$output operators. With $\overline{\mathcal{BD}}(m_1 \times n_1, \ldots, m_N \times n_N)$ we indicate the set of non-square block-diagonal matrices with block sizes $m_i \times n_i$, $i = 1, \ldots, N$. For a transfer matrix G, $\|G\|_\infty$ denotes its H_∞ norm.

2. Preliminaries

2.1 Passivity results

The approach to stability analysis and controller design presented here exploits a generalization of the passivity framework in Miller et al. (1999)-Miller et al. (2004), which is based upon the concepts of output strict passivity (OSP) and input strict passivity (ISP) (Byrnes & Lin (1994); Lozano et al. (2000)). We find it convenient to employ a slightly different characterization of the concepts OSP and ISP in both the continuous and the discrete-time context. Let us introduce the following two definitions.

Definition 1. (continuous-time passivity). Let Σ be a continuous-time dynamical system with input vector $u(t) \in \mathbb{R}^m$, output vector $y(t) \in \mathbb{R}^m$, and state vector $\psi(t) \in \mathbb{R}^n$. If there exists a continuously differentiable positive definite function $V(\psi) : \mathbb{R}^n \to \mathbb{R}$ (called the *storage function*) and $m \times m$ symmetric matrices Δ and Φ such that along all system trajectories $(\psi(t), u(t), y(t))$, $t \in \mathbb{R}$, the following inequality holds

$$\dot{V}(\psi(t)) \le y(t)^T u(t) - y(t)^T \Delta y(t) - u(t)^T \Phi u(t),$$

then, system Σ is *passive* if $\Delta = \Phi = 0$, *output strictly passive with level* Δ ($\Delta-$OSP) if $\Delta > 0$, $\Phi = 0$, *input strictly passive with level* Φ ($\Phi-$ISP) if $\Delta = 0$, $\Phi > 0$, respectively.

Definition 2. (discrete-time passivity). Let Σ_d be a discrete-time dynamical system with input vector $u(k) \in \mathbb{R}^m$, output vector $y(k) \in \mathbb{R}^m$, and state vector $\psi(k) \in \mathbb{R}^n$. If there exists a positive definite function $V(\psi) : \mathbb{R}^n \to \mathbb{R}$ and $m \times m$ symmetric matrices Δ and Φ such that along all system trajectories $(\psi(k), u(k), y(k))$, $k \in \mathbb{N}$, the following inequality holds

$$\begin{aligned} \Delta V(\psi(k)) &= V(\psi(k+1)) - V(\psi(k)) \\ &\leq y(k)^T u(k) - y(k)^T \Delta y(k) - u(k)^T \Phi u(k), \end{aligned} \tag{1}$$

then the system is passive if $\Delta = \Phi = 0$, output strictly passive ($\Delta-$OSP) if $\Delta > 0,\ \Phi = 0$, input strictly passive ($\Phi-$ISP) if $\Delta = 0,\ \Phi > 0$, respectively.

Remark 1. Note that Definitions 1 and 2 differ from the standard notions of OSP/ISP in that the weights Δ and Φ are symmetric matrices instead of scalars.
Note that Δ and Φ need not necessarily be positive definite in this context: indeed, a dynamical system will be said to lack OSP (ISP) when the above definitions hold for non-positive definite Δ (Φ).

Let Σ_d be a discrete-time time-invariant linear system defined by the state space representation (A, B, C, D), where $A \in \mathbb{R}^{n \times n}$, $B \in \mathbb{R}^{n \times m}$, $C \in \mathbb{R}^{m \times n}$, $D \in \mathbb{R}^{m \times m}$. A straightforward extension of the standard Kalman-Yacubović-Popov lemma (Byrnes & Lin (1994)) applies.

Lemma 1. *System Σ_d is passive ($\Delta-$OSP,$\Phi-$ISP) if and only if there exists a symmetric matrix $P \in \mathbb{R}^n$ such that the following two matrix inequalities hold:*

$$\begin{gathered} P > 0 \\ \begin{bmatrix} A^T P A - P + C^T \Delta C & A^T P B - \frac{C^T}{2} + C^T \Delta D \\ B^T P A - \frac{C}{2} + D^T \Delta C & B^T P B - \frac{D + D^T}{2} + D^T \Delta D + \Phi \end{bmatrix} < 0. \end{gathered} \tag{2}$$

In order to address our problems, we find it convenient to look for an alternative formulation of the above result in which some of the quantities involved, in particular matrices B, D, and Δ^{-1}, appear linearly in the matrix inequalities that define the passivity condition (2). This can be accomplished via a Schur complement argument, as the following result shows.

Lemma 2. *Let $\Delta > 0$. System Σ_d is passive ($\Delta-$OSP, $\Phi-$ISP) if and only if there exist a symmetric matrix $Q \in \mathbb{R}^n$ and a matrix $R \in \mathbb{R}^{(n+2m) \times n}$ satisfying the constraints*

$$\begin{aligned} &(a) \quad Q > 0 \\ &(b) \quad \begin{bmatrix} Q & R^T \\ R & S \end{bmatrix} > 0 \\ &(c) \quad R = \begin{bmatrix} \frac{C}{2} \\ A \\ C \end{bmatrix} Q \end{aligned} \tag{3}$$

where

$$S = \begin{bmatrix} \frac{D^T + D}{2} + \Phi & B^T & D^T \\ B & Q & 0 \\ D & 0 & \Delta^{-1} \end{bmatrix}.$$

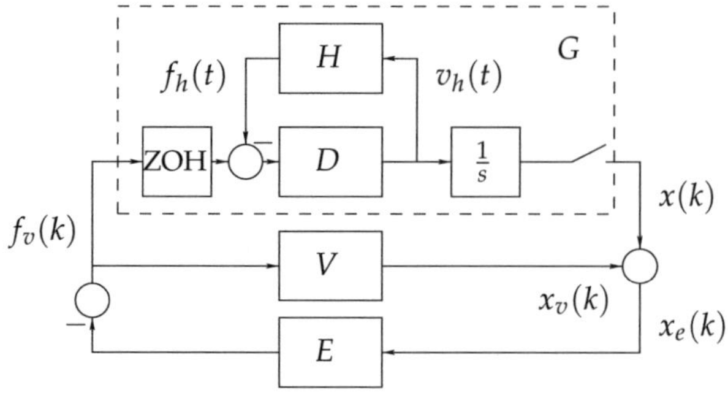

Fig. 1. Haptic loop

Proof. By pre- and post- multiplication of (3)(b) by the positive definite nonsingular matrix $\begin{bmatrix} Q^{-1} & 0 \\ 0 & I_{n+2m} \end{bmatrix}$ we get that (3)(b)-(3)(c) are equivalent to

$$\begin{bmatrix} Q^{-1} & \frac{C^T}{2} & A^T & C^T \\ \frac{C}{2} & \frac{D+D^T}{2}+\Phi & B^T & D^T \\ A & B & Q & 0 \\ C & D & 0 & \Delta^{-1} \end{bmatrix} > 0. \tag{4}$$

Taking the Schur complement with respect to the submatrix $\begin{bmatrix} Q & 0 \\ 0 & \Delta^{-1} \end{bmatrix} > 0$, (4) is in turn equivalent to

$$\begin{bmatrix} Q^{-1} & \frac{C^T}{2} \\ \frac{C}{2} & \frac{D+D^T}{2}+\Phi \end{bmatrix} - \begin{bmatrix} A^T & C^T \\ B^T & D^T \end{bmatrix} \begin{bmatrix} Q^{-1} & 0 \\ 0 & \Delta \end{bmatrix} \begin{bmatrix} A & B \\ C & D \end{bmatrix} > 0$$

which finally is equivalent to (2) once $P = Q^{-1} > 0$.

2.2 Modeling and passivity analysis of multi-contact haptic systems

We characterize multi-contact haptic systems starting from the well-established framework of Colgate & Schenkel (1997), Miller et al. (1999)-Miller et al. (2004). In that framework, a haptic system is modeled as a sampled-data system (with sampling period T) resulting from the interconnection of four main components described by suitable I/O mappings (see Fig. 1): a human operator block H, a haptic device block D, a computer-simulated virtual environment E, and a virtual coupling V, whose role is to act as a controller in order to ensure the stability of the closed-loop. The mappings H and D are continuous-time, while E and V are described by discrete-time dynamical systems.

In this chapter, we fit the above framework to the case of N haptic devices D_i, $i = 1, \ldots, N$, where each device D_i is assumed to have m_i degrees of freedom. One or several human operators are assumed to interact with each device and the N devices are coupled through a $m-$input, $m-$output (with $m = \sum_{i=1}^{N} m_i$) virtual environment E and through a virtual coupling V, which is described by a $m-$input, $m-$output dynamical system as well. In order to simplify our exposition, we assume the absence of delay in the computations and consider

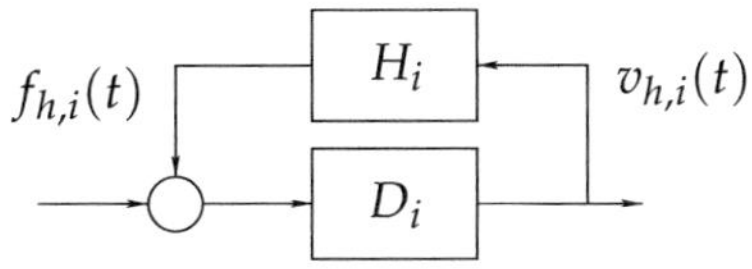

Fig. 2. Human-device interconnection

only the impedance causality representation of the haptic system (see Miller (2000)), although the proposed results are believed to be easily extendable to cover both the delayed case and admittance causality.
The interaction of each device D_i with the respective human operator(s) H_i can be described by the feedback loop in Fig. 2, in which $f_{h,i}(t) \in \mathbb{R}^{m_i}$ represents the generalized force vector and $v_{h,i}(t) \in \mathbb{R}^{m_i}$ is the corresponding generalized velocity vector.
It turns out that the overall system is described by the interconnection in Fig. 1, where

$$\begin{array}{r}H = \text{blockdiag}(H_1, \ldots, H_N) \in \mathcal{BD}(m; m_1, \ldots, m_N) \\ D = \text{blockdiag}(D_1, \ldots, D_N) \in \mathcal{BD}(m; m_1, \ldots, m_N) \\ f_h(t) = [f_{h,1}^T(t) \ \ldots \ f_{h,N}^T(t)]^T \\ v_h(t) = [v_{h,1}^T(t) \ \ldots \ v_{h,N}^T(t)]^T\end{array} \quad (5)$$

and where $x(k) \in \mathbb{R}^m$ and $f_v(k) \in \mathbb{R}^m$ are the sampled generalized device displacement vector and sampled generalized force feedback vector, respectively.

Remark 2. Note that no peculiar structure is enforced a-priori on V and E. However, due to decentralized computation requirements, it is often the case that the haptic device and virtual coupling are lumped together. This requirement can be easily taken into account by assuming that V has a suitable block-diagonal structure as well. Clearly, additional requirements arising from decentralized computation and communication restrictions may enforce different contraints on V. For the sake of simplicity, in the sequel we will assume that V may only be constrained to be block-diagonal, even though the proposed approach is simply generalizable to a wide range of different structures.

Passivity-based stability analysis of haptic systems is typically based on the assumption that both the human and the device can be seen as passive operators; in particular, when an impedance causality model is employed, the device is assumed to be OSP to some extent (Miller et al. (2000)). The OSP level pertaining to a given device can be related to the amount of damping introduced into the system by the device itself. The problem of its computation has been addressed in Miller et al. (1999) for linear devices via a robust stability argument, while in Miller et al. (2004) it is shown, using a standard Lagrangian description of the device, that the OSP level can be related to dissipation in joint space. The latter results are easily generalizable to the OSP notion in Definition 1.
Motivated by the above observations, the following assumption is made.

Assumption 1. (a) Each device block D_i is Δ_{D_i}−OSP, and (b) each human block H_i is a passive continuous-time m_i-input, m_i-output operator.

The following well-known result on passivity of general interconnected systems holds also in view of the OSP notion in Definition 1.

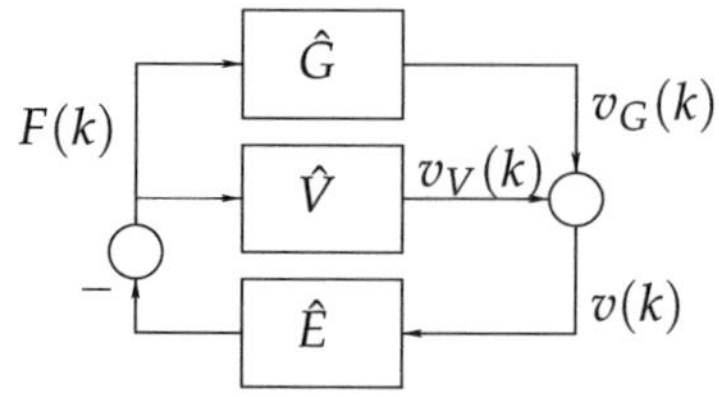

Fig. 3. Transformed haptic loop

Lemma 3. *Let Assumption 1 hold. Then, the feedback interconnection of D_i with H_i is also $\Delta_{D_i}-OSP$.*

Given the block-diagonal structure of the operators D and H and in view of Assumption 1 and Lemma 3, it is almost predictable that their feedback interconnection gives rise to a Δ_D-OSP system where Δ_D has precisely the same structure. Indeed, the following result holds.

Theorem 1. *Let Assumption 1 hold. Then, the feedback interconnection of D and H is Δ_D-OSP where*

$$\Delta_D = \text{blockdiag}(\Delta_{D_1}, \ldots, \Delta_{D_N}). \tag{6}$$

Proof. For each i, a positive definite storage function $V(\psi_i)$ exists such that $\dot{V}_i(\psi_i(t)) < f_{h,i}^T(t)v_{h,i}(t) - v_{h,i}^T(t)\Delta_{D_i}v_{h,i}(t)$, where ψ_i is the state vector of the interconnection of H_i and D_i. Therefore, taking $V(\psi_1, \ldots, \psi_N) = \sum_{i=1}^N V_i(\psi_i)$ one gets that $V(\psi_1, \ldots, \psi_N)$ is positive definite and that

$$\begin{aligned} &\dot{V}(\psi_1(t), \ldots \psi_N(t)) \\ &< \textstyle\sum_{i=1}^N [f_{h,i}^T(t)v_{h,i}(t) - v_{h,i}^T(t)\Delta_{D_i}v_{h,i}(t)] \\ &= f_h^T(t)v_h(t) - v_h^T(t)\Delta_D v_h(t) \end{aligned}$$

with Δ_D as in (6).

Let G denote the discrete-time mapping describing the ZOH-equivalent of the interconnection of H and D (see again Fig. 1), and consider a loop transformation which places the system into the form of Fig. 3, where

$$\hat{G} = \frac{z-1}{Tz}[G+K],\ \hat{V} = \frac{z-1}{Tz}[V-K],\ \hat{E} = \frac{Tz}{z-1}E \tag{7}$$

being K a constant $m \times m$ matrix. Clearly, the loop transformation in (7) is a MIMO version of the one employed in Miller et al. (1999; 2000; 2004). The resulting interconnection of $\hat{G}$, $\hat{V}$ and $\hat{E}$ is a purely discrete-time system in which the transformed components can be characterized in terms of their OSP or ISP passivity levels according to Definition 2, leading to the following result.

Theorem 2. *Consider the haptic loop in Fig. 1 and its transformation in Fig. 3, with $\hat{G}$, $\hat{V}$, $\hat{E}$ as in (7). Suppose that Assumption 1 holds and let*

$$K = \frac{T}{2}\Delta_D^{-1} \tag{8}$$

with Δ_D as in (6). Then, $\hat{G}$ is (discrete-time) $\Delta_{\hat{G}}-OSP$ with

$$\Delta_{\hat{G}} = \Delta_D. \tag{9}$$

Proof. This result extends Lemma 2 in Miller et al. (2004) quite straightforwardly, and the proof is omitted.

Remark 3. It is worth noting that both $\Delta_{\hat{G}}$ and $\hat{G}$ itself have the block-diagonal structure of H and D. This is a simple consequence of (9), (7),(8), and the fact that matrix inversion preserves the block-diagonal structure.

3. LMI stability condition

A generally accepted notion of stability in the haptic context is that the velocity $v_h(t)$ of the device must converge to zero in steady state: in turn, this condition ensures that the system is oscillation free and that all states such as the device position remain bounded.
In Miller et al. (2000) it is shown that if the interconnection of transformed blocks $\hat{G}$, $\hat{V}$, and $\hat{E}$ is asymptotically stable, then the generalized velocity vector $v_h(t)$ presented to the user(s) goes to zero in steady state. Moreover, based on standard passivity results for parallel and feedback interconnected systems, suitable bounds are provided on the (scalar) OSP/ISP levels of the transformed blocks in order to guarantee stability. This way, also the case of non-passive virtual environments (i.e., of virtual environments lacking a certain amount of ISP) can be accounted for.
The following result provides a stability criterion for the haptic system under investigation that generalizes the one in Miller et al. (2000) by exploiting the OSP and ISP notions in Definition 2. The resulting stability conditions are expressed in matrix inequality form.

Theorem 3. *Suppose that there exist symmetric matrices $\Delta_{\hat{V}}$ and $\Phi_{\hat{E}}$ such that*

1. *$\hat{V}$ is $\Delta_{\hat{V}}$−OSP,*
2. *$\hat{E} + \Phi_{\hat{E}}$ is passive, i.e., $\hat{E}$ is $(-\Phi_{\hat{E}})$−ISP.*
3. *the following matrix inequality holds:*

$$\begin{bmatrix} \Delta_D - \Phi_{\hat{E}} & -\Phi_{\hat{E}} \\ -\Phi_{\hat{E}} & \Delta_{\hat{V}} - \Phi_{\hat{E}} \end{bmatrix} > 0 \tag{10}$$

Then, the signal $v_h(t)$ presented to the human operator goes to zero in steady state.

Proof. Let $\psi_{\hat{G}}, \psi_{\hat{V}}, \psi_{\hat{E}}$ be the state vectors of $\hat{G}, \hat{V}, \hat{E}$, respectively. By conditions 1. and 2., there exist positive definite storage functions $V_{\hat{G}}(\psi_{\hat{G}})$, $V_{\hat{V}}(\psi_{\hat{V}})$, and $V_{\hat{E}}(\psi_{\hat{E}})$ such that

$$\begin{array}{r} \Delta V_G(\psi_{\hat{G}}(k)) \leq F^T(k)v_G(k) - v_G^T(k)\Delta_D v_G(k) \\ \Delta V_V(\psi_{\hat{V}}(k)) \leq F^T(k)v_V(k) - v_V^T(k)\Delta_{\hat{V}} v_V(k) \\ \Delta V_E(\psi_{\hat{E}}(k)) \leq -F^T(k)v(k) + v^T(k)\Phi_{\hat{E}} v(k) \end{array}$$

Taking $V_{\hat{G}+\hat{V}}(\psi_{\hat{G}}, \psi_{\hat{V}}) = V_{\hat{G}}(\psi_{\hat{G}}) + V_{\hat{V}}(\psi_{\hat{V}})$ we get

$$\begin{array}{c} \Delta V_{\hat{G}+\hat{V}}(\psi_{\hat{G}}(k), \psi_{\hat{V}}(k)) \leq F^T(k)v(k) - v^T(k)\Phi_{\hat{E}} v(k) - \\ \begin{bmatrix} v_G^T(k) & v_V^T(k) \end{bmatrix} \begin{bmatrix} \Delta_{\hat{G}} - \Phi_{\hat{E}} & -\Phi_{\hat{E}} \\ -\Phi_{\hat{E}} & \Delta_{\hat{V}} - \Phi_{\hat{E}} \end{bmatrix} \begin{bmatrix} v_G(k) \\ v_V(k) \end{bmatrix} \end{array} \tag{11}$$

and hence, by (10)

$$\Delta V_{\hat{G}+\hat{V}}(\psi_{\hat{G}}(k), \psi_{\hat{V}}(k)) \leq F^T(k)v(k) - v^T(k)\Phi_{\hat{E}} v(k)$$

i.e., the parallel interconnection of $\hat{G}$ and $\hat{V}$ is $\Phi_{\hat{E}}-$OSP.
Finally, taking $V(\psi_{\hat{G}}, \psi_{\hat{V}}, \psi_{\hat{E}}) = V_{\hat{G}+\hat{V}}(\psi_{\hat{G}}, \psi_{\hat{V}}) + V_{\hat{E}}(\psi_{\hat{E}})$ it holds that $V(\psi_{\hat{G}}, \psi_{\hat{V}}, \psi_{\hat{E}})$ is positive definite and moreover

$$\Delta V(\psi_{\hat{G}}(k), \psi_{\hat{V}}(k), \psi_{\hat{E}}(k)) < 0$$

i.e., $V(\psi_{\hat{G}}, \psi_{\hat{V}}, \psi_{\hat{E}})$ is a Lyapunov function that proves asymptotic stability of the transformed closed-loop system, and therefore that the velocity vector $v_h(t)$ goes to zero in steady state.

4. Stabilizing structured virtual coupling parameterization

We are now interested in providing a computationally viable parameterization of a class of stabilizing virtual coupling systems that have a given structure. More specifically, we seek the parameterization of a set $\mathcal{V}$ of linear virtual coupling systems V of given order n which share the following properties:

(R1) V stabilizes the haptic loop,

(R2) V has an arbitrarily assigned block-diagonal structure, i.e., $V = \text{blockdiag}(V_1, \ldots, V_{\bar{N}}) \in \mathcal{BD}(m; \bar{m}_1, \ldots, \bar{m}_{\bar{N}})$, where each block V_i is a linear system with state space dimension $\bar{n}_i$, $\sum_{i=1}^{\bar{N}} \bar{n}_i = n$, for given $\bar{N}, \bar{m}_i, \bar{n}_i, i = 1, \ldots, \bar{N}$.

Remark 4. The block-diagonal structure of V need not necessarily be related to the structure of the device block D, although it may be convenient to enforce a virtual coupling structure that reflects actual implementation constraints such as controller decentralization.

Let (A_V, B_V, C_V, D_V) denote a state space representation of V. Requirement (R2) is equivalent to the condition that $A_V \in \mathcal{BD}(n; \bar{n}_1, \ldots, \bar{n}_{\bar{N}})$, $B_V \in \overline{\mathcal{BD}}(\bar{n}_1 \times \bar{m}_1, \ldots \bar{n}_{\bar{N}} \times \bar{m}_{\bar{N}})$, $C_V \in \overline{\mathcal{BD}}(\bar{m}_1 \times \bar{n}_1, \ldots \bar{m}_{\bar{N}} \times \bar{n}_{\bar{N}})$ and $D_V \in \mathcal{BD}(m; \bar{m}_1, \ldots, \bar{m}_{\bar{N}})$.

A straightforward computation yields the following state space representation of the transformed virtual coupling $\hat{V}$:

$$\begin{aligned} A_{\hat{V}} &= \begin{bmatrix} A_V & -\frac{1}{T}B_V \\ 0 & 0 \end{bmatrix}, \quad B_{\hat{V}} = \begin{bmatrix} \frac{1}{T}B_V \\ I_m \end{bmatrix}, \\ C_{\hat{V}} &= \begin{bmatrix} C_V & -\frac{1}{T}D_V + \frac{1}{T}K \end{bmatrix}, \quad D_{\hat{V}} = \frac{1}{T}D_V - \frac{1}{T}K. \end{aligned} \tag{12}$$

We are now ready to state the main design result, which provides the parameterization of a set $\mathcal{V}$ of controllers that satisfy requirements (R1) and (R2).

Theorem 4. *Consider the haptic loop L, let Δ_D be the device OSP level as in (6) and $(A_{\hat{E}}, B_{\hat{E}}, C_{\hat{E}}, D_{\hat{E}})$ be a state space realization of $E(z)\frac{Tz}{z-1}$. Let $P, \Delta_{\hat{V}}, \Phi_{\hat{E}}, \Sigma_{\hat{V}}, Q, Y, A_V, B_V, C_V, D_V$ be any solution of the LMI problem*

$$\begin{aligned} &A_V \in \mathcal{BD}(n; \bar{n}_1, \ldots, \bar{n}_{\bar{N}}) \\ &C_V \in \overline{\mathcal{BD}}(\bar{m}_1 \times \bar{n}_1, \ldots \bar{m}_{\bar{N}} \times \bar{n}_{\bar{N}}) \\ &B_V \in \overline{\mathcal{BD}}(\bar{n}_1 \times \bar{m}_1, \ldots \bar{n}_{\bar{N}} \times \bar{m}_{\bar{N}}) \\ &D_V \in \mathcal{BD}(m; \bar{m}_1, \ldots, \bar{m}_{\bar{N}}) \end{aligned} \tag{13}$$

$$\begin{aligned}
&P > 0\\
&\Delta_{\hat{V}} > 0\\
&\begin{bmatrix} A_{\hat{E}}^T P A_{\hat{E}} - P & A_{\hat{E}}^T P B_{\hat{E}} - \frac{C_{\hat{E}}^T}{2} \\ B_{\hat{E}}^T P A_{\hat{E}} - \frac{C_{\hat{E}}}{2} & B_{\hat{E}}^T P B_{\hat{E}} - \frac{D_{\hat{E}}}{2} - \frac{D_{\hat{E}}^T}{2} - \Phi_{\hat{E}} \end{bmatrix} < 0 \\
&\begin{bmatrix} \Delta_D - \Phi_{\hat{E}} & -\Phi_{\hat{E}} \\ -\Phi_{\hat{E}} & \Delta_{\hat{V}} - \Phi_{\hat{E}} \end{bmatrix} > 0
\end{aligned} \tag{14}$$

$$\begin{aligned}
&Q > 0\\
&\begin{bmatrix} Y & R^T \\ R & S \end{bmatrix} > 0
\end{aligned} \tag{15}$$

where

$$R = \begin{bmatrix} \frac{C_{\hat{V}}}{2} \\ A_{\hat{V}} \\ C_{\hat{V}} \end{bmatrix}$$
$$S = \begin{bmatrix} \frac{D_{\hat{V}} + D_{\hat{V}}^T}{2} & B_{\hat{V}}^T & D_{\hat{V}}^T \\ B_{\hat{V}} & Q & 0 \\ D_{\hat{V}} & 0 & \Sigma_{\hat{V}} \end{bmatrix} \tag{16}$$

being $A_{\hat{V}}, B_{\hat{V}}, C_{\hat{V}}, D_{\hat{V}}$ as in (12), with the further non-convex constraint

$$\Sigma_{\hat{V}} = \Delta_{\hat{V}}^{-1}, \; Y = Q^{-1}. \tag{17}$$

Then, the virtual coupling V defined by the state space representation (A_V, B_V, C_V, D_V) has the structure $\mathcal{BD}(m; \bar{m}_1, \ldots, \bar{m}_{\bar{N}})$ and stabilizes the haptic loop L.

Proof. Constraints (13) enforce that the virtual coupling has the required structure. Moreover, (14) and (15),(16),(17) ensure, respectively, that the OSP level $\Delta_{\hat{V}}$ satisfies the loop stability condition of Theorem 3 for some $\Phi_{\hat{E}}$ and that it can be achieved by a virtual coupling V of the given structure; the latter property follows from Lemma 2.

Remark 5. The set $\mathcal{V}$ parameterized via Theorem 4 clearly does not encompass all linear controllers of the given structure satisfying (R1) and (R2). Nevertheless, the proposed parameterization has the advantage of being linear in the design parameters $(A_V, B_V, C_V' D_V)$. This is a key property that allows for exploiting the proposed parameterization to address performance problems, as it will be further explained in Section 5 below.

4.1 Tackling the non-convex constraint (17)

The cone complementarity linearization algorithm in ElGhaoui et al. (1997) can be employed successfully to reformulate the LMI problem (13)-(16) with the additional non-convex condition (17) as a sequence of LMI optimization problems. We illustrate this reformulation for the basic problem of checking feasibility of (13)-(17), i.e., of checking the existence of a stabilizing controller of the proposed class, although this method can be seamlessly incorporated in several possible performance problems involving the controller parameterization in Theorem 4.

1. Fix a tolerance ε and set $j = 1$.

2. Find a feasible solution W, Z of the relaxed problem (13)-(16) with the convex constraint

$$\begin{bmatrix} W & I \\ I & Z \end{bmatrix} > 0 \tag{18}$$

where

$$W = \begin{bmatrix} \Sigma_{\hat{V}} & 0 \\ 0 & Q \end{bmatrix}, \quad Z = \begin{bmatrix} \Delta_{\hat{V}} & 0 \\ 0 & Y \end{bmatrix}, \tag{19}$$

if no solution exists, then exit and declare the problem infeasible.

3. Fix $W^j = W^{j-1}$, $Z^j = Z^{j-1}$, and find a solution W^{j+1}, Z^{j+1} of the LMI optimization problem

$$\begin{array}{c} \min \ \text{trace}(W^j Z + Z^j W) \\ \text{subject to (13)-(16),(18),(19)} \end{array}$$

4. If $\|W^{j+1}Z^{j+1} - I\| < \varepsilon$ then output the solution, otherwise set $j = j+1$ and go to 3) unless a maximum number of iterations has been reached.

4.2 Spring-damper virtual coupling design

In order to provide a qualitative evaluation of the impact of the virtual coupling on the the sensation felt by the users during haptic interaction, it is an established practice to design the virtual coupling as a discretized spring-damper system Miller (2000); Miller et al. (2000).
In order to generalize this notion to the multi-dimensional case, let us consider a virtual coupling V of the form

$$V = V(z) = \left[\mathbf{K} + \mathbf{B}\frac{z-1}{Tz}\right]^{-1} \tag{20}$$

where $\mathbf{K} \in \mathbb{R}^{m\times m}$ and $\mathbf{B} \in \mathbb{R}^{m\times m}$ will be referred to as the stiffness and damping matrix, respectively. The transfer matrix $V(z)$ in (20) models a network of interconnected virtual springs and dampers that connect the contact endpoints to each other according to the structure of matrices $\mathbf{K}$ and $\mathbf{B}$. Note that enforcing $\mathbf{K}$ and $\mathbf{B}$ to have some block diagonal structure results in the controller V having the same structure.
For this special case, a simple computation shows that a state-space realization of V is of order m and has the form (A_V, B_V, C_V, D_V) where

$$\begin{array}{c} B_V = TA_V \\ D_V = TC_V \end{array} \tag{21}$$

and the pair (A_V, C_V) is related one-to-one to the pair $(\mathbf{K}, \mathbf{B})$ as follows:

$$\mathbf{K} = \frac{1}{T}(I_m - A_V)C_V^{-1}, \quad \mathbf{B} = A_V C_V^{-1}. \tag{22}$$

In (22), note that $(\mathbf{K}, \mathbf{B}) \in \mathcal{BD}(m; \bar{m}_1, \ldots, \bar{m}_{\bar{N}})$ if and only if $(A_V, C_V) \in \mathcal{BD}(m; \bar{m}_1, \ldots, \bar{m}_{\bar{N}})$. Therefore, the parameterization of a set of stabilizing spring-damper controllers having the structure $\mathcal{BD}(m; \bar{m}_1, \ldots, \bar{m}_{\bar{N}})$ is readily obtained from Theorem 4 by taking A_V, B_V, C_V and D_V to be matrices of $\mathcal{BD}(m; \bar{m}_1, \ldots, \bar{m}_{\bar{N}})$ satisfying the linear equations (21). Obviously, the design parameters reduce to A_V and C_V only.

5. A performance problem: virtual coupling transparency

An important performance objective in a haptic system is the transparency of the virtual coupling. When a controller is required in order to guarantee stability, it is desirable that its effect on the dynamics of the virtual environment, as it is seen by the human-device block, be minimized. This amounts to the requirement that the transfer function (admittance) of the $E - V$ loop between the sampled displacement x and the virtual force f_v (see Fig. 1) be as close as possibile to the virtual environment admittance according to some criterion.
We have that

$$f_v = -\mathbf{F}(E, V)x$$

where $\mathbf{F}(E, V)$ is given by

$$\mathbf{F}(E, V) = (I_m + EV)^{-1}E.$$

The problem of designing a stabilizing virtual coupling V ensuring the transparency condition, i.e., $\mathbf{F}(E, V) \approx E$, is most effectively formulated in the context of H_∞ control theory according to two different criteria.
Closed-loop H_∞ design. The transparency problem can be cast as the problem of finding a stabilizing V such that the weighted $\infty-$norm of $(\mathbf{F}(E, V) - E)$ be less than a given (possibly minimum) μ, i.e.,

$$\|\mathbf{W}_1(\mathbf{F}(E, V) - E)\mathbf{W}_2\|_\infty < \mu \tag{23}$$

where $\mathbf{W}_1$ and $\mathbf{W}_2$ are transfer functions that allow for weighing the admittance error differently at different frequencies. A similar formulation was used in Naghshtabrizi & Hespanha (2006).

H_∞ loop shaping. The condition $\mathbf{F}(E, V) \approx E$ can be achieved by "shaping" the loop gain EV so that it is small at given frequencies. This amounts to the requirement

$$\|\mathbf{L}(E, V, \mathbf{W}_1, \mathbf{W}_2)\|_\infty < \gamma \tag{24}$$

where

$$\mathbf{L}(E, V, \mathbf{W}_1, \mathbf{W}_2) = \mathbf{W}_1 EV\mathbf{W}_2 = \mathbf{W}_1 EV\mathbf{W}_2 \tag{25}$$

for given γ and weighing functions $\mathbf{W}_1$ and $\mathbf{W}_2$.
These problems fall into the class of standard H_∞ control problems, and can be solved by means of the combination of LMI-based procedures. The computational details are out of the scope of this chapter, but it is absolutely important to note that the key requirement in these schemes is that a controller parameterization which is linear in V be available, as it is indeed the case with Theorem 4.

6. Examples

Example 1. *We consider a haptic system in which the interaction with a 3−DOF linear virtual environment E is performed through three 1−DOF haptic devices d_x, d_y and d_z.*
According to our characterization, each block of the haptic loop L is described by a m−input, m−output system with $m = 3$.
Let the virtual environment E be the backward Euler discretized version with sample period $T = 0.001s$ of the mechanical system in Fig. 4, where $x_e = [x_{e,1}\ x_{e_2}\ x_{e_3}]^T$ and $f_v = [f_{v,1}\ f_{v_2}\ f_{v_3}]^T$. Assume the parameter values $B_1 = 0.1$, $B_2 = 0.2$, $B_3 = 0.3$, $B = 0.5$, $k_1 = 3800$, $k_2 = 3500$, $k_3 = 3300$, $k = 2600$, $M = 3$, in standard measurement units.
We assume that the three haptic devices are characterized by the OSP levels $\Delta_{d_x} = \Delta_{d_y} = \Delta_{d_z} = 1.37$.

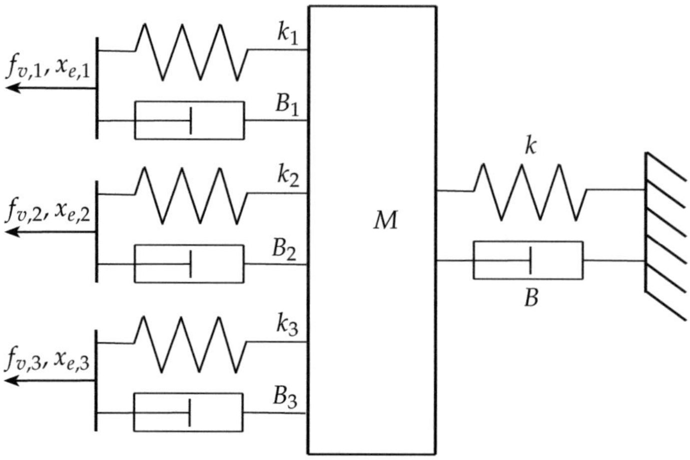

Fig. 4. Example 1: Virtual environment model

These values are computed according to the results in Miller et al. (2004) from the identified dynamics along one axis of Force Dimension's Omega^{TM} *device.*
In the absence of virtual coupling, the haptic system is not stable for all passive human operator blocks as shown by the simulation in Figure 5, in which the human operator is modeled by the following passive continuous-time linear system

$$H(s) = \begin{bmatrix} \frac{0.02(s^2+60s+1000)}{s^2+10.3s+100} & 0.1 & 0.1 \\ 0.1 & \frac{0.02(s^2+60s+1000)}{s^2+10.3s+100} & 0.1 \\ 0.1 & 0.1 & \frac{0.02(s^2+60s+1000)}{s^2+10.3s+100} \end{bmatrix}.$$

We look for a decentralized spring-damper virtual coupling as described in Section 4.2.
A feasible solution is given by

$$\begin{aligned} \mathbf{K} &= \begin{bmatrix} 704.9058 & 0 & 0 \\ 0 & 704.9336 & 0 \\ 0 & 0 & 704.8754 \end{bmatrix}, \\ \mathbf{B} &= \begin{bmatrix} 0.0372 & 0 & 0 \\ 0 & 0.0372 & 0 \\ 0 & 0 & 0.0372 \end{bmatrix}. \end{aligned} \tag{26}$$

Without enforcing the decentralization constraint on V*, we get the following feasible solution.*

$$\begin{aligned} \mathbf{K} &= \begin{bmatrix} 660.4367 & -0.2614 & -0.3282 \\ -0.2614 & 660.4181 & -0.3429 \\ -0.3282 & -0.3429 & 660.4602 \end{bmatrix} \\ \mathbf{B} &= \begin{bmatrix} 0.1674 & -0.0003 & -0.0005 \\ -0.0003 & 0.1685 & -0.0006 \\ -0.0005 & -0.0006 & 0.1675 \end{bmatrix}. \end{aligned} \tag{27}$$

Figures 6 and 7 show simulations of the haptic system with decentralized and centralized virtual coupling as in (26) and (27).

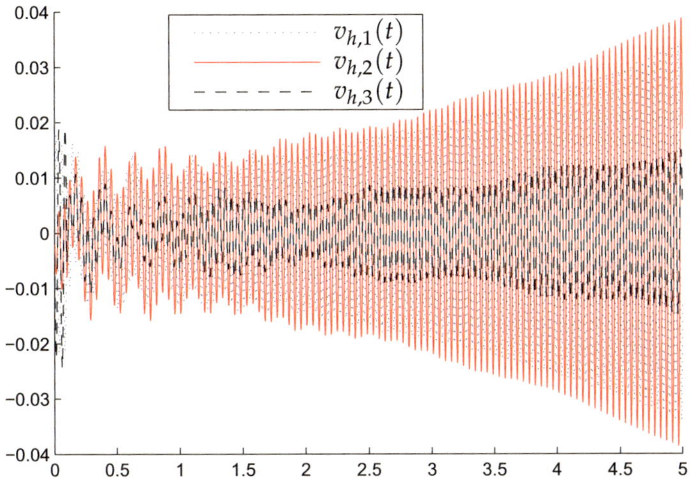

Fig. 5. Example 1: simulation of haptic loop dynamics (velocity vector) without virtual coupling.

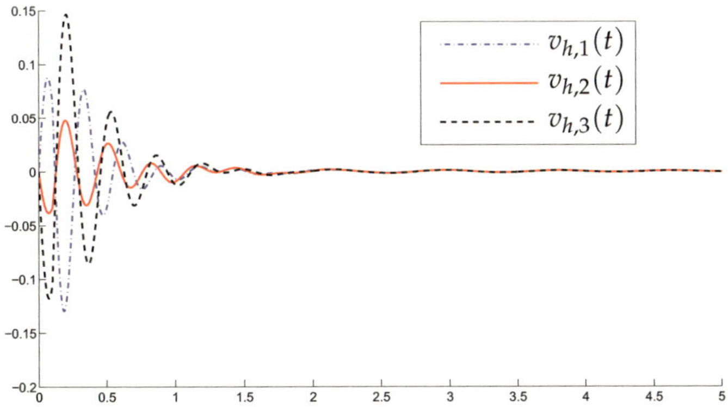

Fig. 6. Example 1, case (i): Simulation of haptic loop dynamics (velocity vector) with decentralized virtual coupling (26).

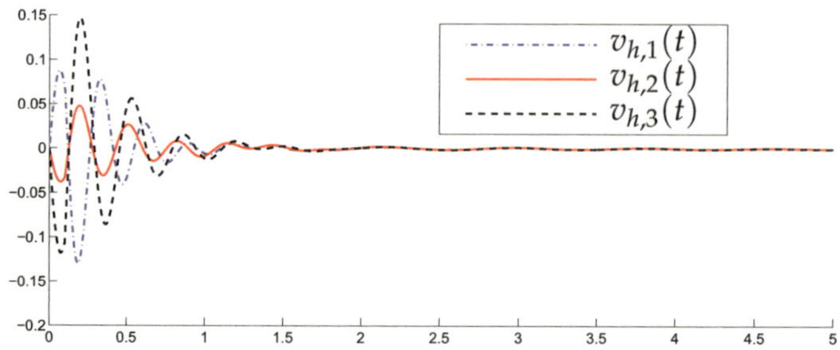

Fig. 7. Example 1, case (i): simulation of haptic loop dynamics (velocity vector) with centralized virtual coupling (27).

Example 2. *Let us consider case (i) in the previous example. For this case, we are interested in computing a (decentralized) spring-damper controller that stabilizes the haptic loop while optimizing controller transparency. To this purpose, we solve the loop shaping problem in (24),(25). In particular, we try to minimize γ such that (24),(25) hold subject to the proposed controller parameterization. As weighing functions we choose*

$$\mathbf{W}_1 = w(z)I_3, \quad \mathbf{W}_2 = I_3$$

where $w(z)$ is the backward Euler discretization of the first-order filter

$$w(s) = \frac{1}{1 + s/\omega_0}, \quad \omega_0 = 125$$

so that the virtual coupling transparency requirement is emphasized in the frequency range 0–20 Hz. By proceeding by bisection on γ and iteratively solving the loop shaping problem, solutions are found down to the value $\gamma = 12.6$, and the corresponding virtual coupling is given by:

$$\begin{array}{c} \mathbf{K} = \begin{bmatrix} 2.7355 & 0 & 0 \\ 0 & 2.7346 & 0 \\ 0 & 0 & 2.7355 \end{bmatrix} 10^3, \\ \mathbf{B} = \begin{bmatrix} -0.2648 & 0 & 0 \\ 0 & -0.2798 & 0 \\ 0 & 0 & -0.2838 \end{bmatrix} 10^{-3} \end{array} . \tag{28}$$

A simulation is shown in Fig. 8.

7. Conclusion

In this chapter, the problem of stability assessment and virtual coupling design for haptic interaction systems involving multiple devices and human operators has been addressed in a passivity-based LMI framework. A class of stabilizing virtual coupling controllers which can be parameterized via a sequence of LMI problems has been introduced. Such a class is quite flexible, since it allows for taking into account decentralization constraints imposed on the control system. Finally, the solution of the controller transparency problem within this class has been outlined.

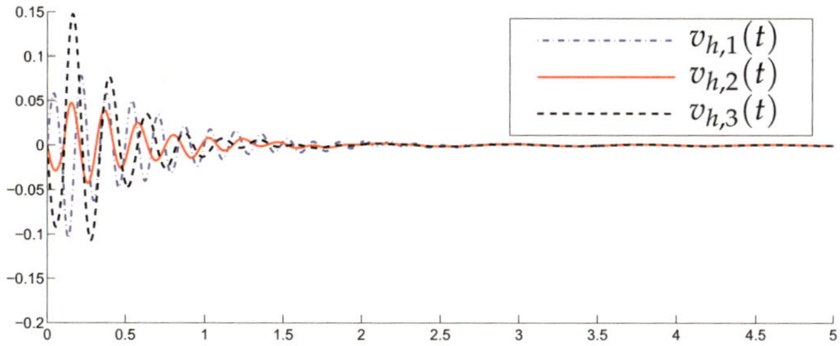

Fig. 8. Example 2: simulation of haptic loop dynamics (velocity vector) with the virtual coupling in (28).

8. References

Barbagli, F., Frisoli, A., Salisbury, K. & Bergamasco, M. (2004). Simulating human fingers: a soft finger proxy model and algorithm, *Proc. Haptics Symposium*, Chicago, IL, USA.

Barbagli, F., Prattichizzo, D. & Salisbury, J. (2005a). *Multi-Point Physical Interaction with Real and Virtual Objects*, Vol. 18 of *STAR, Springer Tracks in Advanced Robotics*, Springer Verlag, Berlin Heidelberg.

Barbagli, F., Prattichizzo, D. & Salisbury, K. (2005b). A multirate approach to haptic interaction with deformable objects single and multipoint contacts, *International Journal of Robotics Research* **4**(29): 703–715.

Byrnes, C. & Lin, W. (1994). Losslessness, feedback equivalence, and the global stabilization of discrete-time nonlinear systems, *IEEE Transactions on Automatic Control* **39**(1): 83–98.

Colgate, J. & Schenkel, G. (1997). Passivity of a class of sampled-data systems: application to haptic interfaces, *Journal of robotic systems* **14**(1): 37–47.

ElGhaoui, L., Oustry, F. & AitRami, M. (1997). A cone complementarity linearization algorithm for static output feedback and related problems, *IEEE Transactions on Automatic Control* **42**(8): 1171–1175.

Lozano, R., Brogliato, B., Egeland, O. & Maschke, B. (2000). *Dissipative systems analysis and control*, Springer Verlag.

Melder, N. & Harwin, W. S. (2003). Improved rendering for multi-finger manipulation using friction cone based god-objects, *Proc. Eurohaptics Conference*, pp. 82–85.

Miller, B. E. (2000). *Stability of haptic systems with nonpassive virtual environments*, Ph.D. Thesis, Nortwestern University.

Miller, B. E., Colgate, J. E. & Freeman, R. (1999). Computational delay and free mode environment design for haptic display, *ASME Dyn. Syst. Cont. Div.*

Miller, B. E., Colgate, J. E. & Freeman, R. (2000). Guaranteed stability of haptic systems with nonlinear virtual environments, *IEEE Transactions on Robotics and Automation* **16**(6): 712–719.

Miller, B. E., Colgate, J. E. & Freeman, R. (2004). On the role of dissipation in haptic systems, *IEEE Transactions on Robotics* **20**(4): 768–771.

Minsky, M., Ouh-Young, M. & Steele, O. (1990). Feeling and seeing: issue in force display, *ACM Trans. Comput.-Human Interactions* **24**(2): 235–243.

Naghshtabrizi, P. & Hespanha, J. P. (2006). Designing transparent stabilizing haptic controllers, *IEEE American Control Conference*, Minneapolis, MI, USA.

Salisbury, J., Conti, F. & Barbagli, F. (2004). Haptic rendering: introductory concepts, *IEEE Computer Graphics and Animation* **24**: 24–32.

Stramigioli, S., Secchi, C., van der Schaft, A. J. & Fantuzzi, C. (2005). Sampled data systems passivity and discrete port-hamiltonian systems, *IEEE Transactions on Robotics* **21**(4): 574–586.

9

Analysis and Experimental Study of a 4-DOF Haptic Device

Ma and Payandeh
Simon Fraser University
Canada

1. Introduction

This chapter presents a new configuration of a haptic device based on a 4-DOF hybrid spherical geometry with a design of a distributed computational platform. The Spherical Parallel Ball Support (SPBS) type device, as it is referred to, consists of a particular design feature with the intersecting joint axes of both active and passive spherical joints. The orientation of the device is determined through the active spherical joint using a special class of spherical 3-DOF parallel geometry. In addition, the passive spherical joint (ball and socket configuration) is introduced in the design to increase the mechanical fidelity of the device. A new forward and inverse kinematics analysis are presented. The study is motivated by deriving a mathematical model and a closed-form solution of the kinematics of the proposed device configuration. A novel desktop computational platform is proposed and studied for creation of haptic feedback. The experimental studies are presented by specifying and demonstrating a virtual wall as a performance-benchmarking tool and aimed to verify a desirable update rate of 1 kHz or more for the haptic effect. A computational algorithm is devised by using a reconfigurable experimental setup that would achieve the desired haptic effect. This framework consists of the 4-DOF prototype, a host computer, and a data acquisition system which uses a microprocessor, a FPGA, integrated circuits and pulse-width-modulation. Such architecture can offer a novel distributed system for tele-operation over the Internet and haptic rendering of deformable objects. Through analysis of the experimental setup, key parameters have been identified for synthesis of a future tele-operation environment.

1.1 Objectives

The major objective of this research is to design, develop and experiment with a novel haptic hardware environment. The design of this architecture and its building blocks are aimed to be reconfigurable, programmable, portable and scalable such that it supports the integration towards a distributed system framwork of a surgical simulator. In this work, we first specified the haptic effect that we wanted to create as an objective. We then demonstrated a virtual wall as a performance-benchmarking set-up and devised a computational algorithm to verify the desirable update rate for the haptic effect using our custom-designed experimental setup and the force-feedback device (Ma & Payandeh, 2008).

The Spherical Parallel Ball Support type device is a prototype based on a 4-DOF hybrid spherical geometry. The orientation of the device is determined by the mobile platform on the active spherical joint using a special class of spherical 3-DOF parallel geometry. In parallel mechanism configuration, the moving end effector is connected to a fixed reference base via multiple kinematic chains. Any two chains thus form a closed kinematic chain which is different in topology in comparison with open loop mechanisms such as the serial robotic arm. Parallel robots (such as the Stewart platform and the Delta robot) usually have wider mechanical bandwidth than traditional articulated robots. This is due to the location of the actuators which can be mounted on the supporting base which as a result can reduce the floating mass of the mechanism. However, it is also known that computational complexities involved in obtaining various kinematic solutions such as forward kinematics can result in more than one unique solution. Our study is motivated by deriving a computational model which can result in a closed-form solution of the kinematics for our proposed haptic device configuration.

In addition, we designed and developed a modular and distributed scheme aiming at a parallelization of the main components of haptic interaction tasks (haptic rendering). We present the design and performance study of a data acquisition system (DAS) which is adapted into our framework. The DAS is reconfigurable and capable of controlling the SPBS haptic device at a fast update rate. The local interconnection framework consists of the host control computer, the custom-designed data acquisition system, and the haptic device. The UDP/IP and TCP/IP socket interface are used for communications between the DAS and a host computer in order to collect performance benchmarking results.

1.2 Contributions

The major contributions of the research are summarized below.
Analysis of a 4-DOF haptic device and derivation of a closed-form solution: a mathematical model and analysis of a new device geometry/configuration is presented. The forward and inverse kinematic solutions and static force mapping are derived.

A distributed computational system framework: a novel desktop computational platform for haptic control of the device is developed. Such architecture can offer a novel distributed system for tele-operation over the Internet and haptic rendering of deformable objects using medical imaging data. In addition, software application development is designed to target multiple operating systems support. This provides the flexibility of the targeted operating systems (Windows, Linux, Solaris, etc.) for running the virtual environment (GUI, graphics, and haptics rendering).

2. Analysis of the Haptic Mechanism

In this section, we present the development and experimental results of the Spherical Parallel Ball Support type mechanism (Li & Payandeh, 2002). The distinctive feature of SPBS is that it uses a 4-DOF hybrid spherical geometry (see Fig. 1). The objective is to take advantage of the spherical 3-DOF parallel geometry as the supporting platform. Hence, the orientation of a stylus is determined by pure rotation of the platform in its workspace while the translational motion of the haptic handle is supported by a prismatic joint. Unlike model presented in (Gosselin & Hamel, 1994), in this design, the rotational axes of the three actuators are coplanar. The center of the sphere is located below the mobile platform where the haptic gripper handle is connected and also located at this center a passive ball/socket supporting joint. This joint is used for supporting both the resultant user interactive forces and also the static weight of the parallel spherical mechanism. The kinematic architecture and geometric parameters of SPBS are presented first. In order to understand the kinematics of the mechanism, a closed-form solution for the forward and inverse kinematics is developed.

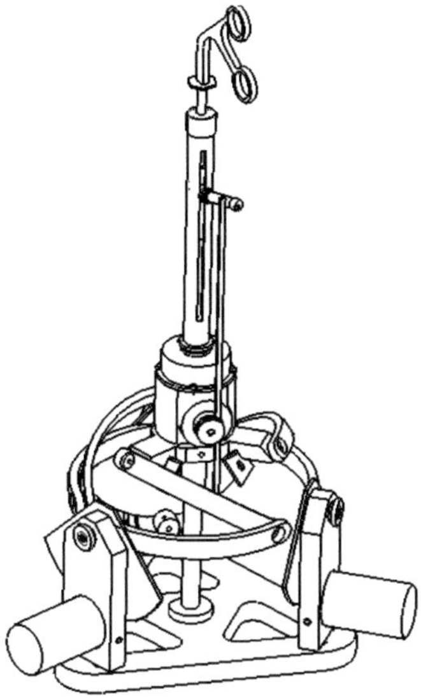

Fig. 1. Design model of the hybrid 4-DOF haptic mechanism.

2.1 Kinematic model

The architecture of SPBS consists of a particular design using an active/passive spherical joint and an active translational joint. The active spherical joint supports a moving platform connected to a fixed base via a spherical parallel mechanism configuration. There are three symmetrical branches which result in a total of nine revolute joints. Each branch has one active joint. Specifically, the mechanical structure of one of the three branches contains an actuator, an active cam, an active link and a passive link. The off-centre gripper handle is attached to the moving platform via a prismatic joint which constitutes to an additional translational degree of freedom. The rotational axes of all nine revolute joints intersect at a common point "O" known as the center of rotation of the mechanism (this point is also the center of the passive spherical joint in the form of a ball/socket configuration). For purposes of legibility only one of the three branches is shown in Fig. 2.

Geometrically, the base and the moving platform can be thought of as two pyramidal entities having one vertex in common at the rotational center "O". The axes of the revolute joints of the base and of the mobile platform are located on the edges of the pyramids. For purposes of symmetry, the triangle at the base of each pyramid is an equilateral triangle.

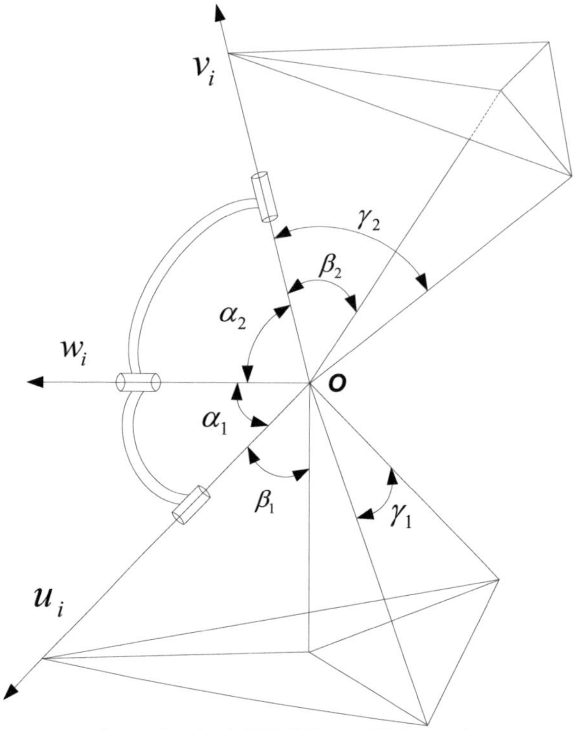

Fig. 2. Geometric parameters of a spherical 3-DOF parallel mechanism.

Let angle γ1 be the angle between two edges of the base pyramid, angle γ2 be the angle between two edges of the mobile platform pyramid, and angle βi i = 1, 2 be the angle between one edge and the vertical axis. The angles are related through the following equation (Craver, 1989):

$$\sin\beta_i = \frac{2\sqrt{3}}{3}\sin\frac{\gamma_i}{2}, \quad i = 1, 2 \tag{1}$$

In addition, angles α1 and α2 represent the radial length associated with the intermediate links. The designs presented in (Gosselin & Hamel, 1994) and (Birglen et al., 2002) use a special class of the geometry which lead to a simplification of the forward kinematics problem. The geometry of SPBS also takes into account some implicit design by explicitly defining coplanar active joints. This results in the following geometric parameters being used in the design of SPBS, namely, α1 = 90°, α2 = 90°, γ1 = 120°, and γ2 = 90°, respectively.

It has been shown that for the general case the forward kinematic problem can lead to a maximum of eight different solutions. One isotropic configuration has been studied in order to obtain an optimized solution of the kinematic problem. Other approaches have been considered in the past using numerical solutions such as artificial neural networks and polynomial learning networks (Boudreau et al., 1998) to solve the kinematic problem. In the following, a new closed-form algebraic solution of the inverse and forward kinematics problem of the configuration used by SPBS is presented.

Let u_i $i = 1, 2, 3$ be a unit vector (see Fig. 2) defining the revolute axis of the *i*th actuator. Let η_i $i = 1, 2, 3$ be an angle measured from u_1 to u_1, u_2 and u_3, respectively. The schematic of SPBS and the reference coordinate frame are shown in Fig. 3. By symmetry, $\eta_1 = 0°$, $\eta_2 = 120°$, and $\eta_3 = 240°$, the following can be defined:

$$u_i = \begin{bmatrix} 0 & -\sin\eta_i & \cos\eta_i \end{bmatrix}^T \tag{2}$$

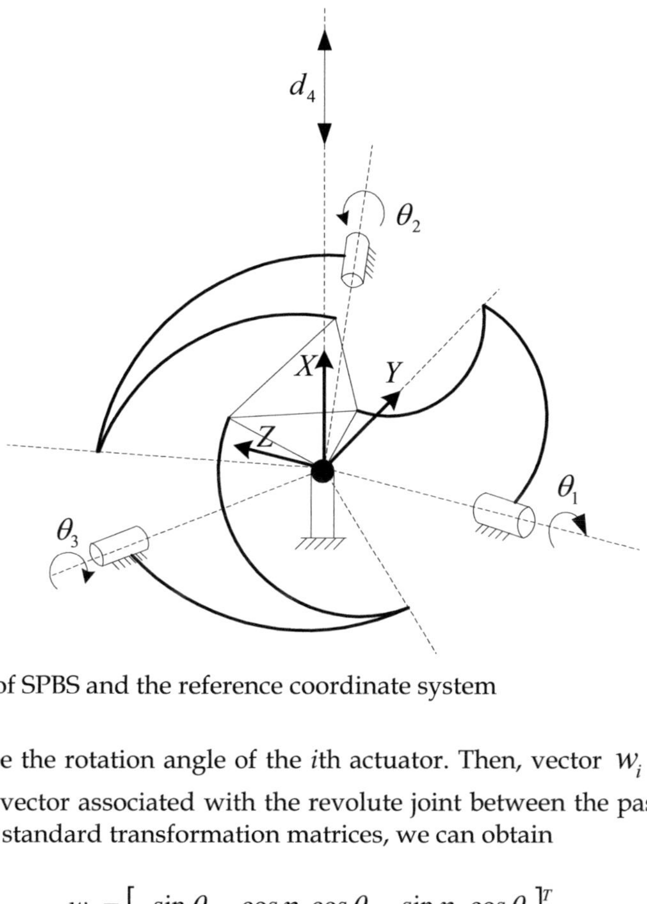

Fig. 3. Schematic of SPBS and the reference coordinate system

Let θ_i $i = 1, 2, 3$ be the rotation angle of the *i*th actuator. Then, vector w_i $i = 1, 2, 3$ can be defined as a unit vector associated with the revolute joint between the passive link and the active link. Using standard transformation matrices, we can obtain

$$w_i = \begin{bmatrix} -\sin\theta_i & \cos\eta_i\cos\theta_i & \sin\eta_i\cos\theta_i \end{bmatrix}^T \tag{3}$$

Similarly, vector v_i i = 1, 2, 3 can be defined as a unit vector along the axis of the ith revolute joint on the mobile platform. Since each of these axes make an angle $\gamma_2 = 90°$ with the others, an orthonormal coordinate frame can be attached to the mobile platform for describing its orientation relative to the reference coordinate frame.

We introduce the rotation matrix Q in order to describe the instantaneous orientation of the mobile platform with X-Y-Z fixed angles rotation. Hence, three successive rotations are defined by a rotation of angle ϕ_3 about the X-axis, a rotation of angle ϕ_2 about the Y-axis, and a rotation of angle ϕ_1 about the Z-axis (see Fig. 4). Let v_{o1} = X, v_{o2} = Y, and v_{o3} = Z, respectively. The orientation of the mobile platform can be expressed as

$$Q = \begin{bmatrix} c\phi_1 c\phi_2 & c\phi_1 s\phi_2 s\phi_3 - s\phi_1 c\phi_3 & c\phi_1 s\phi_2 c\phi_3 + s\phi_1 s\phi_3 \\ s\phi_1 c\phi_2 & s\phi_1 s\phi_2 s\phi_3 + c\phi_1 c\phi_3 & s\phi_1 s\phi_2 c\phi_3 - c\phi_1 s\phi_3 \\ - s\phi_2 & c\phi_2 s\phi_3 & c\phi_2 c\phi_3 \end{bmatrix} \tag{4}$$

$$v_i = Q v_{oi}, \quad i = 1, 2, 3 \tag{5}$$

where $c\phi_i$ and $s\phi_i$ stand for $\cos\phi_i$ and $\sin\phi_i$.

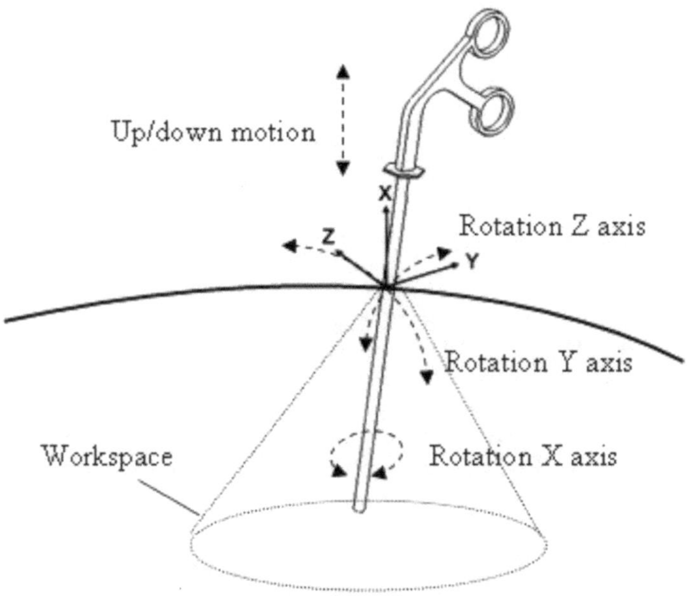

Fig. 4. X-Y-Z fixed angles rotation relative to the reference coordinate system.

2.1.1 Derivation of Inverse Kinematics

Suppose the vector components v_{ix}, v_{iy}, v_{iz} for i = 1, 2, 3 specify a known orientation of the mobile platform relative to the reference frame.

$$v_i = \begin{bmatrix} v_{ix} & v_{iy} & v_{iz} \end{bmatrix}^T \tag{6}$$

The inverse kinematic solution can be obtained through solution to the following equation

$$w_i \cdot v_i = \cos\alpha_2 \tag{7}$$

Since the vectors w_i and v_i, i = 1, 2, 3 are orthogonal when $\alpha_2 = 90°$, the substitution of (3) and (6) with the geometric parameters of SPBS then lead to simple equations in the sine and cosine of the actuated joint angles,

$$\tan\theta_1 = \left(\frac{v_{1y}}{v_{1x}}\right) \tag{8}$$

$$\tan\theta_2 = \left(\frac{1}{2}\frac{\sqrt{3}v_{2z} - v_{2y}}{v_{2x}}\right) \tag{9}$$

$$\tan\theta_3 = \left(\frac{1}{2}\frac{\sqrt{3}v_{3z} + v_{3y}}{v_{3x}}\right) \tag{10}$$

2.1.2 Derivation of Forward Kinematics

The solution of the forward kinematic problem for this configuration is discussed below. Using (4) and (5), expressions of vectors v_i i = 1, 2, 3 as functions of the angles ϕ_1, ϕ_2, and ϕ_3 are obtained. These expressions are then substituted into (7) together with (3). This leads to three equations with the three unknown (ϕ_1, ϕ_2, and ϕ_3) as follows,

$$-s\theta_1 c\phi_1 c\phi_2 + c\theta_1 s\phi_1 c\phi_2 = 0 \tag{11}$$

$$\begin{aligned} &-s\theta_2(c\phi_1 s\phi_2 s\phi_3 - s\phi_1 c\phi_3) \\ &-\frac{1}{2}c\theta_2(s\phi_1 s\phi_2 s\phi_3 + c\phi_1 c\phi_3) \\ &+\frac{\sqrt{3}}{2}c\theta_2 c\phi_2 s\phi_3 = 0 \end{aligned} \tag{12}$$

$$\begin{aligned} &-s\theta_3(c\phi_1 s\phi_2 c\phi_3 - s\phi_1 s\phi_3) \\ &-\frac{1}{2}c\theta_3(s\phi_1 s\phi_2 c\phi_3 - c\phi_1 s\phi_3) \\ &-\frac{\sqrt{3}}{2}c\theta_3 c\phi_2 c\phi_3 = 0 \end{aligned} \tag{13}$$

The solution of these three equations for angles ϕ_1, ϕ_2, and ϕ_3 give the solution of the forward kinematic problem. For the special geometry of our proposed haptic design, a simpler expression for the forward kinematic problem can be obtained. In fact, because of the definition of our fixed reference frame chosen here and the choice of the fixed angles rotation sequence, eq. (11) can be solved for:

$$\phi_1 = \theta_1 \quad or \quad \phi_1 = \theta_1 + \pi \tag{14}$$

Once ϕ_1 is determined, equations (12) and (13) can be rewritten as follows

$$A_1 c\phi_3 + B_1 s\phi_3 = 0 \tag{15}$$

$$A_2 c\phi_3 + B_2 s\phi_3 = 0 \tag{16}$$

where

$$A_1 = s\theta_2 s\theta_1 - \frac{1}{2} c\theta_2 c\theta_1 \tag{17}$$

$$B_1 = -s\theta_2 c\theta_1 s\phi_2 - \frac{1}{2} c\theta_2 s\theta_1 s\phi_2 + \frac{\sqrt{3}}{2} c\theta_2 c\phi_2 \tag{18}$$

$$A_2 = -s\theta_3 c\theta_1 s\phi_2 - \frac{1}{2} c\theta_3 s\theta_1 s\phi_2 + \frac{\sqrt{3}}{2} c\theta_3 c\phi_2 \tag{19}$$

$$B_2 = -s\theta_3 s\theta_1 + \frac{1}{2} c\theta_3 c\theta_1 \tag{20}$$

Since $\cos(\phi_3)$ and $\sin(\phi_3)$ cannot go to zero simultaneously, equations (15) and (16) lead to

$$A_1 B_2 - A_2 B_1 = 0 \tag{21}$$

Substituting (17) to (20) into (21) and rearranging, one can obtain:

$$C_1 (c\phi_2)^2 + C_2 (s\phi_2)(c\phi_2) + C_3 = 0 \tag{22}$$

where

$$\begin{aligned} C_1 &= \frac{1}{2} c\theta_2 c\theta_1 s\theta_3 s\theta_1 + s\theta_2 s\theta_3 c\theta_1^2 \\ &+ c\theta_2 c\theta_3 - \frac{1}{4} c\theta_2 c\theta_3 c\theta_1^2 \\ &+ \frac{1}{2} s\theta_2 s\theta_1 c\theta_3 c\theta_1 \end{aligned} \tag{23}$$

$$C_2 = \frac{\sqrt{3}}{2} s\theta_3 c\theta_1 c\theta_2 - \frac{\sqrt{3}}{2} c\theta_3 s\theta_2 c\theta_1 \tag{24}$$

$$C_3 = -s\theta_2 s\theta_3 - \frac{1}{4}c\theta_2 c\theta_3 \tag{25}$$

Since (23) to (25) are only expressed in terms of the actuated joint angles θ1, θ2, and θ3, these coefficients in (22) can be calculated instantaneously. Four solutions can be obtained algebraically for ϕ_2 from (22). Using the two sets of solutions obtained in (14), a total of eight solutions can be obtained for ϕ_2.

Once angle ϕ_2 is determined, either (12) or (13) can be rearranged to compute ϕ_3 as follows

$$\phi_3 = \tan^{-1}(D_1 / D_2) \tag{26}$$

where

$$D_1 = s\theta_1 s\theta_2 - \frac{1}{2}c\theta_1 c\theta_2 \tag{27}$$

$$D_2 = c\theta_1 s\theta_2 s\phi_2 + \frac{1}{2}s\theta_1 c\theta_2 s\phi_2 - \frac{\sqrt{3}}{2}c\theta_2 c\phi_2 \tag{28}$$

For the sets of solutions of ϕ1, ϕ2, and ϕ3 that can be obtained, the computation of the rotation matrix Q will result in a maximum of eight different X-Y-Z fixed angles rotation matrices with respect to the reference frame. One of these solutions represents the orientation of the mobile platform corresponding to the input actuated joint angles. By taking into account the physical workspace of SPBS given its joint limits, the corresponding orientation can be selected among the solution set with a sufficient conditional check of $v_{1x} > 0$, $v_{2x} > 0$, $v_{3x} > 0$, and $v_{1z} < 0$.

2.2 Jacobians

In robotics, the Jacobian matrix of a manipulator, denoted as J, is generally defined as the matrix representing the transformation between the joint rates and the Cartesian velocities. For the case of a closed-loop manipulator the notion of this mapping for the direct and inverse kinematic problems are interchanged (Angeles & Gosselin, 1990). The Jacobian matrix is defined as:

$$J\omega = \dot{\theta} \tag{29}$$

where ω is the angular velocity of the platform, $\dot{\theta}$ is the actuated joint velocity vector.

An alternative form of (29) with the matrices A and B is rewritten in variant form as,

$$A\omega = B\dot{\theta} \tag{30}$$

where

$$A = \begin{bmatrix} (w_1 \times v_1)^T \\ (w_2 \times v_2)^T \\ (w_3 \times v_3)^T \end{bmatrix} \tag{31}$$

$$B = \begin{bmatrix} (u_1 \times w_1 \bullet v_1) & 0 & 0 \\ 0 & (u_2 \times w_2 \bullet v_2) & 0 \\ 0 & 0 & (u_3 \times w_3 \bullet v_3) \end{bmatrix} \tag{32}$$

Equations (30) to (32) are derived using the general case of the spherical 3-DOF parallel geometry (Angeles & Gosselin, 1990). Similarly, the equations are applicable to the geometry of the SPBS device. Equation (30) shows that the angular velocity of the end-effector can be obtained as an expression of the joint velocities. For haptic rendering purposes, the time derivatives of the rotation angles are used, expressing the angular velocity vector, ω, as

$$\omega = R\dot{\phi} \tag{33}$$

where ϕ is the vector of the Z-Y-X Euler angles, ϕ_1, ϕ_2, and ϕ_3. The matrix R is derived by using the definition of the angular velocity tensor (a skew-symmetric matrix) and taking partial derivatives of the orthonormal matrix in (4). One can obtain,

$$R = \begin{bmatrix} 0 & -\sin\phi_1 & \cos\phi_1 \cos\phi_2 \\ 0 & \cos\phi_1 & \sin\phi_1 \cos\phi_2 \\ 1 & 0 & -\sin\phi_2 \end{bmatrix} \tag{34}$$

Combining equations (29) to (33),

$$\dot{\theta} = JR\dot{\phi} = (B^{-1}A)R\dot{\phi} \tag{35}$$

Equation (35) gives a practical relationship relating the velocities of the active joint rates as a function of an angle set velocity vector.

In addition, we would like to obtain a relationship between the input actuator torques and the output torques exerted on the end-effector about the origin O. In particular, we have the relationship,

$$\text{power} = \text{torque} \times \text{angular speed} \tag{36}$$

where power is in watts, torque is in Nm, and angular speed is in radians per second.

Let w be the torque vector exerted by the end-effector and τ be the active joint torque vector. By using a static equilibrium model and the concept of virtual power, we equate the input and the output virtual powers and obtain the relationship in (39).

$$\mathrm{w}^T\omega=\tau^T\dot{\theta} \tag{37}$$

$$\mathrm{w}^T\omega=\tau^T J\omega \tag{38}$$

$$\tau=J^{-T}\mathrm{w} \tag{39}$$

Equation (39) provides a mapping of the desired output torque vector in Cartesian space to the joint torque vector. As given by equations (30), (31) and (32), an algebraic solution can be used to compute the matrices J, A, and B, respectively. Note that the vectors u_i, w_i and v_i for i = 1, 2, 3, are all known at any instant during the device simulation. The vectors u_i correspond to the reference configuration, whereas the vectors w_i and v_i have been derived in symbolic forms in the previous inverse and forward kinematics sections. The results from this section form a set of basis equations that can be experimented with the prototype.

2.3 Static Relationship

We want to be able to compute the force exerted on the hand of the user holding the tool. A simple point/line model is used for the visualization of the physical tool (handle) of the mechanism. For example, as shown in Fig. 5, the vector r represents the position vector of the handle location at which the user would hold the tip of the tool. The triangular (yellow) surface represent the contacting surface and the force vector F represents the reaction contacting force generated by the computational model.

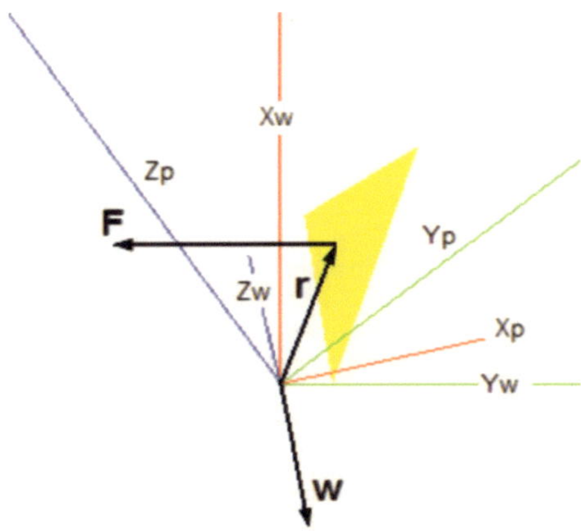

Fig. 5. Representation of contact force and moment vectors.

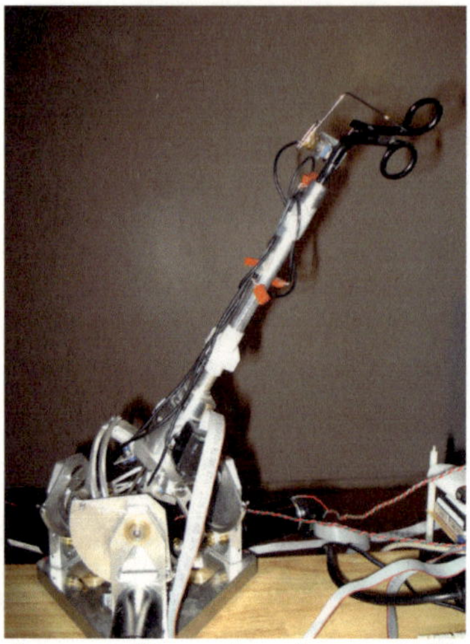

Fig. 6. Haptic device at equilibrium configuration shown in Figure 5.

Fig. 5 and Fig. 6 show an example orientation such that the physical tool is leaning against a virtual wall. The triangle in Fig. 5 illustrates a virtual plane (wall) defined by three arbitrary points in space. The contact point is where the position vector r intersects the plane. The vector F represents the normal force at the contact point having a direction vector perpendicular to the virtual plane. Therefore, by knowing this force vector with respect to the world coordinate frame, the moment of this force vector can be computed by using the vector cross product between r and F. The moment vector w consists of the x-y-z components which are the moments about each principal axis. This moment vector is the desired output torque vector in Cartesian space. Therefore, we can use it to resolve for the joint torque vector by equation (39). The linear force along the handle of the device is independent of the rest of the degrees of freedom and hence is solved separately. Table 1 shows a summary of the computed values of the key parameters used in this equilibrium example.

Parameter Names	Values
Joint angles (degrees)	θ1 = 40.39°, θ2 = 8.42°, and θ3 = 9.43°
Position vector (metres)	r = [0.0748, 0.0250, -0.00797]
Force vector (N)	F = [0, -813.981, 0]
Desired output torque (Nm)	w = [-6.49, 0, -60.88]
Joint torque (Nm)	$\tau = [\,-33.636,\ 1.813,\ 44.873\,]$
Jacobian	$J = \begin{bmatrix} 1.208 & 1.028 & 1.000 \\ 2.152 & -1.025 & -0.224 \\ 0.673 & 0.810 & -0.597 \end{bmatrix}$

Table 1. Numerical values for the example case study.

3. Computational Hardware Design

Haptic displays aim to provide operators with a sense of touch, rendering contact forces as if interactions occurring with real objects. Haptic displays are generally used in conjunction with visual displays, where objects are simulated in a virtual world. The applications of both graphical and haptic displays in virtual reality provide the user with the illusion of touching objects and a heightened sense of presence in the virtual world. The computed interactive force between the user representation and a virtual object is rendered to the user via the haptic device. Due to the elaborate sensory perception of the human hand, which registers even very small oscillations, many research studies have shown that update rates of 1 kHz or above are desired for haptic rendering of any physical rigid contact effects. Therefore, many efforts have been devoted to develop various hardware models, control schemes, and haptic rendering controllers in the past years. Our motivation is to develop a hardware setup which supports the real-time force feedback control of the proposed haptic device.

3.1 Conceptual architecture of the distributed system

Figure 7 shows a conceptual architecture of a distributed system framework. The experimental setup presented in this section includes the 4-DOF SPBS haptic device, a data acquisition system (DAS) and a personal computer (PC). Major processing components are experimented on selected hardware contributing to an integrated VR simulation. The host PC is responsible for haptic rendering and providing a Graphical User Interface. The data acquisition system that consists of a microprocessor, a FPGA, integrated circuits, pulse-width-modulation (PWM) is described in the following.

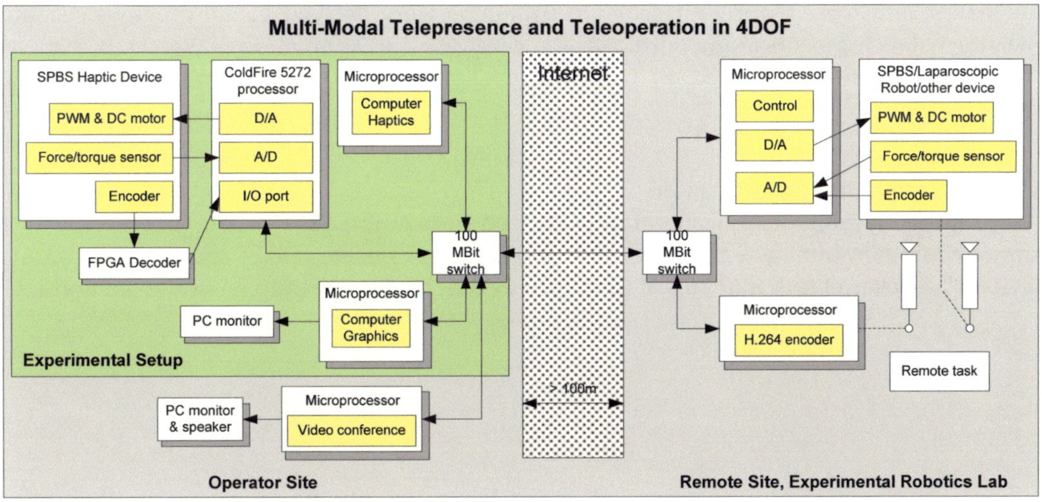

Fig. 7. System architecture of a conceptual microprocessor-based distributed system.

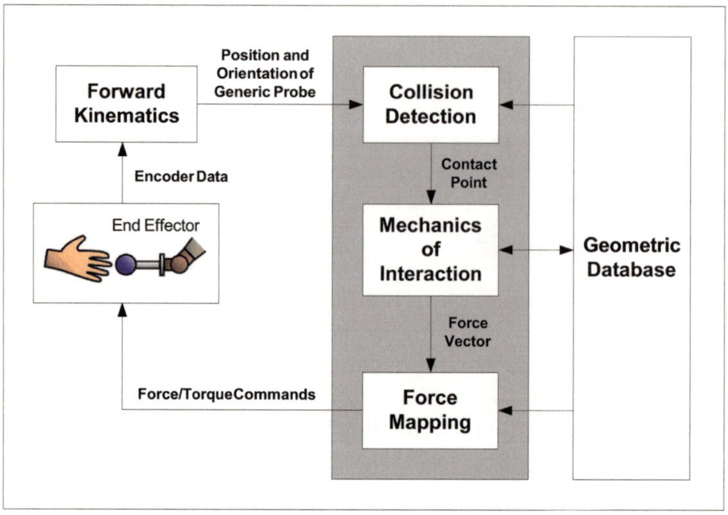

Fig. 8. Typical processes associated in haptic rendering with a force display.

In order to achieve the desired update rates and allow any future expansions, we intend to design and develop the system framework with concepts of concurrency, openness, scalability, and transparency. Potentially we can distribute computational loads, reconfigure, upgrade, and extend for different software and hardware components in order to achieve better system performance. Figure 8 illustrates the main components or processing tasks in a typical simulation hierarchy. The forward kinematics, inverse kinematics, and force mapping (Jacobian) equations were derived in the previous section. The above developments along with collision detection and simulation of materials, such as a virtual wall, are considered as computationally intensive components of any haptic interaction.

3.2 Hardware subsystems design

Our proposed local interconnection framework consists of three major components: the host control computer, our custom-designed data acquisition system (DAS) and the SPBS haptic device. The system block diagram of the experimental hardware setup is shown in Figure 9.

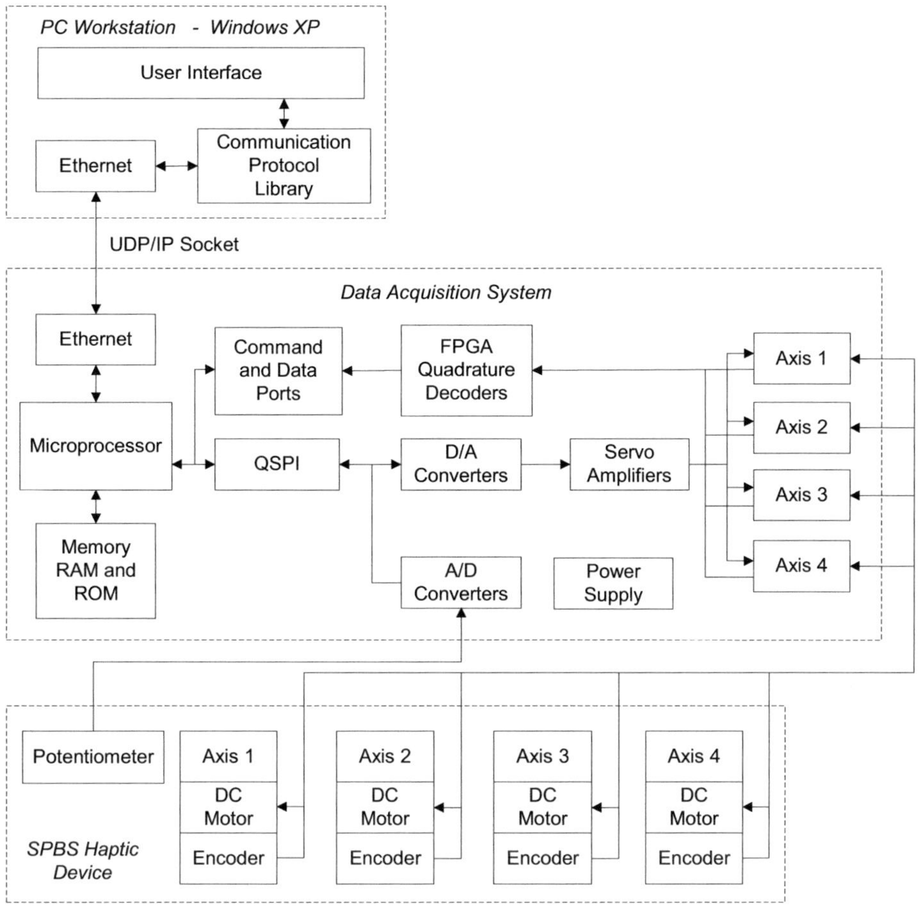

Fig. 9. System block diagram.

The host control computer is the driver for communicating with the DAS. The user perceives force feedback while manipulating the device. The four axes corresponding to the four DOFs are coupled with four DC brush motors. The user's movements with SPBS are acquired by DAS and sent to the host. The host PC provides visual displays and haptic rendering based on local models and simulation laws in the environment. The feedback values are sent back to DAS for real-time control of the motors.

A UDP/IP socket is selected as the primary data communication interface between the host PC and the DAS. The UDP/IP communication is connection-less and is known for having less overhead compared to the TCP/IP communication. The data acquisition system consists of a microprocessor, quadrature decoders, analog-to-digital converter (ADC), digital-to-analog converters (DAC), and servo amplifiers. The DACs provide the feedback voltages through the servo amplifiers to the four motors. We have used the NetBurner MOD5272 development board as the microprocessor unit for controlling data flow. The task of quadrature decoding is distributed and embedded on a Xilinx Spartan-IIE FPGA XC2S200E evaluation kit. The quadrature decoders and ADC serve the purpose of data sampling. A Maxim MAX1203 IC is used for analog-to-digital conversion in this research. The ADC IC is capable of converting an analog voltage input ranged from 0V to 5V into a digital value with 12 bits of resolution. The maximum sampling frequency of the ADC is 2 MHz. By design, the ADC is used with a potentiometer for monitoring the opening and closing of the gripper. In this study, the ADC IC is also configured to collect experimental results (using current monitor output signals).

A quadrature decoder module is implemented to keep track of the motor positions. We used four Maxon DC brush motors for the four axes. Each Maxon motor uses a HEDL 5540 quadrature encoder capable of generating 500 counts per turn. Each encoder line driver requires a line receiver. Hence, two commercial MC3486 ICs are selected for integration with the motors and encoders used in this study. The Spartan-IIE FPGA on the evaluation kit uses a 50 MHz oscillator to drive the system clock. Power for the board is provided by an external +5 VDC regulated supply. The evaluation board provides jumper-selectable reference, output and termination voltages on a bank of the FPGA to facilitate the evaluation of various I/O standards. The LVTTL I/O standard is selected for integration with the ICs and the NetBurner development board used in this research. In addition, the evaluation kit provides 87 general-purpose I/O via two 50-pin connectors. This is sufficient for the current requirements and future exploration. The channels A and B of each quadrature encoder are used. Therefore, four encoders result in eight input bits. A reset signal for the registers is implemented via a push button on the board for clearing all the motor counts. We use a 16-bit data bus and a 2-bit control bus as the interface between the FPGA and the microprocessor module.

The DAS uses the NetBurner development board based on Motorola ColdFire5272 microprocessor. The network capability (TCP/IP and UDP/IP) and general purpose I/O ports are particularly useful for system evaluation in this study. The 10/100 Ethernet provides a standard network interface for connection to the host computer or a hub. The data transmission between the Netburner board and the FPGA is achieved through a 2-bit command port and a 16-bit data port as stated. In addition, the Queued Serial Peripheral Interface (QSPI) hardware on board is able to achieve a data rate up to 33Mbps. The DAS uses the QSPI and communicates with the ADC and DAC ICs by enabling different chip select bits. The UART provides a RS-232 serial interface that can be used for monitoring debug output on the host PC for this study.

The DAC converts the digital data to an analog voltage that feeds into the servo-amplifier. The servo amplifiers are configured to use in current mode, hence desired torque output can be controlled via two reference voltages. The DAC IC used in this project is a Maxim MAX525, which has a serial interface for communicating with the NetBurner board. There are four DAC channels on one IC and each voltage output ranges from 0V to 5V with 12 bits of resolution. The servo-amplifier receives a differential analog input pair. The sign of the differential voltage determines the motor turning direction. The amplitude of the differential voltage determines the motor torque. In our application, we used DC motors with a stall torque rating of 872 mNm. In stall mode, the stall current (and stall torque) is proportional to the applied voltage. Applying twice the voltage results in twice the stall current because when the motor is not rotating (stalled) the armature appears in the circuit as a resistor. Therefore, we can use the rated terminal resistance (0.334 ohms) and the torque constant (19.4 mNm/A) from the motor specification in order to estimate the conversion between our desired torque and the motor current and terminal voltage. For example, if the desired torque is 23.2 mNm, the motor should draw approximately 23.2 / 19.4 = 1.2 A from the power supply. The terminal voltage across the motor leads should be about 1.2 A * 0.334 ohms = 0.4V. In this study, we used a power supply with a 12A nominal output current. Servo amplifiers are the 25A8 models from Advanced Motion Controls. We configured the servo amplifiers to operate in current mode with maximum continuous current rating of 12.5A. Therefore, in our haptic rendering process, we consider a safe operating range for the motors by limiting the torque output to be below 100 mNm.

3.3 Communication Protocols

A simple data packet is used for performance benchmarking of the experimental setup. Figure 10 and Figure 11 show a sample data packet and a control data packet.

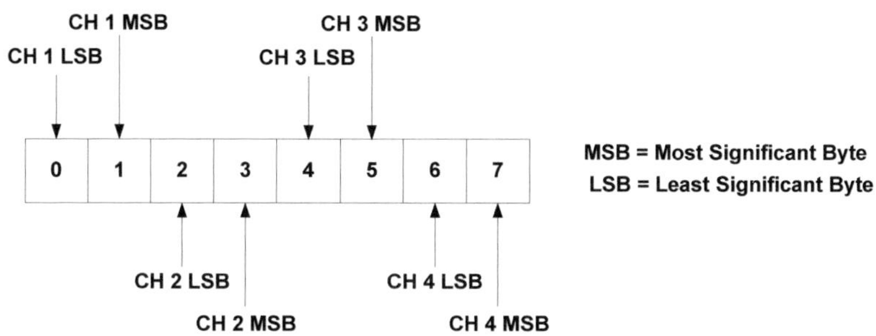

Fig. 10. Sample data packet (8 bytes).

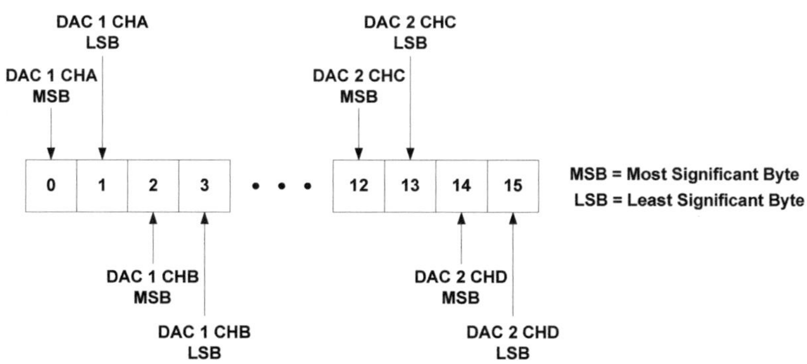

Fig. 11. Control data packet (16 bytes).

3.4 Host Computer

Figure 12 illustrates the high-level design hierarchy of the development of a software application on the host computer. The software applications were targeted and tested on the Windows XP and the Linux operating systems. On Windows XP, Microsoft Visual C++ 6.0 was used as the compiler for building the software application. The WinSock API was used to support UDP/IP and TCP/IP communication with the DAS. On Linux, GNU g++ was used as the compiler for building the software application. The POSIX socket was used similarly on Linux in order to support the communication protocol. The GTK+ software library is used to provide the same look and feel of the GUI on Windows and on Linux.

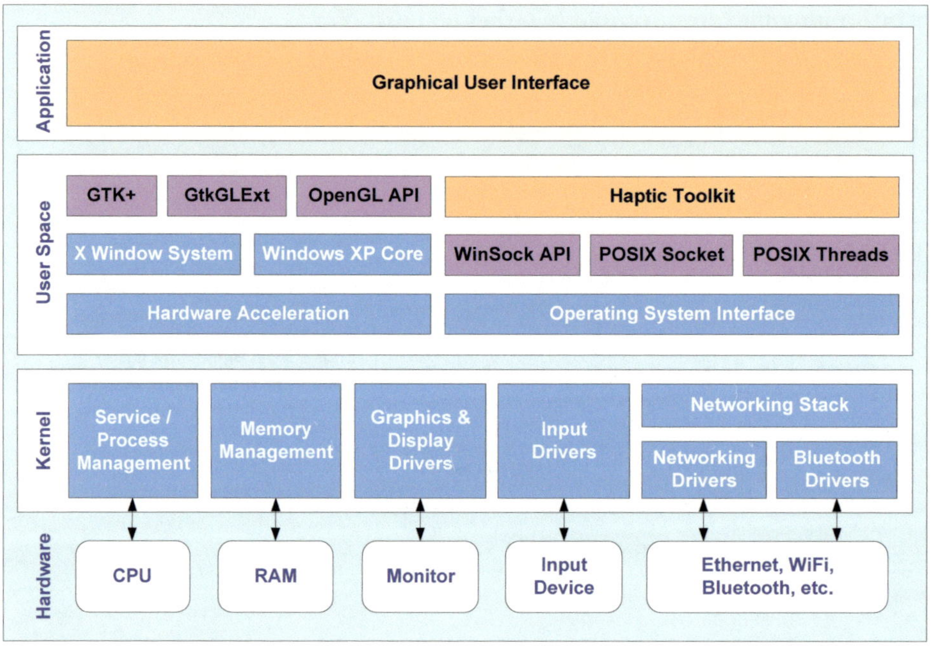

Fig. 12. High-level Design Hierarchy.

4. Experimental Results

Figure 13 shows the sequence diagram of the virtual environment (VE) and the allocation and distribution of the tasks.

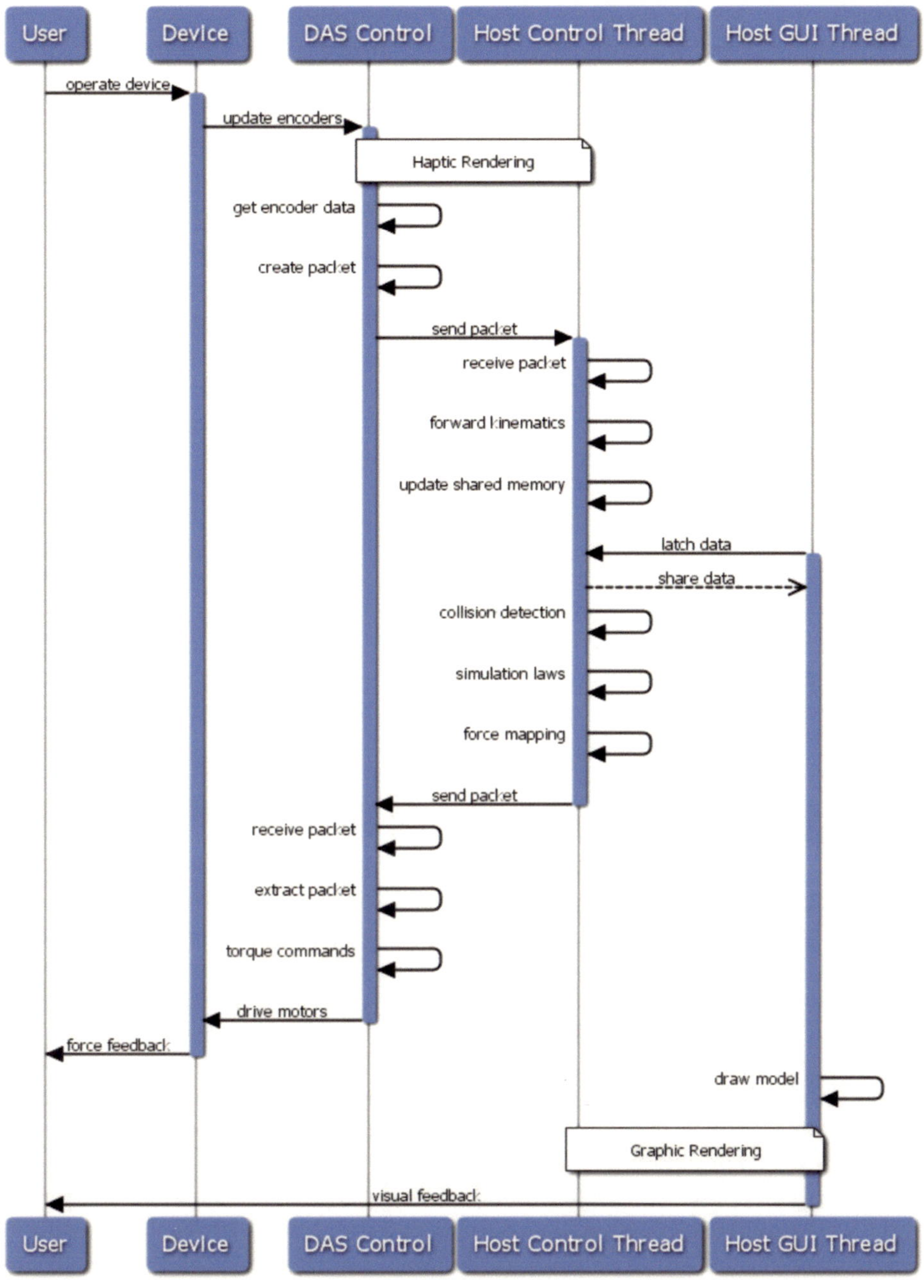

Fig. 13. Sequence diagram of the virtual environment.

As shown, the user and the device represent the human operator manipulating the physical SPBS device while observing the VE and GUI on the PC monitor. The DAS control task represents the control program executing on the NetBurner microprocessor. The multi-threaded software application executing on the host computer consists of two threads. The

GUI thread or task is responsible for graphics rendering such as the user interface, the graphical device model and virtual objects to the operator. The control thread on the host computer runs in the background and is responsible for network communication, kinematics, collision detection, mechanics-based simulation, and force mapping of the control process.

4.1 Performance Benchmarking

Haptic rendering is the process of computing and applying force feedback to the user in response to his/her interaction with the virtual environment. How haptic rendering is implemented should depend on the application requirements, since there is no unique or best solution. Two common approaches are impulsive haptic rendering and continuous haptic rendering (Buttolo & Hannaford, 1997). Impulsive haptic rendering models impulsive collisions such as kicking a ball and hammering a nail. Continuous haptic rendering models extended collisions such as pushing against a wall or lifting an object.

A common question is how fast should we sample, and how will delay affect performances. Previous studies suggest a threshold based on human perception, resulting in a requirement for force reflection bandwidth of at least 30-50 Hz for integrated graphics and impulsive forces [11]. To realistically simulate collisions with rigid objects (i..e. high stiffness such as 1000 Nm^{-1}), desired sampling rates are at least 200 Hz. Many state of the art haptic systems use 1000 Hz sampling rates (Mishra & Srikanth, 2000). In the following, we prepare the experimental setup and the operator positions the tool continuously colliding with a virtual wall in the virtual environment. The GUI thread or the graphics rendering loop (see Fig. 13) is tuned to execute at about 50 Hz. The average sampling rate of the haptic rendering loop can be measured on the host computer or on the NetBurner. We used the continuous haptic rendering model in order to evaluate the performance of the experimental setup.

Table 2 below shows the throughput, sampling rate and tested payload. The sampling rate is defined as how many closed-loop control cycles the host computer can complete in one second. A complete closed loop control cycle requires the host computer to receive a new set of sampled data (motor positions), compute the haptic rendering, and update the control data (voltages). When data is sent over a network, each unit transmitted includes both header information and the actual data being sent. The header identifies the source and destination of the packet, while actual data is referred to as the payload. As indicated in section 3.3, the predefined communication protocol encapsulates the motor positions (the host receives 8 bytes) and control voltages (the host transmits 16 bytes) using a payload of 24 bytes. The performance benchmarking application keeps track of the number of samples/iteration and the actual data size measured in a time interval. The mean sampling rate was the average value over 10 trials. Each trial involved an operator using the device in the virtual environment for a one-minute interval and recorded the sampling rate by using customized firmware on NetBurner. Besides the default size of the data packets, the same experiment was repeated for increasing packet sizes. This allows an observation of the system performance if additional information (such as time stamps) propagated over the networked environment. Table 2 shows the test results with the application executing on Windows XP.

Payload (bytes)			TCP		UDP	
Total	Rx	Tx	Mean Sampling Rate (Hz)	Mean Throughput (Bytes/sec)	Mean Sampling Rate (Hz)	Mean Throughput (Bytes/sec)
24	8	16	768	18432	1105	26520
28	12	16	765	21420	1063	29764
32	16	16	765	24480	1020	32640

Table 2. Communication Performance Statistics (TCP and UDP) in Windows XP.

Comparing the performance of the TCP communication protocol to the UDP, the UDP achieves the desired 1 kHz update rates. The connection-less UDP socket with less overhead outperforms the connection-oriented TCP socket for the intended application of the system. Note that as the size of the data packets increases, the mean sampling rate decreases. Table 3 shows the results by repeating the same experiment on a Linux environment.

Payload (bytes)			UDP (Windows XP)		UDP (Linux)	
Total	Rx	Tx	Mean Sampling Rate (Hz)	Mean Throughput (Bytes/sec)	Mean Sampling Rate (Hz)	Mean Throughput (Bytes/sec)
24	8	16	1105	26520	1181	28344
26	10	16	1083	28158	1161	30186
28	12	16	1063	29764	1134	31752
30	14	16	1042	31260	1108	33240
32	16	16	1020	32640	1084	34688
36	18	18	999	35964	1063	38268
40	20	20	980	39200	1039	41560
44	22	22	959	42196	1019	44836
48	24	24	941	45168	998	47004

Table 3. Communication Performance Statistics (Windows XP and Linux).

4.2 Kinematics Verification

Other tests have been conducted using the hardware setup, the SPBS device, and a Pentium 4 PC running the software application on Windows XP. As shown in Figure 14, the measured length from the origin (centre of rotation) to the tip of the handle is 0.35m. By moving the tip of the handle to test point 1, the measured coordinate on the device in the physical workspace is (0.346, 0.050, 0.000) ± 0.001m.

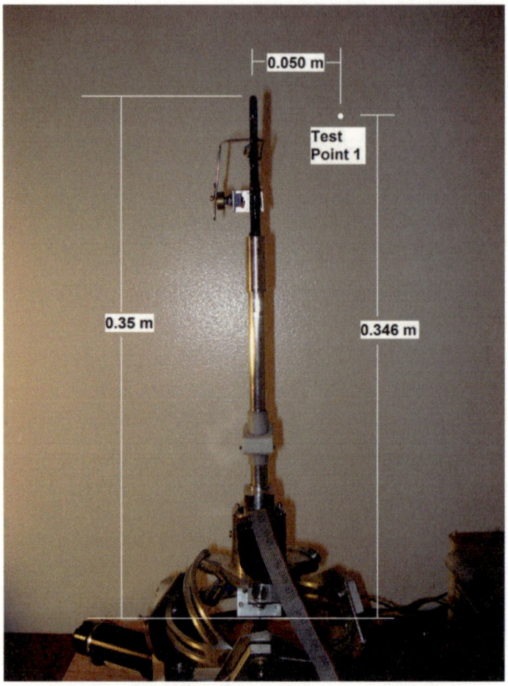

Fig. 14. Measured test point in physical workspace.

Comparing to the model rendered in the virtual environment, as the operator positioned the device to the test point, the calculated coordinate based on measured motor angles, forward kinematics, and a proper scaling of the model is (0.346, 0.050, 0.000).

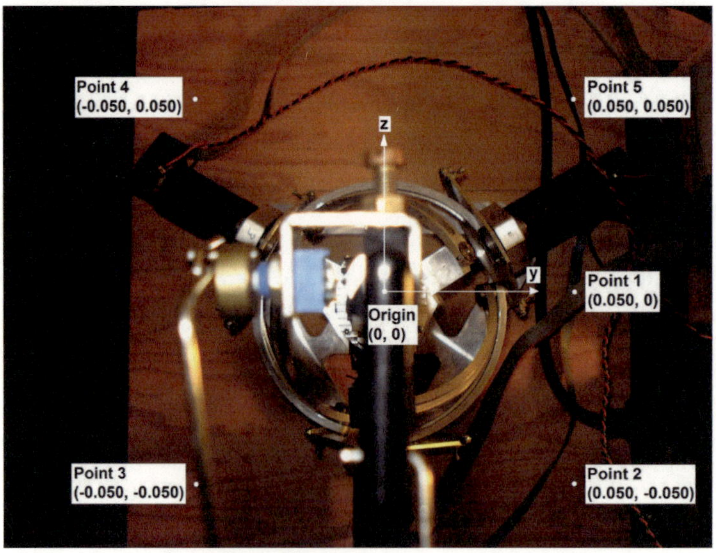

Fig. 15. Test points in physical workspace.

By adjusting the position of a camera along the positive x-axis, Figure 15 shows the top view of the device and the previous test point 1 projected onto this view plane at a distance approximately 0.35m parallel to the y-z plane. Table 4 shows the comparison between the measurements on the actual device and the calculated coordinates on the virtual model as the operator manipulated and positioned the tip of the handle to all the test points shown. Note that the experiments were conducted by the operator determining the position of the tip of the handle and estimating a home reference with all motor angles resetting to zero at the starting origin. The imperfect zero-home reference, estimated location of the handle tip, and camera displacements may introduce source of errors during the experiments.

Test Point	Measured y-z coordinates on physical device (metres)	Calculated y-z coordinates on virtual model (metres)
1	(0.050, 0.000)	0.050, 0.000
2	(0.050, -0.050)	0.050, -0.049
3	(-0.050, -0.050)	-0.049, -0.049
4	(-0.050, 0.050)	-0.049. 0.051
5	(0.050, 0.050)	0.050, 0.051

Table 4. Comparison between measured coordinates and calculated coordinates

4.3 Haptic Feedback

In addition to the observation and tracking of a virtual tool, an example haptic scene is prepared for the operator to experience haptic feedback in the environment. A virtual wall is predefined in the scene prior to the experiment. Figure 16 shows the virtual environment (left) and the home position of the device model (right). The sphere rendered in the left region indicates the haptic interface point in the scene.

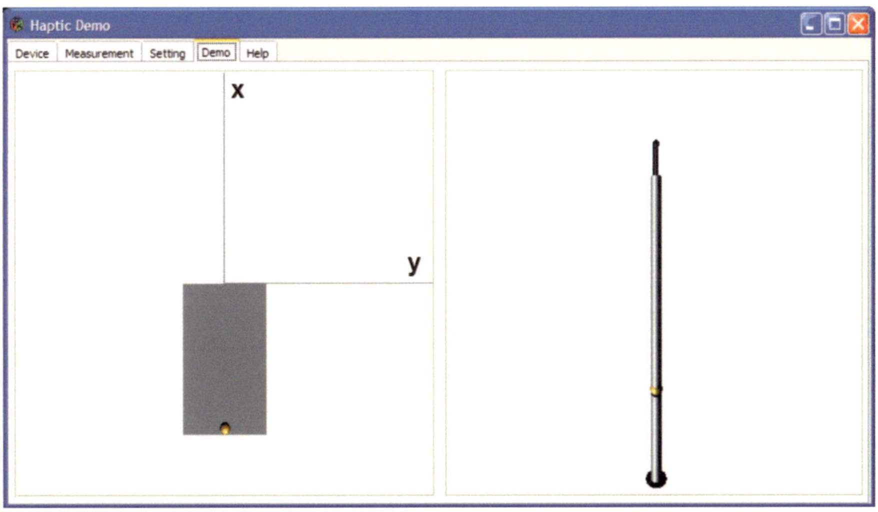

Fig. 16. Virtual environment for haptic exploration (virtual wall into page)

The position of the wall is located at 0.020m into the page (positive z-axis) relative to the origin. The wall (rectangle) is parallel to the x-y plane. The home position of the tool (or straight up) is along the positive x-axis. Figure 16 shows the scene with the camera behind (on negative z-axis) and looking at the origin. The operator performed the experiment by moving the sphere towards the wall along the positive z-axis and colliding the sphere with the virtual wall. Figure 17 shows the position of the sphere as the operator manipulated the tool and moved the sphere accordingly. Figure 18 shows the calculated Cartesian force Fz (Fx = Fy = 0) at the haptic interface point when the sphere collided with the virtual wall.

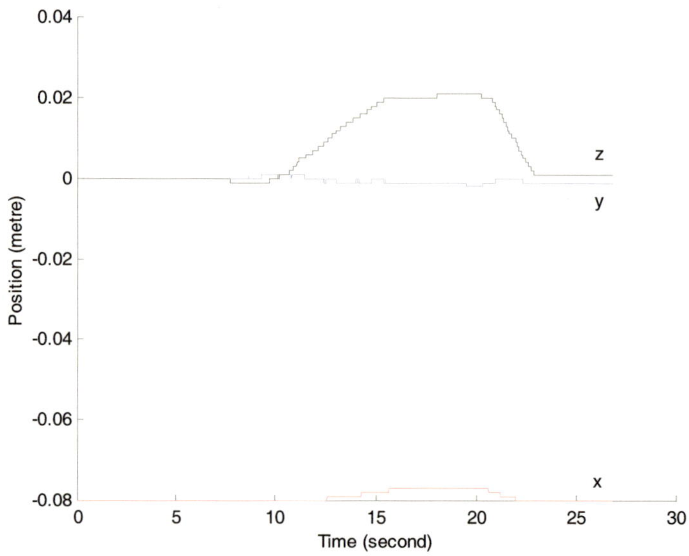

Fig. 17. Position of the sphere with respect to the reference coordinate system.

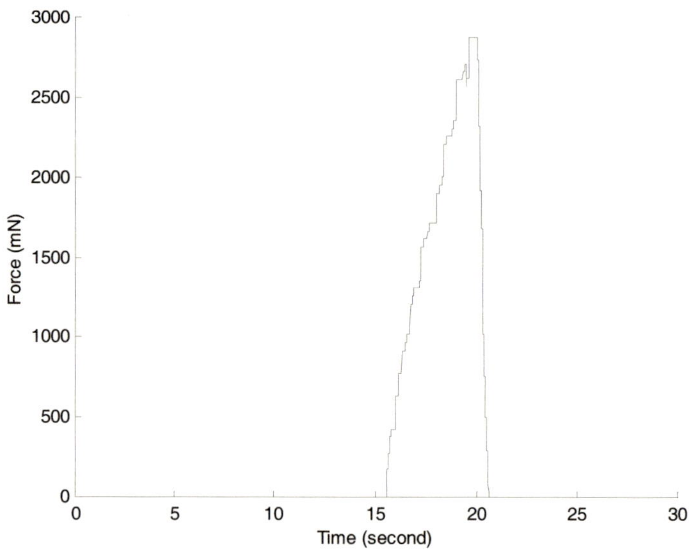

Fig. 18. Cartesian force at the haptic interface point along the z-axis.

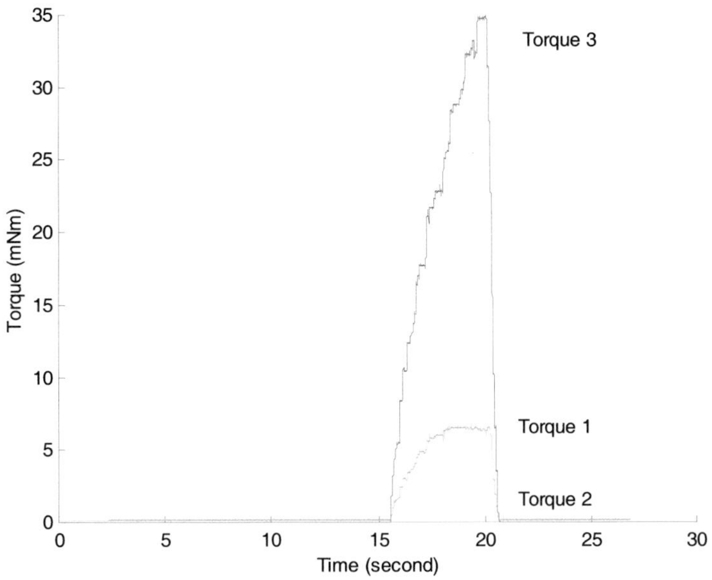

Fig. 19. Measured torque versus time plot.

Figure 19 shows the measured torque versus time plot. The torque was measured by the application of the current monitor output (signals available from the servo amplifiers) and the integration of a low-pass filter circuit and the ADC IC on the DAS. Three axes of the motors were monitored for the torque output during the experiment. The results show the torque experienced by the operator holding the tool and repeatedly colliding with a virtual wall. As seen in the above plots, the period during which the sphere position is at the threshold, i.e. when the spring model is in effect, the force started to increase as the operator attempted to push the sphere further onto the wall. Figure 19 shows the decomposition of the torque into three motor torques felted by the operator. In this example, actuator 1 and actuator 3 were operating in order to generate the reaction force. Using the same virtual scene, the following plots show the experimental results as the operator moved the sphere back and forth from the origin to the wall experiencing a greater reaction force while attempting to penetrate the sphere further into the wall.

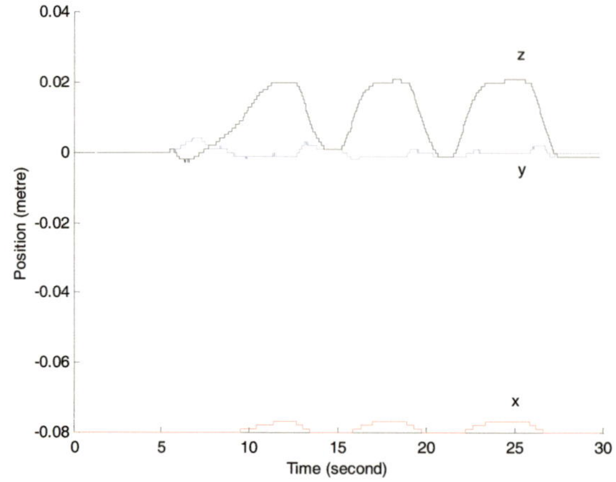

Fig. 20. Position of the sphere with respect to the reference coordinate system.

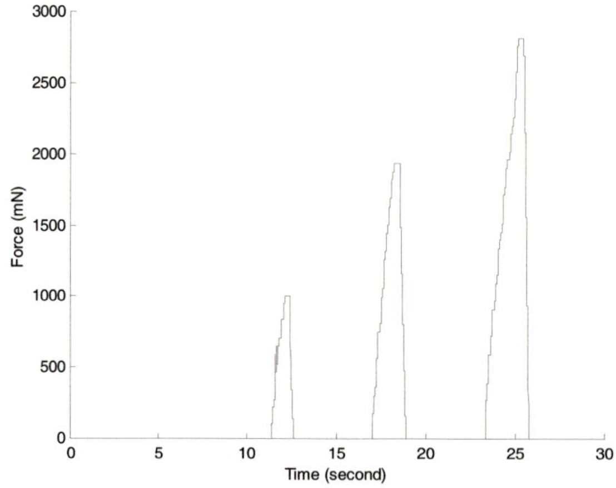

Fig. 21. Cartesian force at the haptic interface point along the z-axis.

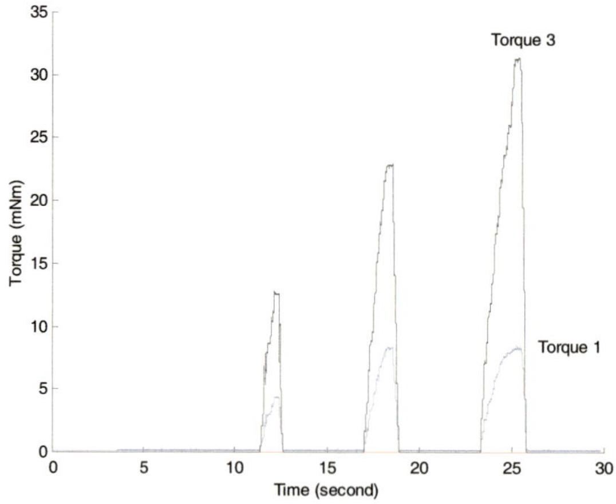

Fig. 22. Measured torque versus time plot.

4. Summary

This chapter presented the design, modelling and hardware integration of a haptic device. The design of the haptic device is based on the notion of the hybrid spherical mechanism which consists of both a passive and active spherical joints. The passive joint is responsible for supporting the static load and user interaction forces whereas the active joint is responsible for creating the haptic feedback to the user. Closed-form solution for kinematic analysis and force mapping of the device is presented. A novel distributed computational platform is also proposed. The platform exploits the notion of scalability and modularity in the design. Performance of the closed loop system is presented in the context of interacting with a rigid environment and achieving a high sampling rate using either the UDP or the TCP communication protocols.

5. References

Angeles, J. & Gosselin, C. (1990). Singularity analysis of closed-loop kinematic chains, *IEEE Transactions on Robotics and Automation*, vol. 6, no. 3, pp. 281-290, 1990

Birglen, L.; Gosselin, C.; Pouliot, N.; Monsarrat, B. & Laliberté, T. (2002). SHaDe, a New 3-DOF Haptic Device, *IEEE Transactions on Robotics and Automation*, vol. 18, no. 2, pp. 166-175, 2002

Boudreau, R., Darenfed, S. & Gosselin, C. (1998). On the Computation of the Direct Kinematics of Parallel Manipulators Using Polynomial Networks, *IEEE Transactions on Systems, Man, and Cybernetics - Part A: Systems and Humans*, vol. 28, no. 2, pp. 213-220, 1998

Buttolo, P., Oboe, R. & Hannaford, B. (1997). Architectures for Shared Haptic Virtual Environments, *Computers & Graphics*, vol. 21, no. 4, pp. 421-429, 1997

Craver, W. (1989). *Master Thesis: Structural Analysis and Design of a Three-Degree-Of-Freedom Robotic Shoulder Module,* The University of Texas at Austin, 1989

Gosselin, C. & Hamel, J. (1994). The Agile-Eye: a High-Performance Three-Degree-Of-Freedom Camera Orienting Device, *Proc. IEEE Int. Conf. Robotics and Automations*, vol. 1, pp. 781-788, 1994

Li, T. & Payandeh, S. (2002). Design of Spherical Parallel Mechanisms for Application to Laparoscopic Surgery, *Robotica*, pp. 133-138, 2002

Ma, A. & Payandeh, S. (2008). Analysis and Experimentation of a 4-DOF Haptic Device, *16th Symposium on Haptic Interfaces for Virtual Environment and Teleoperator Systems*, pp. 351-356, March 2008

Mishra, R. & Srikanth, S. (2000). GENIE - An Haptic Interface for Simulation of Laparoscopic Surgery, *Intelligent Robots and Systems*, vol. 1, pp. 714-719, 2000

10

A Haptically Enhanced Operational Concept for a Hydraulic Excavator

Henning Hayn and Dieter Schwarzmann
Robert Bosch GmbH
Germany

1. Introduction

In mobile hydraulic machines, like excavators, backhoe loaders, wheel loaders, and forklift trucks, haptic human-machine interfaces are not in use. Today, the machines are operated with mechanical-hydraulic joysticks. Each joystick axis controls a single hydraulic actuator. This leads to not very easy to use operational concepts. Since electrohydraulic systems with electronic joysticks are available for serial applications, alternative operational concepts become feasible.
A known alternative is to control the machine using an operating device whose segments resemble the manipulator geometry, as shown in Fig. 1 (Uchino et al., 1977). This operational concept is often called *coordinated control*. Typically, a master-slave system is employed where the operating device (master) outputs the reference position to the position control loop of the machine (slave). This concept promises an intuitive operation of the machine.

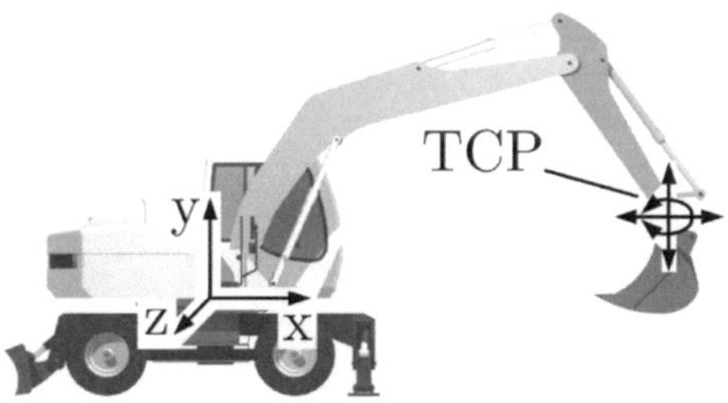

(a) Excavator

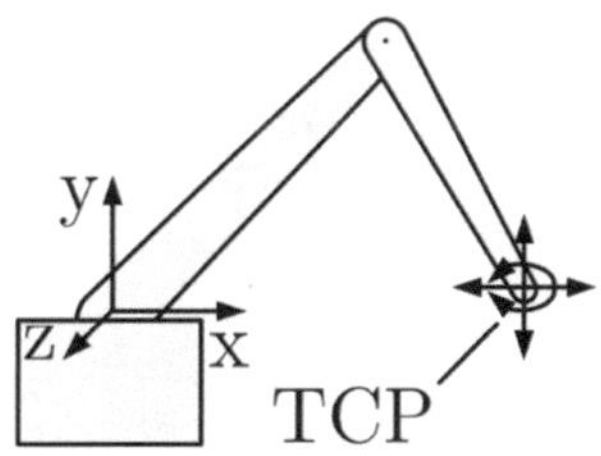

(b) Operating device

Fig. 1. Operating device resembles the manipulator geometry

This concept can be enhanced by haptic assistance systems in order to improve the operator's performance. These haptically enhanced coordinated control operational concepts aim at

- increasing the machine efficiency (handling capacity) by providing driver assistance systems,
- reducing the time needed by the driver to learn the operation of the machine, and
- reducing operating errors especially for unexperienced drivers.

In this work, a SensAble Phantom Omni haptic device is used to generate the position reference signal for the tool center point (TCP) of the hydraulic manipulator of an 18 ton excavator. The two arm segments of the operating device resemble the boom and stick of the excavator, as shown in Fig. 2.

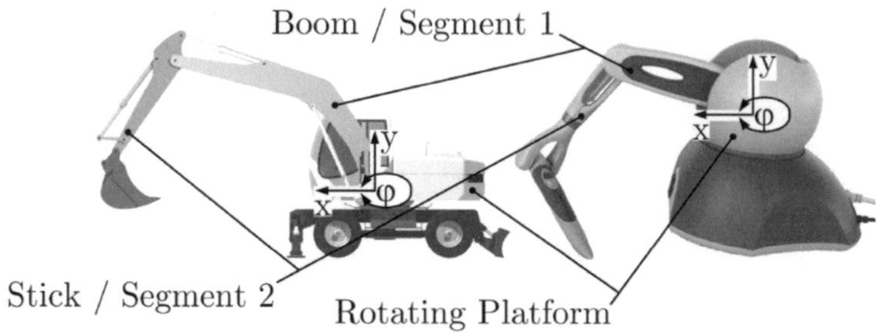

Fig. 2. Analogy of the geometry of a Phantom Omni device and an excavator manipulator

This chapter is organized as follows: Section 2 gives an overview of haptic feedback in mobile hydraulic machines. In Section 3 an alternative operational concept for excavators is proposed. Section 4 discusses the interconnection of the position controllers of the haptic device and the hydraulic excavator leading to a control methodology for bilateral master-slave systems. Section 5 introduces the applied controller design method, namely *internal model control* (IMC), for integrating plants with input constraints. After describing the controller design for the electric actuators of the haptic device and for the hydraulic actuators of the excavator, experimental results are given in Section 6. Section 7 shows the results of initial usability experiments with test drivers and Section 8 offers some conclusions.

2. Haptic Feedback in Mobile Hydraulic Machines

The automation level of available mobile machines is low, with the exception of some special applications like forest machines or robotic cargo loading systems. Due to the increasing use of automation technology, research and development activities focus on new human-machine interfaces and operational concepts. They aim at improving efficiency, safety and comfort. A prerequisite for innovative human-machine interfaces is the availability of electrohydraulics and the corresponding controllers. Then, new functions like driver assistance and safety systems can be integrated in the controller software as well as alternative operating devices. In the future, the level of automation in mobile machines will increase up to complete automation (Haas & Kim, 2002).

The integration of the sense of touch in the human-machine interface promises an easier, faster and more intuitive operation than the typically encountered visual information. Haptic interfaces have advantages, compared to human-machine interfaces that do not integrate the sense of touch, especially if the operator has to work delicately and accurately, or if various materials – for example with different elasticity – are handled.

Haptically enhanced assistance systems can support the driver of a mobile machine in performing his working task by providing tactile sensations via the operating device. Haptic driver assistance systems for hydraulic excavators could for example

- warn the driver of damaging obstacles,
- feed back digging or gripping forces,

- imitate open-center hydraulic systems,
- enable the driver to sense the inertia of the machine's manipulator,
- simplify leveling and slope cutting,
- limit the excavator's workspace,
- guide the bucket on a specific trajectory, or
- assist the collaborative manipulation of a heavy building element by multiple operators.

A significant advantage of haptic systems compared to semi- or fully automated assistance systems is, that the operator always has complete control over his machine. The driver is able to manually overrule the assistance systems, assuming that the human operator is always stronger than the actuators of the haptic device.
The application of haptic technologies in human-machine interfaces of mobile machines is not prior art in series-production vehicles. It can be found in some scientific contributions and sporadic industrial projects, only. One finds that either the machines are controlled with conventional force-feedback joysticks (Cemenska et al., 1989; Parker et al., 1993; Yamada & Muto, 2003; Augustine, 2005) or special haptic operating devices whose segments resemble the manipulator geometry (Ostoja-Starzewski & Skibniewski, 1989; Yoshinada & Takeda, 1990; Kraft, 1991; Kontz, 2007). The same principle is known from industrial robots and similar manipulators. An overview of haptic interface technology for mobile machines, like hydraulic excavators, can be found in Hayn & Schwarzmann (2008).

3. Development of an Intuitive Operational Concept for Hydraulic Excavators

Alternatives to conventional operational concepts are known but did not become widely accepted. The most important reasons are:

- Electrohydraulics was not available for series-production at reasonable prices,
- mechanical-hydraulic components are known for being robust and reliable, and
- the mobile machinery industry has a rather conservative attitude towards alternative operational concepts.

In order to design an intuitive operational concept for the hydraulic manipulator of excavators the coordinated control approach was developed further. It was assumed that operating elements that resemble the manipulator geometry are intuitive and easy to use. These operating elements have the same degree of freedom, the same types of joints and the same moving direction as the machine that has to be controlled. This property is called compatibility of the moving directions (Sachs et al., 1994). This means in detail for the manipulator of an excavator:

- The rotation of the cabin has to be controlled using a rotary operating element,
- the translation of the tool center point has to be controlled using an element which is free-moving within a vertical plane, and
- tilting the bucket has to be controlled using a rotary element.

The realization of this idea was expected to result in an unambiguous, predictable, and consistent, thus intuitive operational concept. When developing new operational concepts for hydraulic excavators it is additionally important to consider the concept being ergonomic and suitable for earthmoving machinery.

After evaluation of different configurations of operating elements on a virtual reality excavator simulator, the concept, shown on Fig. 3(a) as a virtual model, is proposed.
To improve the ergonomics the operating elements are scaled down to allow the manipulation via small motions of the right hand instead of the full arm. The operating elements are integrated into the arm rest to support effortless working. The sizes of the elements were adapted by polystyrene models. Unlike the original coordinated control concept here the operation of the manipulator is shared between both hands. The driver's left hand operates the rotation of the cabin. The right hand operates the position of the TCP in the x-y-plane on Fig. 2 and the bucket. It is possible to invert both elements to facilitate the use by left-handed persons. Fig. 3(b) shows the operating elements from the driver's point of view.

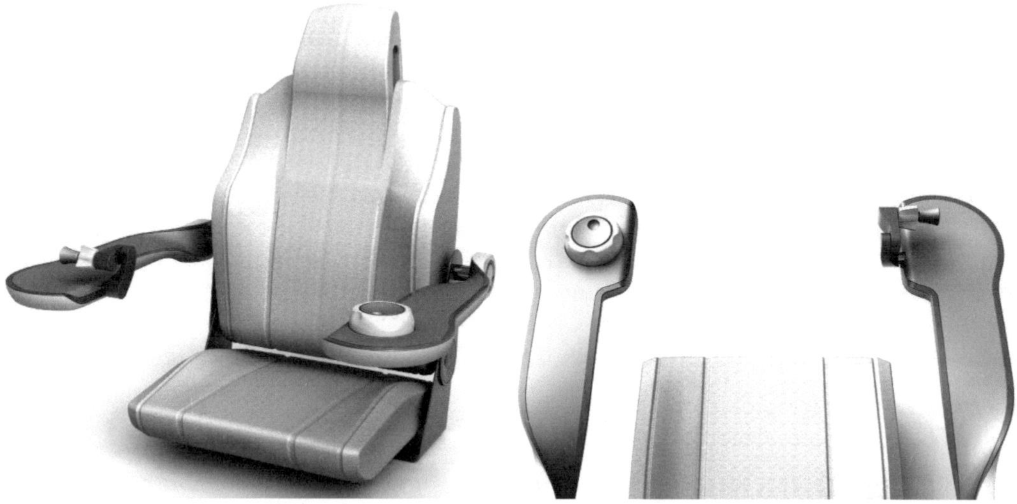

(a) Front view (b) Driver's view

Fig. 3. Intuitive operational concept for hydraulic excavators

The element for the operation of the TCP und the bucket is shown in detail on Fig. 4(a). The two main segments resemble the manipulator geometry. The bucket is controlled by swiveling the light gray, spring centered element. The slew drive for the rotating platform with the cabin is operated with the left hand using the turning knob shown in Fig. 4(b). The turning knob is divided into an inner dark gray disc and an outer light gray wheel. The inner disc can be used to set a desired swing angle. The outer wheel is used to control the yaw rate. The outer wheel allows positioning the rotating platform slowly and sensitively.
The operating elements are intended to be actuated in order to integrate haptically enhanced driver assistance systems according to Section 2.
The concept was tested on a virtual reality excavator simulator and on a real 18 ton wheel excavator. The proposed operational concept, which exists only as a virtual model, was evaluated using commercially available devices, namely a SensAble Phantom Omni device and a 3Dconnexion SpaceBall 5000, that are similar to the operating elements proposed before. The driver's right hand operates the SensAble Phantom Omni device. Unneeded degrees of freedom of the device, like the rotating platform, were locked into position. Instead of the turning knob the 3Dconnexion SpaceBall 5000 was used to set the reference yaw rate. Fig. 5 shows the operating devices mounted in the cabin of the test excavator.

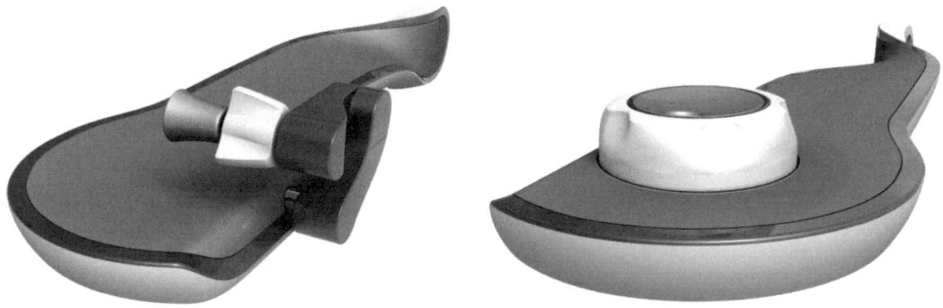

(a) Element to operate the manipulator (b) Turning knob to rotate the cabin

Fig. 4. Enlarged view of the operating elements

4. Haptically Enhanced Master-Slave Control Methodology

4.1 Position Control Concept for Haptic Device and Excavator

The proposed operational concept is a typical bilateral master-slave system. The TCP of the hydraulic manipulator arm (slave) follows the reference signal of the operating element (master) on the right-hand side. However, in the case with an excavator as the slave, two issues appear: First, the human operator needs to sense how far the excavator lags behind the operating device. Without this information, it is difficult to accurately position the machine since the excavator moves significantly slower than the operator can move the operating device. Thus, without some sensory information, the operator cannot know how much lag to expect. Second, and more importantly, if the human operator releases the operating device (in steady-state), the excavator should not start to move. Otherwise, considering the case when the device is not actuated, the handle will fall if the user lets go and, consequently, the boom moves rapidly downwards as it follows the operating device. This behavior has to be avoided at all times. This leads to the assumption that the operating element necessarily has to be actuated. This was important for the technical realization of the proposed operational concept:

- The actuators are used to position-control the operating device in order to permanently synchronize its position with the position of the TCP of the excavator.
- The actuated device gives the possibility to feed back if the driver moves the operating element faster than the excavator can follow. This improves the handling quality of the machine.
- The actuators can be used to implement haptic driver assistance systems.

Fig. 6 shows the block diagram of a haptic human-machine interface for an electrohydraulic excavator including the human operator. Obviously, algorithms for the two controllers Q_{hd} and Q_{ex} have to be designed. The two controlled plants Σ are the haptic device (index hd) and the excavator (index ex). w denotes the reference variable, u the actuating variable and y the control variable, that is the output signal of each system. The physical representation (mechanical, electric, hydraulic) of each signal is given.

A control methodology for the proposed operational concept had to be found. Typical control concepts for bilateral teleoperator systems are based on the two-port network theory (Hannaford, 1989; Zhu & Salcudean, 1995; Salcudean et al., 1997; Tafazoli et al., 2002; Huang, 2004).

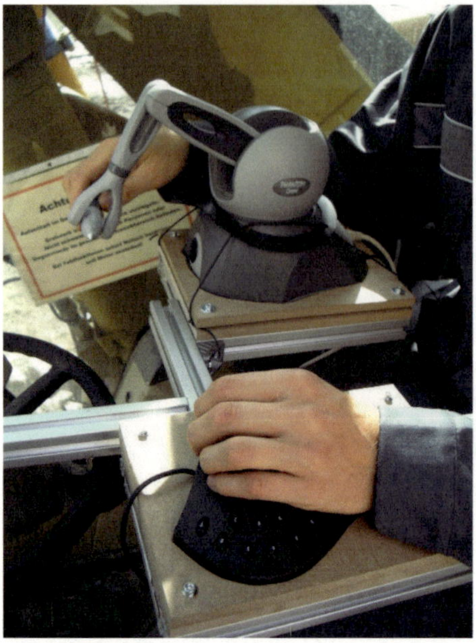

Fig. 5. Test excavator equipped with operating devices

This approach is not applicable to the presented problem because the operating device and the test excavator were not equipped with force sensors. Furthermore, transparency of the bilateral system was not required. Consequentially, an alternative control concept was adopted to solve the above-mentioned problems. The proposed solution is that two position controlled plants (excavator and haptic device) provide the reference position to each other, i.e., each system mirrors the position of the other system. Therefore, the operating device has to be actuated and position-controlled to mirror the current position of the excavator's arm. With this approach, if the user releases the handle in steady-state, it remains at its current position. Additionally, the haptic device will try to counteract the operator if it is moved away from its reference position. The operator can interpret the resulting force of the haptic device as an indication of the lag between the excavator and the operating device due to the inertia of the hydraulic manipulator.

The control methodology for the full master-slave system consisting of the haptic device and the excavator is shown in Fig. 7. Each plant output y_{hd} and y_{ex} is the reference signal for the other system, i.e., each system mirrors the actual position of the other system. This interconnected control loop works because the bandwidths of both systems differ significantly. The operator input w_{op} is modeled as an input disturbance d_{op} of the haptic device.

Position controllers for both systems – haptic device and excavator – are desired. Since the design method internal model control was utilized, as described later in Section 5 and 6, each controller Q consists of an internal model controller C and a prefilter F_{pre}. K_{hd} and K_{ex} are constant transformations

$$w_{\mathrm{ex}} = k_1 \cdot y_{\mathrm{hd}} + k_2 \tag{1}$$

$$w_{\mathrm{hd}} = \frac{1}{k_1} \cdot y_{\mathrm{ex}} - \frac{k_2}{k_1} \quad , \tag{2}$$

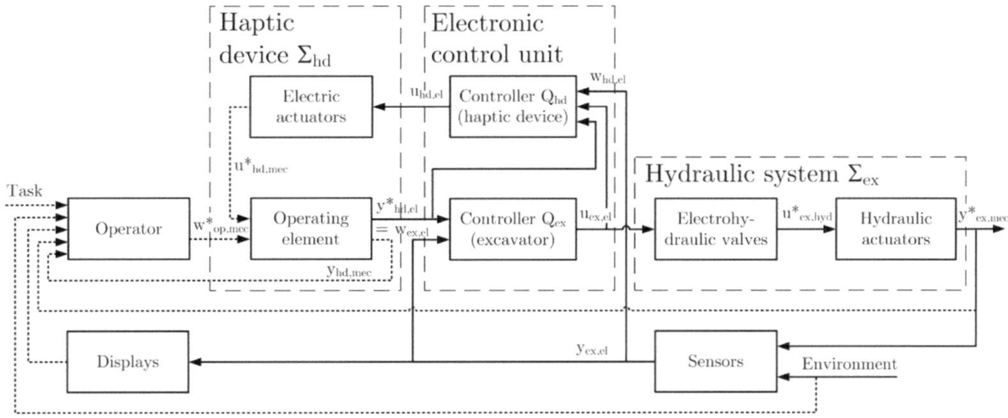

Fig. 6. Haptic human-machine interface of an excavator

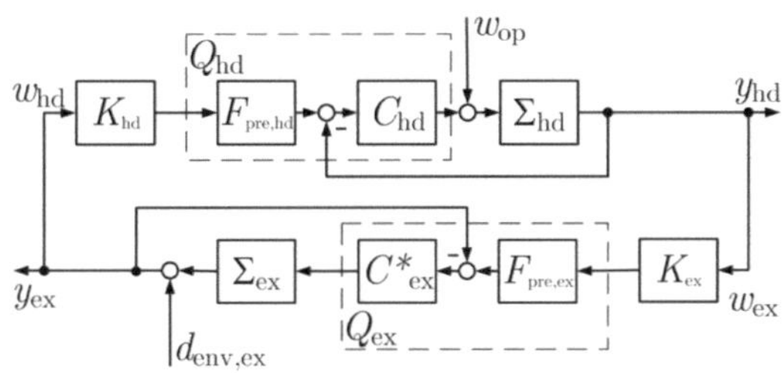

Fig. 7. Master-slave control loop

that convert the dimensions of the workspaces of one device to the other's. Internal stability of the system can be shown examining the poles of the relevant transfer functions.

The reference position is given in cylindrical coordinates: $w_{hd,x}$, $w_{hd,y}$, $w_{ex,x}$, $w_{ex,y}$ for the position of the TCP in a vertical plane (driven by boom and stick) and φ_{set} for the angle of the rotating platform (slew drive). The rotating platforms of both systems are single-input, single-output (SISO) plants. In order to control the position of the TCP, a reference signal generator is used. The reference signal generator converts the desired position into reference variables for the electric joint actuators φ_{ref} and the hydraulic cylinders $l_{ref,z1}$, $l_{ref,z3}$ using the inverse kinematics. In spite of the inaccuracy due to the static computation of the reference variables using the inverse kinematics, this approach provides the advantage that the joint actuators and cylinders can be treated as SISO systems and shows satisfactory experimental results.

Plants with static nonlinearities CC^{-1}, which are the hydraulic actuators including the valves, were treated by approximating them as Hammerstein models. The complete excavator control system is shown in Fig. 8.

4.2 Implementation of Haptically Enhanced Assistance Systems

The proposed control methodology implicates haptic feedback of the inertia of the hydraulic manipulator. Additional driver assistance systems like limiting the excavator's workspace or guiding the bucket on a specific trajectory are desired. These assistance systems can be implemented as virtual fixtures simulating stiff walls (Rosenberg, 1993; Burdea, 1996). Fig. 9 shows virtual walls within the workspace of the SensAble Phantom Omni. The an-

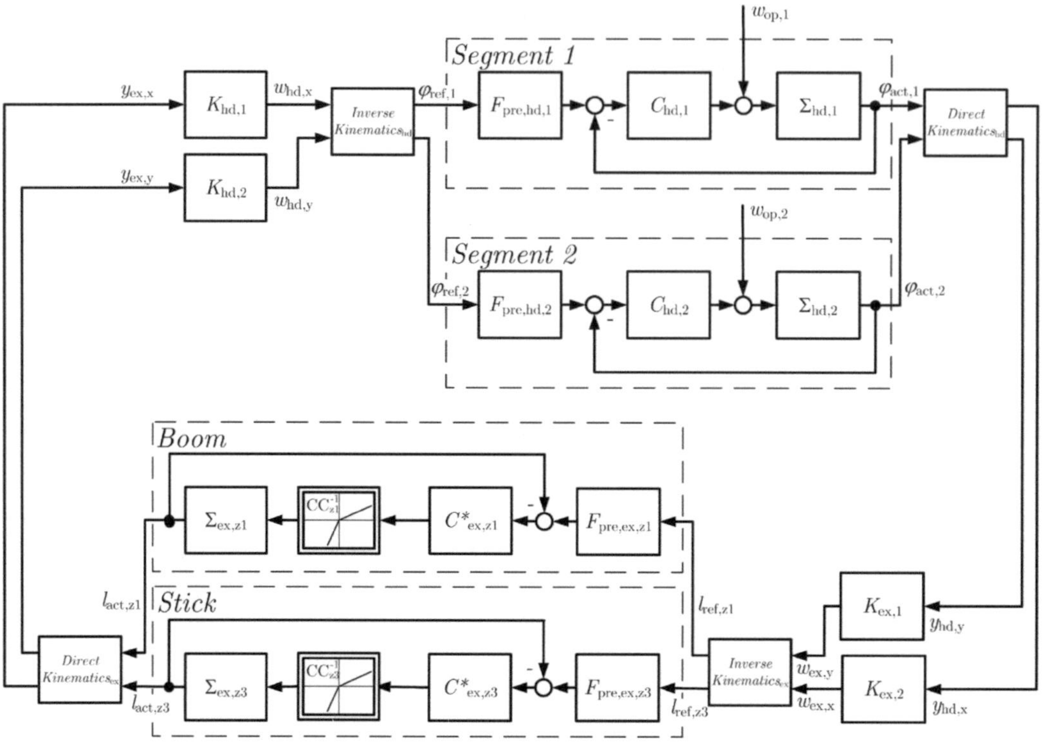

Fig. 8. Control loop implemented on the test excavator using a SISO architecture

gular wall in Fig. 9(a) supports the operator in slope cutting, the vertical wall haptically limits the workspace to protect the cabin of the excavator. Fig. 9(b) shows two walls building a slide rail that give the operator the feeling to be guided on a defined trajectory.
Usually, virtual walls are simulated as spring or spring-damper systems and implemented by adding a virtual force $\mathbf{f}_{\text{virtual}}$ via the controller of the haptic device. In this case, the actuators auf the haptic device are position- not force-controlled. Thus exerting such an external force onto the haptic device will interfere with the position controller which will lead to undesired results as the controller will try to counteract this seemingly undesired disturbance. In order to circumvent this problem, the method to constrain the actuating variable, introduced in Section 5.4, was applied to modulate the input constraints $u_{\text{hd,min}}$ and $u_{\text{hd,max}}$ dynamically to achieve a spring-like behavior. As a result, the position controller is made aware of the desired interference and will exert it on the haptic device itself. In a sense, the dynamic input constraints are used to tell the position controller how to incorporate the desired behavior into the running position control loop. The algorithm to calculate the constraints works as follows:

1. Computation of the spring force $\mathbf{f}_{\text{virtual}}$ which depends on the distance d between the TCP and the virtual wall:

$$\mathbf{f}_{\text{virtual}} = \begin{pmatrix} f_{\text{virtual,x}} \\ f_{\text{virtual,y}} \end{pmatrix} = k_{\text{wall}}\mathbf{n} = k_{\text{wall}} \begin{pmatrix} d_{\text{x}} \\ d_{\text{y}} \end{pmatrix} \quad . \tag{3}$$

   $\mathbf{n}$ is a normal vector with the length d.

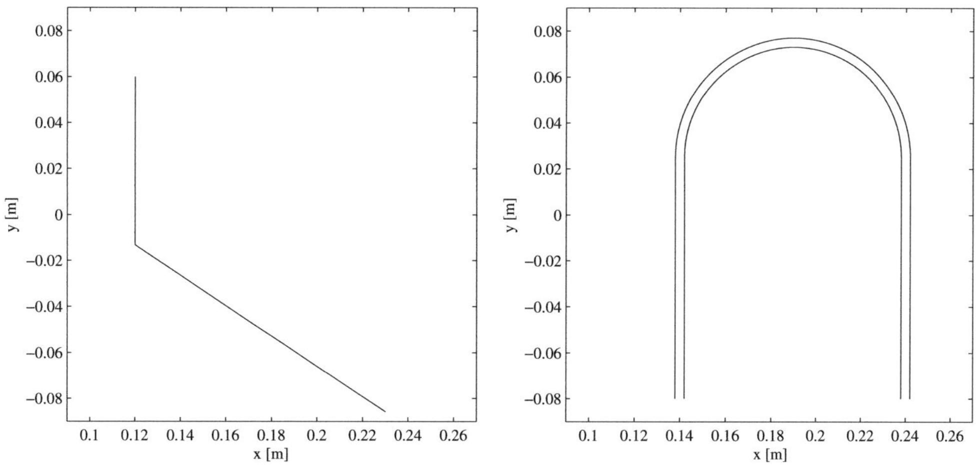

(a) Slope assistance and workspace limitation (b) Trajectory guidance

Fig. 9. Virtual walls within the workspace of the haptic device

2. If the TCP penetrates the virtual wall ($d \leq 0$) two moments M_{virtual} for both segments of the operating element are calculated:

$$M_{\text{virtual},1} = u_{\text{hd,feedback},1} = \frac{k_{\text{wall}}}{l_1} \cdot \frac{d_{\text{x}} \sin\varphi_2 - d_{\text{y}} \sin\varphi_2}{\sin\varphi_1 \sin\varphi_2 + \cos\varphi_1 \cos\varphi_2} \tag{4}$$

$$M_{\text{virtual},2} = u_{\text{hd,feedback},2} = \frac{k_{\text{wall}}}{l_2} \cdot \frac{-d_{\text{x}} \cos\varphi_1 - d_{\text{y}} \sin\varphi_1}{\sin\varphi_1 \sin\varphi_2 + \cos\varphi_1 \cos\varphi_2} \quad . \tag{5}$$

These moments generate the desired force at the TCP. The equation results from the kinematics of the haptic device. l and φ denote the lengths and angles as shown in Fig. 10. These calculated moments and the actuating variable u_{hd} of the electric actuators of the device are proportional ($M_{\text{virtual}} \sim u_{\text{hd}}$). Hence the actuating variable to generate the desired force $\mathbf{f}_{\text{virtual}}$ via these moments is called $u_{\text{hd,feedback}}$.

3. The constraints $u_{\text{hd,min}}$ and $u_{\text{hd,max}}$ of the actuating variables of both segments are

$$u_{\text{hd,min}} = u_{\text{hd,limit,min}} + u_{\text{hd,gravity}} + u_{\text{hd,feedback}} \quad , \tag{6}$$

$$u_{\text{hd,max}} = u_{\text{hd,limit,max}} + u_{\text{hd,gravity}} + u_{\text{hd,feedback}} \quad . \tag{7}$$

$u_{\text{hd,limit}}$ is the physical input constraint of each plant according to Section 5.4. $u_{\text{hd,gravity}}$ is a constant that compensates the influence of gravity on the haptic device even if the control deviation is null. The constraints $u_{\text{hd,min}}$ and $u_{\text{hd,max}}$ are applied according to Equations (30) and (31).

The adopted constraints force the haptic device to behave like a stiff spring if the TCP is within the predefined fixtures. After adjusting k_{wall} in experiments this approach showed good results. The simulated stiff wall can be sensed easily.

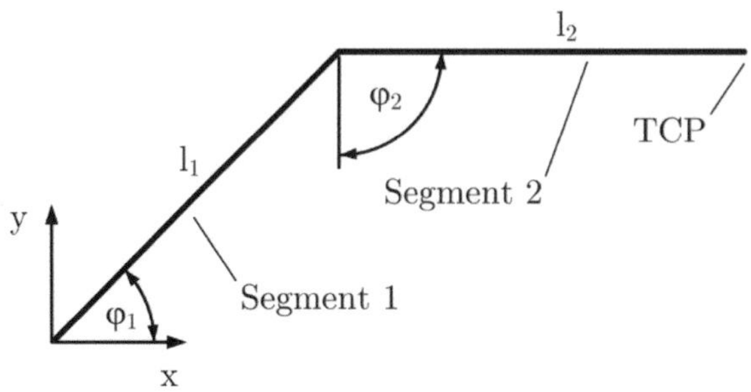

Fig. 10. Kinematics of a SensAble Phantom Omni

5. Internal Model Control of Linear SISO Systems

The proposed control methodology in Fig. 8 demands several controllers, one for each plant in both systems. Since both types of plants (electric joint actuators of the SensAble Phantom Omni device as well as the hydraulic cylinders and the slew drive of the excavator) show an integrating behavior, the same control method, namely internal model control for integrating linear SISO systems, is chosen for all plants. A review of the design is given in the following, starting with non-integrating plants, i.e., plants Σ having i poles p_i with $\mathrm{Re}\{p_i\} < 0$ for all i.

5.1 IMC for Non-Integrating Stable Systems

The main idea of IMC is to include a model $\tilde{\Sigma}$ of the plant Σ into the controller K, as shown in Fig. 11. If $\tilde{\Sigma}$ models the plant Σ exactly and in the absence of disturbances ($d = 0$), the feedback signal equals zero ($y(t) - \tilde{y}(t) = 0$), and the IMC controller Q is a feed-forward controller.

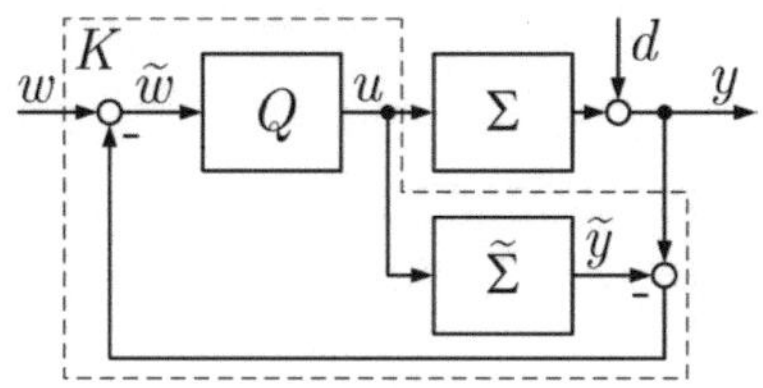

Fig. 11. IMC structure

The IMC controller Q is a series connection of a filter F and the inverse model $\tilde{\Sigma}^{-1}$:

$$Q = F\tilde{\Sigma}^{-1} \quad . \tag{8}$$

For non-integrating plants, in Frank (1974) and Morari & Zafiriou (1989), the following structure for the filter F is proposed:

$$F(s) = \frac{1}{(\frac{1}{\lambda}s + 1)^r} \quad \text{with} \quad \lambda > 0 \quad , \tag{9}$$

where λ is a design parameter and r is the relative degree of $\tilde{\Sigma}$.
The IMC structure can always be converted into the standard control loop shown in Fig. 12 (Schwarzmann, 2007):

$$C = \frac{1}{1-F}Q = \frac{F}{1-F}\tilde{\Sigma}^{-1} = F_{tot}\tilde{\Sigma}^{-1} \quad . \tag{10}$$

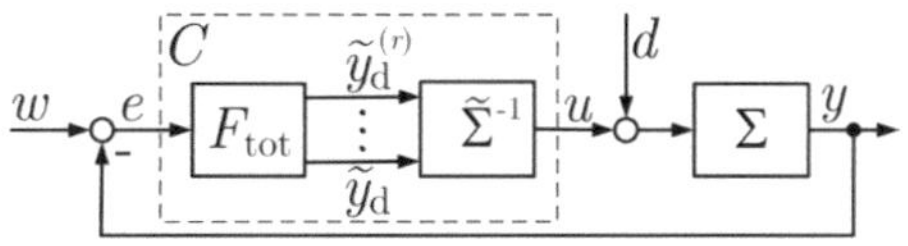

Fig. 12. IMC structure implemented in a standard control loop

The separation of the controller C into a filter F_{tot} and the inverse of a model $\tilde{\Sigma}^{-1}$ is required for the proposed limitation of the controller output u in Section 5.4.

5.2 IMC for Integrating Systems

The previously proposed filter F in Equation (9) and the resulting filter F_{tot} are not sufficient for integrating systems because step input disturbances d lead to a steady-state offset (Morari & Zafiriou, 1989). The filter F_{tot} has to have at least the same relative degree as $\tilde{\Sigma}$ and $i+1$ pure integrators (i.e. poles at zero) in order to design a proper controller C, where i is the number of pure integrators of the plant model $\tilde{\Sigma}$. According to the design procedure presented in Morari & Zafiriou (1989), a system of linear equations has to be solved to determine the filter F for this type of plants. To avoid this difficulty, a modified design rule for F is introduced to design an internal model controller for integrating linear minimum phase systems in a standard control loop. This modified design rule leads to the same result as the proposed solution by Morari & Zafiriou (1989) but in a single step as opposed to solving a system of equations.
To generate the desired filter F_{tot} from the positive feedback loop of F (cf. Equation (10)), F is chosen in such a manner that terms $\delta_i s^i$ up to the i-th order of the denominator polynomial of F are canceled by subtracting the numerator. The corresponding filter F is

$$\begin{aligned} F(s) &= \frac{\frac{\gamma_i}{\lambda^i}s^i + \frac{\gamma_{i-1}}{\lambda^{i-1}}s^{i-1} + \ldots + \frac{\gamma_2}{\lambda^2}s^2 + \frac{\gamma_1}{\lambda}s + 1}{\frac{\gamma_{r+i}}{\lambda^{r+i}}s^{r+i} + \ldots + \frac{\gamma_i}{\lambda^i}s^i + \ldots + \frac{\gamma_1}{\lambda}s + 1} \\ &= \frac{\delta_i s^i + \delta_{i-1}s^{i-1} + \ldots + \delta_2 s^2 + \delta_1 s + 1}{(\frac{1}{\lambda}s+1)^{r+i}} \\ &\text{with} \quad \delta_n = \frac{\gamma_n}{\lambda^n} \quad , \quad 0 \le n \le i \quad . \end{aligned} \tag{11}$$

The numerator of F consists of all terms up to the i-th order of the polynomial of the extended denominator of F ($(\frac{1}{\lambda}s+1)^{r+i}$), which are the last $i+1$ summands of the denominator. λ is a design parameter, r is the relative degree of $\tilde{\Sigma}$, γ and δ are constant coefficients. F_{tot} is then

$$
\begin{aligned}
F_{\text{tot}}(s) &= \frac{F}{1-F} = \frac{\text{numerator}(F)}{\text{denominator}(F) - \text{numerator}(F)} \\
&= \frac{\delta_i s^i + \delta_{i-1} s^{i-1} + \ldots + \delta_2 s^2 + \delta_1 s + 1}{(\frac{1}{\lambda}s+1)^{r+i} - \delta_i s^i - \ldots - \delta_2 s^2 - \delta_1 s - 1} \\
&= \frac{\frac{\gamma_i}{\lambda^i} s^i + \frac{\gamma_{i-1}}{\lambda^{i-1}} s^{i-1} + \ldots + \frac{\gamma_2}{\lambda^2} s^2 + \frac{\gamma_1}{\lambda} s + 1}{\frac{\gamma_{r+i}}{\lambda^{r+i}} s^{r+i} + \ldots + \frac{\gamma_{i+1}}{\lambda^{i+1}} s^{i+1}} \\
&= \frac{\frac{\gamma_i}{\lambda^i} s^i + \frac{\gamma_{i-1}}{\lambda^{i-1}} s^{i-1} + \ldots + \frac{\gamma_2}{\lambda^2} s^2 + \frac{\gamma_1}{\lambda} s + 1}{s^{i+1}(\frac{\gamma_{r+i}}{\lambda^{r+i}} s^r + \frac{\gamma_{r+i-1}}{\lambda^{r+i-1}} s^{r-1} + \ldots + \frac{\gamma_{i+1}}{\lambda^{i+1}})} \quad .
\end{aligned} \tag{12}
$$

This results in the desired number of integrators in F_{tot}. The tuning parameter λ determines the resulting bandwidth of the closed loop. The specified design rule for F_{tot} allows to follow ramp reference signals and removes the steady-state offset in the case of step input disturbances.

5.3 Prefilter Design

A prefilter F_{pre} is introduced to reduce overshoot. This leads to a second degree of freedom to parameterize the behavior of the closed loop.
If $\tilde{\Sigma}$ is an ideal model of the plant Σ, the transfer behavior of the closed loop system is equal to the filter F (see Fig. 11). Hence the desired behavior F_{d} of the system can be forced by the prefilter

$$F_{\text{pre}} = F_{\text{d}} F^{-1} \quad . \tag{13}$$

The desired behavior F_{d} is usually a low-pass filter

$$F_{\text{d}} = \frac{1}{(\frac{1}{\lambda_{\text{d}}}s+1)^{r_{\text{d}}}} \tag{14}$$

with the design parameter λ_{d}. This holds if r_{d} is greater than or equal to the relative degree of F.

5.4 Input Constraints

In technical systems, the actuating variable u is limited: $u \in [u_{\text{min}}, u_{\text{max}}]$. When neglected, this input constraint of the plant can lead to undesirable windup effects. Especially the haptic device shows these effects because of the persistent integration of the position error variable due to the operator holding the handle of the device. If not treated by the control algorithm, the result is a strong integral windup effect if the user releases the handle of the haptic device. Due to the design specifications overshoot is not desired. Therefore, a windup compensation according to Schwarzmann (2007) was designed as follows:
If the IMC controller Q is implemented as a series connection of F and the inverse of the plant model $\tilde{\Sigma}^{-1}$ (cf. Fig. 12), a constraint of the highest derivative $\tilde{y}_d^{(r)}$ of the filter output limits the output u of the controller. Using this structure, the filter F forces a desired behavior $\tilde{y}_d$ of the plant that does not violate the input constraints u_{min} and u_{max} of the plant Σ.
According to Graichen & Zeitz (2006) the inverse of a model $\tilde{\Sigma}$ can be determined as follows: A controllable model $\tilde{\Sigma}$

$$\tilde{\Sigma}: \quad \dot{x} = \boldsymbol{f}(\boldsymbol{x},u), \quad \boldsymbol{x}(0) = \boldsymbol{x}_0, \quad \tilde{y} = h(\boldsymbol{x}) \tag{15}$$

with a relative degree r, defined as

$$r = \arg\min_k \{\frac{\partial}{\partial u} L_f^k h(\boldsymbol{x},u) \neq 0\} \quad , \tag{16}$$

where $L_f h$ means the Lie-derivative of h with respect to f, can be transformed to the nonlinear normal form

$$\tilde{y}^{(r)} = \alpha(\tilde{y},\dot{\tilde{y}},\ldots\tilde{y}^{(r-1)},\boldsymbol{\eta},u) \tag{17a}$$

$$\dot{\eta} = \boldsymbol{\beta}(\boldsymbol{\eta},\tilde{y},\dot{\tilde{y}},\ldots\tilde{y}^{(r-1)},u) \tag{17b}$$

with $\alpha(\cdot) = L_f^r h \circ \boldsymbol{\phi}^{-1}$ and $\beta(\cdot) = L_f \phi_{n,i} \circ \boldsymbol{\phi}^{-1}$ using the state transformation

$$[\tilde{y},\dot{\tilde{y}},\ldots\tilde{y}^{(r-1)},\boldsymbol{\eta}]^T = \boldsymbol{\phi}(\boldsymbol{x}) \quad \text{with} \tag{18a}$$

$$\tilde{y}^{(i)} = L_f^i h(\boldsymbol{x}) = \phi_{i+1}, \quad i = 0,\ldots,r-1 \tag{18b}$$

$$\boldsymbol{\eta} = \boldsymbol{\phi}_\eta(\boldsymbol{x}) \in \mathbb{R}^{n-r} \quad . \tag{18c}$$

The inverse of the model $\tilde{\Sigma}$ is then

$$\tilde{\Sigma}^{-1}: \quad u = \alpha^{-1}(\tilde{y}_d,\dot{\tilde{y}}_d,\ldots\tilde{y}_d^{(r)},\boldsymbol{\eta}) \tag{19a}$$

$$\dot{\eta} = \boldsymbol{\beta}(\boldsymbol{\eta},\tilde{y}_d,\dot{\tilde{y}}_d,\ldots\tilde{y}_d^{(r-1)},u) \quad , \tag{19b}$$

where the function α^{-1} is the solution of Equation (17a) for u.
For linear systems $\tilde{y} = \tilde{\Sigma}u$ without zeros, the controller output $u = \tilde{\Sigma}^{-1}\tilde{y}$ can be described as

$$u = u(\tilde{y}_{\mathrm{d}},\dot{\tilde{y}}_{\mathrm{d}},\ldots,\tilde{y}_{\mathrm{d}}^{(r-1)},\tilde{y}_{\mathrm{d}}^{(r)}) = a_0\tilde{y}_{\mathrm{d}} + a_1\dot{\tilde{y}}_{\mathrm{d}} + \ldots + a_{(r-1)}\tilde{y}_{\mathrm{d}}^{(r-1)} + a_r\tilde{y}_{\mathrm{d}}^{(r)} \quad . \tag{20}$$

For the above-named systems with i integrators at the plant output, the controller output u is not a function of the desired behavior $\tilde{y}_{\mathrm{d}}$ and its first $i-1$ derivatives

$$u = u(\tilde{y}_{\mathrm{d}}^{(i)},\tilde{y}_{\mathrm{d}}^{(i+1)},\ldots,\tilde{y}_{\mathrm{d}}^{(r-1)},\tilde{y}_{\mathrm{d}}^{(r)}) = a_i\tilde{y}_{\mathrm{d}}^{(i)} + a_{i+1}\tilde{y}_{\mathrm{d}}^{(i+1)} + \ldots + a_{(r-1)}\tilde{y}_{\mathrm{d}}^{(r-1)} + a_r\tilde{y}_{\mathrm{d}}^{(r)} \quad . \tag{21}$$

Note that this is an algebraic equation. To obtain the necessary derivatives $\tilde{y}_d^{(r)}$ for the inverse of the model, the filter F was implemented as a state-variable filter (SVF) as shown in Fig. 14. This structure allows to limit the highest derivative $\tilde{y}_d^{(r)}$ in order to constrain the actuating variable u.
The limits $\tilde{y}_{\mathrm{d,min}}^{(r)}$ and $\tilde{y}_{\mathrm{d,max}}^{(r)}$ can be calculated by solving Equation (19a) for $\tilde{y}^{(r)}$ and using Equation (21):

$$\tilde{y}_{\mathrm{d,min}}^{(r)} = \min_{u\in[u_{\min},u_{\max}]} (\bar{\alpha}(\tilde{y}_{\mathrm{d}},\dot{\tilde{y}}_{\mathrm{d}},\ldots,\tilde{y}_{\mathrm{d}}^{(r-1)},u)) \tag{22a}$$

$$\tilde{y}_{\mathrm{d,max}}^{(r)} = \max_{u\in[u_{\min},u_{\max}]} (\bar{\alpha}(\tilde{y}_{\mathrm{d}}d,\dot{\tilde{y}}_{\mathrm{d}},\ldots,\tilde{y}_{\mathrm{d}}^{(r-1)},u)) \quad . \tag{22b}$$

This means that the actuating variable u is constrained exactly to $[u_{\min}, u_{\max}]$ if the highest derivative $\tilde{y}_{\mathrm{d}}^{(r)}$ is restricted to these limits.

6. Controller Design for the Operating Device and for the Excavator

6.1 Design Procedure

The controllers in Fig. 8 were designed utilizing the IMC method. The following procedure was used to design the IMC controllers for the haptic device (electric motors) and the excavator (electrohydraulic valves to control the boom, stick, and bucket cylinders):

1. Take measurements of the static and dynamic behavior of the plant Σ (gain and step response)
2. Parameter identification of the parametric model in Equation (23) for each actuator
3. IMC controller design using the parameterized models
4. Design of a prefilter to minimize overshoot

This approach allows a straightforward controller development. The prefilters in Fig. 8 are needed since a large peak overshoot is not acceptable due to safety reasons: The excavator boom is not allowed to exceed its reference position because it could damage objects close to the bucket. The additional prefilter converts the structure to a two-degrees-of-freedom controller.
To this end, the plant models were chosen as an integrator and a first-order filter:

$$\tilde{\Sigma} = \frac{k}{s(Ts+1)} \quad , \tag{23}$$

where parameter k is the gain and T is the time constant of the low-pass filter. The model parameters were determined by measurements. The controllers C and prefilters F_{pre} were designed according to Section 5.

6.2 Controller Design for the Haptic Device

The actuating variables for the SensAble Phantom Omni haptic device are the motor currents of each joint. The output variables are the joint angles. Fig. 13 shows the step response of the first segment and the actuating variable $u_{\mathrm{hd},1}$. The actuating variable does not return to zero as the effect of gravity requires the electric motors of the haptic device to be actuated permanently to hold their positions.
As mentioned before, the controller of the haptic device requires an anti-windup strategy according to Section 5.4. As a consequence, F_{tot} was implemented as the state-variable filter shown in Fig. 14. The used filter F_{tot}

$$F_{\mathrm{tot}} = \frac{\delta_1 s + 1}{\delta_3 s^3 + \delta_2 s^2} \tag{24}$$

leads to the differential equation

$$y_d^{(3)} + \frac{\delta_2}{\delta_3} y_d^{(2)} = \frac{\delta_1}{\delta_3} u^{(1)} + \frac{1}{\delta_3} u \quad . \tag{25}$$

The system can also be described in controllable standard form (Lunze, 2006) as

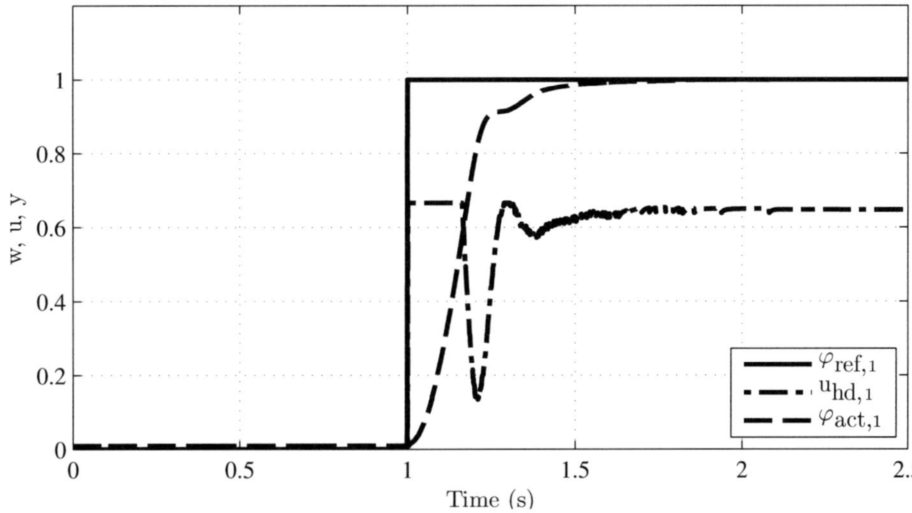

Fig. 13. Step response of the first segment of the haptic device

$$\dot{\boldsymbol{x}}_{tr} = \begin{pmatrix} 0 & 1 & 0 \\ 0 & 0 & \frac{\delta_3 - \delta_1\delta_2}{\delta_3^2} \\ 0 & 0 & -\frac{\delta_2}{\delta_3} \end{pmatrix} \boldsymbol{x}_{tr} + \begin{pmatrix} 0 \\ \frac{\delta_1}{\delta_3} \\ 1 \end{pmatrix} u \tag{26}$$

$$\tilde{y}_d = \begin{pmatrix} 1 & 0 & 0 \end{pmatrix} \boldsymbol{x}_{tr} \tag{27}$$

by using the transformation $\boldsymbol{x}_{tr} = \boldsymbol{T}_R \boldsymbol{x}$ with

$$\boldsymbol{T}_R = \begin{pmatrix} \frac{1}{\delta_3} & \frac{\delta_1}{\delta_3} & 0 \\ 0 & \frac{1}{\delta_3} & \frac{\delta_1}{\delta_3} \\ 0 & 0 & 1 \end{pmatrix} . \tag{28}$$

The transformed system can be implemented as the block diagram shown in Fig. 14. Note the integrator chain at the output of F_{tot}.
The algebraic model of each actuated segment j of the operating element is

$$k_j \cdot \ddot{y}_{hd,j} + \dot{y}_{hd,j} = T_j \cdot u_{hd,j} \quad . \tag{29}$$

Utilizing the algebraic model Σ_{hd} allows to compute the constraints for the highest derivative $\ddot{y}_{hd}$ according to Section 5.4:

$$\ddot{y}_{hd,min} = \frac{1}{k_j}(-\dot{y}_{hd} + T_{1,j} \cdot u_{hd,min}) \quad , \tag{30}$$

$$\ddot{y}_{hd,max} = \frac{1}{k_j}(-\dot{y}_{hd} + T_{1,j} \cdot u_{hd,max}) \quad . \tag{31}$$

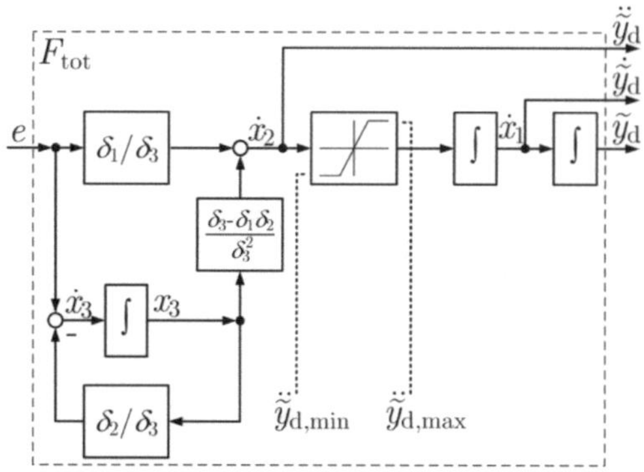

Fig. 14. State-variable filter for the haptic device controller including input constraints

6.3 Controller Design for the Hydraulic Boom

The actuating variables for the hydraulic cylinders of the excavator are the flow rates of the hydraulic oil that the valves distribute to each cylinder or to the slew drive. The output variables are the cylinder positions or the angle of the rotating platform, respectively. Fig. 15 shows the step response of the boom cylinder and the actuating variable $u_{ex,z1}$.

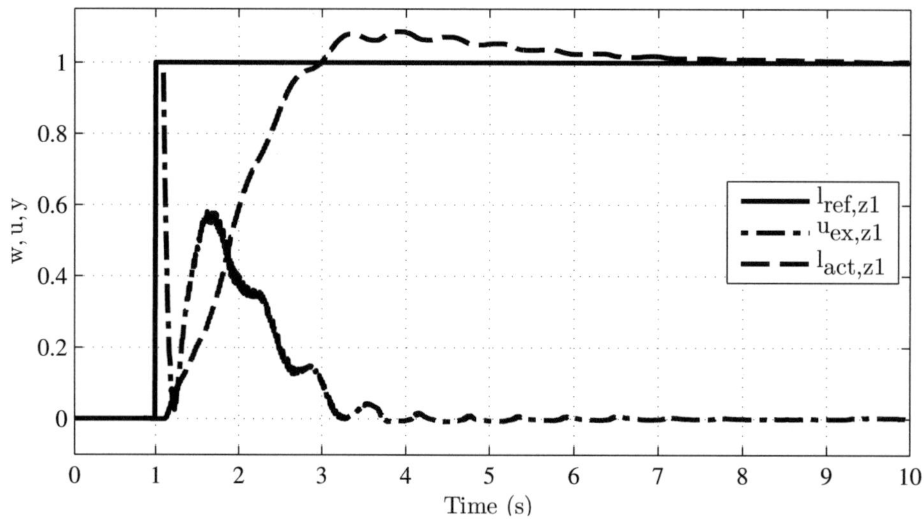

Fig. 15. Step response of the excavator's boom cylinder

Model errors result in an acceptable overshoot. The oscillations of the machine on its tyres can be seen in the measurements.

6.4 Experimental Results

The master-slave control approach introduced in Section 4 shows satisfying results in experiments on the test excavator. The controller for the SensAble Phantom Omni device was running under MATLAB/Simulink. The boom controller was implemented on dSPACE proto-

typing hardware. Position sensors for the hydraulic cylinders and an angular rate sensor for the rotating platform were utilized to measure the actual position of the machine.
The step response of the x-y-controlled hydraulic arm in the horizontal direction x is shown on Fig. 16 (a). The position error in the vertical direction y is less than $\pm$ 0.05 m (cf. Fig. 16 (b)).

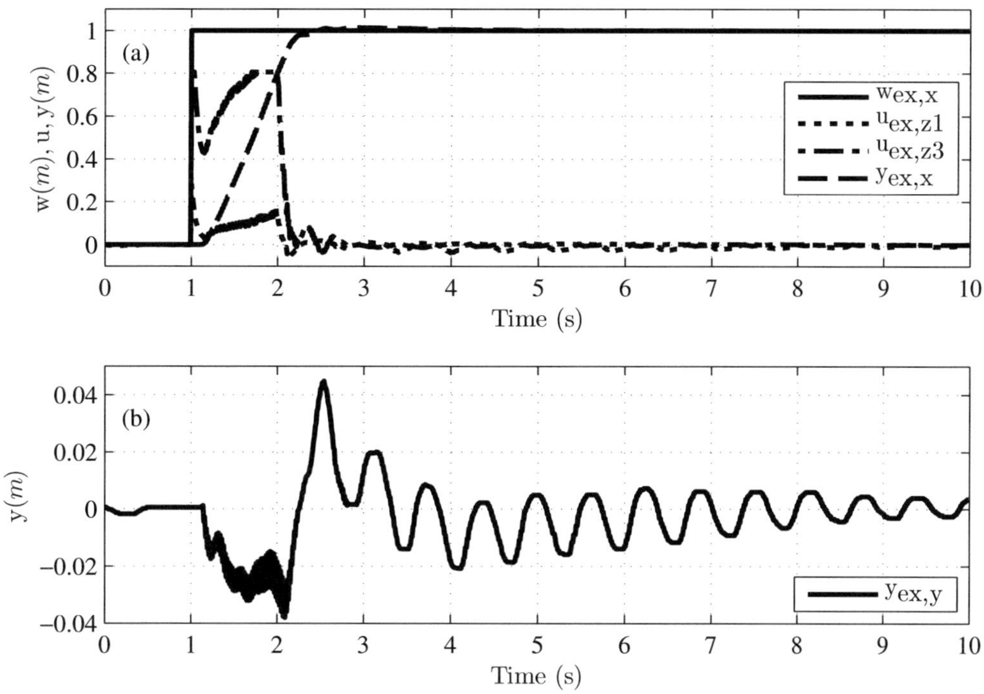

Fig. 16. Step response of the hydraulic arm

The behavior of the interconnected master-slave system is shown on Fig. 17. The position signals $w_{ex,x}$ and $w_{ex,y}$ of the haptic device are low-pass filtered. This was necessary to achieve a smooth reference signal for the excavator. The operator used the haptic device to prescribe the curve in Fig. 18.

7. Evaluation of the Haptically Enhanced Operational Concept

Goal of the proposed operational concept is to improve the handling quality and to simplify the operation — especially for untrained drivers. This target was evaluated by usability experiments with test operators. The configuration using a SensAble Phantom Omni and a 3Dconnexion SpaceBall 5000, as shown in Fig. 5, was used to proof this concept. Twelve male test operators without any relevant experience with hydraulic excavators performed a predefined working task. They were filmed to analyze the working cycle times and operating errors. Finally the test persons were surveyed using a questionnaire.

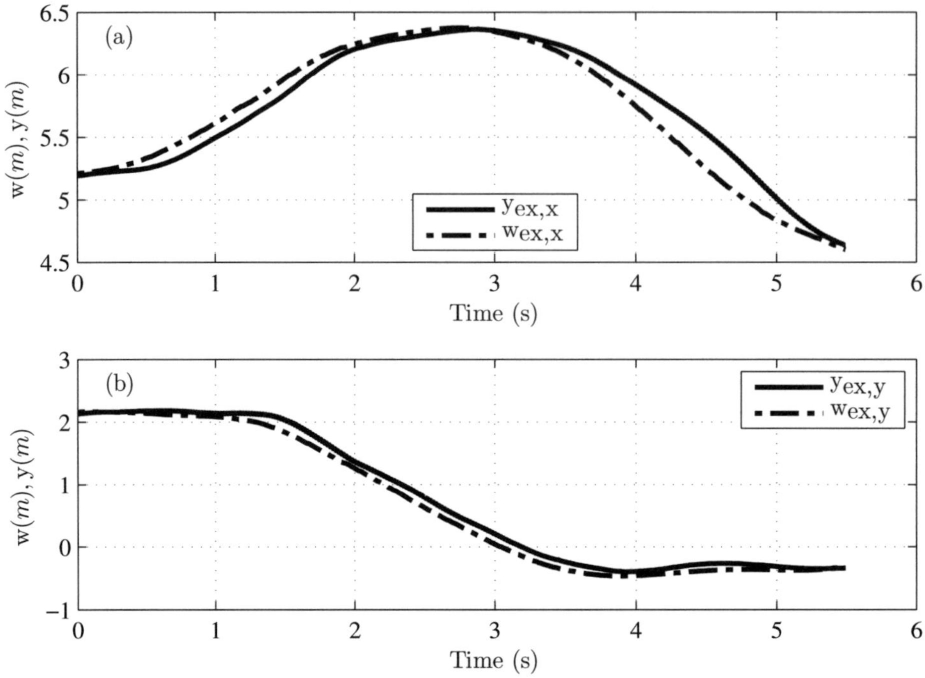

Fig. 17. Position on x- and y-axis of the excavator and the haptic device over time

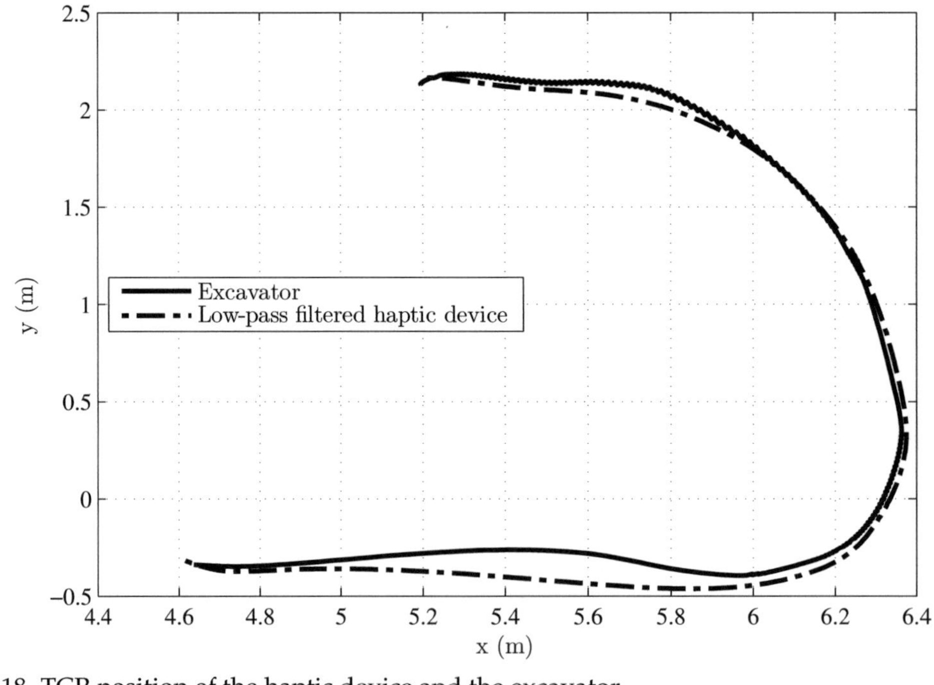

Fig. 18. TCP-position of the haptic device and the excavator

7.1 Intuitive Operational Concept

The test operators started with performing a typical working task using the standard joysticks. After this run, they performed the same tasks using the new concept. The time to complete a working cycle and the operating errors were compared. An operating error is a motion of the excavator's TCP into the wrong direction due to a wrong operator input. These errors were easily seen due to the predefined task. Reasons for errors are confusions of operating elements or joystick axes. The typical working cycle consisted of

- loading the bucket with soil,
- rotating the cabin about 90° and lifting the bucket over an obstacle,
- unloading the soil,
- moving back to the initial position and starting the next cycle.

Before starting, the test operators got a brief instruction to the hydraulic excavator and the operational concepts. Since some learning effects can be observed already after a short time only the first two cycles of each operator were analyzed. It was assumed that short cycle times and less operating errors are indicators for an intuitive operational concept. A paired t-test was calculated for the cycle times ($t(11) = -3.324; p = 0.007$) and for the operating errors ($t(11) = -6.588; p = 0.000$). The results in Fig. 19 show significant differences between both operational concepts. The cycle time and especially the number of errors are significantly lower. These results coincide with related studies by Wallersteiner et al. (1993) and Lawrence et al. (1990). The survey showed that the inexperienced operators subjectively benchmark the coordinated control concept better than the standard control concept regarding usability and training time.

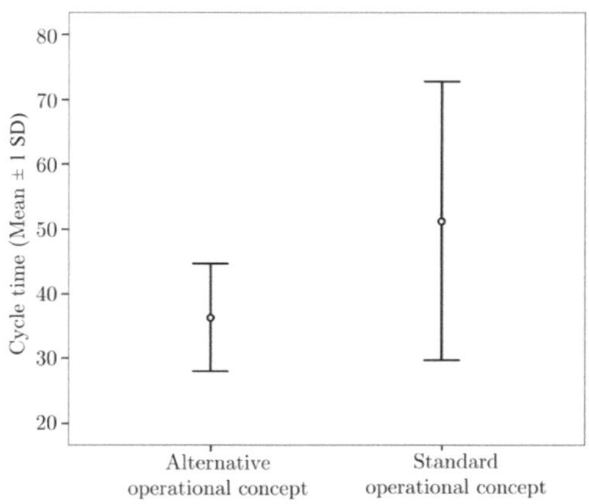

(a) Cycle time

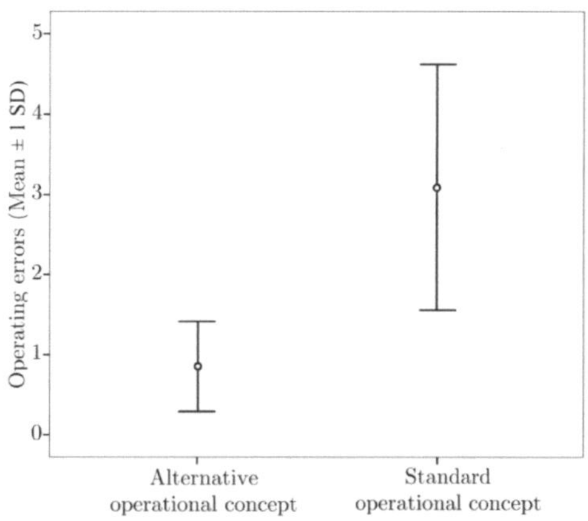

(b) Operating errors

Fig. 19. Evaluation of the proposed operational concept

7.2 Haptically Enhanced Driver Assistance Systems

Fig. 20 illustrates the implemented haptic driver assistance systems for slope leveling and trajectory guidance according to Fig. 9. Fig. 20(a) shows the position y_{ex} of the hydraulic manipulator's TCP. It was necessary to filter the signal y_{hd} in order to eliminate the high-frequency jittering of the operator's hand before using it as reference signal w_{ex} for the excavator. Note that the operator can easily follow the predefined slope without penetrating the virtual fixtures. The repeat accuracy is less than 0.1 m. In the workspace right of the virtual wall the operating device can move freely. A measurement of the trajectory guidance system is shown in Fig. 20(b). The operator is guided on a predefined trajectory. A noticeable high force is needed to leave this path.

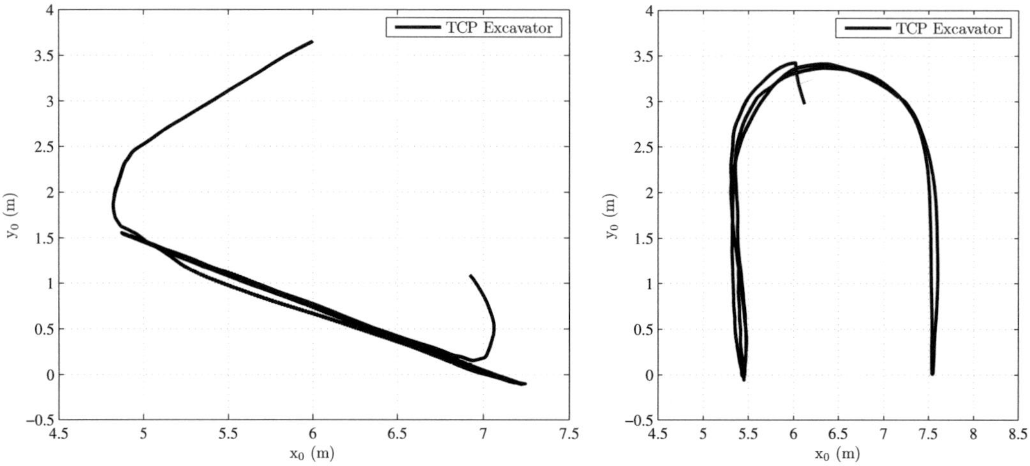

(a) Slope assistance (b) Trajectory guidance

Fig. 20. Measurements of the implemented haptic driver assistance systems

The test operators evaluated the haptically enhanced assistance systems as very expedient and helpful.

8. Conclusion

An intuitive operational concept for a hydraulic excavator was proposed. A conceptual design for an alternative operating device for excavators was developed. In order to implement this concept on a test excavator, an IMC-based control methodology was used and extended where necessary. An introduction to internal model control with input constraints for a haptic device and a feedback control methodology for a master-slave system were presented. An anti-windup approach for models with pure integrators is proposed. This approach is extended to implement haptic feedback. The application was tested in experiments using a SensAble Phantom Omni device and a hydraulic test excavator.
This work shows a straightforward control method to manipulate a machine using an active operating device that resembles the boom geometry. The approach can be applied to similar master-slave systems, e.g. for teleoperation.
The user is able to feel the inertia of the excavator's manipulator and thus gets feedback on the interaction of the bucket with the environment. Haptically enhanced assistance systems for tactile workspace limitations, leveling of soil and guidance on specific trajectory are integrated.
Future work has to be the development of working prototypes of the proposed operating elements, including actuators. These prototypes have to be robust and suitable for mobile

machines. Extensive usability tests should be performed with that system to ensure the concept.
Additionally, the haptic device and the test excavator could be equipped with force sensors to allow testing of further bilateral control concepts.

9. References

Augustine, A. W. (2005). Tactile feedback system for a remotely controlled work machine, *Patent US 6836982 B1*, Caterpillar Inc.

Burdea, G. C. (1996). *Force and Touch Feedback for Virtual Reality*, John Wiley & Sons, Inc., New York.

Cemenska, R. A., Schneider, M. P. & Buege, T. J. (1989). Force feedback lever, *Patent US 4800721*, Caterpillar Inc.

Frank, P. M. (1974). *Entwurf von Regelkreisen mit vorgeschriebenem Verhalten*, G. Braun Verlag, Karlsruhe.

Graichen, K. & Zeitz, M. (2006). Inversionsbasierter Vorsteuerungsentwurf mit Ein- und Ausgangsbeschränkungen, *Automatisierungstechnik* **54**(4): 187–199.

Haas, C. T. & Kim, Y.-S. (2002). Automation in infrastructure construction, *Construction Innovation* **2**: 191–210.

Hannaford, B. (1989). A design framework for teleoperators with kinesthetic feedback, *IEEE Transactions on Robotics and Automation* **5**(4): 426–434.

Hayn, H. & Schwarzmann, D. (2008). Haptic feedback for mobile machines, *6th International Fluid Power Conference*, Vol. 1, Institut für Fluidtechnik, Technische Universität Dresden, Dresdner Verein zur Förderung der Fluidtechnik e. V. Dresden, Dresden.

Huang, P. (2004). *Regelkonzepte zur Fahrzeugfhrung unter Einbeziehung der Bedienelementeigenschaften*, PhD thesis, TU Mnchen.

Kontz, M. E. (2007). *Haptic Control of Hydraulic Machinery Using Proportional Valves*, PhD thesis, G.W. Woodruff School of Mechanical Engineering, Georgia Institute of Technology.

Kraft, B. W. (1991). Force feedback control for backhoe, *Patent US 5019761*.

Lawrence, P., Sauder, B., Wallersteiner, U. & Wilson, J. (1990). Teleoperation of forest harvesting machines, *in* J. Coutteau (ed.), *Proceedings of the Symposium Robotics in Forestry - Forest Operations in the Age of Technology*, number SR-75, Vaudreuil, Quebec, pp. 36–39.

Lunze, J. (2006). *Regelungstechnik 1 - Systemtheoretische Grundlagen, Analyse und Entwurf einschleifiger Regelungen*, Springer-Verlag, Berlin, Heidelberg.

Morari, M. & Zafiriou, E. (1989). *Robust Process Control*, Prentice-Hall, New Jersey.

Ostoja-Starzewski, M. & Skibniewski, M. (1989). A master-slave manipulator for excavation and construction tasks, *Robotics and Autonomous Systems* **4**: 333–337.

Parker, N. R., Salcudean, S. E. & Lawrence, P. D. (1993). Application of force feedback to heavy duty hydraulic machines, *IEEE International Conference on Robotics and Automation*, Atlanta, pp. 375–381.

Rosenberg, L. B. (1993). Virtual fixtures: Perceptual tools for telerobotic manipulation, *Proceedings of the Virtual Reality Annual International Symposium*, pp. 76–82.

Sachs, S., Teichert, H.-J. & Rentzsch, M. (1994). *Ergonomische Gestaltung mobiler Maschinen*, ecomed-Verlag, Landsberg.

Salcudean, S., Tafazoli, S., Hashtrudi-Zaad, K. & Lawrence, P. D. (1997). Evaluation of impedance and teleoperation control of a hydraulic mini-excavator, *in* A. Casals &

A. T. de Almeida (eds), *Experimental Robotics V, Proceedings of the Fifth International Symposium*, Barcelona, pp. 187–198.

Schwarzmann, D. (2007). *Nonlinear Internal Model Control with Automotive Applications*, Logos Verlag, Berlin.

Tafazoli, S., Salcudean, S. M., Hashtrudi-Zaad, K. & Lawrence, P. D. (2002). Impedance control of a teleoperated excavator, *IEEE Transactions on Control Systems Technology* **10**(3): 355–367.

Uchino, H., Takada, M., Shimizu, T., Shibayama, M. & Furuno, F. (1977). System for controlling a power shovel, *Patent US 4059196*, Hokushin Electric Works.

Wallersteiner, U., Lawrence, P. & Sauder, B. (1993). A human factors evaluation of two different machine control systems for log loaders, *Ergonomics* **26**(8): 927–934.

Yamada, H. & Muto, T. (2003). Development of a hydraulic tele-operated construction robot using virtual reality (new master-slave control method and an evaluation of a visual feedback system), *International Journal of Fluid Power* **4**(2): 35–42.

Yoshinada, H. & Takeda, S. (1990). Master/slave type manipulator, *Patent US 4893981*, Kabushiki Kaisha Komatsu Seisakusho.

Zhu, M. & Salcudean, S. E. (1995). Achieving transparency for teleoperator systems under position and rate control, *Proc. Intl. Conf. Intelligent Robots and Systems*, Pittburgh, PA, pp. 7–12.

11

Five Fingers Haptic Interface Robot HIRO: Design, Rendering, and Applications

Osama Halabi and Haruhisa Kawasaki
Iwate University, Gifu University
Japan

Introduction

Haptic interfaces are devices that allow human-machine interaction through force and touch. Combined haptic and visual interfaces have been around for decades. Yet, despite an enormous increase in research activity in the last few years, the science of haptics is still a technology in its infancy. The majority of commercially available haptic devices operate based on a principle of point interaction. Thus, contact between the operator and the simulated virtual environment occurs only at an arbitrary single point, typically the tip of a stylus or thimble used for interaction. Many literatures have identified the importance of multifinger display in the field of haptics (Wall et al., 2001).

Haptic interfaces have been utilized in the area of tele-manipulation (Ivanisevic et al., 2000) (Dubey et al., 2001) (Elhajj et al., 2001) (Ando et al., 2001), interaction with micro/nano scale phenomenon (Guthold et al., 2000) (Marliere et al., 2004), medical training and evaluation (Basdogan et al., 2001) (Bardorfer et al., 2001) (Langrana et al., 1994). Multifinger haptic interface has a higher potential for the above mentioned applications than that of a single point haptic interface. A number of multifinger haptic interfaces (Kawasaki et al., 1993) (Ueda et al., 2004) (Walairacht et al., 2001) (Bouzit et al., 2002) (Yoshikawa et al., 2000) (CyberGlove Systems, 2009) have been developed. However, the issue of developing a haptic interface opposite to the human hand that reflects the force feeling to the finger tips was never addressed. The haptic interface is demanded to be safe, work in wide operation space, and able to present not only force at the contact points but also the weight feeling of the virtual objects. Also impose no oppressive feeling to the operator's hand. Moreover, the haptic interface itself imposes no weight feeling. In this chapter the new developed five-fingers Haptic Interface RObot (HIRO II) based on HIRO (Kawasaki et al., 2003) (Alhalabi et al., 2004) that addresses these issues is introduced. HIRO II is a new haptic device that enables users to interact and feel the virtual object safely and it does not impose any weight on the users hand since it is not wearable device nor it is cumbersome. Two main important issues were in mind while designing HIRO II, multiple interaction points and reflecting forces directly to the human fingertips where other haptic devices failed to provide suitable solutions. In addition, user's safety and ease of attachment issues have been also considered while designing HIRO II.

The first goal is to design a generic architecture that will support both haptic and graphic requirements by proposing a multi-layer architecture that can be used in a networked haptic environment to achieve shared virtual haptic interaction over the network.
It has been clearly shown that it is necessary to run the simulation and the graphics loops of virtual environments (VE) systems asynchronously in order to maintain reasonable display update rates (around 30Hz) in the presence of long simulation computation. Such a decoupling is even more critical for force display, where high update rate is required to produce high-quality forces (Gossweiler et al., 1993) (Adachi et al., 1995) (Mark et al., 1996) (Balaniuk, 1999).
We can decouple the simulation and haptic loops on a single machine by using multiple processes (Adachi et al., 1995) (Balaniuk, 1999). This is the approach of most commercial devices. It is often more practical to dedicate one real-time machine to the haptic servo loop, and use other machine(s) for the rest of the virtual environment tasks (simulation, high-performance graphics, etc.). Our approach was to decouples haptic and graphics rendering, running each on a separate machine allowing a high degree of independence between haptics and graphics. This strategy allows each machine to be well matched to its task. It also allows for flexible system configuration, which is particularly useful in a research environment.
The second goal of this research is to utilize the new HIRO in application that specifically sensitive to multifinger interaction, such as medical palpation and surgery. Therefore, interacting with soft deformable object is necessary. Most high-precision techniques for deformable objects tend to be computationally expensive, making high control rates (> 1 KHz) difficult to reach. Different solutions proposed to solve this problem as will be discussed in details later section (Balaniuk, 1999) (Barbagli, 2002) (Mendoza, 2001) (Cavusoglu, 2000). Most of these methods deal with intermediate representation or local models in the haptic loop to obtain force at a high update. Contribution to the literature, however, to the best of our knowledge, concern only single-point contact. Multiple points of contact used in touching deformable objects must consider individual effect of each point on the other points and how the object should be deformed based on all fingers interaction. Using a local model is not a solution because the entire model, or sufficiently large independent part of it, must be dealt with to take into account the effects of each finger on the model and on the other fingers. To do so, we take an "elementary displacement" approach in finite element modeling.
To verify the presented methods and approaches, Future Haptic Science Encyclopedia was developed and presented as a new potential application that benefit greatly from the haptic research to achieve a new level of realism. Also, to fully demonstrate the potentiality of the new haptic interface and to verify the proposed architecture and techniques for force calculation and collision that specifically considered multipoint contact haptic interaction. Moreover, a physically-based modeling technique for displaying forces and deformations has been used to achieve interaction with relatively large deformable objects in real time, where it is computationally expensive and the haptic update rate may drop below the requirement.

1. HIRO-II Design

1.1 Basic Design

A multifinger haptic interface joined to an arm can provide a wide operation space. But, most of them are mounted on the back of the human hand like the CyberForce (CyberGlove Systems, 2009). Fixing the haptic interface to the hand gives oppressive feeling to the operator since the interface binds the human hand firmly. In order to reduce the oppressive feeling and increase safety, a three-finger haptic interface opposite to human hand has been presented by our group (Kawasaki et al., 2003). Later, we developed a new Haptic Interface RObot named HIRO II to present force feeling to all human hand fingers. Fig. 1 shows the developed five-finger haptic interface, and how it is connected to the operator's hand. The haptic interface consists of an interface arm, a haptic hand with five haptic fingers, and a controller. When the operator moves his/her hand, the haptic interface follows the motion of operator's fingers and present the force feeling. The operator feels just a little oppressive feeling because the coupled part between the human hand and the haptic interface is only the fingertips of the operator.

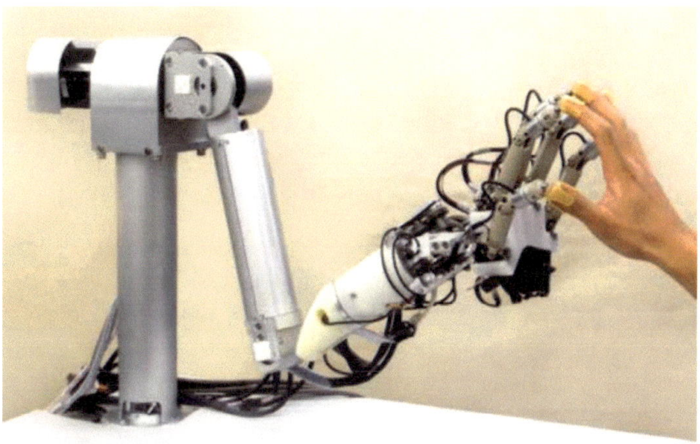

Fig. 1. The Developed five-finger haptic interface: HIRO II

1.2 Haptic hand

The haptic hand starts from the wrist but does not include it, and ends with the fingertips. This includes a hand base, and five haptic fingers as shown in Fig. 2. The haptic fingers are designed to be similar to the human fingers in geometry and motion ability. Table 1 shows specifications of the haptic hand.

Hand	Number of fingers	5	
	Degree of freedom	15	dof
	Weight	0.73	Kgf
Finger	Degree of freedom	3	dof
	Weight	0.13	Kgf
	Work space of thumb	713	cm^3
	Work space of finger	535	cm^3
	Output force	3.5	N (max)
	Velocity	0.23	m/s (max)

Table 1. Specifications of the haptic hand

The developed haptic finger is shown in Fig. 3. The design of the finger is based on an anthropomorphic robot hand, named Gifu Hand III (Mouri et al., 2002). Each finger has 3 joints allowing 3 DOF. The first joint allows abduction/adduction. The second joint allows flexion/extension. The third joint allows flexion/extension. All joints are driven by DC servomotors with gear transmissions and rotary encoders. The motion ranges of the 1st to the 3rd joints are -30 ~ 30, -25 ~ 94, and -10 ~ 114 [deg], respectively. Thumb is almost same as the finger except for a reduction gear ratio and movable ranges of joint 1 and joint 2. The motion ranges of the 1st to the 2nd joints of the thumb are -40 ~ 40 and -25 ~ 103 [deg]. Workspaces of thumb and hand are shown in Fig. 4(a) and Fig. 4(b). Volumes of the workspace of the thumb and fingers are 535 and 713 [mm^3], respectively.

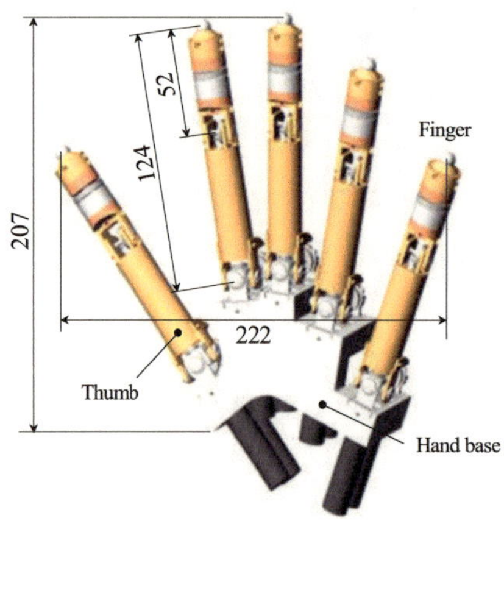

Fig. 2. Haptic hand design

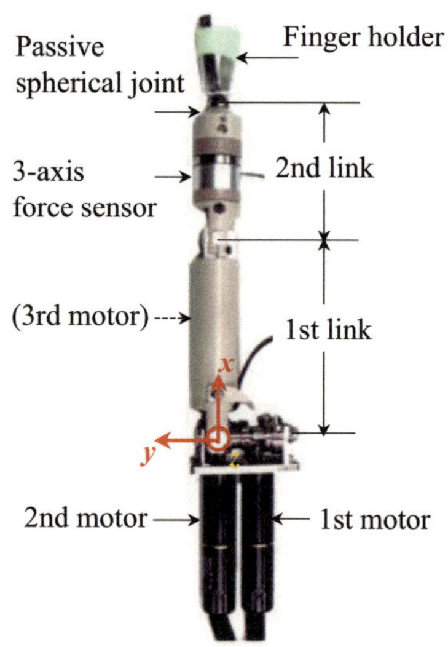

Fig. 3. Haptic finger

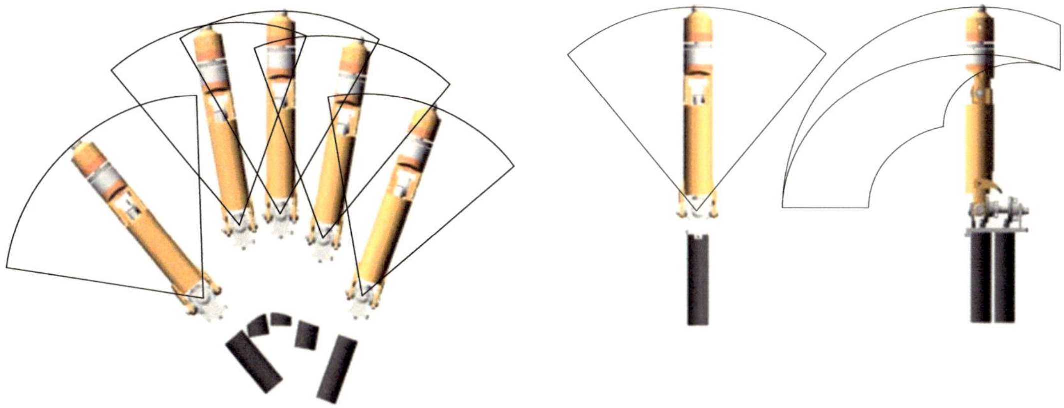

(a) (b)

Fig. 4. The workspaces of the thumb and the hand

The thumb is designed to work in wide space because the workspace of the human's thumb is larger than that of other fingers. Finger layout of the haptic hand is designed to maximize the product space between the workspace of the haptic hand and the human hand. Fig. 5 shows an optimum pose of the haptic finger for the human index finger. The size is decided based on a practical statistics conducted on Japanese males. The lengths of distal, middle, and proximal phalanxes are 39, 20, and 26 [mm], respectively. The workspace of the human index finger and the haptic finger is 281 and 535 [cm^3], respectively. The product space at the optimum pose of the haptic finger is 259 [cm^3]. The allocation of fingers in haptic hand was designed taken in consideration the above geometrical relation.

In the second link of each finger, a 6-axes force sensor (NANO sensor by BL AUTOTEC. LTD.) is installed. The force sensor is used to control the human fingertip force. On the force sensor, a finger holder is mounted through a passive spherical joint attached to the force sensor by permanent magnet as shown in Fig. 6. The operator inserts his/her fingertips into the finger-holders to operate the interface. The passive spherical joint attached by the magnet has two roles: First, the adjustment of differences between the human and haptic fingers orientations. Each human finger has 6 DOF and each haptic finger has 3 DOF, therefore, additional passive 3 DOF are needed. Second, to ensure the operator's safety by enabling him/her to remove their fingers easily and quickly should instability or malfunctions occurs.

The maximum output torques of the 1st, 2nd, and 3rd joints are 0.81, 0.43, and 0.2 [Nm] respectively, which are equivalent to fingertip force of 6.5, 3.5, and 3.8 [N] respectively. The maximum velocities of the 1st joint to 3rd one are 1.9, 3.5, and 9.2 [rad/s] respectively, which are equivalent to fingertip velocities of 0.23, 0.43, and 0.48 [m/s] respectively. These specifications show that the haptic fingers can follow the human fingers motion in any task implementation.

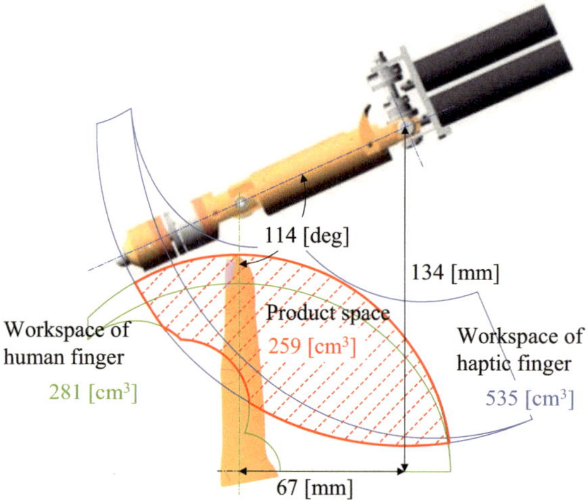

Fig. 5. Optimum pose of the haptic finger for the human finger

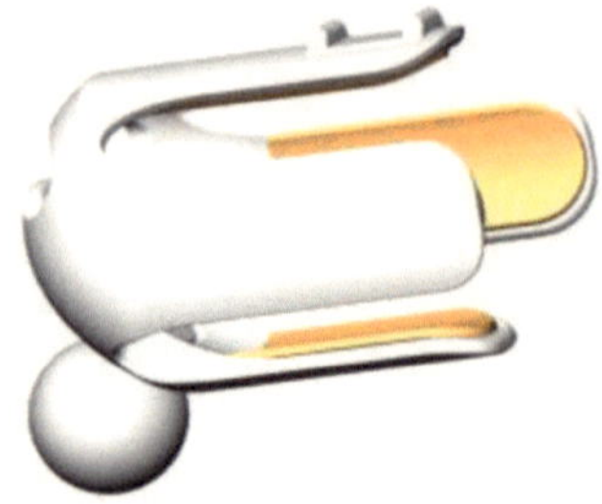

Fig. 6. Finger holder

1.3 Interface arm

The interface arm is designed to be as close as possible to the human arm in geometry and motion ability as shown in Fig. 7. The upper joint of the interface arm is the shoulder joint. The shoulder joint motion is simplified to 2 DOF because the contribution of the third DOF to the arm flexibility is too limited compared to the complexity of realizing it. The two possible DOF are the shoulder flexion/extension and shoulder adduction/abduction, and the neglected DOF is the shoulder radial/lateral rotation. The middle joint of the interface arm is the elbow joint with 1 DOF, which generates the elbow flexion/extension. The lower joint of the interface arm is the wrist joint with 3 DOF. The first DOF is the forearm supination/pronation, the second DOF is the wrist flexion/extension, and the third DOF is the wrist abduction/adduction. The interface arm has therefore 6 joints allowing 6 DOF. The interface arm has a similar size to the human arm, and its joints motion ranges are compatible with it.

The lengths of the upper arm and the forearm are 0.3 and 0.31 [m], respectively. The arm joints are actuated by AC servomotors equipped with rotary encoders and gear transmissions. The movement angles of the 1st to 6th joint ranges are (-180, 180), (0, 180), (-90, 55), (-180, 180), (-55, 55), and (-90, 90) [degrees]. Fig.8 shows the movement space and the workspace of the haptic arm. The workspace is about 400x800x300 [mm]. Table 2 shows the specifications of the arm. The weight of the whole mechanism is 40% reduced compared with HIRO (Kawasaki et al., 2003). Maximum output force is 45 N and maximum velocity at the haptic hand base is 0.4 [m/s].

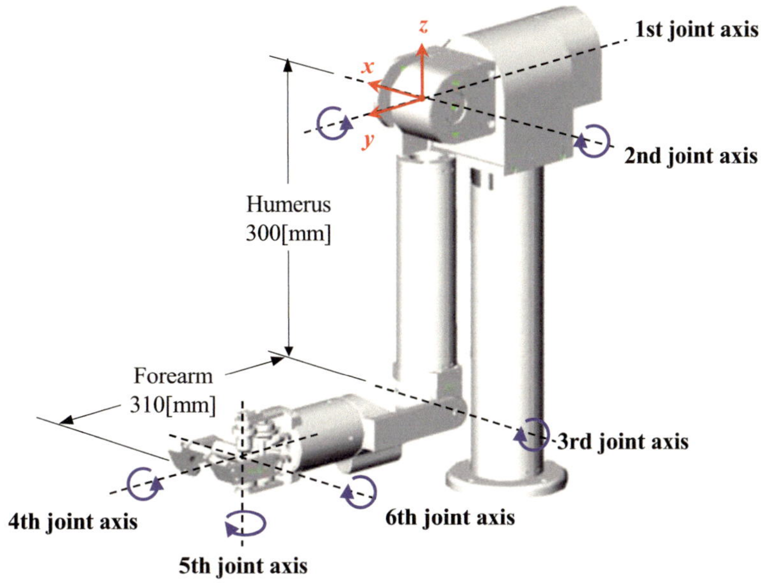

Fig. 7. Arm Design

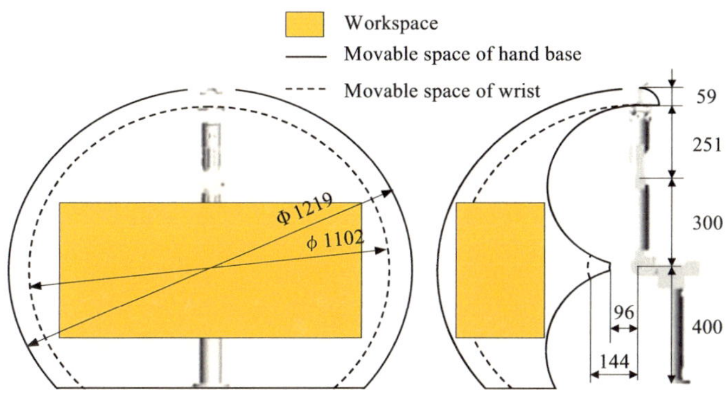

Fig. 8. Workspace of the haptic arm

Degree of freedom	6	
Output force	45	N
Output moment	2.6	Nm (max)
Transnational velocity	0.4	m/s (max)
Rotational velocity	1.4	rad/s (max)
Weight	6.9	Kgf

Table 2. Specifications of the haptic

Haptic rendering

1.4 Multipoint haptic interaction

The goal of haptic rendering is to display the shape surface of arbitrary 3D objects in real time through a haptic interface. Initial haptic rendering methods focused on displaying object primitives. Later Zilles and Salisbury (Zilles & Salisbury, 1999) developed a more sophisticated constraint-based method to render generic polygonal meshes. Pervious methods are not sufficient to model the haptic interaction with more complex category of haptic interfaces like gloves and haptic hands. Popescu and his colleges (Popescu et al., 1999) used a haptic interaction mesh (a set of points used for haptic rendering) that accounts for the hand interaction model. The method provided better representation of finger haptic interaction but still can only covers a certain patch of the fingertip. The proposed haptic interaction technique considers the exact point of the fingertip that touched the virtual object and the orientation relative to the virtual object. For the sake of simplicity, we restrict ourselves to static environment composed of deformable objects and rigid hand. The haptic rendering was implemented by first checking for collision detection between the fingertips of the simulated fingers and the virtual objects. Since the finger is considered to be non-deformable, the fingertip's displacement vector $\vec{d}$ components $\vec{d}x$, $\vec{d}y$, $\vec{d}z$ is measured between the "ideal haptic interface point" (IHIP) on the surface and the centroid of the collided polygon of each fingertip. The concept of calculating the displacement vector can be seen from Fig. 9. This displacement vector is applied on the centroid of the collided polygon of the virtual deformable object and treated as the fingertip penetration distance (Alhalabi et al., 2004).

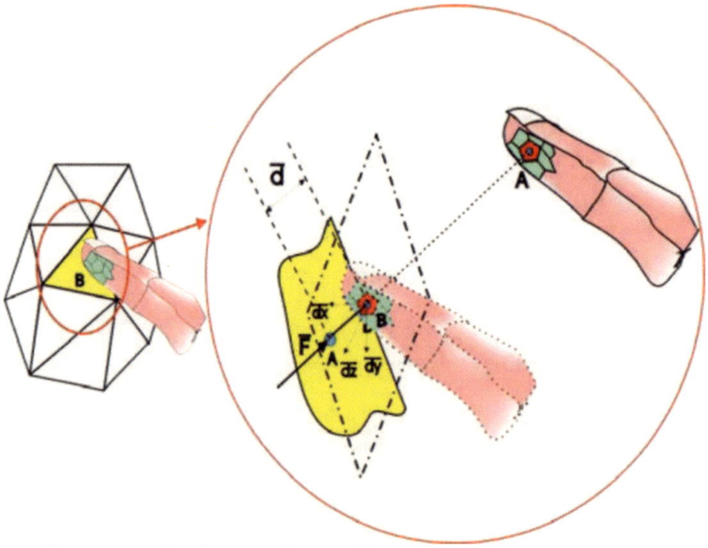

Fig. 9. Penetration distance calculation after collision detection

1.5 Haptic rendering with deformable objects

A real-time dynamic analysis of force-reflecting deformable objects using finite-element techniques is quite difficult with the computational power available. In a Virtual

Environment (VE) simulation of interaction with deformable bodies, most high-precision techniques for deformable objects tend to be computationally expensive, making it difficult to reach high control rates (> 1 KHz). It is not possible to increase the update rate of the physical model to the haptic rate with its full complexity due to computational limitations. Among the many solutions proposed to solve this problem, one applies the same force between model updates, or to low-pass filter this generated force to the bandwidth of the model update rate. These effectively reduce the haptic update rate to the visual update rate, impairing the fidelity of haptic interaction — a point especially grave when high frequency interaction forces are required, for example, in nonlinear contact phenomena.

Many solutions have been proposed based on the intermediate representation or local model representation concept, where the basic idea is to use a simple implicit function that approximates, to a good extent, a small part of the object being touched. More specifically such intermediate representation or local model represents that part of the object closest to the current position of the haptic interface. Past implementations of local models, typically god-object (Zilles et al., 1996) or proxy (Ruspini et al., 1997), have been implemented using different techniques. Theses approaches are typically used for single point of contact haptic interaction with rigid objects. Adachi et al. used a plane that always tangent to the virtual object surface (Adachi et al., 1995), as an intermediate representation, as did Mark et al. in (Mark et al., 1996). Balaniuk in (Balaniuk et al., 1999) used a spherical local model. These two concepts — intermediate representation and the local model — have been adopted by many researchers for particular cases of deformable objects. Barbagli et al. (Barbagli et al., 2002) presented techniques that based on the concept of local model adapted to deformable objects. (Mendoza & Laugier, 2001) proposed a local model based on the topology of the virtual object being used by taking a set of facets where interaction is taken place around a long virtual probe. Cavasoglu and Tendick (Cavasoglu & Tendick, 2000) used a linearization of the non-linear deformable model to obtain a simpler model. None of these approaches has, however, fully exploited the entire model in haptic control, but dealt only with small representations of the model. All available literature is concerned only with single-point contact. When multiple points of contact are involved in touching deformable objects, the effect of individual points on the other points must be considered, as well as how the object is to be deformed based on all fingers interaction. Using a local model is not sufficient to solve this problem, because the entire model or a sufficiently large independent part of it must be dealt with to consider the effects of individual fingers on the model and on other fingers.

The physically based modeling technique we propose for displaying force and deformation involving interaction with multipoint contact overcomes the difficulty of real-time dynamic analysis of force-reflecting deformable objects using finite-element techniques, which is quit difficult given the available computational power. To do so, we take an "elementary displacement" approach in finite element modeling.

1.5.1 Elementary displacement approach

Tissues are in general heterogeneous, exhibiting non-linear, anisotropic elastic and viscous behavior. Combination models of this quickly becomes complex and requires a huge calculation core that tend to eliminate the possibility of real-time simulation. Solving this problem requires that we make a number of simplifications. We chose the linear elastic deformation model known as Hook's law. Although this model is only valid for very small

deformation and strain, it is widely used in surgical simulators, where it has been proven to provide satisfactory results.
Consider an elastic solid Ω in three-dimensional space $\chi = [x, y, z]$ with boundary conditions in terms of given force and displacement on the surface *A*. The strain energy of the solid is defined as:

$$E_{strain} = \frac{1}{2} \iiint_{\Omega} \varepsilon^T \ \sigma dx \tag{1}$$

where $\varepsilon^T = [\varepsilon_x \ \varepsilon_y \ \varepsilon_z \ \gamma_{xy} \ \gamma_{xz} \ \gamma_{yz}]^T$ is a strain vector. By defining a displacement vector $U = [u \ v \ w]^T$, the strain vector is rewritten as $\varepsilon = BU$ where

$$B = \begin{bmatrix} \frac{\delta}{\delta x} & 0 & 0 \\ 0 & \frac{\delta}{\delta y} & 0 \\ 0 & 0 & \frac{\delta}{\delta z} \\ \frac{\delta}{\delta y} & \frac{\delta}{\delta x} & 0 \\ \frac{\delta}{\delta z} & 0 & \frac{\delta}{\delta x} \\ 0 & \frac{\delta}{\delta z} & \frac{\delta}{\delta y} \end{bmatrix} \tag{2}$$

Stress vector σ is related to the strain vector through Hook's law by $\sigma = D\varepsilon$. Matrix D reads as:

$$D = \frac{E}{(1+v)(1-2v)} \begin{bmatrix} 1-v & v & v & 0 & 0 & 0 \\ v & 1-v & v & 0 & 0 & 0 \\ v & v & 1-v & 0 & 0 & 0 \\ 0 & 0 & 0 & \frac{1-2v}{2} & 0 & 0 \\ 0 & 0 & 0 & 0 & \frac{1-2v}{2} & 0 \\ 0 & 0 & 0 & 0 & 0 & \frac{1-2v}{2} \end{bmatrix} \tag{3}$$

where *E* is Young's modulus of elasticity and υ is the Poisson ratio.
Using these relations, we rewrite strain energy and add work done by given external force *f* to yield the potential energy function:

$$\Pi(U) = \frac{1}{2} \iiint_{\Omega} U^T B^T DBU dx - \iint_{A} f^T U dx \tag{4}$$

After discretizing solid Ω by volumetric finite elements and equating the first variation of the potential energy to zero we arrive to a static equilibrium equation of the discrete element:

$$0 = \iiint_{\Omega^e} B^{eT} DB^e U^e dv - f^e = K^e U^e - f^e \tag{5}$$

where matrix B^e depends on the type of chosen finite element. Then we assemble global matrices from already obtained element matrices in Eq. (5) describing the solid Ω by a large sparse system of linear equations $KU = F$.

For haptics, we are interested only in visible nodes deformations and interaction with contact nodes, so we need not to consider the motion of nodes that are not visible, i.e., internal, or forces applied at nodes that are not in direct contact with the fingertips. We tried several different solvers and approaches, including model matrices condensation, the use of pre-calculated stiffness matrix inverse updates, and found that they are too slow for our desired discretization level. Very good performance has been achieved when implementing "the elementary displacement" approach, which takes the advantage of the model linearity where the principle of superposition is valid. In off-line calculation, all possible loading cases for elementary (usually unitary) displacements are examined; calculated deformation and equivalent force at controlled points are saved to files. Data about deformation is stored as a set of 3×3 $[T^d_{nk}]$ tensors, expressing the relation between the displacement of node n and elementary displacement $d_k = [d_{xk}\ d_{yk}\ d_{zk}]$ imposed at node k. In the same way the components of elementary equivalent force are stored in 3×3 $[T^f_k]$ tensors. Since only surface nodes are considered, the amount of stored data is dramatically reduced.

In real-time calculation, pre-calculated results are scaled based on robot fingertips movement and added. Displacement d_n of model node n, for example, induced by constraint d^*_k applied to node k is obtained by the following linear equation:

$$d_n = \left[T^d_{nk}\right] \left|\frac{d^*_k}{d_k}\right| \tag{6}$$

for any node $k \neq n$, where $\left|\frac{d^*_k}{d_k}\right|$ denotes component-by-component vector division. HIRO II has five points of contact, so more than one node is in touch at the same time and more than one node could be moved. In this case the total displacement of a node is the sum of all displacements induced by touched nodes m:

$$d_n = \sum_{l=1}^{m} \left[T^d_{nkl}\right] \left[\tilde{d}_{kl}\right] \tag{7}$$

where $\left[\tilde{d}_{kl}\right]$ is corrected displacement of the touched node (Cotin et al., 1999). The force associated with the touched node k is determined as:

$$f_n = \left[T^f_{nk}\right] \left[\tilde{d}_k\right] \tag{8}$$

The finite element method in combination with the *"elementary displacement"* approach is successfully implemented and tested in breast palpation application (Alhalabi et al., 2005) (Daniulaitis et al., 2004). We are currently dealing with models, containing from 500 to 600 surface nodes, simulated at above 1600 Hz frequency. Further refinement of the mesh and increasing node number do not affect significantly the sense of touch, but dramatically increases the memory required to store elementary displacement and force, which makes simulation impractical.

1.5.2 Elementary displacement approach evaluation

We have carefully tested and compared the elementary displacement approach with different approaches to confirm its performance and ensure that it can generates realistic force with high update exceeding 1 KHz required to produce force in the haptic loop. Fig. 10 shows the relationship between node number and calculation frequency for three approaches. Clearly the elementary displacement approach is superior to other approaches and calculates force at high frequency.

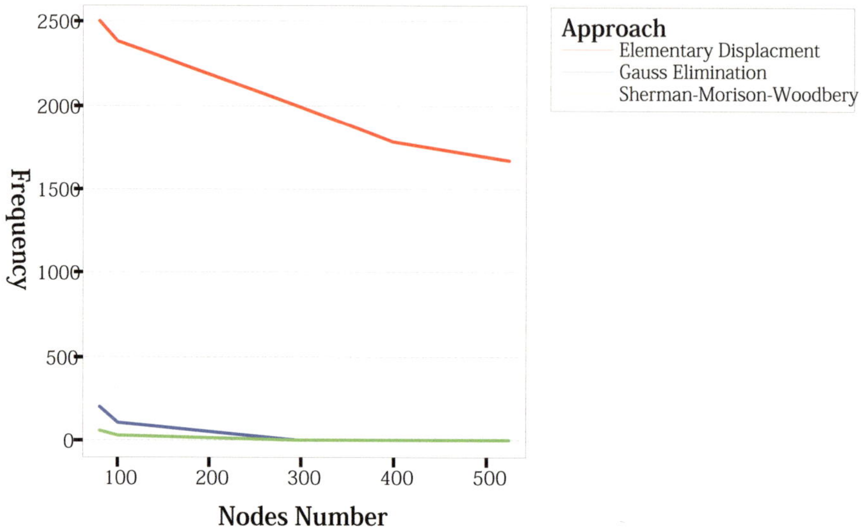

Fig. 10. Frequency-node number curve

Applications

1.6 Future Haptic Science Encyclopedia (FHSE)

We developed a future haptic science encyclopedia (FHSE) to explore the high potential and usability of HIRO II, while testing the proposed architecture and verifying force and deformation calculation. The FHSE enables users to experience many different virtual worlds such as the scientific, historical, and astronomical worlds. Three kinds of encyclopedia — "Planets in the solar system", "the Dinosaur's world", and "the Microscopic world" — were implemented and tested as details in the next section. The interesting feature of FHSE is that it is considered a complete VR interface where the user only uses HIRO II to interact and move between and around scenes. Controls introduced in this system include virtual buttons, levers, and arrows without the need to use devices such as joysticks and keyboards (Fig. 11). These controls reflect force similar to that induced by the actual control (switches, buttons, and levers), making interaction easier, realistic, and enjoyable. A message board for users explains the current scene and the next action to take. Sound guidance conveying most of the content of displayed messages is also provided to make it easier for users to concentrate on the message board during interaction, so both visual and audio messages are available to supply the adequate information at any time of interaction. This gives participants more confidence to move around without outside help and the ability to adapt to the system quickly.

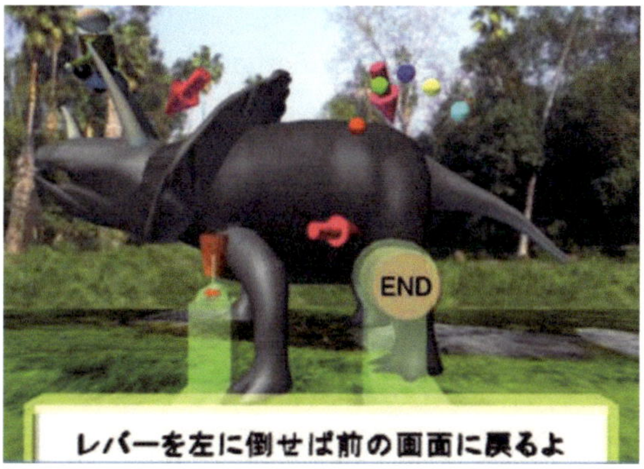

Fig. 11. Selection by control levers, buttons, and arrows

1.6.1 Hardware setup

The system consists of VR station PC (graphic station), where the VR simulation is running and control PC for controlling the haptic interface. The VR station PC is 2.8 GHz equipped with 1.5 GB memory and high performance stereoscopic graphic card (NVIDIA quadro FX1300) where all running on windows 2000. The control PC for controlling the haptic interface is a real time OS (ART-Linux) to ensure 1 KHz update rate of haptic and control thread. To provide better sense of immersion, the operator asked to wear HMD (Head Mounted Display). Since the whole system was to be exhibited at the World Expo 2005. It was very important to provide 3D graphics not only to the user but also to the whole audiences to enable them to share and enjoy the demonstration with the subject. Therefore a large screen was chosen to display the stereoscopic scenes. The audiences wear polarized glasses which is very light and easy to wear. The system architecture is shown in Fig. 12.

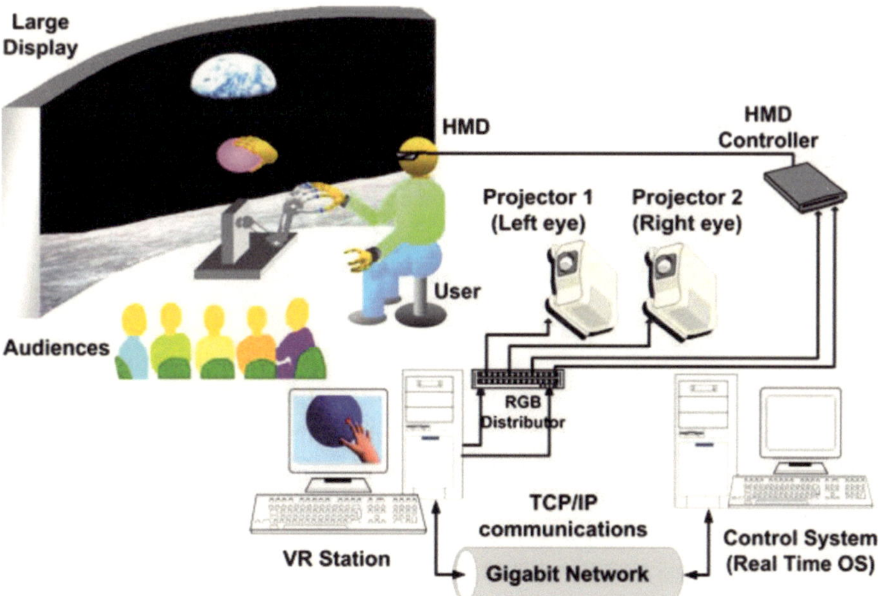

Fig. 12. The system architecture

1.6.2 The solar system

In this world, users experience the effect of different gravity conditions between the Moon and Mars on ball or weight by lifting virtual objects and feeling differences in weight and dynamics. Fig. 13 shows the ball grasped and lifted on the Moon. Physical laws of motion are applied to enable five-finger grasping, and to calculate correct force such as gravity, inertia, and friction.

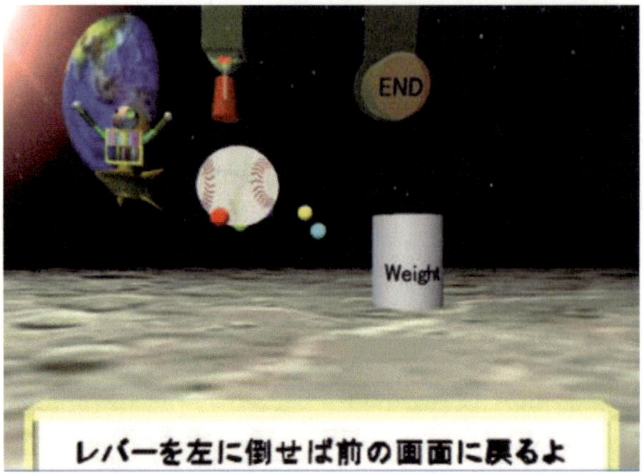

Fig. 13. Ball grasped and lifted on the Moon

1.6.3 The dinosaur's world

This world provides a unique experience by taking users to a mysterious vanished world and letting them touch and feel dinosaurs. A 5-ton triceratops 8 meters long is simulated divided into three touchable parts – head, tail, and leg. Each part is a deformable model implemented using physical modeling as described in the previous section. The physical model has been scaled down so that the hand can easily reach and touch it (Fig. 14).

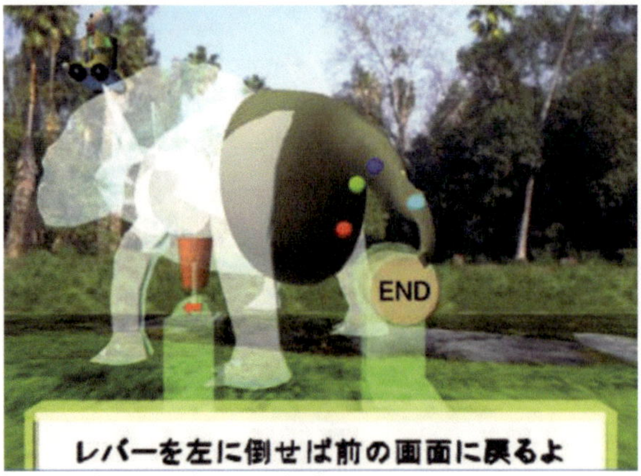

Fig. 14. Tail deformed according to the user's fingers interaction

1.6.4 The microscopic world

In this simulation, users explore the micro world of one-celled called Daphnia longispina 1.5 mm (Fig. 15).

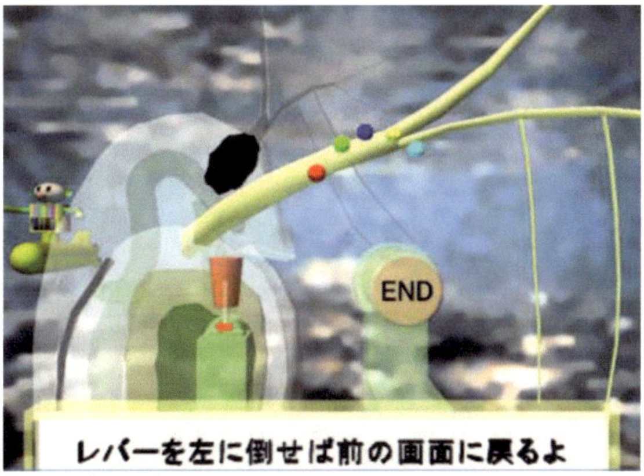

Fig. 15. Interaction with Daphnia horn

Users touch either the horn or the belly of the Daphnia through a selection screen. Physical models have been scaled up so that each part can be touched easily. Animation reflecting real movement of the Daphnia is also simulated.

1.7 Experimental results

World Expo 2005 was a great chance to demonstrate HIRO II and FHSE. Thousands of people had the chance to watch demonstrations, and many had the opportunity to try it. Participants were asked to navigate around the FHSE freely by choosing the world they wanted to explore. No time limit was imposed on each trial or in each world, although, a maximum 10 minutes was set for those trying out the FHSE. Subjects were asked to fill out a questionnaire at the end of their experience. The questionnaire recorded data on HIRO II and FHSE. Data presented here is based on results for 30 subjects from different backgrounds and of different aged. There were sufficient variations in age that questionnaire reflected a wide spectrum of subjects.

1.7.1 Human performance

To facilitate effective, efficient, and safe operation of any VE system, the measurement of human performance should be a consideration throughout the system's life cycle. Subjective and objective evaluations were conducted. Since we are presenting FHSE as a complete VE interface in which making selections and moving between scenes is achieved by what we called controls, it is important to evaluate these controls in providing a suitable approach for users to interact inside the VE. The subjective evaluation was based on three factors—ease of use of controls in selection and transition between scenes, naturalness of control manipulation, and measuring how far subjects were satisfied with such interaction. These were measured on a scale of 1-7 scale. Results showed that books and buttons were easy and natural to use and subjects were very satisfied with them (Fig. 16), followed by arrows, then levers, which presented some difficulty in manipulation. Table 3 shows the samples, mean, and standard deviation for each control based on individual factors.

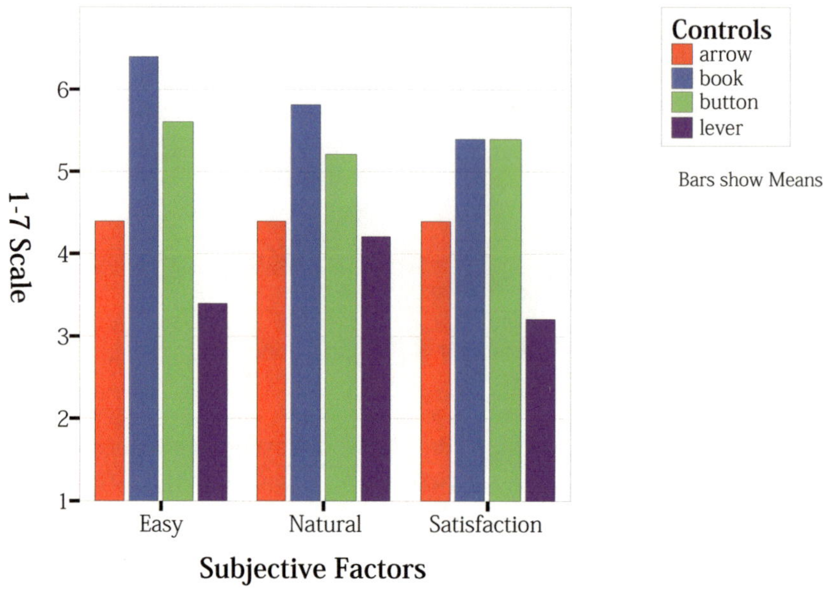

Fig. 16. Subjective evaluation of controls

	Arrow			Book			Button			Lever		
	Count	Mean	Std Deviation	Count	Mean	Std Deviation	Count	Mean	Std Deviation	Count	Mean	Std Deviation
Easy	5	4.40	2.41	5	6.40	.55	5	5.60	1.14	5	3.40	1.67
Natural	5	4.40	1.52	5	5.80	.45	5	5.20	.45	5	4.20	1.10
Satisfaction	5	4.40	1.14	5	5.40	.89	5	5.40	.55	5	3.20	1.64

Table 3. The number of samples, mean, and standard deviation for each control based on individual factors

The objective evaluation is based on an errors factor. When subjects tried to hit a control and missed, it was considered an error. Fig. 17 shows the error evaluation based on misses. Errors were mostly committed in hitting the lever, with few errors in hitting other controls. The reason is due to the need for proper location perception of the lever in 3D space, because it must be pushed from one side—something that not all subjects could easily perceive the right location from the first time. This was also reflected by objective results. Nevertheless, providing the same scenario for all subjects in which they had to hit each control more than 10 times, it is clear that the arrow, book, and button were satisfactory, but the lever requires modification to be used more intuitively. Table 4 shows the Mean and Standard Deviation of error for each control.

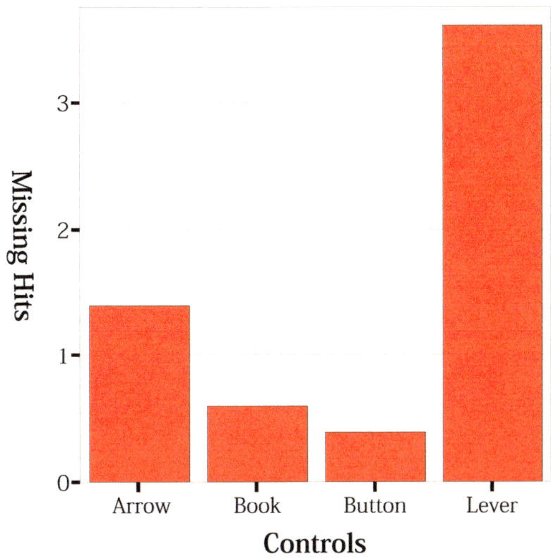

Fig. 17. Control error (bars show means)

	Count	Mean	Std Deviation
Arrow	5	1.40	1.52
Book	5	.60	.89
Button	5	.40	.89
Lever	5	3.60	1.14

Table 4. The number of samples, mean, and standard deviation of error for each control

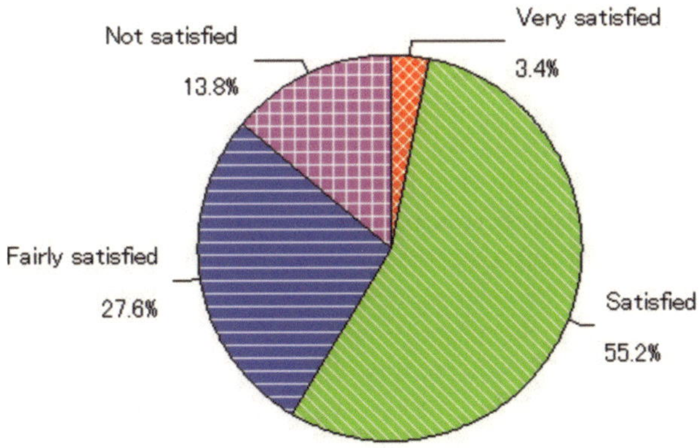

Fig. 18. Overall FHSE simulation evaluation

1.7.2 Overall evaluation

Only 13.8% of subjects were not satisfied with the Future Science Encyclopedia, while 55.2% were satisfied, 27.6% fairly satisfied, and 3.4% very satisfied (Fig. 18). Interestingly for the FHSE, most subjects were very interested in the microscopic world, which was tried by over 51.1%. While, 40.4% expressed interest in the dinosaur world, but only 8.5 % were interested in the solar system.

Summary

Multifinger haptic interface is the ultimate human haptic interface that would provide natural manipulation and feeling to the tip of each finger, same as the real hand interaction with the real world in daily-life tasks. This chapter introduced the second version of HIRO, including the hardware design, the control algorithm, and the software design including the system architecture, haptic rendering, and practical VR application. The hand with the arm provides a large workspace and reflects exactly the human hand movement as you are looking to your hand and arm in the mirror, with some differences related to hardware limitations and control methods that yet need to be improved.

A comprehensive haptic system through demonstration of the future haptic science encyclopedia is presented. The architecture used was a multi-layer network framework that decoupled the haptic from graphic on to separate machines. The architecture maintained the high update rate needed for the haptic servoloop. Also, an accurate collision detection algorithm that considers the shape of human fingertips is developed. A physically based modeling using the finite element method (FEM) combined with an elementary displacement approach proved to ensure stable interaction and realistic forces calculation for a relatively complex deformable model in real time. The approach takes into considerations interaction with multipoint contacts where other approaches failed to achieve such interaction due difficulty in calculating forces at 1 KHz.

The FHSE application was demonstration at World Expo 2005. People enjoyed the demonstration, where the majority were satisfied with the system as it provided a unique experience.

Finally, combining technologies such as virtual reality and haptic robotics enables us to extend the capabilities and effectiveness of simulators. We anticipate that the proposed system will bring the notice of many researchers to the feasibility of implementing multifinger haptic interfaces. Although, every one agree on the importance of such interface, but many obstacles are still preventing the advancement of this research field. This chapter provided a complete picture on how this could be achieved. The greatest lesson of such project was the collaboration between robotics community and virtual reality community is necessary to achieve a better and comprehensive sophisticated haptic robot. Eventhough , I was the leader of the software development side including the haptic rendering and VR application, I was involved from the beginning in the process of designing the hardware and the control algorithms as well, useful feedback was the result of such collaboration.

There are a number of future directions that can apply to this research. First, it is desirable to test the presented architecture in the presence of large delay and apply some techniques to compensate it. Second, develop more robust control algorithm for the arm movements to reflect the exact motion of the human hand, this will make the interface manipulation very natural. Also, make the hardware itself smarter and safer.

References

Adachi, Y., Kumano, T., Ogino, K., Intermediate representation for stiff virtual objects, *Proceedings of IEEE Virtual Reality Annual Intl. Symposium*, Research Triangle Park, N. Carolina; pp. 203-210, 1995

Alhalabi, M. O., Daniulaitis, V., Kawasaki, H. & Hori, T. Medical Training Simulation for Palpation of Subsurface Tumor Using HIRO. *Proceedings of worldHAPTICS*, Italy, pp. 623-624. 2005

Alhalabi, M. O., Danyilaitis, V., Kawasaki, H., Tanaka, Y., Hori, T., Haptic Interaction Rendering Technique for HIRO: an Opposite Human Hand Haptic Interface Robot, *Proceedings of EuroHaptics*, pp. 459-462, Germany, 2004

Ando, N., Korondi, P., & Hashimoto, H., Development of Micromanipulator and Haptic Interface for Networked Micromanipulation, *IEEE/ASME Trans. on Mechatronics*, vol. 6, no. 4, pp. 417-427, 2001

Balaniuk, R., Using fast local modeling to buffer haptic data, *Proceedings of Fourth PHANTOM Users Group Workshop-P UG99*, 1999

Barbagli, F., Prattichizzo, D., Salisbury, K., Multirate analysis of haptic interaction stability with deformable objects, *Proceedings of 41st IEEE conference on Decision and Control*, pp. 917-922, 2002

Bardorfer, A., Munih, M., Zupan, A., & Primozic, A., Upper Limb Motion Analysis Using Haptic Interface, *IEEE/ASME Trans. on Mechatronics*, vol. 6, no. 3, pp. 253-260, 2001

Basdogan, C., Ho, C. H., & Srinivasan, M. A., Virtual Environments for Medical Training: Graphical and Haptic Simulation of Laparoscopic Common Bile Duct Exploration, *IEEE/ASME Trans. on Mechatronics*, vol. 6, no. 3, pp. 269-286, 2001

Bouzit, M., Burdea, G., Popescu, G., & Boian, R., The Rutgers Master II - New Design Force-Feed back Glove, *IEEE/ASME Trans. on Mechatronics*, Vol. 7, No. 2, pp.256-263, 2002

Cavusoglu, M., C., Tendick, F., Multirate simulation for high-fidelity haptic interaction with deformable objects in virtual environments, *Proceedings of IEEE Int. Conf. Robot. Autom*, pp. 2458–2464, 2000

Cotin, S., Delingette, H., & Ayache, N., Real-Time Elastic Deformations of Soft Tissues for Surgery Simulation, *IEEE Transactions on Visualization and Computer Graphics*, Vol. 5 (1), pp. 62-73, 1999

CyberGlove Systems, http://www.cyberglovesystems.com/products/hardware/cyberforce.php, Retrived August, 2009

Daniulaitis, V., Alhalabi, M. O., Kawasaki, H., Tanaka, Y. & Hori, T, Medical palpation of deformable tissue using physics-based model for Haptic Interface RObot (HIRO), *Proceedings of IROS2004*, Japan, pp. 3907-3911, 2004

Dubey, R. V., Everett, S. E., Pernalete, N., &. Manocha, K. A., Teleoperation Assistance Through Variable Velocity Mapping, *IEEE Trans. on Robotics and Automation*, vol. 17, no. 5, pp. 761-766, 2001

Elhajj, I., Xi, N., Fung, W. K., Liu, Y. H., Li, W. J., Kaga, T., & Fukuda, T., Haptic Information in Internet-Based Teleoperation, *IEEE/ASME Trans. on Mechatronics*, vol. 6, no. 3, pp. 295-304, 2001

Gossweiler, R., Long, C., Koga, S., Pausch, R., DIVER: A Distributed Virtual Environment Research Platform, *Proceedings of IEEE1993 Symposium on Research Frontiers in Virtual Reality*, San Jose, Calif., pp. 10-15, Oct. 25-26, 1993

Guthold, M., et. al., Controlled Manipulation of Molecular Samples with the Nanomanipulator, *IEEE/ASME Trans. on Mechatronics*, vol. 5, no. 2, pp. 189-198, 2000

Ivanisevic, I., & Lumelsky, V. J., Configuration Space as a Means for Augmenting Human Performance in Teleoperation Tasks, *IEEE Trans. on SMC*, Part B, vol. 30, no. 3, pp. 471-484, 2000

Kawasaki, H., & Hayashi, T., Force Feedback Glove for Manipulation of Virtual Objects, *Jour. Of Robotics and Mechatronics*, Vol. 5, No.1, pp. 79-84, 1993

Kawasaki, H., Takai, J., Tanaka, Y., Mrad, C., & Mouri, T., Control of Multi-Fingered Haptic Interface Opposite to Human Hand, *Proceeding of the 2003 IEEE/RSJ Int. Conf. on Intelligent Robots and Systems (IROS2003)*, Las Vegas, pp. 2707-2712, 2003

Langrana, N. A., Burdea, G., Lange, K., Gomez, D., & Deshpande, S., Dynamic force feedback in a virtual knee palpation, *Artificial Intelligence in Medicine*, Vol. 6, pp. 321-333, 1994

Mark, W., Randolph, S., Finch, M., Van Verth, J., Taylor, R., Adding force feedback to graphics systems: Issues and solutions, *Proceedings of SIGGRAPH'96*, pp. 447-452, 1996

Marliere, S., Urma, D., Florens, J., & Marchi, F., Mult-sensorial interactio with a nano-scale phenomenon: the force curve, *Proceeding of EuroHaptics*,pp.246-252, 2004

Mendoza, C., Laugier, C., Realistic haptic rendering for highly deformable virtual objects, *Proceedings of Virtual Reality Conference*, pp. 264-269, 2001

Mouri, T., Kawasaki, H., Yoshikawa, K., Takai, J., & Ito, S., Anthropomorphic Robot Hand: Gifu Hand III, *Proceedings of Int. Conf. ICCAS2002*, Korea, pp. 1288-1293, 2002

Popescu, V., Burdea, G., & Bouzit, M., Virtual Reality Simulation Modeling for a Haptic Glove, *Proceedings of Computer Animation'99 Conference*, Geneva, Switzerland, pp. 195-200, 1999

Ruspini, D. C., Kolarov, K., Khatib, O., The haptic display of complex graphical environments. *Proceedings of SIGGRAPH conference*, ACM SIGGRAPH, pp. 345-352, 1997

Ueda, Y., Maeno, T., Development of a Mouse-Shaped Haptic Device with Multiple Finger Inputs, *Proceeding of Int. Conf. on Intelligent Robots and Systems*, pp. 2886-2891, 2004

Walairacht, S., Ishii, M., Koike, Y., & Sato, M., Two-Handed Multi-Fingers String-based Haptic Interface Device, *IEICE Trans. on Information and Systems*, Vol. E84D, No. 3, pp. 365-373, 2001

Wall, S. A., Harwin, W. S., Design of a Multiple Contact Point Haptic Interface, *Proceedings of Eurohaptics 2001*, University of Birmingham; 2001

Yoshikawa, T., & Nagara, A., Devevopment and Control of Touch and Force Display Devices for Haptic Interface, *Proceedings of SYROCO*, pp. 427-432, 2000

Zilles, C. & Salisbury, J., A constraint-based god-object method for haptic display. *Proceedings of IEE/RSJ International Conference on Intelligent Robots and Systems*, Human Robot Interaction and Cooperative Robots, Vol. 3; 146-151. 1996

Zilles, C., & Salisbury, K., A Constraint-based God-object Method For Haptic Display. *Proceedings of IEEE International Conference on Intelligent Robots and Systems '95*, Pittsburgh, PA, Vol. 3, pp. 146-151, 1995

12

Optimal Design of Haptic Interfaces

Volkan Patoglu and Aykut Cihan Satici
Sabancı University
İstanbul, Turkey

1. Introduction

Haptic interfaces are computer-controlled motorized devices that physically interact with human operators to render presence of computationally mediated environments. Ideal haptic devices are desired to withstand human applied forces with very high stiffness and be capable of displaying a full range of impedances down to the minimum value humans can perceive. The performance of a haptic interface under closed loop control is measured by the *transparency* of the display, that is, by quantifying the correspondence between the desired and actually rendered impedance values. During haptic rendering, the haptic interface is coupled to the control system and its existence results in parasitic effects on the displayed impedances, deteriorating the perfect transparency. Therefore, independent of the control algorithm, both the kinematic and dynamic performance of the haptic device have an impact on the overall performance of the haptic display.

Robotic manipulators with parallel kinematic chains are popular among haptic interfaces due to their inherent advantages in satisfying requirements of haptic applications with respect to their serial counterparts. Parallel mechanisms offer compact designs with high stiffness and have low effective inertia since their actuators can be grounded in many cases. In terms of dynamic performance, high position and force bandwidths are achievable with parallel mechanisms thanks to their light, but stiff structure. Besides, parallel mechanisms do not superimpose position errors at joints; hence, can achieve high precision.

Despite these favorable characteristics of parallel mechanisms, optimal design of such mechanisms with closed kinematic chains is significantly more challenging. Parallel mechanisms have smaller workspace with possible singularities within the workspace and their kinematic, dynamic, and singularity analysis are considerably harder than that of serial manipulators. Due to the additional complexities involved, the dimensional synthesis of parallel mechanisms is still an active area of research.

Optimum design of parallel mechanisms, even for a single objective function, is challenging due to the nonlinear, large scale nature of such mechanisms (Lee & Kim, 2006) and non-convex properties of performance indices with respect to the design variables (Qi & Womersley, 1996). Many different optimization approaches applicable to nonlinear, non-convex optimization problems such as genetic algorithms (Lee et al., 2001; Lee & Kim, 2006; Stuckman & Easom, 1992; Zheng & Lewis, 1994), simulated annealing (Risoli et al., 1999), Bayesian techniques (Stuckman & Easom, 1992; Stuckman et al., 1991), Monte-Carlo simulations (Stuckman & Easom, 1992; Zheng & Lewis, 1994), controlled randomized searches (Lou et al., 2008), performance charts (Liu & Wang, 2007), workspace atlases (Liu et al., 2006), and branch and bound methods (Stocco et al., 1998) have been applied to design optimization of parallel mechanisms. In general, deterministic methods can get stuck at a local optimum, heuristic methods cannot guarantee optimality of the converged solution, while branch and bound type methods are only as accurate as the discretization selected.

While designing the geometry of a haptic interface, various performance criteria such as kinematic and dynamic isotropy, singularity-free workspace, sensitivity, and transmission capability have to be considered *simultaneously*. The performance with respect to any of these criteria cannot be improved without deteriorating another; hence, design trade-offs are inevitable. Determination of optimal dimensions with respect to many design criteria is a difficult problem and should be handled with multi-objective optimization methods so that trade-offs can be assigned in a systematic manner.

As emphasized earlier, an optimal design of a haptic interface can only be achieved by considering many competing objectives. There exists several studies in which multiple design criteria have been addressed for this purpose. The studies that can be categorized under *scalarization methods* address the multi-criteria optimization problem in an indirect manner, by first transforming it into a (or a series of) single objective (scalar) problem(s). Among these approaches, Hayward *et al.* define the relationship between multiple criteria and utilize sensitivities of these criteria to conduct a hierarchical optimization study (Hayward et al., 1994). Multiple objectives are considered sequentially in (Alici & Shirinzadeh, 2004; Krefft et al., 2005; Risoli et al., 1999; Stocco et al., 1998) by searching for parameter sets resulting in near optimal kinematic performance and then selecting the design exhibiting the best dynamic performance from this reduced parameter space. Task-priority (Chen et al., 1995), probabilistic weighting (McGhee et al., 1994), composite index (Lee et al., 2001), and tabular methods (Yoon & Ryu, 2001) are among the other scalarization approaches that consider multiple criteria. Scalarization methods possess the inherent disadvantage of their aggregate objective functions requiring preferences or weights to be determined *apriori, i.e* before the results of the optimization process are actually known (de Weck, 2004). Since assigning proper weights or prioritizing different criteria is a problem dependent, non-trivial task, these techniques fall short of providing a general framework to the design of the parallel mechanisms.

The alternative approach is classified as *pareto methods*, which incorporate all optimization criteria within the optimization process and address them simultaneously to find a set of non-dominated designs in the objective space. Pareto methods allow the designer to make an informed decision by studying a wide range of options, since they contain solutions that are optimum from an *overall* standpoint; unlike scalarization techniques that may ignore this trade-off viewpoint. In literature Krefft *et al.* applied a modified genetic algorithm (GA) based Pareto method to design parallel mechanisms (Krefft & Hesselbach, 2005a; Krefft et al., 2005). Similarly, in (Stan et al., 2006) GA is applied to multi criteria optimization of a 2-DoF parallel robot. Finally, in (Unal et al., 2008a;b) authors proposed a multi-objective design framework for optimization of parallel mechanisms based on Normal Boundary Intersection (NBI) method (Das & Dennis, 1996). The proposed framework has been applied to design of rehabilitation robots (Erdogan et al., 2009; Unal & Patoglu, 2008b), robotic exoskeletons (Satici et al., 2009; Unal & Patoglu, 2008a), and compliant micro mechanisms (Tokatli & Patoglu, 2009). This framework is computational efficient, applicable to other performance indices, and easily extendable to include further design criteria that may be required by the application.

In this chapter, the multi-objective design framework for optimization of parallel mechanisms, first proposed by the authors in (Unal et al., 2008a;b) is reviewed. Global kinematic and dynamic performance of parallel mechanisms defined over a pre-specified singularity free workspace are maximized simultaneously and the Pareto-front curve for these two criteria is obtained. Firstly, the global optima of non-convex min-max performance criteria are solved independently from each other, using a modified branch and bound algorithm, called culling algorithm (Stocco et al., 1998). Once optimal solutions of each single criteria optimization problem are obtained, Normal Boundary Intersection (NBI) method (Das & Dennis, 1996), which performs a deterministic geometric search within the objective space, is utilized to efficiently compute uniformly distributed design solutions on the Pareto-front curve.
The chapter is organized as follows: Section 2 identifies and categorizes relevant design objectives for haptic interfaces. Section 3 introduces the sample mechanism used for the analysis, a 3-degrees of freedom (DoF) Modified Delta Mechanism. Section 4 formulates the optimization problems, while Section 5 explains the optimization methods used to address the single and multi-criteria optimization problems. Section 6 presents and discusses the results of the optimization problems. Finally, Section 7 concludes the chapter.

2. Design Objectives

Following the terminology of Merlet (Merlet, 2006), one can categorize the performance requirements of a mechanism into four distinct groups: *Imperative* requirements that must be satisfied for any design solution, *optimal* requirements for which an extremal value of the index is required, *primary* requirements which take place in the specifications but can be modified to some extent to ensure a design solution, and *secondary* requirements which do not appear in the specifications but can be utilized to choose between multiple design solutions.
Ensuring the safety and complying with the ergonomic needs of the human operator are two imperative design requirements every haptic interface must satisfy. Safety is typically assured by the selection of back-drivable actuation and power transmission[1] with force/torque limits implemented in software, while predetermined ergonomic workspace volumes are imposed at the kinematic synthesis level. The absence of singularities in the workspace is another imperative design requirement that ensures the forward and inverse kinematics of the robot be solved uniquely at each point within the workspace.
Both kinematic and dynamic performance of parallel mechanisms are to be optimized to achieve haptic devices with low parasitic effects. Specifically, to achieve high force bandwidths and a uniform "feel" for the device, kinematic/dynamic isotropy and stiffness of the device have to be maximized while its apparent inertia is being minimized . To quantify performance, several design matrices, including Jacobian and inertia matrices, are studied and to date many scalar performance indices have been proposed. These indices either quantify the directional independence (uniformity) of configuration dependent design matrices or represent a distance to a singular configuration. Since singular values of a matrix provide a versatile metric to quantify its properties, most of the indices are derived as a function of these values. These performance metrics are further discussed in the next subsection.
A common primary requirement for haptic interfaces is the workspace volume index (Merlet, 2006), the ratio between the workspace volume and the volume of the robot. Even though predetermined workspace volumes are generally imposed as imperative requirements, a large

[1] In this chapter, we limit our discussion to impedance type devices due to their widespread use, even though admittance type devices can also be treated using an analogous framework.

workspace volume index is still desired to reduce the collisions of the device with the operator or the environment. The footprint area is yet another primary requirement commonly imposed during design.

Finally, the secondary requirements include low backlash, low-friction, high back-drivability, and low manufacturing costs. Friction, backlash, and back-drivability are mainly influenced by the selection of the actuators and the transmission, while choice of link lengths may have an influence on manufacturing costs.

2.1 Measuring Kinematic and Dynamic Performance

To measure kinematic performance, properties of the Jacobian matrix (J) are studied. Condition number, proposed by Salisbury and Craig (Salisbury & Craig, 1982), describing the worst-case behavior at a given configuration is one of the most commonly used kinematic performance measures. Given as the ratio of the minimum and maximum singular values of the Jacobian matrix, this measure locally characterizes directional isotropy for both force/motion transmission accuracy and actuator utilization of a manipulator. Another popular index, manipulability, measures the ease of arbitrarily changing the position and orientation of the end effector and is calculated by taking the product of singular values of the Jacobian matrix (Yoshikawa, 1985b). Sensitivity characterizes the precision of a manipulator by measuring the change in end-effector configuration with respect to small perturbations of joint angles and is given by the sum of the absolute values of the Jacobian matrix elements in a single row (Grace & Colgate, 1993). Finally, minimum singular value of the Jacobian matrix is also proposed as a kinematic performance measure (Klein & Blaho, 1987) quantifying the skewness of the velocity response.

All of the mentioned indices are *local* measures of kinematic performance; therefore, are not constant over the entire workspace. Extensions of these indices have been proposed to characterize the performance of a manipulator over the entire workspace. Gosselin and Angeles proposed *global* condition indices based on the integral of local kinematic performance measures over the workspace (Gosselin & Angeles, 1991). However, being average values, these indices fail to capture possible low performance configurations (near singular points) within the workspace. Moreover, integrating a local measure can be computationally expensive. Mean of the minimum singular value has also been proposed as global measure in order to characterize the path velocity of parallel robots (Krefft & Hesselbach, 2005b). Since mean values are not sufficient to guarantee homogeneity of performance, standard deviation of the minimum singular value has also been introduced as a measure (Krefft & Hesselbach, 2005b). Other global indices include global payload index that measures the force transmission capability (Ozaki et al., 1996). Finally, the global isotropy index ($\mathcal{GII}$), introduced in (Stocco et al., 1998) by Stocco *et al.*, is a workspace inclusive worst-case kinematic performance measure that is intolerant of poor performance over the entire workspace. $\mathcal{GII}$ is calculated as the ratio of the minimum of the smallest singular value and the maximum of the largest singular value of the Jacobian matrix over the workspace.

In this chapter, a global performance index is chosen to quantify the kinematic isotropy of haptic interfaces since the objective of the design problem is to minimize the parasitic effects of the manipulator over the workspace. Even though any global index can be utilized within the framework presented, the conservative workspace inclusive worst-case performance measure that is intolerant of poor performance over the entire workspace, $\mathcal{GII}$, is preferred. As a global worst case performance measure, maximizing $\mathcal{GII}$ corresponds to designing a mechanism with best worst-case kinematic performance. Moreover, an optimal $\mathcal{GII}$ results in a uniform

Jacobian matrix, while also increasing the efficiency of utilization of the actuators. $\mathcal{GII}$ can be mathematically expressed as

$$\mathcal{GII} = min_{\gamma_0,\gamma_1 \in W} \frac{\underline{\sigma}(J(\boldsymbol{\alpha},\gamma_0))}{\overline{\sigma}(J(\boldsymbol{\alpha},\gamma_1))} \tag{1}$$

where J represents the Jacobian of the manipulator, $\underline{\sigma}$ and $\overline{\sigma}$ are the minimum and maximum singular values of the Jacobian matrix, γ_0 and γ_1 are the configurations in the workspace that result in the extreme singular values, $\boldsymbol{\alpha}$ is the column matrix of design variables, and W represents the workspace.

Dynamic performance is measured in a similar manner to the kinematic performance, but properties of the inertia matrix (M) capturing the relation between actuator force/torque and end-effector acceleration, are studied. The goal for improving dynamic performance is to minimize inertial effects that conflict with high acceleration demands. To characterize *local* dynamic performance Asada defined the effective inertia matrix expressing the homogeneity of the moment of inertia of the non-redundant manipulators and introduced the concept of generalized inertia ellipsoid (Asada, 1983). Yoshikawa proposed a dynamic manipulability measure (Yoshikawa, 1985a), which is an extension of manipulability concept and measures the degree of arbitrariness in changing end-effector accelerations. Dynamic manipulability is calculated as the product of singular values of M^{-1} matrix. Angeles *et al.* defined the dynamical conditioning index which measures dynamical coupling and numerical stability of the generalized inertia matrix of manipulators (Ma & Angeles, 1990). Finally, swiftness, a measure to characterize the attitude of the manipulator to produce high end-effector accelarations, is proposed by Di Gregorio *et al.* which can also be applied to planar manipulators with non-homogeneous generalized coordinates (Gregorio & Parenti-Castelli, 2005).

Similar to the case of local kinematic performance indices, extensions to local dynamic indices have been proposed to characterize the performance of a manipulator over the entire workspace. Calculating the mean value and standard deviation of the local dynamic indices are among the most commonly used approaches to achieve a global dynamic performance index. A global dynamic index ($\mathcal{GDI}$) is introduced in (Stocco et al., 1998) to quantify the global worst-case performance of a manipulator. $\mathcal{GDI}$ measures the largest effect of mass on the dynamic performance by calculating the maximum largest singular value over the workspace of the effective mass matrix at the end-effector and is computed as the inverse of the maximum of the largest singular value.

To be consistent with the metric chosen for the kinematic performance, the workspace inclusive best worst-case performance measure ($\mathcal{GDI}$) is used to quantify dynamic performance. As mentioned earlier, any dynamic index could be utilized in the framework introduced, but this decision is conservative and intolerant of poor performance over the entire workspace. As a global worst-case performance measure, maximizing $\mathcal{GDI}$ results in reduced maximum largest singular value of the effective mass matrix, decreasing the inertial interference by the system. $\mathcal{GDI}$ can be mathematically expressed as

$$\mathcal{GDI} = min_{\gamma \in W} \frac{1}{1+\overline{\sigma}(M(\boldsymbol{\alpha},\boldsymbol{\beta},\gamma))} \tag{2}$$

where M represents effective inertia matrix of the manipulator as seen at the end effector, $\overline{\sigma}$ is the maximum singular value of the effective inertia matrix, γ is the configuration in the workspace that results in the maximum singular value, $\boldsymbol{\alpha}$ is the column matrix of design variables, and W represents the workspace.

In general, since entries of the Jacobian and the inertia matrices may not be homogenous in units, proper normalization is necessary such that the measures defined on these matrices are meaningful. Among several approaches proposed in literature, normalization with a characteristic length (Khan & Angeles, 2006; Krefft & Hesselbach, 2005b) or a nominal link length (Lee et al., 2001), and partitioning the matrices into translational and rotational parts (Krefft & Hesselbach, 2005b; Lee & Kim, 2006) are the most popular choices. Normalization is not necessary for the sample problem presented in this chapter, as it possesses only a translational workspace.

3. Modified Delta Mechanism

The optimization framework reviewed in this chapter is demonstrated over a spatial 3-DoF Modified Delta parallel mechanism (see Figure 1). The method discussed in this chapter constitutes a general framework for optimal dimensional synthesis of mechanisms and is by no means limited to the sample mechanism studied.

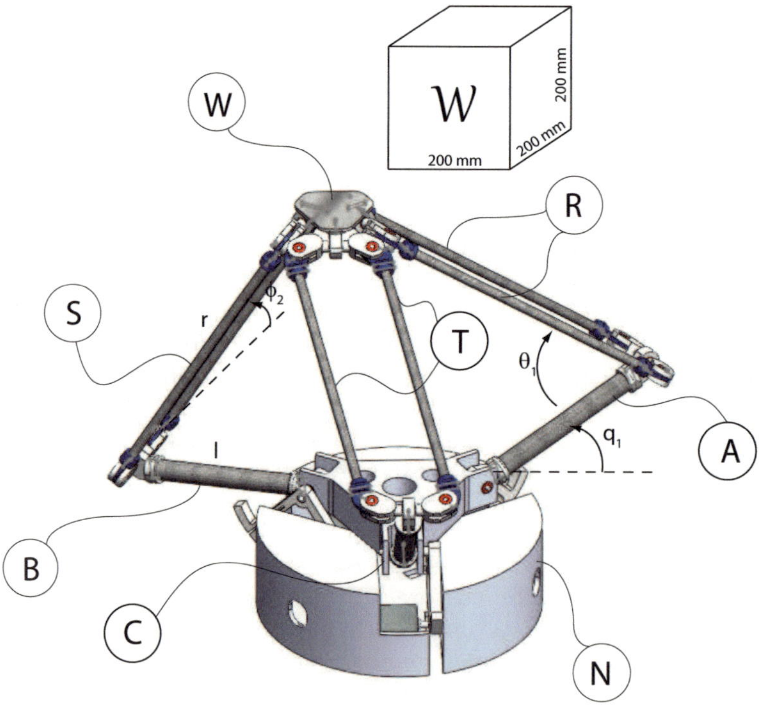

Fig. 1. The Modified Delta Mechanism

The Modified Delta Mechanism, first introduced by Clavel (Clavel, 1988), and further analyzed in (Pierrot et al., 1990), consists of eight bodies: a base platform N, three lower links A, B, C, three upper links R, S, T, and a moving platform W. The end-effector held by the operator is rigidly attached to the moving platform W. The three lower links are connected to the base platform via revolute joints whose axes of rotation are oriented along the tangents of N.

The upper three links are coupled to the lower links via revolute joints. Each of them is a planar four-bar parallelogram, which can perform one DoF motion constrained in its plane. The moving platform is connected to these three upper links by means of revolute joints whose axes of rotation are again oriented along the tangents of W. In this chapter, the analysis is limited to a symmetric modified delta mechanism where the revolute joints at the base and at the moving platform are spaced at 120° along the circumference of each platform whose radii ratio is 0.5. Moreover, the lengths of each of the lower links and similarly that of each of the upper links are considered to be the same. The modified delta mechanism has three translational DoF (x, y, z) of the moving platform W with respect to the Newtonian reference frame N. The controlled DoF are the three revolute joints, with which the lower three links are connected. Kinematic and dynamic models of the Modified Delta mechanism are further detailed in (Li & Xu, 2005; Pierrot et al., 1990; Tsai et al., 1996).
A modified delta mechanism can be characterized by lengths l and r of its two links, since the rest of the mechanism is designed to be symmetric. To quantify the orientation of each link, joint angles $q_i, \theta_i, \phi_i, (i = 1...3)$, are introduced. The workspace of the mechanism is selected to be a cube of length 200mm, and is placed at a fixed location in global coordinate frame: $[x, y, z]^T = [0 - 200,\ 0 - 200,\ 200 - 400]^T$ mm as presented in Figure 1. Table 1 presents the design variables $\boldsymbol{\alpha}$ and design parameters $\boldsymbol{\beta}$ (parameters that do not change during the design process) for the modified delta mechanism.

	Symbol	Definition	Unit
α_1	l	Length of the lower links	mm
α_2	r	Length of the upper links	mm
β_1	$x = 0 - 200$	Workspace along x-direction	mm
β_2	$y = 0 - 200$	Workspace along y-direction	mm
β_3	$z = 200 - 400$	Workspace along z-direction	mm

Table 1. Design variables α and parameters β for the Modified Delta Mechanism

4. Optimization Problem

As discussed in Section 2, two objective functions characterizing the kinematic and dynamic performances of the mechanism are considered in this chapter. The objective of optimization is to maximize the worst kinematic isotropy of the mechanism ($\mathcal{GII}$) while simultaneously minimizing the effective mass (maximum singular value of the effective mass matrix or $\mathcal{GDI}$). In this study, it is assumed that the inertia of the mechanism is only due to those of each link; thus, other inertial factors such as inertia of the actuators etc. are neglected. The negative null form of the multi-objective optimization problem can be stated as

$$\begin{aligned} max\ \mathbf{F}(\boldsymbol{\alpha}, \boldsymbol{\beta}, \boldsymbol{\gamma}) \\ \mathbf{G}(\boldsymbol{\alpha}, \boldsymbol{\beta}) \leq 0 \\ \boldsymbol{\alpha}_a < \boldsymbol{\alpha} < \boldsymbol{\alpha}_u \end{aligned} \tag{3}$$

where $\mathbf{F}$ represents the column matrix of objective functions that depend on the design variables $\boldsymbol{\alpha}$, parameters $\boldsymbol{\beta}$, and workspace positions $\boldsymbol{\gamma}$. Symbol $\mathbf{G}$ represents the inequality constraint function that also depends on design variables and parameters. Finally, $\boldsymbol{\alpha}_l$ and $\boldsymbol{\alpha}_u$ correspond to the lower and upper bounds of the design variables, respectively.
For the modified delta mechanism, the column matrix $\mathbf{F}$ is simply given as

$$\mathbf{F} = \begin{bmatrix} \mathcal{GDI} \\ \mathcal{GII} \end{bmatrix} \tag{4}$$

The constraints on the other hand, are implicitly imposed during the kinematic analysis of the parallel mechanism, which is carried out using numerical integration.

5. Methods

In the previous section, the formulation for the multi-criteria optimization problem for best worst-case performance of a haptic interface is described. Before addressing the multi-criteria optimization problem, the nature of the problem with respect to the selected performance criteria is to be studied. Inspecting the performance criteria, one can conclude that both $\mathcal{GII}$ and $\mathcal{GDI}$ are non-convex with respect to the design variables. Moreover, as workspace inclusive measures, their calculation requires searches over the workspace. As discussed in the introduction, several methods have been proposed to solve for the single criteria optimization problem of parallel manipulators. In general, descent methods suffer from getting trapped at local optima while heuristic methods cannot guarantee optimality of their solution. Feasibility and efficiency of a branch-and-bound type method, called *culling algorithm*, is advocated in the literature to address single objective min-max problems (Stocco et al., 1998).
In this chapter, a modified version of the culling algorithm is used to independently solve for the optimum designs with respect to $\mathcal{GII}$ and $\mathcal{GDI}$. The culling algorithm improves the computational efficiency of a brute-force method by reducing (culling) the amount of searches required through effective performance comparisons. The algorithm capitalizes on the fact that as a worst-case measure, once the global performance index for certain reference parameters is calculated conducting a search over the entire workspace, reduction of the feasible parameter set can be performed without performing any other searches over the workspace. Specifically, after a global index value is calculated for the reference parameters, comparisons with local indices at *only* a single configuration in the workspace. Hence, searches over workspace is significantly reduced as they are conducted only when it is necessary to calculate new reference global index values. Comparing all set of design variables to find the best worst-case index, the algorithm will converge to an optimum solution within the discretization accuracy. As the culling method substantially reduces the amount of workspace searches required by a brute-force method, it is a faster and more efficient algorithm to address min-max type problems.
Since the performance of the culling algorithm is highly dependent on the initial reference values assigned, a fast gradient-based optimization method, sequential quadratic programming (SQP), is used to solve for a local extrema that will serve as a good initialization value. This modification increases the efficiency of the algorithm by resulting in a higher culling rate at the first iteration. Once a solution is obtained, another SQP is invoked to converge to a guaranteed optima within the discretization region.
If the multi-criteria optimization problem is treated as multiple single objective problems where objective functions are handled independently, optimal solution for one criteria may result in an unacceptable design for the other. To achieve a "best" solution with respect to multiple criteria, the trade-off between objectives need to be quantified. Scalarization approaches assume apriori knowledge of this trade-off and convert the multi-criteria problem into a single objective one by assigning proper weights or priorities to each performance index. On the other hand, Pareto methods do not require any apriori knowledge about the design trade-offs and solve for the locus of all dominant solutions with respect to multiple objective functions, constituting the so-called the Pareto-front hyper-surface. Hence, designers

can make a more realistic choice between multiple "best" solutions and avoid the challenge of synthetically ranking their preferences.

There exists several methods to obtain the Pareto-front hyper-surface, among which Normal Boundary Intersection (NBI) method is one of the most featured. As the Pareto-front hyper-surface is a geometric entity in the objective space forming the boundary of the feasible region, NBI approach attacks the *geometric problem* directly by solving for single-objective constrained subproblems to obtain uniformly distributed points on the hyper-surface. NBI solves for subproblems which only depend on the defined optimization model, that is, chosen objective functions and design constraints since these equations map the feasible design space onto the attainable objective space. Given independent optimal solutions for each objective function (solutions of each single objective problem), called shadow points, NBI first constructs an hyper-plane in the objective space by connecting these shadow points with straight lines. Then, this hyper-plane is divided into grids that control the resolution of solutions on the Pareto-front hyper-surface. For each point on the grid, a geometric subproblem is solved to find the *furthest* point on the line that extends along the surface normal passing through the grid point and is in the feasible domain of the objective space. Hence, NBI obtains the Pareto-front by reducing the problem to many single-objective constrained subproblems. Number of subproblems can be adjusted by defining resolution of the grid that maps to the number of points on the Pareto-front hyper-surface. As the number of points increases, the computational time increases linearly, but since the method assumes spatial coherence and uses the solution of a subproblem to initialize the next subproblem, convergence time for each subproblem may decrease resulting in further computational efficiency.

NBI method results in exceptionally uniformly distributed points on the Pareto-front hyper-surface without requiring any tuning of the core algorithm. Moreover, once shadow points are obtained, NBI solves for the geometric problem directly utilizing a fast converging gradient-based method, evading the computationally demanding aggregate optimization problems required in most of the scalarization methods. Therefore, NBI method promises to be much faster and more efficient than other methods to obtain a well represented Pareto-front hyper-surface including aggregate methods such as weighted sums and evolutionary optimization approaches such as GA.

It should also be noted that the NBI method can solve for points on the non-convex regions of Pareto-front hyper-surfaces, a feature that is missing from the weighted sum methods. Compared to weighted sum techniques, NBI achieves higher solution efficiency as it does not suffer from clumping of solution in the objective space. NBI is also advantageous over other methods as it trivially extends to handle any number of objective functions. Compared to Multi-Objective Genetic Algorithm (MOGA) (Fonseca & Fleming, 1993) that requires problem dependent fitness and search related tuning and several steps to reach convergence, a standard NBI approach can map the Pareto-front hyper-surface with higher accuracy and uniformity, while also inheriting the efficiency of gradient-based methods.

Relying on gradient techniques, NBI assumes sufficient smoothness of the geometric problem at hand, but it has also been demonstrated that the method performs remarkably well even for non-smooth geometries (Rigoni & Poles, 2005). In the presence of non-continuous regions, multiple initializations of the NBI method may be required for efficiently generating the Pareto-front hyper-surface. For the case of strongly discontinuous geometries, hybridization with MOGA-II to supply feasible initialization points at each continuous sub-region can be employed, as proposed in (Rigoni & Poles, 2005). It is noted that since NBI relies on equality constraints, it is possible for NBI not to find a solution on the true Pareto-front hyper-surface, converging to a local optima. In such a case, post processing on the solutions of NBI subproblems can be employed to filter out undesired dominated solutions.

6. Results and Discussion

Table 2 presents the results of the modified culling algorithm for the single objective problems, for best kinematic and dynamic isotropy, respectively. These results are obtained by conducting a global search over the entire parameter space with discretization step sizes of 0.5mm and 20mm for the parameter and workspace, respectively, and by performing several local searches with finer discretizations at the neighborhood of the results suggested by the global search.

	Best Design for Kinematic Isotropy	Best Design for Dynamic Isotropy	Unit
$\mathcal{GII}$	0.36228	0.27348	–
$\mathcal{GDI}$	0.18726	0.37294	–
l	484	300	mm
r	583	382	mm

Table 2. Results of independent optimizations with respect to $\mathcal{GII}$ and $\mathcal{GDI}$.

Figure 2 presents the single objective surfaces plotted with respect to the design variables. While, subfigures 2(a) and 2(b) depict GII and GDI individually, in subfigures 2(c) and 2(d) functions are plotted on top of each other. In subfigure 2(c), both functions are supposed to be maximized, while in subfigure 2(d), a simple transformation is performed to revert the maximization into a minimization problem. As is evident from these figures, optimal values for each of these objective functions imply poor performance for the other objective function. Therefore, the trade-off curve has to be characterized, from which a sensible design choice can be made.

To characterize the trade-off between the single objective solutions, Pareto-front curve for the bi-objective optimization problem is constructed in Figure 3. Two different techniques are employed to form the Pareto-front curve, namely NBI method and aggregated performance index method. For the NBI method, a grid size of ten points is selected. In Figure 3 the distribution of points on the Pareto-front curve is marked by dots. For the second method, an aggregated performance index ($\mathcal{API}$) is defined as the weighted linear combination of $\mathcal{GII}$ and $\mathcal{GDI}$. In particular, $\mathcal{API} = \lambda\, \mathcal{GII} + (1 - \lambda)\, \mathcal{GDI}$, where $0 \leq \lambda \leq 1$ denotes the weighting factor. Ten aggregated optimization problems are solved for ten equally spaced weighting factors utilizing the modified culling algorithm with discretization step sizes of 0.5mm for the parameter space and 20mm for the workspace. Circles in the Figure 3 denote the distribution of aggregate solutions on the Pareto-front curve and are marked with their corresponding weighting factor.

As expected, NBI method generates a very uniform distribution of points on the Pareto-front curve while the solutions of the aggregate problem are clumped at certain locations of the curve. To obtain a uniform distribution using the aggregated index approach, proper weights should be assigned. However, the characteristics of the weight distribution is not known before the problem is solved. Moreover, the aggregate performance index relies on the relatively costly culling algorithm to solve for each point on the Pareto-front curve and the accuracy of the solution is limited by the discretization step size chosen. In the Figure 3, the same solutions are obtained for different weighting factors, particulary for weighting factors $\lambda = 0.1$ to

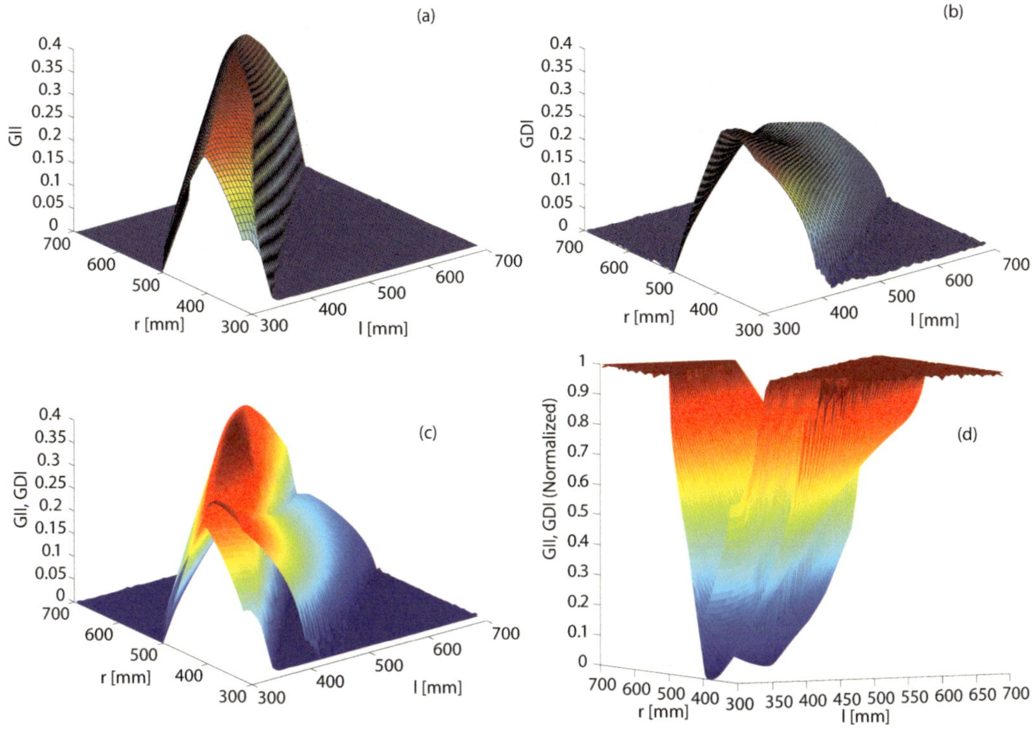

Fig. 2. Functions to be optimized depicted as surfaces. Subfigures (a) and (b) are GII and GDI respectively, while (c) and (d) represent both of them cast as minimization and maximization problems.

$\lambda = 0.3$. Moreover, a large portion of the Pareto front is missed between $\lambda = 0.7$ to $\lambda = 0.8$, due to the course discretization used. Unfortunately, solving for each aggregate performance index for all weighting factors is a computationally demanding task, limiting the density of discretization. NBI method possesses an inherent advantage in terms of computational cost, as it attacks the direct geometric problem to obtain the Pareto-front curve and utilizes continuous, computationally efficient gradient methods for the solution.

In addition to the efficiency offered via the uniform distribution of solutions on the Pareto-front curve, NBI approach results in *orders of magnitude* improvement in the computation time, especially for the design problem at hand, as depicted in Figure 4. All of the simulations presented in Figure 4 are performed using a 64 bit Windows XP workstation that is equipped with double Quad Core 3.20GHz 1600MHz Rated FSB Intel Xeon processors with 2x6MB L2 cache, and 8GB (4x2048) 800MHz DDR2 Quad Channel FBD RAM.

As can be observed from Figure 4, the aggregate problem scales geometrically with the discretization step size, rendering an accurate solution of even ten points on the Pareto-curve almost impossible for the simple sample problem at hand. On the other hand, NBI method with a 10^{-8} tolerance solves for points on the Pareto-front curve very effectively, in about half the time of the weighted-sum approach with 2.5mm step size. Even though the accuracy of solutions obtained by the NBI method is dependent on the constraint tolerance set for the algorithm, convergence for NBI with all the tolerance values 10^{-6} and 10^{-8} are shown to be

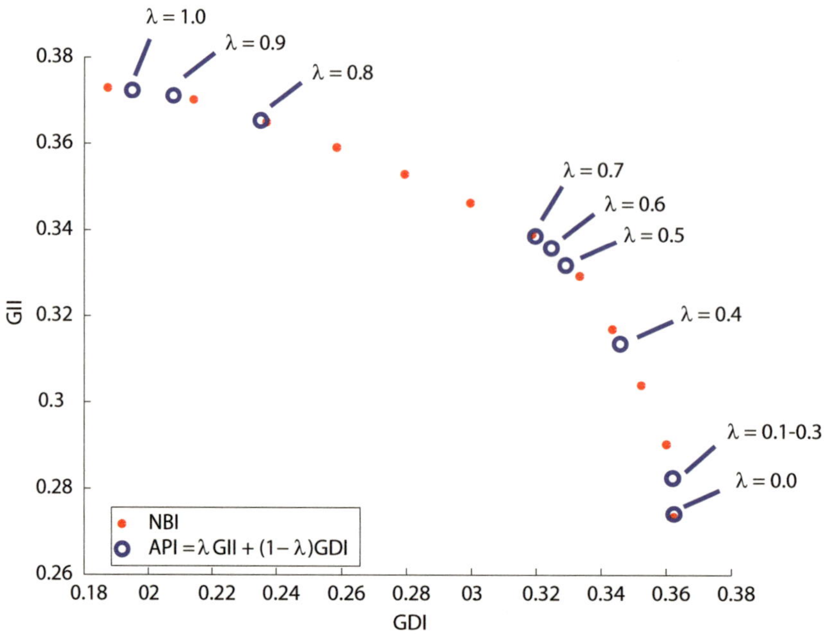

Fig. 3. Comparison of NBI and aggregated performance index methods. Symbol λ is the weighting factor.

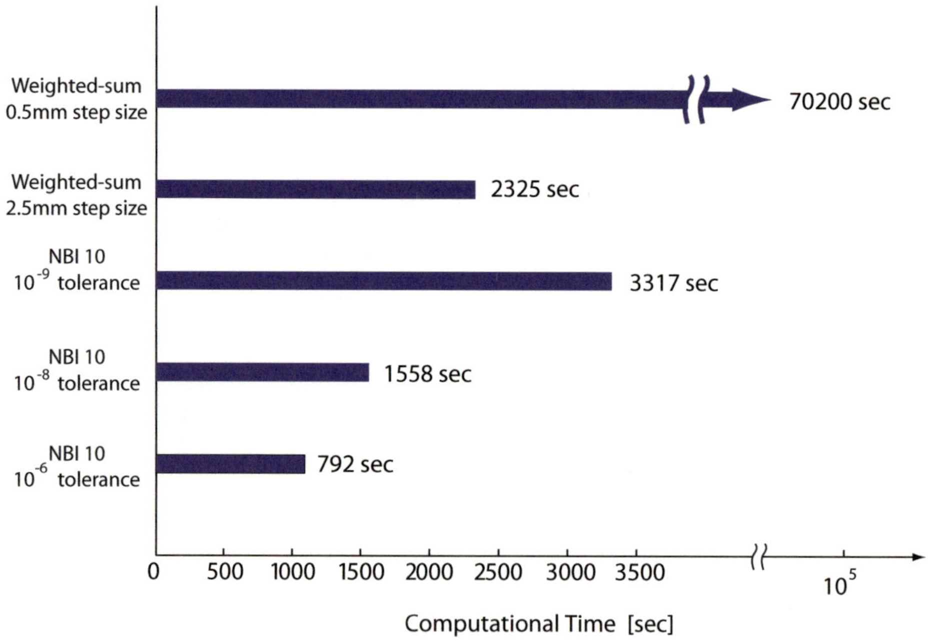

Fig. 4. Computational effort of NBI method with respect to different tolerances and weighted sum method with respect to different discretizations.

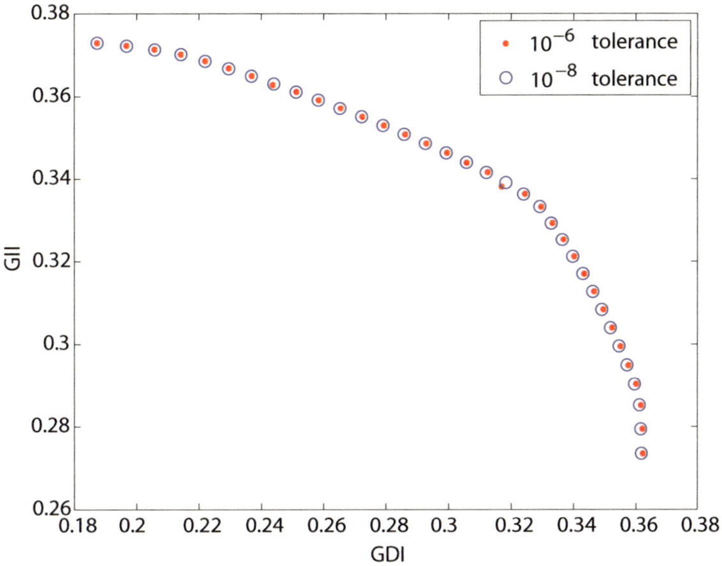

Fig. 5. Distribution of NBI solutions with two different tolerances: 10^{-6} and 10^{-8}

acceptable in Figure 5. Since NBI employs a local search algorithm that is dependent on the initial conditions, convergence can be poor at certain trials as can be observed for a point in Figure 5. However, poor convergence of certain points is not an uncorrectable drawback, as solution for those points can be repeated with different initializations and tighter tolerances. The computational time for NBI method scales linearly with tolerance values as it does with number of points selected for the grid.

To allow for further comparisons of the Pareto methods with other scalarization approaches proposed in the literature, a sequential optimization is implemented for the sample problem as suggested in (Stocco, 1999). In this method, firstly parameter sets resulting in the best $\mathcal{GII}$ values for each discrete value of the parameter l are calculated using the culling algorithm. The change in $\mathcal{GII}$ values and the other link lengths are plotted in Figure 6 with respect to the independent parameter l. In this plot, one can observe that $\mathcal{GII}$ value increases monotonically with increasing l until some point, specifically at $l = 484$, $r = 583$, after which, it becomes a monotonically decreasing function of l.

Assigning l as the independent variable, the sequential method uses the set of "optimal" solutions with respect to $\mathcal{GII}$ as the feasible search domain to conduct another single criteria optimization, this time with respect to $\mathcal{GDI}$. In other words, the parameter set resulting in the best $\mathcal{GDI}$ value is selected from the Figure 6, utilizing the culling algorithm. The result of the sequential optimization approach is plotted in Figure 7 with respect to a dense Pareto-curve obtained using the NBI approach. The plot is re-scaled to have the abscissa represent the maximum singular value of the inertia matrix, which has dimensions of kg, to facilitate the selection of the final design. The process has, of course, turned the max-max problem into a min-max one, where the maximum singular value of the mass matrix over the workspace is intended to be minimized, and $\mathcal{GII}$ is to be maximized. As a result the Pareto curve is reflected about the vertical axis. Inspecting the plot, one can conclude that the "best" solution obtained using the sequential optimization approach is *dominated* – is a point not lying on

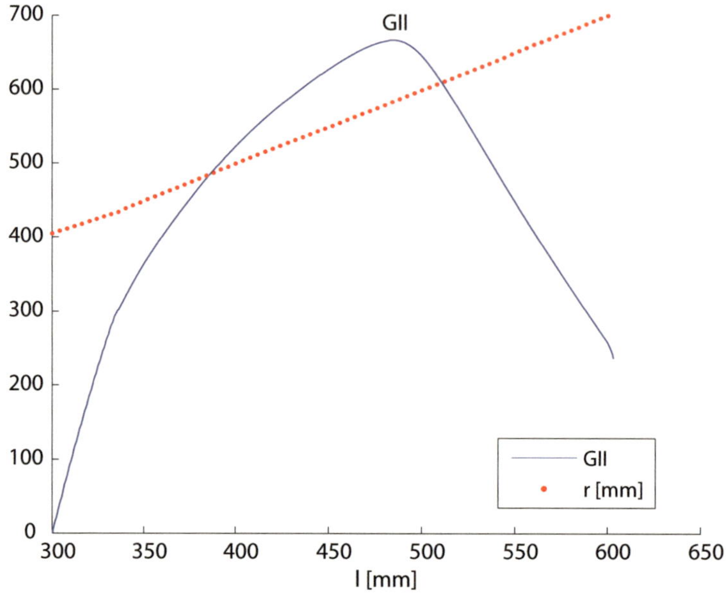

Fig. 6. The parameter sets with best $\mathcal{GII}$ values for each discrete value of l.

the Pareto front, meaning there exists solutions for which one can improve $\mathcal{GII}$ while keeping $\mathcal{GDI}$ constant or vice versa. In fact, improvements up to 10% in the $\mathcal{GII}$ value and up to 12% in the maximum singular value are possible by choosing one of the designs that lies on the Pareto-front boundary found by the intersection of the Pareto curve and vertical and horizontal line, respectively, passing through that point.

As emphasized earlier, any point on the Pareto-front curve is a non-dominated solution. Hence it is up to the designer to choose the "best" design for the application at hand, considering the characteristics of the trade-off mapped out by the Pareto-front boundary. The Pareto methods not only allow additional constraints be considered for the final decision but also let the designer adjust these constraints while simultaneously monitoring their effect on the set of non-dominated solutions. For the sample problem analyzed, a design is selected by imposing three additional physical constraints on the Pareto-front curve: a footprint constraint, a limit on the largest singular value of the mass matrix, and a threshold for the $\mathcal{GII}$ value. The footprint constraint of 400mm x 400mm eliminates the top 13 points of the Pareto curve. The second constraint, specifically the largest singular value of the mass matrix to be less than 250g, eliminates the 14th point in the solution set. Letting $\mathcal{GII}$ possess at least a value of 0.34, takes out 16 non-dominated solutions on the left. Finally, a selection is made among the remaining solutions in the set, by considering ease of manufacturing. The design is marked with a star in Figure 7. The link lengths corresponding to this design choice are $l = 390$mm and $r = 470$mm as also depicted in Figure 7.

7. Conclusions

A general framework suitable for optimization of haptic interfaces, in particular haptic interfaces with closed kinematic chains, with respect to multiple design criteria is presented. Optimization problems for haptic interfaces with best worst-case kinematic and dynamic per-

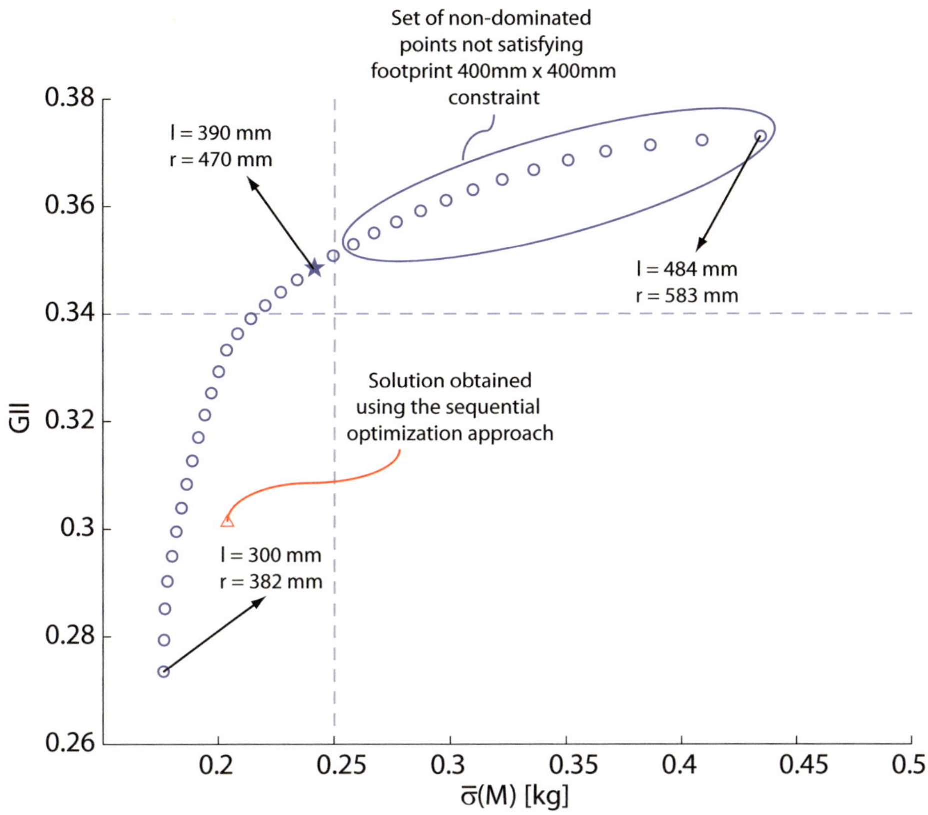

Fig. 7. Comparison of sequential approach with the Pareto-front curve. Effects of additional constraints imposed on the problem and link lengths corresponding to "best" designs.

formance are formulated. Non-convex single objective optimization problems are solved with the modified culling algorithm, while NBI method is used to obtain the Pareto-front curve to present the designer with a wide range of alternative solutions. Computational efficiency of NBI method is demonstrated over aggregating approaches such as weighted sums. The optimality of the design using Pareto methods is shown over prioritization approaches. Dimensional synthesis of a high performance haptic interface utilizing the Pareto-front curve is demonstrated.

Acknowledgements

The authors gratefully acknowledge Gullu Kiziltas Sendur and Ramazan Unal for their valuable contributions at several stages of the framework presented.

8. References

Alici, G. & Shirinzadeh, B. (2004). Optimum synthesis of planar parallel manipulators based on kinematic isotropy and force balancing, *Robotica* **22**(1): 97–108.

Asada, H. (1983). A geometrical representation of manipulator dynamics and its application to arm design, *ASME Journal of Dynamic Systems, Measurement, and Control* **105**(3): 131–135.

Chen, W., Zhang, Q., Zhao, Z. & Gruver, W. A. (1995). Optimizing multiple performance criteria in redundant manipulators by subtask-priority control, *IEEE International Conference on Systems, Man and Cybernetics*, Vol. 3, pp. 2534–2539.

Clavel, R. (1988). Delta: a fast robot with parallel geometry, *18th Int. Symposium on Industrial Robots, Lausanne, Switzerland*, pp. 91–100.

Das, I. & Dennis, J. E. (1996). Normal-boundary intersection: A new method for generating the pareto surface in nonlinear multi-criteria optimization problems, *SIAM Journal on Optimization* **8**(3): 631–65.

de Weck, O. L. (2004). Multiobjective optimization: History and promise, *China-Japan-Korea Joint Symposium on Optimization of Structural and Mechanical Systems*, Invited Keynote Paper.

Erdogan, A., Satici, A. C. & Patoglu, V. (2009). Design of a reconfigurable force feedback ankle exoskeleton for physical therapy, *ASME/IFToMM International Conference on Reconfigurable Mechanisms and Robots, ReMAR 2009.*, pp. 400–408.

Fonseca, C. M. & Fleming, P. J. (1993). Genetic algorithms for multiobjective optimization: Formulation, discussion and generalization, *Multiobjective evolutionary algorithms: Empirical Genetic Algorithms*, pp. 416–423.

Gosselin, C. & Angeles, J. (1991). A global performance index for the kinematic optimization of robotic manipulators, *ASME Journal of Mechanical Design* **113**(3): 220–226.

Grace, K. & Colgate, J. (1993). A six degree-of freedom micromanipulator for ophthalmic surgery, *IEEE International Conference on Robotics and Automation*, Vol. 1, pp. 630–635.

Gregorio, R. D. & Parenti-Castelli, V. (2005). On the characterization of the dynamic performances of planar manipulators, *Meccanica* **40**(3): 267–279.

Hayward, V., Choksi, J., Lanvin, G. & Ramstein, C. (1994). Design and multi-objective optimization of a linkage for a haptic interface, *Advances in Robot Kinematics*, pp. 352–359.

Khan, W. A. & Angeles, J. (2006). The kinetostatic optimization of robotic manipulators: The inverse and the direct problems, *Transaction of ASME Journal of Mechanical Design* **128**(1): 168–178.

Klein, C. A. & Blaho, B. E. (1987). Dexterity measures for the design and control of kinematically redundant manipulators, *The International Journal of Robotics Research* **4**(2): 72–83.

Krefft, M. & Hesselbach, J. (2005a). Elastodynamic optimization of parallel kinematics, *IEEE International Conference on Automation Science and Engineering*, pp. 357–362.

Krefft, M. & Hesselbach, J. (2005b). Elastodynamic optimization of parallel kinematics, *IEEE International Conference on Automation Science and Engineering*, pp. 357–362.

Krefft, M., Kerle, H. & Hesselbach, J. (2005). The assesment of parallel mechanisms – it is not only kinematics, *Production Engineering* **12**(1): 173–173.

Lee, J. H., Eom, K. S., Yi, B.-J. & Suh, I. H. (2001). Design of a new 6-DoF parallel haptic device, *IEEE International Conference on Robotics and Automation*, Vol. 1, pp. 886–891.

Lee, S.-U. & Kim, S. (2006). Analysis and optimal design of a new 6-DoF parallel type haptic device, *IEEE/RSJ International Conference on Intelligent Robots and Systems*, pp. 460–465.

Li, Y. & Xu, Q. (2005). Dynamic analysis of a modified delta parallel robot for cardiopulmonary resuscitation, *Intelligent Robots and Systems, 2005. (IROS 2005). 2005 IEEE/RSJ International Conference on*, pp. 233–238.

Liu, X.-J. & Wang, J. (2007). A new methodology for optimal kinematic design of parallel mechanisms, *Mechanism and Machine Theory* **42**: 1210–1224.

Liu, X.-J., Wang, J. & Zheng, H.-J. (2006). Optimum design of the 5R symmetrical parallel manipulator with a surrounded and good-condition workspace, *Robotics and Autonomous Systems* **54**(3): 221–233.

Lou, Y., Liu, G. & Li, Z. (2008). Randomized optimal design of parallel manipulators, *Automation Science and Engineering, IEEE Transactions on* **5**(2): 223–233.

Ma, O. & Angeles, J. (1990). The concept of dynamic isotropy and its applications to inverse kinematics and trajectory planning, *IEEE International Conference on Robotics and Automation*, Vol. 1, pp. 481–486.

McGhee, S., Chan, T. F., Dubey, R. V. & Kress, R. L. (1994). Probability-based weighting of performance criteria for a redundant manipulator, *ICRA*, pp. 1887–1894.

Merlet, J.-P. (2006). Design, *Parallel Robots, 2nd Edition*, Springer, p. 303.

Ozaki, H., Wang, H., Liu, X. & Gao, F. (1996). The atlas of the payload capability for design of 2-DoF planar parallel manipulators, *IEEE International Conference on Systems, Man, and Cybernetics*, Vol. 2, pp. 1483–1488.

Pierrot, F., Reynaud, C. & Fournier, A. (1990). Delta: a simple and efficient parallel robot, *Robotica* **8**(2): 105–109.

Qi, L. & Womersley, R. S. (1996). On extreme singular values of matrix valued functions, *Journal of Convex Analysis* **3**(1): 153–166.

Rigoni, E. & Poles, S. (2005). NBI and MOGA-II, two complementary algorithms for multi-objective optimizations, *Practical Approaches to Multi-Objective Optimization*.

Risoli, A., Prisco, G. M., Salsedo, F. & Bergamasco, M. (1999). A two degrees-of-freedom planar haptic interface with high kinematic isotropy, *IEEE International Workshop on Robot and Human Interaction*, pp. 297–302.

Salisbury, J. K. & Craig, J. J. (1982). Articulated hands: Force control and kinematic issues, *The International Journal of Robotics Research* **1**(1): 4–17.

Satici, A. C., Erdogan, A. & Patoglu, V. (2009). Design of a reconfigurable ankle rehabilitation robot and its use for the estimation of the ankle impedance, *IEEE International Conference on Rehabilitation Robotics, ICORR 2009*, pp. 257–264.

Stan, S.-D., Maties, V. & Balan, R. (2006). Optimal design of 2 DoF parallel kinematics machines, *Applied Mathematics and Mechanics*, pp. 705–706.

Stocco, L. J. (1999). *Robot design optimization with haptic interface applications*, PhD thesis, The University of British Columbia.

Stocco, L., Salcudean, S. E. & Sassani, F. (1998). Fast constrained global minimax optimization of robot parameters, *Robotica* **16**(6): 595–605.

Stuckman, B. & Easom, E. (1992). A comparison of bayesian/sampling global optimization techniques, *IEEE Transactions of Systems, Man and Cybernetics* **22**(5): 1024–1032.

Stuckman, B., Evans, G. & Mollaghasemi, M. (1991). Comparison of global search methods for design optimization using simulation, *IEEE Winter Simulation Conference*, pp. 937–944.

Tokatli, O. & Patoglu, V. (2009). Multicriteria design optimization of a compliant micro half-pantograph, *ECCOMAS Multibody Dynamics*.

Tsai, L.-W., Walsh, G. & Stamper, R. (1996). Kinematics of a novel three dof translational platform, *Robotics and Automation, 1996. Proceedings., 1996 IEEE International Conference on*, Vol. 4, pp. 3446–3451 vol.4.

Unal, R., Kiziltas, G. & Patoglu, V. (2008a). A multi-criteria design optimization framework for haptic interfaces, *IEEE International Symposium on Haptic interfaces for virtual environment and teleoperator systems, Haptic Symposium 2008*, pp. 231–238.

Unal, R., Kiziltas, G. & Patoglu, V. (2008b). Multi-criteria design optimization of parallel robots, *IEEE International Conference on Cybernetics and Intelligent Systems and IEEE International Conference on Robotics, Automation and Mechatronics, CIS-RAM*.

Unal, R. & Patoglu, V. (2008a). Optimal dimensional synthesis of a dual purpose haptic exoskeleton, *Lecture Notes in Computer Science, Springer*.

Unal, R. & Patoglu, V. (2008b). Optimal dimensional synthesis of force feedback lower arm exoskeletons, *IEEE RAS and EMBS International Conference on Biomedical Robotics and Biomechatronics, BioRob 2008*, pp. 329–334.

Yoon, J. & Ryu, J. (2001). Design, fabrication, and evaluation of a new haptic device using a parallel mechanism, *IEEE/ASME Transactions on Mechatronics* **6**(3): 221–233.

Yoshikawa, T. (1985a). Dynamic manipulability of robotic mechanisms, *Journal of Robotic Systems* **2**(1): 113–123.

Yoshikawa, T. (1985b). Manipulability of robotic mechanisms, *The International Journal of Robotics Research* **4**(2): 3–9.

Zheng, Y. & Lewis, W. (1994). Several algorithms of global optimal search, *Advances in Enginering Software* **22**(2): 87–98.

Transparent and Shaped Stiffness Reflection for Telesurgery

Bert Willaert, Pauwel Goethals, Dominiek Reynaerts,
Hendrik Van Brussel and Emmanuel B. Vander Poorten
Department of Mechanical Engineering, K.U.Leuven
Belgium

1. Introduction

The motivation behind the work presented in this chapter is minimal access *tele*surgery with reliable haptic feedback. Minimal access surgery (MAS) is performed via small incisions in the body, through which long rigid instruments are inserted along with a camera. Telesurgery refers to surgical operations performed by robotic instruments, the *slave*, commanded by a surgeon through one or more complex robotic joysticks, the *master*. Nowadays, the only commercially available master-slave system for minimal access surgery is the Da Vinci Surgical System, which is frequently used for MAS (Hockstein et al., 2007). The benefits of telesurgical laparoscopy over conventional laparoscopy include increased number of degrees of freedom, elimination of tremor, 3D visualization, possible motion scaling and an ergonomic position for the surgeon (Corcione et al., 2005; Nguan et al., 2008). Moreover, the master-slave concept enables the surgeon to be outside the direct environment of the patient. In 2001 e.g., the first transatlantic surgical operation, a laparoscopic cholecystectomy, was performed on a patient in Strasbourg, France by a surgeon situated in New York, United States (Marescaux et al., 2001).

Unfortunately, current telesurgical systems do not provide haptic feedback, which means that the surgeon loses his/her sense of touch. This decreases the efficiency of the surgeon and can result in collateral tissue damage (Bethea et al., 2004; De et al., 2007; Famaey et al., 2009). Several studies have shown that haptic feedback would be able to increase the precision of telesurgery and lower the interaction forces with the tissue (Deml et al., 2005; Tholey et al., 2005; Wagner et al., 2002). However, achieving a system with haptic feedback that accurately represents the feeling of soft tissue, while maintaining stability under all circumstances, is nontrivial and remains a big challenge. A first issue, which is not discussed in this chapter, concerns the design of a robust accurate force-measurement system that integrates well in the surgical environment (Peirs et al., 2004; Seibold et al., 2005; Willaert et al., 2009a; Zemiti et al., 2006). A second issue concerns the control itself of such a master-slave system. During MAS, the environment of interest consists mainly of soft tissue although also interactions with hard contacts can occur (i.e. contact with bone or another instrument). Based on the raw data acquired by Walraevens et al. (2008) (cardiovascular tissue) and by Rosen et al. (2008) (abdominal organs) one can estimate that the maximum stiffness is in the order of 1500 N/m when interacting with soft tissue. When contacting bone, the stiffness can be up to 8000 N/m (Bankman et al., 1990). The design of haptic teleoperation controllers for interaction with these types of environments is receiving growing interest from the research community (Cavusoglu et al., 2002; De Gersem et al., 2005a; Malysz & Siroupour, 2007; Misra & Okamura, 2006; Tavakoli et al., 2006) and forms the topic of this chapter.

To situate the controllers studied in this chapter among the large spectrum of bilateral teleoperation controllers, we distinguish three main concepts based on the rendering of the haptic feedback. Controllers of the first concept send all sensory data directly from the master to the slave and vice versa. All implementations of the "four-channel" controller (Lawrence, 1993; Yokokohji & Yoshikawa, 1994) are examples of such controllers. Controllers of the second concept still exchange the sensory data directly between master and slave, but the sensory data are also used to create a model of the environment and/or human operator. That model is used to adapt one or more parameters of the controller online. Preusche et al. (2002) use an estimate of the environment stiffness to adapt the stiffness of the position controller of the slave, while (Love & Book, 2004) use this estimate to change the extra damping of the master. Controllers of the third concept provide model-based haptic feedback and no sensory data is sent explicitly to the master. The sensory data of the slave are used to create a model of the environment and that model is sent back to the master to create the haptic sensation. Depending on the application, this model can have different levels of complexity. Hashtrudi-Zaad & Salcudean (1996) assume a mass-spring-damper model for the environment while the models of Funda & Paul (1991) and of Mitra & Niemeyer (2008) only describe a rigid wall at a variable location.

The main goal of this chapter is to discuss and demonstrate some major benefits of the third control concept, especially when used for telesurgery: (1) Model-based controllers are well-suited to deal with some typical problems associated with most modern surgical robots. As mentioned by Funda & Paul (1991); Hashtrudi-Zaad & Salcudean (1996); Ji et al. (2005); Kuan & Young (2003); Mitra & Niemeyer (2008); Tzafestas et al. (2008), a teleoperation system with model-based haptic feedback is more robust with respect to communication time delay. The increased robustness is even not restricted to the problem of communication time delay. This chapter shows that model-based controllers also offer also an increased robustness with respect to the restricted position tracking of the slave and the presence of low-pass filters. Note that elimination of surgical tremor by filtering the commands of the surgeon is often mentioned as one of the benefits of telesurgery (Hockstein et al., 2007; Okamura, 2004), but the use of such a filter can be conflicting with the requirement of reliable haptic feedback. To show the beneficial properties of the third concept, this chapter describes a practical implementation of a controller of this concept, which will be referred to as the Stiffness Reflecting controller (SRC). Based on experiments, the robustness of this controller over a controller of the first concept, namely the classical Direct Force Feedback controller (DFF), is demonstrated. (2) An additional benefit, next to the increased robustness, is that model-based haptic feedback offers the possibility to *shape* the reflected environment impedance. A generalized version of the SRC was originally proposed in order to maximize the stiffness discrimination ability of the surgeon during telesurgery (De Gersem et al., 2005b). A psychophysics experiment demonstrated that human stiffness perception for interactions with soft environments follows Weber's law (Weber, 1834), i.e. the change in stiffness that can just be discriminated is a constant fraction of the nominal stiffness, this fraction being 8-12 % (De Gersem, 2005c). To increase the stiffness discrimination ability, this generalized version of the SRC, applies a nonlinear shaping function to the estimated stiffness before reflection to the master. This principle of *enhanced sensitivity* (De Gersem et al., 2005a;b; Malysz & Siroupour, 2007; Son & Lee, 2008), allows the human operator to feel a difference in stiffness that is smaller than one he/she can detect by manual palpation. This chapter describes a practical implementation of the generalized version of the SRC (gSRC) and shows the feasibility of enhanced sensitivity based on a set of psychophysical user tests.

The layout of this chapter is as follows: Section 2 describes the concept of transparency and discusses the relevance of transparency for the application of telesurgery. Section 3 describes both the Stiffness Reflecting Controller with its generalized form and the Direct Force Feedback controller. The implementation of these controllers on an experimental setup is described in Section 4. Experiments comparing the performance and the stability of these controllers are described and discussed in Section 5, while the experiments on enhanced sensitivity are described and discussed in Section 6. The chapter ends with a discussion in Section 7 and a conclusion in Section 8.

2. Transparency for telesurgery

In literature, several definitions and indices for transparency have been proposed. According to Handlykken & Turner (1980) the ideal teleoperation system behaves as a massless infinitely stiff connection between the end-effector of the master and the slave. In that case, the system is completely transparent and the human operator feels as if directly manipulating the remote environment. Yokokohji & Yoshikawa (1994) state that the ideal response is obtained when the positions and forces at the master (x_h, F_h) and slave (x_e, F_e) are identical:

$$\forall t : \begin{cases} x_e(t) = x_h(t) \\ f_h(t) = f_e(t) \end{cases} . \tag{1}$$

Lawrence (1993) looks at the impedance Z_{th} "felt" by the human operator. The subscript *th* denotes 'transmitted to the human operator'. For an environment impedance Z_e, the transparency condition can be written as:

$$Z_{th} = Z_e. \tag{2}$$

Note that impedance is defined as $\frac{F}{v}$. Elaborating on this last definition (2), this section explains the concepts of *stiffness transparency* and *enhanced stiffness sensitivity*.

2.1 Stiffness Transparency

The perception and differentiation of the tissue's stiffness is essential during surgical palpation tasks (De Gersem et al., 2005a). Palpation is the technique of examining parts of the body by touching and pressing them. For example when performing tasks such as quality verification of a suture, localization of arteries or veins beneath fatty or surrounding tissue (Scott & Darzi, 1997), or identification of primary and metastatic cancer (Ota, 1995), stiffness discrimination is important. Therefore, this chapter focusses on the reflection of the stiffness properties of the environment through a bilateral teleoperation controller.

The concept of Stiffness Transparency defines how accurately the human operator feels the environment stiffness (k_e) through the teleoperation system. An indicative measure, is the difference ξ between the real environment stiffness and the stiffness felt by the human operator when manipulating the master quasi-statically. This can be expressed in the frequency domain for a known environment stiffness k_e as:

$$\xi = \lim_{s \to 0}(s.Z_{th}(s, k_e)) - k_e. \tag{3}$$

When experimental data are available, ξ can also be expressed in the time-domain:

$$\xi(t) = \frac{\triangle F_h(t)}{\triangle x_h(t)} - k_e(t). \tag{4}$$

In literature, experimental results are typically shown with a position versus time and a force versus time plot, following the definition of the ideal response of Yokokohji & Yoshikawa (1994). However, from such plots, it is difficult to analyse what the human operator feels. For this purpose, it is more useful to present the experimental data on force versus position plots, as done by De Gersem et al. (2005a); Mahvash & Okamura (2007); Tzafestas et al. (2008); Willaert et al. (2008b). Both ways of plotting the experimental data in the time-domain are employed in this chapter. Note that the frequency domain analysis is most appropriate to see all linear dynamics felt by the human operator, while the time domain analysis can also show the effect of nonlinear phenomena present in the teleoperation system.
Inspired by the idea of Impedance Reflection (De Gersem et al., 2005b; Hannaford, 1989; Hashtrudi-Zaad & Salcudean, 1996), Willaert et al. (2008b) presented the Stiffness Reflecting Controller (the SRC) for the purpose of stiffness transparency. This is a controller of the third concept for which haptic feedback is generated through reflection of the estimated environment stiffness to the master. The implementation of this controller will be discussed in detail in Section 3.

2.2 Enhanced Stiffness Sensitivity

As stated above, differentiation of tissue stiffness is important during surgical procedures. Since human perception of stiffness is limited both by absolute and differential thresholds, a perfectly stiffness-transparent system might not be sufficient for some differentiation tasks. To overcome the absolute thresholds, existing linear scaling techniques can be used, while for the differential thresholds, these techniques offer no solution. The problem of the differential thresholds is addressed in this chapter. Inspired by the idea of Impedance Shaping (Colgate, 1993), De Gersem et al. introduced the idea to overcome the differential thresholds by means of teleoperation control (De Gersem et al., 2005a;b). As stated in the introduction, the minimal change in stiffness that can be discriminated by a human operator is a constant fraction c of the nominal stiffness. For soft environments this fraction c was found to be 8-12 % (De Gersem, 2005c). To increase the stiffness discrimination ability, a relative change δk_e around the nominal environment stiffness $k_{e,n}$ should induce a higher relative change in stiffness felt by the operator:

$$\delta k_{th} = \frac{\Delta k_{th}}{k_{th,n}} > \frac{\Delta k_e}{k_{e,n}} = \delta k_e. \tag{5}$$

Introducing an extra design parameter σ, and requiring that

$$\delta k_{th} = \sigma \, \delta k_e, \tag{6}$$

makes that a tissue with stiffness $k_e = (k_{e,n} + \Delta k_e)$ feels different from $k_{e,n}$ if and only if $\delta k_e \geq \frac{c}{\sigma}$. Requiring that

$$k_{th} = K \, k_e^{\sigma}, \tag{7}$$

yields that one can discriminate environments with a difference in stiffness σ times smaller than the human differential threshold for stiffness discrimination. The factor σ can be interpreted as the sensitivity factor for discrimination. K serves as a scaling factor. Here it is used to keep the absolute value of k_{th} at a similar value as k_e. As stated above, this chapter

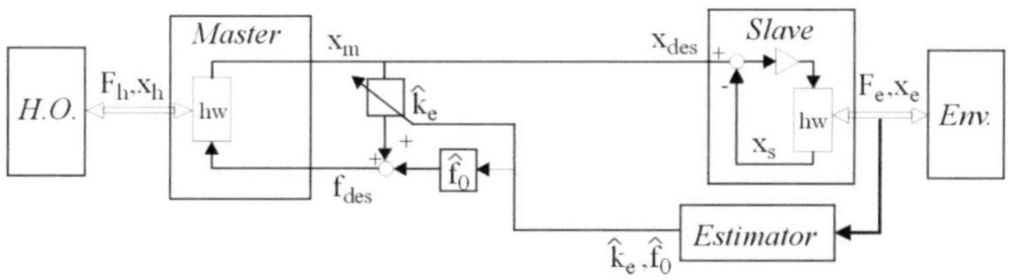

Fig. 1. The Stiffness Reflecting Controller (SRC), reflecting the estimated stiffness of the environment to an impedance controller at the master side.

only addresses the differential thresholds, although, through the parameter K, the presented controller can also be employed to overcome absolute thresholds. The implementation of the control law realizing expression (7) will be discussed in the following section.

3. Controller Definition

This section describes the definition of controllers designed for stiffness transparency and enhanced stiffness sensitivity. Experimental validation of the quality of these controllers takes place in Sections 5 and 6. The first controller is the Stiffness Reflecting controller presented by Willaert et al. (2008b). The second controller is the generalized form of the Stiffness Reflecting Controller proposed by De Gersem et al. (2005b). Both controllers will be compared to the classical Direct Force Feedback controller (DFF), described in the latter part of this section. Earlier work on soft tissue telemanipulation already described the potential of the DFF for telesurgery (Cavusoglu et al., 2002; De Gersem et al., 2005a). All controllers described are to be used with a master device of the impedance type, i.e. a system with low mass and low friction (e.g. the PHANToM). However, the implementations of the controllers can be modified in such a way that they can also be used with a master of the admittance type. For the hardware of master and slave, 1-d.o.f rigid-body models are supposed, obeying the following equations of motion:

$$F_h + \tau_m = M_m\ddot{x}_m + B_m\dot{x}_m, \tag{8}$$

$$\tau_s - F_e = M_s\ddot{x}_s + B_s\dot{x}_s, \tag{9}$$

$$Z_m = M_m s + B_m, \quad Z_s = M_s s + B_s, \tag{10}$$

with Z_m and Z_s representing the impedances of the master and the slave robot. Remark that for a rigid body model the positions x_m and x_s (the position at the motors) correspond to respectively x_h and x_e (the position of the end-effectors).

3.1 The SRC scheme

The Stiffness Reflecting Controller (SRC) originates from the idea to reflect the estimated stiffness of the environment to an impedance controller at the master side. In the SRC, depicted in Fig. 1, the slave is under position control following the master's position. While the slave follows the master, an estimator estimates the *local* remote environment stiffness k_e and the offset force f_o. These parameters are related to the position of the slave x_e and the measured interaction force F_e by the following local, linearized force-position relationship:

$$F_e = f_o + k_e.x_e. \tag{11}$$

Note that the relationship $F_e = k_e(x_e - x_0)$ is not linear in the parameters to be estimated (k_e, x_0). Fig. 2 shows the relation between the different parameters on a force-position curve.

The estimates $\hat{k}_e$ and $\hat{f}_o$ are used to determine f_{des}, the force input for the master:

$$f_{des} = \hat{f}_o + \hat{k}_e.x_m + c.\hat{k}_e.\dot{x}_m. \tag{12}$$

The last term in expression (12) is a stiffness dependent damping term (gain: $c.\hat{k}_e$), which has a significant positive effect on the stability as discussed in Section 4.1. As the considered master is of the impedance type, the force f_{des} is applied in open loop to the master. To summarize, the control inputs for the master and the slave become:

$$\tau_m = -f_{des}, \tag{13}$$

$$\tau_s = K_p(x_m - x_s) - K_v\dot{x}_s. \tag{14}$$

Based on this control law, the impedance "felt" by the human operator can be approximated by:

$$Z_{th} \approx M_m s + (B_m + c.\hat{k}_e) + \frac{\hat{k}_e}{s}. \tag{15}$$

As a consequence, the difference between the stiffness the human operator feels when manipulating the master quasi-statically and the real environment stiffness is:

$$\xi = \lim_{s \to 0}(s.Z_{th,k_e}(s)) - k_e = \hat{k}_e - k_e. \tag{16}$$

Depending on the correctness of the estimate, this difference approaches zero and thus the human operator feels approximately the correct environment stiffness.

The stiffness estimator used in this work is an Extended Kalman Filter. This is a well-known and widely-used recursive algorithm to estimate time-varying parameters, taking into account uncertain system dynamics and uncertainty caused by measurement noise (Kalman, 1960). For a compact tutorial on the Kalman Filter, see De Schutter et al. (1999). At each time-step, a new estimate and an associated uncertainty are calculated, given the previous estimate with its associated uncertainty and given the latest measurements. Within the Kalman filter formalism, the system's *process* and *measurements equations* are described as follows:

$$\mathbf{y}_i = A.\mathbf{y}_{i-1} + B.\mathbf{u}_{i-1} + \rho_p, \tag{17}$$

$$\mathbf{z}_i = H_i.\mathbf{y}_i + \rho_m, \tag{18}$$

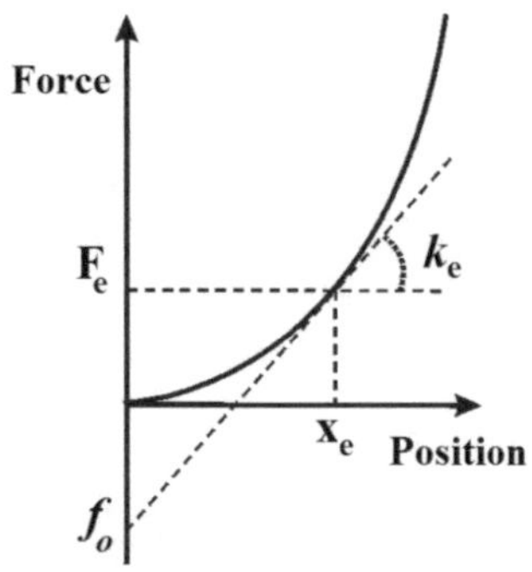

Fig. 2. The relation between the *local* stiffness k_e, the offset force f_o, the position x_e and the force F_e.

with $\mathbf{y}_i$ the state vector, $\mathbf{u}_i$ the control input and $\mathbf{z}_i$ the measurement vector at time step i. ρ_p is the process model uncertainty or process noise and ρ_m is the measurement model uncertainty. Applied to the estimation of the environment stiffness, the unknown parameters k_e and f_o form the state variables $\mathbf{y}_i = [f_o, k_e]^T$. Based upon the idea that the stiffness varies only slowly during surgical manipulation, the process is modelled as a random walk process with process noise ρ_p and no control input $\mathbf{u}_i$. So, equation (17) reduces to:

$$\mathbf{y}_i = \mathbf{y}_{i-1} + \rho_p. \tag{19}$$

ρ_p represents Gaussian process uncertainty with zero mean and covariance matrix Q. Large values for the covariance matrix Q result in faster convergence (e.g. when going from non-contact to contact state), but have the drawback that the estimates become more volatile. The approach to determine sensible values for the covariance matrix of the process noise is discussed in more detail in Section 4.1. The measured position $x_{e,i}$ and the interaction force $F_{e,i}$ do not allow direct estimation of f_0 and k_e as these two unknowns are related only by the single equation (11) to x_e and F_e. In order to decouple both estimates, the measurement equation at each time step is constructed as follows, based upon the measured position ($x_{e,i}$) and force ($F_{e,i}$) and the with j time steps T_S delayed position measurement ($x_{e,i-j}$) and force measurement ($F_{e,i-j}$):

$$F_{e,i} = f_o + k_e.x_{e,i}, \tag{20}$$

$$k_e = \frac{\Delta f}{\Delta x} = \frac{F_{e,i} - F_{e,i-j}}{x_{e,i} - x_{e,i-j}}. \tag{21}$$

To obtain the estimates $\hat{k}_e$ and $\hat{f}_o$, the explicit measurement equation of (18) should be reorganized into the following implicit measurement equation:

$$h(\mathbf{y}_i, \mathbf{z}_i) + \rho_m = 0 \qquad \text{with} \tag{22}$$

$$h(\mathbf{y}_i, \mathbf{z}_i) = \begin{bmatrix} F_{e,i} - F_{e,i-j} - k_e(x_{e,i} - x_{e,i-j}) \\ F_{e,i} - f_o - k_e.x_{e,i} \end{bmatrix}. \tag{23}$$

Since the measurement equation is nonlinear, an Extended Kalman Filter is used. The resulting estimates $\hat{k}_e$ and $\hat{f}_o$ form the environment model (12) that is used to create the haptic feedback at the master.

3.2 The gSRC scheme

The gSRC scheme is a generalized version of the SRC scheme. The control inputs for the master and the slave are the same as in (13) and (14), with a generalized f_{des}:

$$f_{des} = f_{th,o} + k_{th}.x_m + c.\hat{k}_e.\dot{x}_m. \tag{24}$$

The parameters $f_{th,o}$ and k_{th} are now a function of the estimated parameters $\hat{k}_e$ and $\hat{f}_o$, rather than being the estimates themself. To realize enhanced stiffness sensitivity following (7), k_{th} is calculated as $K\hat{k}_e^{\sigma}$. The parameter $f_{th,o}$ can be obtained using the requirement that any zero interaction force ($F_e = 0$) at the slave side should give a zero transmitted force ($f_{des} = 0$). Using (24) and supposing quasi-static manipulation, the requirement $f_{des} = 0$ can be written as:

$$f_{th,o} = -K\hat{k}_e^{\sigma} x_m. \tag{25}$$

The position tracking behaviour of the slave can be described using linear techniques. If the hardware of the slave is described by its impedance Z_s and the local position controller by C_s, the relation between x_m and x_e can be written as:

$$\begin{aligned} X_e &= h_1\, X_m - h_2\, F_e, \qquad (26)\\ \text{with} \quad h_1 &= \frac{C_s}{Z_s + C_s}\\ h_2 &= \frac{1}{Z_s + C_s}. \end{aligned}$$

For low-frequency manipulation, h_1 can be considered as 1 and h_2 as constant. The position tracking in time domain can now be written as:

$$x_e = x_m - h_2 F_e. \qquad (27)$$

For the considered case that the interaction force is zero ($F_e = 0$), above expressions simplify to their first term. Combining the equations (11), (25) and (27) results in:

$$\begin{aligned} f_{th,o} &= -K\,\hat{k}_e^{\sigma}\, x_e\\ &= -K\,\hat{k}_e^{\sigma-1}(\hat{k}_e\, x_e)\\ &= K\,\hat{k}_e^{\sigma-1}\,\hat{f}_o. \qquad (28) \end{aligned}$$

Fitting the last expression (28) into (24) results in:

$$f_{des} = K\,\hat{k}_e^{\sigma-1}\,\hat{f}_o + K\,\hat{k}_e^{\sigma}\, x_m + c\,\hat{k}_e\,\dot{x}_m. \qquad (29)$$

Note that if h_2 is small, the slave tracking is robust with respect to external forces. In that case, using expression (28) is still acceptable for reasonably small F_e.
The parameters $f_{th,o}$ and k_{th}, being function of the estimated parameters $\hat{k}_e$ and $\hat{f}_o$, form the model that is used to create the haptic feedback at the master, following (24).

3.3 The DFF scheme

The Direct Force Feedback controller (DFF) is a combination of a position controller at the slave side and a force controller at the master side. The input for the slave's position controller is the measured position of the master and the input for the master's force controller is the measured interaction force at the slave side F_e. Compared to the position-controller of the SRC scheme a velocity-feedforward term is added to the position controller of the slave, as this implementation of the DFF has better stability properties (Willaert et al., 2009b). The control inputs for the motors of the master and the slave become:

$$\tau_m = -F_e, \qquad (30)$$

$$\tau_s = (K_v s + K_p)(x_m - x_s). \qquad (31)$$

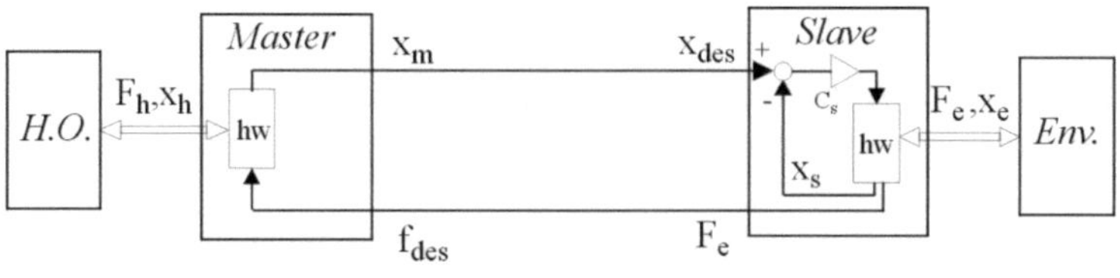

Fig. 3. The Direct Force Feedback Controller.

Model		Controller	
M_m:	0.64 kg	K_v:	80 Ns/m
B_m:	3.4 Ns/m	K_p:	4000 N/m
M_s:	0.61 kg		
B_s:	11 Ns/m		

Table 1. Parameters of the teleoperation system

Based on this control law, the impedance felt by the human operator can be calculated:

$$Z_{th} = \frac{(M_m s^2+B_m s)(M_s s^2+(B_s+K_v)s+(K_p+k_e))+k_e(K_v s+K_p)}{s(M_s s^2+(B_s+K_v)s+(K_p+k_e))}. \tag{32}$$

As a consequence, the difference between the stiffness the human operator feels when manipulating the master quasi-statically and the real environment stiffness is:

$$\xi = \lim_{s\to 0}(s.Z_{th}(s,k_e)) - k_e = (\frac{K_p k_e}{K_p + k_e}) - k_e. \tag{33}$$

Therefore, the human operator feels the series connection of the real environment stiffness and the stiffness of the position controller, i.e. a stiffness smaller than the actual environment stiffness.

4. Controller Implementation

This section describes the implementation on a 1-d.o.f experimental master-slave setup of the controllers defined above. The experimental setup, shown in figure 4 consists of two current-driven voice coil motors recycled from hard disk drives. On both devices, one-dimensional force sensors are mounted, measuring the interaction forces between slave and environment and between the human operator and the master (noise level: ± 0.05 N). Linear encoders offer accurate position measurements (resolution: 1μm). A rigid-body model for the master and the slave is chosen as the structural resonance frequencies are above 100 Hz. The controllers are implemented on a dSPACE board, in a real time loop with a frequency of 1 kHz ($T_s = 1\ ms$). Table 1 summarizes the parameters for the hardware, based on a linear model identification of the setup, and the parameters for the DFF controller, employed during the experiments. The implementations of the SRC and the gSRC are described in more detail in two following sections.

4.1 The SRC scheme

This section describes the practical implementation of the controller defined in Section 3.1. Firstly, the position controller, see eq. (14), is tuned following standard techniques in order to obtain a good and stable step response. The resulting parameters can be found in Table 1.
Next, the parameters of the Extended Kalman filter, i.e. the estimator, are tuned. The behaviour of this filter depends on the process noise ρ_p, the measurement model uncertainty ρ_m and the delay (expressed as a number of time samples: $j \cdot T_s$) between the used measurements. The covariance matrix for the measurement model uncertainty ρ_m is fixed a priori based on

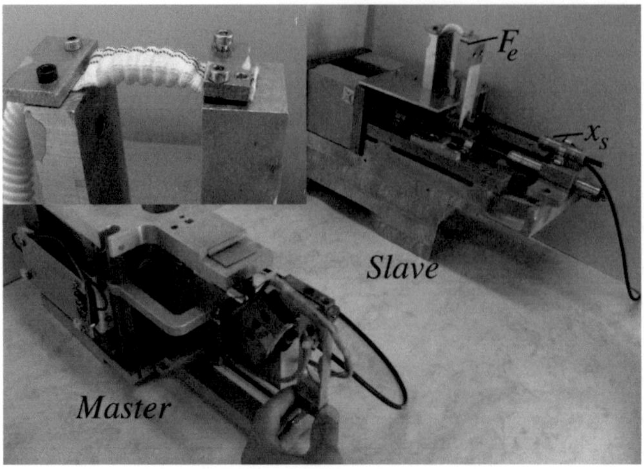

Fig. 4. The experimental 1 d.o.f. master-slave system. In detail a Dacron cardiovascular prosthesis at the slave side.

the sensor specifications:

$$R = \begin{bmatrix} (0.002\ mm)^2 & 0 & 0 & 0 \\ 0 & (0.002\ mm)^2 & 0 & 0 \\ 0 & 0 & (0.05\ N)^2 & 0 \\ 0 & 0 & 0 & (0.05\ N)^2 \end{bmatrix} \tag{34}$$

The process noise is a vector with zero mean and a covariance matrix Q:

$$Q = \begin{bmatrix} (q_1\ N)^2 \\ (q_2\ N/m)^2 \end{bmatrix} \tag{35}$$

A number of simulation runs and experiments were performed to determine sensible values for q_1, q_2 and j. Figures 5(a) and 5(b) show the simulation data (x, F) used as input to tune the estimator. White-noise is added to the force measurement signal ($\pm 0.02\ N$). Figure 5(c) shows the estimates $\hat{k}_e$ and $\hat{f}_o$ for $j = 12$ and different values of $q1 = q2 = q$. Figure 5(d) shows these estimates for $q_1 = q_1 = 0.03$ and different values of j. From these figures, one can see that:

- Larger values q_i of the covariance matrix of the process noise ρ_p result in a faster (and more correct) response to a change in environment stiffness. This is obvious as the process is defined as a random walk process in eq. (19). However, larger values of q_i also mean that the estimator is more reactive to measurement noise. This results in more volatile estimates, which might be transferred to the human operator and disturb his/her perception of the remote environment. Therefore, tuning the covariance matrix of the proces noise boils down to finding a compromise between having *sufficiently* smooth transients and *sufficiently* fast convergence to correct estimates $\hat{k}_e$ and $\hat{f}_o$. Note that this compromise depends strongly on the signal-to-noise ratio of the position and force measurements at the slave. The better the signal-to-noise ratio of the measurements, the larger the values q_i that can be chosen.

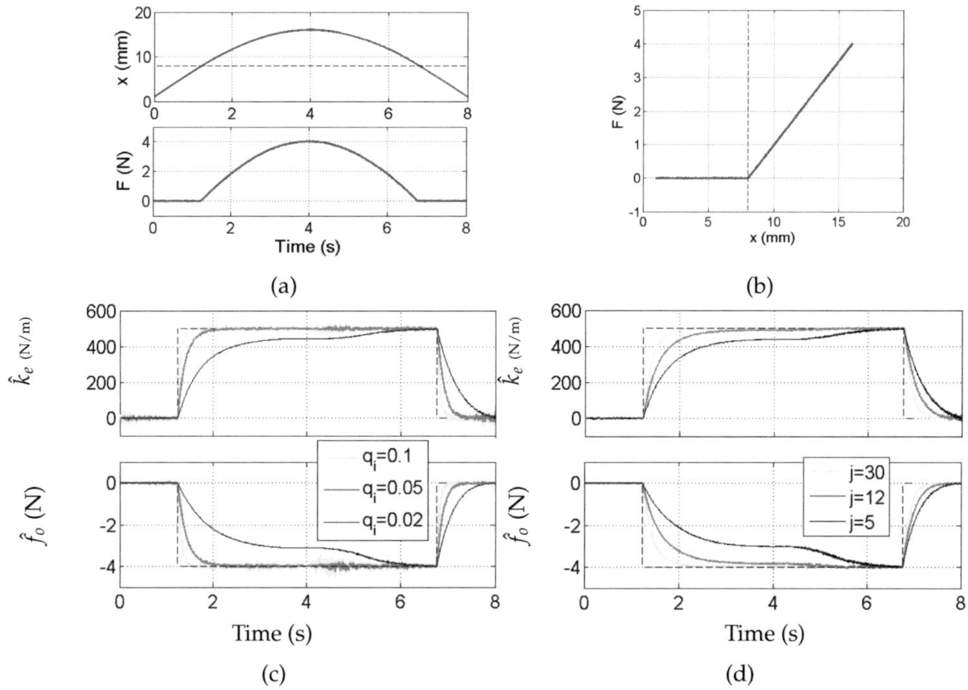

Fig. 5. The motion and force profiles (a), simulating an interaction with a perfect spring, with stiffness $k_e = 500$ N/m (b), used to analyse the behaviour of the estimator. The estimates $\hat{k}_e$ and $\hat{f}_o$ are displayed for this simulation data for (c) $j = 12$ and different values of $q_1 = q_2 = q_i$ and (d) for $q_1 = q_2 = 0.03$ and different values of j. The theoretically correct value is indicated as a dashed line in (c) and (d).

- A larger time shift $j \cdot T_s$ between the two data sets $(x_{e,i}, F_{e,i})$ and $(x_{e,i-j}, F_{e,i-j})$, also results in a faster (and more correct) response to a change in environment stiffness. This can be explained as follows: the update equation of the form $\hat{y}_i = \tilde{y}_i + K_k(c - h(\tilde{y}_i, z_i))$ contains an error term $(c - h(\tilde{y}_i, z_i))$ described by (23). For a particular velocity the absolute values of both $(F_{e,i} - F_{e,i-j})$ and $(x_{e,i} - x_{e,i-j})$ are larger for a longer delay $j \cdot T_s$ in contact mode. Thus, the first error term in (23) increases as the delay increases, which results in a faster response. However, also here a compromise is at hand, as the very initial response to a change in environment stiffness is slower for a larger value j. Note that this is only problematic for very abrupt changes in environment stiffness. The initial contact with a perfectly linear spring shows such an abrupt change. When contacting soft tissue in a surgical scenario, the initial contact is typiccaly not problematic, due to the low stiffness of soft tissue at small strain. On the other hand, the change in environment stiffness at the moment of motion reversal could be problematic. Both cases are shown in figure 6.

Based on these findings and trials on the experimental setup, the covariance matrix has been set to:

$$Q = \begin{bmatrix} (0.1\ N)^2 & \\ & (0.1\ N/m)^2 \end{bmatrix}, \tag{36}$$

and the time shift between the two data sets is set to $(12 \cdot T_s)$. Ideally, the estimator uses position measurements and force measurements acquired at the end-effector of the slave. Here, the force measurement is actually done at the end-effector (F_e) and the position measurement

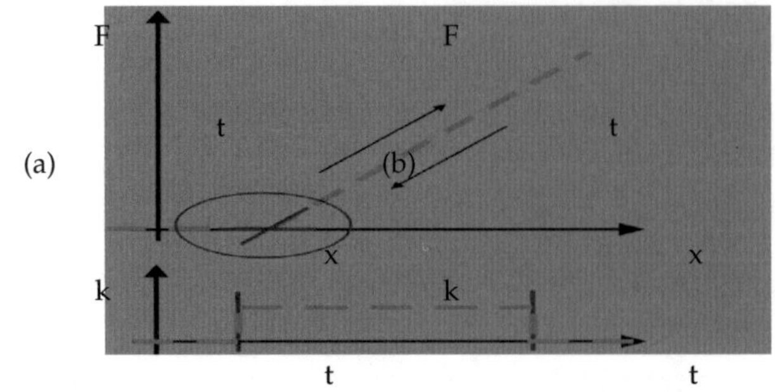

Fig. 6. Abrupt changes in stiffness (a) at the initial contact with a linear spring and (b) at the reversal of motion when manipulating soft tissue.

is done at the motor of the slave (x_s instead of x_e). For the 1 d.o.f. master-slave setup used here, this is only a theoretical difference as both the slave and the master behave as a rigid-body for frequencies below 100 Hz ($x_s \approx x_e$).
Note that in order to have a smooth feeling in free motion ($F_e \approx 0$) and to avoid problems with transition from free motion to contact, f_{des} is set to zero as long as the measured interaction force F_e is smaller than 0.2 N.

The last aspect of the implementation of the SRC, discussed in this section, is its stability. The analysis of the stability of this controller is not straightforward. Due to the presence of the Extended Kalman Filter, classical tools such as closed-loop stability and frequency-domain passivity cannot be used. De Gersem et al. (2005b) suggest that the SRC decouples the master and the slave. In practice, however, this is only partially true due to the existence of estimation errors and estimation lag. Especially when contacting hard objects, i.e. for a sudden change in environment stiffness, stability can be problematic with the SRC. For an intuitive understanding of the stability properties of the SRC, one can observe that the stability properties of this controller shift from those of a haptic controller for interaction with a virtual wall to those of a Direct Force Feedback teleoperation controller (DDF), depending on the ratio $\frac{q_1}{q_2}$. Figure 7 shows the effect of varying q_2 for a fixed q_1. From this figure, it is clear that for decreasing

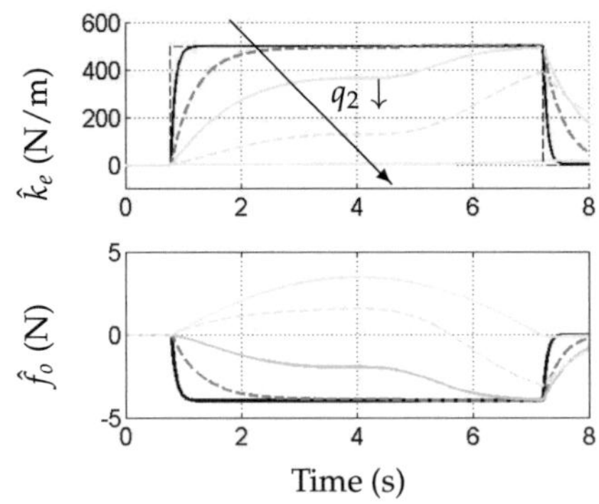

Fig. 7. The estimates $\hat{k}_e$ and $\hat{f}_o$ for the simulation data in figure 5(a) for decreasing values of q_2 (0.1-0.02-0.005-0.003-0.001) while q_1 is kept constant ($q_1 = 0.1$).

values of q_2, the error on the estimate of the environment stiffness increases. Stated differently, the estimate $\hat{k}_e$ tends more and more to zero than to the correct environment stiffness, while the estimate $\hat{f}_o$ tends towards F_e. For the limit case $\hat{k}_e \approx 0$ and $\hat{f}_o \approx F_e$, the force input to the master does no longer depend on the position of the master x_m and the SRC behaves exactly as the DFF. This shows that the decoupling of the master and the slave is not absolute but depends on the properties of the estimator. The gain in robustness, mentioned in the introduction, proper to controllers of the third concept, depends on how well master and slave are decoupled. In order to maximize the decoupling, both q_1 and q_2 have to be large.
An extra measure to improve the overall stability of the system, while only minimally compromising the transparency, is the addition of a damping at the master proportional to the estimate of the environment stiffness: $c.\hat{k}_e.\dot{x}_m$ (see (12)). This extra damping term has a significant positive effect on the range of environment stiffnesses the system can stably interact with. Based on experimental testing, the factor c is set to 0.015 as further increasing of this factor did not result in further improvement of the system's stability. For all parameters described above, the experimental setup is stable for interaction with stiffnesses up to at least [7000-8000] N/m.

4.2 The gSRC scheme

This section describes the practical implementation of the controller defined in Section 3.2. Except for the parameters of the estimator, the implementation is the same as described in the former section. The tuning of the estimator has to be revised as the function $K\hat{k}_e^\sigma$ has an amplifying effect on the noise of the estimate $\hat{k}_e$. Figure 8 shows $\hat{k}_e$ and $K\hat{k}_e^\sigma$ for $\sigma = 3$ and $K = \frac{1}{500^2}$, for the parameters selected above ($q_i = 0.1$ and $j = 12$). The input for the estimator employs the same simulation data as shown in figure 5(a). From this figure, it is clear that the signal-to-noise ratio of $K\hat{k}_e^\sigma$ is worse than the signal-to-noise ratio of $\hat{k}_e$. This is actually obvious as the goal of the function $K\hat{k}_e^\sigma$ is to increase the relative differences in stiffness. Based on this finding, the values of the covariance matrix Q should be reduced in the case that $\sigma > 1$. Here, the covariance matrix has been set to:

$$Q = \begin{bmatrix} (0.03\ N)^2 & \\ & (0.03\ N/m)^2 \end{bmatrix}. \tag{37}$$

In order to maintain a sufficiently fast (and correct) response of the estimator, the delay between the two data sets has to be increased if the values of the covariance matrix Q decrease

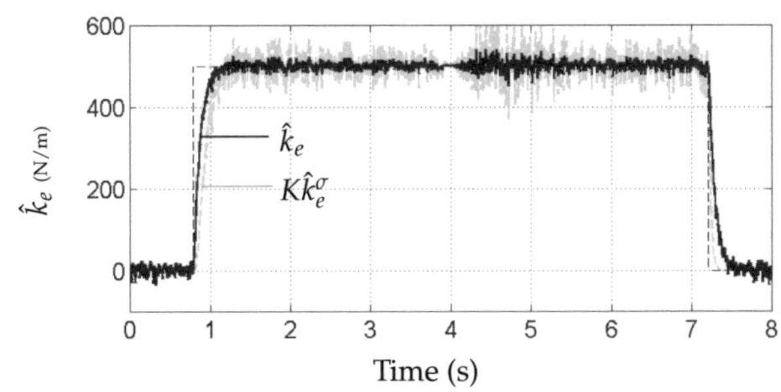

Fig. 8. The estimate $\hat{k}_e$ and $K\hat{k}_e^\sigma$ for the simulation data in Figure 5(a) but with white-noise added to the force measurement signal ($\sigma = 3$ and $K = \frac{1}{500^2}$).

(see 5(c) and 5(d)). The time shift between the two data sets is set to $(30 \cdot T_s)$. With these values, the stiffness presented to the human operator k_{th} $(= K\hat{k}_e^{\sigma})$ behaves sufficiently smooth and accommodates sufficiently fast to changes in the environment stiffness for $\sigma \in [1-3]$. The scaling factor K has to be used to maintain the absolute value of the stiffness presented to the human operator at a similar value as the real environment stiffness. Hereto, the nominal environment stiffness has to be known or estimated a priori.

5. Experimental results: part I

As stated in the introduction, controllers of the third concept show better robustness compared to controllers of the first concept. The experiments described in this section compare the Stiffness Reflecting Controller (SRC), a controller of the third concept to the Direct Force Feedback Controller (DFF), a controller of the first concept. A number of experiments are performed on the experimental master-slave setup described in Section 3: a comparison of the two controllers (subsection 5.1), a comparison of the two controllers when a low-pass filter with cutoff frequency of 3.2 Hz is present (subsection 5.2), and a comparison of the two controllers when a 100 ms time delay was introduced on both the control and the communication channel (subsection 5.3). Moreover, a last experiment shows the interaction with a nonlinear environment, having the material properties of typical cardiovascular tissue (subsection 5.4).

5.1 SRC vs. DFF

During this experiment, a linear tension spring ($k_e = 1100$ N/m) is manipulated. Figure 9(a) and 9(b) show the experimental data acquired during this manipulation for respectively the DFF and the SRC. For the DFF, as mentioned in Section 3.3, the stiffness felt by the operator is the series connection of the environment stiffness (k_e) and the stiffness of the position controller (K_p) following expression (16). Linear curve fitting shows that the stiffness presented to the operator is ± 850 N/m. This approximates the expected value of $(\frac{1}{ke} + \frac{1}{Kp})^{-1}$. Thus, despite good force tracking and acceptable position tracking the stiffness felt by the operator is significantly lower than the real environment stiffness. For the SRC, however, the stiffness felt by the operator is nearly the correct environment stiffness, although neither the positions nor the forces do correspond well. This example stresses the importance of displaying force position plots when analyzing stiffness transparency.

5.2 SRC vs. DFF: a low-pass filter in the loop

During this experiment, the same linear tension spring ($k_e = 1100$ N/m) is manipulated, but a low-pass filter (cut-off frequency: 3.2 Hz) has been added to the control channel, i.e. the position of the master is filtered before it is used as position command at the slave. In literature, the use of low-pass filters for elimination of surgical tremor is often mentioned as one of the benefits of telesurgery (Hockstein et al., 2007; Okamura, 2004). Moreover, low-pass filters can also be used to avoid excitation of the structural resonance frequencies of the slave. However, one should realize that such low-pass filters can jeopardize the implementation of haptic feedback, especially for controllers of the first and the second concept. For the DFF e.g., a low-pass filter in the loop has a negative effect on both the transparency and the stability of the overall system. Fite et al. (2001) show that the introduction of a lead filter has a positive effect on the stability of the overall system while Willaert et al. (2009b) show that velocity-feedforward to the slave also improves the stability. Both approaches decrease the total phase-lag of the position controller in the loop. In contrast to this, the introduction of a low-pass filter in the control channel increases the total phase-lag and thus, has a negative effect on the

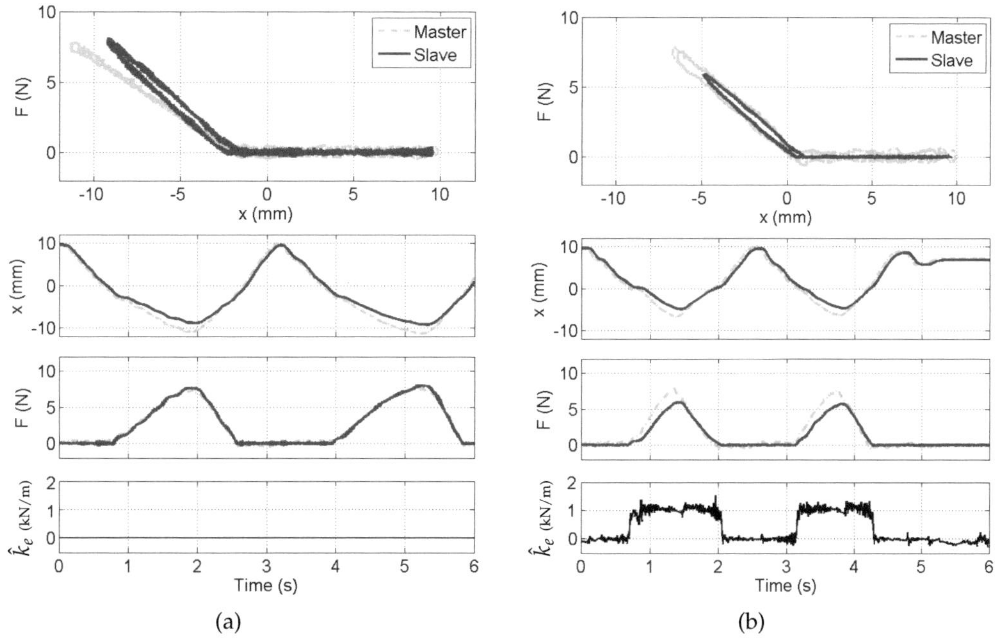

Fig. 9. Manipulation of a linear spring ($k_e = 1100$ N/m) for (a) the DFF and (b) the SRC.

system's stability.

Figure 10(a) shows the experimental data acquired during this manipulation with a low-pass filter in the loop for the SRC. One can see that the remote environment is presented well to the human operator. Moreover, the stability is not jeopardized by the presence of the low-pass filter in the loop. With the DFF, however, the effect of the low-pass filter is clearly felt by the human operator and only for small environment stiffnesses ($k_e < 200$ N/m), the human operator is able to keep the system stable.

5.3 SRC vs. DFF: time-delay in the loop

During this experiment, the same linear tension spring ($k_e = 1100$ N/m) is manipulated, but 100 ms time delay has been introduced into the control and the communication channel. This means a round-trip time delay of 200 ms. Time delay is often mentioned as an important aspect of telesurgery (C.R.Doarn et al., 2007; Lum et al., 2009; Rayman et al., 2006), although the current practice is that both the master and the slave are located in the same surgical room. As mentioned in the introduction, different controllers of the third concept have been presented in order to provide useful haptic feedback for time-delayed systems (Funda & Paul, 1991; Hashtrudi-Zaad & Salcudean, 1996; Ji et al., 2005; Kuan & Young, 2003; Mitra & Niemeyer, 2008; Tzafestas et al., 2008). Note that the estimates $\hat{k}_e$ and $\hat{f}_o$ are transferred from the slave to the master through the communication channel. Figure 10(b) shows the experimental data acquired during this manipulation with time-delay in the loop for the SRC. One can see that the human operator can feel the correct environment stiffness. As the stiffness is rendered at the master with a rest position corresponding to the real rest position, the human operator initially overshoots this rest position due to the time delay. The size of this overshoot depends on the round-trip time delay and the velocity of the master ($\dot{x}_m = \pm 21$ mm/s at the first contact and $\dot{x}_m = \pm 30$ mm/s at the second contact). Especially in constrained environments,

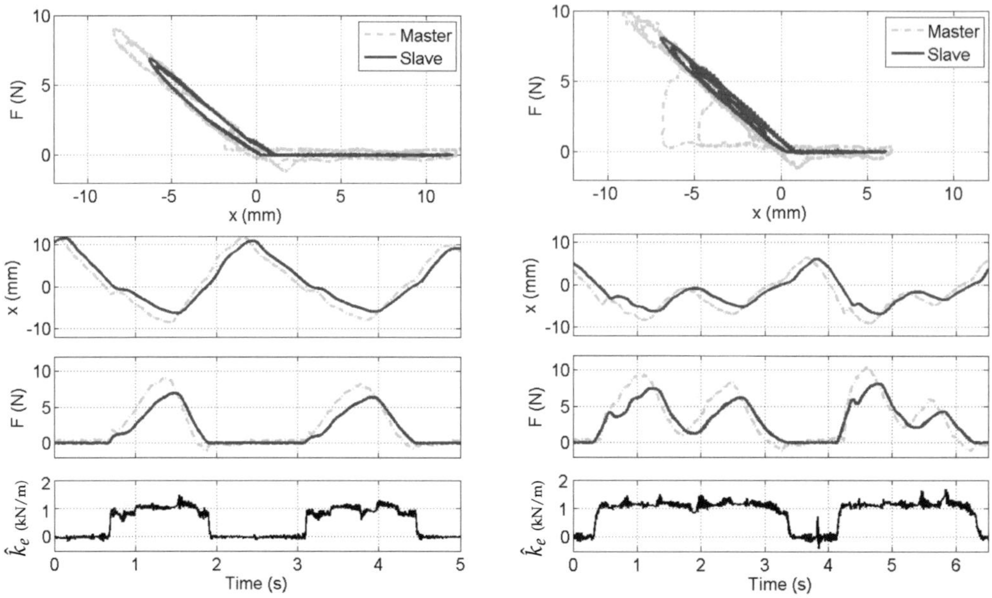

Fig. 10. Manipulation of a linear spring (k_e = 1100 N/m) for the SRC with (a) a low-pass filter in the loop (3.2 Hz) and (b) time-delay in the loop ($T_{d,1}$ = $T_{d,2}$=100 ms).

this approach has the advantage that the human operator can directly be aware of the relative distance between different objects. With the DFF, the effect of the time-delay is similar to the effect of the low-pass filter. The time-delay is clearly felt by the human operator and only for small environment stiffnesses, the human operator is able to keep the system stable. Note that no figures are shown for the DFF with a low-pass filter or time-delay in the loop.

5.4 SRC vs. DFF: representation of a nonlinear environment

During this experiment, a material with nonlinear material properties is manipulated. Instead of real soft tissue as in (Willaert et al., 2008b), a Dacron cardiovascular prosthesis is used, i.e. a material with longitudinal material properties similar to cardiovascular soft tissue (Grande-Allen et al., 2001). The detail in figure 4 shows how the Dacron prosthesis is clamped as a whole and stretched in the longitudinal direction. Figure 11(a) and 11(b) show the experimental data acquired during this manipulation for respectively the DFF and the SRC. The force-position plots demonstrate that the nonlinear behaviour of the material is well reflected to the master for both controllers. But as mentioned before, the stiffness perceived with the DFF is always lower than the actual stiffness. This problem does not occur when using the SRC. This data shows that the localized linear model (11) is able to reflect a nonlinear environment reliably to the master. Note that only at the moment of motion reversal, the stiffness felt at the master is inaccurate. This due to a combination of a position tracking lag of the slave with respect to the master and an estimation lag for the abrupt change in environment stiffness as explained in Section 4.1.

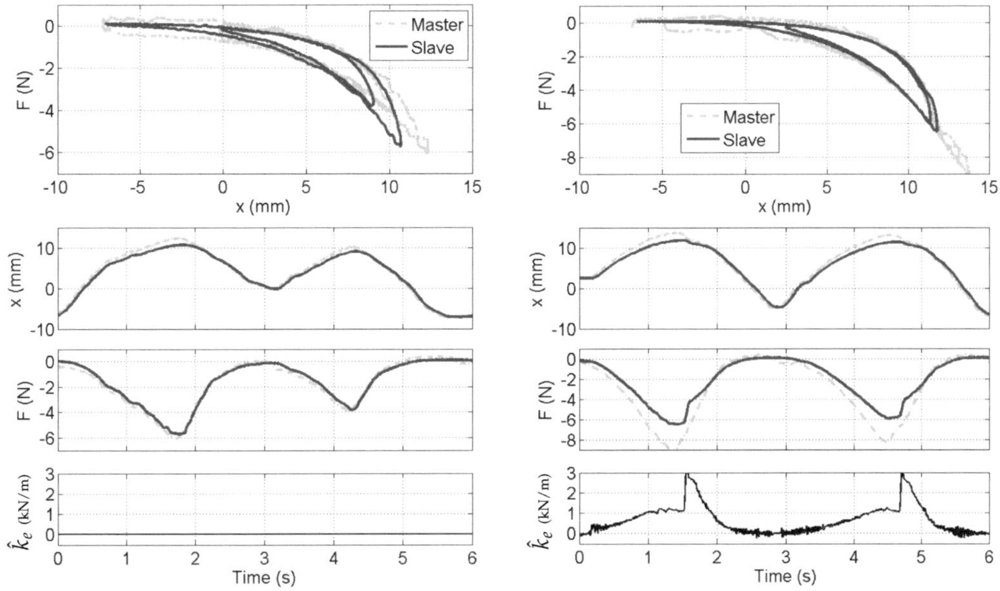

(a) (b)

Fig. 11. Manipulation of a nonlinear material for (a) the DFF and (b) the SRC.

6. Experimental results: part II

The experiments, described in this section, show the potential of the generalized Stiffness Reflecting Controller (gSRC). Firstly, an interaction with a linear spring is described (subsection 6.1). Next, a psychophysical experiment is described, demonstrating the feasibility of enhanced stiffness sensitivity (subsection 6.2).

6.1 the gSRC: stiffness shaping for interaction with a linear spring

During this experiment, a linear tension spring (500 N/m) is manipulated. The stiffness presented to the operator is shaped following expression (7) with $\sigma = 3$ and $K = 4.5 * 10^{-6}$. As a consequence, the stiffness felt by the operator should be 562 N/m. Fig. 12 shows the experimental data. Linear curve fitting on these data shows that the stiffness felt by the operator is 568 N/m, which only minimally deviates from the desired value of 562 N/m.
However, one can see a clear error during the initial contact. It takes about 0.5 *sec* before the correctly *shaped* stiffness is felt by the operator. This behaviour can be explained by the combined effect of the estimator tuned to be less reactive (smaller process noise) and the following: when the slave makes contact with a spring, the estimated stiffness $\hat{k}_e$ converges from 0 to k_e, the real stiffness of the environment, during a periode of time (here in about 0.5 *sec*, see Fig. 12). The stiffness presented to the operator, follows expression (7) and, as mentioned in Section 4.1,K serves as a scaling factor to keep k_{th} at a similar value as k_e. Thus, typically $K \simeq \frac{1}{\bar{k}_e^{(\sigma-1)}}$, with $\bar{k}_e$ an *a priori* determined estimate of the real environment stiffness. As a result, the nonlinear mapping delays the convergence of k_{th} to the correctly *shaped* stiffness:

$$k_{th} \simeq \frac{\hat{k}_e(t)^{\sigma}}{\bar{k}_e^{(\sigma-1)}} < \hat{k}_e(t) \quad \text{for} \quad \left\{ \begin{array}{l} \hat{k}_e(t) < \bar{k}_e \\ \sigma > 1 \end{array} \right.$$

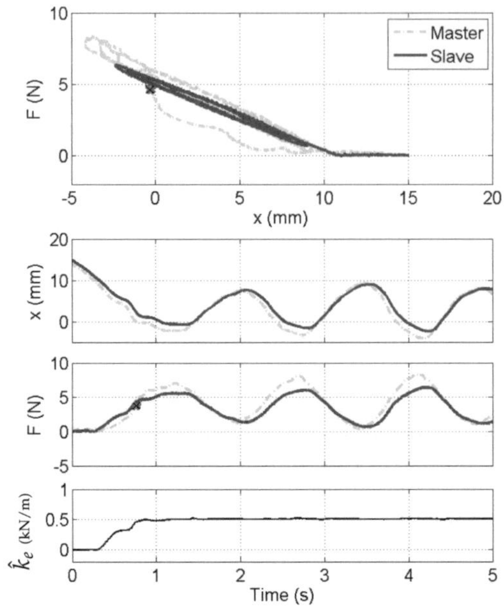

Fig. 12. Manipulation of a linear spring with shaped stiffness reflection: the force-position curve, the force vs. time, the position vs. time and the estimated environment stiffness $\hat{k}_e$ for the SSRC with $\sigma = 3$ and $K = 4.5$. The green dot (x) shows two data-points from the same time step.

6.2 the gSRC: a psychophysical experiment

During a psychophysical experiment six different subjects performed a stiffness differentiating task. They were asked to interact with two different springs through the master slave system, after which they had to say which spring was the stiffest. A two-alternatives forced choice procedure was employed. During the tests, the subjects could not see the slave and received no feedback from the examinator about their performance. Each subject did a total of 18 comparisons: 6 times with $\sigma = 1$, 6 times with $\sigma = 2$ and 6 times with $\sigma = 3$. These 18 test were randomized. The subjects were not informed about when and how many times each condition occurred.

The two springs had a stiffness of 182 N/m and 197 N/m. This is a relative difference of 7.6%, which lies below the practical discrimination threshold (i.e. 8%-12%). For $\sigma = 1$, K is set to 1, this is the special case of the gSRC, corresponding to the SRC. Enhanced stiffness sensitivity is offered for the cases $\sigma = 2$ and $\sigma = 3$. Then, K is set to 0.0053 and 0.028 respectively, in order to have the perceived stiffness in the range of the real environment stiffness. Table 2 shows how each spring is presented at the master side under the three different conditions. Moreover, Table 2 shows the average percentage of correct answers for each test condition. For $\sigma = 1$, the subjects were right 53 % of the time. This corresponds to pure guesswork. For $\sigma = 2$ and $\sigma = 3$ however, i.e. with enhanced sensitivity, the average percentage of correct answers is 80 % and 94 % respectively. This demonstrates the ability to shape the reflected stiffness through a master-slave setup in such a way that the operator's discrimination ability is augmented. Moreover, this confirms the finding in De Gersem et al. (2005a) that the mini-

	$\sigma = 1$	$\sigma = 2$	$\sigma = 3$
Spring 1	182 N/m	175 N/m	169 N/m
Spring 2	197 N/m	205 N/m	214 N/m
δ	7.6 %	14.6 %	21 %
P	53 %	80 %	94 %

Table 2. Results of the Psychophysical Experiment. δ is the relative difference between the two springs felt at the master, P is the percentage of correct differentiation.

mal difference in stiffness that can just be discriminated is larger than 8%-12% of the nominal stiffness.

7. Discussion

The main goal of this chapter is to demonstrate the potential benefits of controllers of the third concept, i.e. controllers with model-based haptic feedback, especially for telesurgical applications. Hereto, this chapter describes the practical implementation of the Stiffness Reflecting Controller. The experiments described in Section 5 support the claim that such controllers show good robustness properties. It is shown that, for the SRC, the compliance of the position controller does not influence the stiffness felt by the operator. It is also shown that the introduction of a low-pass filter or non-negligible time-delay only minimally affects the transparency and stability for the SRC. Although not explicitly demonstrated in this chapter, controllers of the third concept can also behave more robust with respect to other hardware-related issues of surgical slave robots that traditionally restrict the applicability of bilateral controllers on such robots. Willaert et al. (2009b) show e.g. that the inertia of the slave has a large influence on the stability properties of the DFF controller and conclude that the slave inertia should be as low as possible. Since current commercial surgical robots are mostly not lightweight robots, the SRC can be a useful controller for these robots. Another, hardware aspect of current surgical robots is the restricted structural stiffness, which influences both transparency and stability (Christiansson & van der Helm, 2007; Tavakoli & Howe, 2009). For the DFF and a slave with flexibilities, the stiffness that the human operator feels is a series connection of the real environment stiffness, the stiffness of the position controller and the structural stiffness of the slave. In this work, the estimation of the environment stiffness is based on the force measurement at the end-effector (F_e) and the position measurement at the motor ($x_s \approx x_e$). As the 1 d.o.f master and slave behave as a rigid-body for frequencies below 100 Hz, the correct environment stiffness can be estimated. For flexible multi-d.o.f. systems, however, the estimation of k_e should be based on the force measurement at the end-effector (F_e) and the position measurement at the end-effector ($x_e \neq x_s$). In future research, it will be investigated how the position of the end-effector can be measured or estimated. By doing so, the SRC can be made insensitive to both the compliance of the position controller and the compliance of the slave robot itself.

Based on the detailed stability analysis of the DFF and the experiments presented here, it is clear that, compared to the DFF, the SRC will have significantly better stability properties when implemented on multi-d.o.f master-slave setups. But, a detailed analysis of the stability properties of the SRC is not straightforward due to the presence of the Extended Kalman Filter. Thanks to the introduction of a stiffness-depending damping term (see 12), the SRC implemented on the setup described in this chapter is stable for environment stiffnesses up to

8000 N/m. However, for real hard contacts, stability cannot be guaranteed for the SRC. Some time-domain stabilization approaches could be added to the SRC to maintain stability, also when contacting such real hard objects (Franken et al., 2009; Hannaford & Ryu, 2001; Ryu et al., 2007; Willaert et al., 2008a).

Next, some other points of attention related to the SRC are discussed. Firstly, the master described in this chapter is of the impedance type and the desired force f_{des} is sent in open loop. As a consequence the operator always feels the full dynamics (damping/friction and mass) of the master. As damping/friction can deteriorate the haptic feedback, it should be restricted. This can be done through mechanical design or by using friction compensation techniques (Tjahjowidodo et al., 2007). Here, the friction level of the master of the experimental setup is $\pm 0,5\ N$. Although the friction is clearly visible on the figures, this is only hardly perceived by the operator.

Secondly, with the SRC, the interaction force at the master side F_h is typically larger than the interaction force at the slave side F_e. This is a consequence of the position tracking error. The larger the proportional gain K_p can be, the smaller the difference between F_h and F_e. For an infinitely stiff position controller, the transparency will be similar for both the SRC and the DFF, in case no low-pass filter or time-delay is introduced. The fact that the interaction force F_h is larger than the interaction force F_e should not be too problematic since in surgery, especially during palpation, the perception of the absolute force is less important than the perception of stiffness. Moreover, a larger F_h is in a sense safer as the environment will be subjected to lower forces than the ones applied by the operator.

8. Conclusions

The development of a telesurgical system providing reliable force feedback forms a real challenge. First, such a development requires the design of an appropriate master and slave, applicable in the surgical theatre, and the development of robust force measurement systems. Second, a reliable controller, providing a transparent and guaranteed stable system is required. The latter is addressed in this chapter.

Based on the idea that the perception of stiffness of tissues plays an essential role in the decision making process during surgery, this chapter explains the concepts of stiffness transparency and enhanced stiffness sensitivity. A practical implementation of a model-based haptic feedback approach is presented and discussed, referred to as the (generalized) Stiffness Reflecting Controller (SRC). The SRC employs a spring with variable stiffness and rest position as model for the environment. It was shown, that such a model-based haptic feedback has good robustness properties with respect to time-delay. However, the robustness of this approach is not restricted to time-delay. The experiments presented in this chapter demonstrate that the SRC is also very suitable to realize good stiffness transparency for both linear and nonlinear environments, even when the slave shows limited responsiveness in terms of position tracking. This limited responsiveness can originate from either the hardware of the slave (e.g. a large inertia), the control of the slave (e.g. restricted gains) or a low-pass filter in the control channel (e.g. to avoid the transmission of surgical tremor). A topic to address in the future, is how model-based haptic feedback can be employed to increase the robustness with respect to flexibilities of current surgical slave robots.

Next to the increased robustness, the approach of model-based haptic feedback offers the possibility to *shape* the environment stiffness before it is reflected to the human operator. Human stiffness perception is limited by both absolute and differential thresholds. Enhanced stiffness sensitivity allows to overcome the differential threshold through master-slave control in order to increase the stiffness discrimination ability of the human operator. This chapter describes a practical implementation of the generalized version of the Stiffness Reflecting Controller realizing enhanced stiffness transparency. The psychophysical experiments with this controller demonstrate the feasibility of enhanced stiffness sensitivity for linear environments. Further investigations are necessary to determine how to enhance sensitivity when contacting objects with nonlinear stiffness properties.

Acknowledgement

This work was supported by a PhD grant from the Institute for the Promotion of Innovation through Science and Technology in Flanders (I.W.T.-Vlaanderen), one I.W.T project (IWT/OZM/080086) and by the K.U.Leuven BOF-IDO/05/008 project as well as by an FP7-People Marie Curie Reintegration Grant, PIRG03-2008-231045.

9. References

Bankman, I., Gruhen, K., Halperin, H., Popel, A., Guerci, A. & Tsitlik, J. (1990). Identification of dynamic mechanical properties of the human chest during manual cardiopulmonary resuscitation, *IEEE Transactions on Biomedical Engineering* **37**(2): 211–217.

Bethea, B., Okamura, A., Kitagawa, M., Fitton, T., Cattaneo, S., Gott, V., Baumgartner, W. & Yuh, D. (2004). Application to haptic feedback to robotic surgery, *J Laparoendosc Adv Surg Tech A.* **14**: 191–195.

Cavusoglu, M., Sherman, A. & Tendick, F. (2002). Bilateral controller design for telemanipulation in soft environments, *IEEE Transactions on Robotics and Automation* **18**(4): 641–647.

Christiansson, G. & van der Helm, F. (2007). The low-stiffness teleoperator slave - a trade-off between stability and performance, *Int. Journal of Robotics Research* **26**(3): 287–299.

Colgate, J. E. (1993). Robust impedance shaping telemanipulation, *IEEE Transactions on robotics and automation* **9**(4): 374–384.

Corcione, F., Esposito, C., Cuccurullo, D., Settembre, A., Miranda, N., Amato, F., Pirozzi, F. & Caiazzo, P. (2005). Advantages and limits of robot-assisted laparoscopic surgery, *Surgical Endoscopy* **19**: 117–119.

C.R.Doarn, K.Hufford, Rosen, T. L. J. & B.Hannaford (2007). Telesurgery and robotics: A roundtable discussion., *Telemed J E Health* **13**(4): 369–380.

De Gersem, G., Van Brussel, H. & Tendick, F. (2005a). Reliable and enhanced stiffness perception in soft-tissue telemanipulation, *The international Journal of Robotics Research* **24**(10): 805–822.

De Gersem, G., Van Brussel, H. & Vander Sloten, J. (2005b). Enhanced haptic sensitivity for soft tissues using teleoperation with shaped impedance reflection, *Proceedings of the World Haptics Conference*, Pisa, Italy.

De Gersem, G. (2005). *Kinaesthetic feedback and enhanced sensitivity in robotic endoscopic telesurgery*, PhD thesis, Katholieke Universiteit Leuven.

De, S., Rosen, J., Dagan, A., Hannaford, B., Swanson, P. & Sinanan, M. (2007). Assessment of tissue damage due to mechanical stresses, *The Int. Journal of Robotics Research* **26**(11-12): 1159–1171.

De Schutter, J., Greeter, J. D., Lefebvre, T. & Bruyninckx, H. (1999). Kalman filters: a tutorial, *Journal E* **40**(40): 52–59.

Deml, B., Ortmaier, T. & Seibold, U. (2005). The touch and feel in minimally invasive surgery, *Proceedings of International Workshop on Haptic Audio Visual Environments and their Applications*, Ontario, Canada, pp. 33–38.

Famaey, N., Verbeken, E., Vinckier, S., Willaert, B., Herijgers, P. & Vander Sloten, J. (2009). In vivo soft tissue damage assessment for applications in surgery. Submitted to Medical Engineering and Physics.

Fite, K., Speich, J. & Goldfarb, M. (2001). Transparency and stability robustness in two-channel bilateral telemanipulation, *Journal of Dynamic Systems, Measurement, and Control* **123**: 400–407.

Franken, M., Stramigioli, S., Reilink, R., Secchi, C. & Macchelli, A. (2009). Bridging the gap between passivity and transparency, *Proceedings of Robotics: Science and Systems*, Seattle, USA.

Funda, J. & Paul, R. (1991). Efficient control of a robotic system for time-delayed environments, *Fifth International Conference on Advanced Robotics (ICAR)*, Pisa, Italy, pp. 219–224.

Grande-Allen, K. J., Cochran, R. P., Reinhall, P. G. & Kunzelman, K. S. (2001). Finite-element analysis of aortic valve-sparing: influence of graft shape and stiffness., *IEEE Trans Biomed Eng* **48**(6): 647–659.

Handlykken, M. & Turner, T. (1980). Control system analysis and synthesis for a six degree-of-freedom universal force-reflecting hand controller, *Proceedings of the IEEE Conference on Decision and Control*, pp. 1197–1205.

Hannaford, B. (1989). A design framework for teleoperators with kinesthetic feedback, *IEEE Transactions on Robotics and Automation* **5**(4): 426–434.

Hannaford, B. & Ryu, J. (2001). Time domain passivity control of haptic interfaces, *Proceedings of the IEEE International Conference on Robotics and Automation*, Seoul, Korea, pp. 1863–1869.

Hashtrudi-Zaad, K. & Salcudean, S. (1996). Adaptive transparent impedance reflecting teleoperation, *Proceedings of The IEEE International Conference on Robotics and Automation*, Minneapolis, Minnesota, pp. 1369–1374.

Hockstein, N., Gourin, C., Faust, R. & Terris, D. (2007). A history of robots: from science fiction to surgical robotics, *Journal of Robotic Surgery* **1**: 113–118.

Ji, H., Song, A., Liu, W. & Li, J. (2005). Dynamic vr modeling for force-reflecting teleoperation with time delay, *Proceedings of the IEEE International Conference on Information Acquisition*, Hong Kong, China, pp. 32–36.

Kalman, R. (1960). A new approach to linear filtering and prediciton problems, *Journal of Basic Engineering* pp. 35–45.

Kuan, C.-P. & Young, K.-Y. (2003). Challenges in vr-based robot teleoperation, *Proceedings of the IEEE International Conference on Robotics and Automation*, Taipei, Taiwan, pp. 4392–4397.

Lawrence, D. (1993). Stability and transparency in bilateral teleoperation, *IEEE transactions on robotics and automation* **9**(5): 624–637.

Love, L. & Book, W. J. (2004). Force reflecting teleoperation with adaptive impedance control, *IEEE Transactions on Systems, Man and Cybernetics - Part B: Cybernetics* **34**(1): 159–165.

Lum, M. J., Rosen, J., Lendvay, T. S., Sinanan, M. N. & Hannaford, B. (2009). Effect of time delay on telesurgical performance, *Proceedings of the International Conference on Robotics and Automation*, Kobe, Japan.

Mahvash, M. & Okamura, A. (2007). Friction compensation for enhancing transparency of a teleoperator with compliant transmission, *IEEE Transactions on Robotics* **23**: 1240–1246.

Malysz, P. & Siroupour, S. (2007). Stable non-linear force/position mapping for enhanced telemanipulation of soft environments, *Proceedings of the International Conference on Robotics and Automation*, Roma, Italy, pp. 4307–4312.

Marescaux, J., Leroy, J., Gagner, M., Rubino, F., Mutter, D., Vix, M., Butner, S. E. & Smith, M. K. (2001). Transatlantic robot-assisted telesurgery, *Nature* **413**: 379–380.

Misra, S. & Okamura, A. (2006). Environment parameter estimation during bilateral telemanipulation, *Proceedings of Symposium on Haptic Interfaces for Virtual Environment and Teleoperator Systems*, Virginia, USA, pp. 301–307.

Mitra, P. & Niemeyer, G. (2008). Model-mediated telemanipulation, *Int. Journal of Robotics Research* **27**(2): 253–262.

Nguan, C., Girvan, A. & Luke, P. (2008). Robotic surgery versus laparoscopy; a comparison between two robotic systems and laparoscopy, *Journal of Robotic Surgery* **1**: 263–268.

Okamura, A. (2004). Methods for haptic feedback in teleoperated robot-assisted surgery, *Industrial Robot: An international Journal* **31**(6): 499–508.

Ota, D. (1995). Laparoscopic colectomy for cancer: a favorable opinion, *Ann. Surgical Oncology* **2**: 3–5.

Peirs, J., Clijnen, J., Reynaerts, D., Brussel, H. V., Herijgers, P., Corteville, B. & Boone, S. (2004). A micro-optical force sensor for force feedback during minimally invasive robotic surgery., *Sensor and Actuators A* **115**: 447–455.

Preusche, C., Ortmaier, T. & Hirzinger, G. (2002). Teleoperation concepts in minimal invasive surgery, *Control Engineering Practice* **10**(11): 1245–1250.

Rayman, R., Croome, K., Galbraith, N., McClure, R., Morady, R., Peterson, S., Smith, S., Subotic, V., Wynsberghe, A. V. & Primak, S. (2006). Long-distance robotic telesurgery: a feasibility study for care in remote environments, *Int J Med Robotics Comput Assist Surg* **2**: 216–224.

Rosen, J., Jeffrey, D., De, S., Sinanan, M. & Hannaford, B. (2008). Biomechanical properties of abdominal organs in vivo and postmortem under compression loads, *Journal of Biomechanical Engineering* **130**(2): 1–17.

Ryu, D., Song, J.-B., Choi, J., Kang, S. & Kim, M. (2007). Frequency domain stability observer and active damping control for stable haptic interaction, *Proceedings of the IEEE International Conference on Robotics and Automation*, Roma, Italy, pp. 105–110.

Scott, H. & Darzi, A. (1997). Tactile feedback in laparoscopic colonic surgery, *The Britisch Journal of Surgery* **84**: 1005.

Seibold, U., Kübler, B. & Hirzinger, G. (2005). Prototype of instrument for minimally invasive surgery with 6-axis force sensing capability, *Proceedings of the IEEE International Conference on Robotics and Automation*, Barcelona, Spain, pp. 496–501.

Son, H. I. & Lee, D. Y. (2008). Enhancement of kinesthetic perception for microsurgical teleoperation using impedance-shaping, *Proceedings of the 30th Annual Int. IEEE EMBS Conference*, Vancouver, B.C., Canada, pp. 1939–1942.

Tavakoli, M. & Howe, R. (2009). Haptic effect of surgical teleoperator flexibility, *Int. Journal of Robotics Research* .

Tavakoli, M., Patel, R. & Moallem, M. (2006). A haptic interface for computer-integrated endoscopic surgery and training, *Virtual Reality* **9**: 160–176.

Tholey, G., Desai, J. & Castellanos, A. (2005). Force feedback plays a significant role in minimally invasive surgery, *Annals of surgery* **241**(1): 102–109.

Tjahjowidodo, T., Al-Bender, F., Van Brussel, H. & Symens, W. (2007). Friction characterization and compensation in electro-mechanical systems, *Journal of Sound and Vibration* **308**: 632–646.

Tzafestas, C., Velanas, S. & Fakiridis, G. (2008). Adaptive impedance control in haptic teleoperation to improve transparency under time-delay, *Proceedings of the IEEE International Conference on Robotics and Automation*, Pasadena, CA, USA, pp. 212–219.

Wagner, C. R., Stylopoulos, N. & Howe, R. D. (2002). The role of force feedback in surgery: Analysis of blunt dissection, *The 10th Symp. on Haptic interfaces for virtual environment and teleoperator systems*, Orlando.

Walraevens, J., Willaert, B., De Win, G., Ranftl, A., De Schutter, J. & Vander Sloten, J. (2008). Correlation between compression, tensile and tearing tests on healthy and calcified aortic tissues, *Medical Engineering & Physics* **30**: 1098–1104.

Weber, E. H. (1834). De pulsu, resorptione, auditu et tactu, *Annotationes Anatomicae Et Physiologicae* pp. 19–135.

Willaert, B., Vander Poorten, E., Reynaerts, D. & Van Brussel, H. (2008a). A pragmatic method for stable stiffness reflection in telesurgery, *Haptics: Perception, Devices and Scenarios (6th Int. Conf, Eurohaptics)*, Madrid, Spain, pp. 73–82.

Willaert, B., Vander Poorten, E., Reynaerts, D. & Van Brussel, H. (2008b). Reliable stiffness reflection for telesurgery, *ICRA 2008 Workshop on new vistas and challenges in Telerobotics*, Pasadena, CA, USA.

Willaert, B., Reynaerts, D., Van Brussel, H. & Vander Poorten, E. (2009a). Extracorporeal force measurement system for robot-assisted mis with 3d force feedback, *ICRA 2009 Workshop on Advanced Sensing and Sensor Integration in Medical Robotics*, Kobe, Japan.

Willaert, B., Corteville, B., Reynaerts, D., Van Brussel, H. & Vander Poorten, E. (2009b). Bounded environment passivity of the classical position-force controler, *Proceedings of the IEEE International Conference on Intelligent Robots and Systems*, St. Louis, MO, USA, p. 4622 - 4628

Yokokohji, Y. & Yoshikawa, T. (1994). Bilateral control of master-slave manipulators for ideal kinesthetic coupling, *IEEE transactions on robotics and automation* **10**(5): 605–620.

Zemiti, N., Ortmaier, T., Vitrani, M. & Morel, G. (2006). *A Force Controlled Laparoscopic Surgical Robot without Distal Force Sensing*, Springer Berlin / Heidelberg, chapter V. Medical Robotics in Experimental Robotics IX, pp. 153–164.

14

Mechanism Design of Haptic Devices

Han Sung Kim[1]
Kyungnam University[1]
Republic of Korea[1]

1. Introduction

The mechanism of a haptic device should have low inertia, high stiffness, large force reflection capability, good kinematic conditioning as well as large workspace, back-drivable, low friction, and small weight.

The first step of mechanism design is to select a proper mechanism structure (or type synthesis). For required DOF, several mechanism structures including serial-, parallel-, and hybrid-kinematic manipulators can be considered through type synthesis. Based on the previous review on haptic mechanisms (Martin and Savall, 2005), most successful haptic mechanisms are parallel-type and at least hybrid-type, due to low moving inertia, large force reflection and high stiffness. One of major disadvantages of parallel-kinematic manipulators may be smaller workspace compared to serial-kinematic counterparts. Joint and actuator types are also very important in type synthesis of haptic mechanisms. Most commercial haptic mechanisms use only revolute joints and rotary actuators, since those types can provide smaller friction, better back-drivability, and larger workspace than prismatic joints and linear actuators. In addition to linkage-type haptic devices, wire actuation (Agronin, 1987) and magnetic levitation (Berkelman et al., 1996) are also developed. In order to give broad information on mechanism structures to readers, novel mechanisms employed in haptic devices are classified by DOFs presented in Table 1 and the characteristics of each mechanism is briefly explained.

The second step of mechanism design is the dimensional synthesis of a selected mechanism structure. In the design of kinematic dimensions, workspace and other kinematic performances need to be considered together. The kinematic performance measures may be the manipulability, the inverse of condition number, the minimum force output, and so forth, which can be derived from the manipulator's Jacobian matrix. In general, workspace is inversely proportional to force transmission capability, accuracy and stiffness, which are closely related to the manipulability. Therefore, compromise between workspace volume and one of the kinematic performances related to manipulability should be included in the kinematic optimization.

This chapter is organized as follows. In section 2, novel mechanism structures employed in haptic devices are explained. In section 3, the methodologies of kinematic analysis and optimization are presented. In section 4, example of kinematic analysis and design of the Delta haptic device is illustrated.

2. Mechanism Structures

In this section, a state of the art in mechanisms of haptic devices is presented from planar to spatial mechanisms. Once required degrees of freedom (DOF) of a haptic device is specified, several feasible mechanisms to satisfy specified DOF can be synthesized (Tsai, 2001; Kong & Gosselin, 2007; Gogu, 2008). The degrees of freedom, F, of a mechanism can be easily calculated by well-known Grubler's formula as (Tsai, 1999)

$$F = \lambda(n - j - 1) + \sum_{i=1}^{j} f_i \tag{1}$$

where

λ : degrees of freedom of the space

n : number of links including the fixed link

j : number of joints

f_i : degrees of relative motion by joint i.

However, degrees of freedom can be simply calculated for serial- and parallel-kinematic manipulators as follows:

$$\begin{aligned} F &= \sum_{i=1}^{j} f_i && \text{for serial manipulators} \\ F &= \lambda - \sum_{i=1}^{m} c_i && \text{for parallel manipulators} \end{aligned} \tag{2}$$

where c_i denotes the total number of independent constraints of the ith leg consisting of a parallel manipulators with m legs. Note that for serial manipulators, the first term in Eq. (1) always becomes zero. For example, 5-bar can be considered as a planar parallel manipulator with two legs, then $F = \lambda - (c_1 + c_2) = 2$ where $\lambda = 3$, $c_1 = \lambda - 3 = 0$, and $c_2 = \lambda - 2 = 1$. Another example is a spatial parallelogram with two *S-S* (spherical-spherical) chains. The parallelogram has $F = \lambda - (c_1 + c_2) = 4$, since $\lambda = 6$ and $c_i = \lambda - 5 = 1$ for $i = 1, 2$. Note that one rotational DOF along the leg is passive DOF (Tsai, 1999).

Table 1 shows mechanism structures of developed haptic devices and mechanism structures are classified by DOFs.

<table>
<tr><td rowspan="2">2-DOF</td><td colspan="2">[Spherical 5-bar]
- Spherical Remote-Center-of-Motion Manipulator for MIS (Angerilli et al., 2001)
- Immersion Impulse Engine 2000 (Rosenberg & Jackson, 2002)</td></tr>
<tr><td>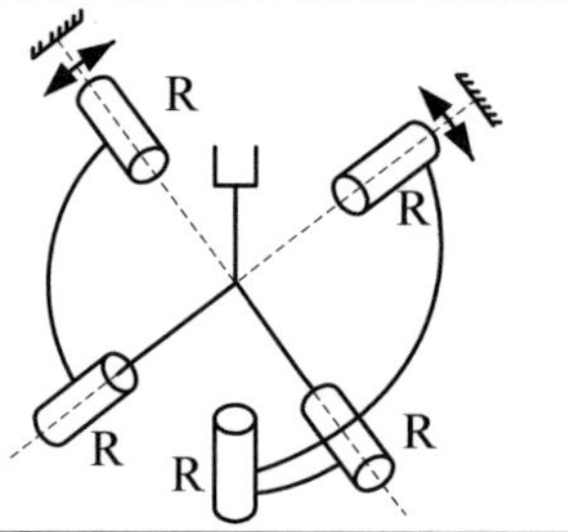
</td><td>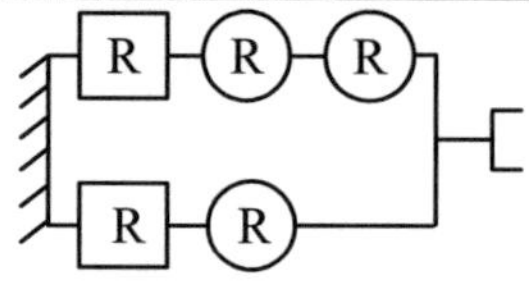

Shortly,
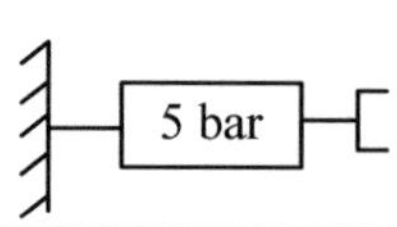
</td></tr>
</table>

2-DOF	**[Planar 5-bar]** - The Pantograph (Campion et al., 2005)	
	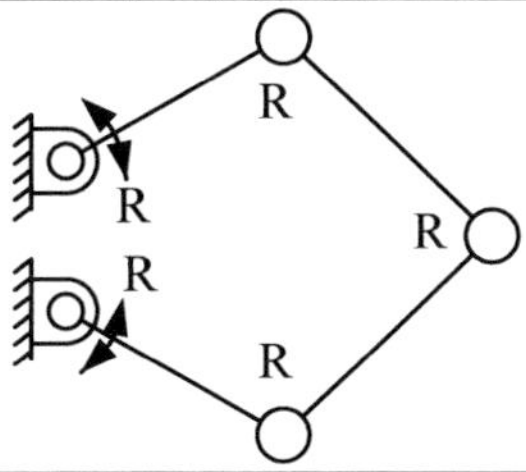	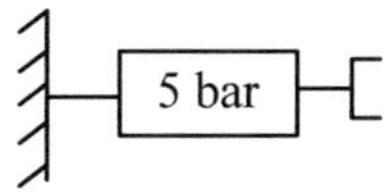
3-DOF	**[Spherical mechanism]** - SHaDe (Birglen et al., 2002)	
	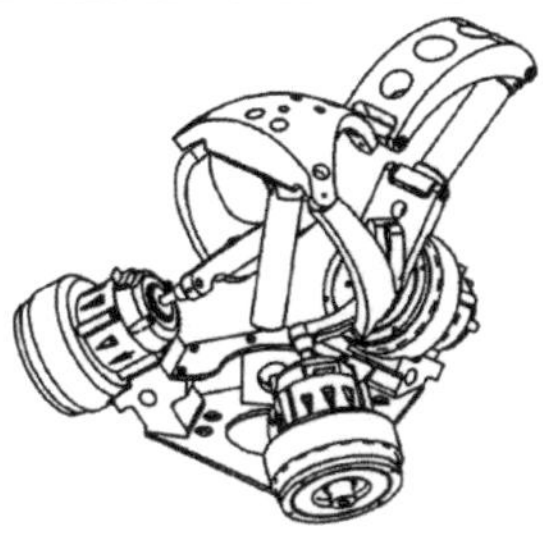	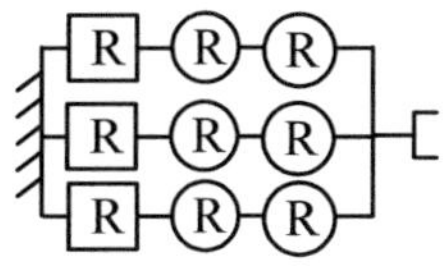
3-DOF	**[Two Planar 5-bars]** - 3-DOF Planar Pantograph Interface (Sirouspour et al., 2000)	
	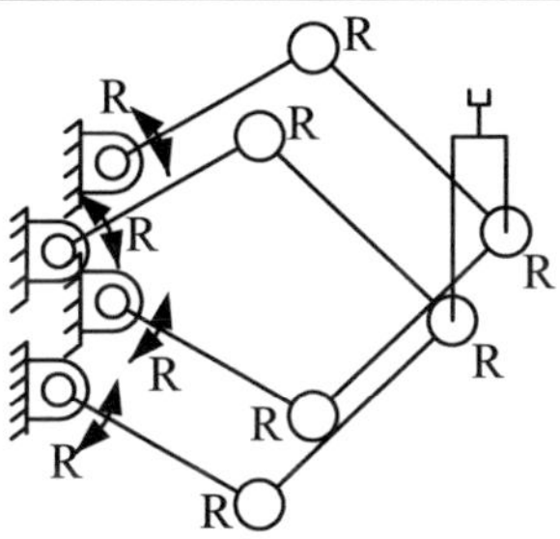	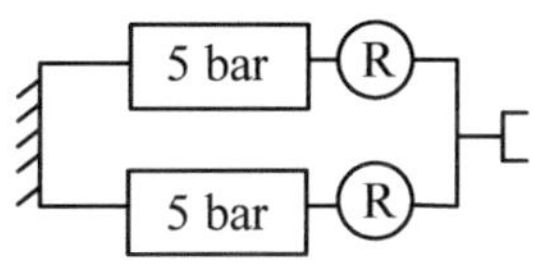
3-DOF	**[Spatial Parallelograms]** - Delta Haptic Device (Grange et al., 2001, http://www.forcedimension.com)	
	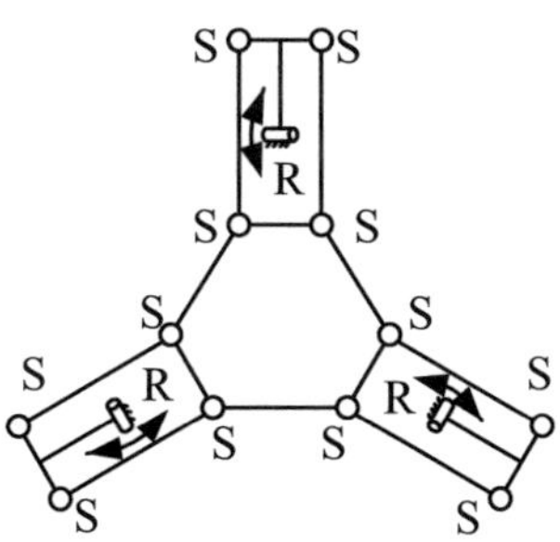	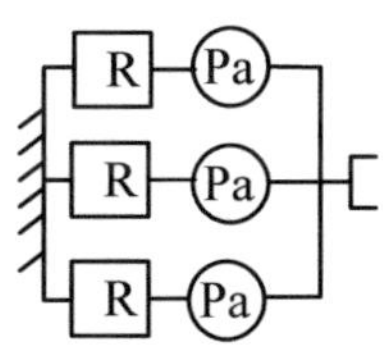 where, 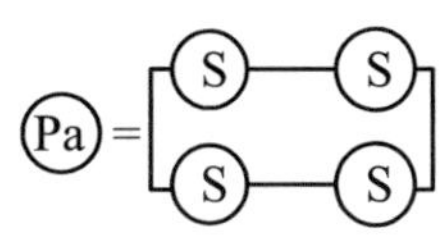

<table>
<tr><td rowspan="2">3-
DOF</td><td colspan="2">[Wrist Mechanism for the Delta Haptic device]
- Connecting the wrist on the Delta haptic device for 6-DOF motion.
- Instead of the linkages of S-P-S chains, wires are used.</td></tr>
<tr><td>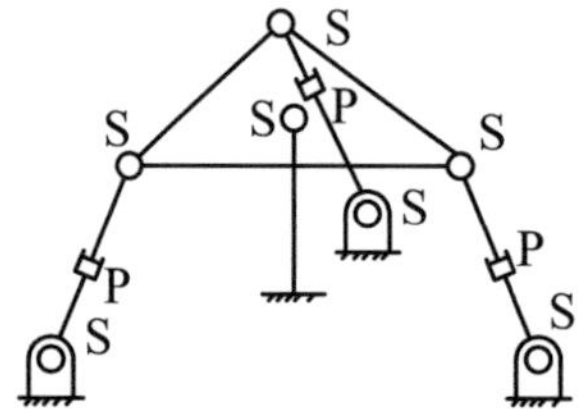
</td><td>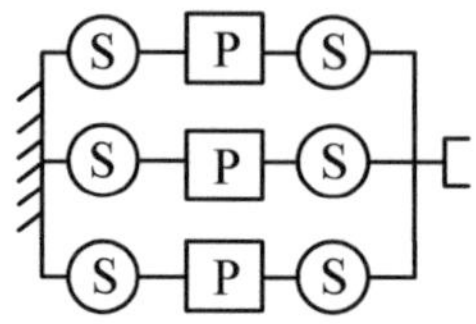
</td></tr>
<tr><td rowspan="2">3-
DOF</td><td colspan="2">[Hybrid Manipulator]
- PHANTOM Desktop/Omni (Cavusolgu et al., 2002; http://www.sensable.com)</td></tr>
<tr><td>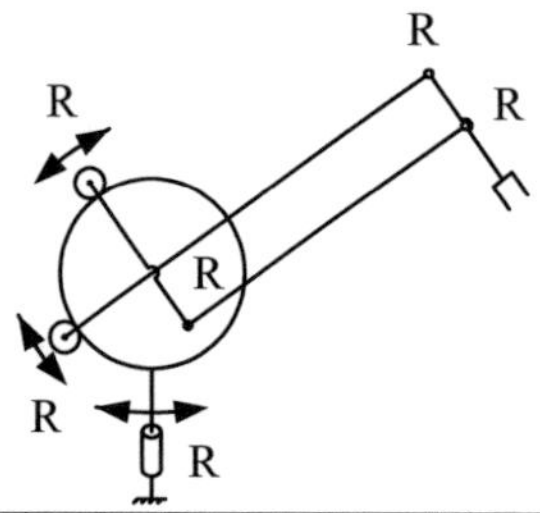
</td><td>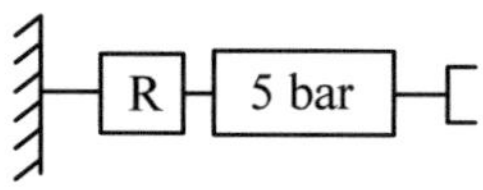
</td></tr>
<tr><td rowspan="2">5,6-
DOF</td><td colspan="2">[Two PHANTOMs Configuration]
- Connecting two PHANTOM devices by a 5- or 6-DOF serial Chain
(Wang, 2001; Iwata, 1993)</td></tr>
<tr><td>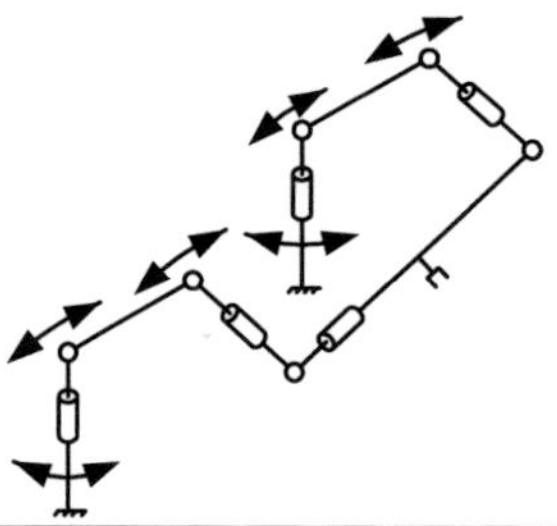</td><td>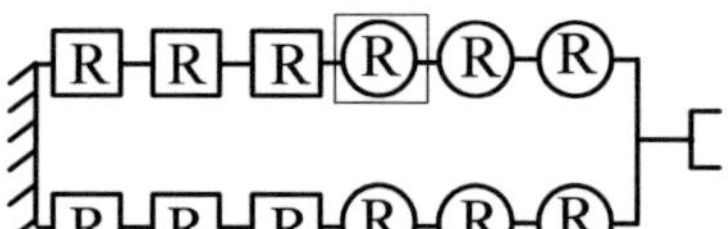

where, (R) may be actuated for 6-DOF</td></tr>
<tr><td rowspan="2">5,6-
DOF</td><td colspan="2">[Twin Pantographs]
- 5-DOF Haptic Wand (Stocco, 2001, http://www.quanser.com)</td></tr>
<tr><td>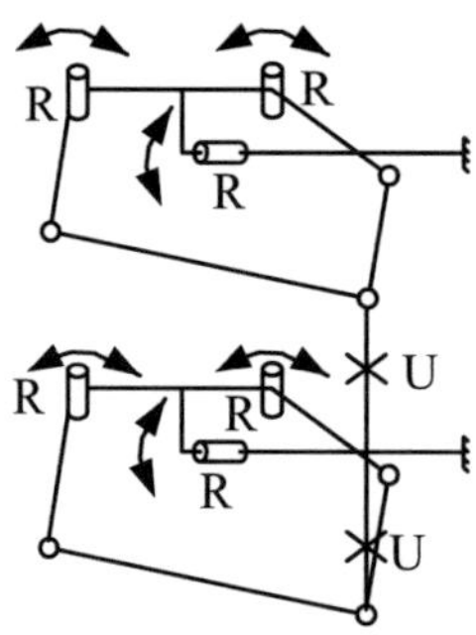
</td><td>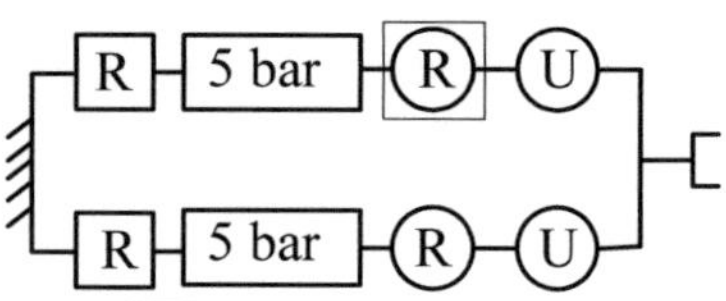

where, (R) may be actuated for 6-DOF</td></tr>
</table>

6-DOF	**[Serial Manipulator]** - PHANTOM Premium 1.5/6DOF (Chen, 1999; Cohen & Chen, 1999) - Actually, it is a hybrid-kinematic manipulator.	
	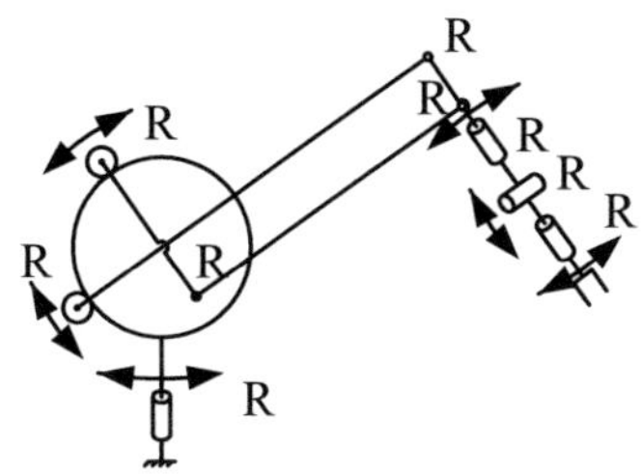	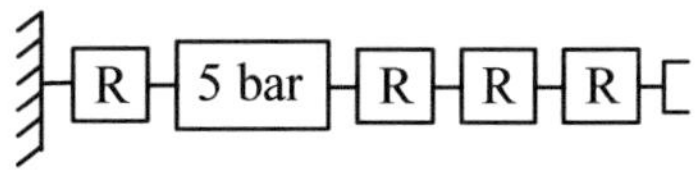
6-DOF	**[Hybrid Manipulator]** - Compact 6-DOF Haptic Interface (Tsumaki et al., 1998; Yoon, 2003)	
	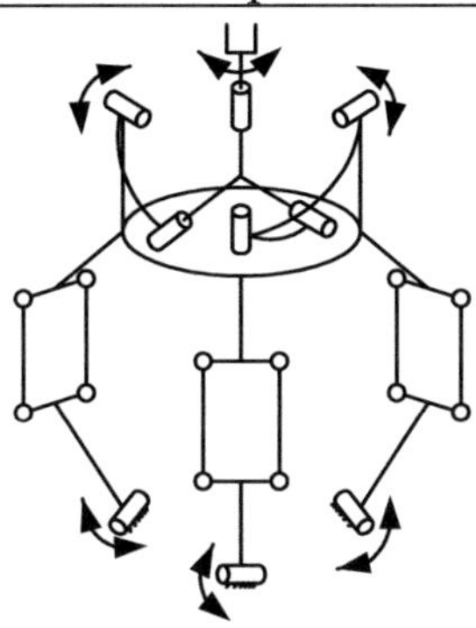	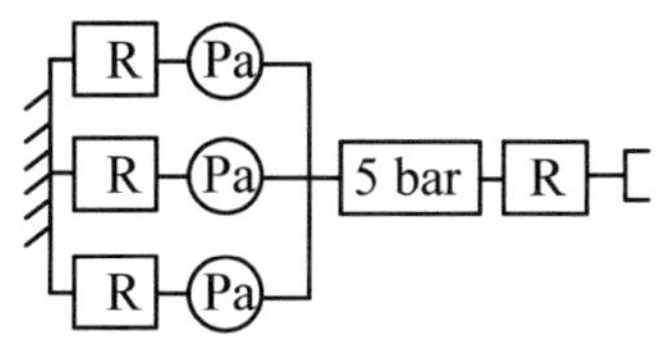
6-DOF	**[Three Pantographs]** (Long & Collins, 1992)	
	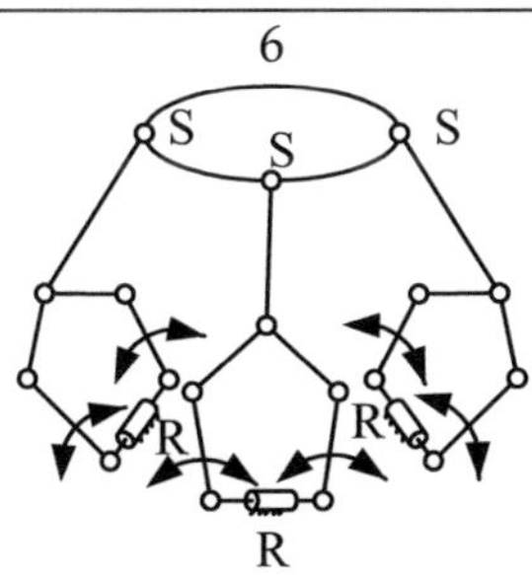	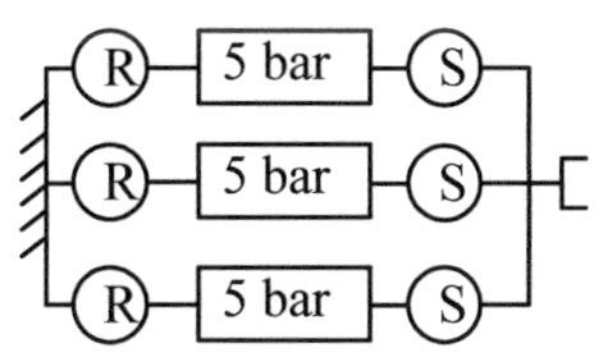
6~10 DOF	**[Serial Manipulators]** - ViSHaRD6 (Ueberle & Buss, 2002) - ViSHaRD10 (Ueberle et al, 2004) - Freedom6s (http://www.mpb-technologies.ca) - Freedom-7 (Hayward, 1995; Hayward et al., 1997)	

Table 1. Mechanism structures of currently developed haptic devices

3. Kinematic analysis and optimization

The overall process of haptic rendering is shown in Figure 1. First, according to operator's movement, the controller of a haptic device system measures joint displacements and calculates the tip (or end-effector of a haptic device) position and velocity by forward kinematics and velocity relation, respectively. Then, the position and velocity commands are sent to virtual environments or real tele-operated robots and the contact force between tool and environment is calculated or measured. Finally, the required actuation force to realize the contact force is calculated through the statics relation of a haptic device. Note that scaling or mapping between the measured and commanded positions/forces may be required.

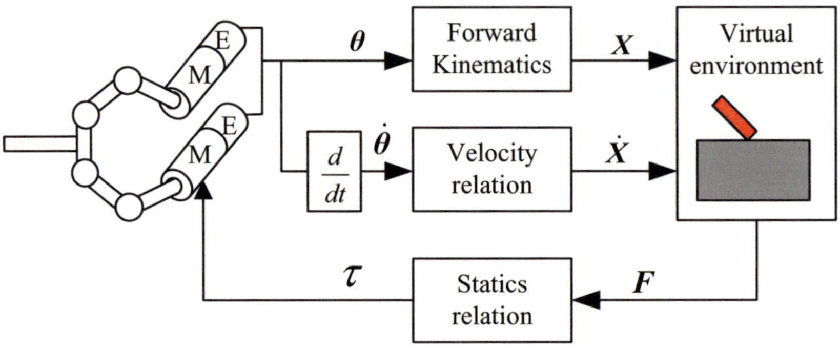

Fig. 1. Schematic diagram of haptic rendering cycle

3.1 Kinematic analysis

In this subsection, brief explanation of the kinematic analysis will be given. For the haptic rendering cycle, the analyses of forward/inverse kinematics and velocity/statics relations are required. The analysis of inverse kinematics is not directly used in the cycle; however it is required in the calculation of the Jacobian matrix especially for parallel manipulators.

In general, the forward kinematics of an n-DOF serial manipulator can be calculated by multiplying the Denavit-Hartenberg homogeneous transformation matrices, ${}^{i-1}T_i(\theta_i)$, from the base coordinate system to the end-effector coordinate system in series.

$$ {}^0T_n = {}^0T_1(\theta_1)\,{}^1T_2(\theta_2)\cdots{}^{n-1}T_n(\theta_n) \tag{3} $$

The velocity and statics relations of an n-DOF serial manipulator are given by

$$ \dot{\boldsymbol{X}} = J\dot{\boldsymbol{\theta}} \text{ and } \boldsymbol{\tau} = J^T\boldsymbol{F} \tag{4} $$

where $\dot{\boldsymbol{X}} = [\boldsymbol{v}^T, \boldsymbol{\omega}^T]^T$ when $\boldsymbol{v}$ and $\boldsymbol{\omega}$ denote the linear and angular velocity vectors and $\boldsymbol{F} = [\boldsymbol{f}^T, \boldsymbol{m}^T]^T$ when $\boldsymbol{f}$ and $\boldsymbol{m}$ are the force and moment vectors. The column vectors of Jacobian matrix consist of the joint screws expressed in the axis coordinates (Duffy, 1996).

$$J = \begin{bmatrix} \boldsymbol{r}_1 \times \boldsymbol{s}_1 & \cdots & \boldsymbol{r}_n \times \boldsymbol{s}_n \\ \boldsymbol{s}_1 & \cdots & \boldsymbol{s}_n \end{bmatrix} \tag{5}$$

where $\boldsymbol{s}_i$ denotes the unit direction vector of the ith joint axis and $\boldsymbol{r}_i$ is the position vector from the end-effector to the ith joint axis.

On the other hands, the forward kinematics of an n-DOF parallel manipulator is not straightforward and has multiple solutions in general. However, the inverse kinematics is much simpler and can be analyzed by using vector-loop equations. The velocity and statics relations of an n-DOF parallel manipulator are given by

$$\dot{\boldsymbol{\theta}} = J^T \dot{\boldsymbol{X}} \text{ and } \boldsymbol{F} = J\boldsymbol{\tau} \tag{6}$$

where $J = J_x J_\theta^{-1}$. Here, J_θ is the diagonal matrix and becomes an $n \times n$ identity matrix if actuators are linear. The column vectors of J_x consist of the joint screws expressed in the ray coordinates (Duffy, 1996).

$$J_x = \begin{bmatrix} \boldsymbol{s}_1 & \cdots & \boldsymbol{s}_n \\ \boldsymbol{r}_1 \times \boldsymbol{s}_1 & \cdots & \boldsymbol{r}_n \times \boldsymbol{s}_n \end{bmatrix} \tag{7}$$

3.2 Kinematic optimization

In the preliminary design of a haptic device, large workspace volume, high force transmission capability, high accuracy and high stiffness are essential considerations. In general, the workspace is inversely proportional to force transmission capability, accuracy and stiffness, which are closely related to the manipulability. Therefore, compromise between workspace volume and one of the performances related to manipulability are required in the kinematic optimization.

First, the closed form solution for workspace cannot be obtained for most spatial manipulators. Usually, workspace is calculated numerically by using the inverse kinematics considering actuator strokes and joint limits.

Some kinematic performance measures such as manipulability, force/velocity transmission capability, accuracy and stiffness can be derived from the manipulator's Jacobian matrix. Some of well-known kinematic performance measures are

- manipulability: the product of the singular values of the Jacobian matrix (Yoshikawa, 1985)
- mechanism isotropy: the inverse of the condition number of the Jacobian matrix or the ratio of the smallest to the largest singular value of the Jacobian matrix (Salisbury & Craig, 1982)
- minimum force (or velocity) output: the smallest singular value or the force (or velocity) output in the worst direction (Kim & Choi, 2001).

One of the measures can be used as LDI (Local Design Index), which means the kinematic performance at one configuration in workspace. The average value of LDI over whole workspace can be obtained by (Gosselin and Angeles, 1989; Kim and Tsai, 2003)

$$\mathrm{GDI}(\boldsymbol{\beta}) = \frac{1}{W} \int_W \mathrm{LDI}(\boldsymbol{\beta})\, dW \tag{8}$$

where W and dW denote the total workspace volume and a differential workspace, respectively, and $\boldsymbol{\beta}$ denotes design variables or kinematic dimensions. The sum of LDI over workspace can be normalized by the workspace size, which yields a kinematic performance measure independent of different workspace volume of design candidates. Therefore, it is usually called GDI (Global Design Index). However, maximizing the GDI alone usually leads to very small workspace, while maximizing workspace generates poor kinematic performances. Hence, the optimal design problem may be formulated as

$$\begin{aligned} &\text{Maxmimize: } \mathrm{GDI}(\boldsymbol{\beta}) \\ &\text{Subject to } \ : W \geq W_{\min} \end{aligned} \tag{9}$$

where $W_{\min}$ denotes the minimum required workspace volume. The physical meaning is to maximize the average value of a selected kinematic performance measure over whole workspace while guaranteeing the minimum required workspace volume.

4. Example of the kinematic optimization of a Delta haptic device

In this section, the kinematic analysis and optimization methods for a haptic device are illustrated with the Delta haptic device. As explained in section 2, the Delta mechanism consists of three *R-Pa* (Revolute-spatial Parallelogram) legs. Since each leg has one rotational constraint (or rotation about the normal vector of the plane made by each parallelogram), the combined effects result in three constraints of the rotation of the moving platform. Therefore, the moving platform has three translational degrees of freedom.

As shown in Figure 2, fixed reference frame (x, y, z) is attached to the center O of the fixed base. Local fixed frame (x_i, y_i, z_i) is attached to the fixed base at point A_i. The moving frame (u, v, w) is also attached the center P of the moving platform. The angle, ϕ_i, is defined as the angle from the x-axis to the x_i-axis. In Figure 3, the joint angles, $\theta_{1i}, \theta_{2i}, \theta_{3i}$ for the ith leg are defined. A vector-loop equation can be written for each leg:

$$\overline{A_i M_i} + \overline{M_i B_i} = \overline{OP} + \overline{PB_i} - \overline{OA_i} \quad \text{or} \quad l_{1i}\boldsymbol{u}_{1i} + l_{2i}\boldsymbol{u}_{2i} = \boldsymbol{p} + \boldsymbol{b} - \boldsymbol{a}\,. \tag{10}$$

The vector-loop equation can be expressed in local frame (x_i, y_i, z_i) as

$$\begin{bmatrix} l_{1i}c\theta_{1i} + l_{2i}s\theta_{3i}c(\theta_{1i} + \theta_{2i}) \\ l_{2i}c\theta_{3i} \\ l_{1i}s\theta_{1i} + l_{2i}s\theta_{3i}s(\theta_{1i} + \theta_{2i}) \end{bmatrix} = \begin{bmatrix} b_{xi} \\ b_{yi} \\ b_{zi} \end{bmatrix} \tag{11}$$

where

$$\begin{bmatrix} b_{xi} \\ b_{yi} \\ b_{zi} \end{bmatrix} = \begin{bmatrix} c\phi_i & s\phi_i & 0 \\ -s\phi_i & c\phi_i & 0 \\ 0 & 0 & 1 \end{bmatrix} \begin{bmatrix} p_x \\ p_y \\ p_z \end{bmatrix} + \begin{bmatrix} b-a \\ 0 \\ 0 \end{bmatrix} \tag{12}$$

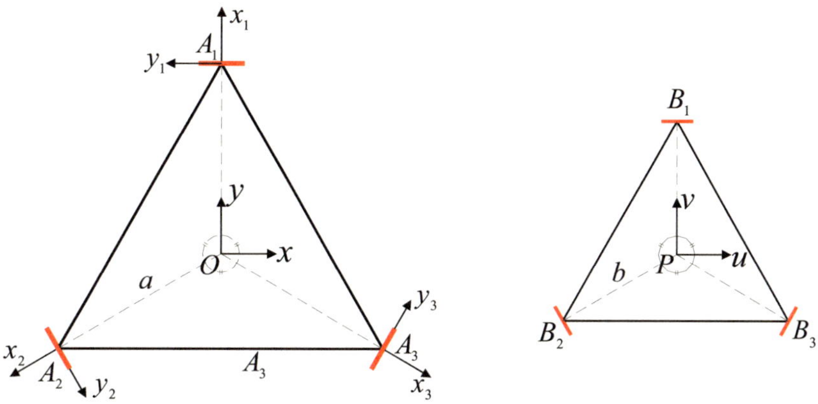

(a) Fixed base (b) Moving platform

Fig. 2. Top views of the Delta manipulator

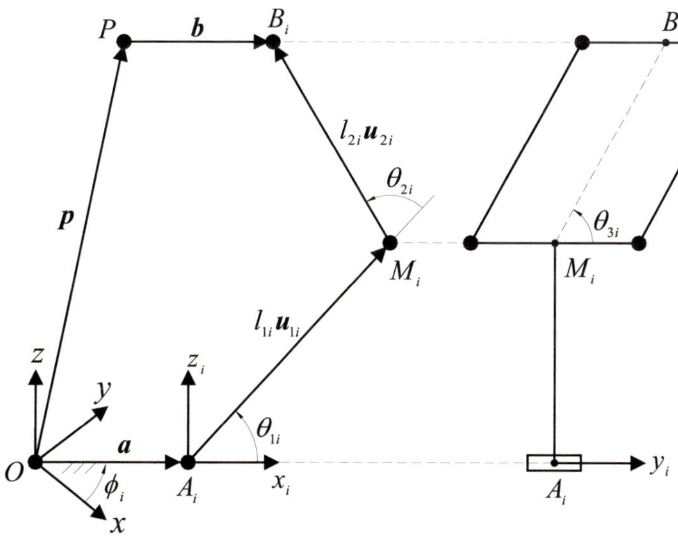

Fig. 3. Vector-loop diagram of the ith leg

The problem of inverse kinematics is to find the actuated joint angle, $\theta_{11}, \theta_{21}, \theta_{31}$ for given the position vector, $\boldsymbol{p}$, of the moving platform. From the second element of Eq. (11), θ_{3i} is obtained by

$$\theta_{3i} = \cos^{-1}\frac{b_{yi}}{l_{2i}}. \tag{13}$$

Summing the squares of b_{xi}, b_{yi}, and b_{zi} in Eq. (11) and solving for θ_{2i} yields

$$\theta_{2i} = \cos^{-1}\kappa \tag{14}$$

where $\kappa = (b_{xi}^2 + b_{yi}^2 + b_{zi}^2 - l_{1i}^2 - l_{2i}^2)/(2l_{1i}l_{2i}s\theta_{3i})$. Note that θ_{3i} and θ_{2i} has two solutions, respectively, however only positive values are selected. Once θ_{3i} and θ_{2i} are determined, θ_{1i} can be obtained from Eq. (11) by

$$\theta_{1i} = \text{Atan2}(-g_{2i}b_{xi} + g_{1i}b_{zi},\ g_{1i}b_{xi} + g_{2i}b_{zi}) \tag{15}$$

where $g_{1i} \equiv l_{1i} + l_{2i}c\theta_{2i}s\theta_{3i}$ and $g_{2i} \equiv l_{2,i}s\theta_{2i}s\theta_{3i}$.
The forward kinematics problem is to find the position vector, $\boldsymbol{p}$, of the moving platform for given the actuated joint angle, $\theta_{11}, \theta_{21}, \theta_{31}$. Geometrically, the point, *P*, is calculated as the intersection point of three spheres centered at M_i', which is located at a distance b from M_i in the direction of $\overline{B_iP}$. The detailed derivation can be referred to that of the Maryland Manipulator (Tsai, 1999).
The Jacobian matrix can be derived by differentiating Eq. (10) as

$$\boldsymbol{v}_p = l_{1i}(\boldsymbol{\omega}_{1i} \times \boldsymbol{u}_{1i}) + l_{2i}(\boldsymbol{\omega}_{2i} \times \boldsymbol{u}_{2i}) \tag{16}$$

where $\boldsymbol{v}_p$ is the linear velocity of the moving platform and $\boldsymbol{\omega}_{ji}$ is the angular velocity of the *j*th link of the *i*th leg. To eliminate the passive joint rate, dot-multiplying both sides of Eq. (16) by $\boldsymbol{u}_{2i}$ yields

$$\boldsymbol{u}_{2i} \cdot \boldsymbol{v}_p = l_{1i}\boldsymbol{\omega}_{1i} \cdot (\boldsymbol{u}_{1i} \times \boldsymbol{u}_{2i}) \tag{17}$$

Expressing the vectors in Eq. (17) in the local frame (x_i, y_i, z_i) gives

$$ {}^{i}\boldsymbol{\omega}_{1i} = \begin{bmatrix} 0 \\ -\dot{\theta}_{1i} \\ 0 \end{bmatrix}, \quad {}^{i}\boldsymbol{u}_{1i} = \begin{bmatrix} c\theta_{1i} \\ 0 \\ s\theta_{1i} \end{bmatrix}, \quad {}^{i}\boldsymbol{u}_{2i} = \begin{bmatrix} s\theta_{3i}c(\theta_{1i}+\theta_{2i}) \\ c\theta_{3i} \\ s\theta_{3i}s(\theta_{1i}+\theta_{2i}) \end{bmatrix}, \quad {}^{i}\boldsymbol{v}_{p} = \begin{bmatrix} v_{px}c\phi_i + v_{py}s\phi_i \\ -v_{px}s\phi_i + v_{py}c\phi_i \\ v_{pz} \end{bmatrix} \tag{18} $$

Substituting Eq. (18) into Eq. (17) and applying the result for i=1, 2, and 3, the velocity relation can be derived by

$$ J_x^T \boldsymbol{v}_p = J_q \dot{\boldsymbol{\theta}} \quad \text{or} \quad \dot{\boldsymbol{\theta}} = J^T \boldsymbol{v}_p \tag{19} $$

where $J = J_x J_\theta^{-1}$,

$$ J_x = \begin{bmatrix} j_{1x} & j_{2x} & j_{3x} \\ j_{1y} & j_{2y} & j_{3y} \\ j_{1z} & j_{2z} & j_{3z} \end{bmatrix}, \text{ and } J_q = \begin{bmatrix} l_{11}s\theta_{21}s\theta_{31} & 0 & 0 \\ 0 & l_{12}s\theta_{22}s\theta_{32} & 0 \\ 0 & 0 & l_{13}s\theta_{23}s\theta_{33} \end{bmatrix} \tag{20} $$

where

$$ \begin{aligned} j_{ix} &= c(\theta_{1i}+\theta_{2i})s\theta_{3i}c\phi_i - c\theta_{3i}s\phi_i \\ j_{iy} &= c(\theta_{1i}+\theta_{2i})s\theta_{3i}s\phi_i + c\theta_{3i}c\phi_i \\ j_{iz} &= s(\theta_{1i}+\theta_{2i})s\theta_{3i} \end{aligned} \tag{21} $$

The design variables of the Delta manipulator can be radii of the fixed base and the moving platform, (a,b), and lengths of lower and upper legs, (l_{1i},l_{2i}). For symmetrical design, all the legs are set to be identical, i.e., $l_j = l_{ji}$ for $i = 1,2,3$. Therefore, the design variables become

$$ \boldsymbol{\beta} = [a,b,l_1,l_2] \tag{22} $$

Furthermore, the design variables may be normalized by a characteristic length, a, as

$$ \tilde{\boldsymbol{\beta}} = [\frac{b}{a},\frac{l_1}{a},\frac{l_2}{a}] \tag{23} $$

In this optimal design problem, the minimum force output is selected as a LDI. The physical meaning of the index corresponds to the maximum magnitude of the force vector which can be generated in all directions at the end-effector for given unit magnitude of actuator forces (Kim and Choi, 2001). The problem of determining the extreme magnitudes of the force vector at the end-effector when the magnitude of actuator forces is constrained can be formulated as follow:

$$\begin{aligned} &\text{Maximize}: \|\boldsymbol{F}\|^2 = \boldsymbol{F}^T\boldsymbol{F} \\ &\text{Subject to}: \|\boldsymbol{\tau}\|^2 = \boldsymbol{F}^T(JJ^T)^{-1}\boldsymbol{F} = 1 \end{aligned} \tag{24}$$

Applying the Lagrange multipliers yields the following eigenvalue problem:

$$(JJ^T)\boldsymbol{F} = \alpha_f^2\boldsymbol{F} \tag{25}$$

The minimum force output for given unit magnitude of actuator forces can be obtained as the square root of the minimum eigenvalue of JJ^T. Hence, the optimal design problem is formulated as

$$\begin{aligned} &\text{Maxmimize}: \ \text{GDI}(\tilde{\boldsymbol{\beta}}) = \frac{1}{W}\int_W \text{LDI}(\tilde{\boldsymbol{\beta}})\, dW \\ &\text{Subject to} \quad : W \geq W_{\min} \end{aligned} \tag{26}$$

In this numerical example, the ranges of the normalized design variables and the minimum workspace volume are set to

$$0.1 \leq \frac{b}{a} \leq 1.0,\ 0.5 \leq \frac{l_1}{a} \leq 2.5,\ 0.5 \leq \frac{l_2}{a} \leq 2.5, \text{and } W_{\min} = 0.008\,m^3$$

where $a = 100\,mm$.

Figure 4 shows the workspace volume and LDI with respect to l_1 and l_2 when $b = 20\,mm$. As expected, the workspace volume is increasing as l_1 and l_2 are larger, however the LDI is larger when l_1 is smaller, because actuated force at M_i is larger when l_1 is smaller. Genetic algorithm in Matlab is used to search optimal design variables based on Eq. (26). The result is obtained by

$$b = 17.3, l_1 = 73.2, l_2 = 209.5\,mm.$$

Figure 5 shows the mechanism at (0, 0, 200) *mm* and the workspace volume of the optimized Delta haptic device.

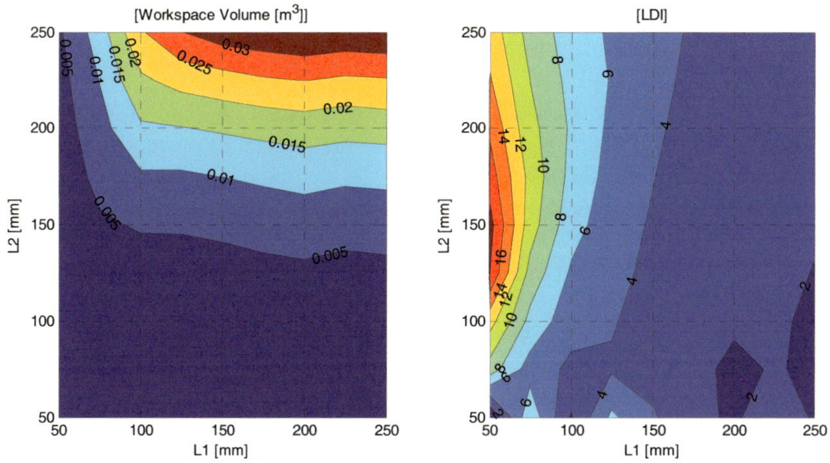

Fig. 4. Contour plots of workspace and LDI with respect to l_1 and l_2 for $b = 20\,mm$

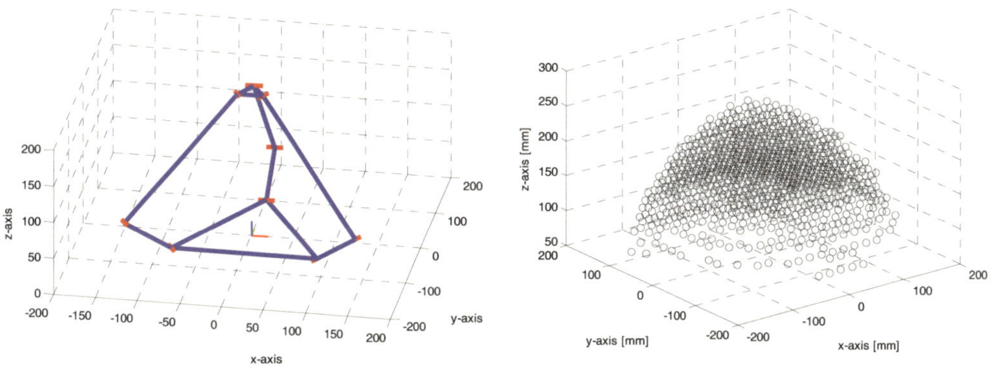

Fig. 5. Configuration at (0, 0, 200) *mm* and workspace volume of the optimized Delta haptic device

5. Conclusions

This chapter discuss recent development of novel mechanism structures used in haptic device. The kinematic analysis methods of serial- and parallel-kinematic manipulators for haptic rendering cycle are presented and some important kinematic measures are suggested. The procedure of kinematic optimization of haptic mechanisms is presented. Example of the Delta haptic device shows the effectiveness of the kinematic optimization.

6. References

Martin, J. & Savall, J. (2005), Mechanism for Haptic Torque Feedback, *Proceedings of the First Joint Eurohaptics Conference and Symposium on Haptic Interfaces for Virtual Environment and Teleoperator System*.

Agronin, M. L. (1987), The Design of a Nine-string Six-degree-of-freedom Force-feedback Joystick for Telemanipulation, *Proceedings of the NASA Workshop on Space Telerobotics*, pp. 341-348.

Berkelman, P. J.; Butler, Z. & Hollis, R. L. (1996), Design of a Hemispherical Magnetic Levitation Haptic Interface, *Proceedings of the ASME Dynamics Systems and Control Division*, Vol. 58, pp. 483–488.

Tsai, L. W. (1999), *Robot Analysis: The Mechanics of Serial and Parallel Manipulators*, John Wiley & Sons, Canada.

Tsai, L. W. (2001). *Mechanism Design: Enumeration of Kinematic Structures According to Function*, CRC press.

Kong, X. & Gosselin, C. (2007). *Type Synthesis of Parallel Mechanisms*, Springer, Netherlands.

Gogu, G. (2008). *Structural Synthesis of Parallel Robots*, Springer, Netherlands.

Angerilli, M.; Frisoli A. & Salsedo, F. & Marcheschi, S. & Bergamasco, M. (2001), Haptic Simulation of an Automotive Manual Gearshift, *Proceedings of the IEEE International Workshop on Robot and Human Interactive Communication*.

Rosenberg, L. B. & Jackson, B. G. (2002), Force Feedback Device Including Flexure Member Between Actuator and User Object, *United States Patent 6437771*.

Campion, G.; Wang, Q. & Hayward, V. (2005), The Pantograph Mk-II: A Haptic Instrument, *Proc. IROS 2005, IEEE/RSJ Int. Conf. Intelligent Robots and Systems*, pp. 723-728.

Birglen, L.; Gosselin, C. & Pouliot, N. & Monsarrat, B. & Laliberte, T. (2002), SHaDe, A New 3-DoF Haptic Device, *IEEE Transactions on Robotics and Automation,* Vol. 18, pp. 166-175.

Sirouspour, M. R.; DiMaio, S. P. & Salcudean, S. E. & Abolmaesumi, P. & Jones, C. (2000), Haptic Interface Control - Design Issues and Experiments with a Planar Device, *Proceedings of the IEEE International Conference on Robotics & Automation*.

Grange S.; Conti F. & Helmer P. & Rouiller P. & Baur C. (2001), The Delta Haptic Device as a Nanomanipulator, *SPIE Microrobotics and Microassembly III*, Boston, MA.

Cavusoglu, M. C.; Feygin D. & Tendick, F. (2002), A Critical Study of the Mechanical and Electrical Properties of the PHANToM Haptic Interface and Improvements for High-Performance Control, *The MIT Press Journals*, Vol. 11, No. 6, pp. 555-568.

Wang S. (2001), *Role of torque in haptic perception of virtual objects,* Thesis S M, Dept of Mechanical Engineering, Massachusetts Institute of Technology.

Iwata H. (1993), Pen-Based Haptic Virtual Environment, *Proceedings of the IEEE Virtual Reality Annual International Symposium*, Seattle, Washington, pp. 287- 292.

Stocco, L. J.; Salcudean, S. E. & Sassani, F. (2001), Optimal Kinematic Design of a Haptic Pen, IEEE/ASME Transactions on Mechatronics, Vol. 6, No. 3, pp. 210-220.

Chen, E. (1999), Six Degree-of-Freedom Haptic System For Desktop Virtual Prototyping Applications, *Proceedings of the International Workshop on Virtual Reality and Prototyping*, Laval, France, pp. 97-106.

Cohen A. & Chen, E. (1999), Six Degree-of-Freedom Haptic System as a Desktop Virtual Prototyping Interface, *Proceedings of the ASME Winter Annual Meeting, Dynamics Systems and Control*, Nashville, Tennessee, Vol. 67, pp. 401-402.

Tsumaki, Y.; Naruse, H. & Nenchev, D. N. & Uchiyama, M. (1998), Design of a Compact 6-DoF Haptic Interface, *Proceedings of the IEEE International Conference on Robotics & Automation*, pp. 2580-2585.

Yoon, W. K.; Suehiro, T. & Tsumaki, Y. & Uchiyama, M. (2003), A Compact Modified Delta Parallel Mechanism Design based on Stiffness Analysis, *Proceedings of the 2003 IEEE/ASME International Conference on Advanced Intelligent Mechatronics*, pp. 1262-1267.

Long, G. L. & Collins, C. L. (1992), A Pantograph Linkage Parallel Platform Master Hand Controller for Force- Reflection, *Proceedings of the IEEE International Conference on Robotics and Automation*, Nice, France, pp. 390-395.

Hayward, V. (1995), Toward a Seven Axis Haptic Interface, *Proceedings of the IROS International Workshop on Intelligent Robots and Systems*, Vol. 2, pp. 133-139.

Hayward, V.; Gregorio, P. & Astley, O. R. & Greenish, S. & Doyon, M. (1997), Freedom-7: A High Fidelity Seven Axis Haptic Device With Application To Surgical Training, *Proceedings of the ISER 6th International Symposium on Experimental Robotics*, Vol. 5.

Ueberle, M. & Buss, M. (2002), Design, Control, and Evaluation of a New 6 DOF Haptic Device, *Proceedings of the IEEE International Conference on Intelligent Robots and Systems*, Lausanne, Switzerland, pp. 2949-2954.

Ueberle, M.; Mock, N. & Buss, M. (2004), ViSHaRD10, a Novel Hyper-Redundant Haptic Interface, *Proceedings of the IEEE 12th International Symposium on Haptic Interfaces for Virtual Environment and Teleoperator Systems*, Chicago, Illinois, USA, pp. 58- 65.

Duffy, J. (1996), *Statics and Kinematics with applications to Robotics*, Cambridge University Press, pp. 89-156.

Yoshikawa, T. (1985), Manipulability of Robotic Mechanisms, *International Journal of Robotics Research*, Vol. 4, No. 2, pp. 3-9.

Salisbury, J. K. & Craig, J. J. (1982), Articulated Hands: Force Control and Kinematics Issues, *International Journal of Robotics Research*, Vol. 1, No. 1, pp. 4-17.

Kim, H. S. & Choi, Y. J. (2001), Forward/Inverse Force Transmission Capability Analyses of Fully Parallel Manipulators, *IEEE Transaction on Robotics and Automation*, Vol. 17, No. 4, pp. 526-530.

Kim, H. S. & Tsai, L. W. (2003), Design Optimization of a Cartesian Parallel Manipulator, *Journal of Mechanical Design*, Vol. 125, No. 1, pp.43-51.

Gosselin, C. & Angeles, J. (1989), The Optimum Kinematic Design of a Spherical Three-Degrees-of-Freedom Parallel Manipulator, *ASME Journal of Mechanisms, Transmissions and Automation in Design*, Vol. 111, No. 2, pp. 202–207.

15

Haptic-Based 3D Carving Simulator

Gabriel Telles O'Neill, Won-Sook Lee and Jeff William
University of Ottawa
Canada

Abstract

We aim to add realistic force-feedback to the process of real-time volume removal from a 3D mesh object. We refer to this volume removal as "3D carving". 3D carving is particularly applicable to the computer simulation of surgical procedures involving bone reductions that are performed with a motorized burr tool; however the methods and algorithms presented here are generic enough to be used for other purposes, such as modeling, destructible objects & terrains in games, etc.

The system represents the volume of the virtual objects using a voxel-set during carving process. A polygonal mesh is created from this voxel-set to display a smoother rendition of the virtual object. Out system also employs the novel Dynamic Ball-Pivoting Algorithm to generate quick mesh updates when voxel-set revisions occur. The advantages of this being that minor changes to the voxel-set only require minor changes to the mesh, whereas the standard Ball-Pivoting Algorithm approach is to perform a global re-meshing.

In our haptic carving system interactions with the aforementioned voxel-set can provide output force-feedback to the system operator. A pen-based haptic tool is used to act as a 3D mouse in order to "feel" the surface of the model as well as to remove select volume segments of the object. Two collision detection schemes are presented here which allow users to feel the surface of virtual objects either using the voxels alone or by using supplemental information from the polygonal mesh. When the burr-tool has its "cutting mode" enabled, which sections of an object's volume are to be removed is decided by evaluating that volume's proximity to the center of the burr.

1. Introduction

Traditionally, the majority of computing applications have relegated their output to what can be seen or heard- modalities consistent with the hardware available on the average desktop computer. However, the advantage gained from incorporating the sense of touch to computing applications has recently increased in practicality as the hardware supporting virtual touch decreases in cost and becomes more accessible. Haptic devices are a relative new technology that provides humans a tactile interface to elements in a virtual world. Even as a fledgling field it has already shown promise in virtual-reality systems, design of computer-generated objects, medicine, robotics and gaming.

In some cases, pre-existing audio-visual systems seeking to enhance the realism of a user's experience can do so by replacing one of the system's input devices (e.g. a mouse) with one of these haptic devices. The system to be described here is an example of this.
The graphical simulation system is to demonstrate their Dynamic Ball Pivoting Algorithm (DBPA) 0. The aim was to develop a system for the real-time visualization of removing volume for an object model. In the DBPA system, an object's volume is represented using voxels, but an associated triangle mesh is also maintained for display purposes since direct visualization of voxels is unrealistic and unappealing. Tasks such as simulating the drilling or carving of bone during medical procedures, boring wood, biting food and chiselling marble can all be observed in real time by the operator of the DBPA system.
Our haptic simulation system was built on-top of the DBPA system; where control of the volume-removing element was given to a haptic device, whereas the graphical simulation system itself was mouse-driven. The result is a means to carve, drill and trim a three dimensional object stored inside the computer while observing the removal of sections of volume and receiving corresponding force feedback immediately.
While this system's general scope is that of virtual-reality, it has been designed with the ultimate goal of being used as a training environment for surgeons in order to help them accumulate experience and muscle memory useful in actual operations involving bone reductions. For example, motivational surgery around which this new system was designed was a minimally invasive procedure to correct femoroacetabular impingements (FAIs). FAIs describe a condition where there exists an overgrowth of bone on either a patient's femur neck or around the hip socket. These overgrowths often cause discomfort and chafe during normal hip exercise, producing premature cartilage damage and labral tears, which lead to further medical complications and pain. These impingements can be treated by using a motorized burr tool to grind away the excess bone and reshape the affected regions for a better fit between the femur head and hip socket. As such, a virtual burr with a spherical head, fashioned to resemble the one depicted in Fig. 1 (without the hood), is used as the default tool for volume removal inside our simulation.

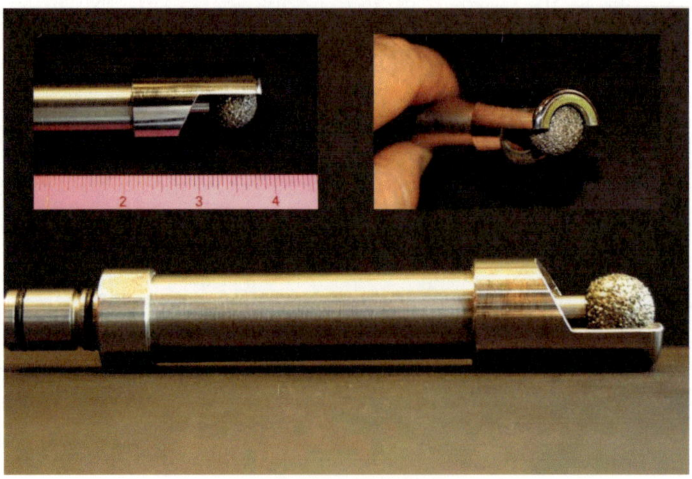

Fig. 1. An example of a motorized burr tool with a hood

In our system, the force-feedback and the intersection points between the burr and object's volume can be computed using one of two methods. The first being the voxel-set, which most directly represents to object's volume, and the second being the set of triangles that compose the polygonized mesh generated by the DBPA. Volume is removed from an object by isolating sections of voxels intersecting with the virtual burr and eliminating them from voxel-set. When voxels do get removed from the virtual model, the affected regions of the corresponding triangle mesh are updated and re-displayed.

2. Related Work

Increasing interest has developed over the past decade on developing carving simulators with faithful haptic feedback for various medical fields. Of these the most technically successful appear to be dental training systems. These systems are designed to allow dental students to practice certain procedures on a virtual set of teeth such as drilling operations and filling cavities with amalgam. In these simulators, the manner in which collision detection and the resulting haptic force-feedback is calculated is intrinsically linked to how the system's designers chose to represent the volume of their carvable objects.

In Kim and Park's dental simulator 0, their model's volume was represented using a Computational Solid Geometry (CSG) point-set. CSG expresses an object as the combination from a set of solid primitives. These primitives can be parametric equations of a quadric surface (e.g. planes, spheres, cones, cylinders, or paraboloids), or simple, regular prisms (e.g. cubes). The primitives will form the leaves of a binary tree, in which internal nodes represent rigid transformations (translations, rotations, or scalings) of the children nodes, or represent regularized Boolean set operations (union, intersection, or difference) on the left or right sub-tree. Performing volume removal (cutting, drilling, etc.) using CSG is a relatively simple matter of representing the object that will have its volume removed as a CSG sub-tree whose parent is a difference operation with the second sub-tree being the union of all instalments of volume that have been "cut". However a major drawback of this approach is that the volume to be "cut" must first be converted to a CSG representation, which is difficult and non-automated for complex objects such as human bones. A second drawback is that the method does not scale well as the number of volume removals increases. This is because the tree representing each "cut" must be added to the main tree of the object. As a result, successive cuts to an object's volume will make the tree representation grow large quickly. Using this CSG model, the two researchers chose to implement collision detection by calculating the distance from an offset field surrounding the surface of the virtual teeth to the center of the user's dental tool. If the tool's center passed the offset field, the haptic device controlling the dental tool would provide force-feedback in the direction of the field's implicit surface normal. The force's direction is used to calculate the tool's virtual contact point with the object's surface. This contact point is then used to calculate the force vector by using a spring-damper model based on Hooke's law.

Similarly, Yau et al. 0 also used a spring-damper model to calculate the force vector sent to the haptic device of their dental training system. However, instead of representing the volume of their objects using CSG, an adaptive voxel model is used. These researchers used an implicit function to define their cutting tools, which in turn were used to decide exactly what volume was to be removed from the model. As the voxels used to represent the object are of varying sizes in this scheme, if the tool comes into contact with a large voxel,

recursive subdivision must be performed on that voxel until the voxels in contact with the tool are small enough for removal. Any voxel whose volume is found to be completely "inside" the tool will subsequently be remove from the model.
A real-time haptic and visual bone dissection simulator00 was also proposed by Agus et al., aimed as being used as a training tool for temporal bone surgery. This system most closely resembles our own as it generates its object volume through the voxel discretization of 3D Computed Tomography (CT) or Magnetic Resonance Imaging (MRI) data. In addition to bone matter, secondary visual effects such as bone dust, debris, and water are realized using a particle system to potentially heighten the realism of surgeon's experience.

3. Graphical Carving System

Graphical simulation system is necessary before detailing our own hi-fidelity haptic feedback improvements. The development goal of this graphical carving system, DBPA, is the real-time visualization of volume removal for an object model. Updates in a model's volume resulting from simulated operations such as drilling, carving, boring, biting and chiselling the object are performed and displayed back to the operator at a rate that appears instantaneous to them. This method uses voxels (of a constant size) as a volumetric representation of the object. Since renderings composed of voxels appear very blocky, they fail to provide the realistic visual interface necessary for a surgical training simulator. A further presentation step is required: from the object's voxel-set, the system generates a much nicer looking polygon mesh to visualize the object model before, during, and after cutting. Triangulation is achieved using the Dynamic Ball Pivoting Algorithm0, which is an extension of Ball Pivoting Algorithm (BPA)0.
The objects to be carved are represented by three major data structures: a voxel-set used for volume representation, a triangle mesh used for display purposes, and a modified BPA front-end used for updating the display mesh when the voxel-set is altered. Each surface voxel in the voxel-set is also linked to its corresponding vertex in the triangle mesh. The mesh is defined such that vertices are shared between adjacent edges, and edges are shared between adjacent triangles.

3.1 Initialization

To start, the system needs one of the following inputs:

1) *A solid pre-modeled as a voxel-set*

This option is designed to facilitate the insertion of 3D CT or MRI data into the program for patient/ object specific simulation.

2) *A polygon model*

The model provided will then subsequently be reduced to a voxel-set. Afterwards, the voxel in which each vertex of the bounding box finds itself is found in order to determine the voxel-space volume that binds the triangle. Then, for each voxel within the volume, the fast 3D triangle-box overlap test from Akenine-Möller 0. All intersecting voxels form a boundary around the mesh volume. The volume inside the boundary is then filled using a 3D scanline filling algorithm.

Either way, once the voxel representation of the solid is determined, the system then computes the corresponding polygonal mesh using the BPA. The algorithm is intended for 3D data-acquisition of real-world objects, but Williams et al 0 found it to be equally well suited for generating a triangle mesh from a voxel-set by using the centers of the voxels as the point set.

3.2 Carving Out Volume

Within the system, carving is performed by manipulating a virtual tool which resembles the motorized burrs used by medical professionals. In practice, burrs are used by surgeons to dexterously grind way at bone surfaces with a rotating, abrasive head while gripping the tool's handle. In this system, the tool is implemented as a spherical cutting head which is attached to a non-cutting handle. When the user moves the cutting tool over the object being carved, voxels are removed and the mesh is updated.

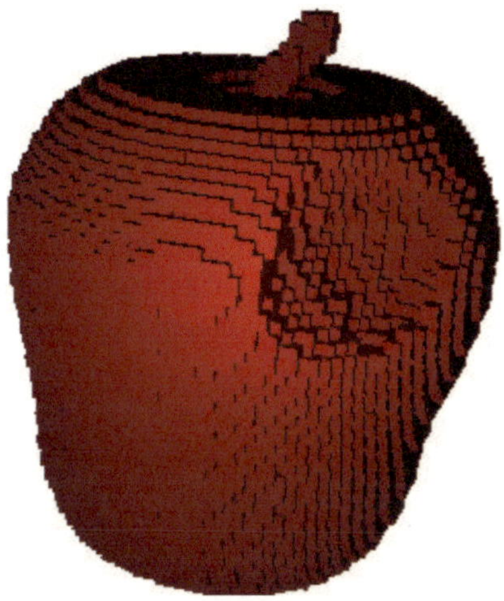

Fig. 2. Unmeshed voxelized apple with carved hole

Whenever the tool's position is changed, the system uses the geometric equation for the tool's head to determine if there are the voxels whose centers are within its boundary. If so, they are removed from the voxel-set. When voxels are removed from the set, the triangle mesh must be updated to reflect the changes. The DBPA is responsible for these updates and, for each voxel *v* removed from the set, performs the following procedure:

1) *If v was not a surface voxel*

   no additional steps need to be taken.

2) *Otherwise, if v was a surface voxel*

   It must have a corresponding mesh vertex with adjacent triangles. The voxel's removal indicates the removal of a vertex from the mesh, thus all triangles adjacent to that vertex become invalid and must also be removed. After removal, a new loop in the front-end is created that bounds the removed triangles. Care is taken when adding the loops to ensure that the BPA front invariant property is preserved while iteratively removing voxels and their associated mesh triangles. Adding these loops sometimes cause undesirable adjacent edges which are removed using the BPA's "glue" operation.

In order for the DBPA to work properly, certain additional information must be stored at each edge in the front. When the BPA processes a front, it pivots a ball around each edge in that front until it strikes a point. This calculation requires not only the coordinates of the pivotal edge's vertices, but also (1) the "ball-center" (coordinates of the center of the BPA ρ-ball when it had previously struck the point that generated the triangle) and (2) the coordinates of the point (vertex) opposite to front edge in its binding triangle. In order to have this information available, newly created triangles in the mesh also store their respective ball-centers. Also, when an edge is added to the front, the front's corresponding edge will store both the ball-centre and opposite-point as additional data.

3.3 Texturing Meshes

To further enhance the visual fidelity of carvable objects, this system has the option of applying textures to the voxels. An alternative to flatly colouring the voxels, a 2D texture can be applied over the exterior of the shape while a 3D texture can be specified for the object's interior. The 2D texture is applied during the initialization stage and is attached directly to the triangle mesh that represents the whole, un-carved object. Once object carving is underway, the new triangles created through the DBPA are mapped to the contents of the 3D texture. Examples are shown in Fig. 3 and Fig. 4.

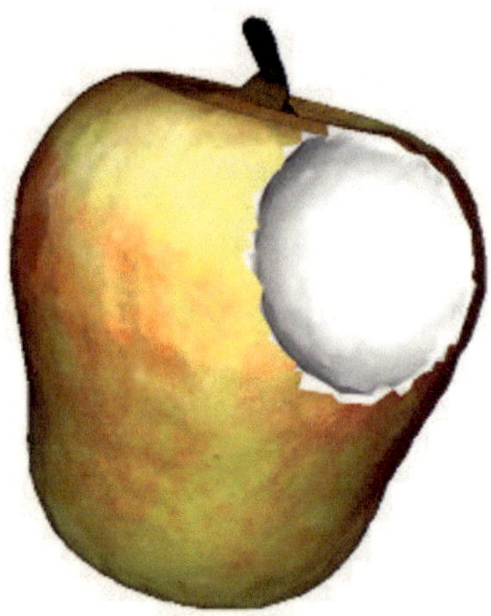

Fig. 3. Meshed apple with external texture

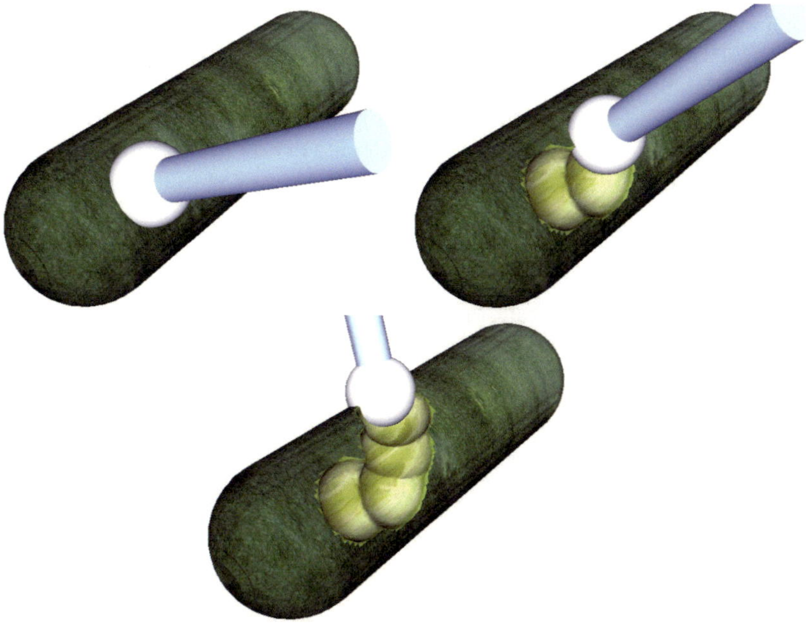

Fig. 4. Demonstration of carving an externally and internally textured object. The cucumber uses an external 2D texture as well as an internal 3D texture

4. Haptic system

While the DBPA 0 has the graphical solution using OpenSceneGraph (OSG), the haptic simulation system chooses the NOVINT Falcon™ along with its stock API to implement our conjoined haptic solution. The Falcon is a pen-based haptic device intended as a joystick or mouse substitute. It allows a user to control an application in a three dimensional space while also providing him or her with high-fidelity force-feedback. When a user holds the Falcon's grip and moves the cursor to interact with a virtual scene, motors in the device turn on and are updated at precise rate of 1000Hz, allowing the operator to feel texture, shape, weight, dimension, and dynamics.

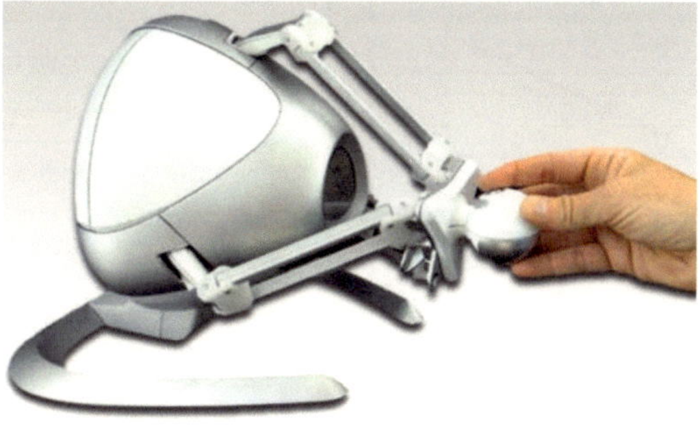

Fig. 5. NOVINT Falcon, reprinted from the NOVINT website

Our system's interface with the Falcon was the Haptic Device Abstraction Layer (HDAL) which is NOVINT's pre-packaged API. HDAL lacks the higher-level functions that other haptic APIs (such as Sensable's OpenHaptics or H3D.org's HAPI) have, which means that most operations such as force calculations and button status lack automation and need be calculated manually. Also, because the haptic device needs to be updated a thousand times a second, all operations performed inside the HDAL's regular maintenance loop need to be performed in under 1 ms in order to maintain "high-fidelity" haptic force feedback. The implication here is that special effort must be taken in order to ensure that the haptic loop's tasks are performed as efficiently as possible to guarantee that the device operator does not sense that the haptic output feels "choppy".

4.1 System Overview

The sequence of steps used to implement this model-cutting strategy is illustrated in Fig. 6. This activity diagram serves as an overview of the new haptic system's two intercommunicating threads of execution. The two concurrent threads begin executing at runtime. There is an OSG thread responsible for what the user sees, and a haptic thread responsible for what the user feels.

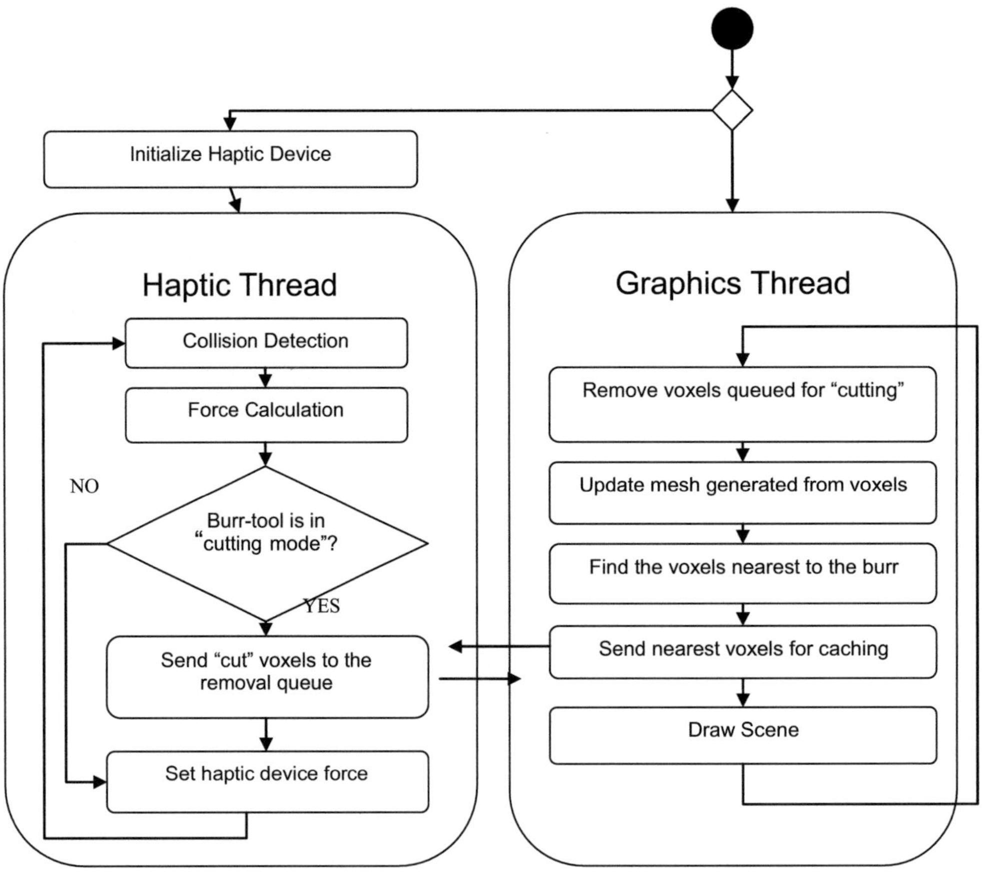

Fig. 6. Activity Diagram for the new haptic system

The haptic thread implements one of two collision detection methods which in turn provide input values for the force calculation step. The first collision detection method uses only the object's voxel representation to detect collisions and scale to force feedback while the second method takes advantage of the polygon mesh created from the voxel-set to perform these tasks. The former has shown to be useful in quickly evaluating the effects of new features to system but suffers from a somewhat "blocky" contact with the volume. The latter method provides a smoother contact force while passing over the object but in turn requires the management of a set of triangles from the mesh in addition to a cache of voxels.

4.2 Graphics Thread

Our system adds a double-ended queue to the Graphics OSG thread. Named the "removalQueue". This structure contains the coordinates of voxels which ought to be removed from the object during the next execution loop. This queue is populated by the haptic thread when it has been decided that certain sections of volume have been "cut" during the user's operation of the burr-tool. At the start of each OSG loop, the queue will be emptied and all corresponding voxels in the model will be removed. In addition, the polygonizer will be informed of any change to the voxel set so that it can re-mesh the isolated changed regions rather than re-polygonizing the whole model.

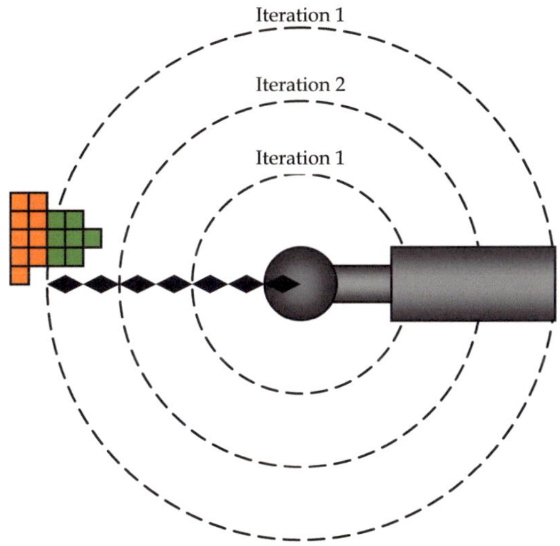

Fig. 7. A 2D slice showing how nearby voxel are found

In order to minimize the number of voxels the haptic thread needs to investigate for collisions, only the nearest voxels to the burr's head are sent for caching to the haptic class. The nearest voxels are found using an iterative, step-based approach: if the burr radius is designated the symbol *r*, the loop will first look for any voxels within 3r of the burr-head center, then 5r, then 7r, etc. until it finds at least one voxel which it can send to the haptic thread for caching. If no voxels are found within 23r of the voxel head, the searching quits. It was determined through experimentation that after 23r, the voxel set is sufficiently far enough from the burr-tool that that, even at high speeds, the tool was unlikely to come into contact with the objects in between cache updates. If the haptic thread's collision detection is to be performed using the voxel-only method, this step ends here. Otherwise, all the triangles part of the mesh within the same "nearest distance" to the burr head are also sent to the haptic thread to be part of its cache.

4.3 Haptic Thread

It is worth mentioning that since the 3D space coordinates, roll, pitch and heading of the voxel model can be altered in the scene to get a better view of the object from all angles, conversion from local to world coordinates (and back) is required. Upon entering the haptic loop, the burr's position is converted to the model's local coordinate system to simplify the calculation of burr-to-voxel distances. Conversely, the initial force feedback direction is calculated in the voxel model's local coordinate system, so it is converted to world coordinates before being sent to the haptic device as a force command.

4.3.1 Collision Detection (with only voxels)

Detecting a collision between the burr and the voxel model (or between a prospective anchor and the voxel model) is fairly simple for a spherical burr head.

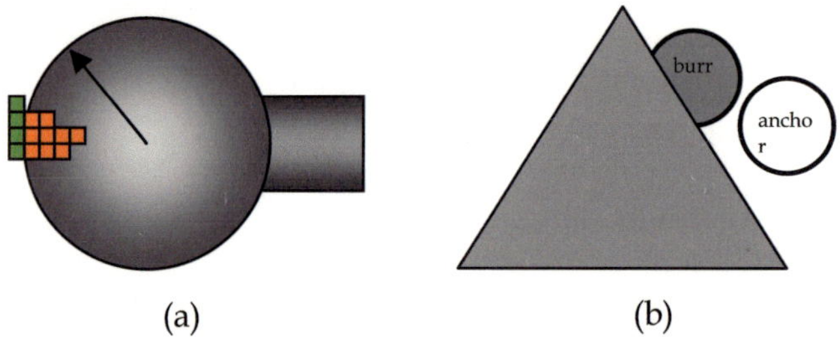

Fig. 8. (a) Voxels causing a collision to be detected (b) Example positioning of a burr head and anchor point as a collision is being detected

An iterator is created to traverse the set of cached voxels. While doing so, if the distance from a voxel to the center of the burr-head is less than or equal to the burr's radius, then a collision has occurred and the iteration is halted. If the iterator has traverses the voxel cache completely, no collision has occurred. As shown in Fig. 8(a), the coloured squares represent the set of voxels cached by the haptic class, but only the voxels marked as orange squares would cause a collision to occur. If no collision has occurred for any of the nearby voxels, then the "anchor" is set to the burr head's current position. This anchor represents an approximation of closest point to the burr head that does not intersect with any voxels. This becomes important later when the next collision does occur, since this system scales the magnitude of the force feedback based on the distance between the burr center and the anchor center.

When a collision has been detected, the first thing the haptic thread will do is to determine if there is an alternate anchor point within "anchor drag" distance which is closer to the burr head than the current anchor point.

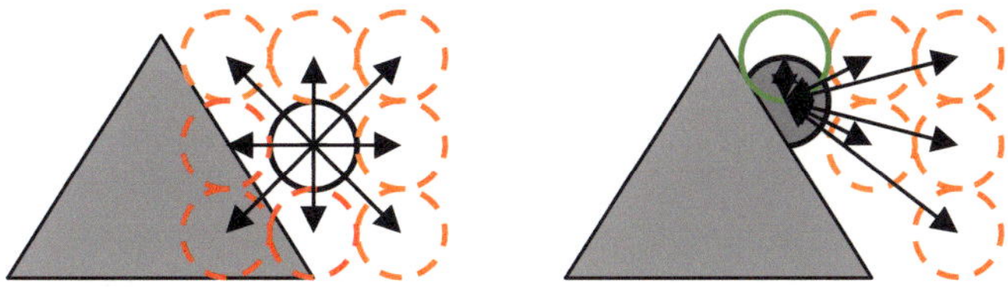

(a) (b)

Fig. 9. (a) A 2D slice of 8 new anchor candidates placed around the original anchor (b) Distances from the candidate anchors to the burr-head

Twenty-six new anchor candidates are generated by applying a fixed "anchor drag" distance in each combination of *x/y/z* direction around the old anchor. New anchor positions that collide with one or more voxel points are disqualified from being candidate anchor points (coloured red in Fig. 9(a)). The reason why the anchor is permitted to "drag" in any direction is to let the burr tool slide across the surface of the voxel model after it has collided. This allows the operator to get an impression of the model landscape. If a drag feature were not implemented, the burr-tool would be virtually glued to a spot on the model where it collided and would only relinquish its spot when the burr tool was fully pulled away.
As shown in Fig. 9(b), the candidate anchor with the shortest distance to the burr-head's current position, circled here in green, becomes the new anchor point. With the anchor point established, the following two values are computed:

$$forceVector \leftarrow anchor\ center - burr\ center$$

$$linkDist \leftarrow distance\ between\ anchor\ center\ and\ burr\ center$$

4.3.2 Collision Detection (with triangle mesh)

Using the cache of nearest triangles to the burr head allows us calculate the force vector and link distance without have to evaluate candidate anchor points. First the nearest triangle to the burr head is identified from the triangle cache (coloured red in Fig. 10). The plane on which this nearest triangle lies is determined and the distance from the burr center to that plane is calculated.

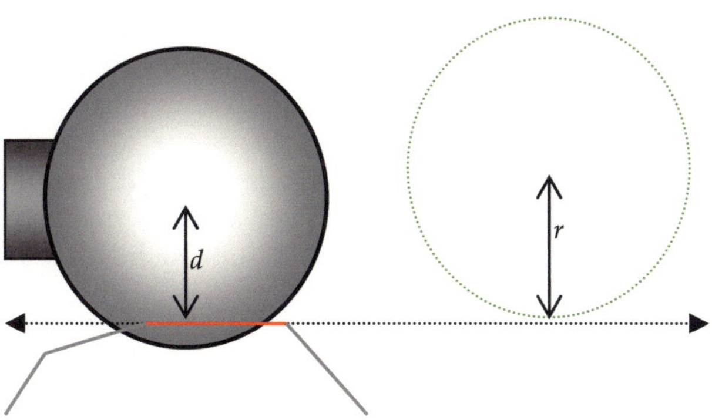

Fig. 10. A 2D slice of a collision between the burr head and some triangles from the mesh

If the distance from that burr center to the plane is greater than the burr's radius ($d > r$), no collision has occurred. Otherwise, a collision is recorded and the following two values are computed:

$$forceVector \leftarrow nearest\ triangle's\ normal$$

$$linkDist \leftarrow burr\ radius - burr\ centre's\ distance\ from\ the\ plane$$

4.3.3 Force Calculation

Finally, the actual calculation for the local force is computed using equation (1).

$$\vec{F}_t \leftarrow matUltStrength * scaleFactor * linkDist * forceVector \tag{1}$$

This above force equation is inspired by Hooke's Law (*Force* = $-k \times x$). However, instead of using the spring constant k, this equation uses a material's "ultimate strength". The ultimate strength of a material being defined as the "maximum stress a material can withstand". Some examples which were used as material parameters in our system can be found in Table 1.

Material	**Ultimate Strength (S_u) 10^6 N/m^2**
Steel (ASTM-A36)	400
Bone (limb)	170
Wood (Douglas fir)	50

Table 1. Comparative ultimate strength values0

In the previous equation, *forceVector* is the 3D directionality component along which the (local) force feedback will be aligned, *linkDistance* is the depth to which the burr has been pushed into the object's volume and is used to scale the magnitude of the force according to how strongly a user is pushing into the volume of the model, *materialUltStrength* is the ultimate strength of the material from which the model is made, and *scaleFactor* is a downscaling factor to place the final force magnitudes within range of the NOVINT Falcon's capabilities.

In order to ensure a smoother transition from one force to the next, a force-filter, as implemented by Yau et al.0, is adopted by applying a damper to our spring system. This is applied to the local force by using the method described in Equation (2) where δ is a predefined threshold for the force change.

$$\Delta\vec{F} = \vec{F}_t - \vec{F}_{t-1}$$
$$\begin{cases} \vec{F}_t' = \vec{F}_{t-1} + \delta \times \dfrac{\Delta\vec{F}}{\left\|\Delta\vec{F}\right\|} & \left\|\Delta\vec{F}\right\| > \delta \\ \vec{F}_t' = \vec{F}_t & \left\|\Delta\vec{F}\right\| \le \delta \end{cases} \tag{2}$$

Following this method, the new force is converted back into the global coordinate system, where a few force effects are added (e.g. a slight vibration in the tool tip to simulate the rotating nature of the burr) and finally, this force value is sent to the Falcon as an output force command.

4.3.4 Voxel Cutting

Any voxel whose distance to the center of the burr head is less than or equal to ¾ of the burr radius is considered "cut". To cut a voxel, first, its coordinates will be pushed to the back of the OSG removal queue. Second, its unique identifier (based on its position in the voxel model) is placed in a hash-map so that the haptic thread will no longer process that voxel for collisions while waiting for the OSG thread to send it an updated cache of the nearby and uncut voxels.

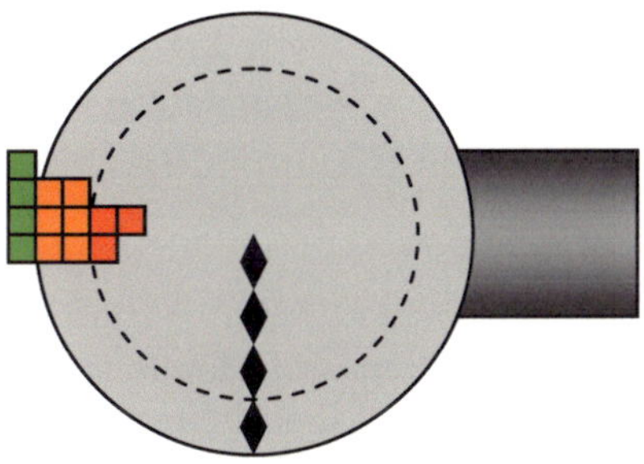

Fig. 11. Distinction between simply colliding (orange) and colliding & cut (red) voxels

5. Results

The results thus far have been promising. The surface features of our apple, femur and pelvis models can easily be felt using either collision detection method. Surface contact is definitely smoother using the mesh collision detection scheme. However, carving and, even more so, drilling operations tend to perform more reliably using the anchor based, voxel-only method at the moment. Using a material's ultimate strength has also shown to be useful in providing the user with haptic feedback on how difficult it is to cut different materials.

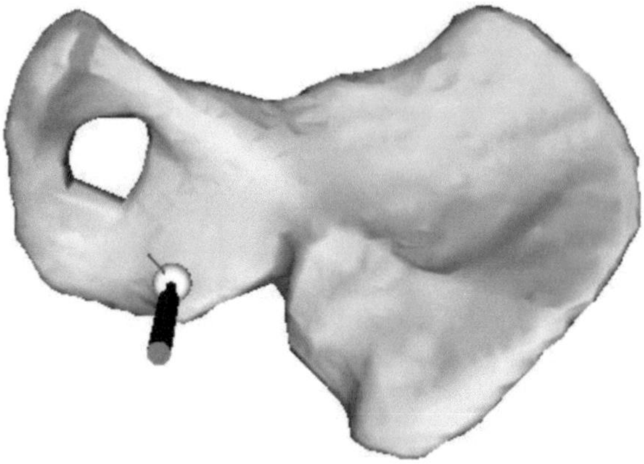

Fig. 12. A burr-tool receiving force-feedback from a polygonized pelvis model where the force (direction and strength) is displayed with a blue line

At present, users are unable to distinguish between most different types of material textures while using the voxel-only approach to collision detection. This is largely due to the discrete nature of voxels promoting a "blocky" surface contact with the spherical burr. This issue could be partially addressed by increasing the voxel density used to represent and object volume. However, this solution becomes resource demanding past a certain point. The collision detection method that exploits the mesh feels much smoother when passing over flat and rounded surfaces with the burr; however different material haptic surface textures have not yet been convincingly implemented.

6. Discussion

Both the Dynamic Ball Pivoting Algorithm and Haptic system need to mature into more robust versions of their current selves before their inherent potential can truly shine through. Also, while basing the haptic class' force equation on Hooke's law is convenient, it is also inaccurate. A more involved and realistic model would be to use a material's full stress-strain curve0 to dictate the amount of force required to remove volume from the model. However, such a change would require a means to measure to amount of force the user is exerting on the haptic device.

A question that has come up before is: why we bother with the anchor-based method for finding the force direction when we could use the nearest colliding voxel or use the summation of the direction vectors of all voxels colliding with the burr-head instead? The reason for this is that the nearest-voxel or voxel-summation methods have shown to perform erratically whenever the burr-head is placed in a tight corner or inside a pit. On the other hand, the anchor-based method has shown to perform as expected in both these situations as well as on normal surface curvatures.

7. Conclusion and Future Work

This new system adds a sense of touch to the process of removing volume from voxelized objects and is built on top of William et al.'s graphical carving simulator. Two components operate in unison in order to make this work: an OpenSceneGraph thread and a haptic thread. The former is responsible for clearing voxels queued for removal, redrawing the scene and providing the haptic thread with a subset of the object data; the voxels and triangles most likely to be relevant during collision detection are cached here. The latter deals with issuances of both the direction and magnitude of force as well as evaluating which sections of volume should be removed from the object.

There are certainly a great many directions where the haptic portion of the system can be improved and extended in the future. One area that would improve the program's use would be to have a more modular approach to the cutting tools. Tools other than a burr with a spherical head are likely to be useful to surgeons. The head may instead be an ellipsoid, conical or cylindrical. The cutting tool could also be something non-motorized such a scalpel which would require the distinction between cutting surfaces and non-cutting surfaces to be made.

At the moment, models have a global ultimate strength value meaning that all the voxel will have the same stiffness. In many cases, such as our target example; operating on human bone, this is unrealistic as their exteriors are made of dense cortical bone while their interior is composed of much softer bone marrow. Assigning each voxel its own density value is our next step. This will also allow us to examine a voxel removal strategy whereby the act of "cutting" an object will incrementally reduce the voxels density and voxels finding themselves with a density of zero are considered wholly "cut". The same idea can be extended to the mesh-based collision detection. The hope is that this will allow a user to feel a more progressive entry into an object while it is being cut.

8. References

[1] Williams J, Telles O'Neill G, Lee WS. Interactive 3d haptic carving using combined voxels and mesh. Haptic Audio visual Environments and Games, 2008. HAVE 2008; pp 108-113, DOI: 10.1109/HAVE.2008.4685308

[2] Kim L, Park SH. Haptic interaction and volume modeling techniques for realistic dental simulation. The visual Computer: International Journal of Computer Graphics. Volume 22, Issue 2, 2006; pp 90-98, DOI: 10.1007/s00371-006-0369-8

[3] Yau HT, Tsou LS, Tsai MJ. Octree-based Virtual Dental Training System with a Haptic Device. Computer-Aided Design & Applications. Volume 3, 2006; pp 415-424

[4] Agus M, Giachetti A, Gobbetti E, Zanetti G, Zorcolo A. Real-time haptic and visual simulation of bone dissection. Presence: Teleoperators and Virtual Environments; special issue: IEEE virtual reality 2002 conference; Volume 12, Issue 1, 2003; pp 110-122

[5] Agus M, Giachetti A, Gobbetti E, Zanetti G, Zorcolo A. Adaptive techniques for real-time haptic and visual simulation of bone dissection. Virtual Reality, 2003. Proceedings. IEEE; pp 102-109, DOI: 10.1109/VR.2003.1191127

[6] Bernardini F, Mittleman J, Rushmeir H, Silva C, Taubin. The ball-pivoting algorithm for surface reconstruction. Visualization and Computer Graphics, Volume 5, Issue 4, 1999; pp 349-359, DOI: 10.1109/2945.817351

[7] Akenine-Möller T. Fast 3D triangle-box overlap testing. International Conference on Computer Graphics and Interactive Techniques. ACM SIGGRAPH 2005
[8] Halliday, Resnick, Walker. Data from Table 13-1. Fundamentals of Physics, 5E, Extended, Wiley, 1997
[9] Tensile Properties. NDT Resource Center; 2005. Available: http://www.ndt-ed.org/EducationResources/CommunityCollege/Materials/Mechanical/Tensile.htm (Accessed: Tuesday, April-15-08)

16

Manipulation of Dynamically Deformable Object using Impulse-Based Approach

Kazuyoshi Tagawa
Ritsumeikan University
Japan

Koichi Hirota
University of Tokyo
Japan

Michitaka Hirose
University of Tokyo
Japan

1. Introduction

Recent advancement of network and communication technologies has raised expectations for transmission of multi-sensory information and multi-modal communication. Transmission of haptic sensation has been a topic of research in tele-robotics for a long period. However, as commercial haptic device prevails, and as internet spreads world-wide, it became possible to exchange haptic information for more general communication in our daily life.

Although a variety of information is transmitted through haptic sensation, the feeling of a soft object is one that is difficult to transmit through other sensations. This is because the feeling of softness is represented only by integrating both the sense of deformation by somatic sensation and intensity force by haptic sensation. Feeling of softness is apt to be considered as static information that represents static relationship between deformation and force. Our previous study on implementing a static deformation model suggested that the dynamic aspect of deformation has an important effect on the reality of interactions.

A static model can not represent behavior of an object while the user is not interacting with the object. For example, it is unnatural that an object model immediately returns to its original shape just after user releases hand or finger. Also, resonant vibration of object during the interaction is often perceived through haptic sensation. These differences of dynamic model from static model are considered to become more recognizable to user as more freedom of interaction is given.

In this chapter, an outline of our approach to implement a deformable model that is capable of representing dynamic response of deformation is presented. Supplemental idea that realizes non-grounded motion of the deformable model is also stated; manipulation of deformable object becomes possible by this idea. In the next section, a survey of background research is stated and positioning and purpose of our research is clarified. Formulation of IRDM and non-grounded object motion is discussed in section 3 and 4 respectively. Experimental results and evaluation of the proposed approach is stated in section 5. Finally, advantages and problems of the approach are discussed, and conclusion is given in section 7.

2. Related Works

2.1 Presentation of force

Presentation of the sensation of force in a virtual environment has been studied since the early stages of researches in virtual reality, and investigation has been made in both hardware and software aspects by G.Burdea (1996). Model and simulation that is used to compute force is one important part of software research, and computation of this sort is collectively called Haptic Rendering by K.Salisbury et al. (1995). Representation of deformable object has been a topic of research, because interaction with deformable objects is a quite common experience.

2.2 Motion and manipulation

The free motion of an object is computed simply by solving equations regarding the motion of the object. Computation of motion becomes difficult in cases when constraints on motion are applied by contact with other objects or user's body. A taxonomy of methodology that deals with the constraints has been presented by J.E.Colgate et al. (1995). Typically there are two approaches: one is an approach that solves equation of motion with constraint condition, and another is an approach that introduces penalty force. In computer graphics, the former approach has been presented by D.Baraff (1989), and advantage of the latter approach has been discussed by B.Mirtich & J.Canny (1995).
In haptic rendering, one of major applications of computation of motion is presentation of behavior of object while it is manipulated. Object manipulation by the user frequently causes complicated constraint conditions, and it is usually difficult to solve equations of motion with these constraints. Hence, the approach of penalty force is preferred in hatic rendering researches; Borst & Indugula (2005); K.Hirota & M.Hirose (2003); S.Hasegawa & M.Sato (2004); T.Yoshikawa et al. (1995).

2.3 Deformation model

2.3.1 Model-based approach

Visual representation of deformation has been a major topic in computer graphics. In the early stages, there was research on geometric deformation including Free Form Deformation (FFD) by T.W.Sederberg & S.R.Parry (1986). Nature of this approach that it is not based on physics-based model cause advantage and disadvantage. The nature provides more freedom in deformation including unrealistic deformation. On the other hand, notion of deforming force is not supported by the approach, and interaction force can not be defined.
Finite element method (FEM) and boundary element method (BEM) has been used in the field of computational dynamics, and there is research that introduces these methods to improve reality in computer graphics, such as Terzopoulos et al. (1987). These methods provide the means to implement precise models strictly based on dynamics of continuum. However, generally it is difficult to perform real-time simulation using models of practical complexity; although computation cost is drastically reduced by using static linear model by James & Pai (1999); K.Hirota & T.Kaneko (2001), as stated in section 1, the approximation also reduce reality of deformation. There are studies that accelerate the computation by both using advanced hardware such as GPU by Goeddeke et al. (2005) and improvement of the model structure.

Some other models such as sprig-mass network model (or, Kelvin model) and particle model are other candidates. Sprig-mass network is a model that approximates elasticity by using the network of spring. There is research that has applied this model to represent breakage in computer graphics by Norton et al. (1991), and also employed for haptic rendering. This model is preferably solved using an explicit method that apparently attains higher update rate of computation. However, it should be noted that deformation on each update cycle is not necessarily a precise solution of the model. This problem of solving method deteriorates reality of dynamic deformation. The particle model is considered to have similar problem of computation, however, the model is advantageous in that it is capable of representing plasticity and relatively large deformation of object which FEM model has difficulty of handling.

2.3.2 Record reproduction-based approach

One approach to solve the problem of computation cost is generating the response of objects based on measured or precomputed patterns of deformation rather than simulating it in real time. This idea has already been applied to presentation of high-frequency vibration of surface that is caused by collision with other object.

Wellman & Howe (1995) carried out pioneering research of this approach. In their research, the vibration of a real object that is caused by tapping was measured and approximately represented by fitting decaying sinusoidal wave, and the vibration wave was retrieved in virtual tapping operation. It was proved that this feedback of vibration is helpful to for users to discriminate materials.

Okamura et al. (1998) expanded this approach to other types of interaction including stroking textures and puncture; their approach is called *reality-based modeling*. Also, in their successive research in Okamura et al. (2000), they proposed an approach to optimizing parameters of vibration based on psychological evaluation on reality.

A similar research has been carried out by Kuchenbecker et al. (2005), where transient force at the beginning of contact is precomputed and then retrieved in interaction.

Above researches were focusing on improving realty of the sensation of contact and not dealing with macro deformation. On the other hand, in application that requires a realistic representation of deformation, approaches to measuring characteristics of deformable objects based on measurement are investigated.

Pai et al. (2001) proposed an approach to constructing virtual object model based on measurement on real object; regarding deformation model, stiffness matrix for linear elastic model is estimated based on force-deformation relationship while interacting with the real object. Also, real-time presentation of deformation is realized using an accelerated computation method for linear elastic model by James & Pai (1999).

It is generally accepted notion that the update rate of approximately 1kHz is required for usual haptic rendering, and at lowest several hundred hertz even in case of presenting a low stiffness object. One of solution for the problem is employing pre-recording or pre-computing approach.

James & Fatahalian (2003) have proposed an approach that uses precomputed trajectory of object state in state space; state transition sequences at a given initial state and force conditions are pre-computed, and there transition sequences are reproduced when these initial conditions are satisfied. In the research, however, little discussion has been made regarding increase in interaction patterns; it is not clear if this approach is applicable to realize arbitrary interaction with deformable objects.

In this chapter, as a novel approach that accommodates large DoF of interaction, impulse response deformation model (IRDM) is presented. IRDM is based on the idea of defining the relationship between input force and output deformation using impulse response; by assuming linear time-invariant model and precomputing impulse response of the system, resulting deformation is computed by convolution of input force and the impulse response.

2.4 Separate computation of deformation and motion

Use of a floating coordinate system is a common approach to define movable objects in virtual environments; scene graph is considered as a generic expansion of this approach, and it has been employed to various graphic and haptic rendering systems such as *GHOST SDK Programmer's Guide* (2002); Rohlf & Helman (1994).

In this chapter, a supplemental idea that realizes non-grounded motion of the deformable model is also presented. A floating coordinate system is introduced to our approach, and motion and deformation is simulated by motion equation and IRDM, respectively.

3. Impulse response deformation model (IRDM)

In this section, details of impulse response deformation model (IRDM) is discussed.

The idea of the IRDM is based on the premise that the model is linear, which means that the influences caused by impulse forces on different degrees of freedom or at different times are independent of each other, and the resulting deformation is computed as the sum total of the influences. The linearity regarding degree of freedom is a frequently employed assumption. For example, a linear elastic model is based on this idea. Also, the approach to compute the response of the system by the convolution of impulse response and input signals is commonly used. This approach implicitly premises temporal linearity.

Although, in a precise sense, real material is not thought to have exact linearity, in most applications, this assumption will provide more merit in reducing computational cost than the demerit of increasing inaccuracy. In a case where the assumption is not employed, the response of the object for the entire combination of the object status (i.e. position in phase space) and interaction status (i.e. boundary condition) must be defined. If these statuses are discretely described, the number of combinations of the discrete status is thought to explode even in models of relatively small complexity.

3.1 1 DoF model

Let us think of a continuous system with one force input and one displacement output. The impulse response of the system is defined as temporal sequence of deformation after the impulse force was inputted into the system. If the system is linear, then the resulting displacement $u(t)$ in response to arbitrary force input sequence $f(t)$ is obtained using the impulse response of the system $r(t)$ as follows:

$$u(t) = \int_0^\infty r(s) f(t-s) ds. \tag{1}$$

When $f(t)$ is a Dirac delta function, resulting $u(t)$ becomes identical with $r(t)$.

In the case of the discrete system, the formula is transformed as follows:

$$u^{[t]} = \sum_{s=0}^{T-1} r^{[s]} f^{[t-s]}, \tag{2}$$

where the variable inside bracket is the index of discretized time step. Also, in the formula, the length of time sequence of impulse response has been limited to finite time step T.
Generally, in case of interaction with a deformable object, the interaction point indicated by the haptic device causes boundary condition that fixes displacement on the point, and interaction force on the point unknown and left to be solved.
In the equation above, $f^{[t]}$ is unknown and $u^{[t]}$ is given, hence $f^{[t]}$ is obtained by:

$$u^{[t]} = r^{[0]} f^{[t]} + \tilde{u}^{[t]}, \tag{3}$$

where $\tilde{u}^{[t]}$ represents current (i.e. at time step t) displacement that has been caused by past sequence of force, which is defined by:

$$\tilde{u}^{[t]} = \sum_{s=1}^{T-1} r^{[s]} f^{[t-s]}. \tag{4}$$

In practical computation of interaction, all past sequence of force is known, and value of $\tilde{u}^{[t]}$ is computable. By solving Equation 3 for $f^{[t]}$, the interaction force is obtained.

3.2 Multiple DoF model

Let us suppose a system with n DoF. In the discussion below, force inputs and displacement outputs are noted using $n \times 1$ vecors $F^{[t]}$ and $U^{[t]}$. Also, impulse response of the system is represented by $n \times n$ matrix $R^{[s]}$. Similarly to 1 DoF model, the input-output relationship is formulated by:

$$\begin{aligned} U^{[t]} &= \sum_{s=0}^{T-1} R^{[s]} F^{[t-s]} \\ &= R^{[0]} F^{[t]} + \tilde{U}^{[t]}, \end{aligned} \tag{5}$$

where

$$\tilde{U}^{[t]} = \sum_{s=1}^{T-1} R^{[s]} F^{[t-s]}. \tag{6}$$

In usual haptic interaction, it is a peculiar case that fixed boundary condition is applied to all DoF of the model; in most cases, the number of haptic interaction points are limited to a small number, hence the DoF with a fixed boundary condition is also limited to similar number. Interaction forces on these fixed DoFs become unknown, and also displacements on other DoFs are unknown.
The difference of boundary conditions is more clearly represented by transforming Equation 6 as follow:

$$\begin{pmatrix} U_o^{[t]} \\ U_c^{[t]} \end{pmatrix} = \begin{pmatrix} R_{oo}^{[0]} & R_{oc}^{[0]} \\ R_{co}^{[0]} & R_{cc}^{[0]} \end{pmatrix} \begin{pmatrix} F_o^{[t]} \\ F_c^{[t]} \end{pmatrix} + \begin{pmatrix} \tilde{U}_o^{[t]} \\ \tilde{U}_c^{[t]} \end{pmatrix}, \tag{7}$$

where suffix o and c indicate values on free and fixed nodes, respectively. The equation is solved for unknown values $F_c^{[t]}$ and $U_o^{[t]}$ as follows:

$$F_c^{[t]} = (R_{cc}^{[0]})^{-1} (U_c^{[t]} - \tilde{U}_c^{[t]}), \tag{8}$$

$$U_o^{[t]} = R_{co}^{[0]} F_c^{[t]} + \tilde{U}_o^{[t]}. \tag{9}$$

3.3 Interpolation of force on triangular patch

In the implementation of the algorithm that will be discussed in section 5, the proposed computation method is adapted to models whose geometry is represented by triangular mesh. Suppose the contact point p is found on a patch that has vertices p_1, p_2, and p_3, and the interface point is causing displacement $\boldsymbol{u}_p$. In our implementation, firstly, the reacting force in the case when the displacement is caused on each of these vertex nodes. Such force is computed using equation 8; we describe these forces as $\boldsymbol{F}_{p_1}$, $\boldsymbol{F}_{p_2}$, and $\boldsymbol{F}_{p_3}$. Next, by multiplying a weighting factor to each of them, we determined the force applied to those nodes:

$$\boldsymbol{f}^{[t]}_{p_1^{[t]}} = \alpha_{p_1}\boldsymbol{F}_{p_1}, \quad \boldsymbol{f}^{[t]}_{p_2^{[t]}} = \alpha_{p_2}\boldsymbol{F}_{p_2}, \quad \boldsymbol{f}^{[t]}_{p_3^{[t]}} = \alpha_{p_3}\boldsymbol{F}_{p_3}, \tag{10}$$

where α_{p_1}, α_{p_2}, and α_{p_3} are the area coordinates (or barycentric coordinate), and has relationship as $\alpha_{p_1} + \alpha_{p_2} + \alpha_{p_3} = 1$. Using the result, the feedback force is computed as reaction of the sum of the forces applied to the nodes:

$$\boldsymbol{F}_p = -(\boldsymbol{f}^{[t]}_{p_1^{[t]}} + \boldsymbol{f}^{[t]}_{p_2^{[t]}} + \boldsymbol{f}^{[t]}_{p_3^{[t]}}). \tag{11}$$

The result of this implementation when the interface point is interacting on a node is identical with the result of equation 8. Also, the resulting feedback force is continuous on the boundary of a triangular patch, or on edges and nodes.
Finally, the displacement on entire nodes of the model is computed by:

$$\tilde{\boldsymbol{u}}^{[t]}_{k^{[t]}} = \sum_{s=0}^{T-1}\sum_{i=1}^{3} R^{[s]}_{p_i^{[t-s]}k^{[t]}} \boldsymbol{f}^{[t-s]}_{p_i^{[t-s]}}. \tag{12}$$

3.4 Complexity of computation

Generally, computation of Equation 8 becomes easy if the number of fixed DoF (i.e., DoF with fixed boundary condition) is small. In cases where DoF of a model is n and number of fixed DoF is n_c, $R^{[0]}_{cc}$ becomes a $n_c \times n_c$ matrix. If the inverse of the matrix is computed using simple Gauss elimination method, the order of the computation is $O(n_c^3)$. On the other hand, the order of computation cost of $\tilde{U}_c$ and $\tilde{U}_o$ are estimated to be $O(n_c^2 \cdot T)$ and $O(n \cdot n_c \cdot T)$ respectively, considering that all of $F^{[t]}$ other than n_c components is 0 for all past and present time t.
Amount of memory that is required to store impulse response matrix is $O(n^2 \cdot T)$, and $O(n_c \cdot T)$ to store past force boundary conditions.

4. Simulation of motion

Impulse response data of IRDM is obtained through simulation of deformation caused by impulsive force. This process of precomputation causes problems in cases when the object is not fix on the ground. Interaction with non-grounded objects causes motion of the entire body of the object that lasts for a long time, and representation of the motion of an entire body is not suited for IRDM.
Let us think a method to deal with non-grounded deformable objects using IRDM. For example, in a case where a deformable object is manipulated and pinched by the user, it becomes unclear whether the displacement on the surface is derived from motion of object as a whole or deformation of the object. It is impossible to represent the motion component that causes

permanent displacement using the IRDM model. Therefore, a computation method that separates these components apart and simulates motion and deformation is necessary.
In this section, a supplemental idea that realizes non-grounded motion of the deformable model is presented.
As stated in section 3, the IRDM is based on the premise that the model is linear, however, in a precise sense, motion and deformation of deformable object must be solved as a non-linear coupled problem. For example, a spinning object is deformed by centrifugal force, the deformation can cause change in an inertia moment, and the change affects the motion of rotation. It is impossible to represent this non-linear coupled model using a linear model.
Fortunately, this non-linearity is not considered to be significant in usual interaction using hand, hence in our approach, it is assumed that motion and deformation can be separately computed. Deformation and rigid motion of an object imposed by interaction force are computed separately, and then the resulting behavior is obtained by adding then together. The deformation and motion are simulated by using IRDM and solving equation of motion respectively.

4.1 Separate simulation of motion and deformation

Our approach to integrate motion and deformation models is illustrated in Figure 1. In the pre-computation process, as stated previously, the behavior of deformable objects in response to impulsive forces is simulated using FEM program. Since the object is non-grounded or floating in space, the impulsive force causes translational and rotational motion of the entire body as well as deformation from its original shape. Our approach deals with the components of motion and deformation separately. The component of deformation is represented by IRDM; the component of motion is approximately retrieved by solving equations of motion, hence there is no need of recording the component. In the interaction process, components of motion and deformation are computed separately based on common interaction force and then added together to obtain the resulting behavior.

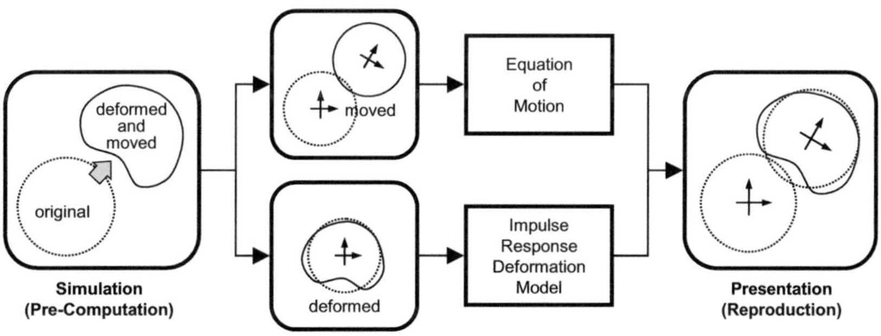

Fig. 1. Integration of motion and deformation model

4.2 Process of pre-computation

As stated in section 4.1, objects motion consists of translation and rotation. Regarding translation, the motion of the center of gravity of the object is equal to the motion of point mass that has identical mass with the object. Because of this equivalence, the translation of object is obtained by computing the center of gravity at each time step.

Regarding the rotation of the object, an estimation algorithm based on geometric matching was employed. The algorithm seeks rotation that minimizes the mean square error of node positions when the deformed object is approximately represented by a non-deformed model. The deformation component is obtained by subtracting the translational and rotational component motion from the result of the simulation. By performing the process to all combinations of DoF, the impulse response matrix $\boldsymbol{R}^{[s]}$ is determined.

4.3 Process of presentation

As stated above, the deformation component and interaction force is computed using IRDM. Then based on the interaction force, the component motion is computed by numerically solving initial-value problem of the motion equation (i.e., Newton's and Euler's equations):

$$m\frac{d\boldsymbol{V}}{dt} = \sum \boldsymbol{F}_{ext} \tag{13}$$

$$\boldsymbol{\omega} \times (\boldsymbol{I}\boldsymbol{\omega}) + \boldsymbol{I}\frac{d\boldsymbol{\omega}}{dt} = \sum \boldsymbol{\tau}_{ext}. \tag{14}$$

where M is the mass of the entire body, $\boldsymbol{I}$ is inertia tensor, $\boldsymbol{V}$ and $\boldsymbol{\omega}$ are velocity and angular velocity of the rigid body respectively, and $\boldsymbol{F}_{ext}$ and $\boldsymbol{\tau}_{ext}$ are external force and torque around the center of gravity that are operated by the user. As stated above, in our approach, mutual influence between rotation and deformation of the object is ignored. The computation cost of IRDM is dominant in the total computation cost of this approach; hence the computational advantage of IRDM is also inherited to this approach.

5. Experiment

This section describes experiments that evaluate feasibility and computation cost of deformation and interaction using IRDM.

5.1 Deformation

5.1.1 Pre-computation

Pre-computation is the process that computes impulse response data though deformation simulation; impulsive force is applied to each of all degrees of freedom and deformation response on each of all degrees of freedom is recorded. Impulse response matrix R is obtained as a collective of the data. Dynamic deformation of the model is simulated by using the FEM model that consists of tetrahedral elements.

Three models of different complexity, as shown in Figure 2 were used for the evaluation: *cat*, *bunny*, and *cuboid*; complexity of these models are summarized in Table 1. Fixed boundary condition was applied to nodes on the bottom surface patches of the models; in order to fix the models to the ground. Height of the *cat* and *bunny* models is approximately 20cm, Height and width of the *cuboid* model is 20cm and 10cm respectively. Physical parameters of all of these models were defined as: Young's modulus $E = 2000\text{N}/\text{m}^2$, Poisson's ratio $\nu = 0.49$, and density $\rho = 110\text{kg}/\text{m}^3$.

Impulse response was recorded for one second at a sampling rate of 500 Hz, hence each impulse response wave in the impulse response matrix consists of 500 point sample values. Time step of FEM simulation was changed accordingly to the velocity of object deformation from 0.1 to 2 ms. Computation time of FEM simulation that is required to obtain the entire impulse response matrix for each model is shown in Table 1, where in house FEM routine by Pentium 4 3.0GHz processor was used.

An example of impulse response of *cuboid* model is shown in Figure 3, where an impulsive downward force has been applied on the node that is indicated by an arrow. Surface elastic wave starts to diffuse from the node and propagate to entire body within approximately 16 ms.

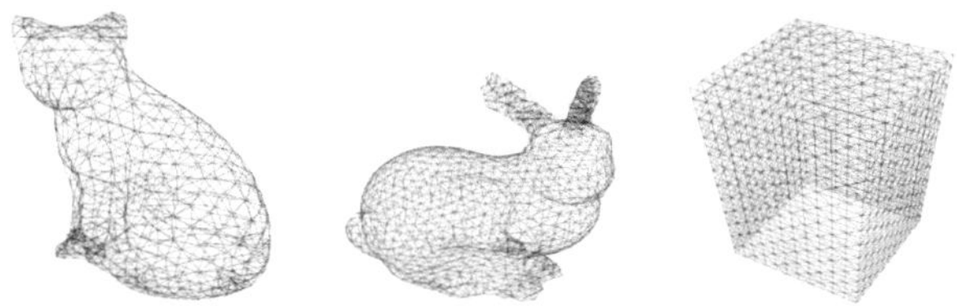

(a) cat (b) bunny (c) cuboid

Fig. 2. Experimental models

	cat	bunny	cuboid
free nodes (n)	359	826	1068
triangle patches	1796	3592	2178
entire nodes	690	1894	3312
tetrahedral elements	2421	8283	13310
pre-computation time (hr)	13.3	126.2	508.7
data size (GB)	4.3	22.8	38.2

Table 1. Complexity of models

5.1.2 Interaction

Experiments to evaluate interaction with models were carried out. Blockdiagram of the experimental system is shown in Figure 4. The system consists of PC1 (CPU:Itanium2 1.4GHz$\times$4, memory:32GB, OS:Linux) that is in charge of model computation, PC2 (CPU:Pentium3 500MHz$\times$2, OS:Windows) that serves as controller of two PHANToM devicesMassie (1996); All computation related to the IRDM model is performed by PC1. Computation of force and deformation are executed asynchronously using thread mechanism; these computations are noted as force process and deformation process respectively in the rest of this paper.

In the force process, firstly interaction point information is received from the Ethernet interface, next collision of the point with the surface of object model is detected, then interaction force on the point is computed, history of interaction force is updated, and finally the interaction force is output to the sent to PC2 through the Ethernet interface. Collision between the interaction point and the object surface is computed using an algorithm that is similar to God-Object MethodZilles & Salisbury (1995); this algorithm fits with our implementation because it eliminates ambiguity of the interaction point and provides unique displacement value. This force process is repeatedly executed every 2 ms, or at a rate of 500 Hz.

Deformation process computes deformation of an object using the history of force computed by the force process. As stated before, the impulse response matrix is a relatively large data set, and the matrix must be held on the main memory while force and deformation processes are executed. As suggested by Table 1, the data size of the *cuboid* model exceeds the size of

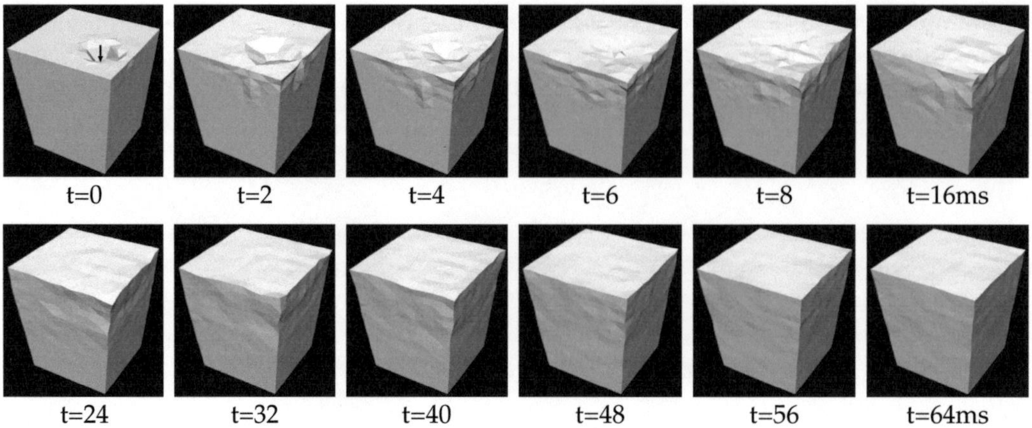

Fig. 3. Examples of impulse response

main memory of PC1, hence only half of the data where interaction force is applied to nodes on the upper half of the model were loaded on the main memory, and the area of interaction by the user was limited to these upper half nodes.
Program of force and deformation processes running on PC1 was optimized by performance using Intel Compiler and Performance Libraries. Deformation process was implemented using Math Kernel Library, parallelized by OpenMP Compiler, and three CPUs were allotted to the computation.
PC2 serves as a local controller of the PHANToM device, it simply works as bidirectional translator between the PHANToM device and Ethernet (TCP/IP) connection with PC1. Control of the device is implemented using GHOST library; control process of the library is executed at 1kHz, and in the process, the latest data that is received from the Ethernet interface is set to output force and the current position of interface point received from the device is sent back to the Ethernet interface.

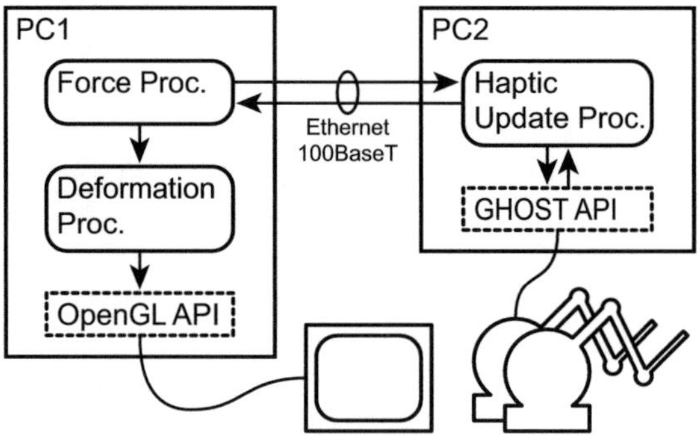

Fig. 4. System block diagram

5.1.3 Experimental Results

Figure 5 shows examples of interaction with a deformable object, where dynamic deformation is presented by a sequence of images. Since it was impossible to store images in real time, these images were generated off-line using the history of the interaction force; the arrow in the first image of each sequence indicates the point of application of force.

In figure 5(a), relatively quick motion of the *cat* model after releasing force that had been applied on a node. Figures 5(b) and (c) show the vibration of the *bunny* model that is caused by different interaction; the model was released after being pulled near and right in (b) and (c) respectively. It should be noted that different a vibration mode is presented according to different ways of interaction.

Figure 5(d) shows the deformation of *cuboid* model by step input of displacement; the force is applied to a node that is identical with the node where impulse force was being applied in Figure 3. Also, interaction force during the operation is plotted in Figure 6(a). Because of the nature of the dynamic model, interaction force gradually approaches a balance point while vibrating around the point.

Interaction using two interaction points is presented in Figure 5(e), where the user is pushing on the left and right side of the face of the *cat* model. Interaction force during the operation is plotted in Figure 6(b). As displacement on the right side increases, interaction force on the left side is also increasing.

Finally, change of interaction force while the user traced the back of the *cat* model from neck to tail is plotted in Figure 6(c). The plot suggests that interaction force is smoothly changing all through the interaction. Although invisible from the plot, subtle vibration is felt during contact with the object. The vibration is considered as an artifact that derives from sampling rate of IRDM model, which is 500Hz in our current implementation. The vibration is thought to be diminished by raising the sampling rate of the model in future implementation.

Evaluation of computation time is listed in Table 2. Computation of the interaction force comprises the evaluation of 8 for 3 to 9 times. Overhead of collision detection, communication, and graphic rendering is not included in values on the table. The computation of force is sufficiently fast for haptic presentation in that it is performed within 0.5ms per cycle even in case of using two interaction points.

Regarding deformation computation, real-time update of graphics at full video rate was not attained. For example, in the case of the *bunny* model, the update rate deteriorated to approximately 10 Hz. In spite of the low update rate, interaction was not felt greatly unreasonable subjectively, probably because the interaction is depending on information of force that is presented with less delay time.

	cat	bunny	cuboid
Computation of interaction force			
one-point	78	105	97
two-points	285	436	286
Computation of object deformation			
one-point	13040	33578	42614
two-points	26451	67339	85705

Table 2. Computation time (μs)

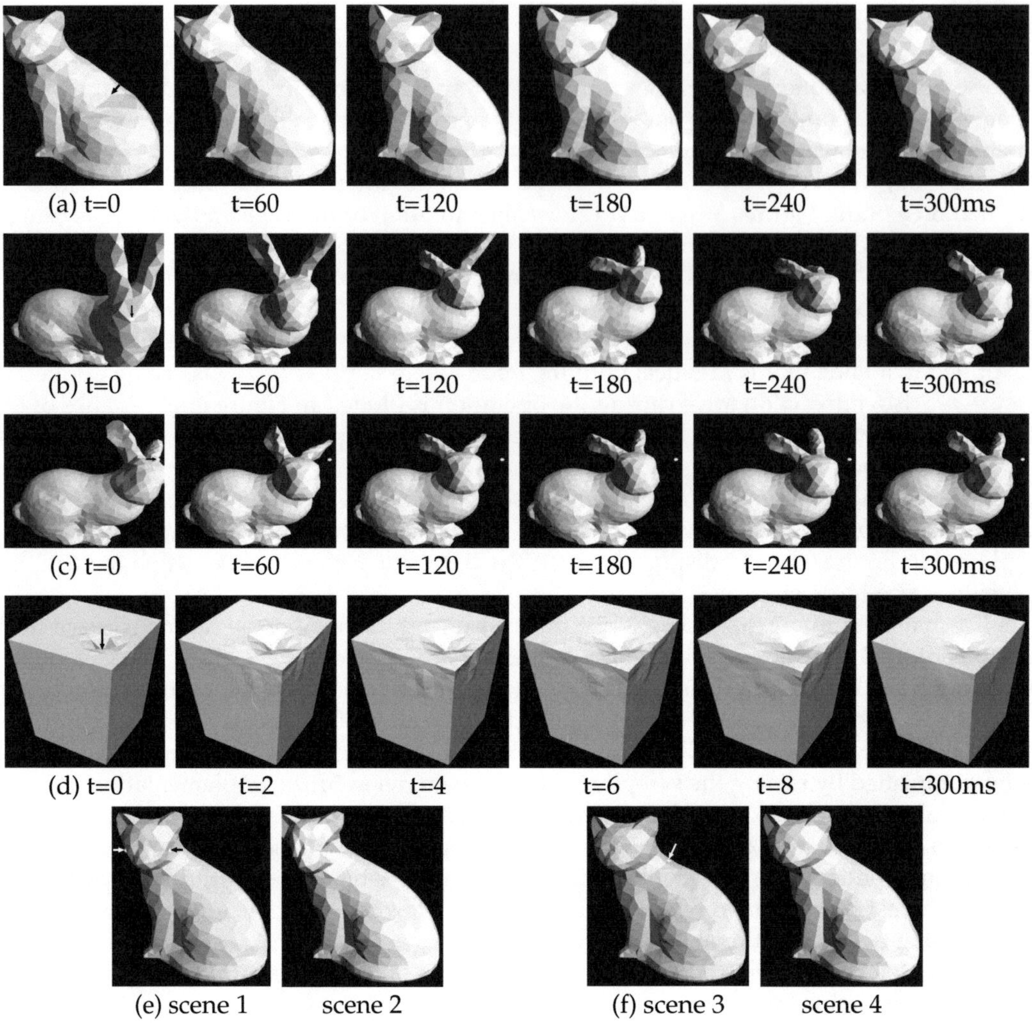

Fig. 5. Examples of dynamic deformation

5.2 Manipulation

5.2.1 Pre-computation

A *cube* model, 12cm on a side, as shown in Figure 7 was used for the evaluation; complexity of the model is summarized in Table 3. Physical parameter of the model was defined as: Young's modulus $E = 2000\text{N/m}^2$, Poisson's ratio $\nu = 0.49$, and density $\rho = 110\text{kg/m}^3$.

The computation time of FEM simulation that is shown in Table 3, where commercial FEM software (RADIOSS, Altair Engineering) with a Dual-Core Xeon 3.0GHz processor was used. Components of solid body motion and deformation were separated using the algorithm described in section 4 , and deformation component was stored as impulse response data.

Figure 8(a) shows that impulsive force is applied to the *cube* model; horizontal rightward force on the figure has been applied. Since the cube is floating, it starts moving while causing similar

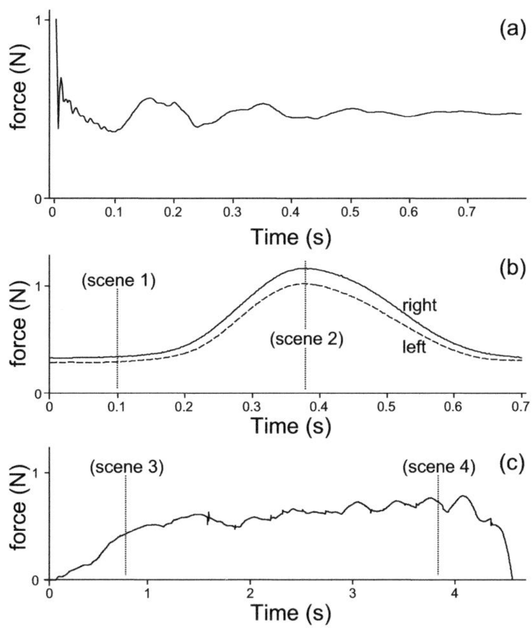

Fig. 6. Interaction force

deformation to the *cuboid* model. Figure 8(b) shows motion and deformation components separately extracted from (a).

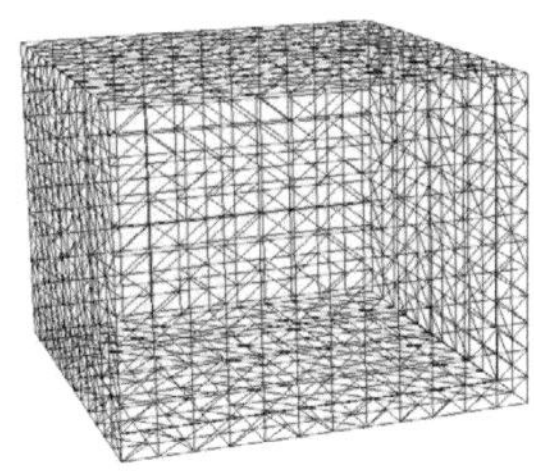

Fig. 7. Experimental model

5.2.2 Experimental Results

Figure 9 shows an example of a manipulating object; similarly to Figure 5, it presents sequences of images that were generated off-line.

In Figure 9(a), the user is picking up the top of a *cube* model and swinging right and left. Interaction force and motion of center of gravity of the object during the operation is plotted in Figure 10. The center of gravity motion is approximately sinusoidal, hence if the object is rigid, interaction force is expected to show similar sinusoidal change. However, the actual force is apparently causing oscillation at a different frequency. This fact suggests that the object is vibrating at its natural vibration frequency.

free nodes (n)	866
triangle patches	1728
entire nodes	1360
tetrahedral elements	5309
pre-computation time per d.o.f. (s)	1462
data size per d.o.f. (MB)	9.9

Table 3. Complexity of model

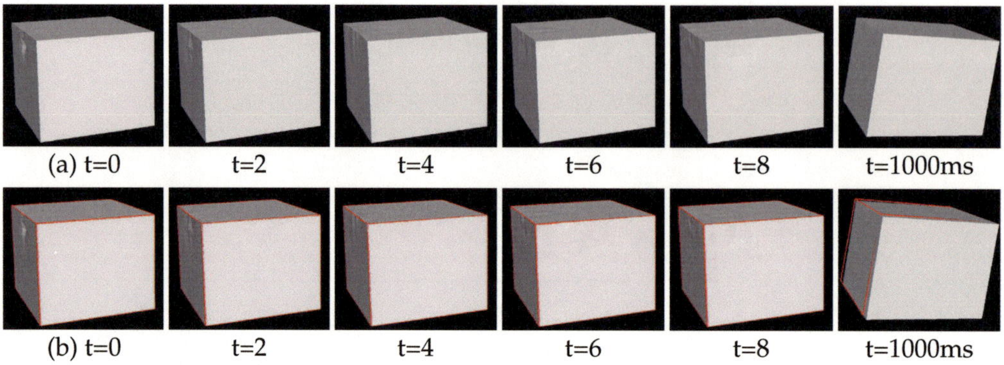

Fig. 8. Example of impulse response

Figure 9(b) shows a case where the user is tapping on a node of the *cube* model. The effect of both impact of collision and inertia of the object is reflected in the deformation and motion of the object; also, similarly to interaction with grounded models, relatively quick deformation is represented.
Figure 9(c) presents another example of interaction where the user is swirling the object along an elliptic orbit whose lengths of major and minor axes were approximately 6cm and 3cm respectively. Deformation that is caused by centrifugal force is represented naturally. Also, in the author's subjective impression, interaction force was realistic and reasonable.

6. Disucssion

6.1 Computation cost

As stated previously, computation complexity of the proposed method is independent of the DoF of the entire model n and proportional to the DoF of fixed boundary condition n_c. Experiments above have proved that, in cases when n_c is small, it was possible to compute interaction force in real time. Computation cost of deformation is $O(n^1)$ and the feature of the approach was also verified through experiments.
In cases of solving deformation by FEM, its computation cost depends on the algorithm of the solver program. The order of the computation of simple Gauss elimination method is $O(n^3)$, and even in case of using iterative algorithm such as Gauss-Seidel method, the order of computation is approximately $O(n^2)$. This fact suggests that our approach is advantageous as n becomes large.
Actually at present complexity of the model, the computation time that was required for pre-computation process suggests that it is difficult to perform the FEM simulation in real time,

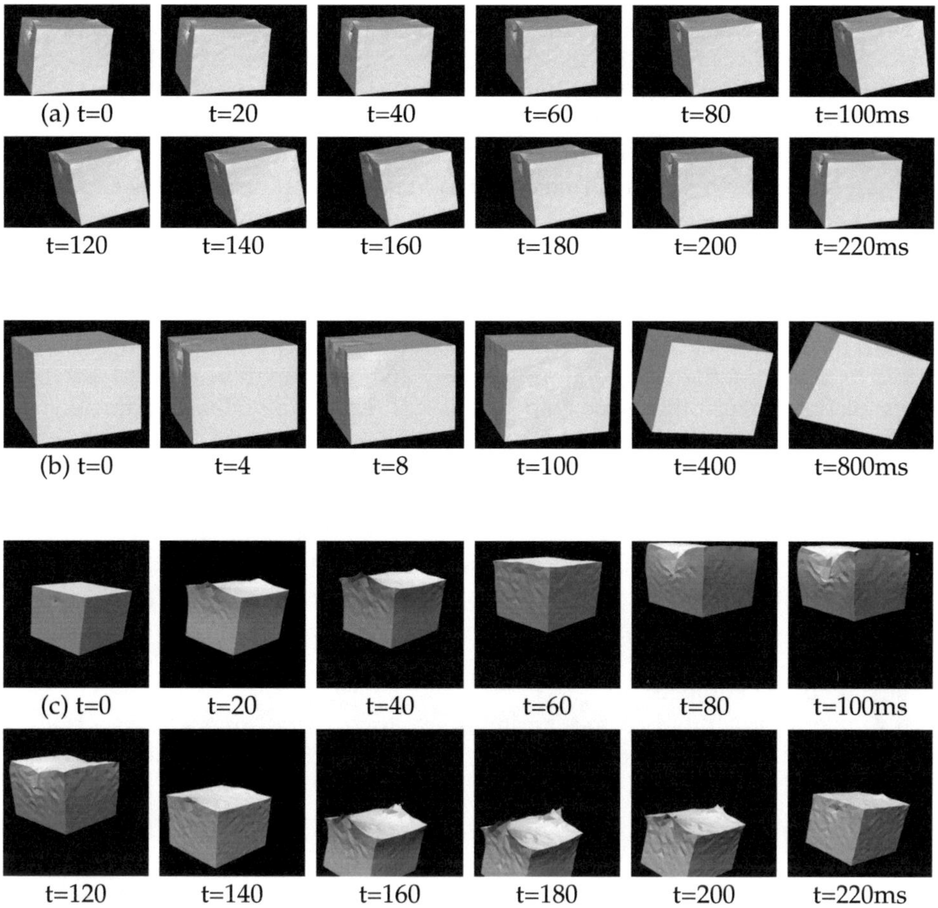

Fig. 9. Example of dynamic motion and deformation

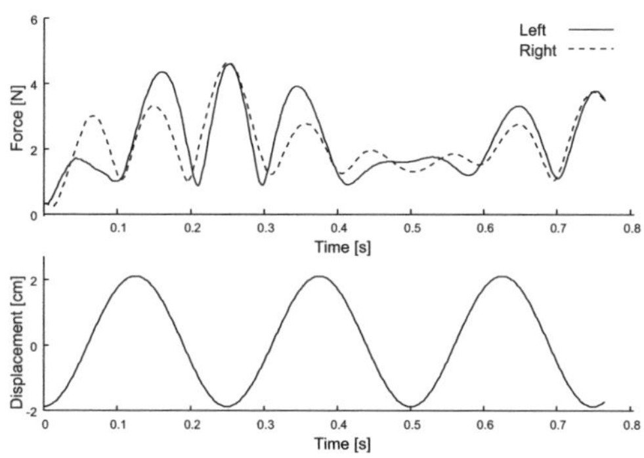

Fig. 10. Interaction force

although the FEM program that was employed for the computation was not aimed at real-time simulation.

One idea to reduce deformation computation cost is approximately generating deformed shape using reduced number of nodes; reduction of the number of nodes almost proportionally reduces computation cost, and interpolation using curved surface contributes to presentation of smooth surface. Another idea is accelerating the computation process using an advanced computing environment such as GPU. Our preliminary study is suggesting that the computation of the IRDM model is well suited to parallel computation using GPU.

6.2 Memory consumption

Regarding memory consumption, IRDM of present implementation requires a relatively large amount of memory and not applicable to practical application. Data compression method to solve this problem has been investigated, and our preliminary experiment suggests that it is possible to compress the data to approximately one-hundredth of original size by taking advantage of similarities of impulse response waves related to nodes that are geometrically close each other.

This compression method is expected to expand the area of application. For example, the size of IRDM data of the *cat* model is approximately 4GB. Since the data must be held in main memory during interaction, the computer that is available for the interaction is limited to relatively high specification machines. Also, the data size is somewhat too large to transmit over the Internet. If the data is compressed to 40MB, it is easily handled using most current computer systems and network connections.

6.3 Evaluation using subjects

Finally, evaluation of reality becomes an important topic of research, and as a basis for the research, methodology to quantify reality of dynamic interaction with deformable object must be established.

7. Conclusion

In this chapter, a novel approach to implement real-time interaction with deformable objects was presented. A core idea of the approach is modeling deformation using a set of impulse response data and computing deformation by convolution of interaction force with the model. The idea was experimentally implemented and evaluated through experiments. Also, an extension of the model to represent non-grounded object is discussed, by which manipulation of deformable object was enabled.

Finally, it should be noted that our approach is just one implementation of precomputation-based deformation model. A model of this kind has problem of trade-off between number of precomputed interaction and reality of presentation. The problem may be alleviated by introducing assumptions that effectively prevent combinational explosion of interaction patterns and by compressing precomputed data based on similarity of response. Further investigation is needed to find better representation of precomputation-based models. We hope that this paper will stimulate the discussion for such investigation.

8. References

B.Mirtich & J.Canny (1995). Impulse-based simulation of rigid bodies, *Proc. Symp. Interactive 3D Graphics* pp. 181–188.

Borst, C. & Indugula, A. (2005). Realistic virtual grasping, *Proc. IEEE VR 2005* pp. 91–98.

D.Baraff (1989). Dynamic simulation of non-penetrating rigid bodies, *Computer Graphics* **23**(3): 223–232.

G.Burdea (1996). *Force and Touch Feedback for Virtual Reality*, A Wiley-Inter-Science Publication, New York.

GHOST SDK Programmer's Guide (2002). SensAble Technologies, Inc.

Goeddeke, D., Strzodka, R. & Turek, S. (2005). Ergebnisberichte des instituts fur angewandte mathematik, *Nummer 292, FB Mathematik, Universitat Dortmund* .

James, D. L. & Fatahalian, K. (2003). Precomputing interactive dynamic deformable scenes, *Proc. ACM SIGGRAPH 2003* pp. 879–887.

James, D. & Pai, D. (1999). Artdefo, accurate real time deformable objects.

J.E.Colgate, M.C.Stanley & J.M.Brown (1995). Issues in the haptic display of tool use, *Proc. IROS95* pp. 140–145.

K.Hirota & M.Hirose (2003). Dexterous object manipulation based on collision response, *Proc. IEEE VR 2003* pp. 232–239.

K.Hirota & T.Kaneko (2001). Haptic representation of elastic object.

K.Salisbury, D.Brock, T.Massie, N.Swarup & C.Zilles (1995). Haptic rendering: Programing touch interaction with virtual objects, *Proc. Symp. Interactive 3D Graphics* pp. 123–130.

Kuchenbecker, K., Fiene, J. & Niemeyer, G. (2005). Event-based haptics and acceleration matching: Portraying and assessing the realism of contact, *Proc. WHC 2005* pp. 381–387.

Massie, T. H. (1996). *Initial Haptic Explorations with the Phantom: Virtual Touch Through Point Interaction*, Master Thiese at M.I.T.

Norton, A., Turk, G., Bacon, B., Gerth, J. & Sweeney, P. (1991). Animation of fracture by physical modeling, *Visual Computer* **7**: 210–219.

Okamura, A. M., Dennerlein, J. T. & Howe, R. D. (1998). Vibration feedback models for virtual environments, *Proc. IEEE ICRA* pp. 2485–2490 (Vol.3).

Okamura, A. M., Hage, M. W., Cutkosky, M. R. & Dennerlein, J. T. (2000). Improving reality-based models for vibration feedback, *Proc. ASME DSCD* **DSC-Vol.69-2**: 1117–1124.

Pai, D. K., van den Doel, K., James, D. L., Lang, J., Lloyd, J. E., Richmond, J. L. & Yau, S. H. (2001). Scanning physical interaction behavior of 3d objects, *Proc. ACM SIGGRAPH 2001* pp. 87–96.

Rohlf, J. & Helman, J. (1994). Iris performer: a high performance multiprocessing toolkit for real-time 3d graphics, *Proc. ACM SIGGRAPH 94* pp. 381–394.

S.Hasegawa & M.Sato (2004). Real-time rigid body simulation for haptic interactions based on contact volume of polygonal objects, *Computer Graphics Forum* **23**(3): 529–538.

Terzopoulos, D., Platt, J., Barr, A. & Fleischer, K. (1987). Elastically deformable models, *Computer Graphics* **21**(4): 205–214.

T.W.Sederberg & S.R.Parry (1986). Free-form deformation of solid geometric models, *Computer Graphics* **20**(4): 151–161.

T.Yoshikawa, Y.Yokokohji & nad X.Z.Zheng, T. (1995). Display of feel for the manipulation of dynamic virtual objects, *Trans. ASME J. DSMC* **117**(4): 554–558.

Wellman, P. & Howe, R. D. (1995). Towards realistic vibrotactile display in virtual environments, *Proc. ASME DSCD* **DSC-Vol.57-2**: 713–718.

Zilles, C. & Salisbury, K. (1995). A constraint-based god object method for haptic display, *Proc. IROS '95* pp. 145–151.

17

Haptic Interaction with Complex Models Based on Precomputations

Igor Peterlík and Luděk Matyska and Jiří Filipovič
Masaryk University
Czech Republic

1. Introduction

The real-time haptic interaction with deformable objects is an important area of research with wide range of applications in medicine and industry. The development of computer-based medical training systems (medical simulators) is perhaps the most challenging task, as it requires physically-based modelling to mimic the behaviour of soft tissues. Such models are usually based on the mathematical formulations emerging from the theory of elasticity, resulting in non-linear boundary-value problems defined over complex domains. Numerical techniques such as the finite element method, which are needed to solve these problems, are computationally expensive and therefore, their employment in the real-time interaction is not straightforward, especially in haptics, where the refresh rate over 1 kHz is required.

There have been several approaches proposed so far to address the issue of coupling the heavy computations with high refresh rate of the haptic loop. Basically, two main classes of solutions can be identified: either simplified models based on linearization or reduction are used, or some precomputation is employed before the real-time interaction takes place. In the first part of this chapter, an overview of the methods proposed in last decade is presented. Some of them are described in detail to emphasize the key concepts which are used frequently in haptic soft-tissue modeling nowadays.

In the second part of the chapter, an approach based on precomputation and interpolation of precomputed data is presented. The technique consists of two procedures: first, it is a construction of a discrete set of data, which can be performed in reasonable time on today's computers. Second, it is a fast approximation of an arbitrary deformation which is needed during the real-time interaction from the data constructed by the first procedure.

In the text, both procedures are described conceptually emphasizing the computational aspect. An algorithm of distributed state-space search used for the precomputation procedure is presented and then, three different types of the interpolations are studied and compared w. r. t. the main features which are employed in the real-time interaction phase. After general description, the evaluation of the method is briefly given using a set of experiments being done with a finite element 3D model of liver.

Finally, possibilities to couple the precomputation with interpolation, leading to a system capable of real-time interaction without off-line computations, is shortly discussed. The chapter is concluded with summary of main features and advantages of the presented systems for haptic interaction with complex models.

2. Methods for Haptic Rendering of Deformable Objects

2.1 Overview of Modelling Methods

The methods in the area of the deformation modelling can be ranged into two main groups which are denoted as non-physical and physical. The **non-physical methods** are used mainly in the computer graphics, as they are very fast and efficient. Two well-known representatives are spline modelling and free form deformations. In **spline modelling**, the curves and surfaces are represented by a set of control points and the shape of the objects is modified by changing the position of the points. The main idea of **free form deformations** is to deform the shape of the object by deforming the space in which the object is embedded. Generally, the non-physical methods are not suitable in the case when the physically realistic behaviour of the deformations is desired. In this case, the physical modeling is the only alternative.
The **physical methods** are based on the mathematical models usually formulated by *partial-differential equations* (PDE). However, the main issue of this method is represented by the fact that the resulting problem formulation is complex and the analytical solution is computationally expensive or even infeasible. To address this issue, the models are simplified to cover the essential observations and the equations are solved numerically. Bellow, the main methods used in the physical modelling are presented with a brief description.

Mass-spring damper method (MSD). The mass is concentrated in a number of nodes which are connected by springs, usually modelled as linear. When a force is applied to a node, it starts to move and pass the force via springs to the neighbouring nodes. From the computational point of view, the method is very simple and the cost of the calculation is low. Although the method is based on physical model, the major drawback of MSD systems is the insufficient approximation of real material properties. They also suffer from inaccuracy of the approximation in the case when the geometry of the object is complex.

Finite difference method (FDM). The continuous derivative which appears in the PDE-based formulations is replaced with a finite difference approximation, which is computed in points organized in regular grid which spans over the domain of the object. The technique is very accurate and efficient for the objects with regular geometry. Nevertheless, in case of complex shape of the domain, the discretization becomes extremely dense, resulting in a huge computational complexity.

Boundary element method (BEM). The differential problem is converted to the integral form, where under special conditions, the integration over the volumetric domain can be substituted by the integration over its boundary. The models based on this model cannot cope with any phenomena related to the volume of the body because of the reduction presented above, so e. g. the applied volume forces or heterogeneity of the body cannot be considered.

Finite element method (FEM). Finite elements are widely used for modelling of soft tissues, since they are directly based on the theory of the elasticity and provide very good approximation for the complex geometries. The method generally consists of discretization of the domain and mathematical re-formulation of the boundary-value problem resulting in large systems of algebraic equations. The finite element method seems to be superior to the other methods when the modelling complex bodies with non-trivial physical properties is considered. It is also suitable when volumetric operations such as cutting and tearing are to be modelled, as the entire domain of the body is included in the formulation.

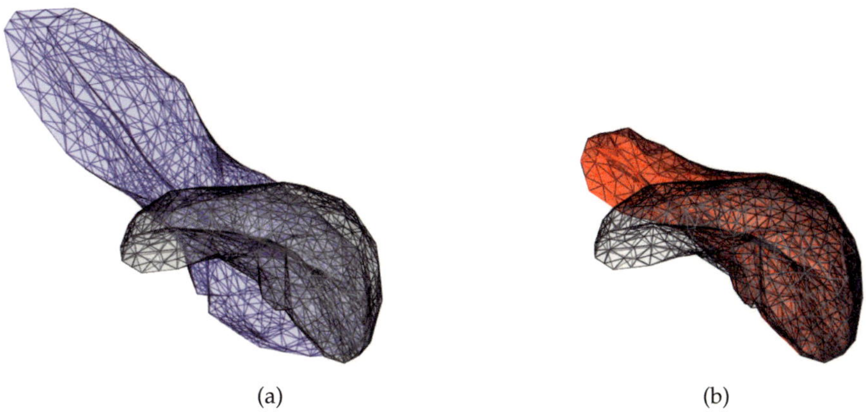

Fig. 1. Deformations of FE mesh of human liver (rest position depicted in gray) for (a) linear elasticity model, (b) non-linear Mooney-Rivlin model with complete strain tensor. In both cases, the same force was applied to a node in the left part of the body.

In the following text, we focus on the methods which are based on the physical approach. More precisely, the finite element (FE) models are briefly introduced and the most important methods employing the real-time haptic interaction are surveyed.

2.2 Overview of FE models

The physically based deformation modeling is based on relation derived within the frame of elasticity theory. A detailed description of the mathematical formulation can be found for example in Ciarlet (1988); J.T.Oden (1972); Wriggers (2008). The realistic behaviour of the objects modelled by the finite element method is usually validated w. r. t. the real measurements. In the following text, only some basic terms are informally introduced in order to identify the main issues which are associated with real-time haptic modeling of soft tissues.

When speaking about the modeling of deformations, two types of non-linearities are usually considered. First, the **geometric non-linearity** introduces non-linear relation between the displacement and strain. In case when the non-linear term in the definition of the strain tensor is neglected, only small deformations are rendered correctly. For larger deformations, the volume of the deformable object is not preserved and the overall behaviour of the object is not realistic. Therefore, geometrically non-linear model must be used when large deformations take place. The difference in behavior between geometrically linear and non-linear model is demonstrated in Fig. 1.

Second, **physical non-linearity** is introduced if non-linear relation between the stress and strain is used. The visual difference between physically linear and non-linear model is not so apparent, nevertheless, this type of non-linearity heavily affects the force response of the body and it plays an important role for realistic simulation of the soft tissues (see Misra et al. (2007)). Physically non-linear model is represented by Mooney-Rivlin material employing the non-linear incompressibility condition.

Putting it all together, both non-linearities are of a great importance when realistic modelling is required, since the geometrically linear model cannot handle large deformations properly, whereas physically linear model is limiting w. r. t. the material properties. Nevertheless, both geometrically and physically linear models have been extensively used in the past because of

lower computational cost, so they represent the first efforts in the area of haptic deformation modeling. Also, the linear models turn out to be sufficient for modeling of deformations in various laparoscopic simulators where mostly the small deformations are encountered.
Therefore, the survey of methods being proposed for the haptic deformation modeling aims at linear models first. Then, techniques proposed to combine the computationally demanding non-linear models with real-time haptic interactions are presented. In both cases, the methods employing various types of precomputations are emphasized, nevertheless some other important approaches are mentioned as well.

2.3 Linear Models

The pioneering approach in the area of soft tissue modelling is presented in Bro-Nielsen & Cotin (1996). Several important concepts proposed there have been successfully re-used since then. First, the model is completely based on physical formulation of deformations. The finite element method is used to reformulate the relations from the theory of elasticity, using the discretization of the domain by 3D tetrahedral mesh and approximation of the solution with linear shape functions over the elements, arriving to the system of linear equations

$$\mathbf{Ku} = \mathbf{f} \tag{1}$$

where $\mathbf{u}$ represents the vector of nodal displacements, $\mathbf{f}$ denotes the external forces (and applied loads) and $\mathbf{K}$ is a linear mapping between the two quantities. In this case, $\mathbf{K}$ is given by a $3n \times 3n$ matrix where n is the number of nodes in the FE mesh. It is important to realize that in the case of linearity of the system 1, the matrix $\mathbf{K}$ is invariant w. r. t. the displacement $\mathbf{u}$. The simulation is **driven by forces**, i. e. the force is regarded as the input and finite element method is used to compute the deformations.
The main goal of the proposal is to increase the speed of the simulation as much as possible at the cost of time consuming precomputation phase performed before the simulation, memory requirements and lower accuracy of the simulation. Three concepts are proposed to increase the speed of the computations shifting it towards the real-time scene. First, a concept of **condensation** is applied to the system: the nodes of the mesh are divided into *surface* and *internal* and the linear system is reordered as follows:

$$\begin{bmatrix} \mathbf{K}_{ss} & \mathbf{K}_{si} \\ \mathbf{K}_{is} & \mathbf{K}_{ii} \end{bmatrix} \begin{bmatrix} \mathbf{u}_s \\ \mathbf{u}_i \end{bmatrix} = \begin{bmatrix} \mathbf{f}_s \\ \mathbf{f}_i \end{bmatrix}. \tag{2}$$

Using the blocked system above, $\tilde{\mathbf{K}}$ and $\tilde{\mathbf{f}}$ are defined as

$$\tilde{\mathbf{K}}_{ss} = \mathbf{K}_{ss} - \mathbf{K}_{si}\mathbf{K}_{ii}^{-1}\mathbf{K}_{is} \qquad \tilde{\mathbf{f}}_s = \mathbf{f}_s - \mathbf{K}_{si}\mathbf{K}_{ii}^{-1}\mathbf{f}_i \tag{3}$$

and a reduced system $\tilde{\mathbf{K}}_{ss}\mathbf{u}_s = \tilde{\mathbf{f}}_s$ involving only the m nodes is solved during the simulation, so that $\tilde{\mathbf{K}}_{ss}$ is $3m \times 3m$ matrix for $m \ll n$. It is emphasized that although the size of the system is given only by the surface nodes, the behaviour of the system is the same as in the case of the volumetric FE model. Besides the static scenario, the dynamic system is considered as well employing *mass matrix* $\mathbf{M}$ and damping matrix $\mathbf{D}$:

$$\mathbf{M}\ddot{\mathbf{u}} + \mathbf{D}\dot{\mathbf{u}} + \mathbf{Ku} = \mathbf{f}. \tag{4}$$

It is shown that the condensation can be used also for the dynamic system in combination with the finite difference scheme applied for time integration.

Second, another improvement of the method is given by the fact that the reduced linear system is not solved by some conventional iterative method such as Conjugate Gradients, but **direct inversion** of the stiffness matrix is used. And this is the place where the precomputations are employed: since the matrix is constant, the inverse $\mathbf{K}^{-1}$ can be precomputed and stored explicitly before the interaction starts. The authors admit that the direct inversion can introduce numerical errors and moreover, the resulting inverse is no more a sparse matrix. Nevertheless, the trade-off between the precomputation overhead, memory requirements and accuracy on one side and speed of the computations on the other is acceptable. Third, a concept of **selective matrix vector multiplication** is employed: since the force vector $\mathbf{f}$ contains only a small number of non-zero elements, the product $\mathbf{K}^{-1}\mathbf{f}$ is done selectively, i. e. only for the non-zero positions of the vector $\mathbf{f}$. It is shown however, that this approach can be applied only in the case of static model, since in the dynamic case, the corresponding force vector is not sparse any more due to the finite difference scheme.

Putting it all together, the computation of deformations based on static finite element model using the condensation, precomputation of direct inverse of the stiffness matrix and selective multiplication is denoted as **fast finite elements**. The method is used for the visual simulation of human leg with 700 surface nodes (as the number of internal nodes does not affect the speed of the simulation) achieving 20 frames per second. Further, the authors proposed a parallelized version of the technique based on domain decomposition. However, the parallel implementation employing iterative solution method (preconditioned CG) turned out to be too slow to achieve a real-time performance. Another extension proposed by the author in (Bro-Nielsen, 1996) is represented by cutting in finite element system which is performed by removing an element from the FE mesh. Such a modification requires precomputation of the stiffness matrix inverse which is computationally demanding and cannot be done in real-time. Nevertheless, much more efficient solution is proposed by the authors based on Woodbury formula as shown in (Hager, 1989).

The concept of condensation of linear FEM introduced above is used also in (Frank et al., 2001). The nodes are divided into two categories — those with given boundary conditions and other nodes which are not directly involved in the interaction. A cube model composed of linear tetrahedra is used for testing: besides a mesh with 375 DOFs, meshes with higher resolution are used, both increasing the order of the elements (*p-resolution*) and decreasing the element size (*h-resolution*). The reduced system is solved by direct (Cholesky) and iterative methods (Conjugate Gradients, Preconditioned-Jacobi and Preconditioned SSOR). It is shown that only for the coarsest model, the haptic refresh rate (500 Hz) can be achieved using the Conjugate Gradients method. Beside the conventional solvers, full multi-grid method is used exploring the hierarchy of meshes.

The method based on condensation and precomputation of the inverse of the stiffness matrix is also used in work published in (Gosline et al., 2004). The simulation of the fluid pockets inside a soft tissue is developed using static linear elasticity and static fluid analysis. The speed of the simulation is improved significantly by condensation and off-line precomputation of the inverse matrices needed for solving of the reduced system. The needle insertion is then simulated on a single machine using a model with 82 surface nodes achieving refresh rate of more than 500 Hz.

The condensation technique is also explored in (Chai et al., 2001) where a step towards non-linear models is proposed. The soft tissue is divided into two parts: first, a small area that is in direct contact with operation tool is modeled more accurately, so the stiffness matrix corresponding to the nodes from the area is updated during the interaction. The rest of the

body is considered as linear, so the corresponding part of the stiffness matrix is constant and the condensation and inverse precomputation can be applied. The authors state that real-time refresh rate is achieved in their setting for a body with 6601, including 861 nodes in the "operational part" of the body, however, no further quantitative results are provided.
The combination of precomputation and condensation is proposed in Nikitin et al. (2002). In the off-line mode, the global stiffness matrix K was assembled and further, the block $(K)_S$ with rows corresponding to the visible surface nodes was inverted obtaining $(K^{-1})_S$. By this simplification, time as well as storage were reduced significantly.
A novel approach to soft tissue modelling was proposed in Cotin et al. (1996). The model introduced in the paper is based on linear elasticity, so small deformations are modelled realistically. The equations are reformulated using the finite element method; the domain of the body is discretized by tetrahedral FE mesh. The simulation is proposed as being **driven by displacements**: the displacements of the fixed nodes are given as input (so called applied loads) whereas the response forces are computed by the FEM together with the overall deformation. Mathematically, the method of Lagrange multipliers is used to obtain the reaction forces corresponding to the applied loads as shown in (Cotin et al., 1999). The method results in augmented system $\hat{\mathbf{K}}\hat{\mathbf{u}} = \hat{\mathbf{f}}$ defined as

$$\begin{bmatrix} \mathbf{K} & \mathbf{A} \\ \mathbf{A}^\top & \mathbf{0} \end{bmatrix} \begin{bmatrix} \mathbf{u} \\ \boldsymbol{\lambda} \end{bmatrix} = \begin{bmatrix} \mathbf{f} \\ \mathbf{u}^* \end{bmatrix} \tag{5}$$

where $\mathbf{u}^*$ is a vector of pseudo-loads given by the prescribed displacement of touched nodes and $\mathbf{A}$ is a rectangular constraint sparse matrix containing non-zero elements only at the positions corresponding to the nodes with prescribed displacements. Further, the vector $\boldsymbol{\lambda}$ represents the Lagrange multipliers that is obtained by the solution of the system. The method is suitable for the haptic interaction using impedance-control devices, as the multipliers $\boldsymbol{\lambda}$ directly represent the response force associated with the pseudo-loads given by $\mathbf{u}^*$.
In order to speed up the rate, the linearity of the model is explored resulting in **superposition principle**. For each free surface node k that is not fixed by a boundary condition, an elementary displacement is applied and two quantities are precomputed: first, for each other free node $n \neq k$ the displacement induced by the applied load in node k is computed and stored as tensor $[\mathbf{T}^{\mathbf{u}}_{\mathbf{nk}}]$. Second, elementary response force at node k is calculated and stored as tensor $[\mathbf{T}^{\mathbf{f}}_{\mathbf{k}}]$. All the tensors are computed by solving the linear system using the conjugated gradient method. During the interaction, both the actual deformation of the body and reaction force are calculated from the precomputed tensors using the superposition principle, i. e. the deformation in node n and force in node k are computed as

$$\mathbf{u}_n = \sum_{l=1}^{M} [\mathbf{T}^{\mathbf{u}}_{\mathbf{nl}}][\mathbf{u}^*_l] \qquad \mathbf{f}_k = [\mathbf{T}^{\mathbf{f}}_{\mathbf{k}}][\mathbf{u}^*_k] \tag{6}$$

where $\mathbf{u}^*_k$ is corrected applied load computed from the actual prescribed displacement of the node k. Computing time of 7 ms is reported using the superposition principle for a model with 1400 nodes and 6500 tetrahedra after 8 hours of precomputations of the tensors corresponding to the elementary displacements.
The model presented above is based on static equilibrium and the simulation of the dynamic behaviour is replaced by a **quasi-static** approach: the deformation at time t is computed as static solution of the boundary-value problem utilizing the boundary conditions imposed in time $t-1$. Due to the precomputation of the tensors, any modifications of mesh topology (e. g.

tearing or suturing) are not possible. Therefore in Cotin et al. (2000a), a dynamic **tensor-mass** model is proposed allowing for topology changes. In this case each tetrahedron is associated with data structure containing tensors corresponding to its vertices and edges. The mass and damping matrices in the dynamic Eq. 4 are considered as diagonal (simplification known as **mass lumping** that allows to decouple the motion of the nodes, so the dynamic Eq. 4 can be integrated separately for each node of the FE mesh.

The fourth-order Runge-Kutta integration method is used to solve the dynamic equation in each step of the simulation. The actual force is calculated from the tensors, which are used to determine the local stiffness between the adjacent tetrahedra. The tensors are also computed separately for each tetrahedron directly during the haptic loop. The cutting and tearing is implemented by tetrahedra removal. In this case, only the tensors corresponding to the adjacent elements are updated. The refresh rate of 40 Hz for mesh with 760 vertices and 4000 edges is reported on computer equipped with 233 MHz Alpha processor.

Since the mass-tensor model is computationally more expensive than the previous one based on the precomputations, **hybrid approach** combining both is proposed in Cotin et al. (2000b). The part of the tissue where the operation takes place is modelled by the dynamic mass-tensor model allowing cutting, whereas the rest of the body is modeled by the quasi-static model based on the precomputation of the elementary displacements. The model is further extended in Picinbono et al. (2002) by introducing anisotropic properties To achieve the haptic refresh rate, **force extrapolation** is proposed when the forces updated at the frequency of 500 Hz are generated from the simulation based on the hybrid model running at 30 Hz. Linear extrapolation is employed, so the force estimation $\mathbf{f}^e(t)$ at time t, $t_n \leq t < t_{n+1}$ is computed as

$$\mathbf{f}^e(t) = \mathbf{f}_n + \frac{t - t_n}{t_n - t_{n-1}}(\mathbf{f}_n - \mathbf{f}_{n-1}). \tag{7}$$

In Delingette & Ayache (2005), the methods based on hybrid model and further extensions are summarized and the successful implementation of hepatic surgery simulator **Laparoscopic Impulse Engine** is reported.

In (James & Pai, 2002), a unified treatment of the elastostatic simulation is proposed based on Green functions. It is shown that any deformation simulated by the linear model can be computed using the Green functions as a basis. Algorithm for precomputation of the Green function based on capacitance matrices is presented and example for boundary elements is derived.

A model based on linear static elasticity is presented in Popescu & Compton (2003). To achieve the high refresh rate needed for the real-time haptic interaction, **small-area paradigm** is introduced, being an extension of the displacement-driven interaction based on the solution of the augmented system $\hat{\mathbf{K}}\hat{\mathbf{u}} = \hat{\mathbf{f}}$ defined by 5. It is assumed that the area affected by the haptic device is small, i. e. the vector of prescribed displacements $\mathbf{u}^*$ has only m elements where m is a small number. Moreover, no external forces are applied on the tissue, so the vector $\mathbf{f}$ is zero. Since linear elasticity is considered, the stiffness matrix $\mathbf{K}$ is constant (as well as its inverse) and only the constraint matrix $\mathbf{A}$ varies within the augmented matrix $\hat{\mathbf{K}}$ during the interaction. However, the system 5 can be inverted as

$$\begin{bmatrix} \mathbf{u} \\ \boldsymbol{\lambda} \end{bmatrix} = \begin{bmatrix} \mathbf{K} & \mathbf{A} \\ \mathbf{A}^\top & \mathbf{0} \end{bmatrix}^{-1} \begin{bmatrix} \mathbf{f} \\ \mathbf{u}^* \end{bmatrix} = \begin{bmatrix} \tilde{\mathbf{P}} & \tilde{\mathbf{Q}} \\ \tilde{\mathbf{R}} & \tilde{\mathbf{S}} \end{bmatrix} \begin{bmatrix} \mathbf{0} \\ \mathbf{u}^* \end{bmatrix} \tag{8}$$

where

$$\tilde{\mathbf{P}} = \mathbf{K}^{-1} - (\mathbf{K}^{-1}\mathbf{A})(\mathbf{A}^\top\mathbf{K}^{-1}\mathbf{A})^{-1}(\mathbf{A}^\top\mathbf{K}^{-1}) \quad (9)$$

$$\tilde{\mathbf{Q}} = (\mathbf{K}^{-1}\mathbf{A})(\mathbf{A}^\top\mathbf{K}^{-1}\mathbf{A})^{-1} \quad (10)$$

$$\tilde{\mathbf{R}} = (\mathbf{A}^\top\mathbf{K}^{-1}\mathbf{A})^{-1}(\mathbf{A}^\top\mathbf{K}^{-1}) \quad (11)$$

$$\tilde{\mathbf{S}} = (\mathbf{A}^\top\mathbf{K}^{-1}\mathbf{A})^{-1}. \quad (12)$$

Having the vector $\mathbf{u}^*$ of the prescribed displacements, the corresponding force response stored in $\boldsymbol{\lambda}$ is computed as $\boldsymbol{\lambda} = \tilde{\mathbf{S}}\mathbf{u}^*$. The matrix $\tilde{\mathbf{S}}$ can be computed in real-time: using the relation 12, a submatrix $\tilde{\mathbf{S}}^{-1} = \mathbf{A}^\top\mathbf{K}^{-1}\mathbf{A}$ of $\mathbf{K}^{-1}$ is extracted. The small area paradigm implies that $\tilde{\mathbf{S}}^{-1}$ is a small $m \times m$ matrix that can be inverted easily by some direct method to obtain $\tilde{\mathbf{S}}$.
The computational framework is set as follows: first, the sparse matrix $\mathbf{K}$ is assembled using finite element method and its inverse $\mathbf{K}^{-1}$ is computed and stored. During the interaction, the reaction force $\boldsymbol{\lambda}$ is computed on high-frequency by inverting the small submatrix of $\mathbf{K}^{-1}$ and multiplying by $\mathbf{u}^*$. The overall deformation is computed by analogy using the definition of the matrix $\tilde{\mathbf{Q}}$. The implementation of the model showed good results: using Silicon Graphics Onyx2 with 8 CPU running at 250 MHz, the computation of the mesh deformation was 0.0277 s and 0.0493 s respectively, for the models with 6,000 and more than 10,000 elements, with 30 vertices included in the touched area.
Another area of research is represented by exploration of linear viscoelastic models and their employment in haptic rendering and interaction. A robust adaptive method for simulating dynamic deformations of a viscoelastic object in real time is described in Debunne et al. (2001). The explicit FEM is assembled and solved for each element independently through a local approximation. The method further employs the adaptive refinement in order to increase the quality of modeling in the vicinity of the interaction.
An algorithm for real-time haptic interaction with linear viscoelastic model is presented in Sedef et al. (2006). The viscoelastic materials are regarded as *materials with memory* as the time-dependent response history is recorded that is evident from the constitutive relation between the stress and strain. Using relations from the linear elasticity and generalized Maxwell solid, the model of linear viscoelasticity is derived resulting in linear time-dependent equation

$$\mathbf{f}_{int}^{n+1} = \mathbf{K}\mathbf{u}^{n+1} + \mathbf{h}_H^{n+1} - \mathbf{K}_H\mathbf{u}^n \quad (13)$$

where $\mathbf{u}^{n+1}$ and $\mathbf{u}^n$ are the vectors of nodal displacement in current and previous time steps, $\mathbf{u}$ and $\mathbf{u}_H$ are the constant stiffness matrix and history stiffness matrix and finally, $\mathbf{h}_H^{n+1}$ is the history vector at the current step computed from the recursive formula for the internal stress variables. The algorithm is divided into two parts: first, the stiffness matrix $\mathbf{K}$ is assembled and inverted and history stiffness matrix $\mathbf{K}_H$ is calculated. Second, the time step loop calculations are executed where in each step $n+1$, the actual history vector $\mathbf{u}_H^{n+1}$ is calculated together with the actual force response $\mathbf{f}^{n+1}$ and displacement field $\mathbf{u}^{n+1}$. Despite the precomputation of the matrix inverse $\mathbf{K}^{-1}$, the calculations proposed for a single time step are still too expensive to be performed in real-time at haptic refresh rate. Therefore, another precomputation is proposed exploiting the linearity and superposition principle. For each surface node, two sets of data are precomputed: first, force response of the node and displacement response of the neighbouring nodes corresponding to unit displacement applied for 30 second to given surfaces node. Second, a unit step force is applied to each surface node for 10 ms and the recovery displacement response is recorded for the node and its neighbours lasting 30 seconds.

Above, several techniques used for haptic interaction with linear deformation models have been briefly described. It can be concluded that linearity of the mathematical model can be explored very efficiently to achieve the real-time performance as proposed in the papers referenced above. However, as stated before, the linear models provides only limited accuracy and are not generally suitable for large-deformation physical modelling. Therefore, the techniques employing non-linear models proposed recently are briefly introduced in the next section.

2.4 Non-linear models

The shortcomings of linear models are studied in (Picinbono et al., 2001) showing that it is not invariant w. r. t. the rotations and therefore, large deformations cannot be modelled realistically. Therefore, the **non-linear mass-tensor** model is proposed as an extension of the linear version described in the previous section. Geometrical non-linearity is introduced by complete Green-StVenant strain tensor establishing second order relation between strain and displacement. The relation between the stress and strain is, however, linear so material non-linearity is not considered. In order to improve the behaviour of the tissue, anisotropic term is added to the definition of the elastic energy. The formula determining the force applied in a vertex i of a tetrahedron $\mathbf{T}$ is composed of sum of linear, quadratic and cubic term w. r. t. the displacement:

$$\mathbf{f}_p^{\mathbf{T}_i} = 2\sum_j \mathcal{B}_{pj}^{\mathbf{T}_i}\mathbf{u}_j + \sum_{j,k}\left[2(\mathbf{u}_k \otimes \mathbf{u}_j)\mathcal{C}_{jkp}^{\mathbf{T}_i} + (\mathbf{u}_j\mathbf{u}_k)\mathcal{C}_{pjk}^{\mathbf{T}_i}\right] + 4\sum_{j,k,l}\mathcal{D}_{jklp}^{\mathbf{T}_i}\mathbf{u}_l\mathbf{u}_k^\top\mathbf{u}_j \tag{14}$$

The linear term is treated as shown in the previous section: for each tetrahedron, local 3×3 *stiffness tensors* $\mathcal{B}_{pj}^{\mathbf{T}_i}$ are computed for vertices and edges and the results are accumulated to the global stiffness tensors. It is shown that the higher-order terms can be treated similarly: *stiffness vectors* $\mathcal{C}_{jkp}^{\mathbf{T}_i}$ are computed for vertices, edges and triangles in case of the quadratic term whereas *stiffness scalars* $\mathcal{D}_{jklp}^{\mathbf{T}_i}$ are calculated for vertices, edges, triangles and tetrahedra. The structures are then used during the simulation to compute forces for each vertex, edge, triangle and tetrahedron. The Newtonian differential equation

$$\mathbf{M}\ddot{\mathbf{u}} + \mathbf{D}\dot{\mathbf{u}} + \mathbf{K}(\mathbf{u}) = \mathbf{f} \tag{15}$$

is used as follows: the mass matrix $\mathbf{M}$ and damping matrix $\mathbf{D}$ are replaced by diagonal matrices m_i and γ_i and $\mathbf{f}$ is computed using the Eq. 14. Finally, the equation is decoupled for each vertex separately resulting in

$$m_i\ddot{\mathbf{p}}_i = \gamma_i\dot{\mathbf{p}}_i + \mathbf{f}_i \tag{16}$$

where $\mathbf{p}_i$ is the actual position of a vertex. The explicit integration scheme is used to update the vertex position $\mathbf{p}^{t+1}$ in the following step:

$$\left(\frac{m_i}{\Delta t^2} - \frac{\gamma_i}{2\Delta t}\right)\mathbf{p}_i^{t+1} = \mathbf{f}_i + \frac{2m_i}{\Delta t^2}\mathbf{p}_i^t - \left(\frac{m_i}{\Delta t^2} + \frac{\gamma_i}{2\Delta t}\right)\mathbf{p}_i^{t-1} \tag{17}$$

that can be computed in the time step providing the force $\mathbf{f}_i$ is computed from the stiffness data according to 14.

The modifications of the mesh topology caused by cutting or tearing are implemented by removing the involved tetrahedra and updating the stiffness data of adjacent elements. In order to increase the performance, a **non-linear model with threshold** is proposed: the model is treated as non-linear only if the current deformation exceeds a defined threshold. Otherwise, linear elasticity is preserved requiring much less computations of the stiffness data. The refresh rate is then increased to 20 Hz from 8 Hz for a model with 6342 tetrahedra Picinbono et al. (2003).

The geometrically non-linear dynamic model of soft tissue with physically linear isotropic material is studied in (Zhuang & Canny, 1999). The finite element method is used to discretize the continuous elasticity problem resulting in time-dependent non-linear Eq. 15 with both **M** and **D** constant mass and damping matrices and $\mathbf{K}(\mathbf{u})$ stiffness matrix which only depends on the actual displacement vector **u**. Newmark explicit integration method is used to reformulate the nonlinear Eq. 15 to obtain three linear equations

$$\mathbf{u}_{n+1} = \mathbf{u}_n + \dot{\mathbf{u}}_n \Delta t_n + \frac{1}{2}\ddot{\mathbf{u}}_n \Delta t_n^2 \tag{18}$$

$$(\mathbf{M} + \frac{1}{2}\Delta t_n \mathbf{D})\ddot{\mathbf{u}}_{n+1} = \mathbf{f}_{n+1} - \mathbf{K}(\mathbf{u}_{n+1}) - \mathbf{D}(\dot{\mathbf{u}}_n + \frac{1}{2}\ddot{\mathbf{u}}_n \Delta t_n) \tag{19}$$

$$\dot{\mathbf{u}}_{n+1} = \dot{\mathbf{u}}_n + \frac{1}{2}(\ddot{\mathbf{u}}_n + \ddot{\mathbf{u}}_{n+1})\Delta t_n. \tag{20}$$

The computational bottleneck disallowing the real-time computations is given by the Eq. 19 where inverse of the matrix $(\mathbf{M} + \frac{1}{2}\Delta t_n \mathbf{D})$ is needed. Two variants are proposed in (Zhuang & Canny, 2000): first, mass-lumping approximation is used resulting in diagonalization of both mass matrix **M** and damping matrix **D**. Although the approximate version of matrix **M** is acceptable, diagonalization of **D** results in loss of viscous property of the material. Therefore, another approach is proposed based on precomputation exploring the fact that both **M** and **D** are constant and Δt_n is the only varying term depending on the stability of the explicit integration method. The main idea is to restrict the time step Δt_n to small set of values $\{\Delta t_i\}$ and to precompute $(\mathbf{M} + \frac{1}{2}\Delta t_i \mathbf{D})^{-1}$ for each Δt_i. Further optimizations are suggested to minimize the number of floating-point operations needed for the calculations of the equations derived by the Newmark method. The total length of 0.06 s needed for a single time step is reported in (Zhuang, 2000) for a uniform mesh with 1331 elements. The haptic refresh rate is achieved by the force interpolation using two adjacent simulation steps.

Both geometrically and physically non-linear model was presented in (Wu et al., 2001). The finite element formulation is given for the Mooney-Rivlin and Neo-Hookean materials using the complete non-linear strain tensor. Dynamic scenario is considered based on the Eq. 15 where both mass and damping matrices are diagonalized. The explicit integration scheme is used in the simulation. The main contribution is represented by implementation of on-line mesh refinement using **dynamic progressive meshes**. To achieve the real-time refresh rate, all the invariant components of the model, such as constant matrices **M** and **D**, Jacobian matrix **J** needed for the calculation of the stress, are precomputed off-line together with their inverses. Moreover, the constant data structures needed for the mesh refinement and coarsening are identified and precalculated. For a model of tissue with 2200 vertices, refresh rate of 20 frames per second is reported using Pentium III PC running at 800 MHz. The stability of the explicit integration is improved by **multigrid method** proposed in (Wu & Tendick, 2004). A multigrid time integrator is developed to perform the integration of the Eq. 15 using *restriction*, *interpolation* and *solution* operator to implement the projections between multiple unstructured independent meshes. Finally, the parallel version of the multigrid-based simulation is described in (Wu et al., 2004). The performance of the solver is evaluated together with the stability of the simulation showing promising results suitable for the real-time processing.

A new approach based on precomputation is proposed (Barbič & James, 2005) based on **formal model reduction** of StVenant-Kirchhoff. The reduction, which is suitable for large deformations but only a small local strain, is based on projection of the displacement vector $\mathbf{u}$ with $3n$ elements onto vector $\mathbf{q}$ with r elements where $r \ll 3n$ using time-independent basis represented by a $3n \times r$ matrix $\mathcal{P}$: $\mathbf{q} = \mathcal{P}\mathbf{u}$. The nontrivial task of generation of the basis $\mathcal{P}$ is studied in detail and method based on combination of *linear vibration modes* and mass-scaled PCA is suggested. The reduced equation of motion is derived resulting in

$$\ddot{\mathbf{q}} + \tilde{\mathbf{D}}(\mathbf{q}, \dot{\mathbf{q}}) + \tilde{\mathbf{R}} = \tilde{\mathbf{f}} \tag{21}$$

where $\tilde{\mathbf{D}}$ and $\tilde{\mathbf{R}}$ are r-dimensional vectors representing the reduced forces. Further, it is shown that for the StVenant material, the components of the reduced internal forces $\tilde{\mathbf{K}}$ are cubic polynomials in $\mathbf{q}$:

$$\tilde{\mathbf{R}} = \mathbf{P}^i \mathbf{q}_i + \mathbf{Q}^{ij}\mathbf{q}_i\mathbf{q}_j + \mathbf{S}^{ijk}\mathbf{q}_i\mathbf{q}_j\mathbf{q}_k \tag{22}$$

where $\mathbf{P}^i$, $\mathbf{Q}^{ij}$ and $\mathbf{S}^{ijk}$ are constant polynomial coefficients that can be efficiently precomputed; e. g. for object with 14,444 elements, the time of 97.4 minutes needed for the precomputations on single 3 GHz Pentium workstation is reported. The polynomial coefficient can be used also to compute the derivative of $\tilde{\mathbf{R}}$ w. r. t. $\mathbf{q}$ corresponding to the reduced tangent stiffness matrix. During the simulation, the reduced Eq. 21 is integrated in time using implicit integration Newmark method. In each time step, only single Newton-Raphson is executed instead of iterating until convergence is achieved. The Newton-Raphson method requires calculation of reduced stiffness and tangent stiffness matrix that is done using the precomputed coefficients $\mathbf{P}^i$, $\mathbf{Q}^{ij}$ and $\mathbf{S}^{ijk}$ and dense linearized $r \times r$ system is solved. The model reduction is applied to objects having between 2000 and 14500 element resulting in systems with $r \in \{12, 15, 30\}$. The refresh rate ranging between 45 Hz to 470 Hz is achieved using GPU acceleration. The approach based in the modal reduction is reused in (Barbič & James, 2008) where contact modeling is analyzed for 6DoF haptic rendering of object with complex geometry.

The approach published in (De et al., 2006) is based on non-linear elasticity and mesh-free discretization known as **point-associated finite field**. Instead of FE discretization, the PAFF-based discretization of the domain provided by scattered points is used together with interpolation generated by least-squares method. Comparing to standard FEM, PAFF introduces additional error in the simulation. Moreover, the non-linearity of the tissue in the vicinity of the operation tool is considered, whereas linear model is employed on the rest of the body. Likewise in FEM, the PAFF discretization leads to a system of non-linear algebraic equation that can be solved by Newton-Raphson methods where in k-the iteration, the correction of the displacement vector $\Delta\mathbf{u}^{(k)}$ is computed by solving a linearized system and the displacement vector is updated, i. e.

$$\mathbf{K}_T(\mathbf{u}^{(k-1)})\Delta\mathbf{u}^{(k)} = \mathbf{f} - \mathbf{K}(\mathbf{u}^{(k-1)}) \tag{23}$$

$$\mathbf{u}^{(k)} = \mathbf{u}^{(k-1)} + \Delta\mathbf{u}^{(k)} \tag{24}$$

where the tangent stiffness matrix $\mathbf{K}_T$ dependent on $\mathbf{u}$ is composed of the constant stiffness matrix $\mathbf{K}_0$ from the linear small deformation problem and varying component $\mathbf{K}_S(\mathbf{u})$. Clearly, the iterative calculations composed of assembling and inverting the large matrix $\mathbf{K}_T$ cannot be done in real-time and therefore it is assumed that there is a scalar s such that $\mathbf{K}_T = s\mathbf{K}_0 + \Delta\mathbf{K}_S$

and s can be found easily minimizing the Frobenius norm $\|\mathbf{\Delta K}_S\|_F$. Then, the time-consuming solution given by Eq. 23 can be replaced by computation $\mathbf{\Delta u}^{(k)} = \frac{1}{s}\mathbf{K}_0^{-1}(\mathbf{f} - \mathbf{K}(\mathbf{u}^{(k-1)})$. Since the matrix $\mathbf{K}_0$ is constant, its inverse can be precomputed before the iteration starts. The total length of computations needed to calculate the scalar s is about 0.14 s on Pentium 4 running at 2 GHz, provided the inverse $\mathbf{K}_0^{-1}$ has been already precomputed taking about 20 minutes.
Another approach based on standard finite element method is presented in (Deo & De, 2009). First, commercial software is used to compute a set of deformations corresponding to a selected boundary-value problems. The precomputed data are then used for training of *radial basis function networks*, i. e. neural networks being associated to each node of the FE mesh. The neural network is then used to determine the reaction force for given node displaced by the surgical tool. The error of the approximation given by a network composed of 50 neurons after training on 3000 precomputed sample is given being 5% when processing 5000 samples not included in the training set. The real-time computation of the force response takes about 1.5 μs for a 3D model having 2839 elements after 19 hours of precomputations.
A novel algorithm for non-linear real-time FE modelling is presented in (Taylor et al., 2007). It is based on **total Lagrangian explicit dynamics** (TLED) (Miller et al., 2007). The algorithm is composed of two phases: first, all the element shape function derivatives are precomputed together with the mass matrix. Second, the real-time simulation is executed where in each time step, prescribed displacements are applied to the model and total nodal forces are precomputed together with strain-displacement matrix and stresses. These are incorporated in the central difference method to compute the update displacement vector. The algorithm is re-implemented within the SOFA framework (Allard et al., 2007) on nVidia GPU accelerators using CUDA programming language as shown in (Comas et al., 2008). The performance of the CUDA-based implementation is demonstrated on medical application—cataract surgery. Employing the FE model simulating non-linear, viscoelastic and anisotropic behaviour of the lens, undergoing large deforamations, one step of the TLED algorithm is reported to run at 284 Hz and 87 Hz for two models of lens having 4058 and 47633 elements, respectively.

In this section, the algorithms employing non-linear models for modelling the deformations in real-time have been briefly presented. Also in this case, several techniques rely heavily on the precomputations, so the time-consuming computations needed for realistic non-linear modeling are performed separately from the high-frequency haptic loop. However, it turns out that the techniques are often restricted to a certain type of a material (e. g. for which the model reduction can be performed) or they are limited by the instability in the case when explicit time-integration schemes are employed.

3. Haptic Interaction Based on Precomputation of Configuration Spaces

3.1 Approximation from Discretized Spaces

Similarly as in the case of the algorithms surveyed in the section 2, our algorithm is focused on the solution of the problem how to combine the high refresh rate of the haptic interaction and computationally expensive finite element calculations which are needed to computed the deformations and response forces. There are two main goals in the design of the algorithm:

1. the deformation model is based on non-linear static finite element formulation and there are no *a priori* assumptions about the complexity of the mathematical model, however, the topological changes are not considered;

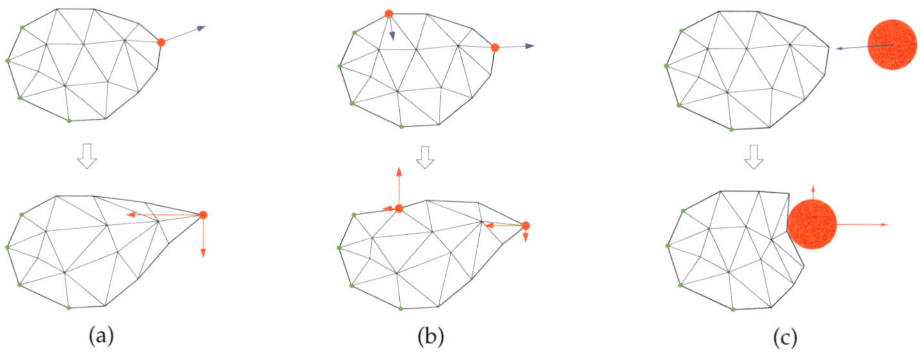

Fig. 2. Interaction modes: (a) point interaction, (b) multi-point interaction, (c) probe interaction

2. the computations needed for rendering the response force can be done within the haptic loop computed on today's computers.

The algorithm is designed for the **displacement-driven interaction**: it is supposed that the positional data $\mathbf{p}$ provided by the haptic device are somehow mapped to a non-homogeneous boundary conditions $\mathbf{b}_N$ which are applied within the boundary-value problem being solved to obtain the response forces and the overall deformation of the object. The positional data $\mathbf{p}$ are therefore regarded as a **control parameter** of the simulation and mathematically, it is represented by a vector which fully determines the position and the orientation of all the haptic devices involved in the simulation. The mapping between the positional data $\mathbf{p}$ and the non-homogeneous boundary conditions $\mathbf{b}_N$ depends on the type of the interaction between the haptic device and deformable body. We distinguish two basic types of the interaction depending on this coupling as follows.

Single-point interaction: the haptic device is represented by a single point in 3D space called *haptic interaction point* (HIP), so the positional data $\mathbf{p}$ are given by the spatial coordinates of the point. If the point collides with the deformable object, it snaps to a vertex of the FE mesh representing the body. Without loss of generality, it is assumed that HIP snaps to the closest vertex of the mesh which becomes **active node**. The mapping between the positional data $\mathbf{p}$ and the non-homogeneous boundary conditions $\mathbf{b}_N$ is straightforward: the displacement of the active node is given directly by the actual position of the haptic device. The scenario is depicted by Fig. 2(a).

An extension of the approach can be proposed: e. g. **multiple-point interaction** is considered if there are at least two HIPs (manipulated by e. g. two haptic devices) each being attached to one active node. In this case, the control parameter $\mathbf{p}$ contains the prescribed positions of all the active nodes which are attached to the corresponding HIPs and the mapping to the boundary conditions is again straightforward. The scenario is illustrated by Fig. 2(b).

Probe interaction: the HIP is represented by a **probe** which moves in the space. If the probe collides with the FE mesh, the nodes in collision are identified and the boundary conditions are assembled. Mathematically, the positional data $\mathbf{p}$ are given by the position

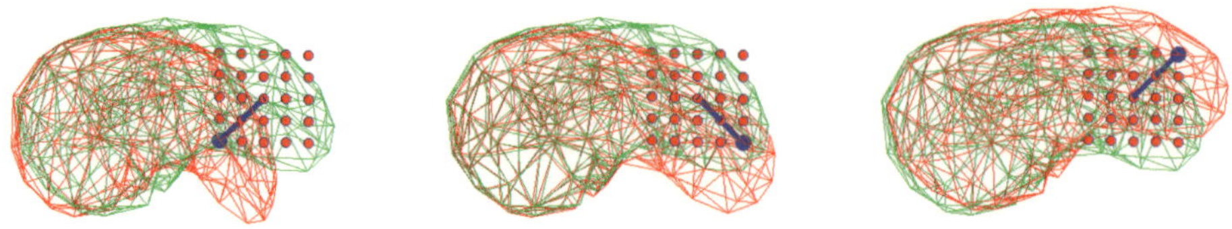

Fig. 3. Three configurations of the deformable body stored in the grid. Two-dimensional projection is used for the simplicity.

of the probe. However, the mapping between $\mathbf{p}$ and non-homogeneous boundary conditions $\mathbf{b}_N$ is not straightforward anymore, as the displacements of the nodes being in collision with the probe are not a priori known. To obtain the boundary conditions, some advanced methods developed in the contact modelling can be applied, e. g. using the **gap function** as studied in Saupin et al. (2008). The scenario with spherical probe being manipulated by a 3DoF haptic device sourcing its position in 3D space is depicted by Fig. 2(c). Alternatively, the probe with more complicated or irregular shape can be employed, e. g. representing a surgical tool. In this case, not only the position but also the orientation of the probe can be given by the positional data $\mathbf{p}$.

Let us now focus on the single-point interaction, so the vector $\mathbf{p}$ represents directly the prescribed positions for some given set of nodes. Therefore, given a FE mesh discretizing the body being fixed in the space, the finite element method is used to compute a generally non-linear mapping $\mathbf{p} \rightarrow (\mathbf{h}, \mathbf{u})$ where $\mathbf{h}$ and $\mathbf{u}$ are the response forces and nodal displacements corresponding to the prescribed positions $\mathbf{p}$. It is supposed that the mapping $\mathbf{p} \rightarrow (\mathbf{h}, \mathbf{u})$ is unique, i. e. for given prescribed positions $\mathbf{p}$, the boundary-value problem has a unique solution. This is given by the ellipticity of the problem being considered. Formally, the state of the model in a given step of the simulation is fully given by a configuration C which is defined as a triple $\langle \mathbf{p}, \mathbf{h}, \mathbf{u} \rangle$.

If the vector of the prescribed positions is updated, i. e. $\mathbf{p} \rightarrow \mathbf{p}'$ due to the change in the position of HIP, the corresponding response forces $\mathbf{h}'$ and the deformation $\mathbf{u}'$ of the body are computed, i. e. the *transition* $C \rightarrow C'$ between the two configurations is constructed. Exploiting this concept, the haptic interaction can be regarded as travelling through configuration space when each step is given by a transition between two configurations. Finally, the set of all configurations with defined mapping $C \rightarrow C'$ is denoted as a configuration space $\mathcal{C}$. Apparently, $\mathcal{C}$ is infinite and continuous, however, it is *bounded*: i. e. only configurations having the amplitude of reacting forces $|\mathbf{h}|$ lower than some finite constant F_{max} are included in the space. This is given by the physical limitation of each haptic device, as the force which can be displayed by the device is bounded by some F_{max} which ranges from 10 N to 20 N for today impedance-control devices.

In terms of the configuration spaces introduced above, the main idea of our approach is to construct a discretization — a finite subspace $\mathcal{D} \subset \mathcal{C}$, so that $\mathcal{D}$ can be constructed in finite time and stored. Considering the single-point interaction, it is assumed that the discretization is provided by a regular uniform grid $\mathcal{G}$ where each point $\mathbf{g} \in \mathcal{G}$ is given by three spatial coordinates (g_x, g_y, g_z). The center of the grid is denoted as $\mathbf{g}_0$ and there are two parameters determining the distributions of the grid points: $r_{\mathcal{G}}$ is the radius of the grid, i. e. the distance between the grid center and the outermost grid point, and $d_{\mathcal{G}}$ is the distance between two

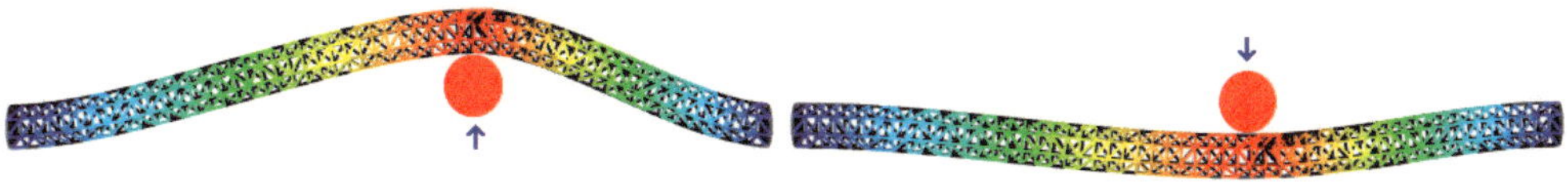

Fig. 4. Two deformations of the object for the identical position of the probe (depicted by the filled red circle) showing the non-flatness of the probe interaction model. On the left, the probe comes from the space below the deformable body, on the right it comes from the space above the body (the directions are depicted by the blue arrows.

adjacent grid points being measured along the coordinate axes. It is important not to confuse the regular uniform grid $\mathcal{G}$ with the unstructured finite element mesh of the deformable body. Provided the active point has been already selected, the grid $\mathcal{G}$ is employed by the precomputation-approximation scheme which composed of two separated phases as follows:

Off-line phase. The discrete configuration space $\mathcal{D}_\mathcal{G}$ is constructed using $\mathcal{G}$: the active node is placed to each grid point $\mathbf{g}$ and the corresponding configuration $C_\mathbf{g} = \langle \mathbf{g}, \mathbf{u}, \mathbf{h} \rangle$ is constructed and inserted into $\mathcal{D}_\mathcal{G}$. In other words, it is simulated that the control parameter is set to each $\mathbf{g}$ and the corresponding response force and deformation are computed. The grid of configurations for the single-point interaction is demonstrated by Fig. 3.

The points of the grid are traversed systematically: having a configuration $C_\mathbf{g}$ stored in the point $\mathbf{g}$, the transitions $C_\mathbf{g} \rightarrow C_{\mathbf{g}'}$ for all adjacent grid points $\mathbf{g}'$ are constructed and this process is recursively repeated until there is a configuration associated to each grid point of the grid $\mathcal{G}$. The algorithm of systematic grid traversal together with distributed version is described in section 3.2.

On-line phase. The haptic interaction is executed for given active node, approximating the response forces and overall deformation for arbitrary position of the haptic device using the precomputed data. More precisely, in each step of the haptic loop, the positional data $\mathbf{p}$ are acquired and the corresponding configuration $\tilde{C}_\mathbf{p} = \langle \mathbf{p}, \mathbf{u}, \mathbf{h} \rangle$ is computed by interpolation from the precomputed configurations stored in $\mathcal{D}_\mathcal{G}$. The interpolation techniques suitable for the real-time interaction are studied in section 3.3.

The concept of the space-division scheme presented above can be used also for other types of the interaction. First, in case of the multi-point interaction, the higher-order grid must be employed; e. g. for two active points A and B, the six-dimensional grid is considered, where each point is given as six-tuple $(g_x^A, g_y^A, g_z^A, g_x^B, g_y^B, g_z^B)$. During the off-line phase, the configurations are computed for all the grid points, i. e. for all the positions of the two points A and B within the positions of the discretized space. In the on-line phase, the response forces are interpolated for each active node separately using the precomputed data.

Second, in case of the probe-interaction, the adaptation is a bit more complex. Let us assume a spherical probe, as shown in the Fig. 3. The position of the probe is given by a three-dimensional vector containing the position of the probe center. Therefore, the space containing the deformable object is discretized by three-dimensional grid in the same way as in the single-point interaction. However, it is important to realise that for one position of the probe, there can be multiple distinct configurations as shown in Fig. 4; the overall deformation and reaction forces depend on the direction $\mathbf{d}$ of the probe motion. Therefore, **enriched regular grid** $\mathcal{G}^*$ is introduced: it is based on the grid $\mathcal{G}$, but additionally, for given grid point $\mathbf{g}$, there are multiple levels $l_1, l_2, \ldots l_L$ corresponding uniquely to particular directions. During the off-line phase, the enriched grid is traversed systematically: being in a configuration $C^l_{\mathbf{g}}$ stored in a grid point $\mathbf{g}$ and a level l, the transition towards a grid point $\mathbf{g}' = \mathbf{g} + \mathbf{d}$ is constructed as follows:

1. the configuration C' corresponding to the position $\mathbf{g}'$ is computed taking into account the original position $\mathbf{g}$ from which the probe has arrived.
2. The configuration C' is stored as $C^{l'}_{\mathbf{g}'}$ where l' is the identifier of the level associated with the direction $\mathbf{d} = \mathbf{g}' - \mathbf{g}$.

Having the configurations stored in the enriched grid $\mathcal{G}^*$, the space can be traversed easily during the on-line phase, since the actual direction can be used to identify the level where the target configuration is stored.

Clearly, the concept of levels can be combined with higher-order grids for the case when there are more positional data identifying the state of the probe. For example if rotations are given for the probe using for example 6DoF device, the 6D enriched grid can be established, where the grid points corresponds to the positional and rotational data and the levels are used to handle the transitions between various positions and orientations of the probe.

In the following section, the algorithms for both the construction of the configuration space and interpolation from the precomputed data are briefly described. For the sake of simplification, the algorithms for single-point interaction are presented. The reader interested in concept of enriched grid used for the real-time haptic interaction with precomputations can find detailed description in Křenek (2003); Peterlík (2009).

3.2 Algorithm for the Space Construction

The generation of the configuration space is a time-consuming procedure, since the configurations for the entire grid must be systematically constructed. The procedure is studied on two levels: first, it is necessary to specify the method of calculation of single configuration C. Second, the algorithm for the overall construction of the configuration space must be given, i. e. the order in which the computations of the transitions are done to generate the entire space.

The computation of one transition $C_A \to C_B$ is performed as follows. According to the assumption formulated in the previous section, the non-linear finite element formulation is employed. The simulation is driven by the control parameter $\mathbf{p}$ which represents the vector of the prescribed positions for a given set of nodes. Provided, the configuration C_A is known as $C_A = \langle \mathbf{p}_A, \mathbf{h}_A, \mathbf{u}_A \rangle$ whereas the new position for the configuration C_B is $\mathbf{p}_B$, the vector of the prescribed displacements in C_A and C_B can be computed easily as $\mathbf{u}^*_A = \mathbf{p}_A - \mathbf{p}_0$ and $\mathbf{u}^*_B = \mathbf{p}_B - \mathbf{p}_0$ where $\mathbf{p}_0$ is the rest position of the active nodes. Within the finite element formulations, the vector $\mathbf{u}^*$ represents a non-homogeneous Dirichlet condition. There are several methods to include the condition into the system—elimination, penalization or Lagrange multipliers. In our case, the method of the Lagrange multipliers is employed, since it directly yields the response forces which are to be determined. The method results in the augmented non-linear system of algebraic equations $\hat{\mathbf{K}}([\mathbf{u}|\boldsymbol{\lambda}]) = [\mathbf{f}|\mathbf{u}^*]$ which must be solved iteratively. In our approach, a technique combining the incremental loading and Newton-Raphson methods is considered. First, using $\mathbf{u}^*_A$ and $\mathbf{u}^*_B$, an **incremental loading** path $\{\mathbf{u}^*_A = \mathbf{u}^*_{(0)}, \mathbf{u}^*_{(1)}, \ldots \mathbf{u}^*_{(M)} = \mathbf{u}^*_B\}$ is constructed and the sequence of non-linear systems $\hat{\mathbf{K}}([\mathbf{u}|\boldsymbol{\lambda}]) = [\mathbf{f}|\mathbf{u}^*_{(i)}]$ with initial estimation $\mathbf{u}^*_{(i-1)}$ is solved for $i = 1, \ldots, M$.

Further, the solution in each step is obtained by **Newton-Raphson method**: having some estimation of both the nodal displacement vector $\mathbf{u}^{(j)}$ and Lagrange multipliers $\boldsymbol{\lambda}^{(j)}$ in the j-th iteration of the method, new estimations are computed as

$$\mathbf{u}^{(j+1)} = \mathbf{u}^{(j)} + \Delta\mathbf{u}^{(j+1)} \tag{25}$$

$$\boldsymbol{\lambda}^{(j+1)} = \boldsymbol{\lambda}^{(j)} + \Delta\boldsymbol{\lambda}^{(j+1)} \tag{26}$$

where both corrections $\Delta\mathbf{u}^{(j+1)}$ and $\Delta\boldsymbol{\lambda}^{(j+1)}$ are computed by solving the linearized system

$$\hat{\mathbf{K}}'([\mathbf{u}^{(j)}|\boldsymbol{\lambda}^{(j)}]) \begin{bmatrix} \Delta\mathbf{u}^{(j+1)} \\ \Delta\boldsymbol{\lambda}^{(j+1)} \end{bmatrix} = \begin{bmatrix} \mathbf{f} \\ \mathbf{u}^*_{(i)} \end{bmatrix} - \hat{\mathbf{K}}([\mathbf{u}^{(j)}|\boldsymbol{\lambda}^{(j)}]) \tag{27}$$

where $\mathbf{u}^*_{(i)}$ is the vector of the prescribed displacement given in the actual step i of incremental loading and $\hat{\mathbf{K}}'([\mathbf{u}^{(j)}|\boldsymbol{\lambda}^{(j)}])$ is the tangent stiffness matrix computed as the spatial derivative of the non-linear mapping $\hat{\mathbf{K}}([\mathbf{u}|\boldsymbol{\lambda}])$. The estimation for the first step of the Newton-Raphson method in the first step of the incremental loading method is taken from the starting configuration C_A: $\mathbf{u}^{(0)}_{(0)} = \mathbf{u}_A$ and $\boldsymbol{\lambda}^{(0)}_{(0)} = \mathbf{h}_A$. There are two criteria for the Newton-Raphson method to stop: first, if the residual given by the right-hand side of the Eq. 27 is less then a chosen ε in some iteration of the Newton-Raphson method, the resulting solution converges and is considered to be a valid data. Second, the iteration process is also stopped after N maximum iterations also if the condition above does not hold. In this case, the calculation is considered as non-convergent and the data is considered to be invalid. After obtaining the results in the last step M of the incremental loading path, new configuration C_B is set as $C_B = \langle \mathbf{p}_B, \boldsymbol{\lambda}_{(M)}, \mathbf{u}_{(M)} \rangle$. It is to be noticed that besides the final configuration C_B the intermediate configurations $C_{(1)}, \ldots C_{(M-1)}$ are computed due to the incremental loading. These can be stored in an additional file, because they can be utilized by a special type of the interpolation as shown in the following section.

On the higher lever, the order in which the transitions are computed is to be specified. In Peterlík (2008), the *layer-based technique* is proposed for the efficient construction of the configuration spaces. Originally, the technique was designed for sequential processing, however, it could be also executed in distributed environment, as the independent transitions within one layer can be computed concurrently. Further, in Filipovič et al. (2009) a distributed algorithm is proposed for state space generation based on client-server scheme. Briefly, the client is represented by a *scheduler process*, whereas on the server side, there is a pool of *solver processes* which compute the transitions simultaneously. All the processes involved in the computations communicate among themselves using message-passing.

The main role of the scheduler is as follows. It maintains two data-structures:

1. table t_C of all configurations which are to be computed. In the table, each configuration is marked either as *unknown*, *assigned* or *computed*;
2. table t_S of all the solver processes being in the pool. Each server is marked either as *idle* or *busy*.

Initially, each configuration is marked as unknown and each solver is marked as idle. In the first step, the scheduler finds such a position $\mathbf{g}$ within the grid $\mathcal{G}$ that there is no collision between the HIP and the FE mesh, i. e. the both the force $\mathbf{h}$ and nodal displacement $\mathbf{u}$ are zero and therefore, the corresponding configuration is marked as known. Then, the algorithm executes as follows:

1. If there is an idle solver S_i, choose an unknown configuration C' such that the transition $C \rightarrow C'$ can be constructed, i. e. the configuration C is marked as computed. If there is such C', send the configuration C to the solver S_i together with the target prescribed displacement, mark C' as assigned and S_i as busy.
2. If there is still some unknown configuration, but no transition can be actually computed, wait until some of the processes completes the computations and sends the notification message. Let's assume, that a solver S_i sends a notification about completing the computation of a configuration C'. In this case, mark S_i as idle and mark configuration C' as computed.
3. Repeat the steps 1. and 2. until all configurations are marked as computed.

On the other side, the protocol of the solver process is simpler: the computation of a transition $C \rightarrow C'$ is initialized by a message from the scheduler, determining the initial configuration C and the target prescribed displacement. After the computation is completed, the configuration is stored and the notification message is sent to the server. Anytime the configuration is needed by some solver, the scheduler can provide the identifier of the solver which keeps the configuration. The concept of notifications is again utilized to obtain the configuration from some solver in order to start the computation of a new transition.
The construction of the configuration space is completed, providing all the configurations are marked as computed. This also implies that all the solvers are also marked as idle and all the configurations have been stored on a disk and can be used for the haptic interpolation being executed in the second phase.

3.3 Real-time Interaction

Basically, the real-time interaction is implemented by a single process called *force interpolator*, which first reads all the precomputed data from the disk and then, for the actual position of the HIP, it identifies the adjacent points of the precomputed configuration space and computes the interpolation to approximate the actual force. The interpolation can be performed inside the haptic loop, as it requires only a small number of operations with data stored in the computer memory.
It is important to note, that the precomputed data are utilized also for the approximation of the object deformation for the visualization purposes. The interpolation of the surface nodes is computed by visual interpolator and rendered by visual thread running at 25 Hz. Albeit the interpolation of larger data set must be performed, the refresh rate of the visual rendering runs on much lower frequency.
In this part we focus on interpolation of the response force during interaction. Without loss of generality, it is assumed that the force is represented by three components Each component (f_x, f_y, f_z) is interpolated from the precomputed forces separately. In the following, two different methods are briefly studied: *polynomial* and *radial-based function* interpolation. For each of them, linear and cubic versions are employed.

Polynomial interpolation. As the polynomial interpolation works with regularly distributed data, only the configurations $C_{\mathbf{g}}$ stored in the points of the 3D grid are used. Having the actual position $\mathbf{p}_A$ of the active node displaced by HIP, the neighboring points $\mathbf{g}_i$ of the 3D grid must be first determined. For the simplest case of *trilinear interpolation*, eight neighboring nodes are needed for the interpolation. The main advantage of the tri-linear interpolation is that the computations are very simple, since only a small number of operations is needed. Precisely, the interpolation of a single force component requires about 250 floating point operations, regardless the size of the grid. Therefore, the interpolation of the force vector can be performed on single-core computer easily. On the other hand, there are some drawbacks of this method. Although the interpolation is continuous, it is not smooth in the moment of switching between cells: the actual values are instantly interpolated from different values. E.g. when traversing the cell boundary via the face, four vertices are switched, whereas when traversing via corner, even seven vertices must be switched resulting in non-smoothness of the interpolation in the moment of cell switching.

Another alternative within the frame of the polynomial method is *tricubic interpolation*. In this case, 64 precomputed configurations are needed for approximating a single value. The resulting tricubic form is $f(x, y, z) = \sum_{i,j,k=0}^{3} a_{ijk} x^i y^j z^k$. where the coefficients a_{ijk} can be calculated from the precomputed forces within the off-line phase of the interaction. Due to the non-linearity of the underlying problem, the convergence for some configurations does not have to be achieved during the off-line phase. Comparing to the tri-linear interpolation, the complexity of cubic interpolation increased, as it requires about 2.000 floating-point operations to be evaluated for the interpolation of one component of the force vector. Nevertheless, this number is again independent on the size and density of the grid. When comparing to the performance of today's processors, the interpolation of the force vector can be easily computed within the haptic loop running on high frequency. The problem with non-smooth behaviour is not solved completely, nonetheless, the smoothness is significantly improved, as in the worst case (HIP crossing the grid point) 27 out of 64 interpolation points remain unchanged. In the best case, when the face is traversed, even 48 out of 64 interpolation points remain unchanged.

Radial-basis function interpolation. There are two reasons why a method interpolating from scattered (irregularly distributed) data is desired:

- both the configurations in the points of the regular grid and in the intermediate states can be utilized and
- before the interpolation takes place, the configurations computed in non-convergent iterations can be excluded from the precomputed data.

To meet these requirements, *radial-basis function* (RBF) interpolation was employed. Briefly, having a set of values $f(\mathbf{x}_j)$ for positions $\mathbf{x}_j$ placed irregularly in space, then arbitrary value of $f(\mathbf{x})$ for a position $\mathbf{x} = (x, y, z)$ is calculated as:

$$f(\mathbf{x}) = \sum_{i=1}^{N-1} w_i \phi(|\mathbf{x} - \mathbf{x}_i|) \tag{28}$$

where ϕ is a chosen function, e. g. $\phi(r) = r$ or $\phi(r) = r^3$ determining linear and cubic interpolation, respectively.

The weights w_i can be computed during the precomputation phase by solving and decomposing a linear system which is assembled by substituting the known values $f(\mathbf{x}_j)$ into Eq.28. Having the weights precomputed, the interpolation for the actual position can be computed quickly even for large number of interpolation points. Unlike the polynomial interpolation, the time complexity of the computations inside the haptic loop linearly depends on the number of nodes in the grid. Nevertheless, the computations can be performed real-time for sufficiently large grids using today computers. As the data can be scattered in the configuration space, an arbitrary subset of the precomputation configurations can be used in order to increase the efficiency and accuracy of the interpolation.

As shown above, polynomial as well as the RBF interpolation can be explored in the on-line phase of the scheme to approximate the actual configuration in real-time using the precomputed data. In the following section, some details concerning the implementation and evaluation of the algorithms presented before are given.

3.4 Evaluation and Discussion

In our prototype implementation, both the scheduler and pool of the solvers were implemented in C++ programming language. The communication between the remote processes was provided by Message-Passing Interface (MPICH implementation ver. 1.2.7 communicating over sockets). The configurations represented by the various deformation of the object were using using GetFEM, an open-source FEM library. The solution of the linearized system computed in each iteration of the Newton-Raphson method was performed by MUMPS linear solver (see P.R.Amestoy et al. (2000)). Further, the force interpolator was implemented for the interpolation techniques presented in section 3.3. The interpolation of the forces was stably running at a frequency of 1,000 Hz on a workstation equipped with 2× Dual Core AMD Opteron 285 processor. Similarly, precomputed nodal displacements were utilized by shape interpolator computing the actual deformation of the body for the visualization purposes running at 25 Hz.

The experiments evaluated in the next part of this section were performed on 3D model of human liver obtained from the INRIA repositories. The model was meshed by TetGEN mesh generation tool resulting in two meshes with 1777 elements (501 nodes) and 10280 elements (2011 nodes), respectively. The real length of the model was about 22 cm. We use both Mooney-Rivlin and StVenant-Kirchhoff material laws; in the case of Mooney-Rivlin, the incompressibility conditions were imposed by mixed formulation.

Extensive testing has been performed to validate the approach based on the precomputation of the configuration spaces. The evaluation can be divided into two parts as follows. First, the accuracy of the methods has been studied. For this purpose, a large number of configurations has been computed and stored for a random values of the positional data. The approximated counterparts have been generated by the interpolation of the precomputed spaces, the forces and displacements have been compared and evaluated. The mean and maximum errors have been calculated using the large set of computed data as shown in Peterlík & Matyska (2008). The tests have been performed for four different densities of the grid and 4 different interpolation methods. It was concluded that the density of the grid is the important factor, nevertheless, it can be compensated by using RBF interpolation which gives good results also for sparse grids. For example, the tri-linear interpolation on the dense grid ($d_{\mathcal{G}} = 6.667\,mm$) results in relative mean error below 1%, which is roughly the same as the results obtained by the RBF cubic interpolation on the sparse grid ($d_{\mathcal{G}} = 20\,mm$). Similar results were obtained also w. r. t. the maximum errors: tri-linear interpolation on the dense grid results in maximum relative error achieving 30%, whereas the RBF interpolation on the coarse grid results in maximum relative error under 20%.

The second part of the testing focused on the precomputation phase. Here, the behaviour of the distributed algorithm was studied w. r. t. the scalability and speed-up. It was shown that the algorithm scales almost linearly for 4, 8, 16, 32 and 64 solver processes in the pool. Furthermore, the experiments with geographically distributed environment were performed using two clusters being located more than 300 km from each other. It was confirmed that the algorithm is resistant to latencies as the scalability was not affected by the distance between the two clusters. Finally, the total length of the computations was studied. The cubic complexity of the computations w. r. t. the resolution of the grid $\mathcal{G}$ was confirmed. Nevertheless, it was shown that also for detailed models, the precomputation can be done in time which is acceptable. For example, using the cluster with 64 CPUs, the construction of the configuration space on grid with 14146 grid points ($d_{\mathcal{G}} = 6.667\,mm$) took less than 3 hours for a model with 10270 elements employing the Mooney-Rivlin material with incompressibility conditions. For the comparison, construction of the space for grid with 514 nodes ($d_{\mathcal{G}} = 20\,mm$) using the same mesh and model took less than 30 minutes.

The quantitative evaluation and detailed discussion of the results obtained for the method presented in this chapter can be find in Peterlík (2009); Peterlík et al. (2010), where also the convergence analyses for various materials, boundary conditions and loading paths are investigated.

So far, the tests have been performed for the single-point interaction, since in that case, only the flat 3D grid is constructed during the off-line phase. It is clear, that other types of the interpolation can be considered, however, at the cost of increased computational complexity: in the case of multiple-point interaction, each degree of freedom yields additional dimension of the grid, whereas the probe interaction introduces additional levels for each grid point. In each case, the number of transitions that must be constructed to traverse the entire configuration space increases rapidly. Therefore, a modification of the approach has been presented in Filipovič et al. (2009). The configuration space is not constructed in advance in a separated phase, however, the new configurations are generated directly during the real-time interaction. The "on-line" version of the space construction assumes the haptic interaction point to be connected to sufficient computational resources such as cluster or grid and it introduces some restrictions concerning the maximum speed of the haptic device during the interaction. On the other side, the time-consuming precomputation phase is not needed anymore and therefore, more complex versions of the grid (additional dimensions and levels) can be considered. A preliminary evaluation of the on-line generation of configuration spaces can be found in Peterlík & Filipovič (2010).

4. Conclusions

In this chapter, we focused on haptic rendering of objects with complex behaviour. The study aimed at deformable bodies which are difficult to model in real-time, provided realistic and physically-based simulation of deformations is desired as in the case of surgical simulators. First, a short overview of the simulation methods was given, emphasizing the computational complexity of the calculations. The two sources of the non-linearity that emerge in the deformation modeling were briefly described and the effect of the linearization was shown. Then, a survey of methods proposed over the last decade was given: it was shown that the precomputation usually plays an important role in design of algorithms combining computationally demanding calculations and real-time response. The key concepts used to overcome the high refresh rate needed for stable haptic rendering were described separately for linear and non-linear models.

In the second part of the chapter, the approach based on the precomputation of the configuration spaces was described. First, the haptic setting was introduced for single-point, multi-point and probe interactions. After introducing the notion of configuration and transition, it was shown that interaction with the deformable objects can be regarded as traveling through configuration spaces. The discretization of such spaces was proposed together with corresponding algorithms for its construction and approximation. The feasibility of the approach

was briefly sketched summarizing the main results of the extensive evaluation. Finally, the on-line version of the algorithm was briefly discussed, showing the direction of further research towards more complex types of interaction between the user and deformable body.
The development in the area of the soft tissues foreshadows that precomputation can still play an important role in the haptic rendering of complex objects. Nevertheless, the algorithms based on direct on-line computations are becoming still more and more attractive, as they allow for flexible modification of the model parameters during the interaction without necessity to recompute the data. The design of such algorithms is also encouraged by the advent of powerful accelerators such as GPGPUs, which significantly increases the performance of single workstation that can be now used for expensive numerical calculations. Therefore, it is possible to conclude that the physically-based deformation modeling in combination with haptic rendering is a promising area where a sharp increase in the quality of simulation can be expected. This will mainly concern the design of visco-elastic materials being in accordance with *in vitro* experiments, heterogeneous models describing the internal structure of the organs, advanced contact modeling considering the interaction between the organs, more precise FE approximations using the meshes composed of large number of special elements, advanced techniques allowing operations such as cutting, tearing or burning the tissue and others.

5. References

Allard, J., Cotin, S., Faure, F., Bensoussan, P.-J., Poyer, F., Duriez, C., Delingette, H. & Grisoni, L. (2007). Sofa an open source framework for medical simulation, *Medicine Meets Virtual Reality (MMVR'15)*, Long Beach, USA.

Barbič, J. & James, D. L. (2005). Real-time subspace integration for st. venant-kirchhoff deformable models, *SIGGRAPH '05: ACM SIGGRAPH 2005 Papers*, ACM, New York, NY, USA, pp. 982–990.

Barbič, J. & James, D. L. (2008). Six-dof haptic rendering of contact between geometrically complex reduced deformable models, *IEEE Trans. Haptics* **1**(1): 39–52.

Bro-Nielsen, M. (1996). *Medical Image Registration and Surgery Simulation*, PhD thesis, IMM Technical University of Denmark.

Bro-Nielsen, M. & Cotin, S. (1996). Real-time volumetric deformable models for surgery simulation using finite elements and condensation, *Computer Graphics Forum* **15**(3): 57–66.

Chai, J., Sun, J. & Tang, Z. (2001). Hybrid fem for deformation of soft tissues in surgery simulation, *MIAR '01: Proceedings of the International Workshop on Medical Imaging and Augmented Reality (MIAR '01)*, IEEE Computer Society, Washington, DC, USA, p. 298.

Ciarlet, P. G. (1988). *Mathematical Elasticity: Three-dimensional elasticity*, Elsevier Science Ltd.

Comas, O., Taylor, Z. A., Allard, J., Ourselin, S., Cotin, S. & Passenger, J. (2008). Efficient nonlinear fem for soft tissue modelling and its gpu implementation within the open source framework sofa, *ISBMS '08: Proceedings of the 4th international symposium on Biomedical Simulation*, Springer-Verlag, Berlin, Heidelberg, pp. 28–39.

Cotin, S., Delingette, H. & Ayache, N. (1996). Real time volumetric deformable models for surgery simulation, *VBC*, pp. 535–540.

Cotin, S., Delingette, H. & Ayache, N. (1999). Real-time elastic deformations of soft tissues for surgery simulation, *IEEE Transactions On Visualization and Computer Graphics* **5**(1): 62–73.

Cotin, S., Delingette, H. & Ayache, N. (2000a). A hybrid elastic model allowing real-time cutting, deformations and force-feedback for surgery training and simulation, *The Visual Computer* **16**(8): 437–452.

Cotin, S., Delingette, H. & Ayache, N. (2000b). A hybrid elastic model allowing real-time cutting, deformations and force-feedback for surgery training and simulation, *The Visual Computer* **16**(8): 437–452.

De, S., Lim, Y.-J., Manivannan, M. & Srinivasan, M. A. (2006). Physically realistic virtual surgery using the point-associated finite field (paff) approach, *Presence: Teleoper. Virtual Environ.* **15**(3): 294–308.

Debunne, G., Desbrun, M., Cani, M.-P. & Barr, A. H. (2001). Dynamic real-time deformations using space & time adaptive sampling, *SIGGRAPH '01: Proceedings of the 28th annual conference on Computer graphics and interactive techniques*, ACM, New York, NY, USA, pp. 31–36.

Delingette, H. & Ayache, N. (2005). Hepatic surgery simulation, *Commun. ACM* **48**(2): 31–36.

Deo, D. & De, S. (2009). Phyness: A physics-driven neural networks-based surgery simulation system with force feedback, *World Haptics Conference* **0**: 30–34.

Filipovič, J., Peterlík, I. & Matyska, L. (2009). On-line precomputation algorithm for real-time haptic interaction with non-linear deformable bodies, *Proceedings of The Third Joint EuroHaptics Conference and Symposium on Haptic Interfaces for Virtual Environments and Teleoperator Systems*, pp. 24–29.

Frank, A. O., A.Twombly, I., Barth, T. J. & Smith, J. D. (2001). Finite element methods for real-time haptic feedback of soft-tissue models in virtual reality simulators, *VR '01: Proceedings of the Virtual Reality 2001 Conference (VR'01)*, IEEE Computer Society, Washington, DC, USA, p. 257.

Gosline, A. H., Salcudean, S. E. & Yan, J. (2004). Haptic simulation of linear elastic media with fluid pockets, *Haptic Interfaces for Virtual Environment and Teleoperator Systems, International Symposium on* **0**: 266–271.

Hager, W. W. (1989). Updating the inverse of a matrix, *SIAM Rev.* **31**(2): 221–239.

James, D. & Pai, D. (2002). Real time simulation of multizone elastokinematic models, *International Conference on Robotics and Automation*, Washington, D.C., USA, pp. 927–932.

J.T.Oden (1972). *Finite Elements of Non-linear Continua*, McGraw-Hill.

Křenek, A. (2003). Haptic rendering of complex force fields, *EGVE '03: Proceedings of the workshop on Virtual environments 2003*, ACM, pp. 231–239.

Miller, K., Joldes, G., Lance, D. & Wittek, A. (2007). Total lagrangian explicit dynamics finite element algorithm for computing soft tissue deformation, *Communications in Numerical Methods in Engineering* **23**(2): 121–134.

Misra, S., Okamura, A. M. & Ramesh, K. T. (2007). Force feedback is noticeably different for linear versus nonlinear elastic tissue models, *WHC '07: Proceedings of the Second Joint EuroHaptics Conference and Symposium on Haptic Interfaces for Virtual Environment and Teleoperator Systems*, IEEE Computer Society, Washington, DC, USA, pp. 519–524.

Nikitin, I., Nikitina, L., Frolov, P., Goebbels, G., Göbel, M., Klimenko, S. & Nielson, G. M. (2002). Real-time simulation of elastic objects in virtual environments using finite element method and precomputed green's functions, *EGVE '02: Proceedings of the workshop on Virtual environments 2002*, Eurographics Association, Aire-la-Ville, Switzerland, Switzerland, pp. 47–52.

Peterlík, I. (2008). Efficient precomputation of configuration space for haptic deformation modeling, *Proceedings of Conference on Human System Interactions*, IEEE Xplore, pp. 225–230. best paper award.

Peterlík, I. (2009). *Haptic Interaction with non-linear deformable objects*, PhD thesis, Masaryk University.

Peterlík, I. & Filipovič, J. (2010). Distributed construction of configuration spaces for real-time haptic deformation modeling, *IEEE Transactions on Industrial Electronics* p. to appear.

Peterlík, I. & Matyska, L. (2008). Haptic interaction with soft tissues based on state-space approximation, *EuroHaptics '08: Proceedings of the 6th international conference on Haptics*, Springer-Verlag, Berlin, Heidelberg, pp. 886–895.

Peterlík, I., Sedef, M., Basdogan, C. & Matyska, L. (2010). Real-time visio-haptic interaction with static soft tissue models having geometric and material nonlinearity, *Computers & Graphics* p. to appear.

Picinbono, G., Delingette, H. & Ayache, N. (2001). Non-linear and anisotropic elastic soft tissue models for medical simulation, *ICRA2001: IEEE International Conference Robotics and Automation*, Seoul Korea. 6 pages.

Picinbono, G., Delingette, H. & Ayache, N. (2003). Non-linear anisotropic elasticity for real-time surgery simulation, *Graphical Models* **65**(5): 305–321.

Picinbono, G., Lombardo, J.-C., Delingette, H. & Ayache, N. (2002). Improving realism of a surgery simulator: linear anisotropic elasticity, complex interactions and force extrapolation, *Journal of Visualisation and Computer Animation* **13**(3): 147–167.

Popescu, D. C. & Compton, M. (2003). A model for efficient and accurate interaction with elastic objects in haptic virtual environments, *GRAPHITE '03: Proceedings of the 1st international conference on Computer graphics and interactive techniques in Australasia and South East Asia*, ACM Press, New York, NY, USA, pp. 245–250.

P.R.Amestoy, I.S.Duff & L'Excellent, J.-Y. (2000). Multifrontal parallel distributed symmetric and unsymmetric solvers, *Comput. Methods in Appl. Mech. Eng.* **184**: 501–520.

Saupin, G., Duriez, C., Cotin, S. & Grisoni, L. (2008). Efficient contact modeling using compliance warping, *Computer Graphics International Conference (CGI) Istambul, Turkey,*.

Sedef, M., Samur, E. & Basdogan, C. (2006). Real-time finite-element simulation of linear viscoelastic tissue behavior based on experimental data, *IEEE Comput. Graph. Appl.* **26**(6): 58–68.

Taylor, M., Cheng, M. & Ourselin, S. (2007). Real-time nonlinear finite element analysis for surgical simulation using graphics processing units, *Medical Image Computing & Computer-Assisted Intervention Conference*, pp. 701–708.

Wriggers, P. (2008). *Nonlinear Finite Element Methods*, 2008 Springer Verlag.

Wu, X., Downes, M. S., Goktekin, T. & Tendick, F. (2001). Adaptive nonlinear finite elements for deformable body simulation using dynamic progressive meshes, *in* A. Chalmers & T.-M. Rhyne (eds), *EG 2001 Proceedings*, Vol. 20(3), Blackwell Publishing, pp. 349–358.

Wu, X., Goktekin, T. & Tendick, F. (2004). An interactive parallel multigrid fem simulator, *ISMS*, pp. 124–133.

Wu, X. & Tendick, F. (2004). Multigrid integration for interactive deformable body simulation, *International Symposium on Medical Simulation (2004).Association for Computing Machinery, Inc*, pp. 92–104.

Zhuang, Y. (2000). *Real-time simulation of physically realistic global deformations*, PhD thesis, Department of Electrical Engineering and Computer Science, UC Berkeley. Chair-John Canny.

Zhuang, Y. & Canny, J. (1999). Real-time simulation of physically realistic global deformation, *IEEE Vis'99 Late Breaking Hot Topics*.

Zhuang, Y. & Canny, J. (2000). Real-time global deformations, *The fourth International Workshop on Algorithmic Foundations of Robotics (WAFR)*, A. K. Peters, pp. 97–107.

18

A Haptic Modeling System

Jeha Ryu and Hyungon Kim
Haptics Lab
Gwangju Institute of Science and Technology, KOREA
E-mail: { ryu, hyungonkim}@gist.ac.kr

Abstract

Haptics has been studied as a means of providing users with natural and immersive haptic sensations in various real, augmented, and virtual environments, but it is still relatively unfamiliar to the general public. One reason is the lack of abundant haptic content in areas familiar to the general public. Even though some modeling tools do exist for creating haptic content, the addition of haptic data to graphic models is still relatively primitive, time consuming, and unintuitive. In order to establish a comprehensive and efficient haptic modeling system, this chapter first defines the haptic modeling processes and its scopes. It then proposes a haptic modeling system that can, based on depth images and image data structure, create and edit haptic content easily and intuitively for virtual object. This system can also efficiently handle non-uniform haptic property per pixel, and can effectively represent diverse haptic properties (stiffness, friction, etc).
Keywords **–** haptics, haptic modeling, virtual reality, augmented reality, depth image

1. Introduction

Haptics has been studied as a means of providing users with natural and immersive sensations of digital content in the fields of medicine [1], education [2], entertainment [3], and broadcasting [4]. Haptic interfaces allow users to touch, explore, and manipulate 3D objects in an intuitive way with realistic haptic feedback and can be applied to create touch-enabled solutions that improve learning, understanding, creativity and communication. In spite of the considerable advantages, however, haptics is still largely unfamiliar to most people, potentially due to the lack of abundant haptic interaction contents in areas of interest to the general public. Audiovisual content, on the other hand, is readily available to the general public in a variety of forms, including movies and music, because it can easily be captured using a camera or microphone and can be created by a wide range of modeling and authoring tools. Haptic content, on the other hand, has not yet reached this ease of use, as there are not many haptic cameras or microphones available and still relatively few easily-useable modeling and authoring tools for creating haptic content.

In the meantime, there are a few tools providing a graphic modeling system with force feedback in the 3D geometric model design process, including geometric modeling, sculpturing, and painting. Among them, Freeform [5] and ClayTools™ [6] are virtual modeling and sculpturing systems that have been commercialized by SensAble Technologies. InTouch [7] and ArtNova [8] are touch-enabled 3D painting and multi-resolution modeling systems, and dAb [9] is a haptic painting system with 3D deformable brushes. These systems, however, use haptic technology purely as an assistant tool for effective and intuitive geometric modeling, sculpturing, and painting. Therefore, these tools cannot exactly be considered to be the haptic modeling tools according to the definitions and scopes in the following section.

Despite their lack of recognition, though, there are a few haptics-based application systems currently in use. FLIGHT GHUI Builder (FGB) [10] and REACHIN [11] Application Programming Interface (API) are both platforms that enable the development of haptic content. FGB is a tool designed specifically for the creation of graphic and haptic user, while REACHIN API is used to develop sophisticated haptic 3D applications and to provide functionalities when editing haptic data. By providing users with a set of haptic/graphic libraries and some haptics-related editing functions in haptic APIs, as in OpenHaptics Toolkit [12] and CHAI3D [13], it is possible to construct application specific haptic models. Tempkin et al. [14] proposed a haptic modeling system called web-based three dimensional virtual body structure (W3D-VBS). This software provides editing functions for haptic properties and can edit a variety of haptic surface properties including stiffness, friction, and damping for tissue palpation. Seo et al. [15] also proposed a haptic modeling system called K-Haptic Modeler™, which provides editing functions for haptic properties by using the K-Touch™ Haptic Application Programming Interface (API) [16] to support the haptic user interface. Eid et al. [17] further suggested a haptic modeling system called HAMLAT in which the authoring tool is composed of the HAMLAT editor, the HAML engine, and a rendering engine.

Most haptic modeling systems, including HAMLAT, OpenHaptics, and K-Haptic Modeler™, are either object or polygon-based: In the object-based modeling system, the haptic properties are applied on a whole object, while in the polygon-based system, they are applied on some parts of an object. It is therefore difficult to edit non-uniform haptic properties on only part of a surface or object. Thus, instead of applying global properties to a model, as in the object-or polygon-based approach, Kim et al. [18, 19] proposed a haptic decoration and local material editing system for enhancing the haptic realism of a virtual object. This system allows a user to paint directly on to the surface of a 3D object and to locally edit and feel haptic material properties (stiffness, friction) in a natural way.

Haptic content typically consists of computer graphic models, created using a general graphic modeler such as MAYA or 3D MAX, with the subsequent addition of haptic data. In graphic modeling, graphic content is created while the quality of work is directly verified visually. Therefore, in order to create a variety of diverse and naturally feeling haptic content, it is necessary to develop haptic modelers which are user-friendly, easy-to-use, general purpose, and efficient. The modeling software and applications must provide sufficient graphic/haptic functionality in the modeling processes, which can then provide on-line feedback of the edited haptic material properties in real time as users edit on the surface of an object. Moreover, the haptic modelers must have ample speed and memory-efficiency to ensure high productivity and to be economical.

The rest of this chapter is organized as follows. Section 2 defines the haptic modeling processes systematically and comprehensively and then summarizes their scopes. A depth image-based haptic modeling algorithm is then proposed for editing non-uniform and diverse haptic properties on the surface of a virtual object in Section 3. This proposed method stores haptic property values into six orthogonal image data structures, called haptic property images, to more efficiently and cost-effectively represent a more realistic feeling of touch. Section 4 suggests a basic framework for a haptic modeling system (a modified K-HapticModeler™) that can create and edit haptic content for virtual objects. The final section provides conclusions and suggests future research items to improve the proposed modeling functions.

2. Haptic Modeling: defintion and scope

A. Definition of Haptic Modeling

There seems to be no formal comprehensive definition of haptic modeling and its scope, although there are many techniques for digital sculpting or performing geometric modeling with a force sensation that can be evoked by some sort of haptic device. We define haptic modeling more formally and comprehensively as follows:

Definition: *Haptic modeling is a series of processes to create haptic content on graphic models that are components of virtual reality (VR), augmented reality (AR), or mixed reality (MR).*

B. Scope of Haptic Modeling

The haptic modeling processes as a whole consist basically of four smaller processes: (i) acquiring haptic data and the subsequent signal/image processing, as well as data management to acquire haptic data from the physical world, (ii) geometric processing to preprocess graphic models, (iii) haptic processing to edit or to author haptic data onto a graphic model, and (iv) haptic modeling to add haptic effects into the overall graphic environment. Here, haptic data may include not only material properties (stiffness and friction), haptic texture (roughness), and force/torque histories, but also motion trajectories such as time histories of acceleration, velocity, and position. Figure 1 shows the scope of the proposed haptic modeling processes.

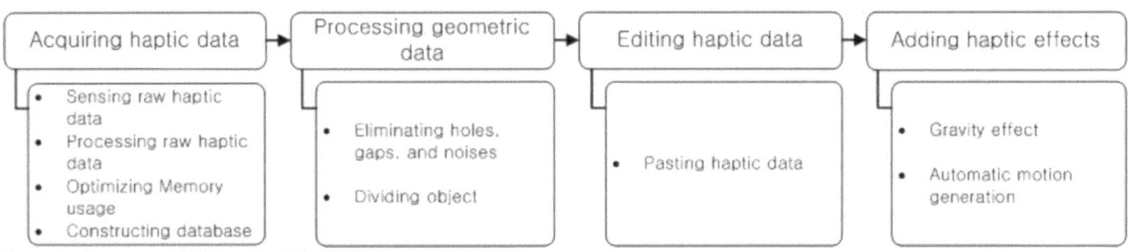

Fig. 1. Scope of Haptic Modeling Processes

a. Acquiring Haptic Data

There are two processes in the acquisition stage of haptic data; (i) the acquisition of haptic data (including signal processing to get true haptic data from noisy raw signals) from the physical world through either a sensing systems or a mathematical modeling technique, and (ii) the construction of a haptic database.

To build realistic haptic contents, haptic data must first be acquired from the real world. Surface material properties (stiffness and friction), haptic texture (roughness), and force

profiles of haptic widgets (buttons, sliders, joypads, etc.) can be obtained through many different kinds of physical sensors, such as a force/torque sensor to get a force/torque time history, while a user is interacting with a real physical object (e.g. physical buttons or sliders) or with a real physical scene (environment). A visual camera may also be used to acquire some of the geometric details of an object surface for haptic texture modeling with subsequent image processing.
After sensor signals are acquired, these raw signals must then be processed to derive haptically useful data. A human perception threshold may be applied in these kinds of processing. For button force history, for example, some identification process may be necessary to find out onset of sudden drop of buttoning force. Motion histories can be captured and stored by visual cameras, inertial sensors, or by motion capture systems. The motion trajectories can also be used for describing ball trajectories and hand writing trajectories. Haptic data may also be modeled by some mathematical functions. Regardless of the means of acquisition, haptic data must be stored efficiently in the memory due to the potentially large size of the dataset. Therefore, it is important to develop an efficient data base management method.

b. Preprocessing Geometric Models

The preprocessing stage requires specific geometric processing for subsequent haptic modeling. For instance, even though a geometric model may seem fine graphically, it may contain many holes, gaps, or noises that have been acquired from 3D scanners, z-Cam™, MRI, CT, etc. These can be felt haptically while users explore the graphic model to receive an unexpected haptic sensation. Therefore, these graphically-unseen-but-haptically-feelable holes, gaps, or noises must be eliminated before any material editing process can begin.
Further preprocessing may be also necessary. In most existing haptic modeling systems, a single set of haptic data is applied to the entire 3D model. However, users may want to model haptic data in one local or special area. In this case, geometric processing for dividing an object into several areas needs to be done before the haptic modeling process. Otherwise, a new method to edit non-uniform haptic properties on the surface of a virtual object should be developed.

c. Editing/Authoring Haptic Data

The editing or authoring of haptic data (surface material properties such as stiffness and frictions, force profiles of haptic widgets, etc.) is a significant part of the haptic modeling process and must be performed as intuitively and quickly as possible, similar to the geometric modeling process.

d. Adding Haptic Effects

Aside from the editing of haptic data onto graphic models, other haptic modeling processes also exist. For example, a gravity or electromagnetic effect may be applied in the whole virtual worlds to simulate weight or inter-atomic interaction force sensation when a user grabs an object or an atom (charged particle) in the gravitational or electromagnetic field. The case of automatic motion generation for a dynamically moving system is another example. If a soccer ball is kicked by an input action from the user and the user want to feel the motion trajectories of the soccer ball, the ball's motion history must be dynamically simulated in real time by the use of numerical integration algorithms.

This chapter discusses only the modeling, more specifically, the haptic editing of graphic objects as discussed in the above step (c). Other steps will be discussed in future publications.

3. A Haptic modeling system

To edit 3D objects haptically, four steps are usually required. First, haptic modeling designers select some 3D object surfaces on which they want to assign haptic property values and, in the second step, they assign the desired haptic property values on the selected surfaces. Third, the user checks whether the touch feeling by the modeled haptic property values is realistic or not. If the feeling is not realistic or appropriate, they should adjust the values on-line by simultaneously changing the values and feeling the surface. Finally, once they are satisfied with the realistic haptic property values for the surfaces, they then store the values and chosen surfaces in a suitable format.

Depending on the method of picking out the surfaces on which the desired haptic property values are pasted, haptic modeling can be classified into three methods: (i) object-based, (ii) polygon-based, and (iii) voxel-based. The object-based haptic modeling method [14, 15] selects the entire surface of a 3D object when assigning haptic property values. Therefore, the entire surface of an object can have only a single uniform haptic property value. A glass bottle, for example, would have a single uniform haptic property value of stiffness, friction, and roughness over the entire surface. Therefore, if a 3D object consists of many parts with different haptic properties, partitioning is required in the preprocessing stage to assign different haptic property values to different parts. The polygon-based haptic modeling method [17] selects some parts of meshes from the whole 3D meshes comprising an object. Therefore, each mesh can have a different haptic property value. If the number of meshes is large for fine and non-uniform specifications of surface haptic properties, however, the size of the haptic property data also increases. Moreover, if a haptic modeling designer wants to model a part smaller than a mesh, subdivision is required. The object and polygon-based haptic modeling methods, therefore, usually cause difficulty when editing non-uniform haptic properties on the selected surfaces. On the other hand, the voxel-based haptic modeling method [18, 19] uses the hybrid implicit and geometry surface data representation. This method uses volumetric data representation and, therefore, in the surface selection process, the selected surfaces need to be mapped into the voxel data. Then the voxel and a single haptic property group that contains diverse haptic properties in a single data structure will be stored. However, the size of the converted volumetric data into surface data by means of a mapping function between the voxel and haptic property values is huge because the data is structured like a hash function. It subsequently needs a large amount of memory (order of N^3) for modeling a very fine non-uniform haptic property.

In summary, for non-uniform haptic property modeling on surfaces of a virtual object, the existing methods require processes that: (i) divide a virtual object into many surfaces or component objects if a visual model consists of many components, (ii) maps between haptic property values and graphical data sets, (iii) converts data because of the dependency on data-representation, such as polygon and voxel. To avoid these additional processes in modeling non-uniform haptic properties, we propose a depth image-based haptic modeling method. In the proposed method, several two dimensional multi-layered image data structures, called haptic property images, store non-uniform and diverse haptic property values. Then, among several images, six orthogonal directional depth images of a 3D object are used to load a haptic property image that corresponds to the current haptic interaction point. Storing and loading haptic property values in this way makes the haptic modeling system more efficient and cost-effective. The proposed method therefore requires no division or partitioning of a virtual object. It is also independent of data-representation of the virtual object and, thus, is not dependent on the complexity of polygonal models.

3.1 Depth Image-based Haptic Modeling

The basic concept of the proposed depth image-based haptic modeling method is inspired by the depth image-based haptic rendering algorithm developed by Kim et al. [20], in which six orthogonal depth images are used for real-time collision detection and force computation. For efficiency and cost-effectiveness, the proposed method uses several layers of six orthogonal image data structures for storing and loading non-uniform and diverse haptic surface property values for the surface of a given 3D model. The six orthogonal depth images are used to identify a position in the six orthogonal image data which corresponds to the ideal haptic interaction point (IHIP), the contact point on the body, and to assign haptic properties to the position of a 3D object. One important assumption in the proposed depth image-based approach is that all points of whole surfaces in an object are mapped to certain positions among the six orthogonal images. Convex objects satisfy this assumption. Concave objects, however, need to be divided into several convex objects in the preprocessing stage, as in [21, 22].

Fig. 2 shows the six orthogonal image planes for an object, which are defined at the top/bottom, left/right, and Front/rear surfaces of a bounding cube. The proposed depth image-based haptic modeling method consists of two parts: (i) an image-based modeling process and (ii) a depth image-based rendering process with the modeled image data. Two steps are therefore needed: an initialization step and a loop step. In the initialization step, a design parameter, such as image resolution, needs to be chosen carefully in order to efficiently assign the haptic property values. Depth images are then acquired from six orthogonal virtual cameras located on the bounding box surfaces, as shown in Figure 2. The haptic property images are image data structures for storing haptic property values for each pixel. In the following loop step, the location of the ideal haptic interaction point (IHIP) in the haptic property images is found by using the six orthogonal depth images in order to assign a haptic property value to a corresponding pixel in the haptic property image. It should be noted that, among the six orthogonal images, up to five haptic property images may be selected for the IHIP. Finally, pixels containing IHIP in the selected haptic property images are assigned haptic property values.

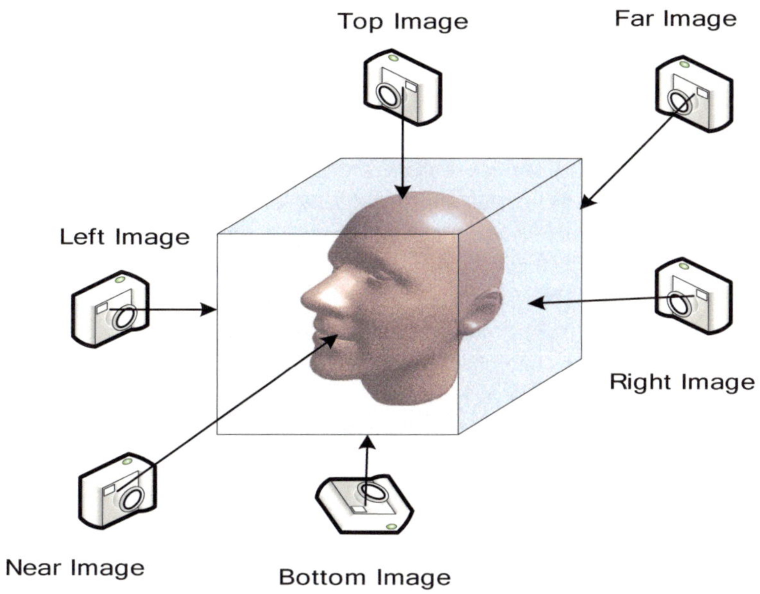

Fig. 2. Six orthogonal image planes for an object with six virtual cameras

A. Initialization Step

The initialization step performs several different functions: (i) it determines six orthogonal haptic property image resolutions, (ii) it initializes six images values to zero values, and (iii) it obtains six orthogonal depth images. The haptic property image is a data structure containing a haptic property value for each pixel. It is therefore needed first in order to determine the resolution of each haptic property image. Since the haptic property image data structure contains haptic property values to describe the six orthogonal surfaces of 3D objects, haptic property images with a higher resolution are able to store finer haptic information and provide a finer touch sensation. Thus, the resolution of the haptic property image determines the quality of the detailed representation of the surfaces. Figure 3 shows several different resolutions for a haptic property image. If the resolution of the image is high, memory usage is also high, possibly creating more work for a haptic modeling designer. Therefore, the image resolution should be carefully determined to match the needs of the designer. Note that each of the six orthogonal haptic property images may all have a different image resolution, depending on the surface details and surface haptic properties.

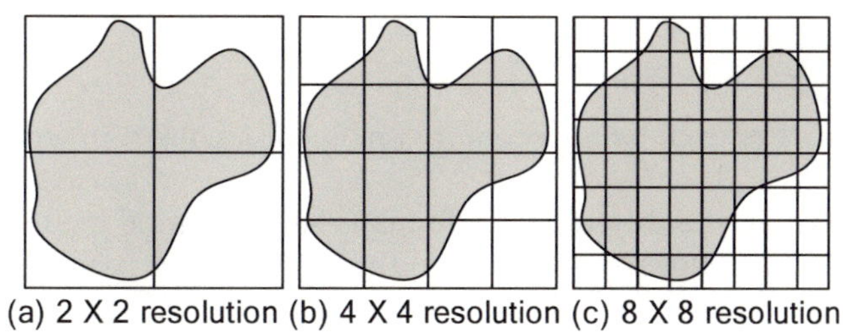

Fig. 3. Resolutions of a haptic property image

Before obtaining the depth images, it is necessary to first create six haptic property images whose pixel values are all set to zero. The desired pixel values in the haptic property images will then be updated by assigning new haptic property values during the modeling stage in the loop process. The next step is to obtain six orthogonal depth images that have the same image resolution as the haptic property images and that have additional depth information from the virtual camera pixel planes to the surfaces of the virtual object. Note that, for simplicity, the resolution of the depth image is selected to be the same as that of a haptic property image. If the resolutions for these two images are not the same, it is necessary to first resolve the resolution difference between them.

In order to set the virtual cameras in the correct positions, a bounding box needs to be constructed. Among various boundary boxes, the axis-aligned bounding box (AABB) is used for its fast computation and direct usage of the depth image-based haptic rendering algorithm [20]. If a virtual camera is located on the surface of the bounding box, then the surface of the object may not be captured because there is no distance between the camera and the surface. Hence, a small margin is necessary between an object and a boundary box. This bounding box with a small margin is called a "Depth workspace". The six orthogonal side surfaces of the cube in Fig. 2 are the locations of the both the haptic property images, as well as the depth images. Figure 2 also shows the location of the six virtual cameras used to obtain the depth images, which will later be used for determining which of the haptic property images correspond to the current contact point (IHIP) during the depth image-based modeling procedure.

B. Loop Step

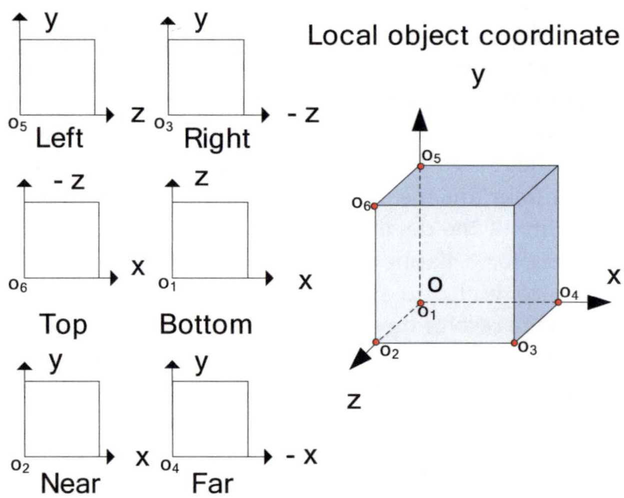

Fig. 4. Local coordinate of each haptic property image for an object in world coordinate

An important problem of the proposed depth image-based haptic modeling method is how to assign haptic property values to the pixels in the haptic property images. For this, we first need to find the pixel positions in all six orthogonal haptic property images. After finding the IHIP, which is the contact point on the surface where the Haptic Interaction Point (HIP; haptic device probe) collides with the surface of a 3D object, the IHIP position is computed in respect to the three dimensional world coordinate system, as had been done in [20]. The corresponding position in each haptic property image can then be obtained by a simple coordinate relationship, as shown in Figure 4. The local coordinate systems of all orthogonal haptic property image planes for an object are also shown. Note that the object's origin in the world coordinate system is located in the left-bottom-far position of an object while each image origin is located at the left-bottom.

Figure 5 shows an example of the contacted IHIP point (red spot) on the human face (just above the left eyebrow) and the associated positions in the six orthogonal depth image planes. Note that, among these six images, only three contain visible images (the three left images corresponding to the front, right side, and top views).

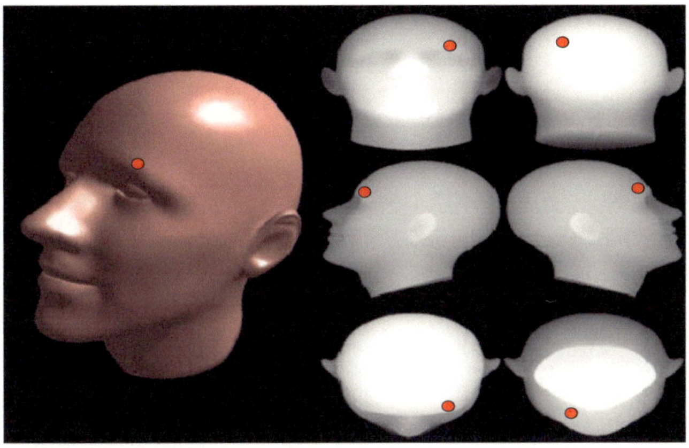

● IHIP position in each Haptic property image

a(object),
b(near image), c(far image), d(right image),
e(left image), f(top image), g(bottom image)

Fig. 5. Example of the IHIP position on each haptic property image corresponding to the IHIP

Second, the haptic property images that contain the IHIP need to be selected. These images are called "True Haptic Property Images." For example, in Figure 5, it is only necessary to select three images as the True Haptic Property Images (the three left images corresponding to the front, right side, and top views). This selection process can be easily done using the six orthogonal depth images and a simple depth comparison algorithm. For example, if the depth value of the far depth image is bigger than the IHIP depth value, then the IHIP z-position is inside of the object's front surface. In this case, the far haptic property image is not a correct True Haptic Property Image. Assume in this depth comparison that the closet depth value is zero and the farthest depth value is one. Once the True Haptic Property Images are determined, the modeling step is finished by assigning a haptic property value to one of the True Haptic Property Image positions, called the True Haptic Property Position. So far, the method of assigning one haptic property value into a few haptic property images has been discussed. However, there are various haptic surface properties which stimulate human sense of touch, such as stiffness, damping, static or dynamic friction values in three directions. To model these diverse haptic surface properties, the proposed algorithm

suggests a concept of multi-layered images, where one image layer is used to represent each haptic property. Interestingly, the proposed modeling method may very easily include some tactile sensation models in a similar way to the haptic surface property model on a per-pixel basis. In other words, vibration effects (in term of vibration time history), for example, can be assigned to each pixel or to a group of pixels of an image to render vibration effects while a user touches a point or a group of points on the surface.
The proposed algorithm is a per-pixel-based method. To assign the same haptic property values on several pixels around the True Haptic Property Position, a user needs to simply choose some surrounding pixels with a brush operation, similar to that in the Photoshop program, and then assign the desired values to the selected pixels. Even though some pixels chosen in this way may not be on the surface of a virtual object, these non-surface pixels are not haptically rendered because they are considered to be non-contacted pixels during the collision detection phase. Therefore, a process to eliminate process these non-surface pixels is not necessary.

3.2 Depth Image-based Haptic Rendering

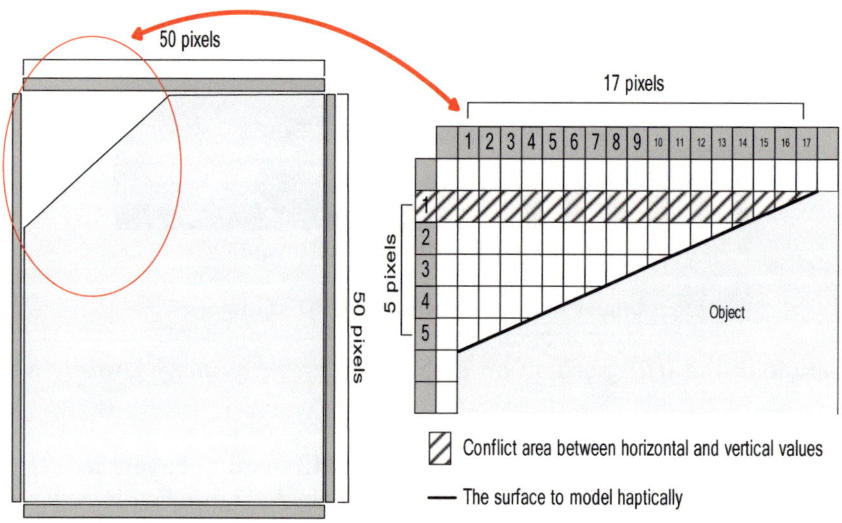

Fig. 6. Conflict problem with multiple haptic property values for single IHIP

In order to haptically render the haptic properties modeled with the proposed depth image-based haptic modeling method, it is only necessary to choose one haptic property image among the three True Haptic Property Images because of a conflict problem. This situation may be explained more clearly with an example. Figure 6 shows two haptic property images in the two dimensional view of a two dimensional object. This problem may be caused either by a difference in the image resolution of the two images, or by a difference in resolution for parts of an object. This example shows that a slope portion of the object is projected into a horizontal image with 17 pixels and, at the same time, into a vertical image with 5 pixels. In this case, a haptic property value is assigned into two images and, when rendering the assigned haptic property value, the haptic renderer cannot determine which image is to be used. Assume for example that one haptic property value are assigned to the

16-th position on the horizontal haptic property image, and another value is assigned to the 15-th position on the same image. In this case, haptic properties on this image are saved correctly; however, at the same time, the two haptic property values are to be saved in the first position on the vertical haptic property image. In this case, only the second haptic property value is saved in the vertical image in the modeling time and use of the haptic property value of the 16-th position in the horizontal image is correct. Therefore, the horizontal image must be selected.

To avoid this conflict problem, we used the contact force vector direction that can be computed in the haptic rendering process while modeling the haptic property values. As shown in Figure 7, all haptic property images have their own normal vectors. A dot product with each normal vector of a True Haptic Property Image and the contact force vector on the contacted point (i.e. IHIP) can identify only one True Haptic Property Image. For example, in Figure 7, the top image is the True Haptic Property Image because the dot product between the contact force vector and the normal vector of the top image is the smallest. When rendering, this haptic property image is identified by this simple dot product operation. For a 45 degree inclined slope, the dot product generates the same values for the two images (for example, the top and left images in Figure 6). In that case, any haptic property image can be chosen as a True Haptic Property Image.

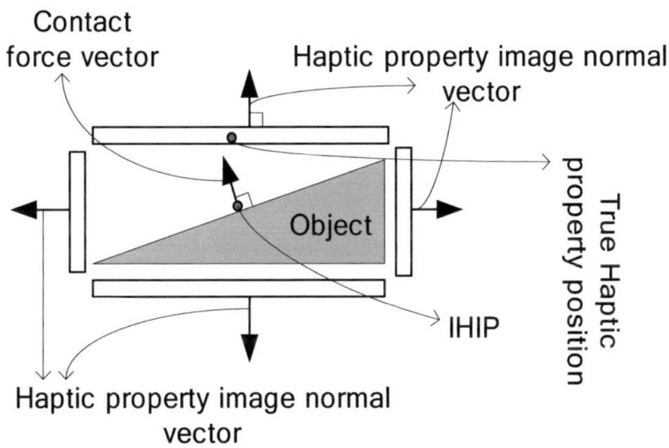

Fig. 7. Identifying a true haptic property image using the contact force vector

Once the desired multiple haptic property images for various properties (stiffness, friction, etc) are constructed from the modeling process by a haptic content designer who is feeling the haptic sensation, haptic rendering for another person (such as a consumer of the modeled haptic contents) can be done, as in the usual rendering process. By a collision detection algorithm, a collision point, which is an Ideal Haptic Interaction Point (IHIP), will search a True Haptic Property Image and the corresponding pixel position in the image. Then, the modeled haptic property value is conveyed to the reaction force computation and is subsequently displayed through a force-reflecting device or tactile property display devices.

A resultant reaction force can be computed by combining the normal reaction force from the stiffness property with several horizontal haptic properties, including friction and damping, as:

$$F_{total} = \sum F_{component} = F_{normal} + F_{friction} + F_{additional} + ... \tag{1}$$

where F_{total} is the total force feedback vector, and $F_{component}$ is each force vector generated by each haptic property. F_{normal} is the normal force vector with a stiffness property that can be generated by a haptic rendering algorithm, such as a penalty method, god object, or virtual proxy algorithm. $F_{frrctoin}$ is the horizontal frictional force vector generated by the friction property on the surface. $F_{addtional}$ is the force vector that is generated either by haptic textures or by any other haptic properties in a similar manner by using the proposed algorithm.

1) Stiffness

In order to calculate the normal force of the contact surface with the objects having non-uniform stiffness parameters, the haptic property image containing surface stiffness parameters is used. Once a collision is detected and the location of the IHIP is determined, the proposed algorithm reads the value of the stiffness corresponding to the surface adjacent to the IHIP by referring to the True Haptic Property Position and Image. Using the stiffness value K, the normal force of the contact surface then calculated using the spring model as

$$F_{stiffness} = K(IHIP_t - HIP_t) \tag{2}$$

where $IHIP_t$ and HIP_t describe IHIP and HIP at time t, respectively. Note that $(IHIP_t - HIP_t)$ is the contact surface normal vector.

2) Viscous Friction

The friction force is applied along the surface tangential direction. Non-uniform frictional force based on the proposed image-based representation can be computed using the following simple viscous friction model as

$$F_{friction} = D_s(IHIP_t - IHIP_{t-1}) / T \tag{3}$$

where D_s is the viscous damping coefficient and T is the haptic rendering rate. Similar to the previous determination of the normal contact force, once a collision is detected and the IHIP is determined, then the proposed algorithm read the viscous damping value corresponding to the IHIP position by referring the haptic property image containing the viscous damping coefficient.

Because haptic rendering should run as quickly as possible (nominally with a 1 KH rate), the proposed depth image-based haptic modeling method must also be performed very fast. On most recent PCs, one estimated time to search the True Haptic Property Image and Position using one IHIP is 0.001 msec. Larger haptic property image sizes take more time to load. Note, however, that loading haptic property images is only a one time event when the application is initialized. Therefore, the haptic property image size is not a serious problem in the proposed haptic modeling paradigm. More memory, however, is required for larger sized haptic property images.

4. Architecture of the haptic modeling System

The K-HapticModeler™, proposed in [15], has been modified for this system by implementing the proposed haptic modeling algorithm. The K-HapticModeler™ provides basic file management functionalities for loading, editing, and saving 3D graphic objects as well as basic graphic model manipulation functions, such as positioning, orienting, and scaling. For haptic modeling, the K-HapticModeler™ provides haptic-specific functionalities through the Haptic User Interface (HUI) for editing surface material properties, such as stiffness, static or dynamic friction, and for editing a pushbutton force profile on a loaded graphic model. It allows users to feel, manipulate, or explore virtual objects via a haptic device.

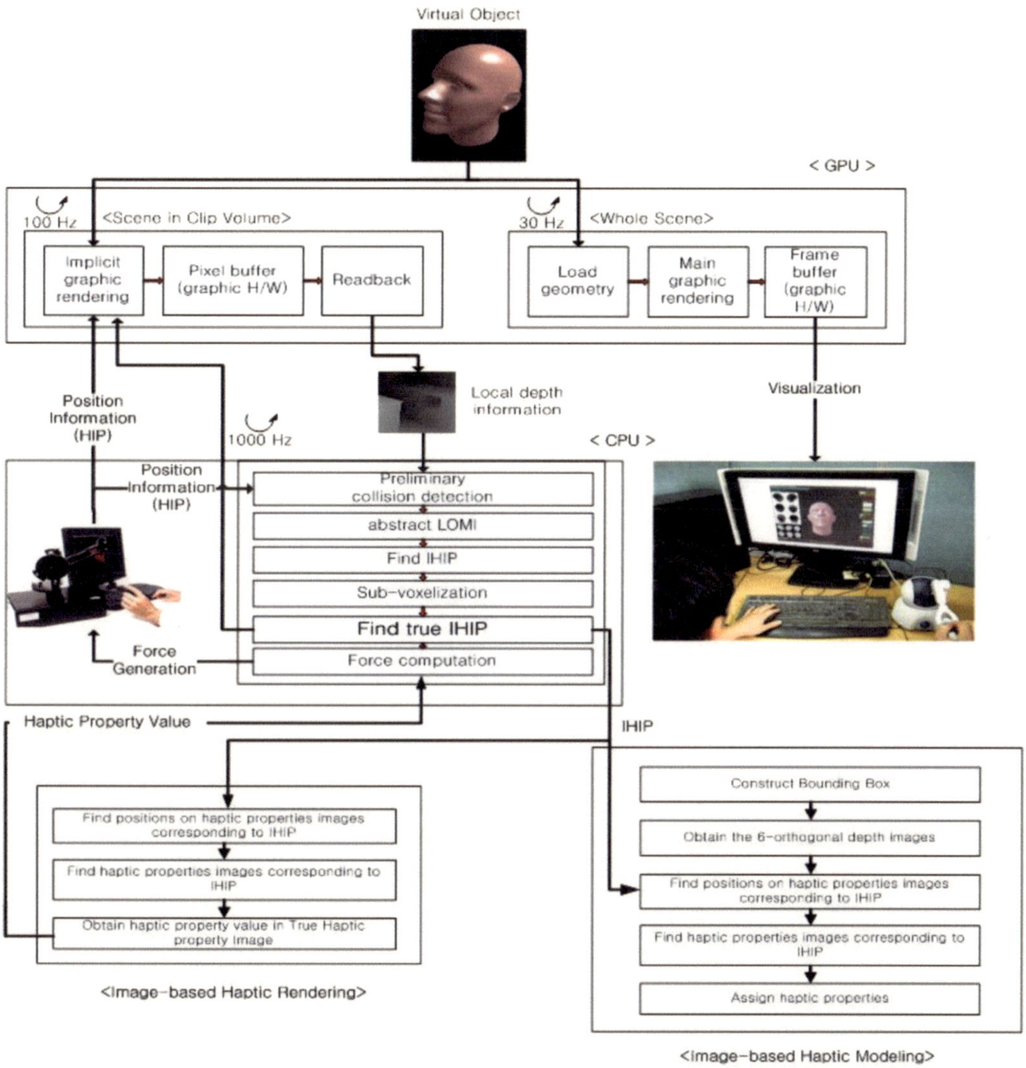

Fig. 8. Overall data flow for depth image-based haptic modeling & rendering

Figure 8 shows the overall data flow for the proposed depth image-based haptic modeling and rendering. The two upper blocks in this figure represent the depth image-based haptic rendering [20]. Note that, in the bottom blocks of this figure, the true IHIP is used both in the proposed depth image-based haptic modeling and rendering processes. For the online feeling of the modeled haptic sensation, the modeled haptic property values are used in the force computation. In order to process a 3D object with haptic properties, the XML file format is used for the entire application architecture, as outlined in Figure 9.

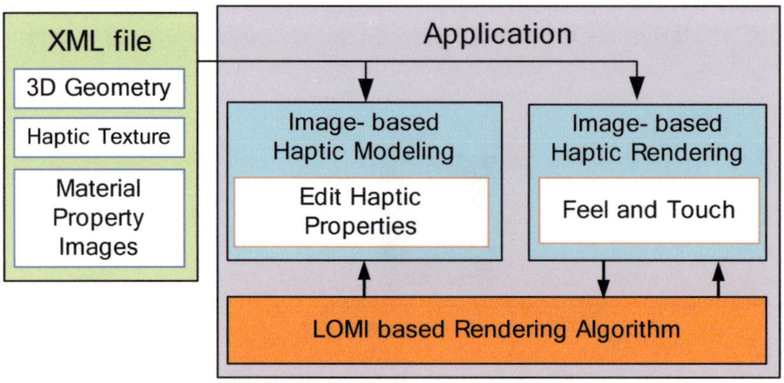

Fig. 9. Haptic modeling application architecture

4.1 XML File Format

Extensible Markup Language (XML) is a simple and flexible text format derived from Solid Graphic Markup Language (SGML) (ISO 8879). It is classified as an extensible language because it allows users to define their own tags. Its primary purpose is to facilitate the sharing of data across different information systems, particularly via the Internet. The proposed haptic modeling application supports the XML file format because it provides a simple interface for dealing with many 3D objects and haptic properties. It allows users to associate meta-information (graphic and haptic information) with 3D objects without converting the representation into a particular 3D format. The tags are described in Table 1. Note that each tag is presented with its identifier (within triangular brackets) followed by the type of the data it stores (within square brackets) and a brief description. By providing access to the XML file format, we can easily save, open, and add content.

Table 1 describes the XML tag definition and description. The Level is the XML data structure hierarchy level and "Note" refers to the number of tags which can be used in each tag. For example, the <object> tag has "multiple" values, meaning that many <object> tags can exist in the <objects> tag. On the other hand, the <type> tag has a "unique" value, meaning that only one <type> tag must exist in the <object> tag. The <objects> tag is used only for notifying root node. Each object in a virtual environment has an <object> tag. "Object" can have multiple haptic properties, so that each <property> tag describes each haptic property type. The <type> tag saves the haptic property type, while the <path> tag in the <property> tag signifies a relative path for the haptic images. The "ref" attribute in the <path> tag describes which image is included among the six haptic property images. By this simple tag combination, the haptic modeling data can be easily expressed.

Tag Name				Description	Note
Level 1	Level 2	Level 3	Level 4		
<objects>				Root Node	Unique
	<object>			each object has object tag	Multiple
		<path>		3D geometry path	Unique
		<texture>		Graphic texture path	Unique
		<property>		Property that a object has	Multiple
			<type>	haptic property type (stiffness, friction)	Unique
			<path>	Path where the haptic property image exist	Multiple
				"Ref" Attribute : left, right, top, down, near, far	Unique

Table 1. XML Tag Definition and Description

4.2 Implementation

The proposed haptic modeling system based on the depth image-based haptic modeling method was implemented on the PHANToM Omni haptic interface [23] using C++ language. The computations were run on a Pentium dual core with a 1.8 GHz CPU and two gigabytes of RAM for haptic rendering, and a Geforce 9600 GT graphic card for graphic rendering. The application was multi-threaded, with the haptic force computation thread running at a higher priority with a 1 KHz rate. The graphic rendering thread ran at 60 Hz rates to display virtual objects. Figure 10 shows a GUI image of the haptic modeling system.

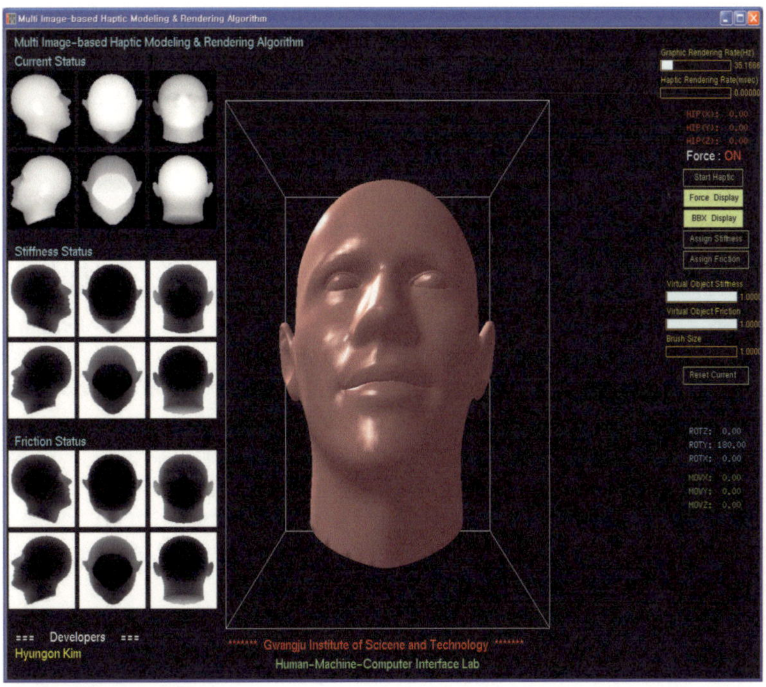

Fig. 10. Haptic Modeling GUI

This system has two main functions:

(i) Load and save haptic data files using XML format

(ii) Edit stiffness and friction haptic properties

To implement these two functions, image GUIs are proposed. The left images in the system, shown in Figure 10, describe the current status, stiffness status, and friction status. The current status GUI shows the area where the haptic modeling designer selected the surface to model. Therefore, after being selected, the area of current status will be updated into stiffness status or friction status.

The center area of the images shown on the right in Figure 10 indicate each haptic property value (in this figure, only stiffness and friction are shown), and brush size. The range of the brush size can be set from 1 to 10, and is editable. These GUIs are created using the Slider technique, so the haptic property values can be changed by clicking a mouse. The selected area will then be assigned by those data. After clicking the buttons in Figure 11, each haptic property will be assigned to each haptic property image. The Start button is for starting the haptic rendering process, while the reset button in the GUI is used to reset the current status images.

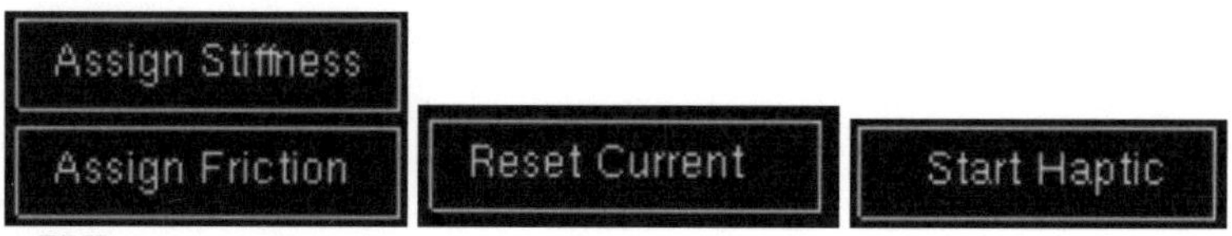

Fig. 11. Button GUI

5. Conclusions, Discussions, and Future Works

This chapter proposes a depth image-based haptic modeling method for effectively performing haptic modeling of 3D virtual objects that provides non-uniform surface haptic property per pixel. Moreover, by adding haptic property images, we can represent diverse haptic properties in a systematic way. Even though we have focused primarily on kinesthetic haptic properties, the proposed method can also be extended for any tactile haptic modeling such as vibration, thermal, and so on. Further, this method is applicable with any geometrical data set (voxel, implicit or mathematical representation, mesh structure) because no pre-processing is required for constructing a hierarchical data structure or data conversion, making this image-based approach highly efficient.

Based on our own systematic and comprehensive definition and scope of haptic modeling, a modified K-HapticModeler™ is proposed as an intuitive and efficient system for haptic modeling of virtual objects. The proposed modified K-HapticMosdeler™ provides basic graphic file management and haptic-specific functionalities, mainly for editing surface material properties of the loaded graphic model with the use of a haptic device. The proposed system, therefore, allows users to perform haptic modeling on graphic models easily, naturally, and intuitively. We believe that any person, even those who are not familiar with haptic technology, would be able to use this system for three-dimensional haptic modeling.

Concave objects, however, cannot be properly modeled by the proposed method because some object surfaces are not visible in all haptic property images. In order to solve this problem, convex decomposition algorithms [21, 22] should be used. Those convex decomposition algorithms, however, may also create unnecessary data sets. Reducing the unnecessary data also is our future work.

The proposed modeling system is now being developed to provide more comprehensive haptic modeling capabilities in more intuitive and efficient ways. Future development will implement each stage of haptic modeling scopes. First of all, methodology for acquiring haptic data further investigated, preprocessors of acquired data, such as segmentation, grouping, and databases, will also be constructed. Furthermore, our basic haptic modeling framework will be extended by comprising various HUI to create haptic content. Finally, we hope to apply our haptic content into a wide range of applications where it may heighten realistic interactions.

Acknowledgment

This research was supported the Ministry of Knowledge Economy (MKE), Korea, under the ITRC (Information Technology Research Center) support program supervised by the NIPA(National IT Industry Promotion Agency)" (NIPA-2009-C1090-0902-0008).

6. References

[1] C. Basdogan, C-H. Ho, Mandayam A. Srinnivasan, "Virtual Environments for Medical Training: Graphical and Haptic Simulation of Laparoscopic Common Bile Duct Exploration", IEEE/ASME TRANSACTIONS ON MECHATRONICS, VOL. 6, NO. 3, pp.269-285, SEPTEMBER, 2001.

[2] J. Minogue, M. G. Jones, "Haptics in Education: Exploring and Untapped Sensory Modality", Review of Educational Research, Vol. 76, No. 3, pp. 317-348, Fall 2006.

[3] B-C. Lee, J. Lee, J. Cha and J. Ryu, "Immersive Live Sports Experience with Vibrotactile Sensation", Tenth IFIP TC13 Int. Conf. on Human-Computer Interaction (INTERACT 2005), LNCS 3585, pp.1042- 1045, Rome, Italy, Sep. 12-16, 2005.

[4] J. Cha, Y. Seo, Y. Kim, and J. Ryu, "Haptic Broadcasting: Passive Haptic Interactions using MPEG-4 BIFS", Second Joint EuroHaptics Conference and Symposium on Haptic Interface for virtual Environment and Teleoperator Systems (WHC'07) pp. 274-279, 2007.

[5] SensAble Technologies, "http://www.sensable.com/ products-freeform-systems.htm"

[6] SensAble Technologies, "http://www.sensable.com/products-claytools-system.htm"

[7] A. D. Gregory, S. A. Ehmann, M. C. Lin,"in Touch: Interactive Multiresolution Modeling and 3D Painting with a Haptic Interface", In the Proceedings of IEEE Virtual Reality Conference 2000.

[8] M. Foskey, M.A. Otaduy, and M.C. Lin, "ArtNova: touch-enabled 3D model design," in Proc. of IEEE Virtual Reality Conf., 2002.

[9] W. Baxter, V. Scheib, M. Lin, and D. Manocha, "DAB: Haptic Paiting with 3D Virtual Brushes," in Proc. ACM SIGGRAPH, pp. 461-468, 2001.

[10] T. Anderson, A. Breckenridge, G. Davidson, "FGB: A Graphical and Haptic User Interface For Creating Graphical, Haptic User Interface", Proc. Forth PHANToM Users Group Workshop, pp. 48-51, Massachusetts, USA, Oct. 9-12, 1999.

[11] Reachin Technologies, "http://www.reachin.se/products/reachinapi/"

[12] SensAble Technologies, "http://www.sensable.com/ products-openhaptics.htm"

[13] CHAI3D, "http://www.chai3d.org"
[14] B. Temkin, E. Acosta, P. Hatfield, E. Onal, and A. Tong, "Web-based Three-dimensional Virtual Body Structures: W3D-VBS", J Am Med Inform Assoc. Sep–Oct; 9(5), pp. 425–436. 2002.
[15] Y. Seo, B-C. Lee, Y. Kim, J-P. Kim, and J. Ryu, "K-Haptic Modeler™: A Haptic Modeling Scope and Basic Framework", IEEE international Workshop on Haptic Audio Visual Environments and their Application, Ottawa, Canada, 2007.
[16] B-C. Lee, J-P. Kim, and J. Ryu, "Development of K-Touch haptic API", Conference of Korean Human Computer Interface, Phoenix Park, 2006.
[17] M. Eid, S. Andrews, A. Alamri, and A. El Saddik, "HAMLAT: A HAML-Based Authoring Tool for Haptic Application Development", Proceedings of the 6th international conference on Haptics: Perception, Devices and Scenarios, 2008.
[18] L. Kim, G. S. Sukhatme, and M. Desbrun, "Haptic Editing of Decoration and Material Properties", Symposium on Haptic Interfaces for Virtual Environment and Teleoperator Systems, 2003.
[19] L. Kim, G. S. Sukhatme, and M. Desbrun, "A Haptic-Rendering Technique Based on Hybrid Surface Representation", IEEE Computer Graphics and Applications, pp. 66-75, March/April, 2004.
[20] J-P. Kim, B-C. Lee, H. Kim, J. Kim, and J. Ryu, "Accurate and Efficient Hybrid CPU/GPU-based 3-DOF Haptic Rendering for Highly Complex Hybrid Static Virtual Environments", PRESENCE, in print, 2009.
[21] S. B. Tor, A. E. Middleditch, "Convex Decomposition of Simple Polygons", ACM Transactions on Graphics. pp. 255-265, 1984.
[22] J-M. Lien, N. M. Amato, "Approximate Convex Decomposition of Polygons", Computational Geometry, Vol. 35, No. 1-2, August, pp.100-123, 2006.
[23] SensAble Technologies, http://www.sensable.com/ products-omni.htm

19

Haptic Data Transmission based on the Prediction and Compression

Yonghee You and Mee Young Sung
Department of Computer Science and Engineering
University of Incheon
South Korea

1. Introduction

Even state-of-the-art haptic technology still suffers from a number of limitations, such as the high price and weight or size of the haptic interface, in addition to the limitations in work space and the lack of force feedback to the body. Moreover, when it comes to networking, the high bandwidths, low network latency, high stability, and the synchronization requirements of haptics are not met yet (Saddik, 2007).

Computer haptics is an emerging area of research that deals with the techniques for generating and displaying the "touch" of virtual environments and objects (Saddik, 2007), (You et al., 2007). Haptic collaborative virtual environment (HCVE) is an enhanced virtual reality space that supports sense of touch, which is called "haptic". In HCVE, remote users connected over networks are able to collaborate by sharing touching experiences in addition to well-established audio and visual interfaces. The success of HCVE largely depends on timely transmission of haptic data despite time-varying network conditions such as delay, loss, and jitter.

One of the important challenges in HCVE data transmission over the Internet is the limited bandwidth. Haptic data is too bulky, relative to the available bandwidth. The situation should improve when better haptic based compression techniques are introduced. The demands for real-time simultaneous recording and transmission of voluminous data produced by multimedia haptics are pushing toward the exploration of haptic data compression. However, despite the stringent need for haptic data compression, the field is still in its infancy and many possibilities have emerged (Saddik, 2007).

The fact that the data generation frequency of haptic interface devices is extremely high, e.g. 1 KHz, makes the realization of successful HCVE more challenging. For seamless haptic data communication even under adverse network conditions, we propose a data compression method which contributes to solve the bandwidth limitations of haptic data transmission over the internet (You et al., 2007). Our method is based on mesh compression.

Some related work is presented in the next section. In section 3, the details of our compression method are described, some experimental results are discussed in section 4, and we conclude our work in section 5.

2. Floating-Point Compression for Haptic Data Transmission

In this section, we briefly describe haptic rendering and some technologies such as haptic data transmission (You et al., 2007) and floating-point compression.

A. Haptic Rendering

Haptic rendering refers to the group of algorithms and techniques that are used to compute and generate forces and torques in response to interactions between the haptic interface avatar inside the virtual environment and the virtual objects populating the environments (Saddik, 2007). The goal of haptic rendering is to enable a user to touch, feel, and manipulate virtual objects through haptic interfaces as realistically as possible (Mark et al., 1996), (Ruffaldi et al. 2006). A force-feedback device can generate kinesthetic information and temporal tactile information. By using these perceptual cues such as shape, stiffness, texture and friction, haptic rendering can render various properties of a virtual object. Unlike visual rendering, a minimum update rate to achieve realistic haptic rendering depends on the properties of virtual objects and a force-feedback device. Recommended update rates are 1 KHz and 5 KHz - 10 KHz for a rigid surface and a textured surface respectively. For a transformable object, it is advised to keep the rate as fast as you can.

B. Haptic Data Transmission

In networked haptic applications, there exist various requirements such as high bandwidths, the low network latency, the high stability, and the synchronization. However, there has been extensive research related to the problems caused by the bandwidth limitations and latency (Hikichi et al., 2001), (Ishibashi & Asano, 2007).
Time-varying network conditions pose challenges to successful communication of haptic data (Hikichi et al., 2001). Adverse network links sometimes cause irregular force-feedback which deteriorates the haptic experiences (You et al., 2007). The transmission of the haptic data, which mainly consists of the position information of haptic device pointers, is basically similar to multimedia streaming. However, it is much more demanding because the haptic rendering rate required for satisfactory haptic experience is quite higher than that of graphic rendering; 1 KHz for haptics, in contrast to 30 Hz for graphics. To meet such challenges, there have been various research efforts. For group synchronization control, Y. Ishibashi et al propose virtual time rendering algorithms (Ishibashi & Asano, 2007). Hikichi et al employ a queue monitoring algorithm (Hikichi et al., 2001) designed for efficient haptic collaboration. However, these approaches have limitations that they are not able to cope with delay, loss and jitter at the same time.

C. Floating-point Number Compression

In some environments, the fast transmission or the storage of large amounts of numerical data are required. Examples involve storing 3D geometry, sending statistical results over a network, and also sending haptic data which is composed of three floating-point numbers x, y and z. Since such data are too bulky, it is necessary to find a way to compress them efficiently in a lossless manner. There are some approaches for compressing the floating-point numbers (IEEE 754, 1985).

Martin Isenburg, Peter Lindstrom, Jack Snoeyink from University of North Carolina have proposed a predictive geometry coding used for 3D mesh compression (Lindstorm & Isenburg , 2006), (Isenburg et al. , 2005), (Isenburg & Alliez, 2002). Paruj Ratanaworabbhan, Jian Ke, and Martin Burtscher have also designed a compression method of scientific floating-point data using a predictor and hash tables (Raranaworabhan et al., 2006). In addition, Costa Touma and Craig Gotsman from Israel Institute of Technology have developed a compression algorithm using entropy coding for triangle mesh compression (Touma & Gotsman, 1998). Even though all of these methods work differently, the main ideas of compression are mostly based on the characteristics of floating-point arithmetic. Those characteristics will be explained in the latter section.

3. Floating-Point Compression for Haptic Data Transmission

In networked haptic virtual environments, there exist various types of haptic devices. Some of those devices called stylus-type generate 3D positional information. The positional information usually consists of x, y and z coordinates which are represented in single precision floating-point numbers. The positions of haptic pointer play an important role to produce the force-feedback, since the position itself or the collision between the haptic pointer and an object are main factors for calculating the magnitude and the direction of force-feedback.

Therefore, we usually need to transmit the positional information at the haptic rendering rate 1 KHz over the network in any networked haptic environment. In this case, we need to send at least 12 bytes per millisecond.

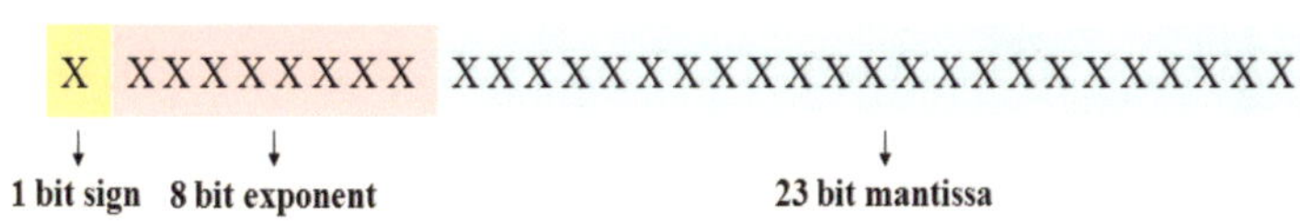

Fig. 1. Configuration of a single precision IEEE floating-point number

Floating-point number	Bit Representation
-81240646	1 10000101 01000100111101100110110
-80.796814	1 10000101 01000011001011111111000
11.638161	0 10000010 01110100011010111101000
11.478516	0 10000010 01101111010100000000000

Table 1. Examples of floating-point numbers in bit representation

Our approach for compressing the haptic data is to compress the bit-representations of single precision floating-point numbers. It is to reduce the size of the haptic data packet (12 bytes) that consists of three floating-point numbers x, y and z. IEEE floating point is the most commonly used representations for real numbers on computers, including Intel-based PC's, Macintoshes, and most Unix platforms. For a single-precision 32-bit IEEE floating-point number, the sign s is a single bit that specifies whether the number is positive (s=0) or negative (s=1), the exponent e is an eight bit number with an added bias of 127 where 0 and

255 are reserved for un-normalized near-zero and infinite values, and the mantissa m is a twenty-three bit number that is used to represent 223 uniformly-spaced numbers within the range associated with a particular exponent (IEEE 754, 1985). Figure 1 shows the configuration of a single precision 32-bit IEEE floating-point number. As shown in Table I, we can recognize that when there are small differences between floating-point numbers. There occur only small changes in mantissa. Due to the configuration of a single precision 32-bit IEEE floating-point number, if the absolute difference between two floating-point numbers is small, the difference in mantissa is also small (IEEE 754, 1985).

We propose an algorithm to compress haptic data using the idea discussed above. If we only transmit the different bits of 3D positions of a haptic pointer, the packet may vary from 0 byte to 12 bytes (0~4 bytes for x, y and z), contrary to the fact that without the compression, we have 12 bytes every millisecond.

As discussed before, the position of the haptic pointer is sampled at 1 KHz and this indicates that the differences between consecutive floating-point numbers are relatively small. Figure 2 is the result from the experiment where we calculated the differences between consecutive positions of the haptic pointers. The number of positions that were used in the experiment was 6000. The maximum difference was 1.937969 while the average difference was 0.390084. This means that the differences are relatively small so changes in mantissa are also small.

From the results of our experiment we found out that if we can make the differences smaller, then the amount of haptic data we need to transmit over a network will be smaller.

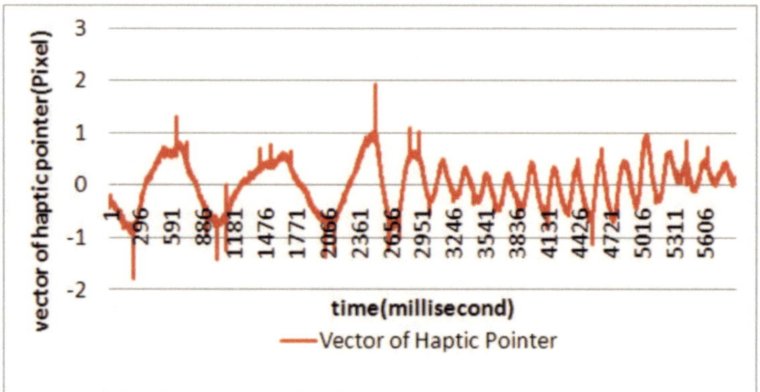

Fig. 2. Differences of consecutive haptic pointers

A. Position Prediction for Haptic Pointer

As discussed above, if we can get smaller differences we have smaller sizes of packets to send. In this section, we describe how the differences can be minimized by prediction.

The haptic pointer, which represents the movement of the haptic device moves freely according to the user's will, so it seems to be impossible to predict the next position based on the previous positions. However, we can predict the next position with a certain acceptable error using the previous vector of the haptic pointer since haptic pointers are sampled very densely.

We propose a simple position prediction method in order to minimize the difference between two floating-point numbers which are used for compression. Our method works as in Figure 3. If we can calculate the previous vector of the haptic pointer, we can predict the next position of the haptic pointer more precisely rather than just using the previous position

The prediction method is executed as follows:

$$x_n^p = x_{n-1} + v_n \tag{1}$$

$$v_n = x_{n-1} - x_{n-2} \tag{2}$$

where x_n^p is the predicted position while x_{n-1} corresponds to the previous position. v_n denotes the velocity of the haptic pointer's position. The velocity v is computed by averaging the previously received positions.

In order to verify the efficiency of applying the linear prediction method to the prediction of haptic pointer, we performed an experiment comparing the error of using the prediction value x_n^p and using the previous position x_{n-1} to compare with the next position x_n. The results of the experiment are shown in Figure 4. If we category one using the previous position as type 1 and the other using its prediction value as type2. The average errors are 0.249083 and 0.038881 for type 1 and type 2 respectively. Since type 2 shows a small error this means that using a linear prediction method will result in the efficiency of compression.

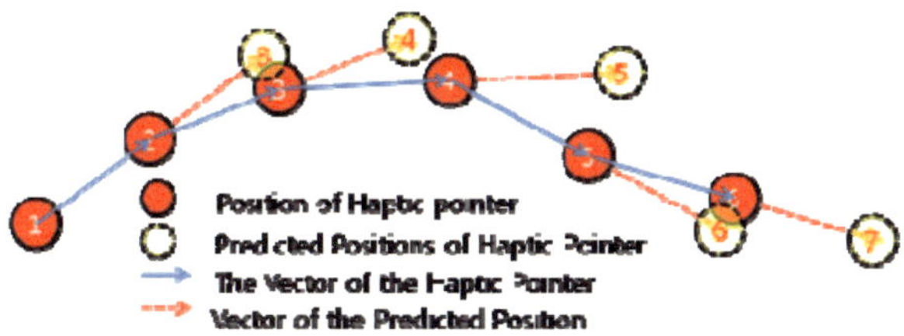

Fig. 3. Prediction of Haptic Pointer

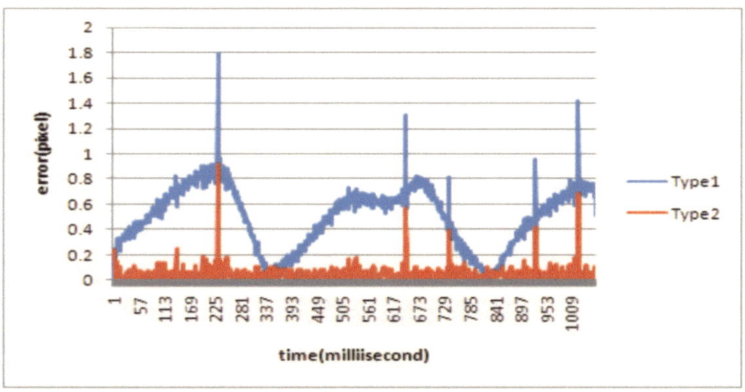

Fig. 4. Results of an Experiment on Prediction of Haptic Pointer

B. Predictive Haptic Data Compression

We compress the floating-point number by extracting the efficient bits from a floating-point number and its prediction, since the small difference in numbers results in a small difference in bit-representation of a floating-point number (IEEE 754, 1985). If the absolute difference between a floating-point number and its prediction value is small, the difference in mantissa is also small and we only need to transmit the difference in bit representation. In this section we examine how the compression of the haptic data proceeds for networked haptic applications. For the ease of explanation, we assume that there is a networked haptic application based on the master-slave model. Figure 5 shows the process of the haptic data

Number of Effcient bits		1~8bit	9~16bits	17~24bits	The whole data
Allocated bytes		1byte	2bytes	3bytes	4bytes
Header	X	0x00	0x40	0x44	
	Y	0x00	0x20	0x22	0x08
	Z	0x00	0x10	0x11	

Table 2. Examples of floating-point numbers in bit representation

transmission.

a) Initialization

To let both the master and the slave have the initiation values, a master sends the whole positional information at least twice. The init value will be stored in Prediction Module for further prediction.

b) Prediction

Prediction Modules in a master and a slave predict the next position based on the previously received position. For example as in Figure 5, the Prediction Module produces the prediction value -77.916992.

c) Encoder

With the actual position from the haptic device and the predicted position, the encoder performs an exclusive-or operation to compress the floating-point number x to the smaller number of bits; for example, the actual number -77.916916 which is 32bit long, can be reduced to 8 efficient bits and only those 8 bits are required to be sent. Encoder also performs the exclusive-or operation iteratively for y and z.

d) Packet Module

Packet Module is responsible for organizing the compressed data into a packet and putting a header onto the packet. Packet Module first calculates the number of the efficient bits of the results from Encoder. In Figure 5, only 11110110 has to be sent to the receiver. However, for the convenience of packetizing, we provide a packetizing policy as in Table 2. If the number of efficient bits are between 1~8, 2~16 and 17~24, we put the efficient bits in 1, 2, and 3 bytes. In addition, if the exponents of the actual position and the predicted position are different, the master transmits all of the positional information without compression for reliability. Packet Module also add to a packet a one byte header which describes the size of the efficient bits for x, y and z.

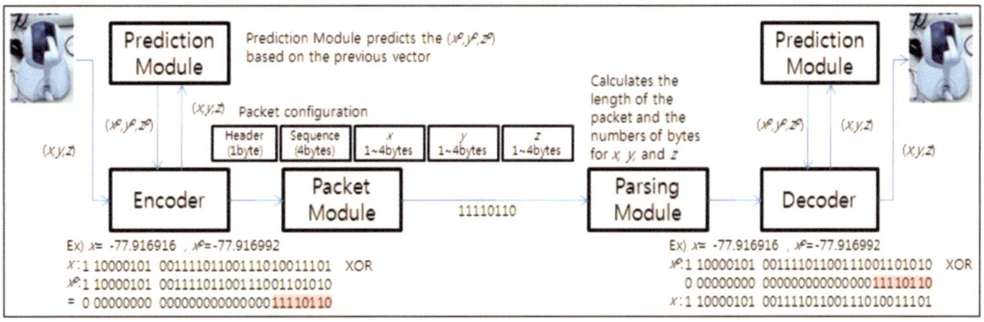

Fig. 5. The Process of the Haptic Data Transmission

e) Parsing Module

Once the slave receives a packet, Parsing Module disassembles the packet into a header and efficient bits of x, y and z.

f) Decoder

Decoder gets a predicted position and performs an exclusive OR operation with the efficient bits of *x*, *y* and *z* added with 0s in the front. Then, we finally regenerate the original position from the relatively small amount of bits.

As discussed above, if we can use the prediction and Exclusive Or operation properly, we don't have to send the 12 bytes(*x*, *y* and *z*) of long floating-point data for bulky haptic data which often cause network delays, losses, and jitters.

4. Experiment

We performed an experiment to evaluate the efficiency of the proposed compression method. In this section, we explain the test application, software configuration, hardware setup, experiment and results.

A. Test Application

The test application used in the experiment is a haptic device tele-operation application. It is composed of two parts: a master and a slave. The master sends the motion data to the slave and the slave outputs the force feed-back according to the motion data which consists of three floating-point numbers. The slave sometimes sends control messages to the master such as connect, ready, NAK and so forth to connect or control errors. The overview of the application is shown in Figure 6. This application is suitable for the test because we can feel the effects of network errors through both the sense sight and touch.

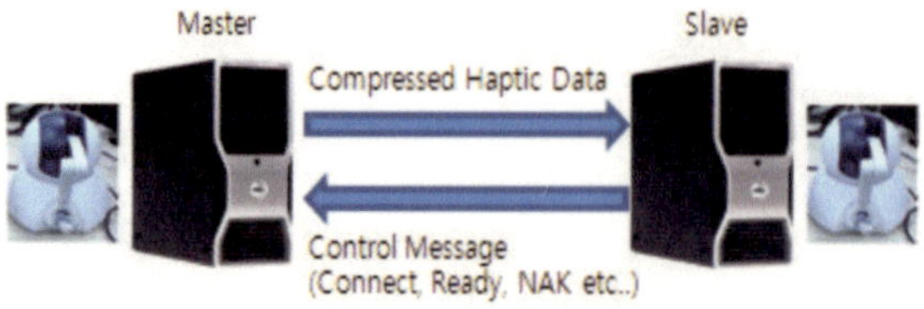

Fig. 6. Overview of the Test Application

B. Software Configuration

The software configuration of the test application is shown in Figure 7. The compression method and network module is developed dependant on C++. The OpenHaptics Toolkit (SDK) from SensAble for haptic rendering from Sensable Technologies, and the QUANTA (The Quality of Service Adaptive Networking Toolkit) are used in the application.

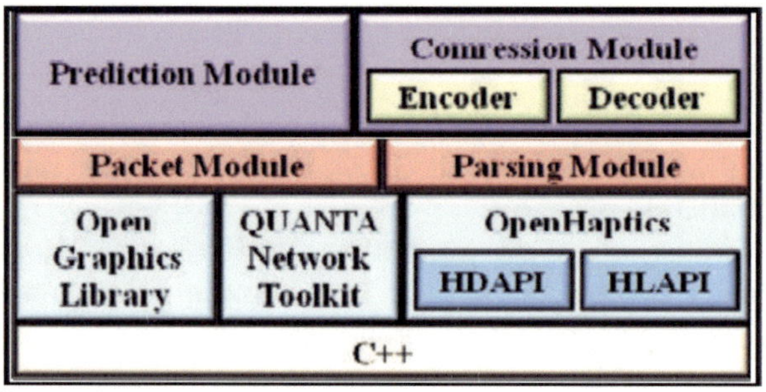

Fig. 7. Software Configuration

C. Hardware Setup

- Sensable PHANToM Omni
- Dell Precision PWS380 Intel® Pentium 4 CPU 3.20GHz, 1.00 GB RAM
- NVIDIA Quadro FX 1400
- Microsoft Windows XP Professional Version 2002 Service Pack 2

D. Experiments

We performed an experiment to evaluate the efficiency of the proposed method. The master mainly transmits its positional information to the slave and the haptic device of the slave follows the motion of the master. In order to assess our method, we measure the size of packets sent in six cases; five cases depending on the motions of the haptic pointer (1: stay static, 2: move slow, 3: draw 8, 4: draw *, 5: move fast and irregularly) and one without compression (6).

Figure 8 shows the result of the transmission experiment for approximately four minutes. If we do not consider the UDP header, the average bandwidths used for the transmission are 7992.59bps (compression ratio 47.06%), 10574.76bps (62.27%), 11201.43bps (65.96%), 11441.18bps (67.37%), 11808.37bps (69.53%), and 16983 bps in the cases of 1, 2, 3, 4, 5, and 6 respectively. The result leads us to confirm that our compression method works efficiently for networked haptic applications.

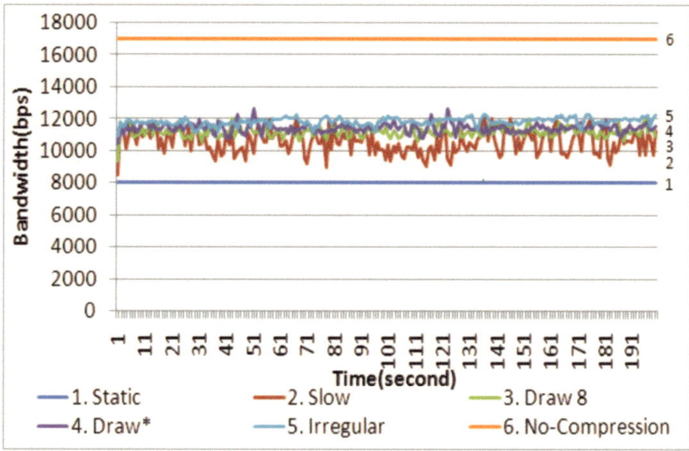

Fig. 8. Results of the experiment

5. Conclusion

We propose a floating-point haptic data compression in order to reduce the bandwidth which sometimes causes packet losses, jitters, and delays when being exceeded. Our compression method is based on the idea that the bit representations of consecutive floating-point numbers change slightly from the most significant bit. The exclusive OR operation helps extract the efficient bits from floating-point numbers and our prediction method produces a smaller difference between two consecutive floating-point numbers. Some experiments on our proposed method lead us to conclude that our method provides relatively high compression ratio, approximately 47.06%~69.53%. This will help the haptic data transmission even under limited bandwidth.

For future work, we plan to work on the QoS algorithms which cope with significant delay, jitter, and loss for haptic applications (Cruz-Neira et al., 1993), (Marsh et al., 2004), (Fujimoto & Ishibashi, 2005).

6. References

Abdulmotaleb El Saddik. (2007). "The Potential of Haptics Technologies," IEEE Instrumentation & Measurement Magazine, IEEE, pp. 10-17

Yonghee You, Mee Young Sung, and Kyungkoo Jun. (2007) "A scheme for Haptic Data Transmission under Various Network Conditions," In Proceedings of IEEE-ICME 2007 (IEEE International Conference on Multimedia & Expo), IEEE, Beijing, China, pp. 2238-2242, July 2-5.

W. Mark, S. Randolph, M. Finch, J. V. Verth, and R. M. Taylor. (1996) "Adding force feedback to graphics systems: Issues and solutions," Proceedings of ACM SIGGRAPH '96 Conference, ACM press, pp. 447-452.

Emanuele Ruffaldi, Dan Morris, Timothy Edmunds, Federico Barbagli and Dinesh K. Pai. (2006) "Standardized Evaluation of Haptic Rendering Systems," In Proceedings of the Symposium on Haptic Interfaces for Virtual Environment and Teleoperator Systems, IEEE, pp. 225-232.

K. Hikichi et al. (2001) "Architecture of Haptics Communication System for Adaption to Network Environments," In Proceedings of IEEE International Conference on Multimedia and Expo Proceedings, IEEE, pp. 744-747.

Yutaka Ishibashi and Toshio Asano. (2007) "Media Synchronization Control with Prediction in a Remote Haptic Calligraphy System," In Proceedings of ACE 2007, ACM press, pp. 79-86.

IEEE 754 (1985) : Standard for binary floating-point arithmetic, IEEE.

Peter Lindstrom and Martin Isenburg. (2006) "Fast and Efficient Compression of Floating-Point Data," In IEEE Transactions on Visualization and Computer Graphics, IEEE, vol. 12, No. 5, pp. 1245-1250.

Martin Isenburg, Peter Lindstrom and Jack Snoeyink. (2005) "Lossless Compression of Predicted Floating-Point Geometry," In Computer-Aided Design, Elsevier Science, volume 37, pp. 869-877.

Martin Isenburg and Pierre Alliez. (2002) "Compressing Polygon Mesh Geometry with Parallelogram Prediction," In Proceedings of Visualization, IEEE, pp. 141-146.

Paruj Ratanaworabhan, Jian Ke, and Martin Burtscher. (2006) "Fast Lossless Compression of Scientific Floating-Point Data," In Proceedings of Data Compression Conference, pp. 133-142.

Costa Touma and Craig Gotsman. (1998) "Triangle Mesh Compression," In Proceedings of Graphics Interface '98, pp. 26-34.

E. He, J. Alimohideen, J. Eliason, N. K. Krishnaprasad, J. Leigh, O. Yu, and T. A. DeFanti. (2003) "Quanta a toolkit for high performance data delivery over photonic networks," In Future Generations Computer Systems, Special Issue: iGRID 2002, FGCS, volume 19, number 6, pp. 919-933.

C. Cruz-Neira, D. Sandin, and T. A. DeFanti. (1993) "Surround-screen projection-based virtual reality: The Design and Implementation of the CAVE," In Proceedings of the 20th annual conference on Computer graphics and interactive techniques, ACM press, pp. 135-142.

J. Marsh, M. Glencross, S. Pettifer, R. Hubbold, J. Cook, and S. Daubrebet. (2004) "Minimizing latency and maintaining consistency in distributed virtual prototyping," In Proceedings of ACM SIGGRAPH Conference on the Virtual Reality Continuum and its Applications in Industry (VRCAI), ACM press, Singapore, pp. 386–389.

M. Fujimoto, Y. Ishibashi. (2005) "Packetization Interval of Haptic Media in Networked Virtual Environments," In ACM NetGames, ACM press, pp. 1-6. Information

Digitizing literacy: reflections on the haptics of writing

Anne Mangen* and Jean-Luc Velay**
*The National Centre for Reading Education and Research, University of Stavanger, Norway
** Mediterranean Institute for Cognitive Neuroscience, CNRS, Université de la Méditerranée, Marseille, France

How utterly bound to the physical world of bodies is writing, one of the most awesome products of the human mind. (Haas 1998)

1. Introduction

Writing is a complex cognitive process relying on intricate perceptual-sensorimotor combinations. The process and skill of writing is studied on several levels and in many disciplines, from neurophysiological research on the shaping of each letter to studies on stylistic and compositional features of authors and poets. In studies of writing and literacy overall, the role of the physically tangible writing device (pen on paper; computer mouse and keyboard; digital stylus pen and writing tablet; etc.) is rarely addressed. By and large, the (relatively young) field of writing research is dominated by cognitive approaches predominantly focusing on the visual component of the writing process, hence maintaining a separation between (visual) perception and motor action (e.g., haptics[1]). However, recent theoretical currents in psychology, phenomenology & philosophy of mind, and neuroscience - commonly referred to as "embodied cognition" - indicate that perception and motor action are closely connected and, indeed, reciprocally dependent.

Today, most of our writing is done with digital writing devices (the computer, the mobile phone, the PDA [i.e., Personal Digital Assistant]), rather than writing by hand. The switch from pen and paper to mouse, keyboard and screen entails major differences in the haptics of writing, at several distinct but intersecting levels. Handwriting is by essence a unimanual activity, whereas typewriting is bimanual. Typically, handwriting is also a slower process than typewriting. Moreover, the visual attention of the writer is strongly concentrated during handwriting; the attentional focus of the writer is dedicated to the tip of the pen, while during typewriting the visual attention is detached from the haptic input, namely the

[1]Haptics is defined as a combination of tactile perception associated with active movements (i.e. voluntary movements generated by central motor commands which, in turn, induced proprioceptive feedback). Haptic perception is involved in exploratory hand movements and object manipulation.

process of hitting the keys. Hence, typewriting is divided into two distinct, and spatiotemporally separated, spaces: the motor space (e.g., the keyboard), and the visual space (e.g., the screen). Another major difference pertains to the production of each character during the two writing modes. In handwriting, the writer has to graphomotorically form each letter – i.e., produce a graphic shape resembling as much as possible the standard shape of the specific letter. In typewriting, obviously, there is no graphomotor component involved; the letters are "readymades" and the task of the writer is to spatially locate the specific letters on the keyboard. Finally, word processing software provides a number of features all of which might radically alter the process of writing for professional as well as for beginning writers.

A large body of research in neuroscience, biopsychology and evolutionary biology demonstrates that our use of hands for purposive manipulation of tools plays a constitutive role in learning and cognitive development, and may even be a significant building block in language development. Furthermore, brain imaging studies (using fMRI, i.e., functional Magnetic Resonance Imaging) show that the specific hand movements involved in handwriting support the visual recognition of letters. Considering the fact that children today or in the near future may learn to write on the computer before they master the skill of handwriting, such findings are increasingly important. In this article we present evidence from experiments in neuroscience and experimental psychology that show how the bodily, sensorimotor – e.g., haptic – dimension might be a defining feature of not only the skill of writing but may in fact be an intrinsic factor contributing to low-level reading skills (e.g., letter recognition) as well, and we discuss what a shift from handwriting to keyboard writing might entail in this regard. In addition, we discuss the ramifications of the recent interdisciplinary paradigm of embodied cognition for the field of literacy studies in general, and for writing research in particular. Specifically, we intend to address the following questions:

- Why, in what ways and with what implications is keyboard writing different than writing by hand?
- What implications might these differences have for children's learning, and for our reading and writing behavior and experience? Entailed in this question complex are, moreover, the wider implications surrounding the role of the hand-brain relationship in learning and cognitive development overall.

2. Reclaiming the haptics of embodied writing

Writing is an immensely important and equally complex and sophisticated human skill commonly ascribed a fundamental role in children's cognitive and language development, and a milestone on the path to literacy. Nevertheless, compared to the vast field of reading research, there has been less scientific attention devoted to the act and skill of writing. As new technologies complement and eventually replace old ones, and we increasingly type and click rather than write with a pen in our hand, however, the distinctive sensorimotor properties of this skill reveal themselves. Writing has always been dependent on technology; indeed, in a very literal sense, writing *is* technology, for "[…] without the crayon or the stylus or the laptop, writing simply is not possible." (Haas, 1996; preface) From using clay tablets and animal skins via the medieval manuscript and the ancient papyrus roll, to the mechanization of writing with the printing press and the current digitization, writers have always had to handle physical devices and then applying these to some substrate. The outcome of the writing process has always relied on the skilful combination of technical/manual skill and intellectual/aesthetic aptitude (Bolter, 2001; Ong, 1982).

However, at least outside the domain of ergonomics, the role and impact of the different technologies employed in the writing process is rarely addressed. Whether focusing on the cognitive aspects of writing, the semiotics of different codes and sign systems of writing, or studying emergent writing skills within a sociocultural paradigm, the technologies in question are by and large - and deliberately or not - treated as transparent. Hence, arguably important questions of how technologies and devices are physically (e.g., haptically) handled during the act of writing, and how these sensorimotor acts might interplay with, and impact, cognition, seem not to be considered scientifically interesting. The haptics of writing is a curiously ignored area of research, both in the field of literacy studies at large, as well as within the field of writing research in particular.

In the theoretically-methodologically inhomogeneous field commonly referred to as digital (or new) literacies, (digital; multimodal) writing is commonly considered a meaning making process situated in specific social and cultural contexts (Barton, 2007; Barton, Hamilton, & Ivanic, 2000; Buckingham, 2003, 2007; Coiro, 2008; Jewitt, 2006; Kress, 2003; Lankshear, 2006; Säljö, 2006). As such, it is argued, it is most appropriately studied within a theoretical-methodological framework defined mainly, if not exclusively, by sociocultural and/or semiotic perspectives. Within such a framework, reflections on the impact of digital technologies on reading, writing and literacy limit themselves to discussing the changing (semiotic; structural; semantic; aesthetic) relations between different sign systems (e.g., image, text, and sound) when displayed on screen.

A major digital literacy scholar, semiotician Günther Kress readily acknowledges the radical changes to writing brought about by digital technology:

The combined effects on writing of the dominance of the mode of image and of the medium of screen will produce deep changes in the forms and functions of writing. This in turn will have profound effects on human, cognitive/affective, cultural and bodily engagement with the world, and on forms and shapes of knowledge. (Kress, 2003, p. 3)

Such changes, argues Kress, forces "an insistence on the very materiality of writing [...], its *stuff* [...]" (p. 32), hence indicating that it is time, after all, for literacy studies to focus on our sensorimotor, bodily engagement with the materialities of reading and writing - e.g., with the technologies involved. According to Kress, we need a new theory of meaning and meaning making that takes into account the materiality of the different semiotic modes (text, image, sound, etc.) and how they relate differently to bodily reception of meaning. What Kress terms the *affective affordances* of sound are very different from those of sight or those of touch, in that "[...] sound is more immediately tangibly felt in the body than is sight, and certainly different felt. A theory of meaning that is inattentive to these will no be able to provide fully satisfactory accounts of the new communicational forms." (p. 46) Such promising foundations notwithstanding, Kress never goes beyond a semiotic perspective which seems, somehow, to be incompatible with a focus on what goes on in the writer's mind and body during writing in different technologies. In order for the field of digital literacies to be able to address the role and potential impact of changing devices of writing, the field would arguably benefit from opening up to recent research on the embodied aspect of digital writing emerging in fields such as cognitive neuroscience, experimental psychology, phenomenology and philosophy of mind. Keyboards and computer mice transform the process and experience of writing to such an extent that we might - indeed, *should* - ask ourselves what such a shift might entail in terms of cognitive and phenomenological implications for the act and skill of writing. Further, we should ask what epistemological implications this shift might have for the field of writing research, and what pedagogical implications it might hold for the teaching of writing both inside and outside of classrooms. Considering the speed and rate at which the technological environments of literacy develop and change, we can no longer afford to ignore the haptics of writing. This article intends to contribute to these vital reflections.

The purpose of this article is twofold. The first purpose pertains to the field of writing research and instruction: by exploring and explicating the critical role of haptics in writing, we discuss and reflect on how new writing technologies and devices, by radically altering the hand movements and hence the haptic feedback, might have an impact on future writing skills. As a corollary, if the technologies of writing do in fact radically alter the acquisition of writing skills, this ought to be reflected in the pedagogies of writing instruction. In the light of emerging knowledge about the implications of the digitization of writing on emergent literacy and early writing acquisition, how can and should writing instruction adjust accordingly? A closely related issue is the current theoretical-methodological state of the art of writing research. The second purpose of this article has to do with an unfortunate but persistent scientific schism between fields such as literacy and media studies on the one side, and on the other side, philosophy of mind, neurophenomenology,[2] and research in the natural sciences dealing with questions that are obviously relevant to the field of literacy, such as cognitive neuroscience and experimental psychology. Considering what we now know about embodied cognition and the role of the body in learning and cognitive development, what theoretical-methodological challenges does this entail for the fields of literacy, reading and writing research? And how might these challenges be met?

3. The neurophysiology and phenomenology of writing

The act of writing is a complex cognitive process relying on intricate perceptual-sensorimotor combinations. As a highly sophisticated and comprehensive way of externalizing our thoughts, giving shape to past memories as well as future plans and dreams, sharing our stories and communicating our emotions and affections, writing always involves the skillful handling of some mechanical/technical device, and necessarily results in a visuographic representation - some kind of (more or less) readable text, in the form of a

[2] Usually applied to the works of the late neurobiologist Francisco Varela et al. (Varela, Thompson, & Rosch, 1991), neurophenomenology is an attempt at combining phenomenology and neuroscience, emphasizing the corporeally embodied nature of cognition and mental experience. Specifically, neurophenomenology explores "the relevance of first-person methods for producing more refined first-person reports in experimental psychology and cognitive neuroscience." (Thompson, 2007, p. 20)

string of letters or symbols. As mentioned, in studies of literacy in general, and of writing (as well as of reading) in particular, the role and potential impact of the technologies employed - whether pen and paper, or keyboard and computer screen - is rarely addressed. A cursory and cross-disciplinary glance at the current state of writing research yields the impression that writing is mainly, if not exclusively, a mental (e.g., cognitive) process (MacArthur, Graham, & Fitzgerald, 2006; Torrance, van Waes, & Galbraith, 2007; Van Waes, Leijten, & Neuwirth, 2006). Cognitive approaches to the study of writing focus predominantly on the visual component of the process, and how it relates to cognitive processing. However, as evidenced by research in neuroscience, and as phenomenologically experienced by the writer him- or herself, writing is a process that requires the integration of visual, proprioceptive (haptic/kinaesthetic), and tactile information in order to be accomplished (Fogassi & Gallese, 2004). In other words, the acquisition of writing skills involves a perceptual component (learning the shape of the letter) and a graphomotor component (learning the trajectory producing the letter's shape) (van Galen, 1991). Research has shown that sensory modalities involved in handwriting, e.g., vision and proprioception, are so intimately entwined that strong neural connections have been revealed between perceiving, reading, and writing letters in different languages and symbol/writing systems. (James & Gauthier, 2006; Kato et al., 1999; Longcamp, Anton, Roth, & Velay, 2003, 2005a; Matsuo et al., 2003; Vinter & Chartrel, 2008; Wolf, 2007) Current brain imaging techniques show how neural pathways can be differentially activated from handling different writing systems: logographic writing systems seem to activate very distinctive parts of the frontal and temporal areas of the brain, particularly regions involved in what is called motor perception. For instance, experiments using fMRI have revealed how Japanese readers use different pathways - when reading kana (an efficient syllabary used mainly for foreign and/or newer words, and for names of cities and persons), the activated pathways are similar to those used by English readers. In contrast, when reading kanji - an older logographic script influenced by Chinese - Japanese readers use pathways that come close to those used by the Chinese. (Wolf, 2007) Our knowledge about the writing body and brain is steadily increasing, and it is unfortunate - and strange - if such knowledge cannot find accommodation in the field of literary and writing studies.

More and more of our current writing is writing with a digital device, whether it is a laptop, a PDA, or a mobile phone. Computers and keyboards are replacing pen and paper at an ever-increasing rate, and children are increasingly being introduced to writing with computers in addition to, and even at the expense of, writing by hand. With new technologies, we are changing the role of the hands, as the haptic affordances of digital technologies are distinctly different than earlier technologies such as pen and paper, the print book, and even the typewriter. We click and scroll with computer mice and tap keys on a keyboard, instead of putting pen to paper. This switch from pen and paper to mouse, keyboard and screen entails major differences in the haptics of writing, at several distinct but intersecting levels. When writing by hand, we use only one hand, whereas typewriting typically involves both hands; handwriting is commonly experienced as a slower and more laborious process than writing with a keyboard. Writing by hand requires the writer to shape each letter, whereas in typewriting, obviously, there is no such graphomotor component involved. Moreover, our visual attention is commonly restricted to precisely the point where the pen hits the paper during handwriting, while during typewriting there is a distinct spatiotemporal decoupling between the visual attention and the haptic input.

Finally, word processing software provides a number of features all of which might radically alter the process of writing for professional as well as for beginning writers – from autocorrect and spell-check options to large-scale genre templates and stylistic features.
Generally speaking, the process of text production, sensomotorically as well as cognitively and phenomenologically, is radically different in a print writing environment compared to a digital environment. Such a change might plausibly have considerable educational implications, the understanding of which mandates a thorough investigation of the currently changing role of haptics in writing. In order to understand why and to what extent the process, skill, and art of writing is being transformed by digital technologies, we must reconceptualize our understanding of writing as incorporating – literally speaking – sensory modalities not commonly addressed in educational research on writing and literacy, such as haptics. Considering the major ongoing changes in how we write, and – perhaps even more importantly – how children, in our age of digital technology, learn to write (and might learn to write in the near future), the haptics of writing is an aspect in urgent need of scientific scrutiny.

4. Writing, body, and technologies

Writing is, by definition, the production of some kind of text on some kind of surface or display, employing some kind of technical device. As mentioned, the role of this technical device – how it is employed and implemented in the writing process, and how it thus impacts the process of writing – has not been the subject of much attention in the field of writing research. Describing writing in the very early years of word processors, Christina Haas observed:

Changing the technologies of writing has profound implications, at least in part, because different technologies are materially configured in profoundly different ways. That is, different writing technologies set up radically different spatial, tactile, visual, and even temporal relations between the writer's material body and his or her material text. […] Hence, the body […] is the mechanism by which the mediation of the mental and the material occurs. (Haas, 1996, p. 5)

More than a decade later, Haas' claim still holds. Overall, contemporary theoretical discussions on writing tend to treat technology as transparent, or simply not interesting in and by itself. However, phenomenological accounts of writing provide some insight into the fundamental *bodiliness* of the writing process, and the role of the material device in the process, and illustrate how writing is inextricably bound to the entire human sensorium – in which our fingers and hands play a vital part. In his early writings, Martin Heidegger (1982 [1942]) underscores the phenomenological impact of, precisely, the physical inscriptions on some tangible material entailed in handwriting, by contrasting handwriting with the impersonalized mechanization of writing introduced by the (mechanical) typewriter. When writing with a typewriter, Heidegger says,

the word no longer passes through the hand as it writes and acts authentically but through the mechanized pressure of the hand. The typewriter snatches script from the essential realm of the hand – and this means the hand is removed from the essential realm of the word. The word becomes something 'typed.' [...] Mechanized writing deprives the hand of dignity in the realm of the written word and degrades the word into a mere means for the traffic of communication. Besides, mechanized writing offers the advantage of covering up one's handwriting and therewith one's character. (1982 [1942], pp. 118-119)

Replacing the mechanical typewriter with the digital computer and its word processing software introduces new features of equally impersonalized and disembodied writing - a writing modality, moreover, that is undoubtedly more phenomenologically monotonous than handwriting.[3] Although digital word processing does provide features intended to resemble a more "personalized" and idiosyncratic mode of writing (e.g., fonts that are supposed to look like handwriting) and thereby attempting to reintroduce the "aura" or "felt origination" (Benjamin, 1969; Heim, 1999) that authentic handwriting entails, the paradoxical experiential outcome of such digital attempts at reproducing *the trace of the tangible* is to even further detach the embodied relation to the inscribing efforts - the writing - from the displayed outcome, thereby adding yet another layer of phenomenological disembodiment. When writing by hand, we experience a direct and phenomenologically unambiguous relation between the act of inscription and the phenomenological correlate of the pen moving across the paper (cf. Mangen, 2009). In the words of neuroscientists, in handwriting, motor commands and kinesthetic feedback are closely linked to visual information at a spatial as well as a temporal level, while this is not the case with typewriting. For instance, neuropsychologist Alexander R. Lurija uses handwriting as an example par excellence of a "kinetic melody" - e.g., an embodied, automatized incorporated skill:

In the initial stages [...] writing depends on memorizing the graphic form of every letter. It takes place through a chain of isolated motor impulses, each of which is responsible for the performance of only one element of the graphic structure; with practice, this structure of the process is radically altered and writing is converted into a single 'kinetic melody', no longer requiring the memorizing of the visual form of each isolated letter or individual motor impulses for making every stroke. The same situation applies to the process in which the change to write a highly automatized engram (such as a signature) ceases to depend on analysis of the acoustic complex of the word or the visual form of its individual letters, but begins to be performed as a single "kinetic melody" [...] The participation of the auditory and visual areas of the cortex, essential in the early stages of the formation of the activity, no longer is necessary in its later stages, and *the activity starts to depend on a different system of concertedly working zones*. (Lurija, 1973, p. 32)

Luria's kinetic melody thus refers to the neurological role of the hand in writing. In *Physical Eloquence and the Biology of Writing*, Robert Ochsner extends Luria's melody to include two additional neurophysiological functions, namely, visual melodies and auditory melodies. These correspond, respectively, to the roles of the eye and the ear in the handwriting process. The visual melody determines how much of the text the eye takes in as feedback, and the auditory melody regulates the inner voice of the writer as it matches vocally

[3] For instance, consider how handwriting might entail and display visible traces - however subtle - of different sensory traits of the writer, such as temper, stress, or nervousness.

subpressed language with the language of a written text. Basic to these functions of the eye and the ear, however, is nevertheless the kinetic melody, which innervates muscles in the hand, wrist, arm and shoulder to produce graphic shapes. (Ochsner, 1990, p. 55)

The increasing disembodiment of writing currently taking place should not be reduced to a matter of interest primarily for philosophers, nostalgics and neo-Luddites,[4] as it points to the importance of acknowledging the vital role of haptics, and the profound and fundamental links between haptics and cognition, in writing. Our body, and in particular our hands, are inscribed in, and defining, the writing process in ways that have not been adequately dealt with in the research literature. The current radical shift in writing environments mandates an increased focus on the role of our hands in the writing process, and - even more importantly - how the movements and performance of the hand relate to what goes on in the brain.

5. Haptics and learning

In his landmark volume *The Hand* - succinctly described by some scholars as "one of the wisest books of recent decades" (Singer & Singer, 2005, p. 113) - neurologist Frank Wilson vigorously claims that "any theory of human intelligence which ignores the interdependence of hand and brain function, the historical origins of that relationship, or the impact of that history on developmental dynamics in modern humans, is grossly misleading and sterile." (Wilson, 1998, p. 7) Nevertheless, the importance of the hand-brain relationship and of the haptic sense modality for learning, and for our experience of and interaction with the lifeworld in general, is not commonly acknowledged or understood.[5] This widespread and largely internalized neglect becomes obvious when we are reminded of how fundamental haptics and the rest of our tactile sensorium were in our life from the moment we are born:

As infants, we tend to learn as much, if not more, about our environment by touching as well as looking, smelling, or listening. Only gradually, and after many warnings by our parents not to touch this or that, we do finally manage to drive the tactile sense underground. But the many do-not-touch signs in stores and especially in museums suggest that apparently we still would like to touch objects in order to get to know them better and to enrich our experience. (Zettl, 1973, p. 25)

Research in experimental psychology, evolutionary psychology, and cognitive anthropology (Bara, Gentaz, & Colé, 2007; Greenfield, 1991; Hatwell, Streri, & Gentaz, 2003; Klatzky, Lederman, & Mankinen, 2005; Klatzky, Lederman, & Matula, 1993; Wilson, 1998) has convincingly demonstrated the vital role of haptic exploration of tangible objects in human learning and cognitive development. In a very literal way, the sense of touch incorporates

[4] Neo-Luddite is a label commonly attached to people who are considered overly sceptical or resistant of technological change.

[5] The pedagogies of Montessori and Steiner might be considered as exceptions in this regard, with their focus on holistic education, eurythmy (a pedagogical program focusing on awakening and strengthening the expressive capacities of children through movement) and on seeing children as sensorial explorers. (Palmer, 2002)

human nature, as eloquently described by Brian O'Shaughnessy: "Touch is in a certain respect the most important and certainly the most primordial of the senses. The reason is, that it is scarcely to be distinguished from the having of a body that can act in physical space." (O'Shaughnessy, 2002, p. 658) During infancy and early childhood, haptic exploration is very important; however, as we grow up, we tend to lose some of the strength and clarity of the sense of touch (and smell, it is argued), so that we somehow have to re-learn how to make use of it.

Metaphors and colloquialisms are additional indicators of the importance of the haptic modality in cognition. Numerous expressions for understanding and comprehension consist of terms and concepts referring to *dexterity*: expressions such as "to get a hold of someone," "to handle a situation," "to grasp a concept" all point to (pun intended) the paramount influence of our hands and fingers in dealing with the environment. Such an intimate connection between the human body - for example, our hands - the lifeworld, and cognition is a hallmark of phenomenology, in particular the somatosensory phenomenology of Maurice Merleau-Ponty:

It is the body that 'catches' [...] 'and 'comprehends' movement. The acquisition of a habit is indeed the grasping of a significance, but it is the motor grasping a motor significance. [...] If habit is neither a form of knowledge nor any involuntary action, then what is it? It is a *knowledge in the hands* [Merleau-Ponty's example is knowing how to use a typewriter], which is forthcoming only when bodily effort is made, and cannot be formulated in detachment from that effort. (Merleau-Ponty, 1962 [1945], pp. 143-144)

Our fingers and hands are highly active and important means of perception and exploration, representing an access to our lifeworld which in some cases could not have been established by any other sense modality. In our everyday whereabouts, however, we are just not used to thinking of the hands as sensory organs significantly contributing to cognitive processing, because most of our day-to-day manipulation is *performatory*, not *exploratory*: "[T]hat is, we grasp, push, pull, lift, carry, insert, or assemble for practical purposes, and the manipulation is usually guided by visual as well as by haptic feedback." (Gibson, 1979, p. 123) Because of this, the perceptual capacity of the hands, and the vital role it plays in cognition, is often ignored - both because we pay more attention to their motor capacities, and because the visual modality dominates the haptic in our awareness.

6. Writing and embodied cognition

During the past decade, intriguing and influential interdisciplinary perspectives have been established between biology, cognitive neuroscience, psychology and philosophy. Jointly advocated by philosophers, biologists, and neuroscientists,[6] the embodied cognition paradigm emphasizes the importance of embodiment to cognitive processes, hence

---

[6] The most prominent philosophers are Andy Clark, Evan Thompson, Alva Noë, and the late Susan Hurley; Francisco Varela and Humberto Maturana are the biologists most frequently associated with embodied cognition, whereas the best known neuroscientists are Antonio Damasio, V. S. Ramachandran, Alain Berthoz and J.Kevin O'Regan.

countering Cartesian dualism[7] and focusing instead on human cognition as inextricably and intimately bound to and shaped by its corporeal foundation – its embodiment. In this current of thought, cognition is no longer viewed as abstract and symbolic information processing with the brain as a disembodied CPU. It is becoming increasingly clear that the body is an active component that adds uniquely and indispensably to cognition, and that human cognition is grounded in distinct and fundamental ways to embodied experience and hence is closely intertwined with and mutually dependent on both sensory perception and motor action. A number of theoretical contributions from adjacent fields can be subsumed under the heading of embodied cognition:

- Motor theories of perception (initially developed for the perception of spoken language by Liberman et al. [1985]): Until fairly recently, perception and action were studied as quite separate entities in the disciplines involved. Now, converging research data from neuroscience and experimental psychology show how our perception is closely correlated with motor actions, to active explorations of our lifeworld, mainly through the always active and intriguingly complex collaboration of sensory modalities. Commonly referred to as *motor theories of perception*, these theories indicate that we mentally simulate movements and actions even though we only see (or only hear; or only touch) them. Research data from cognitive neuroscience and neurophysiology (Fogassi & Gallese, 2004; Jensenius, 2008; Olivier & Velay, 2009) show how motor areas in the brain (e.g., premotor and parietal area; Broca's area) are activated when subjects are watching someone else performing an action, when they are watching images of tools requiring certain actions (e.g., a hammer; a pair of scissors; a pen, or a keyboard; cf. Chao & Martin, 2000), and when action verbs are being read out loud (e.g.; kick; run; shake hands; write; cf. Pulvermüller, 2005), even when no action or movement is actually required from the subjects themselves. Motor theories of perception hence support the so-called sandwich theory of the human mind, which suggests that human cognition is "sandwiched" between perception as input from the world to the mind, and action as output from the mind to the external environment – also called an "action-perception loop".

- The *enactive approach* to cognition and conscious experience (Varela et al., 1991) argues that experience does not take place inside the human being (whether in a "biological brain" or in a "phenomenological mind"), but is something humans actively – e.g., physically; sensorimotorically – enact as we explore the environment in which we are situated. Building in part on J. J. Gibson's ecological psychology (Gibson, 1966, 1979), Varela et al. emphasize the importance of sensorimotor patterns inherent in different acts of exploration of the environment, and they argue that perception and action supply structure to cognition: "Perception consists in perceptually guided action and [...] cognitive structures emerge from the recurrent sensorimotor patterns that enable action to be perceptually guided." (Varela et al., 1991, p. 173)

---

[7] Cartesian dualism refers to the conception of mind and body as distinct, separate entities and treating mental phenomena (e.g., perceptual experience; cognition; reasoning) as being purely matters of mind.

- The theory of *sensorimotor contingency* (Noë, 2004; O'Regan & Noë, 2001). According to the sensorimotor contingency theory, each sensory modality - audio, vision, touch, smell, taste, haptics, kinesthetics - are modes of exploration of the world that are mediated by knowledge of sensorimotor contingencies, e.g., practical and embodied knowledge of sets of structured laws pertaining to the sensory changes brought about by one's movement and/or manipulation of objects. For instance, visual experience depends on one's knowledge of the sensory effects of, say, our eye-contingent operations - e.g., the fact that closing our eyes will yield no visual input. In contrast, closing our eyes will not change the tactile input of experience. This practical, bodily knowledge of sensorimotor contingencies makes us effective in our exploration.

These theoretical developments all have similarities with the by now classical, ecological psychology of J. J. Gibson, in particular his concept of affordances, which are functional, meaningful, and persistent properties of the environment for activity. (Gibson, 1979) Hence, Gibson would say, we attend to the properties and the opportunities for actions implied by these objects, rather than to the physical properties of objects in the environment *per se*. In other words, we see the world as we can exploit it, not "as it is." (ibid.) Embodied cognition, in other words, is theorized as an active, multisensory probing of the surrounding lifeworld. A central and far-reaching corollary of these conceptualizations is that learning and cognitive development is about developing representations about how to physically - haptically - interact with the environment, e.g., how to explore our surroundings by means of all our sensory modalities, rather than about making internal representations - a quasi-photographic "snapshot" - of the environment itself. Thus, learning and cognition are inextricably tied to and dependent upon our audiovisual, tactile, haptic, *probing* of our surroundings. In other words, it is time, as S. Goldin-Meadow claims, "to acknowledge that the hands have a role to play in teaching and learning" (Goldin-Meadow, 2003) - not only in gestures and non-verbal communication, but also, and more specifically, in the haptic interaction with different technologies.

7. From pen and paper to keyboard, mouse and screen: explicating the differences between handwriting vs typing

The important role of the motor component during handwriting can be deduced from experimental data in neuroscience. There is some evidence strongly suggesting that writing movements are involved in letter memorization. For instance, repeated writing by hand is an aid that is commonly used in school to help Japanese children memorize kanji characters. In the same vein, Japanese adults report that they often write with their finger in the air to identify complex characters (a well-known phenomenon, referred to as "Ku Sho"). In fact, it has been reported that learning by handwriting facilitated subjects' memorization of graphic forms (Naka & Naoi, 1995). Visual recognition was also studied by Hulme (1979), who compared children's learning of a series of abstract graphic forms, depending on whether they simply looked at the forms or looked at them as well as traced the forms with their index finger. The tracing movements seemed to improve the children's memorization of the graphic items. Thus, it was suggested that the visual and motor information might undergo a common representation process.

Various data converge to indicate that the cerebral representation of letters might not be strictly visual, but might be based on a complex neural network including a sensorimotor component acquired while learning concomitantly to read and write (James & Gauthier, 2006; Kato et al., 1999; Longcamp et al., 2003; 2005a; Matsuo et al., 2003). Close functional relationships between the reading and writing processes might hence occur at a basic sensorimotor level, in addition to the interactions that have been described at a more cognitive level (e.g., Fitzgerald & Shanahan, 2000).

If the cerebral representation of letters includes a sensorimotor component elaborated when learning how to write letters, how might changes in writing movements affect/impact the subsequent recognition of letters? More precisely, what are the potential consequences of replacing the pen with the keyboard? Both handwriting and typewriting involve movements but there are several differences - some evident, others not so evident– between them. Handwriting is by essence unimanual; however, as evidenced by for instance Yves Guiard (1987), the non-writing hand plays a complementary, though largely covert, role by continuously repositioning the paper in anticipation of pen movement. Even when no movement seems needed (as for instance, in dart throwing), the passive hand and arm play a crucial role in counterbalancing the move of the active arm and hand. The nondominant hand, says Guiard, "frames" the movement of the dominant hand and "sets and confines the spatial context in which the 'skilled' movement will take place." (ibid.) This strong manual asymmetry is connected to a cerebral lateralization of language and motor processes. Typewriting is, as mentioned, a bimanual activity; in right-handers, the left hand which is activated by the right motor areas is involved in writing. Since the left hemisphere is mainly responsible for linguistic processes (in righthanders), this implies inter-hemispheric relationships in typewriting.

A next major difference between the movements involved in handwriting and typewriting, pertains to the speed of the processes. Handwriting is typically slower and more laborious than typewriting. Each stroke (or letter) is drawn in about 100 ms. In typing, letter appearance is immediate and the mean time between the two touches is about 100 ms (in experts). (Gentner, 1983) Moreover handwriting takes place in a very limited space, literally, at the endpoint of the pen, where ink flows out of the pen. The attention of the writer is concentrated onto this particular point in space and time. By comparison, typewriting is divided into two distinct spaces: the motor space, e.g., the keyboard, where the writer acts, and the visual space, e.g., the screen, where the writer perceives the results of his inscription process. Hence, attention is continuously oscillating between these two spatiotemporally distinct spaces which are, by contrast, conjoined in handwriting.

In handwriting, the writer has to form a letter, e.g., to produce a graphic shape which is as close as possible to the standard visual shape of the letter. Each letter is thus associated to a given, very specific movement. There is a strict and unequivocal relationship between the visual shape and the motor program that is used to produce this shape. This relationship has to be learnt during childhood and it can deteriorate due to cerebral damage, or simply with age. On the other hand, typing is a complex form of spatial learning in which the beginner has to build a "keypress schema" transforming the visual form of each character into the position of a given key in keyboard centered coordinates, and specify the movement required to reach this location (Gentner, 1983; Logan, 1999). Therefore, learning how to type also creates an association between a pointing movement and a character. However, since the trajectory of the finger to a given key - e.g., letter - largely depends on its position on the keyboard rather than on the movement of the hand, the relationship between the pointing and the character cannot be very specific. The same key can be hit with different movements, different fingers and even a different hand. This relationship can also deteriorate but with very different consequences than those pertaining to handwriting. For instance, if a key is pressed in error, a spelling error will occur but the visual shape of the letter is preserved in perfect condition. The visuomotor association involved in typewriting should therefore have little contribution to its visual recognition.

Thus, replacing handwriting by typing during learning might have an impact on the cerebral representation of letters and thus on letter memorization. In two behavioral studies, Longcamp et al. investigated the handwriting/typing distinction, one in pre-readers (Longcamp, Zerbato-Poudou et al., 2005b) and one in adults (Longcamp, Boucard, Gilhodes, & Velay, 2006). Both studies confirmed that letters or characters learned through typing were subsequently recognized less accurately than letters or characters written by hand. In a subsequent study (Longcamp et al., 2008), fMRI data showed that processing the orientation of handwritten and typed characters did not rely on the same brain areas. Greater activity related to handwriting learning was observed in several brain regions known to be involved in the execution, imagery, and observation of actions, in particular, the left Broca's area and bilateral inferior parietal lobules. Writing movements may thus contribute to memorizing the shape and/or orientation of characters. However, this advantage of learning by handwriting versus typewriting was not always observed when words were considered instead of letters. In one study (Cunningham & Stanovich, 1990), children spelled words which were learned by writing them by hand better than those learned by typing them on a computer. However, subsequent studies did not confirm the advantage of the handwriting method (e.g., Vaughn, Schumm, & Gordon, 1992).

8. Implications for the fields of literacy and writing research

During the act of writing, then, there is a strong relation between the cognitive processing and the sensorimotor interaction with the physical device. Hence, it seems reasonable to say that theories of writing and literacy currently dominant in the fields of writing research and literacy studies are, if not misguided, so at least markedly incomplete: on the one hand, currently dominant paradigms in (new) literacy studies (e.g., semiotics and sociocultural theory) commonly fail to acknowledge the crucial ways in which different technologies and material interfaces afford, require and structure sensorimotor processes and how these in turn relate to, indeed, how they *shape*, cognition. On the other hand, the cognitive paradigm in writing research commonly fails to acknowledge the important ways in which cognition is embodied, i.e., intimately entwined with perception and motor action. Moreover, media and technology researchers, software developers and computer designers often seem more or less oblivious to the recent findings from philosophy, psychology and neuroscience, as indicated by Allen et al. (2004): "If new media are to support the development and use of our uniquely human capabilities, we must acknowledge that the most widely distributed human asset is the ability to learn in everyday situations through a tight coupling of action and perception." (p. 229) In light of this perspective, the decoupling of motor input and haptic and visual output enforced by the computer keyboard as a writing device, then, is seriously ill-advised.

Judging from the above, there is ample reason to argue for the accommodation of perspectives from neuroscience, psychology, and phenomenology, in the field of writing and literacy. At the same time, it is worth noticing how the field of neuroscience might benefit from being complemented by more holistic, top-down approaches such as phenomenology and ecological psychology. Neurologist Wilson deplores the legacy of the Decade of the Brain, where "something akin to the Tower of Babel" has come into existence:

We now insist that we will never understand what intelligence is unless we can establish how bipedality, brachiation, social interaction, grooming, ambidexterity, language and tool use, the saddle joint at the base of the fifth metacarpal, "reaching" neurons in the brain's parietal cortex, inhibitory neurotransmitters, clades, codons, amino acid sequences etc., etc. are interconnected. But this is a delusion. How can we possibly connect such disparate facts and ideas, or indeed how could we possibly imagine doing so when each discipline is its own private domain of multiple infinite regressions - knowledge or pieces of knowledge under which are smaller pieces under which are smaller pieces still (and so on). The enterprise as it is now ordered is well nigh hopeless. (Wilson, 1998, p. 164)

Finally, it seems as if Wilson's call is being heard, and that time has come to repair what he terms "our prevailing, perversely one-sided - shall I call them cephalocentric - theories of brain, mind, language, and action." (ibid.; p. 69) The perspective of embodied cognition presents itself as an adequate and timely remedy to the disembodied study of cognition and, hence, writing. At the same time it might aid in forging new and promising paths between neuroscience, psychology, and philosophy - and, eventually, education? At any rate, a richer and more nuanced, trans-disciplinary understanding of the processes of reading and writing helps us see what they entail and how they actually work. Understanding how they work, in turn, might make us realize the full scope and true complexity of the skills we possess and, hence, what we might want to make an extra effort to preserve. In our times of steadily increasing digitization of classrooms from preschool to lifelong learning, it is worth pausing for a minute to reflect upon some questions raised by Wilson:

How does, or should, the educational system accommodate for the fact that the hand is not merely a metaphor or an icon for humanness, but often the real-life focal point - the lever or the launching pad - of a successful and genuinely fulfilling life? […] The hand is as much at the core of human life as the brain itself. The hand is involved in human learning. What is there in our theories of education that respects the biologic principles governing cognitive processing in the brain and behavioral change in the individual? […] Could anything we have learned about the hand be used to improve the teaching of children? (ibid.; pp. 13-14; pp. 277-278)

As we hope to have shown during this article, recent theoretical findings from a range of adjacent disciplines now put us in a privileged position to at least begin answering such vital questions. The future of education - and with it, future generations' handling of the skill of writing - depend on how and to what extent we continue to address them.

9. References

Allen, B. S., Otto, R. G., & Hoffman, B. (2004). Media as Lived Environments: The Ecological Psychology of Educational Technology. In D. H. Jonassen (Ed.), Handbook of Research on Educational Communications and Technology. Mahwah, N.J.: Lawrence Erlbaum Ass.

Bara, F., Gentaz, E., & Colé, P. (2007). Haptics in learning to read with children from low socio-economic status families. British Journal of Developmental Psychology, 25(4), 643-663.

Barton, D. (2007). Literacy : an introduction to the ecology of written language (2nd ed.). Malden, MA: Blackwell Pub.

Barton, D., Hamilton, M., & Ivanic, R. (2000). Situated literacies : reading and writing in context. London ; New York: Routledge.

Benjamin, W. (1969). The Work of Art in the Age of Mechanical Reproduction (H. Zohn, Trans.). In Illuminations (Introd. by Hannah Arendt ed.). New York: Schocken.

Bolter, J. D. (2001). Writing space : computers, hypertext, and the remediation of print (2nd ed.). Mahwah, N.J.: Lawrence Erlbaum.

Buckingham, D. (2003). Media education : literacy, learning, and contemporary culture. Cambridge, UK: Polity Press.

Buckingham, D. (2007). Beyond technology: children's learning in the age of digital culture. Cambridge: Polity.

Chao, L. L., & Martin, A. (2000). Representation of manipulable man-made objects in the dorsal stream. NeuroImage, 12, 478-484.

Coiro, J., Leu, D. J., Lankshear, C. & Knobel, M. (eds.) (2008). Handbook of research on new literacies. New York: Lawrence Earlbaum Associates/Taylor & Francis Group

Cunningham, A. E., & Stanovich, K. E. (1990). Early Spelling Acquisition: Writing Beats the Computer. Journal of Educational Psychology, 82, 159-162.

Fitzgerald, J., & Shanahan, T. (2000). Reading and Writing Relations and Their Development. Educational Psychologist, 35(1), 39-50.

Fogassi, L., & Gallese, V. (2004). Action as a Binding Key to Multisensory Integration. In G. A. Calvert, C. Spence & B. E. Stein (Eds.), The handbook of multisensory processes (pp. 425-441). Cambridge, Mass.: MIT Press.

Gentner, D. R. (1983). The acquisition of typewriting skill. Acta Psychologica, 54, 233-248.

Gibson, J. J. (1966). The Senses Considered as Perceptual Systems. Boston: Houghton Mifflin Co.

Gibson, J. J. (1979). The ecological approach to visual perception. Boston: Houghton Mifflin.

Goldin-Meadow, S. (2003). Hearing gesture: how our hands help us think. Cambridge, MA: Belknap Press of Harvard University Press.

Greenfield, P. M. (1991). Language, tools and brain: The ontogeny and phylogeny of hierarchically organized sequential behavior. Behavioral and Brain Sciences, 14, 531-595.

Guiard, Y. (1987). Asymmetric division of labor in human skilled bimanual action: The kinematic chain as a model. Journal of Motor Behavior, 19, 486-517.

Hatwell, Y., Streri, A., & Gentaz, E. (Eds.). (2003). Touching for Knowing (Vol. 53). Amsterdam/Philadelphia: John Benjamins.

Heidegger, M. (1982 [1942]). Parmenides. Frankfurt: Klostermann.

Heim, M. (1999). Electric language : a philosophical study of word processing (2nd ed.). New Haven: Yale University Press.

Hulme, C. (1979). The interaction of visual and motor memory for graphic forms following tracing. Quarterly Journal of Experimental Psychology, 31, 249-261.

Haas, C. (1996). Writing technology : studies on the materiality of literacy. Mahwah, N.J.: L. Erlbaum Associates.

James, K. H., & Gauthier, I. (2006). Letter processing automatically recruits a sensory-motor brain network. Neuropsychologia, 44, 2937-2949.

Jensenius, A. R. (2008). Action - sound: developing methods and tools to study music-related body movement. University of Oslo, Oslo.

Jewitt, C. (2006). Technology, literacy and learning : a multimodal approach. London ; New York: Routledge.

Kato, C., Isoda, H., Takehar, Y., Matsuo, K., Moriya, T., & Nakai, T. (1999). Involvement of motor cortices in retrieval of kanji studied by functional MRI. Neuroreport, 10, 1335-1339.

Klatzky, R. L., Lederman, S. J., & Mankinen, J. M. (2005). Visual and haptic exploratory procedures in children's judgments about tool function. Infant Behavior and Development, 28(3), 240-249.

Klatzky, R. L., Lederman, S. J., & Matula, D. E. (1993). Haptic exploration in the presence of vision. Journal of Experimental Psychology: Human Perception and Performance, 19(4), 726-743.

Kress, G. (2003). Literacy in the new media age. London ; New York: Routledge.

Lankshear, C. (2006). New literacies : everyday practices and classroom learning (2nd ed.). Maidenhead, Berkshire ; New York, NY: McGraw-Hill/Open University Press.

Liberman A.M., Mattingly I.G. (1985). The motor theory of speech perception revised. Cognition, 21, 1-36.

Logan, F. A. (1999). Errors in Copy Typewriting. Journal of Experimental Psychology: Human Perception and Performance, 25, 1760-1773.

Longcamp, M., Anton, J.-L., Roth, M., & Velay, J.-L. (2003). Visual presentation of single letters activates a premotor area involved in writing. NeuroImage, 19(4), 1492-1500.

Longcamp, M., Anton, J.-L., Roth, M., & Velay, J.-L. (2005a). Premotor activations in response to visually presented single letters depend on the hand used to write: a study in left-handers. Neuropsychologia, 43, 1699-1846.

Longcamp, M., Boucard, C., Gilhodes, J.-C., & Velay, J.-L. (2006). Remembering the orientation of newly learned characters depends on the associated writing knowledge: A comparison between handwriting and typing. Human Movement Science, 25(4-5), 646-656.

Longcamp, M., Boucard, C. l., Gilhodes, J.-C., Anton, J.-L., Roth, M., Nazarian, B., et al. (2008). Learning through Hand- or Typewriting Influences Visual Recognition of New Graphic Shapes: Behavioral and Functional Imaging Evidence. Journal of Cognitive Neuroscience, 20(5), 802-815.

Longcamp, M., Zerbato-Poudou, M.-T., & Velay, J.-L. (2005b). The influence of writing practice on letter recognition in preschool children: A comparison between handwriting and typing. Acta Psychologica, 119(1), 67-79.

Lurija, A. R. (1973). The working brain: an introduction to neuropsychology. London: Allen Lane The Penguin Press.

MacArthur, C. A., Graham, S., & Fitzgerald, J. (eds.) (2006). Handbook of writing research. New York: Guilford Press

Mangen, A. (2009). The Impact of Digital Technology on Immersive Fiction Reading. Saarbrücken: VDM Verlag Dr. Müller.
Matsuo, K., Kato, C., Okada, T., Moriya, T., Glover, G. H., & Nakai, T. (2003). Finger movements lighten neural loads in the recognition of ideographic characters. Cognitive Brain Research, 17(2), 263-272.
Merleau-Ponty, M. (1962 [1945]). Phenomenology of perception. London: Routledge.
Naka, M., & Naoi, H. (1995). The effect of repeated writing on memory. Memory & Cognition, 23, 201-212.
Noë, A. (2004). Action in Perception. Cambridge, Mass.: MIT Press.
O'Regan, J. K., & Noë, A. (2001). A sensorimotor account of vision and visual consciousness. Behavioral and Brain Sciences, 24(5), 939-973.
O'Shaughnessy, B. (2002). Consciousness and the world. Oxford: Clarendon Press.
Ochsner, R. (1990). Physical Eloquence and the Biology of Writing. New York: SUNY Press.
Olivier, G., & Velay, J.-L. (2009). Visual objects can potentiate a grasping neural simulation which interferes with manual response execution. Acta Psychologica, 130, 147-152.
Ong, W. J. (1982). Orality and Literacy: The Technologizing of the Word. London & New York: Methuen.
Palmer, J. A. (2002). Fifty Major Thinkers on Education: From Confucius to Dewey. London & New York: Routledge.
Pulvermüller, F. (2005). Brain mechanisms linking language and action. Nature Reviews Neuroscience, 6, 576-582.
Singer, D. G., & Singer, J. L. (2005). Imagination and play in the electronic age. Cambridge: Harvard University Press.
Säljö, R. (2006). Læring og kulturelle redskaper: om læreprosesser og den kollektive hukommelsen. Oslo: Cappelen akademisk forl.
Thompson, E. (2007). Mind in life : biology, phenomenology, and the sciences of mind. Cambridge, Mass.: Harvard University Press.
Torrance, M., van Waes, L., & Galbraith, D. (Eds.). (2007). Writing and Cognition: Research and Applications. Amsterdam: Elsevier.
van Galen, G. P. (1991). Handwriting: Issues for a psychomotor theory. Human Movement Science, 10, 165-191.
Van Waes, L., Leijten, M., & Neuwirth, C. (Eds.). (2006). Writing and Digital Media. Amsterdam: Elsevier.
Varela, F. J., Thompson, E., & Rosch, E. (1991). The embodied mind: cognitive science and human experience. Cambridge, Mass.: MIT Press.
Vaughn, S., Schumm, J. S., & Gordon, J. (1992). Early spelling acquisition: Does writing really beat the computer? Learning Disabilities Quarterly, 15, 223-228.
Vinter, A., & Chartrel, E. (2008). Visual and proprioceptive recognition of cursive letters in young children. Acta Psychologica, 129(1), 147-156.
Wilson, F. R. (1998). The hand : how its use shapes the brain, language, and human culture (1st ed.). New York: Pantheon Books.
Wolf, M. (2007). Proust and the squid: the story and science of the reading brain. New York: HarperCollins.
Zettl, H. (1973). Sight - Sound - Motion. Applied Media Aesthetics. Belmont, CA: Wadsworth Publishing Company, Inc.

21

Kinesthetic Illusion of Being Pulled Sensation Enables Haptic Navigation for Broad Social Applications

Tomohiro Amemiya[1], Hideyuki Ando[2] and Taro Maeda[2]
[1]NTT Communication Science Laboratories, [2]Osaka University
Japan

Abstract

Many handheld force-feedback devices have been proposed to provide a rich experience with mobile devices. However, previously reported devices have been unable to generate both constant and translational force. They can only generate transient rotational force since they use a change in angular momentum. Here, we exploit the nonlinearity of human perception to generate both constant and translational force. Specifically, a strong acceleration is generated for a very brief period in the desired direction, while a weaker acceleration is generated over a longer period in the opposite direction. The internal human haptic sensors do not detect the weaker acceleration, so the original position of the mass is "washed out". The result is that the user is tricked into perceiving a unidirectional force. This force can be made continuous by repeating the motions. This chapter describes the pseudo-attraction force technique, which is a new force feedback technique that enables mobile devices to create a the sensation of two-dimensional force. A prototype was fabricated in which four slider-crank mechanism pairs were arranged in a cross shape and embedded in a force feedback display. Each slider-crank mechanism generates a force vector. By using the sum of the generated vectors, which are linearly independent, the force feedback display can create a force sensation in any arbitrary direction on a two-dimensional plane. We also introduce an interactive application with the force feedback display, an interactive robot, and a vision-based positioning system.

1. Introduction

Haptic interfaces in virtual environments allow users to touch and feel virtual objects. Significant research activities over 20 years have led to the commercialization of a large number of sophisticated haptic interfaces including PHANToM and SPIDAR. However, most of these interfaces have to use some type of mechanical linkage to establish a fulcrum relative the ground (Massie & Salisbury, 1994; Sato, 2002), use huge air compressors (Suzuki et al., 2002; Gurocak et al., 2003), or require that a heavy device be worn (Hirose et al., 2001), thus preventing these mobile devices from employing haptic feedback.

Although haptic feedback provides many potential benefits as regards the use of small portable hand-held devices (Ullmer & Ishii 2000; Luk et al., 2006), the haptic feedback in mobile devices consists exclusively of vibrotactile stimuli generated by vibrators (MacLean et al., 2002). This is because it is difficult for mobile devices to produce a kinesthetic sensation. Moreover, the application of low-frequency forces to a user requires a fixed mechanical ground that mobile haptic devices lack. To make force-feedback devices available in mobile devices, ungrounded haptic feedback devices have been developed since they are more mobile and can operate over larger workspaces than grounded devices (Burdea, 1996). The performance of ungrounded haptic feedback devices is less accurate than that of grounded devices in contact tasks. However, ungrounded haptic feedback devices can provide comparable results in boundary detection tests (Richard & Cutkosky, 1997). Unfortunately, typical ungrounded devices based on the gyro effect (Yano et al., 2003) or angular momentum change (Tanaka et al., 2001) are incapable of generating both constant and directional forces; they can generate only a transient rotational force (torque) sensation. In addition, Kunzler and Runde pointed out that gyro moment displays are proportional to the mass, diameter, and angular velocity of the flywheel (Kunzler & Runde, 2005).
There are methods for generating sustained translational force without grounding, such as propulsive force or electromagnetic force. Recently, there have been a number of proposals for generating both constant and directional forces without an external fulcrum. These includeusing two oblique motors whose velocity and phase are controlled (Nakamura & Fukui, 2007), simulating kinesthetic inertia by shifting the center-of-mass of a device dynamically when the device is held with both hands (Swindells et al., 2003), and producing a pressure field with airborne ultrasound (Iwamoto et al., 2008).

2. Pseudo-Attraction Force Technique

2.1 Haptic interface using sensory illusions

To generate a sustained translational force without grounding, we focused on the characteristic of human perception, which until now has been neglected or inadequately implemented in haptic devices. Although human beings always interact with the world through human sensors and effectors, the perceived world is not identical to the physical world (Fig. 1). For instance, when we watch television, the images (a combination of RGB colors) we see are different from physical images (a composition of all wavelengths of light), and TV animation actually consists of a series of still pictures. Such phenomena are usually interpreted by converting them to subjectively equivalent phenomena. These distortions of human perception, including systematic errors or illusions, have been exploited when designing human interfaces. Moreover, some illusions have the potential to enable the development of new haptic interfaces (Hayward 2008). Therefore, the study of haptic illusions can provide valuable insights into not only human perceptual mechanisms but also the design of new haptic interfaces.

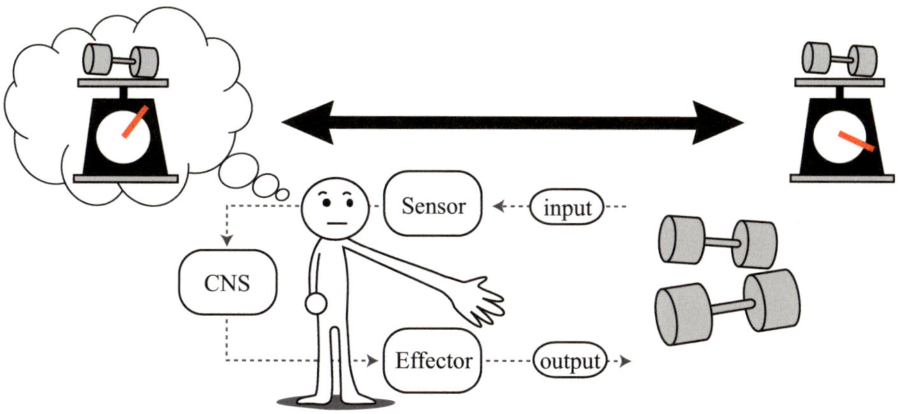

Fig. 1. Difference between perceived world and physical world.

2.2 Principle

The method, which is called the pseudo-attraction force technique, exploits the characteristics of human perception to generate a force sensation, using different acceleration patterns for two directions to create a perceived force imbalance, and thereby produce the sensation of directional pushing or pulling. Specifically, a strong acceleration is generated for a very brief time in the desired direction, while a weaker acceleration is generated over a longer period in the opposite direction. The weaker acceleration is not detected by the internal human haptic sensors, so the original position of the mass is "washed out". The result is that the user is tricked into perceiving a unidirectional force. This force can be made continuous by repeating the motions. Figure 2 shows a model of the nonlinear relationship between physical and psychophysical quantities. If the acceleration patterns are well designed, a kinesthetic illusion of being pulled can be created because of this nonlinearity.

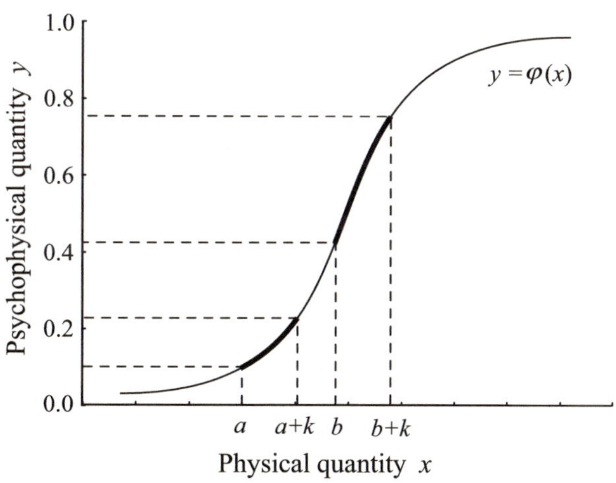

Fig. 2. Nonlinear relationship between physical and psychophysical quantities.

2.3 Implementation

To generate the asymmetric back-and-forth motion of a small, constrained mass, we have adopted a swinging slider-crank mechanism as a quick motion mechanism (Fig. 3). In the mechanism, the rotation of a crank (OB) makes the weight slide backwards and forwards with asymmetric acceleration. The force display is composed of a single degree of freedom (DOF) mechanism. The force vector of the asymmetric oscillation is

$$\mathrm{F}(t) = m\frac{d^2x(t)}{dt^2} \tag{1}$$

where m is the weight. The acceleration is given by the second derivative with respect to time of the motion of the weight x, which is given by

$$x(t) = l_1\cos\omega t + \mu(d - l_1\cos\omega t) + \sqrt{l_3 - \{l_1(\mu - 1)\sin\omega t\}^2} \tag{2}$$

where

$$\mu = \frac{l_2}{\sqrt{l_1^2 + d^2 - 2l_1 d\cos\omega t}}, \tag{3}$$

$x(t) = OD$, $d = OA$, $l_1 = OB$, $l_2 = BC$, $l_3 = CD$, and $\omega t = AOB$ in Fig. 3. ω is the constant angular velocity, and t is time.

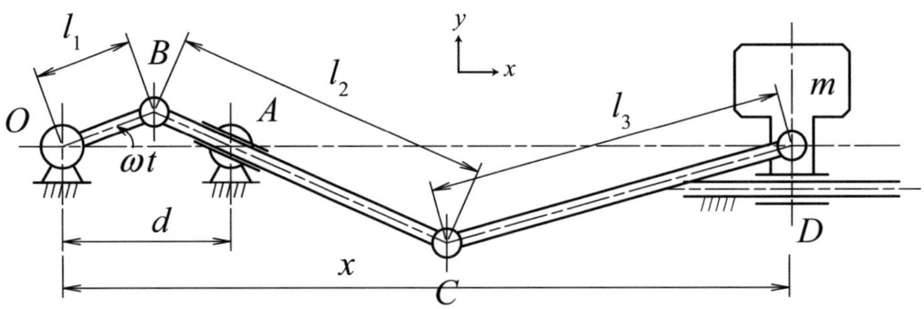

Fig. 3. Overview of the swinging slider-crank mechanism for generating asymmetric oscillation. The slider (weight) slides backwards and forwards as the crank (*OB*) rotates. Point A causes the slide to turn about the same point. Since the relative link lengths (*AB*:*AC*) are changed according to the rotation of the crank, the slider (weight) moves with asymmetric acceleration.

We fabricated a prototype of the force display. In the prototype, d = 28 mm, l_1 = 15 mm, l_2 = 60 mm, and l_3 = 70 mm. The actual acceleration values of the prototype were measured with a laser sensor (Keyence Inc., LK-G150, sampling 20 kHz) employing a seventh order LPF Butterworth filter with a cut-off frequency of 100 Hz (Fig.4).

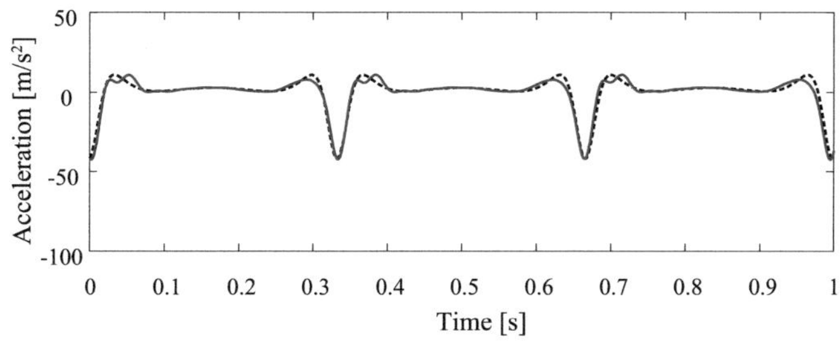

(a) 3 cycles per second

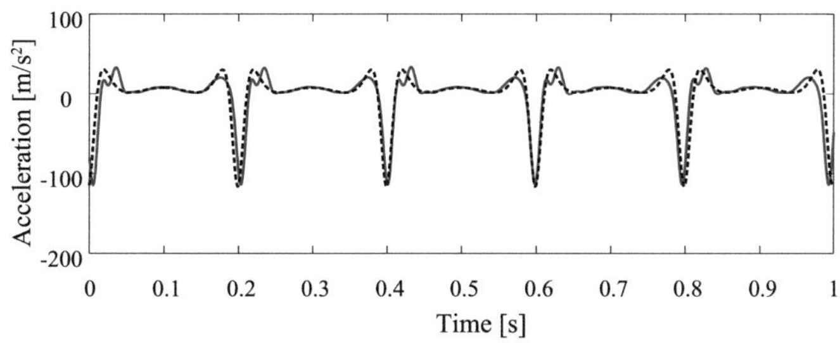

(b) 5 cycles per second

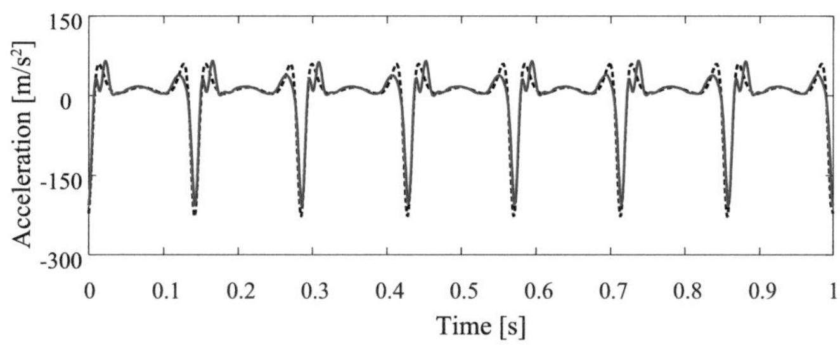

(c) 7 cycles per second

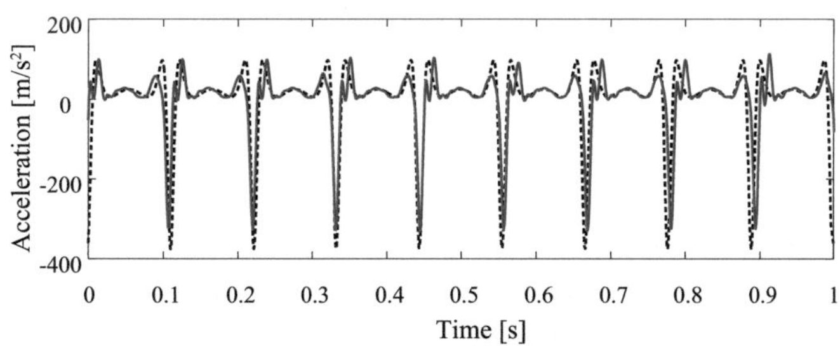

(d) 9 cycles per second

Fig. 4. Actual asymmetric acceleration value with the LPF (blue solid line) vs. the calculated value (black dotted line). Humans perceive a unidirectional force by holding the haptic device. This is because the strong and weak acceleration periods yield different sensations, although the device physically generates a bidirectional force.

3. Requirements for perceiving pseudo-attraction force

There are still many aspects of the perception of the pseudo-attraction force that are not well understood, but knowledge has been accumulating. In this section, we introduce various parameters for eliciting the pseudo-attraction force through experimental results.

3.1 Acceleration profile

First, we determined whether oscillations with asymmetric acceleration elicit the perception of a pseudo-attraction force. Two oscillations with different acceleration profiles were compared as haptic stimuli: asymmetric acceleration (shown in Fig. 4) and symmetric acceleration (control). For the asymmetric acceleration stimuli, the average percentage correct scores (i.e., how often the perceived force direction matched the crank-to-slider direction in Fig. 3) for all subjects were approximately 100% at frequencies below 10 cycles per second when we used a binary judgment task (forward or backward). For the symmetric acceleration stimuli, the scores were between 25% and 75%, which is the chance level. These results show that the symmetric acceleration could not generate a directed force sensation. We performed a binomial test for the average percent correct scores, which showed no significant effect of the control stimuli for any of the frequencies. This means that symmetric acceleration does not elicit the perception of a pseudo-attraction force. Again, no directional force was felt if the mass were merely moved back and forth, but different acceleration patterns for the two directions to create a perceived force imbalance produced the perception of a pseudo-attraction force (Amemiya & Maeda, 2009).

3.2 Frequency of acceleration

Frequency of acceleration plays an important role in eliciting the perception of a pseudo-attraction force. Oscillations with high frequency might create a continuous force sensation, but previous experimental results showed that the performance decreased steadily at frequencies over ten cycles per second (Amemiya et al., 2008). However, low frequency oscillation tends to be perceived as a knocking sensation. If we wish to create a sustained rather than a transient force sensation such as the sensation of being pulled continuously, the frequency should be in the 5 to 10 cycles per second range. In addition, those who experienced the stimuli strongly perceived the sensation at 5 cycles per second independent of other parameters (Amemiya & Maeda, 2009).

3.3 Gross weight of force display

Changes in the gross weight and the weight of the reciprocating mass affects the perceived force sensation. Experimental results have shown that lighter gross weights and a heavier reciprocating mass yield higher percent-correct scores in binary judgment tasks for all frequencies (Amemiya & Maeda, 2009). Considering the Weber fraction of force perception, the differential threshold of force perception is thought to increase as the gross weight increases. In addition, the increase in the gross weight may work as a mass damper, which would reduce the gain of the effective pulse acceleration. The threshold of the ratio of the gross weight and the weight of the reciprocating mass was 16 %, which is a rough standard for effective force perception in the developed prototype.

3.4 Angular resolution

The azimuth accuracy of the perceived force direction versus the stimulated direction generated by an asymmetric acceleration has been examined (Amemiya et al., 2006). The orientation of the force vector was altered from 0 to 360° on the horizontal plane in 15° steps (24 vectors). The subjects were required to reply with one of 360 degrees in a static posture. The results showed that the root mean square of the angular errors between response and stimulus was approximately 20 degrees. When users move or rotate their bodies, i.e., dynamically explore the force vector, their angular resolution would be higher than that in a static posture.

3.5 Cancellation of orthogonal oscillation

If asymmetric oscillation was generated by rotational mechanism such as the slider-crank mechanism, a force perpendicular to the directional one were created because of the motion of the linkages. The side-to-side force prevents the user from sensing the desired direction. The side-to-side force should be cancelled out completely, for instance, by using two identical but mirror-reversed mechanisms (Amemiya et al., 2008).

4. Application

4.1 Overview

For broad social use, we designed an interactive application of haptic navigation based on a pseudo-attraction force display. The scenario was as follows. *A waiter (user) in a cafe wants to deliver a drink ordered by a customer (target). The waiter does not know where the customer is sitting. However, his "smart tray" creates an attraction force centered on the customer and guides the waiter to him/her. Since the guidance is based on force sensation, the guidance information is useful regardless of the waiter's age or language ability. Moreover, since the guidance directions are transmitted via touch, the other senses remain available to the waiter, making it easier for him to move through even the most crowded areas. Finally, the instructions remain entirely private; no one else can discover that the waiter is receiving instructions.*

4.2 System configuration

The system consists of a tray held by the user (waiter), a small bag containing a battery and a control device, and a position and direction identification system based on infrared LEDs and a wide-angle camera (Fig. 5). The force display and infrared LEDs are embedded in the tray. The user's position and posture are detected by placing three super-high luminance infrared LEDs (OD-100, OPTO Diode Corp., peak wavelength 880 nm, beam angle 120 degrees), at the corners of a right-angled isosceles triangle (side length = 100 mm) on the tray. The infrared rays are captured by a ceiling-mounted IEEE1394 black and white CMOS camera (Firefly MV, FFMV-03MTM; Point Grey Research Inc.) with a wide-angle lens (field angle 175 degrees). The positions and orientations of each IR-LED are obtained by binarizing the brightness value from the acquired camera image with OpenCV library, and calculating the position and orientation from the relationship with a right-angled isosceles triangle formed by three dots (Fig. 6).

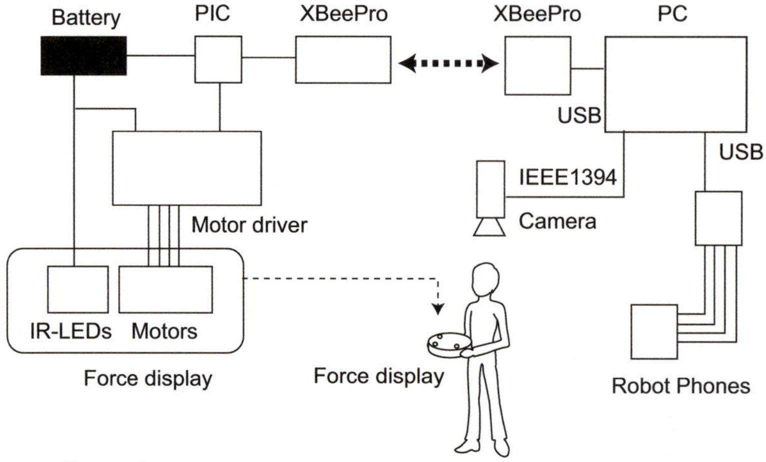

Fig. 5. System configuration.

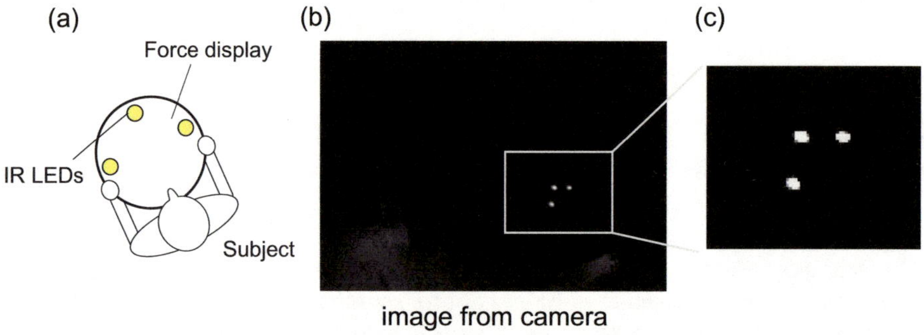

Fig. 6. Vision-based position and posture identification system. The white dots in the camera image are the infrared LEDs.

The user must hold the tray horizontally because of the drink being carried on it. Therefore, the user's posture can be presumed by detecting three IR-LEDs. The image capture rate is about 60 fps. The camera height is about 3.0 m and the camera faces the ground. When three points can be acquired, the position measurement error does not exceed 100 mm. This is sufficient for our demonstration since the distance to the targets is about 1,000 mm.
There are two ways to generate a two-dimensional force vector (Fig. 7), and we fabricate each prototype. A turntable-based force display is one module based on a slider-crank mechanism with a turntable (Fig. 8). The direction of the force display module is controlled with a stepper motor (bipolar, step angle 1.8 degrees, 1/4 micro step drive; KH42HM2-851; Japanese Servo Ltd.). engaged by a belt with a belt pulley installed in the turntable (Amemiya et al., 2009).
A vector-summation-based force display is designed to generate a force sensation in at least eight cardinal directions by the summation of linearly independent force vectors. Four slider-crank mechanism pairs are embedded in the force display in the shape of a crosshair. By combining force vectors generated by each slider-crank mechanism, the force display can create a virtual force in eight cardinal directions on a two-dimensional plane.

The target is several bear-shaped robots (RobotPhone; Iwaya Inc.). As the customer speaks, he also moves his head and hands to communicate with gestures.

4. 3 Demonstration procedure

The user moved towards the target following the direction indicated by the perceived force sensation. The force direction was controlled so that it faced the target (customer) based on the posture detection system. Control instructions were sent from the computer to the microcomputer via a wireless link (XBee-PRO (60 mW) ZigBee module; MaxStream) when required. The user chose one customer by stopping in front of the target. If this choice was correct, the customer (bear-shaped robot) said, ''thank you''; otherwise, the customer said, ''I did not order this'' while moving his head and hands to communicate with gestures.

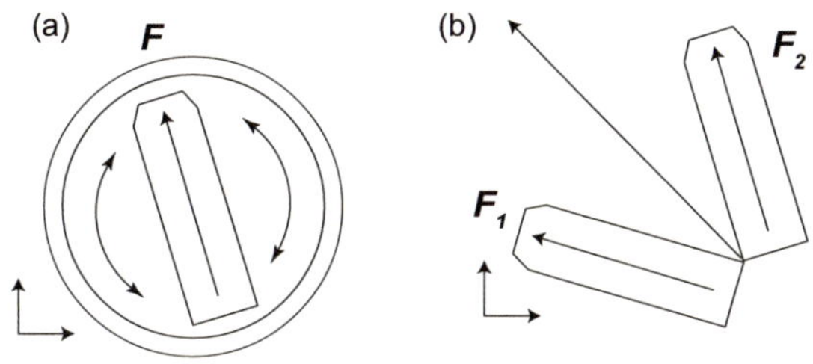

Fig. 7. Two-dimensional force vector. (a) Turntable approach: one module with rotational mechanism. (b) Vector summation approach: modules of linearly independent vectors.

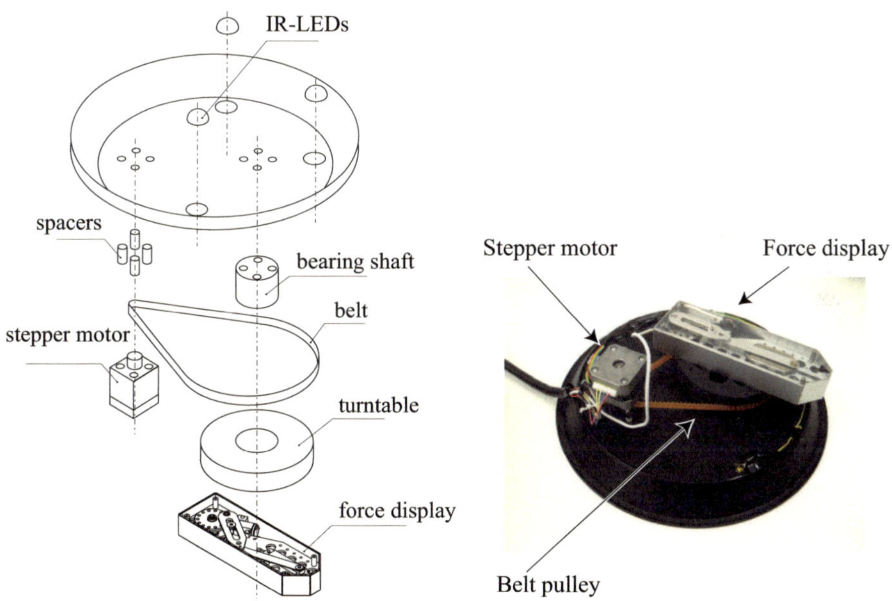

Fig. 8. Overview of the turntable-based force display

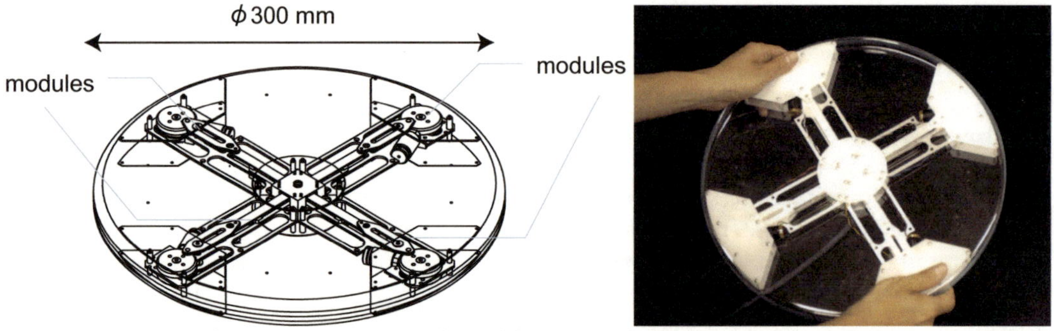

Fig. 9. Overview of vector-summation-based force display

4. 4 Discussion

We demonstrated the above application at an international conference and exhibition. The average rate of correct delivery to the target exceeded 75 % (note that none of the participants received any initial training), indicating that the navigation support provided is effective and appropriate. The results show the usefulness of the proposed technique. The few delivery failures appear to be due to tracking errors in the camera system or a delay between the rotation of the stepper motor and the user's perception of the change. Moreover, we believe the force's amplitude to be attenuated by the connection of the device to the tray, and this attenuation also influenced delivery failure. We sometimes observed that not all the LEDs could be detected since some were occasionally obscured by the participant. System robustness could be improved by adopting a different position and posture identification system. This haptic navigation could be also applied to a navigation system for the visually impaired (Amemiya & Sugiyama 2009).

5. Conclusion and future potential

The developed haptic display based on a pseudo-attraction force technique conveyed a kinesthetic illusion of being pulled or pushed. The ability of the haptic display to realize a wide-area social support system was discussed. Future work will include extending the reach by using a global positioning system to allow outdoor use.

Acknowledgements

We thank Dr. Ichiro Kawabuchi for his assistance. This study was supported by Nippon Telegraph and Telephone Corporation and was also partially supported by the sponsorship of CREST, Japan Science and Technology Agency.

6. References

Amemiya, T.; Ando, H. & T. Maeda T. (2005) Virtual force display: Direction guidance using asymmetric acceleration via periodic translational motion, *Proceedings of World Haptics Conference*, pp. 619-622, IEEE Computer Society.

Amemiya, T.; Ando, H. & T. Maeda T. (2006). Directed force perception when holding a nongrounding force display in the air. *Proceedings of Eurohaptics 2006*. Paris, France. pp. 317-324.

Amemiya, T.; Ando, H. & T. Maeda T. (2007). Hand-held force display with spring-cam mechanism for generating asymmetric acceleration, *Proceedings of World Haptics Conference*, pp. 572-573, March 2007, IEEE Computer Society.

Amemiya, T.; Ando, H. & T. Maeda T. (2008). Lead-Me interface for pulling sensation in hand-held devices, *ACM Transactions on Applied Perception*, Vol. 5, No. 3, pp. 1-17.

Amemiya, T. & Maeda, T. (2008). Asymmetric oscillation distorts the perceived heaviness of handheld objects, *IEEE Transactions on Haptics*, Vol. 1, No. 1, pp. 9-18.

Amemiya, T. & Maeda, T. (2009) Directional force sensation by asymmetric oscillation from a doublelayer slider-crank mechanism, *Journal Computing Information Science in Engineering*, Vol. 9, No. 1, 011001, ASME.

Amemiya, T.; Maeda, T. & Ando, H. (2009). Location-free Haptic Interaction for Large-Area Social Applications, *Personal and Ubiquitous Computing*, Vol. 13, No. 5, pp. 379-386, Springer.

Amemiya, T. & Sugiyama, H. (2009). Haptic Handheld Wayfinder with Pseudo-Attraction Force for Pedestrians with Visual Impairments, *Proceedings of 11th ACM Conference on Computers and Accessibility (ASSETS 2009)*, pp. 107-114, ACM Press.

Burdea, G. C. (1996). Force & Touch Feedback for Virtual Reality, Wiley, New York.

Chang, A. & O'Sullivan, C. (2005). Audio-haptic feedback in mobile phones. *Proceedings of CHI'05 extended abstracts on human factors in computing systems*, pp. 1264-1267, ACM Press.

Gurocak, H.; Jayaram, S.; Parrish, B. & Jayaram U. (2003). Weight sensation in virtual environments using a haptic device with air jets, *Journal of Computing and Information Science in Engineering*, Vol. 3, No. 2. ASME, pp. 130-135.

Hirose, M.; Hirota, K.; Ogi, T.; Yano, H.; Kakehi, N.; Saito, M.; Nakashige, M. (2001). HapticGEAR: The Development of a Wearable Force Display System for Immersive Projection Displays, *Proceedings of Virtual Reality 2001 Conference*, pp. 123–130.

Iwamoto, T; Tatezono, M; Hoshi, T.; Shinoda, H. (2008). Non-Contact Method for Producing Tactile Sensation Using Airborne Ultrasound, *Proceedings of EuroHaptics 2008*, pp. 504-513.

Kunzler, U. & Runde, C. (2005) Kinesthetic Haptics Integration into Large-Scale Virtual Environments, *Proceedings of World Haptics Conference 2005*, pp. 551–556.

Luk, J.; Pasquero, J.; Little, S.; MacLean, K.; Levesque, V. & Hayward, V. (2006). A role for haptics in mobile interaction: Initial design using a handheld tactile display prototype. *Proceedings of conference on human factors in computing systems*, ACM Press, pp. 171-180.

MacLean, K. E., Shaver, M. J. & Pai, D. K. (2002). Handheld Haptics: A USB Media Controller with Force Sensing, *Proceedings of Tenth Symposium on Haptic Interfaces for Virtual Environment and Teleoperator Systems (HAPTICS 2002)*, pp. 311–318.

Massie, T. & Salisbury, J. K. (1994). The phantom haptic interface: A device for probing virtual objects, *Proceedings of the ASME Winter Annual Meeting, Symposium on Haptic Interfaces for Virtual Environment and Teleoperator Systems,* Vol. 55-1, Chicago, IL., 1994, pp. 295-300.

Nakamura, N. & Fukui, Y. (2007). Development of Fingertip Type Non-grounding Force Feedback Display, *Proceedings of World Haptics Conference 2007,* pp. 582-583.

Richard, C. & Cutkosky, M. (1997). Contact Force Perception with an Ungrounded Haptic Interface, *Proceedings of the ASME Dynamic Systems and Control Division,* pp. 181–187.

Sato, M. (2002). Spidar and virtual reality, *Proceedings of the 5th Biannual World Automation Congress,* Vol. 13, pp. 17-23.

Suzuki, Y.; Kobayashi, M. & Ishibashi, S. (2002). Design of force feedback utilizing air pressure toward untethered human interface, *Proceedings of CHI '02 Extended Abstracts on Human Factors in Computing Systems.* ACM Press, 2002, pp. 808-809.

Swindells, C.; Unden, A. & Sang, T. (2003). TorqueBAR: an ngrounded haptic feedback device. *Proceedings of the 5th international conference on multimodal interfaces.* ACM Press, pp. 52-59.

Tanaka, Y.; Masataka, S.; Yuka, K.; Fukui, Y.; Yamashita, J. & Nakamura, N. (2001). Mobile torque display and haptic characteristics of human palm. *Proceedings of 11th international conference on augmented tele-existence,* pp. 115-120.

Ullmer, B. & Ishii, H. (2000). Emerging frameworks for tangible user interfaces. *IBM Syst. J.* Vol. 39, Nos. 3-4, pp. 915-931.

Yano, H.; Yoshie, M. & Iwata, H. (2003). Development of a nongrounded haptic interface using the gyro effect, *Proceedings of 11th international symposium on Haptic Interfaces for Virtual Environment and Teleoperator Systems.* IEEE Computer Society, pp. 32-39.

22

Perceptual Issues Improve Haptic Systems Performance

Marco Vicentini and Debora Botturi
Verona University
Italy

1. Introduction

Since its introduction in the early 50's, teleoperation systems have expanded their reach, to address micro and macro manipulation, interaction with virtual worlds and the general field of haptic interaction. From its beginnings, as a mean to handle radioactive materials and to reduce human presence in dangerous areas, teleoperation and haptics have also become an interaction modality with computer generated objects and environments.

One of the main goals of teleoperation is to achieve *transparency*, i.e. the complete perception by the human operator of the virtual or remote environment with which he/she is interacting (Lawrence, 1993). The ability of a teleoperation system to provide transparency depends upon the performance of the master and the slave, and of its control system. Ideally, the master should be able to emulate any environment, real or simulated, from free-space to infinitely stiff obstacles.

The design of a transparent haptic interface is a quite challenging engineering task, since motion and sensing capabilities of the human hand/arm system are difficult to match. Furthermore, recent studies are providing more and more evidence that transparency is not only achieved by a good engineering design, but also by a combination of perceptual and cognitive factors that affect the operator ability to actually perceive the stimuli provided.

The current knowledge on operator models reflects two separate groups of results. On one hand, there are guidelines for the design of an effective interface, from a human factors points of view, which include perceptual issues related to the cognitive and information processing of the human operators (see Subsection 2.4). On the other hand, there are several operator models related to biomechanical, bandwidth and reaction time issues (see Subsection 2.5).

In this work we survey the main human factors that concur to the effectiveness of a haptic interface, and we present a series of psychophysical experiments, which can enrich performance in haptic systems, by measuring the mechanical effectiveness of the interface, providing a measure of the perception of a human operator. In addition the experiments are useful to represent the complex behavior of the human perception capabilities, and to propose new ways for enhancing the transparency of the virtual environment, by proposing suitable force scaling functions. In addition, our experience with psychophysics procedures highlights the needs of non-classical approaches to the problem, but the design of this type of experiments is not trivial, thus the need of a dedicated software tool or library arises.

The study of the perceptual capabilities is relevant for the design of virtual reality simulators, and for the specification of haptics applications that overcomes current users limitations. Their study is important for improving telepresence in tele-manipulation system. There is a growing need to not only continue to improve hardware platforms and rendering algorithms, but also to evaluate human performance with haptic interfaces.
In a kinesthetic interaction, since the user lacks direct tactile information, the probe of the haptic device has to firmly penetrate the virtual surface before the user, via force feedback, is able to make use of kinesthetic cues and deduce the features of the body. It is necessary to achieve a compromise between accuracy in tissue discrimination, governed by the magnitude of force feedback, and the temporal and displacement extent of surface penetration, which is tightly related to the probability of damaging the tissue.
In the state of the art, we review earlier results on human bandwidth and biomechanical models of an operator involved in manual control, and the methods to identify the range and threshold of human haptic perception. These earlier results point out the lack of analysis of the interplay between different sensing modes of the human perception system, and the need to move from experiments testing a single factor to experiments involving several interplaying factors.
These considerations motivated the development of a series of experiments, carried out in the Altair Laboratory in Verona, combining multiple biomechanical and human factors. In particular, we evaluate those human factors most relevant to surface contact task in low stiffness environments. We address the study of human factors, among over force detection threshold, reaction time, contact velocity, and minimal penetration depth in a contact task with pliable surfaces.
Psychophysical experiments are conducted using different haptic devices. In the first two experiments we measure the absolute force discrimination threshold of the human hand when grasping, a haptic device, both for onset and for sinusoidal force stimuli. We develop a set of compensation rules, capable of granting higher overall accuracy in perceiving haptic virtual environments, by directly involving the results collected in the previous perceptual experiments. The overall goal is accurate rendering of haptic interactions between a tool and any pliable body.

The third experiment combines the just-mentioned factors in a single task of surface detection, in which the subjects are instructed to halt exploration as quickly as they feel the force due to the contact with a virtual object. We measure the penetration depth that can be used to reliably perceive the contact surface, and the enhancement due to the proposed perceptual based scaling method.

The Chapter is organized as following. In the follow up of this Section we present some relevant findings on biomechanical properties of the human arms and the models and guidelines that have been derived. In Section III a series of psychophysical experiments are presented to consider the relevance of perceptual findings for teleoperation systems; in Section IV we justify the needs for a circular approach between perceptual issues and teleoperation system. An overview of a new library for perceptual experiments is presented in Section V. In Section VI conclusions and future works are pointed out.

2. Relevant Findings from Human Factors

In this section, we summarize some of the main findings relevant to the quantitative measures of the human perceptual capabilities. We start from the bandwidth measurements of the human haptic perception. Then, we describe some of the haptics parameters analyzed using one-factor psychophysical methodology. That is, we review the human capabilities on length, angle, force, and stiffness detection and discrimination; we also consider the perception of the peri-personal space and some measures of human performance in bilateral teleoperation. Furthermore, we advance the guidelines that arise from these findings for teleoperation system. Finally, we describe the human models, mostly biomechanical, that these tests have produced.

2.1 Human Response Characteristics

In manual control, the human perception system does not have one single bandwidth (Burdea, 1996). Human bandwidth is a function of the mode in which he/she is operating. Sensation of mechanical vibration of the skin has been reported as high as 10 Khz, but the ability to discriminate one signal from another declines above 320 Hz. In general, the human hand can sense compressive stress (about 10 Hz), skin motion stimulus (30 Hz), vibration (50-400 Hz) and skin stretch (low frequency).
With respect to specific aspects of teleoperation, there are a number of important sensory inputs to the human operator: tactile, proprioceptive, and kinesthetic ones. Because the bandwidth of the muscular actuation is limited at about 10 Hz, Brooks (1990) argues that a hand controller should be asymmetrical in data flow. In fact, a good hand controller must track hand motions up to 5-10Hz, and must be able to feedback to the operator signals as high as 30 Hz for proprioceptive/kinesthetic sensing and possibly up to 320 Hz low-amplitude vibrational information.

2.2 Experiments on Thresholds Detection

To refine the analysis of the above bandwidth characteristics, measures related to the *Just Noticeable Difference (JND),* also called the *Weber fraction,* are used. This measure is the minimal difference between two intensities of stimulation (I vs. I + ΔI) that leads to a change in the perceptual experience. The JND is an increasing function of the base level of input, generally defined as a percentage value by:

$$JND\% = \frac{(I + \Delta I) - I}{I} \times 100 \quad (1)$$

In haptics, the perceptual experience is investigated considering several independent factors. That is, the perception of length, angle, and parallelism, the perception of force vectors, and surface stiffness, the relevance of the peri-personal space, the numerosity judgments are investigated with classical psychophysical methods. Besides, several haptic perceptual illusions and performance in haptic tasks are considered. Several examples of measurements methods and relevant findings are the following.

2.2.1 Length

Length measures are addressed by Durlach et al (1989). They observe that the JND in length measured in discrimination experiments is roughly 1 mm for reference lengths of 10 to 20 mm. It increases monotonically with reference length but violates Weber's law. Similar results are reported by Tan et al. (1992): using a Constant Stimuli paradigm, they find that the JND is not linearly proportional to the reference length L: it is 8.1% for L=10 mm, 4.6% for L=40 mm and 2.8% for L=80 mm.

2.2.2 Angle

The threshold for detecting changes in angle is determined as about 15%, using the magnitude estimation and magnitude production (Newberry et al., 2007). It is argued that both cutaneous and proprioceptive feedbacks are relevant for haptic angle discrimination (Levy et al. 2007).

2.2.3 Force

The JND percentage value for pinching motions between finger and thumb is found to be ranged between 5% and 10% of the reference force (Pan et al., 1991). In a force matching experiment about the elbow flexor muscles, Jones (1989) observes a JND ranging between 5% and 9%. JND is relatively constant over a range of different base force values between 2.5 and 10 N (Allin et al., 2002). Tan et al. (1992) conclude that the force JND is essentially independent from reference force and displacement. It is argued that sensorimotor predictions, visual object information and prior experience influence force perception (Kording et al., 2004).

Detection of force vibration has been studied extensively. The large number of studies results from the large number of variables that can affect the vibratory perception: frequency, duration, direction, contact geometry, contact area, contact force, state of adaptation, skin site, skin temperature, age, and pathology.

In haptics research, the detection thresholds for the somatosensory system have been well characterized in terms of the smallest perceivable amplitude of sinusoidal movements over the frequency range 0.4 and 600 Hz.

The results of these studies are accounted for well by the hypothesis that vibratory detection depends on some critical level of activity in Pacinian afferents at high frequencies (at about 300 Hz, or more) and in a separate set of afferents at low frequencies (at about 40 Hz, or less) which have been identified as Meissner afferents (Johnson et al., 2000) . It is observed a decreasing trend in the relationship between threshold and frequency, especially in the range 2 and 300 Hz (Yang et al., 2004). The relationship between threshold and frequency is the traditional U-shaped function within the range 40 and 300 Hz (Brisben et al., 1999).

2.2.4 Stiffness

Using a contralateral limb-matching procedure, Jones and Hunter (1990) calculate the psychometrical function for stiffness. The JDN for stiffness is 0.23, which is three times that reported for elbow flexion forces and forearm displacement. These findings indicate that perceptions are based on sensory signals conveying force and movement information. Shon and McMains (2004), considering stiffness values over 1000N/m, compute the Weber fraction of 0.67 of the base stimulus, and find an overshoot error from 3 to 13mm for different stiffness values, decreasing when values of stiffness increase.

2.2.5 Velocity

In a force control task, using a reference speed factorially varied in the range 1 and 30 mm/s, Wu et al. (2005) determine the upper bound of human force control ability which occurs at or below a velocity of 20 mm/s. Moreover, they find that performance decreases as the velocity of hand motion increases.

2.3 Perception of the peri-personal space

To address more complex stimuli, researchers developed other testing paradigms that include also the effects of other sensory channels, such as visual and tactile sensing, on the peri-personal space.

2.3.1 Force directions

Barbagli et al. (2006) find discrimination thresholds for force directions to be in the range between 18.4, and 31.9%. The results show that the congruency of visual information significantly affects haptic discrimination of force directions and that the force-direction discrimination thresholds do not seem to depend on the reference force direction. In a similar task, Elhajj et al. (2006) find that humans perceive force direction more accurately between the 60 and 120 degree region than the other regions. The perceptual capabilities are also related to training effects, and fatigue.

2.3.2 Objects spatial properties

These results support the statement that the haptic perception of objects spatial properties is systematically distorted (Fasse et al., 2000). That is, what humans haptically perceive as parallel is often far from physically parallel. These deviations from parallelity are highly significant and very systematic. There exists accumulating evidence, both psychophysical and neuro-physiological, that what is haptically parallel is decided in a frame of reference intermediate to an allocentric and an egocentric one. The results of Kappers and Viergever (2006) show that deviation size varies strongly with condition, exactly in the way predicted by the influence of a hand-centered egocentric frame of reference.

2.3.3 Haptic Illusion

Several haptic illusion are evaluated with psychophysics paradigm, in order to better understand the role of the internal sensorimotor predictions, from both a neural and cognitive prospective, and to create new perceptual experiences. For example, Diedrichsen et al. (2007) report a novel force illusion, in which constant force acting on a hand is perceived to increase when the apparent reason for that force is removed. This illusion arises because of a violation of an internal prediction. When an object is removed from a supporting hand, we expect that the load force generated by the object will be eliminated.

Starting from the peculiarities of the human perceptual system, and, in particular, the sensory saltation illusion, Tan et al. (2000) develop a new haptic interface, capable of presenting haptic information in an intuitive and effective manner. This perceptual phenomenon is a haptic spatiotemporal illusion that, with the appropriate spatial and timing parameters, evokes a powerful perception of directional lines. Their findings show that the saltatory signals share unique and consistent interpretations of directional lines among the group of observers tested.

2.4 Guidelines from Human Factors

Starting from the previous findings in human perception, several works identify the conditions under which haptic interaction displays can enhance the human capabilities, both in accuracy and performance. The results provide a set of guidelines for the effective design of a haptic interface that minimizes perceptual and cognitive aspects of the interface.

Earlier research addresses the teleoperating multifingered robotic hands in which Shimoga (1992) analyzes some specific requirement on the design of dexterous master devices regarding constructional and functional aspects. The constructional issues consist of the isomorphism, portability, motion range capability and accommodation for human hand size variability. The functional issues consist of the bandwidth compatibility with the human hand, which has asymmetric input/output characteristics, the proprioceptive (force limit) compatibility and the consideration of the psychophysics stability of the human hand in sensing force magnitudes and variations.

In their works, Stanney et al. (1998) state that integrating haptic interactions in multimodal systems requires understanding user's sensory, perceptual, and cognitive abilities and limitations. They argue that haptic interaction relates to all the aspects of touch and body movement. This involves not only sensation and perception, but also the motor and cognitive aspects of active movement (that is, self-initiated movement) for which detailed motor plans are created, stored in memory, and compared to receptor feedback from the muscles, joints, and skin. They review several significant human factors issues that could stand in the way of virtual reality realizing its full potential. These issues involve maximizing human performance efficiency in virtual environments, minimizing health and safety issues and circumventing potential social issues through proactive assessment.

Hale and Stanney (2004) indicate a set of guidelines for the design of the kinesthetic (body motion and position) interaction based on a psychophysical motivated approach. (i) To ensure more accurate limb position, use active rather than passive movement. (ii) Avoid minute, precise joint rotations, particularly at distal segments. (iii) Minimize fatigue by avoiding static positions at or near the end range of motion. (iv) Surface stiffness of 400N/m should effectively promote haptic information transfer. (v) End-point forces of 4N should effectively promote haptic information transfer. (vi) Add kinesthetic information to enhance objects spatial location. (vii) Gestures should be intuitive and simple. (viii) Minimize fatigue by avoiding frequent, awkward, or precise gestures. (ix) Avoid precise motion gestures, as making accurate or repeatable gestures with no tactile feedback is difficult.

To the best of our knowledge, the findings on human capabilities in haptics, of which few examples have been summarized above, led to identify guidelines and proposal for the design of new haptic devices. However, complete models of the human operator inclusive of several psychophysics characteristics have been proposed in the literature, to aid in the design of teleoperation systems. The most common models are based on biomechanical concepts, as described next.

2.5 Human Operator Models in Teleoperation

Based on the above findings, a number of biomechanical models have been developed, which are then used to validate manual control as well as perception capabilities of human operators during control task.

One the best known models is the one of McRuer and Krendal (1959), used especially to simulate tracking task of moving targets. The operator's responses, mainly defined as a time delay, will depend upon at least the following factors: the dynamic characteristics of the controlled elements; the type of input or forcing function driving the system; the individual reaction delays, and thresholds during the particular operation; the motivation, attention, previous training, and general psychological and physiological condition of the human at the time of the operation. This model shows a phase shift proportional to the frequency without any associated amplitude change. This human reaction delay of about 150 msec manifests itself as a linear increase in phase with frequency (Sheridan & Ferrell, 1974).

More recently, Townsend and Salisbury (1989), pointed out the difficulties of defining the bandwidth of a force display in terms of a force input-output transfer function, since it depends strongly on the boundary conditions encountered by the device. The performance of a haptic interface is often reported in terms of the dynamic range of impedances it may represent. At the low end, the range is typically limited by inherent dynamics of the interface device, such as inertia and friction. At the high end, the range is typically limited by system stability. A benchmark problem of considerable importance is the implementation of a stiff "wall". A theoretical analysis of stiff wall implementation is presented by Colgate et al. (1993), who develops a criterion for the passivity of a virtual wall in terms of two non-dimensional parameters.

Moreyra and Hannaford (1998) defined a novel method of analysis of haptic perception, the Structural Deformation Ratio (SDR), which makes it relatively easy to quantify some aspects of the high frequency performance of force displays. This model addresses the difficulty of defining the bandwidth of a force display, as pointed out by Townsend and Salisbury (1989).

The inclusion of cognitive effects has been proposed by Corker (1999) using a model of human performance in large scale and complex systems called Man-Machine Integrated Design and Analysis System. This model has long served to engineers in prediction of system performance, and it has also been used to identify performance shortfalls in the human-machine system under a range of anticipated scenarios. This model assumes a functional architecture about the underlying process of human behavior. The human operator model functions as a closed-loop control model with inputs coming from the world and action being taken in the worlds. However, the perceptual module discussed here is composed only by the vision and audition micro-modules, thus lacking a haptic (tactile, kinesthetic, proprioceptive) one.

As summarized in the previous Section, the current knowledge on operator models applicable to force reflecting systems reflects two separate groups of results from haptics and teleoperation. There is the need to merge the two body of knowledge with experiments that would allow to test appropriate combinations of biomechanical and perceptual factors, and to propose methods and instruments which can be relevant for either of them.

3. Current Research

Our research focus is on teleoperation with force feedback. In this area of application there are highly variable forces. For example, in fine manipulation or high dexterity operations very low forces are often involved. Furthermore, these forces are difficult to perceive but very important to accomplish the task. By means of a bilateral teleoperation system we would like to overcome this limitation and provide a perception enhancement that would lead to an increased transparency.
We investigate the haptic perception using psychophysics methods (in particular Threshold detection and Magnitude Estimation). These methods grant precision and thoroughness of results using a high number of trials in an extremely accurate and well-defined setup.
We account for the haptic perception of force, both as onset force as well as sinusoidal waves, in order to quantify how well a user detects changes in force magnitude, and how well one can perceive unappreciable forces.
With the aim of making low force feedback suitable and significant, we incorporate the human perception abilities into the necessary conditions for designing a new scaling function for master-slave systems. That is, after the identification of the JND related to kinesthetic perception, we describe a perceptual-based scaling method that relies on these results and permits to correctly recognize low stimuli generated on the salve side. The validation of the method is made designing a further experiment.

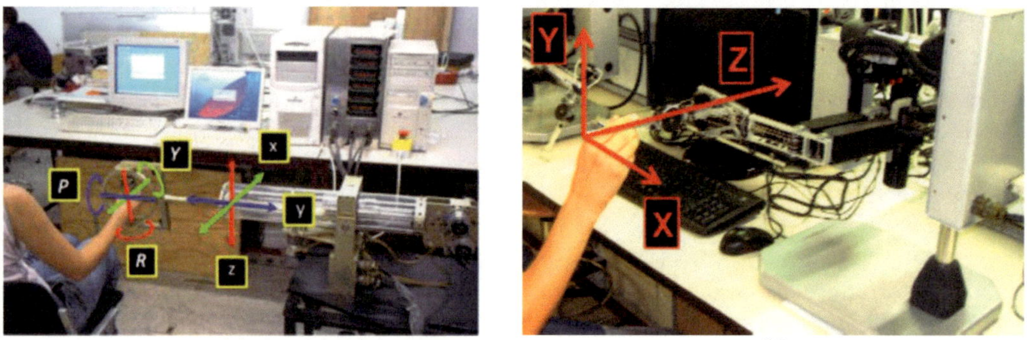

(a) (b)

Fig. 1. The experimental setup with (a) NASA-JPL Force Reflecting Hand Controller haptic device, and (b) MPB's Freedom 7S device.

3.1 Experimental Setup

3.1.1 Involved Haptic Devices

Psychophysical experiments on force perception are conducted using different haptic devices. In the prior experiment, we use a Force Reflecting Hand Controller (FRHC), developed at NASA's Jet Propulsion Laboratory (Bejczy & Salisbury, 1980). It has been refurbished recently, in particular with the addition of a custom designed controller implemented mostly on a NI PCI-7831R FPGA board (National Instruments, Austin, TX), that drives the device motors (Galvan et al., 2006). This device has 6 Degrees-of-Freedom consisting of one translational and five rotational joints (see Figure 1/a). With this structure, an operator can work with full dexterity in a cubic workspace of 30×30×30 cm^3.

In the latter experiments, in order to render the virtual surfaces, we involve a high performance Freedom 7S force-feedback device (MPB Technologies Inc., Montreal, Quebec, see Figure 1/b). The pen-hold grasping configuration is involved by concurrently using the thumb, index, and middle fingers. The range of motion of this device allows for hand movements that pivot at the wrist. In translation, the position resolution is 2 μm; the resolution in force rendering is 40 mN. The update and log rate is > 2 kHz.

3.1.2 Psychophysics Procedure for Threshold Measurement

The Green's (1993) Maximum-Likelihood adaptive procedure of psychophysics measurement, in the 2 alternative forced-choice paradigm, is involved to measure the absolute threshold; this procedure promises highly efficient trial placement and threshold estimation, minimizes the number of trials, and then the session duration.

During each trial, different controllable forces are applied in successive intervals to a single joint, generated by the force-feedback device. Subjects were given a choice of 2 alternatives, and they had to select the one containing the greater one. That is, the subjects know that exactly one alternative contains the stimulus s_i, and that the other has the comparison stimulus s_c.

After each stimuli presentation, a set of candidate logistic psychometric functions is fitted to all the data collected up to that point, and the likelihood associated with each function is computed. Starting from these parameters, a further comparison stimulus is calculated. The final estimate of threshold was extracted from the most likely psychometric function after a number of trials.

3.1.3 Statistical Analysis

Statistical analyses are conducted separately for each subject and for aggregate data. Every group analysis includes a factor for individual subjects so that differences between subjects are not counted as random variation; this makes each analysis more sensitive to the stimulus parameter being varied. Unless otherwise indicated, all statements referring to statistical significance are based on the criterion of probability level $p < 0.001$.

3.2 Force and torque magnitude discrimination thresholds

Our aim is to identify whether force intensities and orientation are associated with different values of JND%. This finding could let us discover a force threshold felt by the human operator and distinguish the most sensitive directions for the arm, and thus allowing us to identify one or more suitable scaling functions for force-feedback in haptic environments.

The purpose of the experiments described here following is to explore the differences in ability of a person to discriminate a wide range of force intensities applied along the axes of a reference frame positioned at the hand-grip.

3.2.1 Experimental Setup

For each joint of the FRHC haptic device, 10 reference forces or torques s_i were identified among the physical stimulus domain. The forces ranged from 0.4 to 9.0 N and the torques from 0.02 to 0.50 Nm. The comparison stimulus presented on the next trial was the sweet-point of the most likely psychometric function (Green, 1993). Each stimulus was applied for 1,200 ms; the interval between different stimuli was 300 ms. No feedback was given during the experiment. The participants had to take a break among runs at about every 7 minutes and whenever needed.

Direction		Reference Stimuli									
		s_1	s_2	s_3	s_4	s_5	s_6	s_7	s_8	s_9	s_{10}
X	Reference [N]	-5.99	-3.28	-1.80	-0.87	-0.54	0.50	0.83	1.79	3.26	5.98
	JND%	15.3	16.3	18.0	18.1	25.7	31.6	22.7	15.7	17.0	9.6
Y	Ref. [N]	-7.21	-3.87	-2.06	-0.80	-0.51	0.41	1.07	2.29	4.07	7.35
	JND%	11.62	12.56	19.29	36.93	25.33	29.58	32.66	24.87	13.25	12.16
Z	Ref. [N]	-8.77	-4.71	-2.52	-1.01	-0.60	0.62	1.01	2.30	4.42	8.33
	JND%	15.73	16.95	19.92	56.47	57.06	48.57	32.47	20.31	12.96	11.25
R	Ref. [Nm×10^{-2}]	-32.93	-16.87	-8.17	-4.50	-2.78	2.59	4.78	10.25	18.22	32.94
	JND%	12.65	23.25	45.06	35.88	41.99	63.02	56.46	31.48	23.85	13.79
P	Ref. [Nm×10^{-2}]	-21.24	-12.02	-9.40	-6.50	-3.60	1.95	6.87	11.37	15.43	29.72
	JND%	11.13	16.20	18.56	17.56	66.73	> 100	46.14	31.61	28.19	14.65
Y	Ref. [Nm ×10^{-2}]	-41.22	-20.86	-15.07	-8.67	-3.50	4.84	11.86	18.86	25.20	47.48
	JND%	12.11	19.30	21.16	24.02	> 100	46.04	30.86	27.48	20.49	12.21

Table 1. Mean values of the threshold and slope distributions estimated for the reference forces s_i for each joint.

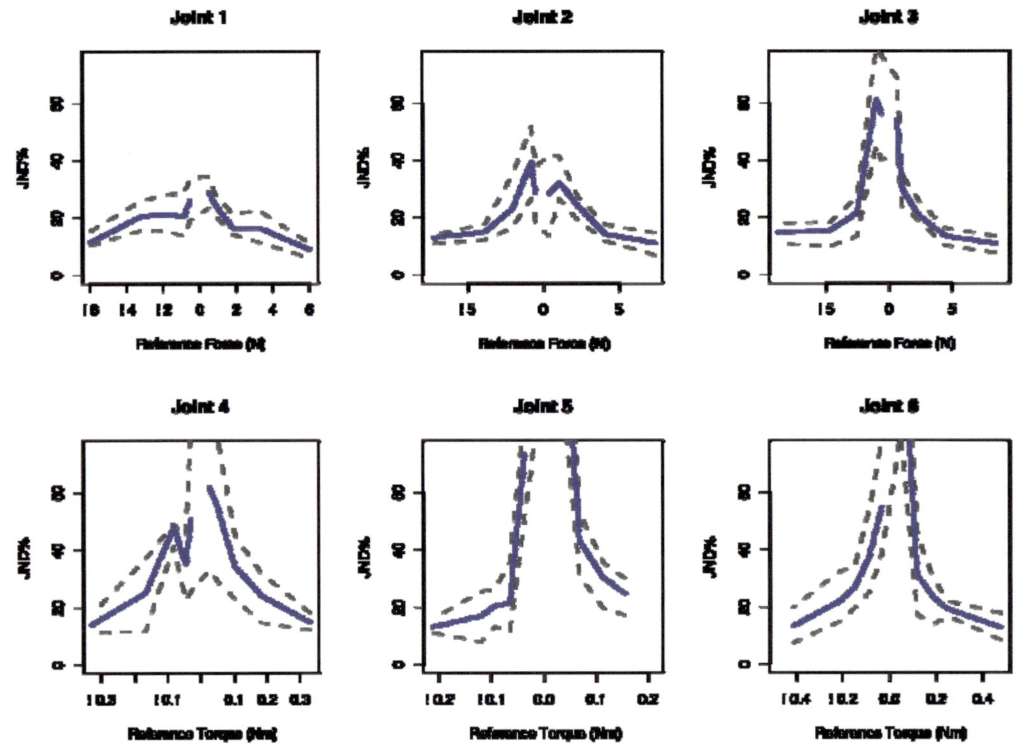

Fig. 2. JND versus reference force and torque. Each point is the participants' threshold. The blue line maps the median values; the dashed grey lines map the lower and the upper hinge.

3.2.2 Results

Data were analyzed in order to estimate the perceptual threshold for the reference stimuli. Results are reported in Table 1. For each joint, a between-subjects ANOVA was conducted to determine if there were significant differences among the perceptual thresholds due to the different reference values with respect for the different subjects' thresholds. Significant differences in the JND along the stimulus continuum were observed for all the translational and rotational axes.

In Figure 2 the force JND is plotted versus the reference force for all the joints. We observed a non-linear relationship between the reference stimuli and the JND. Considering the lower reference stimuli, the force stimulus and the JND appeared to be inversely associated: the lower the force or torque applied, the higher the perceived JND value.

A direct result of this experiment is the identification of force thresholds for each hand direction and many indirect results are coming out from intra- and post-experimental observations. The observation of the asymmetries in the JND plots leads us to an in depth investigation of the human workspace, not considering only the reachability but also the accuracy of each region of the workspace.

The perceptual thresholds for intense stimuli were higher than in the foregoing experiments: our findings provide evidence that the perceptual threshold or torques can be treated as linear for intense values, with an average value of about 15% of the reference force. But, low forces (i.e. below 0.5 N) cannot be perceived adequately with the current setup. Only very large differences between different stimuli are perceived and recognized by the neuro-musculo-skeletal system. Besides, the mechanical capabilities of the involved device do not allow considering these force range. Thus, we do not know exactly how these restrictions are due to the specific 6 DoFs haptic device or to human peculiarities.

3.3 Perception of harmonic forces

To the best of our knowledge, there is only few data on the perception of very low forces, and no available data on the relation between force discrimination threshold and frequencies signals. Therefore, it is necessary to first estimate the absolute detection thresholds for force signal (both presented as onset force, and as a sinusoidal wave), in the form of a force-magnitude versus temporal-frequency function, involving a high precision haptic display.

With this experiment, fully presented in Vicentini & Botturi (2009), we measure the absolute detection threshold (i.e. the smallest amount of stimulus energy necessary to produce a subjective sensation) for the hand in a pen-hold configuration (typical for using haptic devices), for both low force signal and for sinusoidal wave signals. We hypothesize the lowest detection threshold for wave signals. With the validation of our hypothesis, we can assert that there is an intensity range in which low forces are not perceivable, but wave signals, characterized by the same intensity, are. From these results it is possible to identify a particular signal manipulation, which can allow enhancing the perception of sub-threshold force intensities.

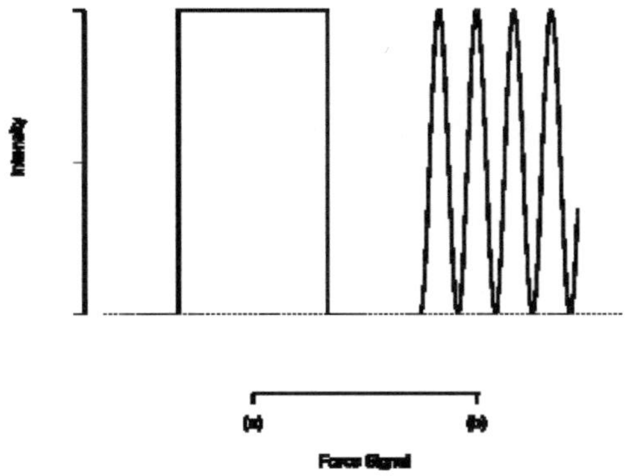

Fig. 3. Prototypical representation of the force signal: (a) onset force, with no frequency components, (b) sinusoidal wave.

3.3.1 Experimental Setup

The experimental design for absolute force detection is defined by the factor force signal, defined by five levels, generated according to (a) an onset force, with no frequency components, or to (b) sinusoidal waves at 40, 100, 300, and 600 Hz (a prototypical representations is depicted in Figure 3). Subjects repeated each session 4 times. The presentation order was fully randomized.

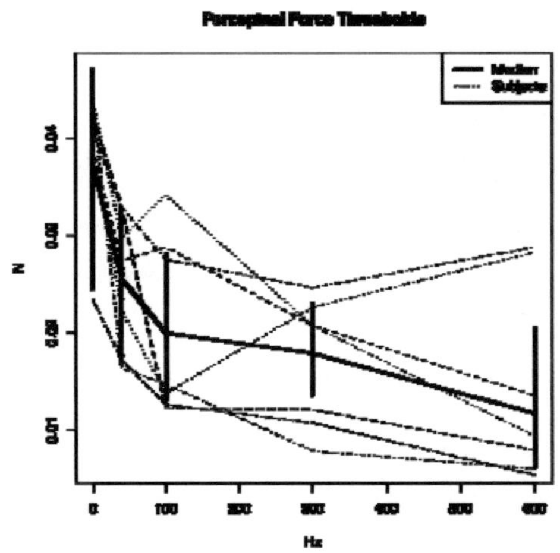

Fig. 4. Median values in absolute force estimation for all the subjects (strong line, with standard error bars), and for each subjects (dotted lines).

3.3.2 Results

Figure 4 reports the median values in absolute force estimation for all the subjects, and for each subjects. It shows the critical values for the minimal force detectable by a subject concurrently using the first three fingers, like grasping a pen. It is evident that the force thresholds decrease in detecting high frequency force signals.

With our experimental setup, when detecting onset force, the discrimination threshold is 39.28 mN (Interquartile Range (IR) from 24.40 to 46.68 mN), for sinusoidal 40 Hz wave is 24.49 mN (IR 16.99 to 32.96 mN), for 100 Hz is 19.65 mN (IR 12.71 to 25.75 mN), for 300 Hz is 17.30 mN (IR 12.22 to 22.76 mN), and for 600 Hz is 8.37 mN (IR 6.17 to 20.55 mN).
An ANOVA (force signals × subjects) was conducted to verify whether the significance of the differences in force thresholds. There are clear differences in absolute force thresholds ($F_{4,106}$=25.62, $p < 0.001$). The Tukey's Honestly Significant Difference post-hoc test (HSD) reveals that the onset force threshold is always greater than the wave signals ones. There is also a significant difference between the 40 Hz force wave and the 300 Hz one: no improvements in force detection are observed for higher values.
As shown in Figure 4, we observe relevant differences among subjects' thresholds. Two subjects report an outlier behavior in force detection of high frequency waves: they show a constant trend in force thresholds for force waves = 300 Hz. That is, while there is a clear difference between onset force and wave signals perception, it is not observable the well-known decreasing trend from 40 to 300 Hz (Brisben et al. 1999).
Starting from these results, we can now assert that there is an intensity range in which low forces are not perceivable, but wave signals, characterized by the same intensity, are. We argue that this perceptual range can be successfully involved to enhance the presence experience, by letting a user to accurately feel the contact with a virtual surface, without involving dedicated display.

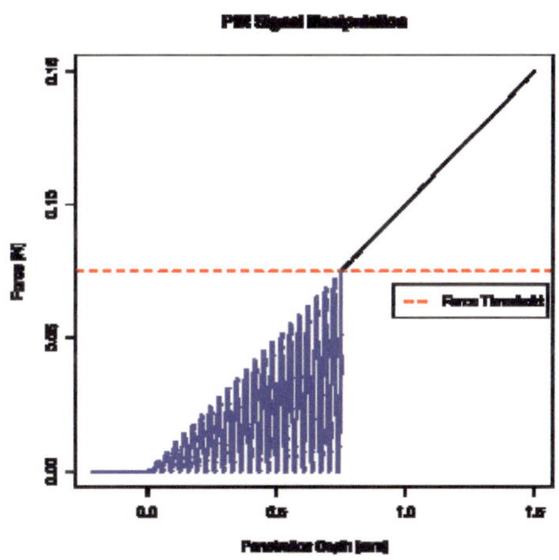

Fig. 5. Force signal manipulation according to Eq. (2) for over-thresholds forces, and to Eq. (3) for intensities under the onset force threshold

4. Signal Manipulation Based on Force Perceptual Thresholds

In this section we show how to build a perceptual-based force signal manipulation that can be embedded in a bilateral teleoperation system in order to improve performance in terms of the amount of force absolute detection that can be perceived by the user. A suitable signal processing is needed to improve the force feedback and moreover the operation performance, without compromising the stability of the teleoperation system.

Our proposal is aimed at augmenting the perception, for a human being, by superimposing, on undetectable force values, frequencies components generated by a common haptic device, without using any specific tactile display, to carry out a teleoperation task.
This is a new approach to force augmentation in teleoperation, since the acquainted concept of signal manipulation in this field concerns mainly constant amplification or variable force scaling. As originally proposed by Okamura et al. (1998), we use stimuli in frequency domain for very low forces. But, now, this concept is used in a standard teleoperation scenario to present only the sub-threshold, not-perceivable forces. Meanwhile, the use of common haptic devices can cover all the force range needed for a contact task with pliable surface.
With the following experiment setup we are aimed at accounting for the effectiveness of the proposed perceptual-based signal manipulation. We define a surface contact task characterized by a low stiffness (pliable) virtual surface; we manipulate the force signal, which is proportional to the penetration in the virtual wall, by substituting the sub-threshold not-perceivable forces with wave force signals, without changing the force intensity. A vibration waveform is superimposed onto the force signal sent to the actuator motors. With this approach, rather than amplifying the sub-threshold forces, we enhance the contact with a pliable surface minimizing penetration depth, according to the "perceptual based" capabilities in high-frequency detection (see Sect. 3.3).

4.1 Experimental setup

The haptic stimulus consists in a virtual surface, placed in at l = 80±10 mm far from the initial position of the red circle. The virtual surface is not visually rendered, so as not to bias the subject with respect to the location of the surface contact point.
Subjects are asked to a) move the probe with the Freedom haptic device along a designed direction until they feel the surface; b) once contact is perceived, subjects are instructed to instantly move backwards.
As depicted in Figure 5, when the tip penetrates the virtual object, force F_p is rendered according to

$$F_p = -k \cdot D_p \tag{2}$$

where k is the stiffness value, D_p is the penetration inside the virtual surface. When signal manipulation is applied, if F_p is smaller than the absolute force threshold for onset force, force F_p is rendered according to

$$F_p = -k \cdot D_p \cdot \left(1 + \sin(2\pi\omega t)\right)/2 \tag{3}$$

where ω is the sinusoidal wave frequency, t is the time.
Two experimental factors (stiffness and signal manipulation) are combined in a 3×3 factorial design. Stiffness values k have been chosen amongst commonly reported values of stiffness for the human body: 300, for a surface similar to the human fat, 700, and 1100 N/m, for a harder surface similar to the human skin or muscle tissue. The further experimental factor is signal manipulation. We test whether there are differences in penetration depth for the following three conditions: a) no signal manipulation, forces are rendered according to Eq.

(2); b) not perceivable forces are rendered according to Eq. (3) and ω = 40 Hz; c) not perceivable forces are rendered according to Eq. (3) and ω = 300 Hz.

4.2 Results

We evaluate the relevance of the position of the virtual surface and of the effective contact velocity on the penetration depth. A robust regression is conducted over the collected data. No significative relevance of the surface position (*t*-value = -1.045, p = 0.296), nor of the effective contact velocity (*t*-value = -1.766, p= 0.059) is observed.

The penetration depth collected within the factorial design is plotted in Figure 6. Data shows that penetration depth inversely decreases as surface stiffness increases. Furthermore, we observe that there is an improvement in the task performance given by the signal manipulation. That is, the penetration inside the virtual surface is always greater when the surface is rendered according to the lone Eq. (2) than when forces are rendered with high frequencies sinusoidal waves, as expressed in Eq. (3). In these latter conditions, we observe an average decreasing in penetration depth equal to 10.33 % with respect to the previously mentioned one.

We employ a two-way ANOVA (stiffness × signal manipulation) to measure the significance of these differences in penetration depth values. The second-order interaction between stiffness and signal manipulation is not significant ($F_{4,1595}$ = 1.33, p = 0.257), while the first order factors are. The relevance of the factor stiffness is confirmed ($F_{2,1595}$ = 160.47, p < 0.001) with an high performance device, and with a less accurate device (Vicentini & Botturi, 2008).

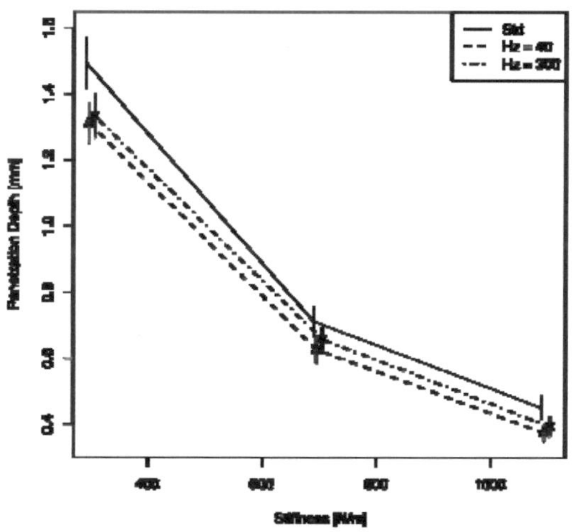

Fig. 6. Penetration depth is plotted against stiffness values for pooled data. The solid lines refer to the no signal manipulation condition, expressed by Eq. (2); the dotted lines refer to the signal manipulation at 40 and 300 Hz, as expressed in Eq. (3).

The lower penetration depth found in this study indicates that the perception of surface contact is impaired with the resolution and the inertial mass of the haptic device.

As hypothesized, the factor signal manipulation is relevant ($F_{2,1595}$ = 6.44, p < 0.002) for the task. There are clear differences in maximal penetration depth due to the involved force

signal processing. The HSD test reports significant differences between the onset force and 40 Hz conditions (p = 0.0018), the onset force and 300 Hz conditions (p = 0.0165), and no significant differences between the 40 Hz and the 300 Hz conditions (p = 0.776).
These results provide evidences on the effectiveness of the proposed perceptual based signal manipulation, especially when a 40 Hz force sinusoidal wave is involved.
The approach here presented is intended to complete the panorama of methods used to improve the human perception in case of environment interaction through devices. Methods based on tactile display (Kontarinis & Howe, 1995; Goethals et al., 2008) are limited to the specific device, which is not able to supply the complete force range of an interaction task. The force scaling method proposed in Vicentini et al. (2007) is useful in case of wide range of forces and in different directions. In this work the device has to support the frequencies signal manipulation but at the same time has to undertake a complete contact task. Therefore usability of those methods is for different purpose, in one case touching mainly virtual surface, in the other contact in classical teleoperation, in our case we propose an interaction with pliable surface.

5. PsychoGear: a Psychophysics Library for Haptics Experiments

Only few works in the literature bring together physiological, perceptual and cognitive factors, such as velocity, force, reaction time, mental workload, EMG measurement, and transmission delay. The main reason is that experiments testing a number of factors are not trivial, and the design implementation has to carefully take over the synchronization and the interface between different stimuli.
We have experienced the difficulties to implement a multi-factorial experimental design, even harder when the subject has to interact with the environment where there are noisy sensors, delayed stimuli and complex devices. The experiments just mentioned show the needs of multi-factorial design, in which several cognitive factors have to be evaluated in order to model the human perception in haptic system.
We are developing PsychoGear, a new psychophysics library to control all the aspects of the experimental setup, maintaining the rigor of the psychophysics methodology within a haptic system. The library will be able to control the experiments by governing stimuli generation and synchronization, data acquisition from different sensorial channels and data logging.

5.1 Features

Our approach follows the research line described in Anderson (2001), that is, to combine multiple psychophysics measurements within a full factorial design. We are working on a modular approach that arises from the decomposition of an experiment in a series of psychophysics methods, each one composed by a variable number of trials. For each trial we consider the presentation of a stimulus, the hardware source, the psychophysics procedure type (classical or adaptive) and the logging of the subject's response.
The focus of the approach described is on the infrastructure, not on a specific method. We want to provide a framework in which including a new experimental method is quick and easy. The user can define the design and choose the parameters without dealing with the underlying code because we have decoupled the programming phase from the utilization one. Moreover, we pursue the code reusability and all the implementations such as trials,

stopping rules, generation of the next stimulus, and data collection are stored in the framework.
With this library the user can concentrate on the design of the experiment putting together methods he/she needs, the programmer can rely on the framework to implement new details, without even know the psychophysics purpose. Finally, we point out in this library the possibility to have multi-factorial design and easy device integration.
As stated above arranging experiments with factorial design is a complex task, in which several cognitive factors have to be evaluated. The design is even harder when the subject has to interact with a real environment. This is a possible scenario when dealing with human perception in a real teleoperation task, taking into account noisy sensors, delayed stimuli and complex devices.
In order to control all the aspects of such a complicated setup maintaining the rigor of the psychophysical methodology and the requests from a teleoperation system, we are working on the development of a new psychophysics library.
Starting from the idea of the Psychophysics Toolbox extensions (Brainard, 1997) developed for MatLab, and the PsychoPy-Psychophysics software in Phython (Peirce, 2007), we are looking at providing C++ classes and methods to cover several aspects, from stimulus presentation and response collection using classical and adaptive procedures, to simple data analysis, such as psychometric function fitting.
We are working on a modular approach that arises from the decomposition of an experiment in a series of psychophysical methods, each one composed of a variable number of trials. For each trial we consider the presentation of a stimulus that may deal with the hardware, both with classical and adaptive procedures, and the log of the subject's response. The novelty of the approach is that we want to provide a framework in which the addition of a new method is easy and immediately integrates with the overall design of the experiment. We do not focus on a specific method but we provide the infrastructure. The aim is to relief the programmer from redefining the experiment when a new psychophysical method is needed and to let the final user to concentrate on the right choice of parameters without dealing with the underlying code.

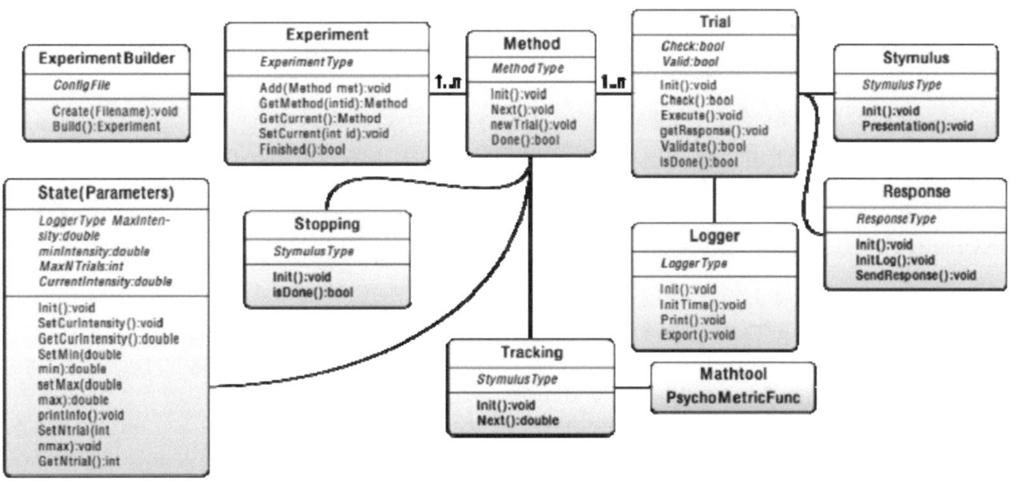

Fig. 7. PsychoGear: Experimental Psychophysics Library UML Class Diagram.

5.2 Class Structure

In Figure 7 we show the object hierarchy: an *Experiment* contains an arbitrary number of methods, each *Method* contains a *State* class, which contains all the parameters needed for a correct execution of all the sub-component, a *Tracking* class, that controls the stimuli intensities, a *Stopping* class, that checks the end of the method, and a *Trial* class, that manages the stimulus presentation, *Stimulus*, the response acquisition, *Response*, and logs the data, *Logger*.

Each class has a simple and easy to use interface. The main component of this framework is the *Method* class that supervises all the different control aspects of the experiment procedure. We have to present a sequence of stimulus intensities, that are known a priori or settled at run time, and for this purpose the *Tracking* class gives basic commands to control the evolution of the stimuli in the procedure.

A very important aspect is the procedure ending management. The *Stopping* subclass checks the end of the procedure and also allows easily change between different stopping rules. Moreover following the psychophysics definition, *Trial* class is implemented with a *Stymulus* subclass, that manages the stimulus presentation, and a *Response* subclass, which controls the responses acquisition. In addition, a *Logger* subclass is implemented to save all the meaningful parameters that describe user activities data.

Besides the psychophysics procedure uses some statistical tools, for example probability distribution and random number generator therefore the *Mathtool* class is implemented to contain all the auxiliary mathematical functions.

It is common to design a real experiment that involves more than a single psychophysics procedure (for example, two staircase procedures with random stimulus presentation). So we need to control which procedure has to be executed, how many trials have to be presented, when the entire experiment finishes. To manage this type of design, the *Experiment* class manages different methods defining a global end criteria and a switching rule between methods in every step of stimulus presentation.

The specific parameters of the classes involved in the experiment are stored in the *State* class. This class contains all the parameters in the same place, so it is easy for every sub-class to access useful sharable information.

When an experiment is clearly designed, it may be seen as a set of psychophysics procedures and parameters (i.e. stimulus intensities, starting values, stopping rule, presentation time). Especially during the pilot testing, the user needs to tune some parameters to fit the current design to the goal of her/his study.

To make this operation easier, we set a unique XML configuration file, where the user can easily choose the components and set the parameters of the experiment. The *ExperimentBuilder* class reads the configuration file and initializes the experiment with the correct sub-classes and parameters.

5.3 Developing new experiments

The proposed psychophysics library takes advantage from the experience of other implementations and the needs of the haptic perception experiments. The novelty of this library is the native management of the psychophysics procedures and of the haptic system; moreover some problems from the existing libraries are solved in this implementation ensuing the software engineer suggestions (i.e. object oriented code organization, haptic device support).

The library architecture is not only due to software engineering, but is meaningful for the organization and the development of every experimental design, in haptic research is even more important, given the complexity of the experiments designs. We are extending the implementation of the basic components, adding, for example, the support for all the fundamental adaptive methods, as discussed in Leek (2001). Once the base code allows a wide set of example and a fast building process we will use them as an "how to" for our library, to allow an easy and fast startup time for new users.
We are also widening the hardware device support and to improve their integration with other source of stimulus devices, i.e. audio/video, with a unified synchronization protocol. We are introducing support for OpenGL to improve the rendering of visual stimuli, and we are working on support for OpenCL to obtain faster parallel computation (i.e. in psychophysics functions fitting evaluation).
Moreover a graphical user interface is being improved to drag and drop the components during the creation procedure and to manage the experiment execution, broadening the PsychoGear library use both for researchers and for students.

6. Conclusion

In this work we present how the results of psychophysics experiments in human perception can improve the telepresence of a haptic system.
In the past, perceptual experiments were carried out to obtain quantitative measurements of human perceptual capabilities. From there, information about peri-personal space and fusion with others sensory channels was extracted and biomechanical models were developed. At the same time, a lot of work was spent about the concept of transparency of teleoperated systems from a pure engineer point of view, i.e. control and mechanical design. We consider these two aspects as the sides of the same coin. We introduce perceptual experiments to support our vista where the two points of view converge and to provide a methodology of research. We introduce two experiments about force perceptual thresholds, both for high and low intensities. We analyze the results and formulate a scaling model based on the perceptual threshold: in a teleoperation system we use stimuli in frequency domain to let the user perceive sub-threshold, not-perceivable forces generated by the interaction with pliable surfaces. That is, rather than amplifying the under threshold forces, we enhance the feeling of contact with any pliable body by minimizing penetration depth, according to the "perceptual based" capabilities in high-frequency detection.
The second step is concerned with validating this scaling method in a task of pliable surface contact. Hence, we analyze the conditions under which haptic displays can enhance human accuracy and performance in a teleoperation task, by presenting an innovative force scaling for bilateral teleoperated system. We focused our attention on human perception capabilities and, we exploit the human ability to perceive low forces as onset or sinusoidal stimuli. We have used acquired data in order to obtain the proper modifications needed to enhance the information contained in the force signal coming back from the environment by defining a function that maps the not-perceivable forces to let the user completely interpret the interaction with the environment.
Data collected from perceptual experiments can provide guidelines for the design of better haptic devices, but we think that these results are also useful in order to obtain one or several models of the human operator from a psychophysical point of view. These models

can go beyond the simple mechanical and muscular representation of the human/machine interaction since they can catch the way human reacts to haptic stimuli and how the sensor fusion strategies works, thus permitting an useful enrichment of force information with visual and acoustic clues.

The main goal refers to the identification of the haptic human space in order to exploit its peculiarities. The measurement of perceptual abilities and the possibility to find relations among perceptual and cognitive factors permit to broaden the concept of transparency and telepresence providing the values to assign to specific parameters in order to maximize the perception with respect to specific tasks.

7. References

Allin, S., Matsuoka, Y., & Klatzky, R. (2002). Measuring just noticeable differences for haptic force feedback: Implication for rehabilitation. *Proceedings of Haptic interfaces for virtual environment & teleoperator systems*, pp. 299-303, Orlando, Florida, USA: IEEE Computer Society.

Anderson, N. H. (2001). *Empirical direction in design and analysis*. Mahwah, NY: Lawrence Erlbaum Associates.

Barbagli, F., Salisbury, K., Ho, C., Spence, C., & Tan, H. Z. (2006). Haptic discrimination of force direction and the influence of visual information. *ACM Transactions on Applied Perception*, 3 (2), 125-135.

Bejczy, A., & Salisbury, K. (1980). Kinematic coupling between operator and remote manipulator. *Advances in Computer Tecnology*, 1, 197-211.

Brainard, D. H. (1997). The Psychophysics Toolbox. *Spatial Vision*, 10, 433-436.

Brisben, A. J., Hsiao, S. S., & Johnson, K. O. (1999). Detection of vibration transmitted through an object grasped in the hand. *Journal of Neurophysiology*, 81, 1548-1558.

Brooks, T. L. (1990). *Telerobot response: Requirements* (Tech. Rep. No. STX/ROB/90-03). Lanham, MD: STX Robotics.

Burdea, G. (1996). *Force and touch feedback for virtual reality*. New York, NY, John Wiley & Sons, Inc.

Colgate, J. E., Grafing, P. E., Stanley, M. C., & Schenkel, G. (1993). Implementation of stiff virtual walls in force-reflecting interfaces. *Proceedings of IEEE Virtual Reality Conference*, pp. 202-208. IEEE Computer Society.

Corker, K. M. (1999). Human performance simulation in the analysis of advanced air traffic management. *Proceedings of Winter simulation conference*, pp. 821-828.

Diedrichsen, J., Verstynen, T., Hon, A., Zhang, Y., & Ivry, R. B. (2007). Illusions of force perception: The role of sensori-motor predictions, visual information, and motor errors. *Journal of Neurophysiology*, 97, 3305-3313.

Durlach, N. I., Delhorne, L. A., Wong, A., Ko, W. Y., Rabinowitz, W. M., & Hollerbach, J. (1989). Manual discrimination and identification of length by the finger-span method. *Perception & Psychophisics*, 46, 29-38.

Elhajj, I., Weerasinghe, H., Dika, A., & Hansen, R. (2006). Human perception of haptic force direction. *Proceedings of IEEE Intl. Conf. on intelligent robots and systems,* pp. 989-993, Los Alamitos, CA: IEEE Computer Society.

Fasse, E. D., Hogan, N., Kay, B. A., & Mussa-Ivaldi, F. A. (2000). Haptic interaction with virtual objects: Spatial perception and motor control. *Biological Cybernetics*, 82 (1), 69-83.

Galvan, S., Botturi, D., & Fiorini, P. (2006). FPGA-based controller for haptic devices. *Proceedings of IEEE Intl. Conf. on intelligent robots and systems*, pp. 971-976, Beijing, China: IEEE Computer Society.

Goethals, P., Lintermans, H., Sette, M. M., Reynaerts, D., & Van Brussel, H. (2008). Powerful compact tactile display with microhydraulic actuators. In M. Ferre (Ed.), *Haptics: Perception, devices and scenarios* (Vol. 5024/2008, p. 447-457). Berlin: Springer.

Green, D. M. (1993). A maximum-likelihood method for estimating thresholds in a yes-no task. *Journal of the Acoustical Society of America*, 93 (4), 2096-2105.

Hale, K. S., & Stanney, K. M. (2004). Deriving haptic design guidelines from human physiological, psychophysical, and neurological foundations. *IEEE Computer Graphics and Applications*, 24 (2), 33-39.

Johnson, K. O., Yoshioka, T., & Vega-Bermudez, F. (2000). Tactile functions of mechanoreceptive afferents innervating the hand. *Journal of Clinical Neurophysiology*, 17 (6), 539-558.

Jones, L. A. (1989). Matching forces: constant errors and differential thresholds. *Perception*, 18 (5), 681-687.

Jones, L. A., & Hunter, I. W. (1990). A perceptual analysis of stiffness. *Experimental Brain Research*, 79 (1), 150-156.

Kappers, A. M. L., & Viergever, R. (2006). Hand orientation is insufficiently compensated for in haptic spatial perception. *Experimental Brain Research*, 173 (3), 407-414.

Kontarinis, D. A., & Howe, R. D. (1995). Tactile display of vibratory information in teleoperation and virtual environments. *Presence*, 4 (4), 387-402.

Kording, K. P., Ku, S., & Wolpert, D. M. (2004). Bayesian integration in force estimation. *Journal of Neurophysiology*, 92, 3161-3165.

Lawrence, D. A. (1993). Stability and Transparency in Bilateral Teleoperation, *IEEE Transactions on Robotics and Automation*, 9 (5), 624-637.

Leek, M. R. (2001). Adaptive procedures in psychophysical research. *Perception & Psychophysics*, 63 (8), 1279-1292.

Levy, M., Bourgeon, S., & Chapman, C. (2007). Haptic discrimination of two-dimensional angles: influence of exploratory strategy. *Experimental Brain Research*, 178 (2), 240-251.

McRuer, D. T., & Krendel, E. S. (1959). The human operator as a servo system element. *Journal of the Franklin Institute*, 267 (5-6), 1-49.

Moreyra, M., & Hannaford, B. (1988). A practical measure of dynamic response of haptic devices. *Proceedings of IEEE Intl. Conf. on robotics & automation*, pp. 369-374.

Newberry, A. C., Griffin, M. J., & Dowson, M. (2007). Driver perception of steering feel. *Institution of Mechanical Engineers, Part D: Journal of Automobile Engineering*, 221 (4), 405-415.

Okamura, A. M., Dennerlein, J. T., & Howe, R. D. (1998). Vibration feedback models for virtual environments. *Proceedings of IEEE Intl. Conf. on Robotics & Automation*, pp. 674-679, Leuven, Belgium: IEEE Computer Society.

Pang, X. D., Tan, H. Z., & Durlach, N. I. (1991). Manual discrimination of force using active finger motion. *Perception & Psychophisics*, 49 (6), 531-540.

Peirce, J. W. (2007). PsychoPy-Psychophysics software in Python. *Journal of Neuroscience Methods*, 162 (1-2), 8-13.

Sheridan, T. B., & Ferrell, W. R. (1974). *Man-machine systems: Information, control, and decision models of human performance*. MIT Press.

Shimoga, K. B. (1992). Finger force and touch feedback issues in decterous telemanipulation. In *Intelligent robotic systems for space exploration* (p. 159-178). IEEE Computer

Society. Shon, Y., & McMains, S. (2004). Evaluation of drawing on 3D surfaces with haptics. *IEEE Computer Graphics and Applications*, 24 (6), 40-50.

Stanney, K. M., Mourant, R. R., & Kennedy, R. S. (1998). Human factors issues in virtual environments: A review of the literature. *Presence*, 7 (4), 327-351.

Tan, H. Z., Lim, A., & Traylor, R. (2000). A psychophysically study of sensory saltation with an open response paradigm. *Dynamic Systems and Control*, 69 (2), 1109-1115.

Tan, H. Z., Pang, X. D., & Durlach, N. I. (1992). Manual resolution of length, force and compliance. *Proceedings of Haptic interfaces for virtual environment & teleoperator systems*, vol. 42, pp. 13-18, Anaheim, CA: ASME Dynamic Systems and Control Division.

Townsend, W. T., & Salisbury, K. (1989). Mechanical bandwidth as a guideline to high-performance manipulator design. *Proceedings of IEEE Intl. Conf. on robotics & automation*, vol. 3, pp. 1390-1395.

Vicentini, M., & Botturi, D. (2008). Overshoot effect in stiffness perception tasks during hand motion with haptic device. In M. Ferre (Ed.), *Haptics: Perception, devices and scenarios* (Vol. 5024/2008, p. 189-198). Berlin: Springer.

Vicentini, M., & Botturi, D. (2009). Signal manipulation based on perceptual thresholds enhances surface experience with common haptic device. *Proceedings of Third joint EuroHaptics conference and symposium on haptic interface for virtual environment and teleoperator systems*, pp. 133-138, Salt Lake City, UT: IEEE Robotics and Automation Society.

Vicentini, M., De Maggio, M. C., Botturi, D., & Fiorini, P. (2007). Evaluation of directional force threshold through psychophysics experiments. *Proceedings of the 4th Intl. Conf. on Enactive Interfaces*, pp. 297-300, Grenoble, France: Association ACROE.

Wu, M., Abbott, J. J., & Okamura, A. M. (2005). Effects of velocity on human force control. *Proceedings of EuroHaptics and Conference and Symposium on Haptic Interfaces for Virtual Environment & Teleoperator Systems*, pp. 73-79, Pisa, Italy: IEEE Computer Society.

Yang, S., Tan, H. Z., Buttolo, P., & Johnston, M. (2004). Detection of torque vibrations transmitted through a passively-held rotary switch. *Proceedings of EuroHaptics 2004*, pp. 217-222, Munich, Germany: EuroHaptics Society.

23

Temporal perception of visual-haptic events in multimodal telepresence system

Zhuanghua Shi, Heng Zou and Hermann J. Müller
Allgemeine und Experimentelle Psychologie
Ludwig-Maximilians-Universität München
80802, München, Germany

1. Introduction

Multidomal telepresence systems have been used in remote or hazardous environments, such as telesurgery, orbit or underwater teleoperation, etc. (Ballantyne, 2002; Draper et al., 1998; Hirzinger et al., 1993). In a typical teleoperation task, local action commands are transmitted to a remote teleoperator, which then executes the commands and sends back multimodal sensory information, such as visual, auditory and haptic signals. Due to the communication, data encoding, and control scheme, time delays of this information feedback are inevitable in multimodal telepresence systems. These delays can vary from dozens of milliseconds to seconds. For example, the feedback latency for an intercontinental teleoperation via the Internet is around 300 ms (Peer et al., 2008), while the latency can be up to 5–10 seconds for teleoperation tasks in space (Hirzinger et al., 1993).

The effects of time delay on performance have been investigated in many studies (Ferrell, 1966; Held, 1993; Jay et al., 2007; Kim et al., 2005; Sheridan & Ferrell, 1963). For example, examining the effect of visual-feedback delay on user's task completion time, Mackenzie and Ware (1993) found that performance was affected by delays exceeding 75 ms, with completion time thereafter increasing linearly with time delay (> 75 ms) and task difficulty. A recent study examining the effects of delayed visual feedback on telerobotic surgery (Kim et al., 2005) revealed a similar picture: completion time increased with time delay and dexterity was affected when the delay was longer than 250 ms; in addition, starting at a delay around 400 ms, the operators came to gradually adopt a move-and-wait strategy. Delays in haptic feedback have been found to have a similar influence on performance. For example, in a positioning task, delayed haptic feedback resulted in an increase in completion times and error rates (Ferrell, 1966). A recent study of the effects of continuous (as opposed to pulse) force feedback with delays revealed task performance to be very sensitive to the haptic-feedback delay: the error rate started to increase at delays of 25 ms and then rose more steeply than with visual-feedback delays (Jay et al., 2007).

Since time delay can vary for different types of information feedback, remote multimodal synchronous events, such as a visual-haptic collision, may be turned into local asynchronous incidents. Furthermore, crossmodal asynchrony may also arise from observer-internal perceptual processes. Crossmodal synchrony and asynchrony perception has beeen shown to depend on many factors ranging from low-level neural encoding and to higher-level cognitive processes. For example, auditory (speech) stimuli are typically processed faster by the brain than visual stimuli, so that observers can detect audiovisual asynchrony more easily when the sound is physically presented before the image (Dixon & Spitz, 1980). Similarly, experiments requiring observers to make temporal-order judgments (TOJ) of visual-haptic events have revealed that the visual-haptic simultaneity window is located asymmetrically around the point of physical synchronicity (Spence et al., 2001). Although there is a large literature on multisensory simultaneity perception, most of these studies have used a purely psychophysical approach in which observers are passively presented with crossmodal events and then have to make temporal-order or asynchrony judgments. There has been considerably less research on the perception of multisensory simultaneity in interactive telepresence systems. However, multisensory perception in such systems may be rather different from the situation in pure psychophysical studies: since the human operator continuously interacts with the remote operator through the human-system interface, perception and action are closely linked. Previous studies have demonstrated that visuo-motor action is an influential factor for perception (Noë, 2005; Witney et al., 1999). Consequently, perception and action must be taken into account together for understanding multisensory temporal perception in telepresence systems.

In this chapter, we present an overview of multisensory temporal perception, with particular focus on crossmodal simultaneity, in telepresence systems, based on relevant work as well as our recent studies of visual-haptic simultaneity in the closed perception-action loop and scenarios with communication delays involving packet loss. Since feedback from the events of touching and manipulating objects is of vital importance for humans performing teleoperation tasks, our studies were mainly concerned with the temporal perception of visual-haptic 'collision' events. Based on experimental findings and relevant models of human sensorimotor control, we then go on to propose a process model for multisensory temporal perception. This model permits some general guidelines to be derived for the optimal (human-factors) design of multimodal telepresence systems.

2. Perception of simultaneity and related psychophysical methods

Crossmodal simultaneity is of vital importance in our daily life. It provides the most salient temporal cue to form coherent percepts of objects and events, and it helps to segregate targets from background (Moutoussis & Zeki, 1997). There are two important parameters characterizing the perception of simultaneity: the point of subjective simultaneity (PSS) and the temporal just noticeable difference (JND). The PSS is the time interval between the onsets of two sensory stimuli at which the two stimuli are reported to be most synchronous. The JND, on the other hand, indicates the resolution of the temporal discrimination. These parameters are typically determined using two different types of task (Spence et al., 2001; Vogels, 2004): temporal-order judgment (TOJ) and synchrony/asynchrony judgment (SAS) task, respectively. In TOJ tasks, the observer is asked to determine the temporal order of two stimuli. The PSS is then defined by the 50%-threshold and the JND is calculated as half the difference between the lower (25%) and upper (75%) bound of the threshold. In contrast, in SAS tasks, the PSS is defined by the maximum of the distribution of 'synchronous' responses (plotted as a function of the stimulus onset asynchrony, SOA, between the two events) and the JND is estimated from the standard deviation of the distribution (see below).

To estimate the PSS and JND, psychometric functions, such as the logistic function, are often applied to model the binomial response data (Collett, 2002) in the TOJ task:

$$P(t) = \frac{1}{1+\exp(\frac{\alpha - t}{\beta})}, \tag{1}$$

where *P(t)* is the probability function of the TOJ response (event A before event B) over the crossmodal SOA *t*; α is a parameter indicating the location of the threshold at 50%; and β is a parameter indicating the slope of the psychometric function. The PSS and JND can be then estimated as follows:

$$\hat{PSS} = \hat{\alpha}, \tag{2}$$

$$\hat{JND} = \ln 3 \cdot \hat{\beta}. \tag{3}$$

In the SAS task, on the other hand, a Gaussian function is often fitted using maximum likelihood estimation (Stone et al., 2001):

$$P(t) = a \cdot \exp\left(\frac{-(t-\mu)^2}{2\sigma^2}\right), \tag{4}$$

where a is the maximum proportion of 'synchronous' responses, μ is the location of the maximum 'synchronous' responses, and σ is the standard deviation of the Gaussian function. The PSS and JND are then estimated as follows:

$$\hat{PSS} = \hat{\mu}, \tag{5}$$

$$\hat{JND} = \sqrt{\ln 4} \cdot \hat{\sigma}. \tag{6}$$

3. Crossmodal simultaneity in multimodal telepresence system

3.1 Influences of visuo-motor action on crossmodal simultaneity

Although crossmodal simultaneity has been intensively investigated (Dixon & Spitz, 1980; Fujisaki et al., 2004; Levitin et al., 2000; Spence et al., 2001; Stone et al., 2001; van Erp & Werkhoven, 2004; Vatakis & Spence, 2006), how crossmodal simultaneity is influenced by time delays and self-generated actions in multimodal human-system interfaces has thus far received only little attention. Recently, in an important study, Vogels (2004) examined the effects of time delay on visual-haptic asynchrony judgments, using a task that involved a visual object touching a virtual wall. Participants were asked to move a joystick such that a visual object approached and then collided with this wall. The SOA between the visual collision and the haptic collision (the latter was rendered by a constant 5.5 N force feedback) were varied across trials. Moreover, a further time delay (of 0 to 80 ms) was randomly added between the action and the feedback to simulate the ubiquitous communication delays in telepresence system. In addition, no visual feedback of the initial (joystick-generated) object movement was provided for a random interval of 50-150 ms. The results showed that, regardless of action-feedback delay, participants could easily detect the visual-haptic asynchrony when the SOA exceeded 50 ms. In another experiment, participants received touch and visual stimulus events passively while holding the joystick steady. The sensitivity for visual-haptic asynchrony (indicated by the standard deviation of the response distribution) was found to vary between 15 and 38 ms, which was smaller compared to that in the active-movement condition. Vogels' study represents a pioneering study of the effects of time delay and visuo-motor movement on visual-haptic simultaneity perception. However, her finding of an advantage, in terms of sensitivity, of passive touch over active movement was likely confounded by the experimental setup (as will be elaborated below). Indeed, there is a large body of evidence showing that active perception yields more information and enhances performance compared to passive perception (Heller & Myers, 1983; Wexler & Klam, 2001). Critically however, in Vogels' study, the space of the hand movement was separated from that of the visual representation - which may have impeded the crossmodal movement prediction and required more attentional resources. As a result, it is likely that, in her setup, the uncertainty of the asynchrony judgments was actually higher in the active-movement condition compared to the passive condition.

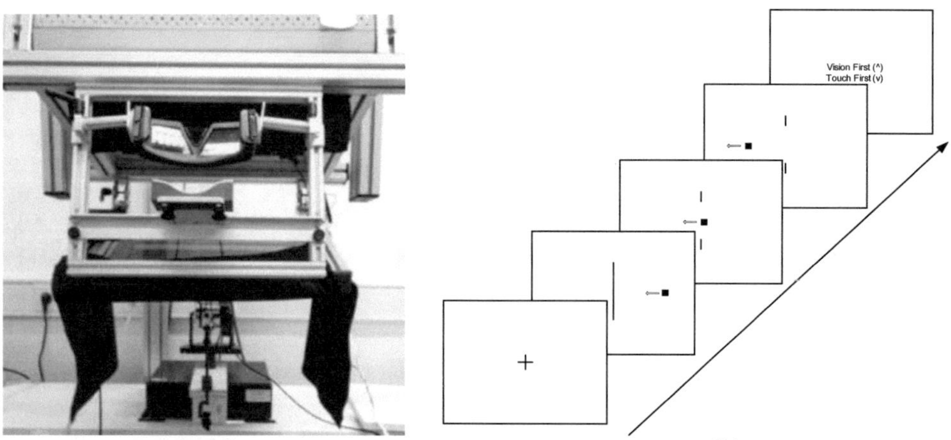

(a) (b)

Fig. 1. (a) Collocated visual-haptic virtual environment used in Shi et al. (2008). Visual stimuli were presented on a CRT monitor and mirrored to the haptic space (below the mirror), where haptic stimuli were generated by means of a PHANToM device. (b) Schematic illustration of a trial sequence in Shi et al. (2008). A small box was moved from the left to the right, or vice versa, either by the participant's active finger movement or automatically by a program-generated (passive) movement. When the moving object approached the middle line (the virtual 'wall'), the line broke into two pieces, signalling a visual collision. Meanwhile, with a varying time delay relative to (i.e., preceding or following) the visual collision, there was a short haptic pulse force feedback in the direction opposite to the movement, signalling the haptic collision. The participant's task was to discriminate which event: the visual or the haptic collision, had happened first.

This potential confounding in Vogels' study by separated manual and visual spaces was addressed in a recent study by the current authors (Shi et al., 2008), who implemented a collocated visual-haptic virtual environment to (re-)examine the influence of the visuomotor closed loop on visual-haptic simultaneity (see Figure 1). The visuomotor closed loop has been demonstrated to be important for controlling fine movements (Keele, 1986). To disassociate the influence of visual-motion feedback and of sensorimotor (hand movement) processing on the crossmodal simultaneity judgments, Shi et al. manipulated these two factors in a full factorial design (manual movement: active vs. passive; visual-motion feedback: with vs. without feedback). One of the resulting conditions simulated a common telepresence scenario: active hand movement with visual-motion feedback; another condition, passive hand movement without visual-motion feedback (except for the visual breaching of the line and the haptic-collision feedback), is comparable to the situation in classical psychophysical studies.

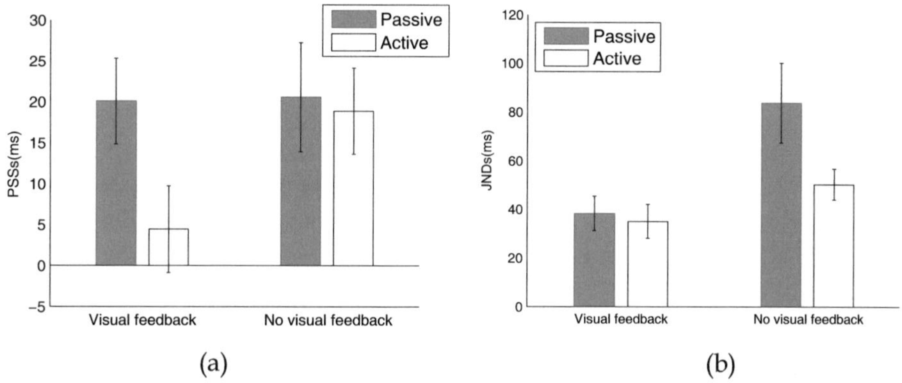

Fig. 2. (a) mean PSSs, and (b) mean JNDs for the four conditions in Shi et al. (2008).

Consistent with the results from classical visual-haptic studies, the PSS was shifted towards event sequences in which the visual stimulus physically occurred first, indicating that the haptic (collision) event was perceived earlier than a synchronous visual (collision) event. On average, the visual event had to occur 20 ms before the haptic event to be perceived as 'synchronous' – a value that is smaller than the typical PSS obtained in classical psychophysical studies (e.g., 50 ms in Spence et al., 2001). Interestingly, in the visuomotor closed-loop condition, the PSS was even smaller: only 4 ms (see Figure 2a). The small PSSs obtained in the interactive environment suggest that additional information, such as sensorimotor and visual-motion information, can help the central nervous system (CNS) to compensate for the difference in crossmodal latencies and improve the temporal-order judgment. More interestingly perhaps, the results of Shi et al. (2008), in contrast to those reported by Vogels (2004), showed that active movement does improve the sensitivity of asynchrony detection: the mean JND was reduced by 18 ms from passive to active visual-haptic collisions. In addition, the visual-motion feedback also greatly improved the sensitivity of crossmodal asynchrony judgments (Figure 2). Thus, the perceptual system can use the movement trajectory and active motor control to predict the forthcoming collision, thus improving the temporal discrimination. The performance improvement conferred by the visuomotor closed loop is consistent with previous studies on spatial positioning, in which the motor command, in conjunction with internal models of both hand and visual feedback, has been demonstrated to be useful for anticipating the resulting load force and the position of the object (van Beers et al., 1999; Wolpert & Ghahramani, 2000; Wolpert et al., 1995). The discrepancy between the studies of Vogels and Shi et al. may come from the different spatial setups. In the latter study, the visual and haptic spaces were collocated in a single space and multisensory events were generated in a natural way, permitting sensorimotor and visual feedback to provide additional sources of information for discerning temporal order.

In summary, these results indicate that the temporal perception of visual-haptic events can be influenced by additional information such as sensorimotor and visual feedback. A similar influence of the perception-action closed loop has also been found in haptic-audio asynchrony detection, and action-to-visual-feedback-delay detection (Adelstein, Begault et al., 2003; Adelstein, Lee et al., 2003). Thus, for the design of telepresence systems, this body of work strongly suggests that the perception-action loop should be taken into account when making considerations as to human operator's capacity for multimodal simultaneity perception.

3.2 Influences of packet loss on visual-haptic simultaneity

In multimodal telepresence system, crossmodal temporal perception is not only influenced by the perception-action loop, but also by inevitable communication delays and disturbances. Telepresence systems operating over large geographical distances are subject to packet loss and network communication delays, so that physically 'synchronous' events may be turned into 'asynchronous' incidents. Packet loss is a common issue in communication network using the DHCP service. Phenomenally, packet loss in video streams reduces image quality and interrupts video continuity. However, how packet loss influences the perception of visual-haptic simultaneity is, as yet, largely unknown. With regard to visual-packet loss, the current authors (Shi et al., 2009) recently examined this issue in a series of experiments. The task in these experiments was similar to the temporal-discrimination task used by Shi et al. (2008, see Figure 1), while adding frame-based packet loss to the visual feedback. The packet loss in the experiments was generated by a 2-state Gilbert-Elliot model (Elliot, 1963; Gilbert, 1960). This model can be wholly described by two transition probabilities between packet loss state (L) and packet no-loss state (N): $P_{n,l}$ and $P_{l,n}$ (See Figure 3). With two probabilities, two important features of the packet loss process, namely: the mean loss rate r_p and the mean burst length l_t, can be easily calculated (Eq. 7 and 8).

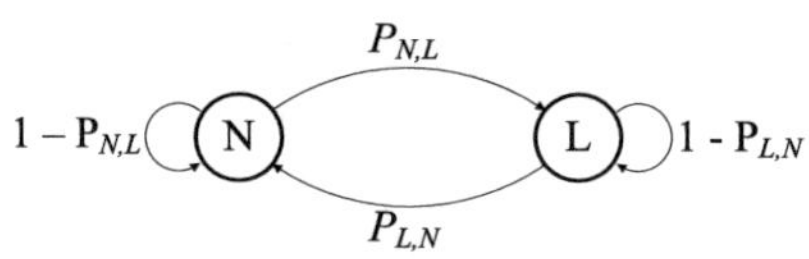

Fig. 3. Illustration of the 2-state Gilbert-Elliot model. 'N' and 'L' denote the states of 'No packet loss' and 'Packet loss', respectively.

$$r_p = \frac{P_{n,l}}{P_{n,l} + P_{l,n}}, \qquad (7)$$

$$l_t = \frac{1}{P_{l,n}}. \tag{8}$$

In Experiment 1 of Shi et al. (2009), four different mean packet loss rates (r_p = 0, 0.1, 0.2 and 0.3), with a constant mean burst length of 33 ms, were examined. The 33-ms burst length was chosen as it is slightly above the critical flicker fusion (CFF) rate, thereby ensuring that, on average, the packet loss was perceivable to the observers. The results demonstrated that visual-haptic simultaneity was influenced by the visual-packet loss rate: with increasing loss rate, the PSS was linearly shifted towards visual delay and away from haptic delay, indicating that observers tended to judge a video stream with packet loss as a delayed video stream. On average, the visual delay increased by 25 ms for each 10%-increment in visual-packet loss. Furthermore, the JND was found to increase when the packet loss rate increased, indicating that the simultaneity judgments became more difficult with higher packet loss rates. In part, these shifts in visual-haptic temporal perception were due to the packet loss disturbing the perception of the visual collision (i.e., the visual collision was 'blacked-out'). More interestingly, however, both trends, in PSSs and JNDs, remained the same even when these parameters were re-estimated based on only those trials on which visual-haptic collision events remained intact (i.e., on which the packet loss did not occur at the visual collision; see Figure 4). Shi and colleagues concluded from these results that visual-haptic simultaneity is influenced by prior exposure to packet loss, more precisely: when the perceptual system adapts to visual feedback degraded by packet loss, the internal estimation of forthcoming crossmodal simultaneity is biased towards visual delay. A similar adaptation effect has also been found in a study concerned with the recalibration of audiovisual asynchrony (Fujisaki et al., 2004). In this study, after exposure to asynchronous audiovisual events for several minutes, observers displayed a shift in their subjective-simultaneity responses toward the particular asynchrony to which they adapted. Our study showed that such recalibration processes can take place even more rapidly: packet loss just prior to the collision already influenced the visual-haptic simultaneity judgment within that trial.

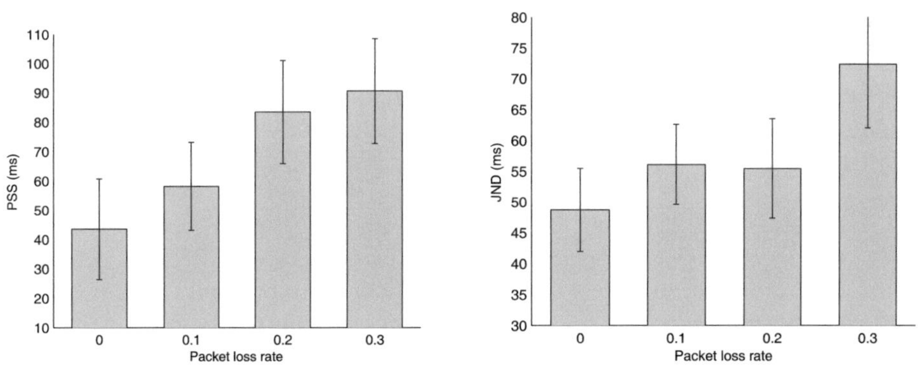

(a) (b)

Fig. 4. (a) PSSs and (b) JNDs as a function of the visual-packet loss rate in Experiment 1 of Shi et al. (2009). The mean values were estimated based on only those trials on which the packet loss did not 'mask' the visual collision.

3.3 Influences of prior information on visual-haptic simultaneity

The study of Shi et al. (2009) suggests that the perceptual system may use past information, such as from visual feedback, to predict the forthcoming events. However, how rapidly past information can be used for this prediction is still an open question. From the perspective of system design, the update rate of the internal temporal percept is an important factor, since it describes the temporal resolution of the dynamic adjustment of crossmodal simultaneity. Thus, to further examine the update rate of prior information on crossmodal temporal perception, we conducted a new experiment on visual-haptic temporal discrimination with packet loss in the visual feedback. In this experiment, we kept the packet loss rate constant at 0.2 for the initial movement prior to the collision event. The experimental design and task were similar to Shi et al. (2009). On a typical trial, the observer moved his/her finger from the left to the right (or vice versa) and made a collision with the 'wall'. When the visual moving object (represented by a small dot, which was controlled by the observer's index finger) approached the wall, visual-packet loss was 'switched off' at certain distances before reaching the wall (i.e., from the respective distance onwards, there was no longer a chance of a packet loss occurring). Four different switch-off distances (i.e., distance from the position of the moving object to the wall at the moment packet loss was switched off) were examined in the experiment: 5, 30, 60 mm, and the whole movement trajectory (in the latter condition, there was no packet loss at any distance; see Figure 5).

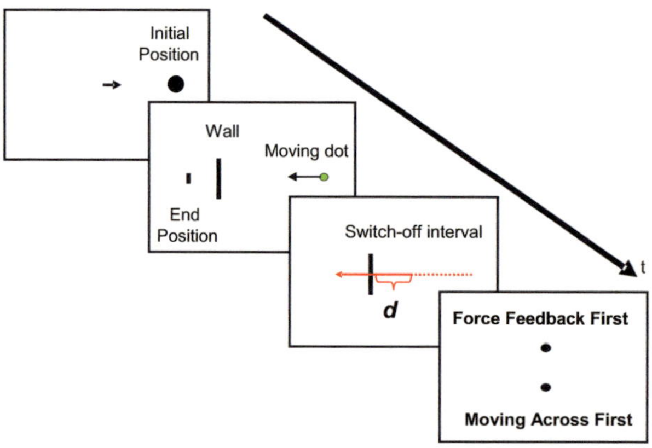

Fig. 5. Schematic illustration of a trial sequence. The movement trajectory is denoted by the long red arrow. The dashed line of the trajectory denotes visual feedback with packet loss, and the solid line visual feedback without packet loss. The packet loss switch-off distance is denoted by ***d***.

The mean PSSs were 106.8, 87.3, and 80.1 ms for switch-off distance of 5, 30, and 60 mm, respectively; the mean PSS for the no-packet-loss condition was 79.5 ms. A repeated-measures ANOVA revealed the effect of switch-off distance to be significant, $F(3,30) = 4.68$, $p<0.01$. A further contrast tested showed the PSS to decrease linearly with increasing switch-off distance, $F(1,10)=5.82$, $p<0.05$. The fact that, with increasing switch-off distance, the PSS approached the level achieved in the no-packet-loss condition suggests that 'no-packet-loss' information between the switch-off and the collision led to a gradual updating of the internal prediction of the forthcoming visual event. To estimate the internal update rate, we converted the switch-off distances into switch-off time intervals using observers' movement speeds; these intervals were, on average, 14 ms, 85 ms, and 172 ms for 5-mm, 30-mm, and 60-mm distances, respectively. The relationship between PSS and switch-off time interval is shown in Figure 6. The 95% confidence intervals revealed that the PSS was significantly larger, relative to the (no-packet-loss) baseline, at a switch-off interval of 87 ms (30-mm distance), while the PSS at a switch-off interval of 172 ms (60-mm distance) was no different from the baseline. This means that a complete update with prior visual feedback took between 85 and 172 ms. In other words, the internal update rate was in-between 6 to 12 Hz.

In summary, the above results demonstrate that prior information does not immediately impact on the internal representation. The internal processing requires some time to update and adapt to changes of the external world. The time required by the internal processing is in the range of a hundred or so milliseconds, which may relate to the short-duration working memory involved in crossmodal temporal processing. In the design of telepresence systems, it would be advisable to use this update rate for the implementation of assistive functions.

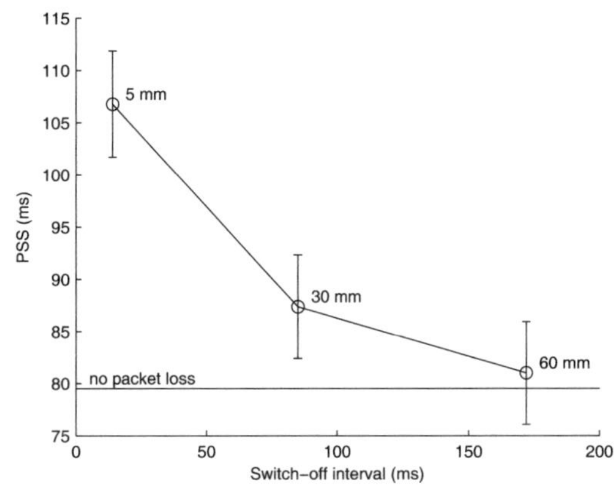

Fig. 6. PSS as a function of the switch-off time interval. The switch-off time intervals were estimated from the movement velocity. Error bars indicate 95% confidence intervals, which were estimated from 1000-sample bootstrapping.

4. Process model of crossmodal temporal perception

The studies discussed above showed that crossmodal simultaneity in an explorative environment is not only influenced by crossmodal temporal inconsistency, but also by many other sources of information, such as the visuomotor movement, the quality of the feedback signal, prior adaptation, etc. A recent study by Adelstein and colleagues (Adelstein, Lee et al., 2003) on head tracking latency also suggested that in virtual environments (with a head-mounted display), observers might use 'image slip' rather than the explicit time delay between input head motion and its displayed consequences to detect the asynchrony. Similarly, it has been found previously in audio-visual simultaneity judgments that, in relatively large environments, the brain may take sound velocity and distance information into account in the simultaneity perception of audio-visual events (Sugita & Suzuki, 2003). All available evidence converges on the view that the CNS may use additional information to predict, or infer, the external forthcoming events. Predicting the next states has been shown to be useful for compensating for the slow speed of updating in the visuomotor control system (Wolpert, 1997; Wolpert et al., 1995). This capacity for prediction has been attributed to an internal model that is assumed to underlie the nervous system's remarkable ability to adapt to unknown or underdetermined changes in the environment (Tin & Poon, 2005).

Inspired by this idea of an internal model for the sensorimotor system, we suggest that dynamic multisensory temporal perception can be described in an analogous way. Figure 6 illustrates such an internal model of multisensory temporal perception. When there are only individual (unrelated) multisensory inputs, the CNS may use the resolution in the individual sensory channels to estimate the onset (or offset) time of events and from this determine crossmodal simultaneity. However, such passive forward estimation may suffer from differences in the neural latencies among different modalities. For example, a auditory event is usually perceived as 'earlier' than a synchronous visual event (Dixon & Spitz, 1980). When additional information is available, such as sensorimotor information, visual-motion trajectories, or visuo-proprioceptive discrepancies, the CNS may use this information to make a fine prediction and provide for crossmodal compensation in anticipating the forthcoming events. Using this model, one can easily explain the small PSS found in the visuo-motor closed-loop condition in Shi et al. (2008). The visuo-motor closed-loop helps the CNS to make a fine prediction of the forthcoming visual events, thus partially compensating for the delay inherent in the visual processing. The prediction mechanism can also be applied to account for the results of the packet loss experiments (Shi et al., 2009). The visual-feedback signal was disturbed by the packet loss, which made the video stream appear stagnant from time to time. Such prior 'delay' information is used by the CNS for predicting the timing of the forthcoming visual-haptic events. As a result, the PSS was shifted towards visual delay. Note, however, that the use of prior information by the CNS to adjust the crossmodal temporal representation is not immediate: the experiment outlined above (in section 3.3) suggests that the update rate of using prior information is only of the order of 6-12 Hz.

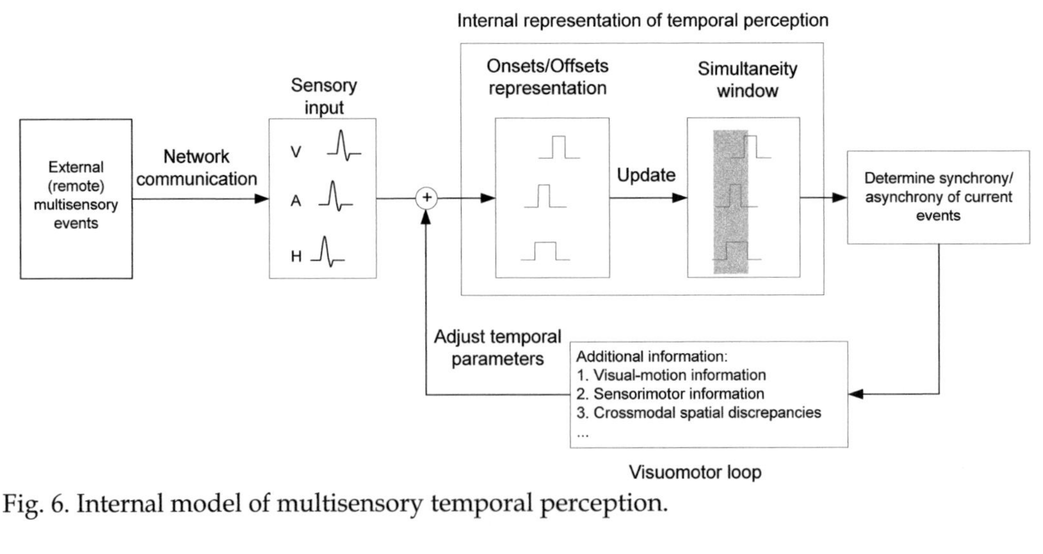

Fig. 6. Internal model of multisensory temporal perception.

5. Conclusion

In summary, we have provided an overview of studies concerned with visual-haptic simultaneity perception in multimodal telepresence system. It is clear that the perception of visual-haptic simultaneity is dynamic. In general, visual events are perceived as 'later' than physically synchronous haptic events. The visual-haptic simultaneity window (indicated by the PSS and JND parameters) may vary from dozens to hundreds of milliseconds. In interactive virtual environments such as telepresence systems, the crossmodal simultaneity window is influenced by other sources of information, such as sensorimotor feedback, packet loss in the feedback signal, and prior adaptation. Packet loss in visual feedback can bias visual-haptic judgments towards visual delay and such biases may influence even the perception of intact (visual-collision) events. In addition, prior information may also influence crossmodal simultaneity, however, this information is effectively taken into account only after one hundred milliseconds or so. Finally, based on the range of empirical evidence reviewed, we proposed that multisensory temporal perception involves an internal process model. The results, and the proposed framework model, can be used to derive guidelines for the design of the multimodal telepresence systems, concerning the crossmodal temporal perception of the human operator.

6. References

Adelstein, B. D., Begault, D. R., Anderson, M. R., & Wenzel, E. M. (2003) Sensitivity to haptic-audio asynchrony, *Proceedings of the 5th international conference on Multimodal interfaces* (pp. 73-76). Vancouver, British Columbia, Canada.

Adelstein, B. D., Lee, T. G., & Ellis, S. R. (2003) Head Tracking Latency in Virtual Environments: Psychophysics and a Model, *Human Factors and Ergonomics Society Annual Meeting Proceedings* (pp. 2083-2087): Human Factors and Ergonomics Society.

Ballantyne, G. H. (2002) Robotic surgery, telerobotic surgery, telepresence, and telementoring. Review of early clinical results. *Surgical Endoscopy 16*(10), 1389-1402.

Collett, D. (2002) *Modelling Binary Data* (2 ed.): Chapman & Hall/CRC.

Dixon, N. F., & Spitz, L. (1980) The detection of auditory visual desynchrony, *Perception* (Vol. 9, pp. 719-721).

Draper, J. V., Kaber, D. B., & Usher, J. M. (1998) Telepresence. *Human Factors 40*(3), 354-375.

Elliot, E. O. (1963) A Model of the Switched Telephone Network for Data Communications, *Bell System Technical Journal* (Vol. 44, pp. 89-109).

Ferrell, W. R. (1966) Delayed force feedback, *Human Factors* (Vol. 8, pp. 449-455).

Fujisaki, W., Shimojo, S., Kashino, M., & Nishida, S. (2004) Recalibration of audiovisual simultaneity. *Nature Neuroscience 7*(7), 773-778.

Gilbert, E. N. (1960) Capacity of a burst-noise channel, *Bell System Technical Journal* (Vol. 39, pp. 1253-1265).

Held, R. (1993) Telepresence, time delay and adaptation. In S. R. Ellis, M. K. Kaiser & A. J. Grunwald (Eds.), *Pictorial communication in virtual and real environments* (pp. 232-246): Taylor and Francis.

Heller, M. A., & Myers, D. S. (1983) Active and passive tactual recognition of form. *Journal of General Psychology 108*(2d Half), 225-229.

Hirzinger, G., Brunner, B., Dietrich, J., & Heindl, J. (1993) Sensor-based space robotics-ROTEX and its telerobotic features, *IEEE Transactions on Robotics and Automation* (Vol. 9, pp. 649-663).

Jay, C., Glencross, M., & Hubbold, R. (2007) Modeling the effects of delayed haptic and visual feedback in a collaborative virtual environment, *ACM Transactions on Computer-Human Interaction* (Vol. 14, Article 8, 1-31)

Keele, S. W. (1986) Motor control. In K. R. Boff, L. Kaufman & J. P. Thomas (Eds.), *Handbook of perception and human performance, Cognitive processes and performance* (Vol. II, pp. 30-60): Wiley.

Kim, T., Zimmerman, P. M., Wade, M. J., & Weiss, C. A. (2005) The effect of delayed visual feedback on telerobotic surgery. *Surgical Endoscopy 19*(5), 683-686.

Levitin, D. J., Maclean, K., Mathews, M., & Chu, L. (2000) The perception of cross-modal simultaneity, *International Journal of Computing and Anticipatory Systems* (pp. 323-329).

Mackenzie, S. I., & Ware, C. (1993) Lag as a determinant of human performance in interactive systems, *CHI '93: Proceedings of the INTERACT '93 and CHI '93 conference on Human factors in computing systems* (pp. 488-493). New York, NY, USA: ACM.

Moutoussis, K., & Zeki, S. (1997) Functional segregation and temporal hierarchy of the visual perceptive systems. *Proceedings of the Royal Society B: Biological Sciences 264*(1387), 1407-1414.

Noë, A. (2005) *Action in Perception*. Cambridge: MIT Press.

Peer, A., Hirche, S., Weber, C., Krause, I., Buss, M., Miossec, S., et al. (2008) Intercontinental cooperative telemanipulation between German and Japan, *Proceedings of the IEEE/RSJ International Conferences on Intelligent Robots and Systems* (pp. 2715-2716).

Sheridan, T. B., & Ferrell, W. R. (1963) Remote Manipulative Control with Transmission Delay, *IEEE Transactions on Human Factors in Electronics* (Vol. 4, pp. 25-29).

Shi, Z., Hirche, S., Schneider, W., & Muller, H. J. (2008) Influence of visuomotor action on visual-haptic simultaneous perception: A psychophysical study, *2008 Symposium on Haptic Interfaces for Virtual Environment and Teleoperator Systems* (pp. 65-70).

Shi, Z., Zou, H., Rank, M., Chen, L., Hirche, S., & Müller, H. J. (2009) Effects of packet loss and latency on temporal discrimination of visual-haptic events. *IEEE Transactions on Haptics*, in press.

Spence, C., Shore, D. I., & Klein, R. M. (2001) Multisensory prior entry, *Journal of Experimental Psychology: General* (Vol. 130, pp. 799-832).

Stone, J. V., Hunkin, N. M., Porrill, J., Wood, R., Keeler, V., Beanland, M., et al. (2001) When is now? Perception of simultaneity, *Proceedings of the Royal Society B: Biological Sciences* (Vol. 268, pp. 31-38).

Sugita, Y., & Suzuki, Y. (2003) Audiovisual perception: Implicit estimation of sound-arrival time. *Nature 421*(6926), 911.

Tin, C., & Poon, C. S. (2005) Internal models in sensorimotor integration: perspectives from adaptive control theory. *Journal of Neural Engineering 2*(3), S147-163.

van Beers, R. J., Sittig, A. C., & Gon, J. J. (1999) Integration of proprioceptive and visual position-information: An experimentally supported model. *Journal of Neurophysiology 81*(3), 1355-1364.

van Erp, J. B. F., & Werkhoven, P. J. (2004) Vibro-tactile and visual asynchronies: Sensitivity and consistency, *Perception* (Vol. 33, pp. 103-111).

Vatakis, A., & Spence, C. (2006) Evaluating the influence of frame rate on the temporal aspects of audiovisual speech perception, *Neuroscience Letters* (Vol. 405, pp. 132-136).

Vogels, I. M. (2004) Detection of temporal delays in visual-haptic interfaces. *Human Factors 46*(1), 118-134.

Wexler, M., & Klam, F. (2001) Movement prediction and movement production. *Journal of Experimental Psychology: Human Perception and Performance 27*(1), 48-64.

Witney, A. G., Goodbody, S. J., & Wolpert, D. M. (1999) Predictive motor learning of temporal delays. *Journal of Neurophysiology 82*(5), 2039-2048.

Wolpert, D. M. (1997) Computational approaches to motor control. *Trends in Cognitive Sciences 1*(6), 209-216.

Wolpert, D. M., & Ghahramani, Z. (2000) Computational principles of movement neuroscience. *Nature Neuroscience 3 Suppl*, 1212-1217.

Wolpert, D. M., Ghahramani, Z., & Jordan, M. I. (1995) An internal model for sensorimotor integration. *Science 269*(5232), 1880-1882.

24

On the Influence of Hand Dynamics on Motion Planning of Reaching Movements in Haptic Environments

Igor Goncharenko, Mikhail Svinin, Shigeyuki Hosoe and Sven Forstmann
3D Incorporated, the Institute of Physical and Chemical Research (RIKEN)
Japan

Abstract

The paper presents an analysis of human reaching movements in the manipulation of flexible objects. Two models, the minimum hand jerk and the minimum driving hand force-change, are used for modelling and verification of experimental data. The data are collected with the haptic system supporting dynamic simulation of the flexible object in real time. We describe some initial experimental results and analyze the applicability of the models. It is found that even for short-term movements human motion planning strategy can depend on arm inertia and configuration. This conclusion is based on the experimental evidence of the multi-phased hand velocity profiles that can be well captured by the minimum driving hand force-change criterion. To support the latest observation, an experiment with reinforcement learning was conducted.

1. Introduction

Recently, reproducing of human-like motions has become a focus of attention in many research fields such as human motor control and perception, humanoid robotics, robotic rehabilitation and assistance (Pollick et al., 2005; Tsuji et al., 2002; Amirabdollahian et al., 2002). In a bio-mimetic analogy, the human arm can be considered as a chain of rigid bodies actuated by driving mechanisms (muscles) and controlled by a computer (central nervous system, CNS), which might by instructive for the design of control systems for advanced manipulators. However, little is known about actual motion strategies planned by the CNS. Human motion planning models available in the literature are mostly remained phenomenological and descriptive – they rely on bulky experimental measurements done with motion capturing systems, encephalographs, feedback force devices, etc. On the other hand, the models based on optimal control methods are very attractive because they take into account trajectory formation, boundary conditions, and dynamic properties of the arm and environment. In addition, minimized performance indexes may have a natural interpretation related to human behaviour.

When humans make rest-to-rest movements in free space, there is, in principle, an infinite choice of trajectories. However, many studies have shown that human subjects tend to choose unique trajectories with invariant features. First, hand paths in rest-to-rest movements tend to be straight (or, slightly curved) and smooth. Second, the velocity profile of the hand trajectory is bell-shaped (Morasso, 1981; Abend et al., 1982). It is well established that for unconstrained reaching movements, the trajectory of human hand can be predicted with reasonable accuracy by the minimum hand jerk criterion (MJC) (Flash & Hogan, 1985). More generally, in the optimization approaches, the trajectory is predicted by minimizing, over the movement time T an integral performance index $\mathcal{J}$ subject to zero boundary conditions imposed on start and end points, corresponding to the rest-to-rest states. The performance index can be formulated in the joint space, in the task space normally associated with the human hand, or in the task space of object coordinates.

When movement is constrained by a 3D curve (door opening is a typical example of constrained movement), there is no uncertainty in spatial trajectory, but the temporal hand velocity profile becomes an important indicative of human hand control. Haptic technologies afford great opportunities for studying human motion planning because virtually any constraints and dynamic environments can be probed for verifying optimality criteria. For example, in studying multi-mass object transport using a PHANToM -based haptic interface (Svinin et al., 2006a; Svinin et al., 2006b), it was shown that the MJC models hand movement much better than the lowest order polynomial model that is common in control of robotic and mechatronic systems with flexible elements. This led to the conclusion that the CNS plans reaching movements in the hand space coordinates rather than in the object space. It was speculated that the trajectories of the human arm in comfortable reaching movements can be predicted without taking into account the inertial properties of the arm, which gave a good reason to believe that the arm dynamics are already "prewired" in the CNS while the object dynamics (the novel environment) are acquired by learning. In (Goncharenko et al., 2006) different curvature types of 3D constraints were considered for the tasks of rest-to-rest rigid body movement and bimanual crank rotation. Among several performance indexes, only two criteria were confirmed to be the best candidates for the description of motion control in the tasks: MJC and the minimum force change criterion (MFCC).

Roughly speaking, the MFCC is a dynamic version of the MJC. While the latter ignores inertial properties of the human arm, the former takes them into account. Both these criteria give very close results for the hand velocity profiles if the stiffness of the haptic device is high enough, or, if the transported object is relatively lightweight. In general, however, the theoretical predictions by these criteria can be very different (Svinin et al., 2006c). It is therefore important to design experiments that would help to distinguish between the two criteria and demonstrate the correct choice of one of them. This constitutes the main goal of this paper: to demonstrate experimentally that the hand mass-inertia properties and configuration cannot be ignored in prediction of human motion planning in highly dynamic environment.

This chapter is organized as follows. The next section formulates the MJC and MFCC for the task of a rest-to-rest transport of a flexible object and introduces a concept of dynamically equivalent configurations. Sections 3 and 4 describe primary experiments with a haptic system for two dynamic configurations. Section 5 describes experiments with reinforcement learning, and the last section concludes the chapter.

2. Optimality criteria for the task of rest-to-rest mass transport

A model of rest-to-rest movements is shown in Figure 1. The object is connected to the hand by a virtual spring of initial zero length. In the initial configuration, the positions of the hand and the object coincide. A human subject is asked to make reaching movement of length L and time T and stop the object without excitation of oscillations. For this task, the MJC and its dynamic constraint are:

$$\mathcal{J}_{MJC} = \frac{1}{2}\int_0^T \left(d^3 x_h / dt^3\right)^2 dt, \tag{1}$$

$$m_o \ddot{x}_o + k(x_o - x_h) = 0, \tag{2}$$

where x_h is the coordinate of the human hand, x_o is the object coordinate, m_o is the mass of the object, and k is the stiffness of the spring. Defining the natural frequency $\omega_o = \sqrt{k / m_o}$ and expressing x_h through x_o using (2), criterion (1) can be rewritten as:

$$\mathcal{J}_{MJC} = \frac{1}{2\omega_o^4}\int_0^T \left(x_o^{(5)} + \omega_o^2 x_o^{(3)}\right)^2 dt. \tag{3}$$

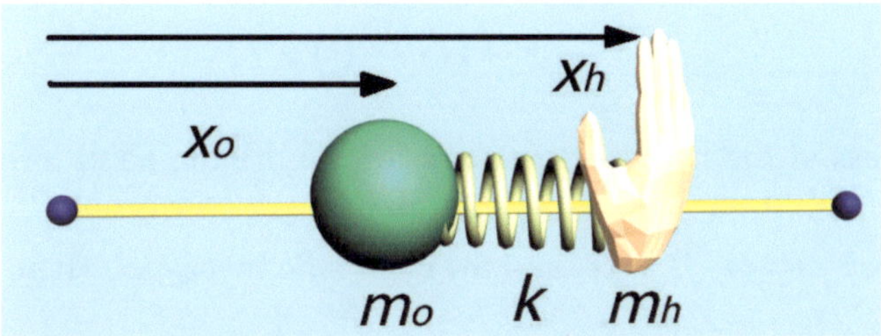

Fig. 1. Model of reaching movement in dynamic environment

The boundary conditions corresponded to rest-to-rest states under the dynamic constraint (2) for both, hand and object, can be also expressed only through x_o:

$$x_o(0) = 0,\ \dot{x}_o(0) = 0,\ \ddot{x}_o(0) = 0,\ \dddot{x}_o(0) = 0,\ \ddddot{x}_o(0) = 0,$$
$$x_o(T) = L,\ \dot{x}_o(T) = 0,\ \ddot{x}_o(T) = 0,\ \dddot{x}_o(T) = 0,\ \ddddot{x}_o(T) = 0.$$

The solution of the problem (1,2) can be represented as a combination of 5-th order polynomial and trigonometric terms as was proven in (Svinin et al., 2006a; Svinin et al., 2006b) .

It was also shown that the hand velocity profile, corresponding to this solution, can have either one phase (bell-shaped) or two phases while the object velocity is always single phased. For example, in Figure 2 the hand velocity for the MJC is shown by thick black line and the object velocity by thin black line. The graphs are given for T=1.15s, k=150N/m, m_o = 3.2kg, L=0.2m.

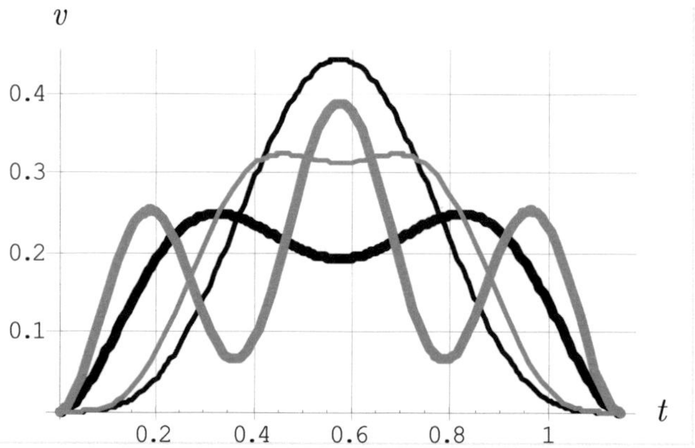

Fig. 2. Velocity profiles for MJC and MFCC

Unlike the MJC, the MFCC takes into account the hand dynamics:

$$\mathcal{J}_{MFCC} = \frac{1}{2}\int_0^T \dot{f}^2 dt, \tag{4}$$

$$m_h \ddot{x}_h + k(x_o - x_h) = f, \tag{5}$$

where m_h is the mass of the hand and f stands for the driving hand force. Again, we can rewrite the criterion (4) to the form similar to (3), taking into account (2), (5), and defining the natural frequency $\omega = \omega_o\sqrt{1+\mu}$, and the mass ratio $\mu = m_o/m_h$. Then,

$$\mathcal{J}_{MFCC} = \frac{1}{2}\left(\frac{m_h m_o}{k}\right)^2 \int_0^T \left(x_o^{(5)} + \omega^2 x_o^{(3)}\right)^2 dt. \tag{6}$$

From (6) and (3) it can be seen that the MFCC converges to the MJC when μ <<1. However, for non-infinitesimal μ, additional parameter m_h influences on the solution for (6) significantly. Namely, there can be more than two phases in the hand velocity profile. In Figure 2 hand velocity for MFCC is shown by the thick grey line, and the object velocity is given by the thin grey line (T=1.15s, k=150N/m, m_o=3.2kg, m_h=0.8kg, L=0.2m). Complete solution and theoretical properties of the MFCC are given in (Svinin et al., 2006c). The portrait of the phase transition for the MFCC is shown in Figure 3, where the numbers inside the areas correspond to the number of phases.

In this figure, point **A** corresponds to the parameters used to calculate profiles shown in Figure 2 (ωT=17.6, $\mu = m_o/m_h$ =4).

Note that one point on the non-dimensional phase diagram can correspond to two different sets of physical parameters. In this connection we can define *dynamically equivalent systems* as systems correspondent to the same point on the phase transition diagram. Define $\kappa = \omega T$.

Assume that we have two sets of parameters. One set $(m_{h1}, m_{o1}, k_{o1}, T_1)$ is characterized by $\mu_1 = m_{o1} / m_{h1}$, $\kappa_1 = T_1\sqrt{k_{o1}(1+\mu_1)/m_{o1}}$ and the other set $(m_{h2}, m_{o2}, k_{o2}, T_2)$ is characterized by $\mu_2 = m_{o2} / m_{h2}$, $\kappa_2 = T_2\sqrt{k_{o2}(1+\mu_2)/m_{o2}}$. Two systems are dynamically equivalent if $\mu_1 = \mu_2$ and $\kappa_1 = \kappa_2$, which gives

$$\frac{m_{o1}}{m_{h1}} = \frac{m_{o2}}{m_{h2}}, T_1\sqrt{\frac{k_{o1}}{m_{o1}}} = T_2\sqrt{\frac{k_{o2}}{m_{o2}}}.$$

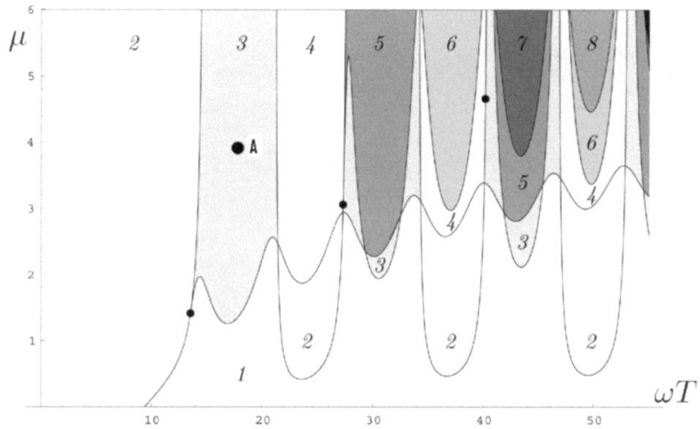

Fig. 3. Diagram of phase transition of the hand velocity profiles for MFCC

3. Experiment plan and setup configuration

It is interesting that for fixed m_h, T, and L velocity profiles yielding solutions for (3) and (6) are exactly the same for various m_o and k, which maintain constant ω and ω_0. Then, to make conclusion in favour of either the MJC or the MFCC for each subject, we may select two different parameter sets, which are dynamically equivalent to the parameters used for hand velocity calculations. The profiles depicted in Figure 2 are clearly two-phased (MJC) and three-phased (MFCC), and their magnitudes are significantly different. Of course, we cannot expect that each subject's "effective" hand mass is close to 0.8kg. Because of the ergonomic of experimental layout forearm mass can partially contribute to the "effective" mass. Standard anthropometric mass of human forearm is 1.48kg (Chandler et al., 1976), however, the uncertainty in m_h can vary from 0.5 to 1.5 kg, or even more if arm joints are not fixed. To avoid this confusion, we completed two experimental series for each subject using the concept of dynamically equivalent systems in the following manner.

Step 1. As a zero-guess, we assume m_h =0.8kg and set other parameters as T=1.15s, k=150 N/m, m_o =3.2 kg, L=0.2m. When a subject completes a long series of trials, we compare his average hand velocity profile with ones shown in Figure 2. If the average profile is three-phased and closely matched to the MFCC curve, we conclude that the MFCC criteria is preferable, and the hand mass is very close to 0.8 kg. Otherwise, the next step is completed.

Step 2. Using a curve matching procedure, we estimate new "effective" m_h, recalculate new dynamically equivalent parameters k and m_o, and ask the subject to repeat the experimental trials. Hand mass and velocities are analyzed again after completing the series.
To analyze human movements, we reconfigure our experimental setup (Figure 4) previously used for multi-mass object movement analysis (Goncharenko et al., 2006). In the setup, a haptic device (1.5/3DOF PHANToM, maximum exertable force 8.5N) was connected to a computer (dual core 3.0 GHz CPU).

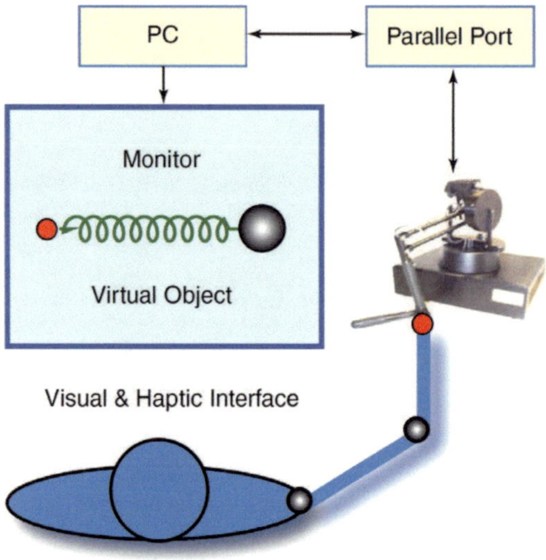

Fig. 4. Experimental setup

Five naïve right-handed male subjects were selected to participate in the experiment. The subjects were instructed to move a virtual flexible object "connected" to the human hand by the PHANToM stylus. The hand & object system was at rest at the start point. The subjects were requested to move the object and smoothly stop both the hand and the object at a target point. The subject made these rest-to-rest movements along a straight line (in the direction from left to right) in the horizontal plane using the PHANToM stylus. The travelling distance was set as L = 0.2m. The object dynamics were simulated using the 4th-order Runge-Kutta method with fixed time step Δt = 0.001s correspondent to the PHANToM cycle. The data regarding the position, velocity of the hand and the simulated object were recorded at 100 Hz. (Stylus position and velocity are measured by the hardware.) PHANToM feedback forces and object acceleration were recorded as well. The subjects were requested to produce the specified reaching movement in a natural way, on their own pace, trying to make as many successful trials as possible. To count successful trials we introduced the following set of tolerances: object and hand final position 0.2±0.005m, object and hand final velocity 0±0.05 m/s, object final acceleration 0±0.16 m/s^2, hand start velocity 0±0.05m/s, trial total time 1±0.2s. The reaching task is successful when the simulation and hardware-measured data obey all the above tolerances, then haptic interaction is stopped and an audio signal prompts the users to proceed with the next trial.

Unlike in our previous experiments with multi-mass objects (Svinin et al., 2006a), the time tolerance is very narrow because the solutions of tasks (1), (4) are sensitive to T. To prompt the subjects that they are within the time window, we implemented additional visual feedback in the system (a colored semaphore). Taking into account that the initial hand speed tolerance is not relevant to the target point, the described task was expected to be difficult and sport-like, without high success rate. In order to collect statistically representative datasets, the subjects were asked to complete 2000 trials each, equally split in two days, but with different object configurations.

4. Preliminary experimental results

When all the subjects completed the first series of 1000 trials on Day 1, parameters m_h, m_o, k, were changed, the setup was reconfigured, and the subjects had to complete new 1000-trial series with new configuration on Day 2. In our previous experiments (Svinin et al., 2006a) a stable growth of motor learning progress (trial success rate) was observed. In this difficult task with the narrow tolerance windows, total success rate was low, about 15% or lower, but still sufficient for statistical analysis (Table 1.). On the average, the second configuration was more difficult for the subjects. There were no obvious learning progress trends inside individual series as well: all the subjects shortly catch their own control strategy after approximately 100-200 first trials, and then the success rate remains various, locally oscillating around 10-15% (see Figure 5 as an example). Sometimes the successful trials followed one-by-one, and sometimes the subjects lost their control strategy for a long period. After 500 trials the subjects took breaks of about 15-20min.

Subject	Day 1 (1000 trials)	Day 2 (1000 trials)
S1	272 (27.2%)	71 (7.1%)
S2	149 (14.9%)	42 (4.2%)
S3	119 (11.9%)	72 (7.2%)
S4	280 (28.0%)	178 (17.8%)
S5	105 (10.5%)	120 (12.0%)

Table 1. Motor learning rate (success, %)

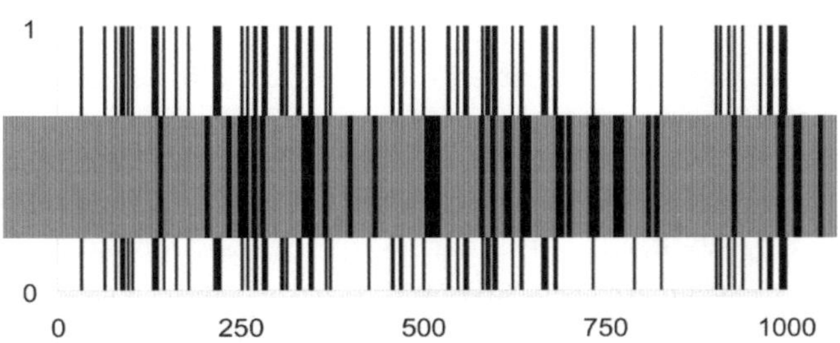

Fig. 5. Individual learning history (subject S3, Day 1)

Reaching time for successful trials varied within the time tolerance window (from 0.8s to 1.2s) on the average was shifted, but very close to 1.15s for each subject (Table 2). It makes it possible to correctly map each individual trial profile to the unified time interval of 1.15s.

Subject	Day 1		Day 2	
	Average	RMS	Average	RMS
S1	1.08s	0.051s	1.17s	0.028s
S2	1.16s	0.027s	1.17s	0.021s
S3	1.12s	0.050s	1.15s	0.034s
S4	1.13s	0.036s	1.16s	0.026s
S5	1.14s	0.038s	1.15s	0.032s

Table 2. Reaching time

We re-estimated new hand mass m_h^* after Day 1 and Day2, using the following curve matching criterion (integral RMS):

$$m_h^* = \arg\min_{m_h} \left(\frac{1}{M} \sum_{j=1}^{M} \sum_{i=1}^{N} \left(v_{pr}(t_i, m_h) - v_j(t_i) \right)^2 \right) \tag{7}$$

where N is the number of measurements in each successful trial, M is the number of successful trials, v_{pr}, v_j are predicted and experimental hand velocities. Therefore, different dynamic configurations (m_h, m_o, k) were used on Day1 and Day2 (Table 3).

	Initial configuration (m_h, m_o, k)	Configuration after Day 1 (m_h, m_o, k)	Hand mass estimated after Day 2
S1	0.8, 3.2, 150	1.3, 5.1, 239	1.5
S2	0.8, 3.2, 150	1.4, 5.4, 253	2.1
S3	0.8, 3.2, 150	1.1, 4.4, 206	1.4
S4	0.8, 3.2, 150	1.1, 4.4, 206	2.3
S5	0.8, 3.2, 150	0.9, 3.6, 169	0.9

Table 3. System configuration parameters for individual subjects

Initially, the subjects were not instructed to fix elbow or shoulder joints. It is interesting, that only subject S5 found his own comfortable arm configuration - he fixed his elbow joint in both experimental days, while other subjects did not fixed. It can partially explain the fact that the estimated hand masses are higher for subjects S1-S4 after Day 1 (Table 3).

After Day 1 subjects S1-S4 demonstrated slightly left-skewed two-phased hand velocity profiles with the maximal magnitude less than 30 cm/s. The profile form cannot be explained quantitatively neither by MJC, nor by the MHCC for the hand mass m_h=0.8 kg. However, matching criterion (7) formally, one can find optimal m_h for MHCC which is significantly different (after Day 1 and Day 2) from the initallly supposed hand mass. Moreover, the matching error is lower for the MHCC than for MJC. Figure 6 (left) shows that the error by the MJC is 0.057 while the error by the MHCC is 0.04 at the optimal "effective" hand mass 1.4kg. In the right part of the Figure 6 the gray thick line shows average experimental hand velocity profile, and two black thick lines depict the profiles predicted by the MJC (two-phased) and the MHCC (three-phased) for m_h=0.8 kg. Finding the optimal "effective" hand masses and using the principle of dynamically equivalent systems, the haptic simulator was reconfigured after Day 1 as ahown in Table 3, and the experiments were repeated on Day 2. Nevertheless, the experimental hand velocity profiles remained two-phased for subjects S1-S4, with the magnitude less than 30cm/s. The second estimation by criterion (7) showed that there is an uncertainty in the "effective" hand masses for subjects S1-S4.

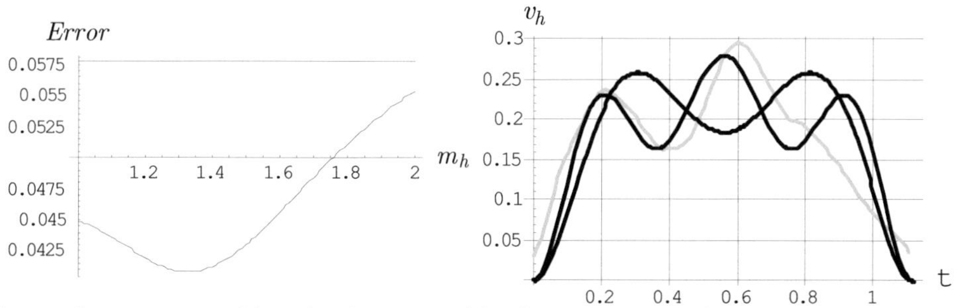

Fig. 6. Matching error and hand velocity profiles for subject S2 (after Day 1)

At the same time, statisticaly representative results for subject S5 (with fixed elbow joint) are strongly in favour of the MFCC. Figure 7 shows the experimental and predicted by the MHCC (at m_h=0.9 kg) hand velocities for subject S5. Thick grey and black lines are the average experimental and predicted profiles, and the thin grey lines depict last 30 successful trials on each experimental day. Matching by the criterion (7) showed that the re-estimated "effective" hand mass (0.9kg) is very close to the initial estimation (0.8kg).

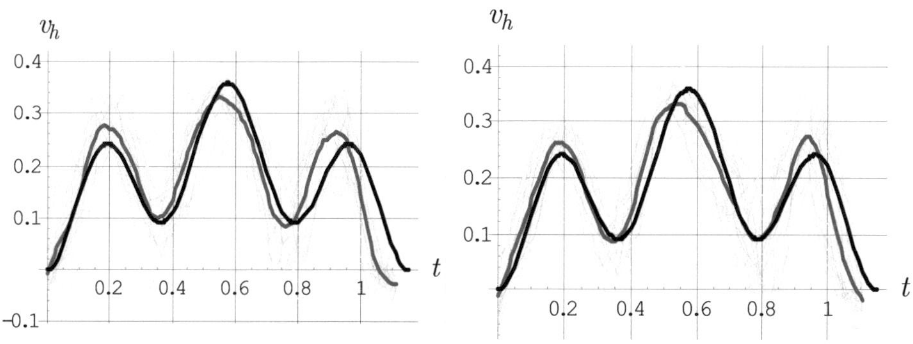

Fig. 7. Hand velocity profiles for subject S5 (left - after Day 1, right – after Day 2)

The only difference between subjects S5 and S1-S4 is that S5 fixed his elbow joint placing the elbow on a stand. Obviously, different muscle groups worked for S5 and S1-S4, and physical limits of S1-S4 could not allow them to reach velocity higher than 30cm/s. Also, the significant difference between hand masses estimated after Day 1 and 2 for S1-S4 means that modelling of the "effective" hand mass via a point mass is dubious for the case of arm configuration without joint fixation.

5. Reinforcement learning and arm configuration

After the course of preliminary experiments it was decided to ask one subject from the group S1-S4 to repeat experiments in order to check if the three-phased hand velocity profiles can be achieved after reinforcement learning. In the reinforcement learning task, the haptic system was repeatedly used in the following teaching mode: it was programmed to drag the subject's hand close to the average trajectory of subject S5. In this case the subject's hand passively followed the driving PHANToM stylus. The teaching mode was supposed to provide motor learning of movement of subject S5.

Subject S3 participated in the experiment on Day 3. First, he completed 1000 trials in the teaching mode (Task A) and then, after 20min break, he was asked to reproduce 1000 times (Task B) the learnt movement in the standard simulator's mode (mass-spring transport) described in the previous sections. In both series, his elbow joint was not fixed. Figure 8 shows the average hand velocity profiles of the subject for this experiment. The black line is the average profile of S3 after Day 1, and the light grey line (two-phased, left-skewed) is the average profile of Task B (after reinforcement learning). Even the subject said that he remembered the desired movement in teaching mode, it can be seen from Figure 8 that the profile of Task B is not tree-phased. Moreover, he found the desired movement less comfortable than his previous self-leant control strategy.

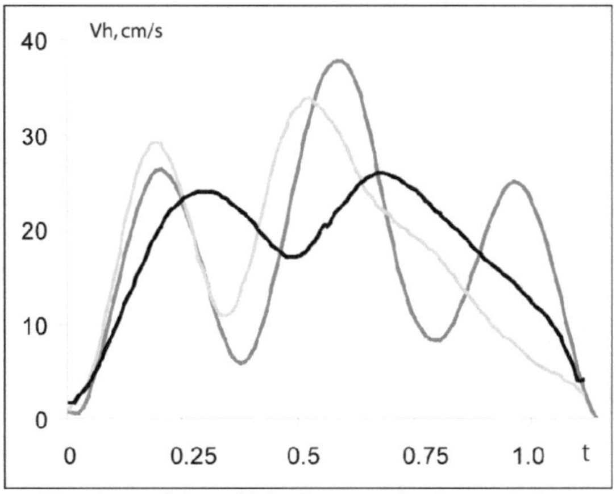

Fig. 8. Hand velocity profiles for subject S3 before and after reinforcement learning

Finally, the subject was asked to complete Task A and Task B with his fixed joint placed on a stand. In this case he found the desired movement much more comfortable and the average hand velocity profile was very close to the profile predicted by the MHCC (Figure 8, three-phased profile). The "effective" hand mass estimated by (7) was 0.85kg.

6. Conclusions

An analysis of human reaching movements in the task of mass transport is presented. Two models, the minimum hand jerk (MJC) and the minimum driving hand force-change (MFCC), are used for modelling and verification of experimental data. The data were collected with a haptic system supporting object dynamics simulation in real time. The importance of the research is that the knowledge of human control strategies may be useful and hopefully beneficial for the design of human-like control algorithms for advanced robotic systems. Perhaps, the main contribution of the paper is that it was demonstrated that human motion planning strategies cannot be captured only by the minimum jerk criterion without taking into account the configuration of the human arm and its inertia. For many reaching tasks the MJC and the MFCC give similar predicted hand motion velocities, and it is important to distinguish between the criteria.

First, we theoretically predicted (with the MJC and the MFCC) a special configuration of the mass-spring system, when the expected hand velocity profiles may differ significantly in terms of magnitudes and phase numbers. With the experiments, it was demonstrated that human arm configuration and ergonomics are important factors for correct theoretical predictions of the hand velocity profiles. Statistically representative results for the case of arm configuration with fixed elbow joint are strongly in favour of the MFCC criterion. Therefore, the hand mass/inertia properties and ergonomics cannot be ignored for hand motion planning in highly dynamic environment. For these skilful tasks a subject forms a unique natural hand velocity profile. Reinforcement learning, "programmed" by another skilful person's profiles, may not provide comfortable control strategies for the subject.

In the future research, it would be worthwhile to analyze the movements for different types of experimental scenarios. Also, it would be interesting to explain our experimental results without arm joint fixation by replacing the equations (2), (5) by models of the arm with two links and joints, including the joint stiffness and viscosity and the dynamics of the the hardware. Also, we found that many of the experimental profiles were slightly skewed to the left. In this respect, studying non-zero boundary conditions (partially, non-zero hand acceleration) of the optimization problems could clarify these effects.

7. References

Abend, W.; Bizzi, E. & Morasso, P. (1982). Human arm trajectory formation, *Brain*, Vol. 105, No. 2, (Jun 1982) pp. 331–348, ISSN: 0006-8950.

Amirabdollahian, F.; Loureiro, R. & Harwin, W. (2002). Minimum jerk trajectory control for rehabilitation and haptic applications, *Proceedings of IEEE International Conference on Robotics and Automation*, pp. 3380–3385, ISBN 0-7803-7273-5, Washington D.C., May 11–15, 2002, IEEE.

Chandler, R.; Clauser, C.; McConville, J.; Reynolds, H. & Young, J. (1976). Investigation of inertial properties of the human body, *Technical report AMRL-TR-74-137, AD-A016-485, DOT-HS-801-430,* Wright Patterson Air Force Base, Ohio, USA, 1976, Washington, DC: US DOT.

Flash, T. & Hogan, N. (1985). The coordination of arm movements: an experimentally confirmed mathematical model, *Journal of Neuroscience*, Vol. 5, No. 7, (Jul 1985) pp. 1688–1703, ISSN: 0270-6474.

Goncharenko, I.; Svinin, M.; Kanou, Y. & Hosoe, S. (2006). Predictability of rest-to-rest movements in haptic environments with 3d constraints, *Journal of Robotics and Mechatronics*, Vol. 18, No. 4, (Aug 2006) pp. 458-466, ISSN : 0915-3942.

Morasso. P. (1981). Spatial control of arm movements, *Experimental Brain Research*, Vol. 42, No. 2, (Apr 1981) pp. 223–227, ISSN: 0014-4819.

Pollick, F. ; Hale, J. & Tzoneva-Hadjigeorgieva, M. (2005). Perception of humanoid movements, *International Journal of Humanoid Robotics*, Vol. 2, No. 3, (Sep 2005) pp. 277–300, ISSN: 0219-8436.

Svinin, M.; Goncharenko, I.; Luo, Z.-W. & Hosoe, S. (2006a). Reaching movements in dynamic environments: how do we move flexible objects?, *IEEE Transactions on Robotics*, Vol. 22, No. 4, (August 2006) pp. 724-739, ISSN: 1552-3098.

Svinin, M.; Goncharenko, I. & Hosoe, S. (2006b). Motion planning of human-like movements in the manipulation of flexible objects, In: *Advances in Robot Control: from Everyday Physics to Human-Like Movement*, Kawamura, S. & Svinin, M. (Eds.), Springer, pp. 263-292, ISBN: 978-3-540-37346-9.

Svinin, M.; Goncharenko, I.; Luo, Z.-W. & Hosoe, S. (2006c). Modeling of human-like reaching movements in the manipulation of flexible objects, *Proceedings of IEEE/RSJ International Conference on Intelligent Robots and Systems (IROS 2006)*, pp. 549-555, ISBN: 1-4244-0258-1, Beijing, China, Oct 9-15, 2006, IEEE.

Tsuji, T.; Tanaka Y.; Morasso, P.; Sanguineti, V. & Kaneko, M. (2002). Biomimetic trajectory generation of robots via artificial potential field with time base generator, *IEEE Transactions on Systems, Man, and Cybernetics. C: Applications and Reviews*, Vol. 32, No. 4, (Nov 2002) pp. 426–439, ISSN: 1094-6977.

25

Haptic touch and hand ability

Miriam Ittyerah
Department of Psychology
Christ University
Bangalore- 560029, India.

Several studies have compared visual perception, tactile (haptic) perception, and visual-haptic perception of stimuli. Often, performance in tasks involving unimodal visual perception exceeds performance in both unimodal haptic and cross-modal tasks. However unimodal haptic comparisons of natural three-dimensional shapes could be as good as visual-haptic and haptic-visual comparisons. Therefore vision and touch may have functionally overlapping, though not equivalent, representations of 3-D space.
The present manuscript argues that vision and touch cannot be equated because the sensitivity and the processes involved in the attainment of information differ between the modalities. Further, vision is useful for haptics only so long as it provides relevant information. The hand is an important source of information in haptic touch. Evidence shows that though one may have a hand preference, the ability of the non preferred hand cannot be undermined as compared to that of the preferred hand. Research indicates that the hands do not differ in tactile ability, and the seemingly lower performance of the non preferred hand is a consequence of its spatial orientation during performance and not an absence of ability.

Haptic touch and hand ability

Several studies have compared visual perception, tactile (haptic) perception, and visual-haptic perception of stimuli (e.g. Easton, Greene, & Srinivas, 1997; Millar, 1981; Abravanel 1971; Lobb, 1965; Rudel & Teuber, 1964). Often, performance in tasks involving unimodal visual perception exceeds performance in both unimodal haptic and cross-modal tasks. But not always: Norman, Norman, Clayton, Lianekhammy, and Zielke (2004), for example, found that unimodal haptic comparisons of natural three-dimensional shapes could be as good as visual-haptic and haptic-visual comparisons. Norman et al inferred that vision and touch have functionally overlapping, though not equivalent, representations of 3-D space.
Underlying much of the research comparing unimodal visual and tactile perception to cross-modal visual-tactile perception is a long-standing theoretical issue: Do perceivers 'naturally' recognize common features of objects perceived through vision and through touch? Or, alternatively, do accurate cross-modal comparisons develop largely or wholly through experience? Molyneux's famous question about the relation between touch and vision – Can a person born blind distinguish between a cube and a sphere after recovering sight in adulthood? – continues to occupy philosophers (Gallagher, 2004).

In this regard, research has shown that very young infants not only show cross-modal transfer of object properties such as texture and hardness (e.g., Meltzoff & Borton, 1979; Gibson and Walker 1984), but also can recognize by sight objects previously presented to touch (Streri, 1987; Streri & Gentaz 2003). These results challenge the empiricist philosophy and modern connectionist models (McClelland & Rumelhart, 1986; Elman, 1996) that assume independent sensory modalities at birth. Presumably, the capacity found in older children and adults to make cross-modal as well as intramodal comparisons evolve from intrinsic capabilities in infants.

Often, studies of cross-modal perception use a sequential design, which places demands on memory, and demands on memory may matter more to unimodal haptic tasks and cross-modal haptic-visual tasks than to visual tasks (Woods, O'Modhrain, & Newell, 2004). Whether simultaneous presentations of stimuli with lesser demands on memory affect processing differently from sequential presentations was a question of interest. Ittyerah and Marks (2008) therefore compared visual, haptic, and visual-haptic discrimination of curvature stimuli when the two stimuli within each pair were presented simultaneously. Figure 1 depicts each of the six stimuli, which differ only in curvature. Stimulus 1 has a difference of 3.81 mm between its midpoint and its height at the ends. Stimulus 2 has a difference of 5.08 mm between its midpoint and the height at its ends and, therefore, has greater curvature than stimulus 1. The remaining stimuli vary similarly, such that stimulus 6 has the greatest curvature and stimulus 1 the least curvature.

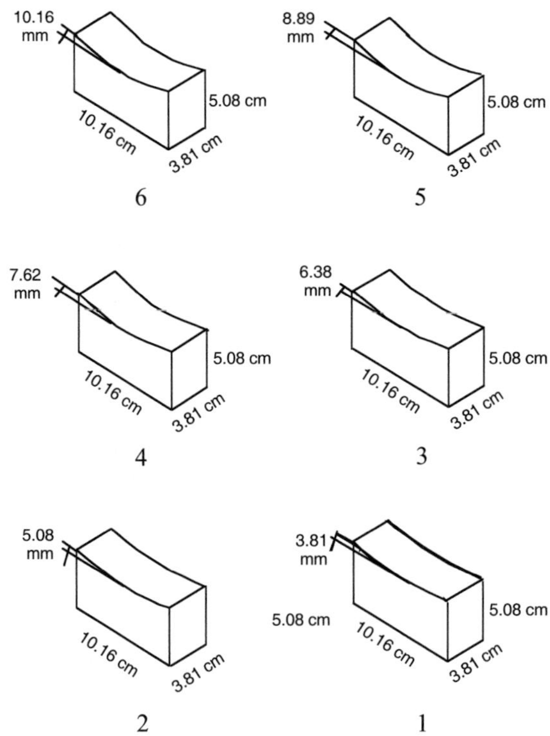

Fig. 1. Dimensions of the six stimuli used in Experiment 1.

With permission from the Editors of Current Psychology Letters. Ittyerah, M. & Marks, L.E. (2008) Intra-modal and cross-modal discrimination of curvature: Haptic touch versus vision. Current Psychology Letters, 24, 1-15.

The findings of Ittyerah and Marks (2008) indicated that when two object surfaces, either the same or different in curvature, were presented simultaneously for comparison, unimodal visual performance exceeded cross-modal performance, which in turn exceeded unimodal haptic performance. Figure 2 shows that the accuracy of responses to same pairs of stimuli is much smaller with haptic comparison than with intramodal visual or with cross-modal comparison. And accuracy of responses to different pairs is also smallest, by and large, with intramodal haptic comparison. As Figure 3 shows, over the three smallest physical differences, where the measures of d′ are most reliable and least susceptible to variability associated with extreme proportions, unimodal visual performance exceeds cross-modal performance by about one d′ unit, essentially, one standard deviation unit, and cross-modal performance similarly exceeds unimodal haptic performance by about one d′ unit.

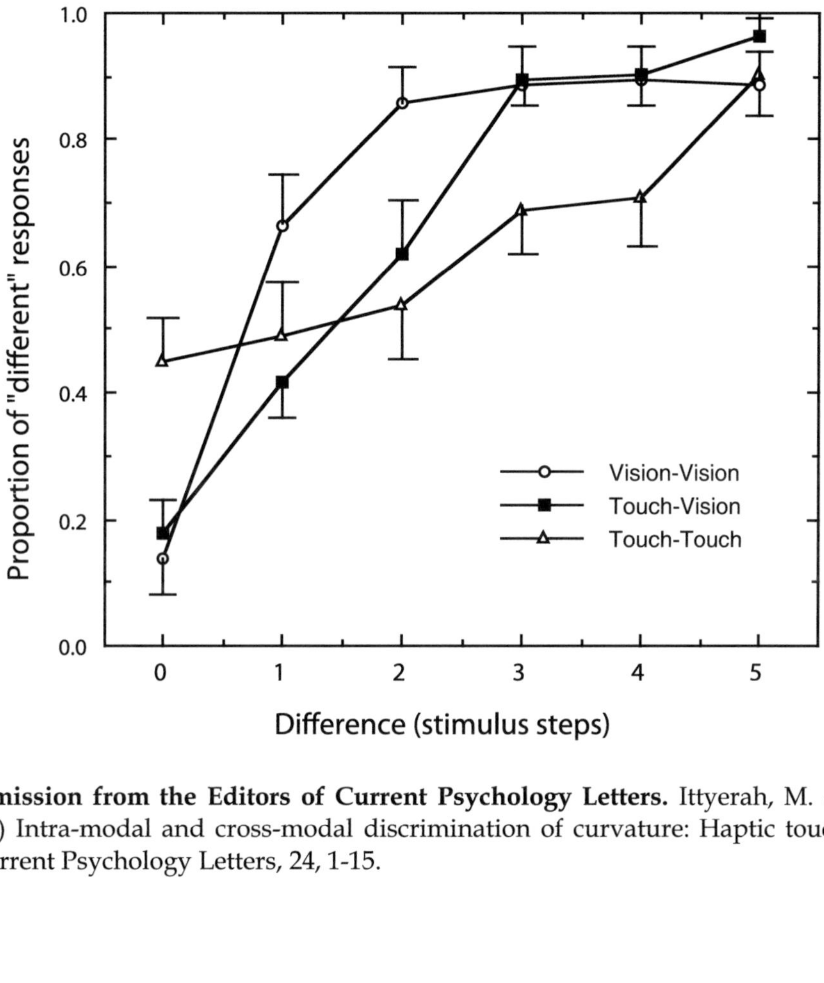

Fig. 2.
With permission from the Editors of Current Psychology Letters. Ittyerah, M. & Marks, L.E. (2008) Intra-modal and cross-modal discrimination of curvature: Haptic touch versus vision. Current Psychology Letters, 24, 1-15.

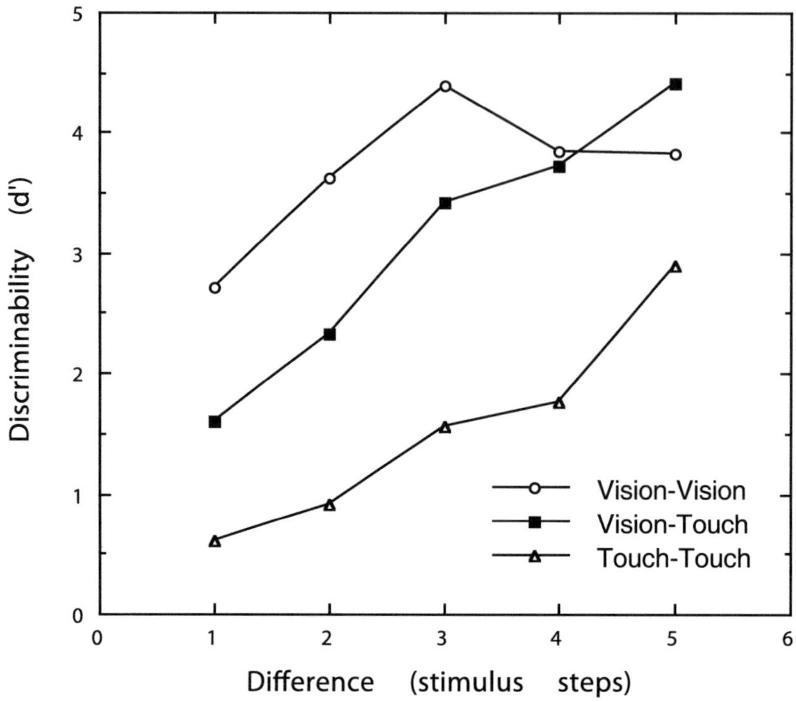

Fig. 3.
With permission from the Editors of Current Psychology Letters. Ittyerah, M. & Marks, L.E. (2008) Intra-modal and cross-modal discrimination of curvature: Haptic touch versus vision. Current Psychology Letters, 24, 1-15.

Haptic perception of form takes place largely by inspection of shapes by the palm and fingers of the hand as they move over the surface of an object. The property of shape or form refers to the spatial layout of the object, which may be specified in terms of contours. An isolated contour may itself be described with respect to its extent and orientation, and interactions among contours, or patterns, may in turn be described in terms of component contours or as combinations of angles, straight or curved surfaces, and other distinctive features. The shapes of many objects may be adequately described in terms of angles and curvatures of various degrees and proportion. In haptic exploration of shapes, the fingers move over the various angles or bend over the curves. The main question of interest is: How do haptic touch and vision compare with regard to people's ability to perceive and remember three-dimensional objects?
A large body of literature concerned with the haptic and visual memory systems has provided two broad accounts. The first is that object memory is multisensory and object representations are shared across modalities if the same object properties are encoded. The second is that objects are stored as modality specific representations that require a recoding from one memory system to another. Such recoding is costly, in time and errors, to cross-modal performance relative to intra-modal performance.
Many recent findings support the idea that visual and haptic memory for objects is shared. For example neuroimaging evidence suggests that the cortical area involved in visual object recognition is also involved in haptic object recognition (Grill-Spector, Kourtzi &

Kanwisheri, 2001). Amedi, Malach, Hendler, Peled and Zohary (2001) reported that activation in the lateral occipital complex (LOC) is not specific to the visual modality. The LOC is also activated during haptic object recognition, though not by auditory information about objects (Amedi, Jacobson, Hendler, Malach & Zohary, 2002). These studies suggest that the LOC is involved in recovering the geometrical shapes of objects (James, Humphery, Gati, Servos, Menon & Goodale, 2002), and behavioural evidence suggests that object representations are shared across modalities (Easton, Greene & Srinivas, 1997; Newell, 2004).

Other studies indicate, however, that tactile memory is not equivalent to visual memory and that information is modality specific. For example, in tests of tactile memory, when a delay intervenes between the presentation of the test stimulus and the test of memory, tactile memory is adversely affected by verbal tasks (counting backwards) interpolated during a 15 sec delay (Gilson & Baddeley, 1969) and by arithmetic tasks after a 5 sec delay (Sullivan & Turvey, 1972). In a study on 3-dimensional object recognition in children, Millar (1974) found that haptic matching performance for nonsense objects was better with an inter stimulus interval (ISI) of 1 sec, than with intervals of 5 and 30 sec, suggesting that haptic memory starts to decay immediately after the exploration of an object.

Other studies report that tactile memory can be sustained for 15 sec (Kiphart, Hughes, Simmons & Cross, 1992) and is vulnerable to articulatory suppression (Mahrer & Miles, 2002). However, performance can also be affected by the task demands or stimulus complexity and the degree of familiarity with the objects being explored (Millar 1981). For example Norman, Norman, Clayton, Lianekhammy and Zielke (2004) observed that accuracy of tactile-visual matching differed across different stimuli, though tactile performance improved with exploration time. Norman et al concluded that observers can match objects known only through touch with other objects known only through vision. Recently, Wood, O'Modhrain and Newell (2004) suggested that tactile-visual object recognition may rely on modality specific representations. Although the effect of delay between cross-modal presentations was the same whether the initial object was coded visually or haptically, recall was better after a 0 sec than a 30 sec delay, indicating delay-induced decay in memory.

In view of the different interpretations, Ittyerah and Marks (2007) tested for inter-modal and intra-modal processes involved in memory for concave curved surfaces that are first presented (perceived) haptically or visually and then later compared to surfaces presented either haptically/visually (unimodal comparison) or visually/haptically (cross-modal comparison). Furthermore, by varying the characteristics of the subjects' activity during a 30-second retention interval (dual task design), we sought to illuminate the underlying mnemonic representation mediating the discrimination.

Dual task paradigms have been used to test for the demands of attention on the primary task (Brown 1958; Peterson & Peterson 1959). The paradigm tests the nature of coding in short term memory by interpolating a secondary task during the delay interval between presentation and recall. Dual task paradigms that test visuo-spatial coding often require movement outputs. For example, tracing, pointing or other gestures are used as secondary tasks. Imagining the task during a delay interval instead of actually performing the task produces similar effects. Millar and Ittyerah (1991) for example, showed modality-specific motor memory in blind conditions not only in actual performance but also in imagined conditions, which excluded any influence of visual knowledge. Thus, it is possible to use movement imagery in the recall of guided movements, as imagined movements biased recall as much as actual movements did. Further, articulatory suppression had no effect on performance, implying little or no role for translation of extent of movement into a verbal format. However, the nature of this modality-specific motor memory is still not well understood. The question arises, for example, whether motor memory is represented spatially in terms of spatial extent or extent of movement. Studies of movement have shown that extent of movement is encoded differently from spatial location in short-term memory (Laabs, 1973; Laabs & Simmons, 1981). Short-term memory could rely, therefore, on kinesthesis even when inputs are not coded spatially, although memory for extent of movement is not very accurate.

Are differences between haptic and visual perception of curvature evident in memory? We (Ittyerah and Marks, 2007) expected that haptic, visual, and cross-modal memory will differ in their sensitivity to the activities in which subjects engage during the interference period. During a delay period of 30 seconds between the presentation of a test stimulus and its recall we introduced any one of the four following activities, such as counting aloud, rehearsing the test stimulus visually or haptically, spacing paper clips in equal distances or moving books from one hand to the other, as well as an unfilled delay that served as a control. We expected that tasks requiring spatial processing may have deleterious effects on performance in both modalities, whereas tasks requiring movement should exert greater effects on haptic memory.

The findings indicated that performance was not only better in haptic than visual conditions, but also that the intervening activities exerted greater effects with haptic than visual presentations. Prior evidence has shown that vision improves shape matching and seems to dominate over touch and haptic inputs that involve touch and movement (Held, 1963, 1965; Rock and Victor 1964). It is also generally agreed that vision is most important in spatial tasks (Sendon 1932, Attneave and Benson 1969). Furthermore, two recent studies suggested that noninformative vision can improve perception by touch (Kennett, Taylor-Clarke and Haggard, 2001; Newport, Rabb and Jackson, 2002). These findings are not consistent, however, with the evidence that people who are totally blind from birth can be equally or more proficient than the sighted on spatial tasks (Hollins 1968; Millar 1994). This evidence implies that proficiency varies with the spatial information that is available from other sources. For example, in a spatial location task of six landmarks, Millar and Al-Attar (2005) found that vision affects haptic processing only if vision adds task relevant information. Touch with diffuse light perception that excluded spatial cues and touch without vision did not differ in accuracy of performance. Millar and Al-Attar concluded that the differences between performance with spatially relevant and spatially irrelevant visual information provide new evidence against the hypothesis that vision affects haptic processing even if it does not add task-relevant information. Therefore, the relatively better performance of tactile compared to visual judgments (Ittyerah and Marks 2007) may reflect differences in the relevance of the delay tasks used to probe the tactile and visual systems.

It is conceivable that the differences in mnemonic representations for haptic and visual curvature are related to differences in haptic and visual perceptual processing. Haptic processing depends on movements of the hand or finger over the stimulus and therefore is subject to spatial constraints on motion, whereas visual processing is often global (Navon, 1977) and the sensory detection and discrimination are limited by the physical properties of the stimuli themselves, such as photon counting at low intensities (De Vries, 1943). In linear movement tasks the demands on memory involve the starting and ending locations of the movement (Laabs & Simmons 1981; Millar 1994). For haptically felt curvature the demands on memory seem to be confined to the slope differences over the far ends of the stimulus (Gordon & Morison 1982; Pont et al, 1998; Pont et al, 1997) for both static and dynamic touch of curved strips (Pont et al 1999). The findings of Ittyerah and Marks (2007) suggest, in turn, that memory for haptic and perhaps for visual representations of curvature, perhaps representations of slope, may be particularly disrupted by tasks that involve spatial processing and movement - as assessed with the dual task paradigm used to test for the demands of attention on the primary task (Brown 1958; Peterson & Peterson 1959). Filling the delay interval with a spatial or a movement task in the haptic and visual modalities produces modality-specific interference (e.g., Logie1986). These results, though specific to the present tasks, may be generalized as being important characteristics in the perception of the curvature of objects. Besides, memory for information from touch and movement has been demonstrated by showing effects of coding texture for unfamiliar shapes and kinesthetic coding for unfamiliar movements (Millar, 1999). This indicates distinct effects for tactile memory. Coding can also involve the mental rehearsal of movements (Millar & Ittyerah, 1991) showing modality specific aspects of the input information. However the informational conditions in which such coding depends differ from those in which visual cues are present. Nevertheless, haptic representations are not recoded into visual coordinates, since impaired memory for recognition in one modality is generally dissociated from performance in the other modality (Farah 1990; Reed, Caselli & Farah, 1996).

Role of vision in tactile tasks

The predominance of studies in reaching and grasping attribute successful performance to the ability of the visual modality for aligning the hand and arm to the size and orientation of the object (Halverson1931, 1932, 1937, Caster 1932, McGraw 1945, Bower 1972, von Hofsten 1982, Jeannerod, 1994; 1997a, b). The role of vision is undoubtedly facilitating, but speculations as to whether it is a necessary modality in the attainment of these specific behaviours can only be examined by comparing congenitally blind children with sighted cohorts. Fraiberg (1968) in extensive work with eight blind infants found that these infants first reached for objects only at the age of ten months, whereas sighted infants on an average reach at the age of five months. Fraiberg (1968) observed that developmental delays in other behaviours of locomotion such as crawling suggested that reaching is the critical skill to locomotion. According to Fraiberg, reaching in blind infants is a two stage process where the initial reaches are to sounding objects pulled from the children's hands and this is followed by reaching to sounding objects held directly before them. Whereas sighted infants spontaneously reach for objects they see, blind infants need to be prompted by sound. If sounding objects are not present, the blind infant may not reach. Therefore reaching is dependent on the awareness of spatial information about the object. Subsequently, Adelson and Fraiberg (1974), Fraiberg (1977) observed that tasks requiring postural control are unaffected, whereas those requiring selfinitiation and mobility are delayed in blind children. Indeed Hatwell (1987) has cogently argued that in instances when blind infants do not use their hands as a perceptual information seeking device (e g. Fraigberg 1977), the reaching behaviour of these infants is mainly a motor executive one where for example the hand is usually used for putting objects in the mouth, and the deficit if any is non-modality specific (e.g. Friedman, 1971). When blind infants reach, this behaviour may be related to their conceptual development (Bigelow 1986). For example, the ear hand coordination for reaching objects in blind children is attained at eight months, whereas eye hand coordination in sighted children is attained by four months. Nevertheless sighted children are not able to reach a hidden object they hear until they are about eight or nine months of age and this is at par with the ages of the attainment of object permanence in blind children. Therefore blind and sighted children do not differ in their understanding of the object concept and vision is neither a necessary modality for the attainment of object permanence and subsequent cognitive development.

Bigelow (1986) found that in instances in which touch and sound are used in analogous tasks, the touch tasks are easier. The infant would rather reach for a toy placed on its chest than for a rattle held before her/him. Children respond to continuous touch before they respond to continuous sound and children reach to cues of previous touch before they reach to cues of previous sound. When touch and sound cues are in conflict, children initially respond to touch cues. Fraiberg (1968; 1977) observed that blind children reached at the body mid-line such as the chest for sounding objects taken from their hands before they reached at mid-line for objects on sound cues alone. Fraiberg concluded that the mid-line is the first space to have subjective reality for blind infants.

There is some evidence that Fraiberg's findings of reaching in blind infants may be operational in sighted infants as well. Wishart, Bower & Dunkheld (1978) studied reaching in sighted infants in dark conditions so that though infants heard the object, they were unable to see the object or know the direction of their reach. Wishart et al (1978) observed that as in the case of blind infants, directional reaches to objects as in off centre positions were more difficult than reaches to objects at the mid-line for sighted infants as well. Therefore there are no fundamental differences in reaching with or without vision. Blind children attain comparable performance with the sighted by relying on self referent cues (Millar, 1981) and self referent cues have been found to be reliable (Stelmach & Larish, 1980). Fraiberg (1968) has shown that this is evident in early infancy when infants reach to their body mid-line for objects they have not seen. Thus the difference between the blind and sighted children may be in the strategies for attaining information and is not a function of visuo-motor control (Jeannrod, 1984, 1994). The fact that blind children between the ages of 6 and 15 years are able to perform acts of reaching, grasping and assessing objects of various sizes using the precision grip (Ittyerah, 1993, 2000, 2009) both with the preferred and nonpreferred hands indicates that though vision may provide complementary information the visual modality is not necessary to perform tactile hand ability tasks because convergent information may be attained from other sources (Millar, 1994). Hatwell (1987) has argued that early in development infants rely on tactile information and perceive objects held in their hands without much assistance from vision. It is only after the age of five or six months that vision dominates and infants become dependent on eye hand coordination. For example when the hands of the infants were occluded by a screen (Streri & Pecheux, 1986 a & b) so that they could not see objects held in their hands, infants displayed a haptic habituation to the familiar stimulus and a novelty response to a new shape as early as four months of age. After five months, there seemed to be an increased synchronization between manual and visual inspection of objects (Rochat 1985). Hatwell (1987) reported that infants aged five to six months displayed suppression in their grasping response when a screen was placed on their shoulders to prevent them from seeing their hands. Although these children did not display any signs of distress nor try to remove the screen, they did not close their hands on the object the experimenter tried to put in it and their hands tended to avoid contact with the object. Over 60% of the infants failed to perform similar unimodal haptic tasks after five months of age or above whereas only 20 % failed to perform unimodal haptic tasks at ages less than four months. Therefore vision clearly dominates at older ages and infant's haptic perceptual abilities begin to be underutilized. Thus early in development, the tactile- haptic system takes precedence over visuo-motor channels for object perception and action.

The relation between hand preference and hand ability

Early reaching behaviours are an indication of hand preference. The difference between handedness and hand ability is that handedness refers to a consistent preference for one hand for executing fairly skilled actions such as writing or sewing. Hand ability refers to the potential capability of each hand in executing the same or different actions and the tacit understanding is that ability for a particular hand action does not differ between the hands. For example, one could write with either hand if encouraged early during development, and differences if any between the hands may be in hand orientation during performance and not in ability (Ittyerah 1996; Ittyerah et al. 2007). The right and left hands of children were able to point at proprioceptive memorized targets, but differed in orientation, in that the right preferred hand was more context oriented and therefore supple, whereas the left nonpreferred hand was more egocentrically oriented and consequently less supple. It may be useful to clarify the notions of hand skill and ability, in order to argue that there is equipotentiality between the hands.
The literature on hand skills may be grouped into three domains of explanation. One view asserts that the preferred hand is the skilled hand (Annett 1972, Annet et al 1979, Honda 1984). Another opinion is that handedness is not a unidimensional variable and hand actions may be grouped according to the muscle groups involved in performing the tasks (Plato et al 1984, Healey et al 1986, Steinhuis and Bryden 1989, 1990). A third opinion holds that the hands may not differ in skill for any action. The performance of both hands may be as good as each other and may depend upon conditions of task demands (Millar 1984, 1987, Ittyerah 1993, 2000, 2009, Millar 2008). It is of interest in this manuscript to examine these differing explanations of hand skill in order to conclude that there is equipotentiality between the hands, although studies of equal ability in the hands may be out numbered by studies that relate hand preference with hand skill.

Is the preferred hand the skilled hand?

Explanations of handedness have indicated a relation between hand preference and hand ability (Annett et. al, 1979, Peters, 1980). They believed that if hand preferences can be coordinated with an independent measure of hand skill, then the understanding of what is handedness can be clarified. Annett (1970b) indicated that the difference between the hands for the peg moving times was highest for the right handers and decreases linearly for the mixed and left handers. Attempts to train the non preferred hand to equal the skill of the preferred hand have not been successful for peg moving (Annett, Hudson & Turner, 1974) nor for finger tapping (Peters, 1976). Annett and Kilshaw (1983) found that degrees of mixed hand preferences between consistent right and consistent left are systematically related to degrees of L-R skill in the peg moving task, and Peters and Durding (1978) found a linear relationship between L-R mean tapping rates and hand preference. These findings led Annett (1985) to conclude that although practice can improve the performance of the non preferred hand, it does not alter the underlying natural asymmetry between the hands. A related notion to the above conclusion is that hand preferences are an out come of eye hand coordination and that eye hand coordination is more efficient on the right than the left side of the body (Woodworth1889, Annett et al, 1979; Peters 1976, 1980; Honda 1984).

Is handedness task specific?

A second group of studies do not consider handedness to be a unidimensional variable, but claim that hand actions may be controlled by groups of muscles that perform various actions and that the more skilled actions such as writing are more lateralized than less skilled actions such as picking up objects(Steinhuis and Bryden 1989, 1990). Reviews of studies on the origin of handedness (Hopkins, 1993) indicate that the earliest signs of hand preference appear to be task specific, in that hand actions are dependent on whether the task involves control of the proximal muscles as for reaching or the control of the distal segments of the hand, as for grasping. Subsequently, Ittyerah (1996) indicated that during development hand preferences may group together into a single category of skill for each hand; the right hand being better at actions of accuracy as in writing or throwing (Healey et al, 1986), and the left hand being more able for acts of strength as in lifting objects (Healey et al, 1986; Peters, 1990).Therefore task demands may dictate hand actions, though the general ability of the hands may not differ.

Do the hands differ in skill?

The question as to whether a particular hand is more skilled than another has not been satisfactorily answered. In nonprehensile tasks such as Braille reading, type writing or piano playing or for prehensile actions of juggling, the hands have a complementary role in task performance. This indicates that the skill is not lateralized, but rather, that task requirements dictate hand actions. For example, there was some initial confusion as to whether Braille is predominantly read by one hand. Superior Braille performance was reported for the left hand (Hermelin & O'Connor, 1971; Rudel, Denckla & Hirsch, 1977), at other times for the right hand (Fertsch, 1947), or for neither hand (Bradshaw, Nettleton & Spehr, 1982; Millar, 1977) and for two handed reading (Foulke, 1982). Millar (1984) has argued that in so far as reading levels are reported, the discrepant findings indicate a pattern that conforms to the notion that highly proficient reading depends mainly on verbal strategies and skill (right hand / left hemisphere advantage); less proficient reading demands attention to spatial coding of the physical characters (left hand / right hemisphere advantage), while early in learning subjects rely on dot density or texture features of Braille characters.

The finding that the general lateralization does not affect ability (Ittyerah 1993, Ittyerah 2000, 2009) indicates, that although one may have a hand preference, there is equipotentiality between the hands. In nonprehensile tasks such as braille reading, Millar (1987) found that fluent braillists use both hands in intermittent alternation for processing text. As to whether this is also true for prehensile actions can be known by testing for hand ability.

Studies in which blind and sighted children were required to match tactile stimuli separately with the left and right hands have indicated that the hands do not differ in tactile ability. Sighted blindfolded and congenitally blind children between the ages of 6 and 15 years were able to match the length, breadth, height and volume of three dimensional bricks of varying sizes with the left and right hands. Results indicated that performance improved with age, though the hands did not differ (Ittyerah, 1993) while performing different manual dexterity tasks such as sorting, finger dexterity and the Minnesota rate of manipulation test. Although there were differences between the groups and ages, the left and right hands of the blind and sighted children did not differ in speed or accuracy (Ittyerah, 2000). However one might argue that the lack of performance differences between the hands for the sighted children may have been a consequence of their temporary blind fold condition that may have interfered with performance, or the lack of differences in the blind children may have been due to a lack of familiarity with the tasks. In a follow up study congenitally blind and sighted blind folded children (Ittyerah 2009) were tested using a sorting task, a stacking task, the finger dexterity test and the Minnesota rate of manipulation test. Performance was assessed for the left and right hands, both before and after a four months practice period. Results indicated an increasing post test gain for all the groups on the tasks with age, though the hands did not differ in performance neither before nor after practice. The consistent results indicate that even if there is a hand preference (Ittyerah, 1993, 1996, 2000, 2009), the general ability of the hands in most tactile tasks does not differ. Thus there is no effect of hand on ability in prehensile tasks as well. The systematic data indicate no significant performance differences between the hands, thus lending support to the present theoretical notion of equipotentiality between the hands. Furthermore, lack of sight does not affect hand ability, just as vision does not determine the direction or the degree of hand preference (Ittyerah, 1993, 2000, 2009).

Visuo-spatial proficiency in the absence of vision

Even if speculations about lack of differences between the hands in the sighted children may be attributed to their temporary blindfold conditions which can be expected to hamper the performance of the preferred hand, there is no reason to expect a similar decline among the blind children who are also mostly right handed. Therefore though vision may provide external references for the sighted, the blind are found to use self reference cues during performance and visuo-spatial proficiency is found to improve under blind conditions as well (Liben, 1988; Millar, 1994). Body centred coding is not confined to the position of the limbs relative to each other or to other body parts. Body centred frames can also be used to code object locations, for example, by coding the hand position which is touching an object by reference to the body midline. When subjects are stationary in blindfold conditions, information is restricted to personal space that is, to spatial locations within the arms reach without moving bodily to another place. Such conditions are of particular interest in studying both short and long term effects of modes of perception on coding.

An absence of differences between the hands both with and without practice, indicates an equally good performance with both hands in the total absence of vision for prehensile movements that involve sorting and stacking of objects, the finer coordination of the thumb and forefinger as in finger dexterity tasks and the general ability of the fingers of both hands in the manipulation tasks. Therefore vision does not affect the general maturation of the child since the blind can gain in proficiency with practice of visuo spatial tasks in the total absence of vision. This proficiency is not only confined to the preferred hand but is also to the same extent in the nonpreferred hand. Findings indicate no effect of hand on ability and suggest equipotentiality between the hands for both prehensile and nonprehensile actions.

The reference hypothesis

The hands are most often used to perceive and discriminate objects by touch. The tactile perception of an object is more accurate with systematic than unsystematic exploration. Accurate haptic coding of information is dependent upon reference frames. The importance of reference frames for accurate coding of movements was emphasized by Jeannerod (1988), Paillard (1991) and Berthoz (1993). Systematic exploration of stimulus characteristics with the hand or fingers requires an anchor or reference point that can be recognized as the end and starting point of the exploratory movement. To know what is to count as spatial processes independent of hand effects, Millar and Al-Attar (2003b) tested two hypotheses. The first hypothesis that the left hand is better for spatial tasks, predicts a left hand advantage for performance in all conditions. The alternate reference hypothesis predicts significantly greater accuracy in haptic recall with explicit additional reference information than in conditions that do not provide additional reference information.

The reference hypothesis assumes that distance and location judgments are spatial tasks. Haptic distance judgments are not solely kinesthetic inputs. Movement distances should be coded spatially if they can be related to reference information (Millar 2008). Millar and Al-Attar (2003a) found that haptic distance judgments do involve spatial coding. Recall of a repeated small distance was disturbed not only by a movement task, but also by a spatial task that required no movements. In a subsequent study (Millar and Al-Attar 2003b) required subjects to recall distance or locations of hapically felt extents. The control condition consisted of scanning the critical distances or locations in presentation and recall without touching any other part of the display or surround. In the experimental or reference conditions, subjects were instructed to use an actual external frame around the stimuli, and also their body midline for reference. The results showed that the added reference information reduced errors very significantly compared to the normal conditions, regardless of whether the left hand scanned the distance in control and frame conditions and right hand was used for the frame, or whether the right hand scanned the distance in control and frame conditions and the left hand was used for the frame. The left and right hands did not differ from each other in accuracy in either control conditions or in reference instruction conditions. The results supported the hypothesis that the use of external frame and body centred reference cues make haptic distance judgments more accurate. The fact that the accuracy of recall with the left hand did not interact differentially with the increase in accuracy with the instructions to use reference cues showed that scanning the distance would involve left hemisphere processing of the movements as well as the spatial aspects of relocating the end position from the new (guided) starting point, and therefore right hemisphere processes also. Cross lateral effects from both right and left hemisphere processes that inhibit or counterbalance each other would explain why the left hand did not perform better than the right and why it did not relate differentially to the advantage in accuracy from instructions to use spatial reference cues. The important finding was that instructions to use body centred and external frame cues for reference improved recall accuracy for both distance and locations, independently of hand performance, task differences and movement effects. Thus reference information can be used as a reliable test of spatial coding.

Millar and Al-Attar (2004) further tested how egocentric and allocentric coding relate to each other. The hypothesis that haptic targets can only be coded spatially in relation to body centred cues would predict that providing haptic cues explicitly from an external surround would not improve recall accuracy beyond the level found with body centred reference cues alone. If on the other hand the difference in spatial coding is due solely to the lack of external reference information that is normally available in haptic task conditions, providing external haptic cues explicitly for reference in a spatial task should improve recall significantly.

Millar and Al-Attar tested subjects with a spatial task that people might actually encounter in daily living. The task was to remember the precise location of five shape symbols as landmarks that had been positioned randomly as raised symbols along an irregular, but easily felt raised line route. This map like layout had an actual tangible rectangular surrounding frame. Each subject was presented with the map like layout placed on the table and aligned to the subject's body midline. The subjects placed the fingertip of their preferred right hand at the start of the route and scanned the route from left to right in all presentation conditions and briefly stopped on each landmark symbol they encountered on the route, in order that they be remembered for the recall tests.

Millar and Al- Attar (2004) found that disrupting body centred cues by rotation increased errors significantly compared to intact body centred coding in the body aligned condition. The critical results were a significant decrease in positioning errors with added external reference information when body centred coding was disrupted by rotation, compared to the rotation condition that lacked external reference information. The condition with intact body centred cues and added external reference information was more accurate in comparison to the body aligned condition without external cues, and more accurate also than the condition with added external information, when body centred coding was disturbed by rotation. Further, accuracy with added external reference information but disrupted body centred coding did not differ from intact body centred coding without external reference information.

The experimental manipulation of separating and combining external and body centred reference showed that external reference cues can also be used with purely haptic information and this seems to be as equally effective for spatial coding as is body centred reference information (Millar and Al-Attar 2004).

In summary haptic touch and hand ability are related. The preferred hand is not necessarily the skilled hand and performance of the left and right hands indicate near equal hand ability. The hands differ in their orientation of performance though haptic perception and identification of objects rely on a frame of reference. Identification of differences in shapes and sizes of objects by touch rely on different reference information. Object identification is possible with either hand early in development in both blind and sighted blindfolded conditions and there is no effect of hand on ability.

References

Abravanel, E. (1971). Active detection of solid-shape information by touch and vision. Perception & Psychophysics, 10, 358-360.

Adelson, E., Fraiberg.S. (1974). Gross motor development in infants blind from birth. Child Development, 45, 114-126.

Amedi, A., Jacobson, B., Malach, R. & Zohary, E. (2002). Convergence of visual and tactile shape processing in the human lateral occipital complex. Cerebral Cortex, 12, 1202-1212.

Amedi, A., Malach, R., Hendler,T., Peled, S. & Zohary, E. (2001). Visuo-haptic object activation in the ventral visual pathway. Nature Neuroscience, 4, 324-330.

Annett, J.; Annett, M.; Hudson, P. T. W.; &Turner, A. (1979) The control of movement in the preferred and non preferred hands. Quarterly Journal of Experimental Psychology, 31, 641-652.

Annett, M. & Kilshaw, D. (1983). Right and left hand skill II: Estimating the parameters of the distribution in L-R differences in males and females. British Journal of psychology, 74,269-283.

Annett, M. (1970b). The growth of manual preference and speed. British Journal of Psychology, 61, 545-558.

Annett, M. (1972). The distribution of manual asymmetry. British Journal of Psychology, 63, 343-358.

Annett, M. (1985). Left, right, hand and brain: The right shift theory. LEA, London. Annett, M. Hudson, P.T.W; &Turner, A. (1974). The reliability of differences between the hands in motor skill. Neuropsychologia, 12,527-531.

Attneave, F. & Benson, B. (1969). Spatial coding of tactual stimulation. Journal of Experimental Psychology, 81, 216-222.

Berthoz, A. (Ed) (1993). Multisensory control of movement. Oxford, UK, Oxford University Press.

Bigelow, A. (1986). The development of reaching in blind children. British Journal of Developmental Psychology, 4, 355-366.

Bower, T.G.R. (1974). Development in infancy. San Francisco: W. H. Freeman.

Bradshaw, J.L., Nettleton, N.C., & Spehr, K.(1982). Braille reading and left and right hemispace. Neuropsychologia, 20: 493-500.

Brown, J.A. (1958). Some tests of the decay theory of immediate memory. Quarterly Journal of Experimental Psychology, 10, 12-21.

Castner, B.M. (1932). The development of fine prehension in infancy. Genetic Psychology Monographs, 12, 105-193.

De Vries, H.L. (1943). The quantum character of light and its bearing upon threshold of vision, the differential sensitivity and visual acuity of the eye. Physica, 10, 553-564.

Easton, R.D., Greene, A.J., & Srinivas, K. (1997). Transfer between vision and haptics. Memory for 2 D patterns and 3 D objects. Psychonomic Bulletin and Review, 4, 403-410.

Elman, J. L. (1996). Rethinking innateness: A connectionist perspective on development. Cambridge, MA: MIT Press.

Farah, M.J. (1990). Visual agnosia: Disoders of object recognition and what they tell us about normal vision. Cambridge, MA: MIT Press.

Fertsch, P. (1947). Hand dominance in reading braille. American Journal of Psychology, 60: 335-349.

Foulke, E. (1982). In W. Schiff & E. Foulke (Eds.) Tactual Perception: A Source Book. Cambridge University Press.

Fraiberg, S(1968) Parallel and divergent patterns in blind and sighted children. Psychoanalytic study of the child, 23, 264-300.

Fraiberg, S. (1977).Insights from the blind. London, UK: Souvenir Press.

Friedman,D.A(1971) Congenital and perinatal sensory deprivation: Some studies in early development. American Journal of Psychology, 127, 1539-1545.

Gallagher, S. (2004). Neurons and neonates: reflections on the Molyneux Problem. In Gallagher, S. (*Ed), How the body shapes the mind.* Oxford: Oxford University Press.
Gibson E.J., & Walker, A. (1984). Development of knowledge of visual- tactual affordances of substance. *Child Development, 55*, 453-460.
Gilson, E.Q., Baddeley, A.D. (1969). Tactile short term memory. Quarterly Journal of Experimental Psychology, 21, 180-184.
Gordon, I.A. & Morrison, V. (1982). The haptic perception of curvature. Perception & Psychophysics, 31, 446-450.
Grill-Spector, K., Kourtzi, Z. & Kanwisher, N. (2001). The lateral occipital complex and its role in object recognition. Vision Research, 41, 1409-1422.
Halverson, H.M. (1937). Studies of grasping responses of early infancy: I, II, III. Journal of Genetic Psychology, 51, 371-449.
Halverson, H.M.(1931). An experimental study of prehension in infants by means of systematic cinema records. Genetic psychology Monographs, 10,107-286.
Halverson, H.M.(1932b). A further study of grasping. Journal of General Psychology, 7, 34-63.
Hatwell, Y. (1987).Motor and cognitive functions of the hand in infancy and childhood. International Journal of Behavioural Development, 20, 509-526.
Healey, J. M., Lederman, J., & Geschwind, N. (1986). Handedness is not an unidimensional trait. *Cortex*, 22, 33-53.
Held, R. (1963). Plasticity in human sensory motor control. Science, 142, 455-462.
Held, R. (1965). Plasticity in sensory motor systems. Scientific American, 213, 84-94.
Hermelin, B., & O'Connor, N. (1971). Functional asymmetry in the reading of Braille, Neuropsychologia, 9, 431-435.
Hofsten, C von. (1982). Eye hand coordination in the newborn. Developmental Psychology, 18, 450-461.
Hollins, M. (1986). Mental haptic rotation: more consistent in blind subjects? Journal of visual impairment and blindness, 80, 950-952.
Honda, H. (1984). Functional between- hand differences and out flow eye position information. Quarterly Journal of Experimental Psychology, 36A , 75-88.
Hopkins, B. (1993). On the developmental origins of handedness. Annual report. Research and clinical centre for child development. Hokkaido University, Sapporo, Japan.
Ittyerah, M & Marks L. E (2008). Intramodal and cross-modal discrimination of curvature: Haptic touch versus vision *Current Psychology Letters*, Vol. 24, Issue 1, 1-15.
Ittyerah, M, Gaunet, F & Rossetti, Y (2007) Pointing with the left and right hands in congenitally blind children. Brain and Cognition, 64 (2) 170-183.
Ittyerah, M. & Marks, L.E. (2007) Perception and Memory in Curvature stimuli. Haptic Touch versus Vision. British Journal of Psychology, 98, 589-610.
Ittyerah, M. (1993). Hand preferences and hand ability in congenitally blind children. *Quarterly Journal of Experimental Psychology*, 46B, 35-50.
Ittyerah, M. (1996). Do the hands differ in skill? *Brain and Cognition*, 32, 2, 291-296.
Ittyerah, M. (2009) Hand ability and practice in congenitally blind children.Journal of Development and Physical Disabilities, 21, 329-344.
James, T.W., Humphery, G.K., Gati, J.S., Savos, P., Menon, R.S. & Goodale, M.A. (2002). Haptic study of three dimensional objects activates extrastriate visual areas. Neuropsychologia, 40, 1706-1714.

Jeanneord, M. (1984). The timing of neural prehension movements. Journal of Motor Behaviour, 16, 235-264.

Jeannerod, M. (1994). The hand and the object: The role of the posterior parietal cortex in forming motor representations. Canadian Journal of Physiology and Pharmacology, 72, 535-541.

Jeannerod, M. (1997a). The cognitive neuroscience of action. Cambridge, Mass: Blackwell Publishers.

Jeannerod, M.(1988). The neural and behavioural organization of goal directed movements. Oxford: Clarendon Press.

Jeannerod, M.(1997b). Grasping Objects: The hand as a pattern recognition device. In Hepp-Reymond, M. C. & Marini, G. (Eds). Perspectives of motor behaviour and its neural basis. Basel, Karger. pp.19-32.

Kennett, S., Taylor, C., & Haggard, P. (2001). Non informative vision improves spatial resolution of touch in humans. Current Biology, 11, 1188-1191.

Kiphart, M.J., Hughes, J.L., Simmons, J.P. & Cross, H.A. (1992). Short term haptic memory for complex objects. Bulletin of the Psychonomic Society, 30, 212-214.

Laabs, G. J. & Simmons, R. W. (1981). Motor memory. In D. Holding (Ed.), Human skills (pp. 119-151). New York: Wiley.

Laabs, G. J. (1973). Retention characteristics of different reproduction cues in motor short-term memory. Journal of Experimental Psychology, 100, 168-177.

Liben, L.S. (1988). Conceptual issues in the development of spatial cognition. In J. Stiles-Davis, M. Kritchevsky, & U. Bellugi (ed.) Spatial Cognition. Hillsdale, New Jersey: LEA.

Lobb, H. (1965). Vision versus touch in form discrimination. Canadian Journal of Psychology, 19, 175-187.

Logie, R.H. (1986). Visuo-spatial processing in working memory. Quarterly Journal of Experimental Psychology, 38A, 229-247.

McClelland, J.M., & Rumelhart, D.E. (1986). Parallel distributed processing: Explanations in the microstructure of cognition. Psychological and biological models, 2. Cambridge, MA: MIT Press.

McGraw, M. B. (1945). The neuromuscular Maturation of the Human Infant. New York: Columbia University Press.

Meltzoff, A.N., & Borton, R. W. (1979). Intermodal matching by human neonates. *Nature, 282*, 403-404.

Millar, S & Al Attar, Z. (2005). What aspects of vision facilitate haptic processing? Brain and Cognition, 59, 258-268.

Millar, S. & Al-Attar (2003a). How do people remember spatial information from Tactile maps? British Journal of Visual Impairment, 21, 64-72.

Millar, S. & Al-Attar (2004). External and body centred frames of reference in spatial memory: Evidence from touch. Perception & Psychophysics, 66, 51-59.

Millar, S. & Al-Attar(2003b). Spatial reference and scanning with the left and right hand. Perception, 32, 1499-1511.

Millar, S. (1974). Tactile short term memory by blind and sighted children. British Journal of Psychology, 65, 253-263.

Millar, S. (1977). Early stages of tactual matching. Perception, 6: 333-343.

Millar, S. (1981). Crossmodal and intersensory perception and the blind. In R.D. Walk & H .C. Pick (Eds.), Intersensory perception and sensory integration (pp. 281- 314). New York: Plenum.

Millar, S. (1987a). The perceptual window in two handed braille. Do the left and right hands process braille simultaneously? Cortex, 23, 111-122.

Millar, S. (1994). Understanding and representing space: Theory and evidence from studies with blind and sighted children. Oxford: Clarendon Press.

Millar, S. (1999). Memory in touch. Psicothema, 11, 747-767.

Millar, S. (2008). Space and Sense. Psychology Press, Hove and New York.

Millar, S., & Ittyerah, M. (1991). Movement imagery in young and congenitally blind children: mental practice without visuo-spatial information. International Journal of Behavioral Development, 15, 125-146.

Navon, D. (1977). Forest before trees. The precedence of global features in visual perception. Cognitive Psychology, 9, 353-383.

Newell, F.N. (2004). Crossmodal object recognition. In C. Spence, G. Calvert & B. Stein (Eds.), Handbook of multisensory integration. Cambridge, MA: MIT Press.

Newport, R., Rabb, B., Jackson, S.R. (2002). Non informative vision improves haptic spatial perception. Current Biology, 12, 1661-1664.

Norman, J.F., Norman, H.F., Clayton, A.M., Lianekhammy, J., & Zielke, G. (2004). The visual and haptic perception of natural object shape. Perception & Psychophysics, 66, 342-357.

Paillard, J. (1991). Motor and representational framing of space. In J. Palliard (ed). Brain and Space. Oxford, Oxford University Press. pp 63–181

Peters, M .& Durding, B.(1978). Handedness measured by finger tapping. A continuous variable. Canadian Journal of Psychology, 32,257-261.

Peters, M. (1980). Why the preferred hand taps more quickly than the non preferred hand. Three experiments on handedness. Canadian Journal Psychology, 34, 62-71.

Peters, M. (1990 c). Phenotype in normal lefthanders. An understanding of phenotype is the basis for understanding mechanism and inheritance of handedness. In Coren (Ed). Left handedness. Behavioural implications and anomalies (pp. 167–192). North Holland: Elsevier Science Publishers.

Peters, M.(1976). Prolonged practice of a simple motor task by preferred and non preferred hands. Perceptual and Motor skills, 43, 447-450.

Peterson, L.R., & Peterson, M.J. (1959). Short-term retention of individual verbal items. Journal of Experimental Psychology, 58, 193-198.

Plato, C. C; Fox, K. M; & Garruto, R.M. (1984). Measures of lateral functional dominance: Hand dominance. Human Biology, 56, 259-276.

Pont, S., Kappers, A.M.L., & Koenderink, J.J. (1997). Haptic curvature discrimination at several regions of the hand. Perception & Psychophysics, 59, 1225-1240.

Pont, S., Kappers, A.M.L., & Koenderink, J.J. (1998). The influence of stimulus tilt on haptic curvature matching and discrimination by dynamic touch. Perception. 27, 869-880.

Pont, S., Kappers, A.M.L., & Koenderink, J.J. (1999). Similar mechanisms underlie curvature comparison by static and dynamic touch. Perception & Psychophysics, 61, 874-894.

Reed, C.L., Caselli, R.J., Farah, M.J. (1996). Tactile agnosia: Underlying impairment and implications for normal tactile object recognition. Brain, 119, 875-888.

Rock, I & Victor, J. (1964). Vision and touch: an experimentally created conflict between two senses. Science, 143, 594-596.

Rudel, R.G., & Teuber, H.L. (1964). Crossmodal transfer of shape information by children. Neuropsychologia, 2, 1-8.

Rudel, R.G., Denckla, M.B.,& Hirsch, S.(1977). The development of left hand superiority for discriminating Braille configurations. Neurology, 27, 160-164.

Sendon. M. Von. (1960). Space and sight: The perception of space and shape in congenitally blind patients before and after operation. London, Methuen.

Steinhuis, R. E. & Bryden, M.P. (1990). Reliability of hand preference items and factors. Journal of Clinical and Experimental Neuropsychology, vol.12. 6, 921-930.

Steinhuis, R.E.& Bryden, M.P.(1989). Different dimensions of hand preference that relate to skill and unskilled activities. Cortex, 25, 289-304.

Stelmach, G, E and Larish, D.D. (1980). Egocentric referents in human limb Orientation. In G.E. Stelmach and J Requin (ed). Tutorials in Motor Behaviour. Amsterdam: North-Holland Publishing Co.

Streri, A. (1987). Tactile discrimination of shape and intermodal transfer in 2- to 3- month old infants. *British Journal of Developmental Psychology, 5,* 213-220.

Streri, A., & Gentaz, E. (2003). Cross-modal recognition of shape from hand to eyes in human newborns. *Somatosensory and Motor Research, 20,* 11-16.

Streri, A., & Pêcheux, M. G. (1986). Tactual habituation and discrimination of form in infancy: A comparison with vision. Child Development, 57, 100-104.

Sullivan, E.V. & Turvey, M.T. (1972). Short term retention of tactile stimulation. Quarterly Journal of Experimental Psychology, 24, 253-261.

Wishart, U.G., Bower, T.G.R. & Dunkeld, J. (1978). Reaching in the dark. Perception, 7, 507-512.

Woods, A.T., O'Modhrain, S., & Newell, F.N. (2004). The effect of temporal delay and spatial differences on cross-modal object recognition. *Cognitive, Affective and Behavioural Neuroscience*, 4, 260-269.

Woodworth, R. S. (1898). The accuracy of voluntary movement. Psychological Review Monograph supplement. No 3.

Force Scaling as a Function of Object Mass when Lifting with Peripheral Fatigue

James C. Larmer, Camille Williams and Heather Carnahan
University of Toronto & University of Waterloo
Canada

1. General Introduction

Fatigue is a relevant and significant factor in many work related settings. Some of these settings include working on an assembly line at a factory, sitting in front of a computer all day or performing long surgeries in the operating room. These types of jobs demand that individuals perform repetitive tasks with either a high or low degree of force intensity for prolonged periods of time without adequate rest breaks (Clarkson et al., 1992; Franzblau et al., 1993). Even under highly repetitive, non-forceful tasks, repetitive strain injuries can result, causing the potential for task performance levels to decrease (Stock, 1991). In addition to the potential long term injury as a result of performing while fatigued, there are immediate performance adjustments that take place when generating motor skills in this state.

Historically, the effects of fatigue on motor performance and motor learning have been of interest. Alderman (1965) found that performance during practice suffered when an interpolated fatiguing protocol was administered when learning two similar motor tasks. However, performance during a retention test after full recovery from fatigue showed no differences between both the non-fatigued and fatigued groups for both motor tasks. Similarly, when participants were fatigued either early or late during practice and then retested in a retention test after full recovery from fatigue, performance during the practice stages of the study was affected and there were no differences between the control and experimental groups during a retention test. These two studies, along with others (Schmidt, 1969; Whitley, 1973), suggest that fatigue is *not* detrimental to the amount learned when practice is performed in a fatigued state. In opposition to these findings, Godwin and Schmidt (1971) found fatigue to be a powerful learning variable as they reported that transfer from a fatigued to non-fatigued condition was only moderate. Many others have supported Godwin and Schmidt's claim by reporting similar findings (Carron, 1972; Carron & Ferchuk, 1971; Pack et al., 1974; Thomas et al., 1975).

Bigland-Ritchie (1984) defined neuromuscular fatigue as any reduction in the force-generating capacity of the total neuromuscular system. Furthermore, Bigland-Ritchie explained that fatigue can occur within the central nervous system (CNS), the neural transmission from the CNS to the muscle, and within the individual muscle itself. The fatiguing protocol employed in this chapter was aimed to elicit task specific local neuromuscular fatigue (peripheral fatigue) of the muscles involved in a precision grasp between the index finger and thumb. The intent of the fatiguing protocol was to produce fatigue-like symptoms that resemble those endured in everyday life, but to produce them in a controlled laboratory environment where their motor effects could be effectively evaluated.

Two main types of peripheral fatigue are found in everyday tasks. Tasks that are of high intensity and short duration cause mainly high-frequency fatigue (HFF) and others that occur at low intensities over a substantial amount of time produce a greater amount of low-frequency fatigue (LFF). To support this definition, electrically stimulating a muscle at frequencies between 50-100 Hz has been shown to produce predominantly HFF whereas stimulating at frequencies of 2-20 Hz produces predominantly LFF (Lehman, 1997). An example of a HFF task may consist of having somebody bench press at 80 % of their maximum voluntary contraction (MVC) as many times as possible. This would send the participant to exhaustion very quickly, but recovery times for HFF tasks are also very rapid. The recovery time can be defined as the time it takes for a participant to recover to 80 % of their MVC (Schwendner et al., 1995). Schwendner et al. (1995) reported recovery times of up to eight minutes following a HFF protocol. The studies conducted in this chapter attempted to induce predominantly LFF as this type of fatigue has been shown to last up to 24 hours post-fatiguing protocol (Edwards et al., 1977) and when present, affects the forces emitted at lower frequencies (Edwards et al., 1977; Fuglevand et al., 1999) which was specific to the low level forces needed to complete the lifting tasks employed in the present studies. In addition, this type of fatiguing protocol satisfied the time constraints of the studies as many samples were collected over a considerable amount of time (approximately 0.5 hours post-fatigue protocol). Alongside fitting the abovementioned criteria, LFF is relevant to many settings such as assembly line work (Dennerlein et al., 2003), typing (Lin et al., 2004; Nakata et al., 1992) and surgery (Uhrich et al., 2002), and therefore, the information gathered about the effects of fatigue at low levels of exertion may help to improve these types of work environments.

Two studies are reported in this chapter. Due to the current lack of research in the area of fatigue related to simple motor control principles, it was the aim of the first study to determine the effects of fatigue on the ability to generate forces appropriate to the mass of lifted objects when using a precision grip. Unvarying visual cues were present in this first study, and therefore, the ability to anticipate object mass was eliminated. The study was designed solely to determine if fatigue altered one's ability to appropriately scale motor output to the varying mass of the lifted objects. The objective of the second study was to address the consequences of fatigue on one's ability to anticipate force and movement generation requirements. Therefore, visual size cues that are congruent with object mass were present in this study. This gave participants the opportunity to anticipate the force and movement characteristics required to lift the various sized boxes and in turn offered insight into whether anticipatory strategies are compromised by fatigue.

It was hypothesized that participants would show a reduction in overall force output after the fatiguing protocol and a reduction in the ability to control fingertip forces throughout the lift. The reduction in force control was expected to be demonstrated by the inability to correctly scale force output from the fingers to the mass of the object being lifted.

2. Study 1

The aim of this study was to examine the effects of neuromuscular fatigue during a precision grasp lifting task when object *mass* is manipulated.

2.1 Rationale

Literature has shown that some basic movement and force patterns are followed when lifting objects that differ in mass (Johansson & Westling, 1984; 1988; 1990). For example, the grip forces emitted by the fingertips increase with the increasing mass of the objects presented (Gordon et al., 1993; Johansson & Westling, 1988; 1990). This is known as force scaling as more force is used to lift and hold heavy objects than light objects. After the grasp has been established and the lift has begun, the grip and load forces have been shown to increase in parallel, with the grip force output being slightly greater than the minimum grip force required to prevent slips. These fundamental measures along with many others have been well documented only in studies with rested participants (e.g., Burgess & Jones, 1997).

The first goal of the present study was to form a template for comparison between a lift under normal and fatigued conditions. After a pre-fatigue test (test 1) was completed, half of the participants completed a fatiguing protocol and were then asked to complete the same lifting task immediately following (post-fatigue test or test 2). The remaining half of the participants, the Control Group, completed the pre- and post-fatigue tests without performing the fatiguing protocol. It was expected that these procedures would show the effects of fatigue on the ability to elicit the appropriate motor output at the object-digit interface based on the mass of the object being lifted.

It was hypothesized that after the fatiguing protocol participants would show a reduction in the overall force output and, in addition, would show alterations in the ability to control finger tip forces throughout the lift. This was to be demonstrated by the inability to correctly scale the force output from the fingers to the mass of the object lifted (e.g., higher forces are normally associated with heavier objects). Thus, it was thought that after the fatiguing protocol, participants may have adopted a cautious strategy when handling objects with a fatigued grip.

2.2 Methods

Participants

Twenty-four naïve, right-handed participants with normal uncorrected or corrected visual acuity and no reported previous history of upper limb neuromuscular injuries participated. The Fatigued Group in this study had 5 males and 7 females (ages 18-27 years) and the Control Group had 6 males and 6 females (ages 21-28 years). The study received ethics approval through the local Office of Research Ethics. Informed consent was obtained from all of the participants prior to their participation.

Apparatus
Five different masses were located centrally inside a uniform object. Therefore, the objects lifted were visually identical. The object mass was varied between 100 g, 200 g, 300 g, 400 g and 500 g. Density also varied, but was similar to 1.0 g^1 cm^{-3} - the density suggested to be common to most everyday handheld objects (Flanagan & Beltzner, 2000; Gordon et al., 1993). Refer to Table 1 for the properties of the objects.

Object	Mass (g)	Length of Side (cm)	Volume (cm^3)	Density (g/cm^3)
1	100	6.7	300.8	0.332
2	200	6.7	300.8	0.665
3	300	6.7	300.8	0.997
4	400	6.7	300.8	1.330
5	500	6.7	300.8	1.662

Table 1. Properties of objects used in Study 1

The object was outfitted with a clasp that attached to the handle. The handle consisted of an area that fastened onto the object and an area where an ATI Gamma Force/Torque transducer system could be mounted between two circular grasping surfaces (ATI Industrial Automation, Gerner N.C., U.S.A.). The force transducer was used to track force changes in the X, Y, and Z axes for the duration of every lift (see Fig. 1). In addition, an Optotrak motion analysis system was used to track the location of the object through space (RMS accuracy to 0.1 mm; resolution to 0.01 mm).

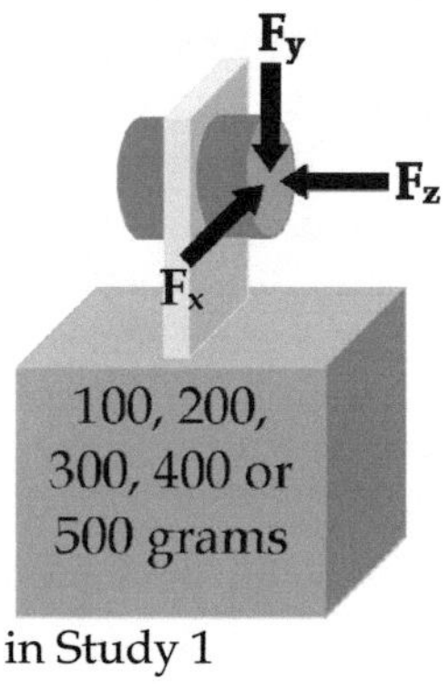

Fig. 1. Diagram of apparatus used in Study 1

Movement task description
Seated participants placed their dominant hand (right hand) in the arm brace located on the table. The arm brace secured the forearm in an attempt to make the lifting task and the fatiguing task as similar as possible. After a tone sounded, the participants lifted the object using a precision grasp (a grasp between the index finger and thumb) at the grasping surface. Participants held the object approximately 1 cm above the table surface for 5 s and then replaced it when told. See Fig. 2 for a schematic representation of the task.

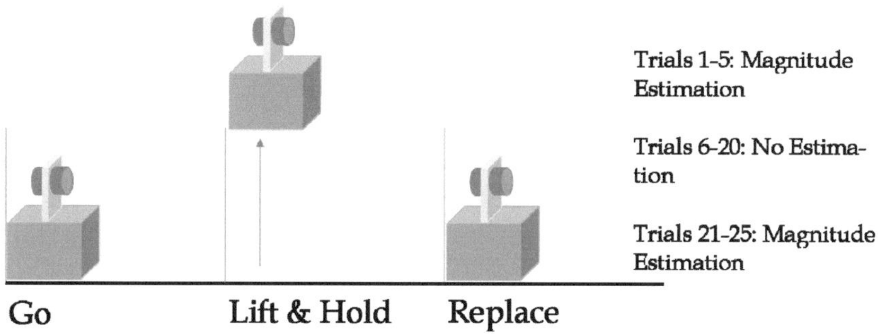

Fig. 2. The order of events during a single lifting trial

Fatiguing protocol

The fatiguing protocol was task specific as it was performed using the same grasping surface participants used to lift the objects during the lifting trials. As such, the width of the grasping area was controlled.

Participants first performed three MVCs. 50 % of the highest registered MVC was the force used in the fatiguing task. After 50 % MVC was calculated, participants completed a fatiguing protocol with a 0.5 duty cycle where they pinched the force transducer for five seconds (contraction time) to 50 % MVC then released it for five seconds (relaxation time) in a continuous cycle for 15 minutes (modified from Fowles et al., 2002). A visual display was available to assist participants with matching the required force output. MVC force output was collected immediately following the 15 minute fatiguing protocol and following the post-fatigue protocol lifting session.

2.3 Procedures

Fatigued group

Pre-fatigue test (test 1). Participants lifted five objects five times each for a total of 25 trials. The objects were presented in a pseudorandom order as each of the five masses was presented once every five trials. Therefore, each mass occurred once in each set of five trials with the first set (trials 1 to 5) and the last set (trials 21 to 25) having the same order of presentation for magnitude estimation purposes. Some example sequences are as follows: (3-1-5-4-2)-(4-5-1-2-3)-(2-4-3-5-1)-(4-5-1-3-2)-(3-1-5-4-2) (numbers 1 through 5 represent the 5 different masses with 1 being the lightest and 5 the heaviest). A 20 s rest period was provided between lifting trials to ensure that fatigue was avoided during the pre-fatigue test (cf. Valero-Cuevas et al., 1998).

Fatigue protocol. Participants were fatigued according to the above mentioned fatiguing protocol.

Post-fatigue test (test 2). An identical procedure to the pre-fatigue test was administered.

Control group

Participants in this group completed the same protocol as the fatigued group; however, these participants spent the 20 minutes between the pre-fatigue and post-fatigue tests of the study resting instead of completing the fatiguing protocol.

2.4 Data analysis

All raw data files were filtered with a second order Butterworth low-pass 15 Hz filter. Forces in the z-axis (F_z), load forces (F_{xy}) and grip rates at different intervals throughout the lift were analyzed. These measures included: peak grip force, peak rate of grip force generation, final grip force (just before participants put the object down), and peak load force. All motor data were analyzed using separate mixed 2 group (control / fatigued) x 2 test (before fatigue break (test1) / after fatigue break (test 2)) x 5 mass (100 g, 200 g, 300 g, 400 g, 500 g) x 5 trial (1 to 5) analyses of variance (ANOVAs), $\alpha = 0.05$. All significant interactions were explored using Tukey's honestly significant difference (HSD) method for post hoc analysis, $\alpha = 0.05$.

Maximum voluntary contraction data was recorded at the end of the test 1 trial set, immediately following the fatiguing protocol and immediately following test 2 for the Fatigued Group. The Control Group provided maximum voluntary contractions at the start of their 20 minute rest break following test 1 and again immediately following the test 2 trial set. A one-way analysis of variance was run on this data with time as a factor for each group. Thus, there were three levels of time for the Fatigued Group and two levels of time for the Control Group.

2.5 Results and Discussion

Grip force

In the analysis of **peak grip force** there was a three way interaction of test by mass by trial, $F(16, 352) = 2.10$, $p < .01$. As seen in Fig. 3, for the first trial of the first test, participants produced the same peak force for the 100 g and 200 g objects, and for the 300 g, 400 g, and 500 g objects. On all subsequent trials, for both tests, participants were generally able to scale forces according to object mass. Also, there was an overall decrease in peak grip force for test 2 in comparison to test 1. There were no statistically significant main effects or interactions with group ($p > .05$), which suggests that the fatiguing protocol had no effect on peak grip force output.

The analysis of **peak rate of grip force production** showed a main effect for mass, $F(4, 88) = 12.12$, $p < .01$, in addition to a test by trial interaction, $F(4, 88) = 6.97$, $p < .01$ (see Fig. 4). The main effect for mass showed that there was a larger rate of grip force production for the 300 g (36.3 N/s, SE = 1.3) and 400 g (38.4 N/s, SE = 1.3) objects in comparison to the 100 g object (31.5 N/s, SE = 1.3). The rate of force production for the 200 g (32.9 N/s, SE = 1.2) and 500 g objects (34.3 N/s, SE = 1.3) did not differ statistically from the others. This was unexpected because no visual cues were available such that participants could anticipate object mass. However, it is possible that at the time of peak grip rate (approximately 30 ms into the lift) enough time was available for haptic inputs to provide some information about object mass (Abbs et al., 1984).

The interaction of test and trial showed that for the first test, peak grip rates were higher for the first and second trials and stabilized on subsequent trials. For the second test, peak grip rate remained stable throughout all trials. This is consistent with the notion that forces produced on initial lifting trials tend to be larger and produced more quickly than on subsequent trials (Johansson & Westling, 1988).

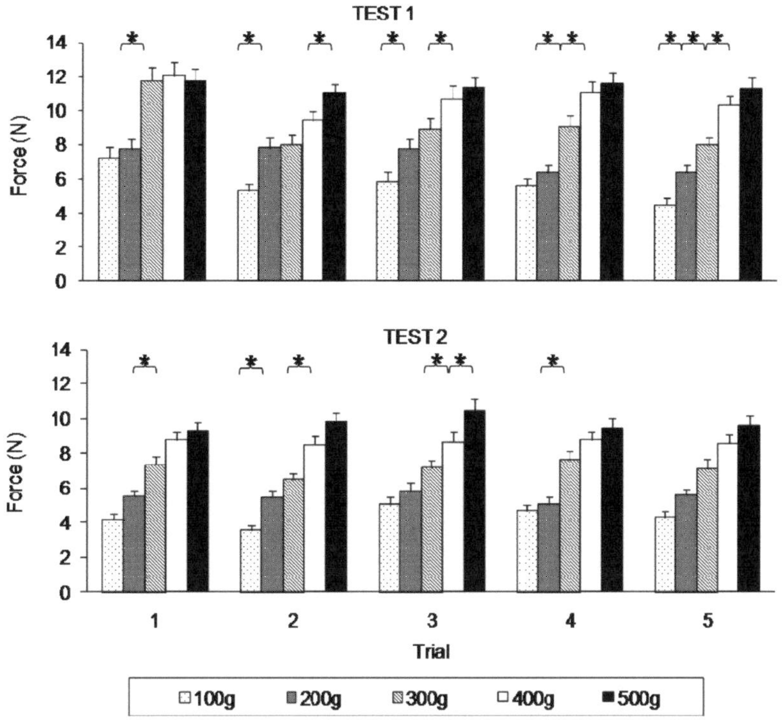

Fig. 3. Test by trial by mass interaction for peak grip force in Study 1 (all asterisks represent significant differences between adjacent masses within each trial set)

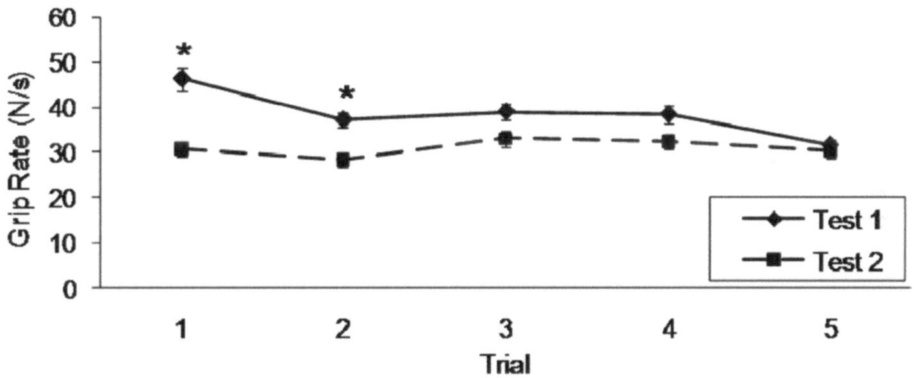

Fig. 4. Test by trial interaction for peak rate of grip force production in Study 1 (all asterisks represent significant differences between trials when compared across tests)

Load force

There was the expected main effect for object mass in the analysis of **peak load force**, F (4, 88) = 1084.5, p < .01 where load force increased as a function of object mass. The group by test interaction, F (1, 22) = 5.9, p < .05, for the analysis of peak load force showed that for the Fatigued Group, peak load force did not differ between test 1 (1.95 N, SE = .05 N) and test 2 (1.95, SE = .04 N). However, for the Control Group, peak load force decreased from test 1 (2.05, SE = .05 N) to test 2 (1.90, SE = .05 N). This is some evidence that the Fatigued Group may have been engaged in some sort of compensatory strategy in response to the muscle fatigue they were experiencing. The group by trial interaction, $F(4, 88) = 3.4$, $p < .01$, depicted in Fig. 5 showed that for the Control Group, peak load force in trial 1 was significantly higher than trials 1 and 2 for the Fatigued Group. However, by trial 2, both groups elicited the same peak load forces.

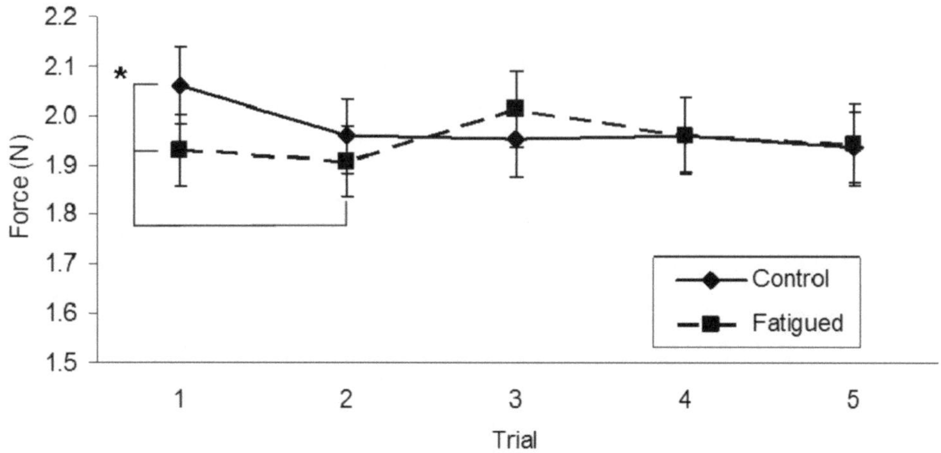

Fig. 5. Group by trial interaction for peak load force in Study 1 (asterisks represent significant differences between groups for each trial)

MVC data

The analysis of the maximum voluntary contraction data revealed that the Fatigued Group had a reduction in maximum force output immediately following fatiguing exercise but recovered to resting levels at the end of the second lifting session ($p < .05$). See Table 2 for means and standard errors.

Fatigued Group			
Time of MVC Test	**Mean (N)**	**SE**	
Prior to Fatiguing Protocol	45.00	2.00	*
Following the Fatiguing Protocol	37.17	1.98	*
At the End of Test 2	43.83	2.49	
Control Group			
In Between Test 1 and Test 2	47.17	2.43	
At the End of Test 2	46.92	2.80	

Table 2. Means and standard errors for MVC data in Study 1 (significant differences have been marked by asterisks)

3. Study 2

The aim of this study was to examine the effects of neuromuscular fatigue during a precision grip lifting task when object *mass* and *size* were manipulated.

3.1 Rationale

Specifically, the purpose of Study 2 was to determine whether fatigue alters the ability of participants to appropriately scale their force characteristics in anticipation when size cues about object mass are provided (Gordon et al., 1993; Wolpert & Kawato, 1998). The intent of this experiment was to answer the following question: Will participants be able to utilize the appropriate sensorimotor representations and therefore, correctly anticipate the mass of the lifted objects after their motor control systems have been compromised by fatigue? It was thought that the same motor representations would be available while in a fatigued state, but it was unclear whether the retrieval of these motor representations would be affected by fatigue.

Similar motor effects to those hypothesized in Study 1 were expected to be present in this study. However, it was thought that, in this study, grip forces would likely remain scaled to object mass after the fatiguing protocol. Force scaling was expected because participants could now use the association of visual size information to object mass along with the pre-fatiguing protocol lifts to formulate the appropriate motor commands. Although scaling was expected to be present, it was still probable that participants would show a reduced force output for all levels of object mass in comparison to the pre-fatigued lifting session. However, the possibility remained that participants would be able to use fatigue as a parameter to update the internal models associated with each of the lifted objects. If this was true, no differences should be found in the motor responses between both control and fatigued groups both in the pre-fatigue test and post-fatigue test lifting conditions. Another measure of particular interest was the rate of grip force generation. It was expected that participants would scale their grip rates as they do their grip forces in this study. Thus, the heavier the object the higher the peak grip rate. This measure happens very early in the lift and can be classified as an anticipatory force control measure as it gives insight into the motor program that was selected for a particular lift based on pre-contact visual information and/or post-contact sensorimotor information from a previous lift (Flanagan et al., 2001; Gordon et al., 1993; Johansson & Westling, 1988). It was expected that, with visual cues, the fatigued group would produce lower overall peak grip rates but would scale them appropriately following fatiguing exercise.

3.2 Methods

Other than the changes listed below, the methods for Study 2 were identical to Study 1.

Participants

Twenty-four naïve, right-handed individuals with normal uncorrected or corrected visual acuity and no reported previous history of upper limb neuromuscular injuries participated (none of whom participated in Study 1). There were 6 males and 6 females (ages 19-28 years) in the Fatigued Group and 6 males and 6 females (ages 22-47 years) in the Control Group.

Apparatus

Five wooden blocks with a common density of 1.0 g^1 cm^{-3} served as the objects to be lifted as this is a good approximation of the densities encountered when dealing with everyday handheld objects (Flanagan & Beltzner, 2000; Gordon et al., 1993). Refer to Table 3 for the masses and sizes of the objects used to achieve the common density.

Object	Mass (g)	Length of Side (cm)	Volume (cm³)	Density (g/cm³)
1	100	4.64	100	1
2	200	5.85	200	1
3	300	6.69	300	1
4	400	7.37	400	1
5	500	7.94	500	1

Table 3. Properties of objects used in Study 2

3.3 Results and Discussion

Grip force

As seen in Fig. 6, the interaction of test by mass by trial, F (16, 352) = 4.71, $p < .01$, revealed that for the first trial of the first test, participants had difficulty scaling their forces as they produced the same peak forces for the 100 g and 200 g objects, and elicited too much force for the 300 g object while scaling forces appropriate to the 400 g and 500 g objects. On all subsequent trials, for both tests, participants were generally able to scale their forces according to object mass. This pattern was very similar to that seen in Study 1. Also, as in Study 1, there was an overall decrease in peak grip force for test 2 in comparison to test 1.

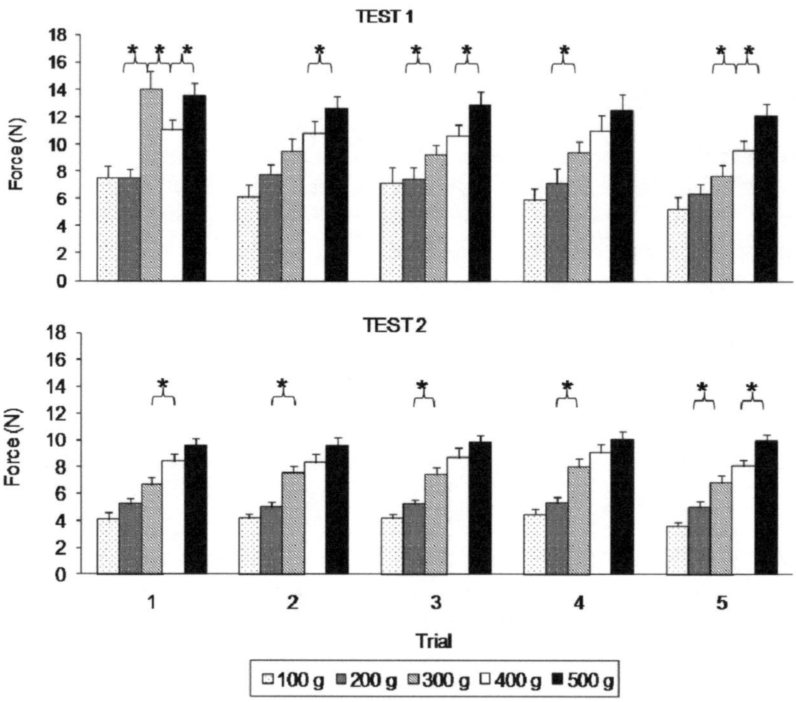

Fig. 6. Test by trial by mass interaction for peak grip force in Study 2 (asterisks represent differences between each mass level within each trial set)

The significant three way interaction of test, trial and group for the analysis of the **peak rate of grip force production,** F (4,88) = 2.98, $p < .05$, showed that peak grip rates increased as object size increased. This was expected as congruent visual information was available in this study such that participants could anticipate object mass. As seen in Fig. 7, the Fatigued Group produced lower peak grip rates on trials 1, 3 and 4 of test 2 in comparison to those same trials in test 1. For the Control Group, only trials 2 and 3 were different in test 2 when compared to those same trials of test 1.

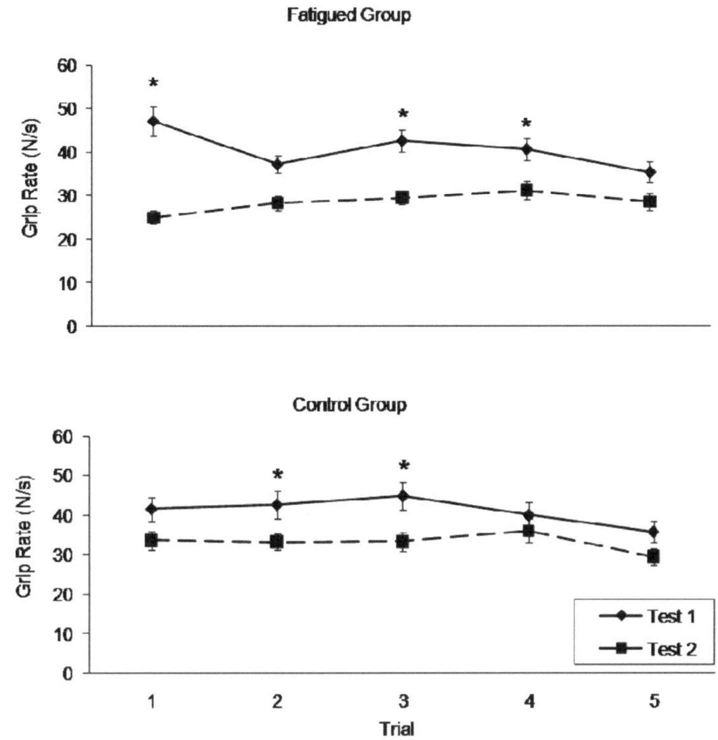

Fig. 7. Group by test by trial interactions for peak rate of grip force production in Study 2 (asterisks represent differences between corresponding trials of test 1 and test 2)

The three-way test by mass by trial interaction, $F(16, 352) = 2.29$, $p < .01$, revealed that for the first trial set of the first test, participants had difficulty scaling their peak grip rates as they produced the same peak grip rates for the 100 g, 200 g, 400 g, and 500 g objects and produced higher peak grip rates for the 300 g object (Fig. 8). However, on all subsequent trials, for both tests, participants were generally able to scale their peak grip rates according to object mass. In addition, overall lower peak grip rates were recorded over all trials and all levels of mass in test 2 (see Fig. 8).

The patterns discussed above and illustrated in the figures provide evidence that participants were successfully able to anticipate the masses of the objects they were lifting after the first trial. This was made possible by providing congruent visual size cues; i.e. the larger objects were heavier. Also, it is important to note the differences between the Fatigued and Control Groups in the group by test by trial interaction. In contrast to Study 1 where no group effects were shown, this study showed the fatiguing protocol to affect the way participants generated peak grip rates.

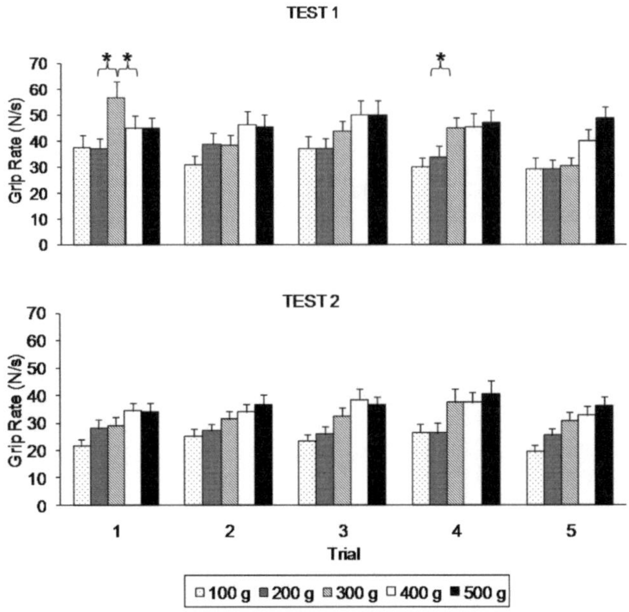

Fig. 8. Test by trial by mass interactions for peak rate of grip force production in Study 2 (asterisks signify differences between masses within each trial set)

Load force

The analysis of **peak load force** showed a two-way interaction of group by mass, F (4,88) = 3.39, $p < .05$, and a three-way interaction of test by mass by trial, F (16, 352) = 1.84, $p < .05$. The group by mass interaction showed that participants in the Fatigued Group produced less peak load force for the 400 g object (see Fig. 9). Although significance was only found between groups for the 400 g object, this finding provides some evidence that the Fatigued Group participants may have had more difficulty lifting the heavier objects. The three-way test by mass by trial interaction mimicked the previous findings with this interaction in that peak load forces stabilized after one exposure to all levels of mass. No differences in peak load forces were experienced in test 2 when compared to test 1 (see Fig. 10).

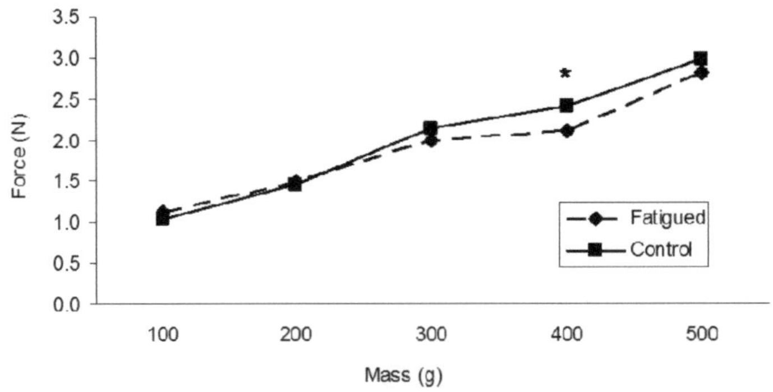

Fig. 9. Group by mass interactions for peak load force in Study 2 (significant differences in load force between groups at each level of mass are shown by an asterisk)

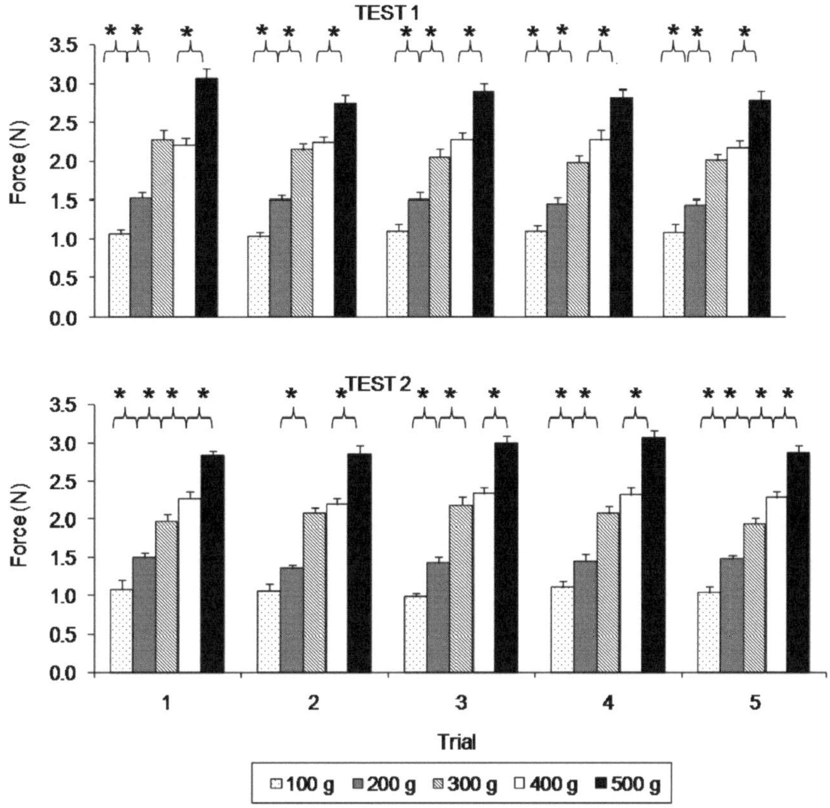

Fig. 10. Test by mass by trial interaction for peak load force in Study 2 (asterisks represent significant differences between masss within each trial set)

MVC data

The analysis of the maximum voluntary contraction data revealed that the Fatigued Group had a reduction in maximum force output immediately following fatiguing exercise but recovered to resting levels at the end of the second lifting session ($p < .05$). See Table 4 for means and standard errors.

Fatigued Group			
Time of MVC Test	**Mean (N)**	**SE**	
Prior to Fatiguing Protocol	46.08	2.28	*
Following the Fatiguing Protocol	38.17	1.80	
At the End of Test 2	41.83	2.58	
Control Group			
In Between Test 1 and Test 2	47.25	3.23	
At the End of Test 2	47.33	1.84	

Table 4. Means and standard errors for MVC data in Study 2 (significant differences have been marked by asterisks)

4. General Discussion

4.1 Summary of Results

Study 1 - Same Sized Objects

Regardless of the group, all participants in Study 1 appropriately scaled their grip forces to the mass of the lifted objects after a quick one trial adaptation. Therefore, after each object had been presented once, participants were able to scale their grip force outputs on subsequent trials. These findings are consistent with previous results by Johansson and Westling (1988) and Gordon et al. (1993). In the pre-fatigue test trials, peak grip rates were higher for the first and second trials and stabilized on subsequent trials whereas for the post-fatigue test, peak grip rate remained stable throughout all trials. Therefore, after a short familiarization period, participants were able to generate grip forces at a suitable rate for the mass of the lifted objects. All of these findings have been reported in previous literature (Gordon et al., 1993; Johansson & Westling, 1984; 1988). In addition, peak grip force outputs were generally lower over all levels of mass in each trial after the 20 minute break.

Peak load force showed that participants in the Fatigued Group produced lower peak load forces on trial one when compared to the Control Group for that same trial. In addition, it was found that the magnitudes of the peak load forces were linked to the masses of the objects in that the 500 g object produced the highest load force. This result is consistent with previous findings (Johansson & Westling, 1984; 1988).

Study 2 – Different Sized Objects

As in Study 1, participants appropriately scaled their peak grip forces to the mass of the lifted objects after the first exposure to all five masses. In addition, peak grip force was reduced immediately following the 20 minute break. Interestingly, after analyzing peak rate of grip force production it was found that participants in the Fatigued Group produced lower peak grip rates following the fatiguing protocol, but recovered by the fifth trial. The Control Group produced slightly lower peak grip rates following their 20 minute rest period; however, the differences were not as profound as those differences shown by the Fatigued Group. These findings suggest that the fatiguing protocol affected the participants' ability to achieve peak grip rate now that they could anticipate object mass. Also, participants in this study were able to scale their grip rates according to the size and mass of the presented objects. Therefore, participants appeared to be anticipating object mass as peak grip rate happens extremely early in the lift (Gordon et al., 1991a; b; c; Gordon et al., 1993; Johansson & Westling, 1984; 1988).

4.2 Revisiting the hypotheses

Study 1 - Same Sized Objects

Was there a reduction in overall force output following the fatiguing protocol? No. Participants in the Fatigued Group were not affected by the fatiguing protocol as no differences were found between test 1 and test 2 for peak grip force, peak rate of grip force generation or peak load force. The Fatigued Group and the Control Group behaved the same way for each of the abovementioned measures in this study.

Was there a reduction in the ability to control force output following fatiguing exercise? No. Following fatiguing exercise, participants appropriately scaled their peak grip and load forces to object mass. Therefore, it appears that participants in this study were able to detect mass differences and adjust their forces accordingly, regardless of their group assignment.

Study 2 - Different Sized Objects

Was there a reduction in overall force output but intact force scaling now that participants could anticipate object mass from visual cues? Or, could participants update their internal representations with their newly fatigued state and thus, compensate for their fatigued state? A reduction in overall force output was shown in this study as participants in the Fatigued Group produced less force during the static hold phase of the lift immediately following the fatiguing protocol.

Why did the fatiguing protocol affect each study differently?

The fatiguing protocol affected participants differently in each of the two studies. In Study 1 where the masses were visually identical, fatigue had no effect on motor control processes; however, in Study 2 where size cues were provided about object mass, significant fatiguing effects were produced. Why? To account for these differences, it is suggested that in the first study, movements were made using on-line feedback rather than anticipatory movement strategies like those used in Study 2. Thus, it appears that when movements are made on-line, any strength decreases that exist due to fatigue are detected and more force is generated. However, when movements are anticipated, the internal model does not take into account muscle fatigue and lower force output results. It is suggested that, in a fatigued state, participants who can anticipate movements use a feed-forward anticipatory strategy and are reluctant to switch to an on-line strategy once the feed-forward model has been selected and initiated.

As mentioned, there were no effects of fatigue for Study 1 and participants recovered from fatigue by the last trial of test 2 in Study 2. It is possible that, in Study 1, larger motor units were recruited to compensate for the effects of neuromuscular fatigue developed in the smaller motor units. Although this allowed for the same forces to be achieved, reduced fine motor control is associated with use of large motor units. Thus, fatiguing effects may have been found if the task involved an increased level of manual manipulation or finger dexterity.

In Study 2 there was no sign of force compensation directly following the fatiguing exercise. It could be argued that the gradual recovery observed over trials in this study was related to the adjustments made by the motor control system to switch from the smaller fatigued motor units to larger ones. Therefore, instead of recovery from fatigue, the adjustments made to achieve baseline levels of force by the end of Study 2 could be a result of compensatory strategies performed by the neuromuscular system to overcome the effects of fatigue. A better understanding of these physiological adjustments could be revealed using physiological stimulation techniques.

It can be disputed that the movements made in Study 1 were not purely on-line as participants were able to use vision to discern characteristics of the boxes they were lifting. Due to the strong influence of vision on human movement, it would be interesting to repeat the same experimental paradigm in the absence of vision. This could be achieved by eliminating vision entirely from Study 1, and by using haptic cues instead of visual cues about object size in Study 2. The influence of vision was quite evident in the present findings; however, would the same results be found if participants could only use their haptic system to anticipate object mass?

To our present understanding, no prior studies have incorporated a Control Group into this type of study design. For example, a study by Cote et al., (2002) suggested that when dealing with local neuromuscular fatigue, the dominant strategy is to maintain the output of the task, but to change the recruitment patterns of the muscles involved in producing the motor task. These researchers had participants saw through logs before and after fatiguing exercise. When differences were detected between the pre-test and post-test data, conclusions were drawn that the changes were due to fatigue. Could it be that participants had time to figure out how to better utilize their body configuration to more efficiently saw the log in the time they had between pre-test and post-test data collections? Adding a Control Group to this study would confirm that the findings were indeed due to fatigue.

Nature of fatiguing protocol

The task specific fatiguing exercise used in this experiment was meant to elicit local neuromuscular fatigue of the index finger and thumb. The fatiguing protocol was to be aggressive enough to elicit an increased level of low frequency fatigue as the effects of this type of fatigue last longer than those of high frequency fatigue (Edwards et al., 1977; Fuglevand et al., 1999; Lehman, 1997; Schwendner et al., 1995). The fatiguing protocol used in this experiment has been validated and used in studies evaluating the vastus lateralis musculature of the leg (Fowles et al., 2002). It would be beneficial to validate the protocol for use with a precision grasp, but because of the complicated anatomy of the human hand, it was difficult to isolate the muscles involved by means of superficial stimulation techniques. Thus, in the future it would be favorable to validate the fatiguing protocol for use specifically on the human hand using fine wire electrode stimulation techniques such as those used by Fuglevand et al. (1999). Adding this component to the present investigations would strengthen the argument that any differences found could indeed be attributed to the neuromuscular changes induced by the fatiguing exercise and not by some other intermediary factor.

Additionally, future studies that use a precision grasp lifting task should attempt to fatigue the wrist as well as the digits involved with the grasp. Incorporating fatigue at the wrist would make the fatiguing task and motor task more closely related as all of the musculature involved with a grasp to lift movement would now be fatigued.

5. Conclusion

Fatigue affected anticipatory and on-line motor control tasks differently. Only the anticipatory task was shown to be affected by fatigue as the motor control observations yielded differences after fatiguing exercise. Participants were unable to update their internal representations to take into account their newly fatigued state and were reluctant to switch to on-line strategies after initiating the lift.

6. References

Alderman, R.B. (1965). Influence of local fatigue on speed and accuracy in motor learning. *Research Quarterly* Vol. 36, 131-140

Abbs, J.H.; Gracco, V.L. & Cole, K.J. (1984). Control of multimovement coordination: Sensorimotor mechanisms in speech motor programming. *Journal of Motor Behavior,* Vol. 16, No. 2, 195-232

Bigland-Ritchie, B. (1984). Changes in muscle contractile properties and neural control during human muscular fatigue. *Muscle and Nerve,* Vol. 7, 691-699

Burgess, P.R. & Jones, L.F. (1997). Perceptions of effort and heaviness during fatigue and during the size-weight illusion. *Somatosensory & Motor Research,* Vol. 14, No. 3, 189-202

Carron, A.V. (1972). Motor performance and learning under physical fatigue. *Medicine & Science in Sports,* Vol. 4, 101-106

Carron, A.V. & Ferchuck, A.D. (1971). The effect of fatigue on learning and performance of a gross motor task. *Journal of Motor Behavior,* Vol. 3, 62-68

Clarkson, P.M.; Nosaka, K. & Braun, B. (1992). Muscle function after exercise-induced muscle damage and rapid adaptation. *Medicine & Science in Sports & Exercise,* Vol. 24, No. 5, 512-520

Cote, J.N.; Mathieu, P.A.; Levin, M.F. & Feldman, A.G. (2002). Movement reorganization to compensate for fatigue during sawing. *Experimental Brain Research,* Vol. 146, 394-398

Dennerlein, J.T.; Ciriello, V.M.; Kerin, K.J. & Johnson, P.W. (2003). Fatigue in the forearm resulting from low-level repetitive ulnar deviation. *AIHA Journal,* Vol. 64, 799-805

Edwards, R.H.T.; Hill, D.K.; Jones, D.A. & Merton, P.A. (1977). Fatigue of long duration in human skeletal muscle after exercise. *The Journal of Physiology,* Vol. 272, 769-778

Flanagan, J.R. & Beltzner, M.A. (2000). Independence of perceptual and sensorimotor predictions in the size-weight illusion. *Nature Neuroscience,* Vol. 3, 737-741

Flanagan, J.R.; King, S.; Wolpert, D.M. & Johansson, R.S. (2001). Sensorimotor prediction and memory in object manipulation. *Canadian Journal of Experimental Psychology,* Vol. 55, No. 2, 87-95

Fowles, J.R.; Green, H.J.; Tupling, R.; O'Brien, S. & Roy, B.D. (2002). Human neuromuscular fatigue is associated with altered Na^+-K^+-ATPase activity following isometric exercise. *Journal of Applied Physiology,* Vol. 92, 1585-1593

Franzblau, A.; Faschner, D.; Albers, J.W.; Blitz, S.; Werner, R. & Armstrong, T. (1993). Medical screening of office workers for upper extremity cumulative trauma disorders. *Archives of Environmental Health,* Vol. 48, No. 3, 164-170

Fuglevand, A.J.; Macefield, V.G. & Bigland-Ritchie, B. (1999). Force-frequency and fatigue properties of motor units in muscles that control digits of the human hand. *Journal of Neurophysiology,* Vol. 81, 1718-1729

Godwin, M.A. & Schmidt, R.A. (1971). Muscular fatigue and learning a discrete motor skill. *Research Quarterly,* Vol. 42, 374-381

Gordon, A.M.; Forssberg, R.S.; Johansson, R.S. & Westling, G. (1991a). Visual size cues in the programming of manipulative forces during precision grip. *Experimental Brain Research,* Vol. 83, 477-482

Gordon, A.M.; Forssberg, R.S.; Johansson, R.S. & Westling, G. (1991b). The integration of haptically acquired size information in the programming of precision grip. *Experimental Brain Research,* Vol. 83, 483-488

Gordon, A.M.; Forssberg, R.S.; Johansson, R.S. & Westling, G. (1991c). Integration of sensory information during the programming of precision grip: comments on the contributions of size cues. *Experimental Brain Research*, Vol. 85, 226-229

Gordon, A.M.; Westling, G.; Cole, K.J. & Johansson, R.S. (1993). Memory representations underlying motor commands used during manipulation of common and novel objects. *Journal of Neurophysiology*, Vol. 69, 1789–1796

Johansson, G.W. & Westling, G. (1984). Roles of glabrous skin receptors and sensorimotor memory in automatic control of precision grip when lifting rougher of more slippery objects. *Experimental Brain Research*, Vol. 56, 550-564

Johansson, G.W. & Westling, G. (1988). Coordinated isometric muscle commands adequately and erroneously programmed for the weight during lifting task with precision grip. *Experimental Brain Research*, Vol. 71, 59-71

Johansson, R.S. & Westling, G. (1990). Tactile afferent signals in the control of precision grip. *Attention & Performance*, Vol. 13, 677–713

Lehman, S.L. (1997). Mechanisms and measurement of muscle fatigue during repeated loading. *Proceedings of Marconi Research Conference*, Marshall, CA.

Lin, M-I.; Liang, H-W.; Lin, K-H.; Hwang & Y-H. (2004). Electromyographical assessment on muscular fatigue - and elaboration upon repetitive typing activity. *Journal of Electromyography and Kinesiology*, Vol. 14, 661-669

Nakata, M.; Hagner, I-M. & Jonsson, B. (1992). Perceived musculoskeletal discomfort and electromyography during repetitive light work. *Journal of Electromyography and Kinesiology*, Vol. 2, No. 2, 103-111

Pack, D.M.; Cotton, D.J. & Biasiotto, J. (1974). Effect of four fatigue levels on performance and learning of a novel dynamic balance skill. *Journal of Motor Behavior*, Vol. 6, 191-197

Schmidt, R.A. (1969). Performance and learning a gross motor skill under conditions of artificially-induced fatigue. *Research Quarterly*, Vol. 40, 85-190

Schwendner, K.I.; Mikesky, A.E.; Wigglesworth, J.K. & Burr, D.B. (1995). Recovery of dynamic muscle function following isokinetic fatigue testing. *International Journal of Sports Medicine*, Vol. 16, 185-189

Stock, S.R. (1991). Workplace ergonomic factors and the development of musculoskeletal disorders of the neck and upper limbs: a meta-analysis. *American Journal of Industrial Medicine*, Vol. 21, No. 6, 895-897

Thomas, J.R.; Cotton, D.J.; Spieth, W.R. & Abraham, N.L. (1975). Effects of fatigue on stabilometer performance and learning of males and females. *Medicine & Science in Sports*, Vol. 7, 203-206

Uhrich, M.L.; Underwood, R.A.; Standeven, J.W.; Soper, N.J. & Engsberg, J.R. (2002). Assessment of fatigue, monitor placement, and surgical experience during simulated laparoscopic surgery. *Surgical Endoscopy*, Vol. 16, 635-639

Valero-Cuevas, F.J.; Zajac, F.E. & Burgar, C.G. (1998). Large indexfingertip forces are produced by subject-independent patterns of muscle excitation. *Journal of Biomechanics*, Vol. 31, 693–703

Whitley, J.D. (1973). Effects of increasing inertial resistance on performance and learning of a training task. *Research Quarterly*, Vol. 44, 1-11

Wolpert, D.M. & Kawato, M. (1998). Multiple paired forward and inverse models for motor control. *Neural Networks*, Vol. 11, 1317–132

Neuromuscular Analysis as a Guideline in designing Shared Control

Abbink D.A. and Mulder M.
Delft University of Technology
The Netherlands

1. Introduction

The challenges in designing human-machine interaction have been around for decades: how to combine the intelligence and creativity of humans with the precision and strength of machines? It is well known that manual control tasks are prone to human errors. The conventional engineering solution is to either fully automate a (sub)task or to support the human with alerting systems. Both approaches have inherent limitations, widely described in literature (e.g., Pritchett, 2001; Sheridan, 2002).
Recently, an alternative solution is receiving increased attention: that of shared control. In the shared control paradigm, an intelligent system continually shares the control authority with the human controller. The idea behind shared control is to keep the human operator in the direct manual control loop, while providing continuous support. Shared control has been investigated for a wide range of applications, for example during the direct control of automobiles (e.g., Griffiths & Gillespie, 2005; Mulder et al., 2008a&b) and aircraft (e.g., Goodrich et al., 2008), or during tele-operated control to support gripping (Griffin et al., 2005), surgery (e.g, Kragic et al., 2005), micro-assembly (e.g, Basdogan et al., 2007) or the steering of unmanned aerial vehicles (e.g., Mung et al., 2009).

There is no strict definition of shared control, but the systems described in literature can be classified in two categories (see Figure 1 for an illustration):

1. "input-mixing shared control", which influences the input to the controlled system
2. "haptic shared control", which influences the forces on the control interface

Shared control of the first category shapes the input to the controlled system to be a mix of the output of the control interface (as a result of human input) and the output of an automation system. An example is the lane-keeping assistance system based on a potential-field approach (Switkes et al., 2006), in which a desired tyre angle is controlled by a steer-by-wire system, which combines the driver's desired steering angle with the steering angle from the assistance system. In other words, when the driver's actions agree with the goal of the assistance system, the system generates no additional steering input. But when the driver disagrees with the assistance system (i.e., steers out of the lane), an additional steering input is generated by the steer-by-wire system so that the command to the tyres will ensure good lane-keeping performance. Note that in this case, there can not be a direct mechanical coupling between steering wheel angle and tyres. It is also important to realize that the driver cannot overrule the system, and may not even be aware of the system's activity, especially when there is no force information.

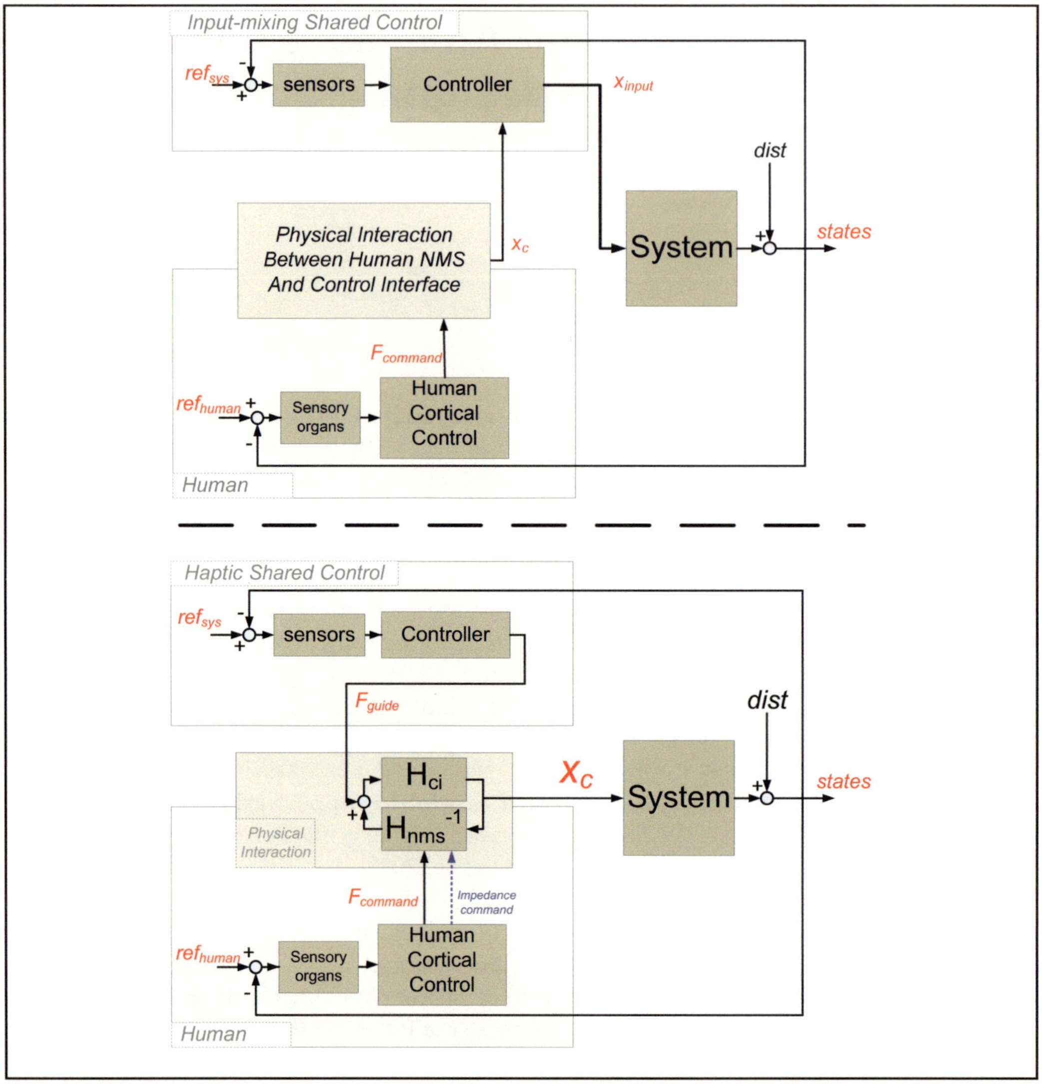

Fig. 1. A schematic, symmetric representation of both categories of shared control: input-mixing (top) and haptic shared control. In both cases, the human and system have sensors to perceive changes in system states (possibly perturbed by *dist*), each having a goal (ref_{human} and ref_{sys}, respectively). During input-mixing shared control, the steering output X_c is weighed by the controller that determines the input to the system. During haptic shared control, both human and system can act with forces on the control interface (with $F_{command}$ and F_{guide} respectively). Through physical interaction, the control interface (H_{ci}) exchanges force and position with the human limb (H_{nms}), of which the neuromuscular impedance can be adapted.

Shared control of the second category allows both the human and the support system to exert forces on a control interface, of which its output (its position) remains the direct input to the controlled system. These systems are sometimes called haptic guidance systems, or force feedback systems and are essentially dynamic extensions from the static 'virtual fixtures' approach (Rosenberg, 1993). A good example is a lane-keeping assistance system in which a motor acts on the steering wheel by adding torques (Griffiths & Gillespie, 2005; Forsyth & MacLean, 2006; Brandt et al, 2008; Mulder et al., 2008b). Note that the relationship between steering angle and tyre angle remains constant, which has been found to be important for vehicular steering (Toffin et al., 2007). Moreover, the driver is not only aware of the system's actions, but can also choose to overrule the system's activity. Part of the driver's neuromuscular response to the feedback forces is passive (due to limb inertia), but it is well known that humans can greatly influence their effective stiffness and damping through muscle (co-)contraction and reflexive feedback.

The influence of neuromuscular adaptability in shared control is acknowledged in most literature, but not well understood. As a result, the tuning of the feedback forces is a trial-and-error process. This process is further complicated by the fact that there is a (probably subject-dependent) trade-off between good performance with a dominant system authority and mediocre performance with less system authority. Although in general the reported shared control systems provided beneficial results such as improved performance and reduced mental load, negative effects were reported as well that seem to indicate that forces were tuned too high. Many subjects did not feel completely in control (e.g., Forsyth & MacLean, 2006), and it was somewhat difficult for subjects to avoid collisions not foreseen by the system (e.g., Griffith & Gillespie, 2005). Lacking quantitative knowledge of neuromuscular response to forces, it is quite difficult to optimally design the feedback forces.

The underlying hypothesis in the current study is that measurements and models of the neuromuscular system will improve the understanding of human response to forces, and thereby, the design of haptic shared control (which will be the focus of this chapter).
Although much relevant knowledge is available in the field of neuroscience, the haptic community has left this knowledge largely unused for shared control design. Therefore, this chapter has the following goals:

1. to provide a brief introduction on human motion control for shared control researchers
2. to provide a novel architecture for shared control systems, based on human motion control models
3. to provide quantitative measurements for the neuromuscular properties for steering
4. to show how much neuromuscular feedback properties influence the steering behaviour during shared control.

In section 2, the brief introduction to human motion control is presented along with the novel shared control architecture. In section 3, the experimental methods will be shown for two experiments that address the third and fourth goal, respectively. Section 4 contains the experimental results. Section 5 will discuss the results, and finally in Section 6 the conclusions will be presented.

2. Neuromuscular control and shared control

2.1 Overview of neuromuscular control

Humans have the ability to adapt their neuromuscular system to the physical environment they interact with, through both feed-forward control and feedback control. For example, humans can learn fast and efficient goal-directed movements, and can realize these same movements with different levels of muscle co-contractions, in order to provide additional stability.

Feedback control of neuromuscular mechanisms, is often called impedance control (Hogan, 1984). Adaptations in impedance control do not only arise from changes in muscle-contraction, but also from changes in afferent feedback. Afferent feedback provides the nervous system with information about muscle stretch and stretch velocity (through muscle spindles) and muscle force (through Golgi Tendon Organs), and has been shown to substantially contribute to impedance control (e.g., Doemges and Rack 1992b, Mugge et al., 2009). Note that afferent feedback is much more energy-efficient than muscle co-contraction.

Impedance control is experimentally investigated by perturbing a limb, and measuring the mechanical and electromyographical responses. Literature shows that these responses are very adaptable, and depend on task instruction (e.g., Hammond 1956; Doemges and Rack 1992b; Abbink 2007), the level of muscle (co-)contraction (Jaeger et al. 1982), the displacement amplitude (Stein and Kearney 1995), the frequency content in the perturbation signal (Van der Helm et al. 2002, Mugge et al. 2007) and the mechanical load which the subject interacts with (De Vlugt et al. 2002).

Goal-directed control is hotly debated in literature, specifically whether it can better be explained by internal model control theories (e.g., Wolpert et al., 1998) or equilibrium-point control theories (e.g., Feldman et al, 1990). Recent studies have provided evidence that internal model control and impedance control can operate as separate mechanisms for motor control (Osu et al., 2002), and are both active during learning of new movements (Franklin et al., 2003). Results show substantial muscle co-contraction when faced with motion tasks in novel environments, which decreases when the task has been learned (after several repetitions), suggesting that impedance control assists in the formation of the inverse model, and provides stability during the learning process. Note that, theoretically, from an energy point of view, it would be optimal to have no co-contraction during well-learned goal directed movements when no perturbations are present. However, it has been suggested that some level of co-contraction is needed to overcome internal perturbations, from sensor and motor control noise (Osu et al., 2004).

This body of knowledge has unfortunately been largely ignored in haptic shared control design. It is common in human manual control literature to disregard impedance control. The neuromuscular system is often described either as a gain, or at best as a second-order low-pass filter, focusing on its role in limiting the position bandwidth of the control interface (e.g., McRuer & Jex, 1967; Keen & Cole, 2006). However, through impedance control of the neuromuscular system, human operators can respond much faster to forces on their control interface than visual or vestibular cues would allow. For example, through muscle co-contraction and reflexive feedback drivers can respond to steering wheel forces that arise from road irregularities, faster (i.e., at a higher bandwidth) than through slower visual feedback.

There are only a few studies that have evaluated neuromuscular feedback in the design of a haptic shared control system: only for car-following (Abbink, 2006) and for unmanned aerial vehicle control (Lam et al, 2009). Unsupported manual control has received slightly more interest: for example, neuromuscular models and measurements have been developed for side-stick control for aircraft (Van Paassen, 1995), gas pedal control (Abbink, 2007) and steering (Pick & Cole, 2007; Pick & Cole, 2008) for automobiles. Typically, the research approach consists of performing a separate experiment in which the response to perturbations is measured, usually during tasks where the subject is instructed to "relax / do nothing", or to "resist the perturbations" during postural tasks. The response is then characterized by a mass-spring-damper model, and subsequently used in model predictions. Recent work has shown that subjects can not only resist forces or relax, they can also decide to actively give way to forces (Abbink, 2006; Abbink, 2007), thereby decreasing their mechanical impedance even below relaxed impedance. Accurate (mechanical and electromyographical) measurements, closed-loop identification and advanced model parameterization techniques have shown that giving way to forces can be accomplished by Golgi Tendon Organ reflex activity (Abbink, 2006; Mugge et al, 2009).

In short, there is ample evidence that:

- manual control tasks require both feed-forward control and impedance control
- impedance control is not only achieved through muscle co-contraction but through afferent feedback as well.

How can we use this knowledge when analysing and designing shared control systems?

2.1 Shared Control based on knowledge of Neuromuscular Control

The main goal of haptic shared control is to keep the human in the loop and provide forces that will continuously assist the human, improving task performance at reduced levels of physical or mental load. Consequently, forces should not be experienced as a perturbation that has to be opposed through impedance control. From an energy perspective it would be optimal if the human is completely relaxed (no muscle co-contractions) in face of forces from the shared control system. However, the forces could also be designed so that subjects can actively give way to them, using their reflexive system for fast responses and little co-contraction. This idea was explored in our group during a research project sponsored by Nissan Motor Co., in which a continuous haptic support system for car following was developed (Abbink, 2006; Mulder et al., 2007). It was designed so that drivers could keep the distance to a lead vehicle constant if they kept the force on the gas pedal constant, thereby reducing control activity and muscle activity while maintaining the same car-following performance. Neuromuscular analyses provided evidence that subjects were indeed giving way (reduced mechanical impedance) when interacting with the haptic support system, and did so using Golgi Tendon Organ activity.

Can we use this kind of analysis already in the design phase of shared control systems? A biologically inspired shared control system would need a good internal representation of the environmental dynamics it is interacting with, more specifically: the impedance of the human operator's limb that is mechanically coupled to the control interface. Then, if the goals of the system and the human coincide, there will be a low-impedance interaction that will be beneficial to the human in terms of performance and control effort.

Moreover, a shared control system that is modelled after human motion control could not only generate forces, but could also adapt its impedance. In this way a smooth shifting of control authority can be realized, the benefits of which have been shown experimentally (Abbink & Mulder, 2009).

The generalized architecture for the proposed haptic shared control is presented in Figure 2.

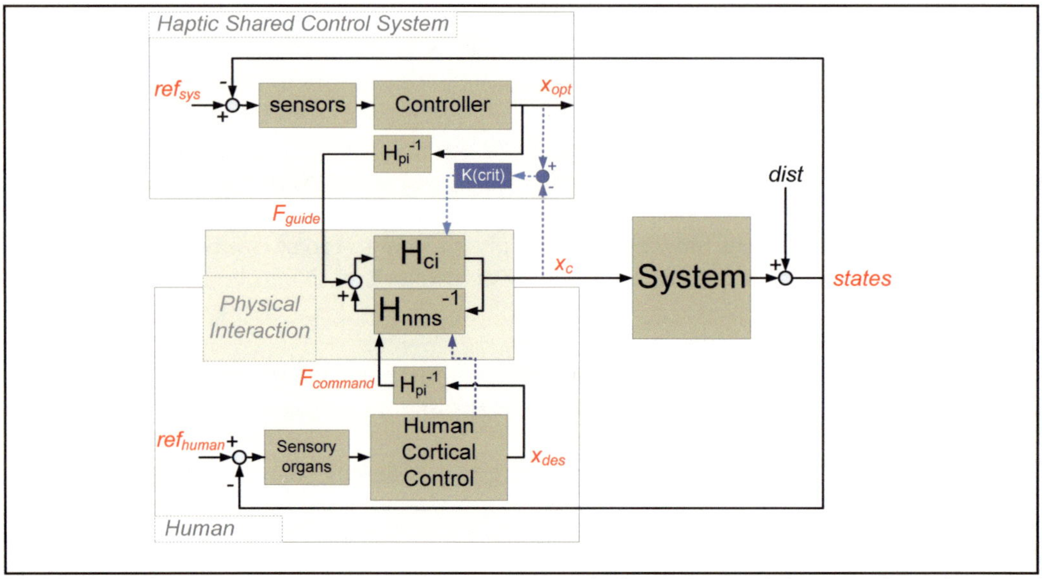

Fig. 2. A schematic, symmetric representation of the proposed haptic shared control architecture based on neuromuscular knowledge. The human operator can generate force ($F_{command}$) and adapt the impedance of her/his neuromuscular system H_{nms} (dotted line). Likewise, the system can not only generate force (F_{guide}) but also adapt the impedance of the control interface H_{ci} (shown by dotted line), for example changes in stiffness based on some criticality function K(crit). Moreover, the system needs to have a good internal representation of the total physical interaction dynamics (H_{pi}) just like the human.

Consider an application for lane-keeping. The support system needs sensor information from the road and car states relative to the road as an input for a control model that continuously calculates the optimal steering angle x_{opt}. Such a control model could be based on potential fields or optimal control, but perhaps an actual representation of a skilled, attentive driver would yield the best driver acceptance.
Note that this optimal control input x_{opt} could be used directly to control the vehicle, which would result in automation. But since the purpose is to share control, x_{opt} will, instead, be translated to a guiding force F_{guide}, which, by itself, would cause the steering wheel to move to that optimal angle x_{opt}. If there would be no driver to hold the steering wheel, the system would need to know only the steering wheel dynamics H_{ci} (in a linear case: stiffness, damping and inertia) to calculate the required guidance force F_{guide}. However, when the driver grips the steering wheel, the driver's neuromuscular dynamics H_{nms} will influence the response to feedback forces and the system should take into account the total physical interaction dynamics H_{pi} (the combined stiffness, damping and inertia of both the driver's

limbs and the steering wheel). The total physical interaction could be measured offline, during other experiments.

Tuning of shared control forces based on neuromuscular measurements

Then, if the system is tuned for the combined physical interaction during a 'relax' situation, drivers can simply hold the steering wheel and if they are indeed relaxed (i.e., do not generate forces or change their impedance) the systems desired steering wheel angel x_{opt} will result from the guidance forces F_{guide}, with an accompanying different vehicle trajectory. The system could also be tuned to only yield the correct x_{opt} during a 'give way' task, in which the driver would need to actively yield to the feedback forces (essentially amplifying them) in order to let the optimal position be reached. Then, smaller feedback forces could be used, and drivers would be more involved in the control loop then when they would only do a 'relax task'.

In either case, if drivers have a different reference trajectory ref_{human} - and therefore a different desired steering wheel angle x_{des} - they can use feed-forward or feedback control to resist the shared control forces.

Adaptive impedance of the shared control

The proposed architecture allows the steering wheel system to respond likewise: when a driver does not respond adequately to a critical situation, the impedance of the steering wheel around x_{opt} can be smoothly and temporarily increased, guiding the driver to more acceptable steering wheel angles, clearly communicating the severity of the situation. Essentially the wheel will act as a predictive display for steering actions that are incorrect from the system's point of view. Clearly, if the impedance is increased to the extent that the driver can not influence the steering wheel angle anymore, this will (temporarily) result in an automation system. For safety reasons, the maximal steering wheel impedance should be limited based on neuromuscular measurements of maximal human impedance (measured during a 'resist forces' task) and maximal steering wheel forces.

The effects of neuromuscular adaptability and adaptive impedance for shared control

In the remainder of this chapter, experimental evidence is provided to illustrate the extent to which drivers can vary their neuromuscular dynamics when interacting with a steering wheel. Also, it will be shown how several tunings for shared control system ('dominant', 'slack') are influenced by different neuromuscular settings ('give way', 'relax', 'resist'), in case feedback forces are given to support the driver during an evasive manoeuvre.

3. Experimental Methods

3.1 Apparatus

The experimental setup used for both experiments consists of a fixed-base driving simulator with an actuated steering wheel (Moog FCS ECoL-8000, "S"-actuator). The base-line steering wheel dynamics consisted of a slight centring stiffness K_{sw}=4.2 Nm/rad, a damping B_{sw} of 2 Nms/rad and an inertia I_{sw} of 0.3 Nms^2/rad, yielding a system with Eigen-frequency 0.6 Hz and relative damping of 0.89. Adaptations to the steering wheel dynamics and feedback forces could be communicated to the control loading computer of the steering wheel at 100 Hz. The steering wheel actuator was force controlled by the control loading computer at an update rate of 2500 Hz. Subjects were asked to be seated in an adjustable car seat and were requested to hold the steering wheel (diameter: 38 cm) with both hands in a "ten-to-two" position (see Figure 3).

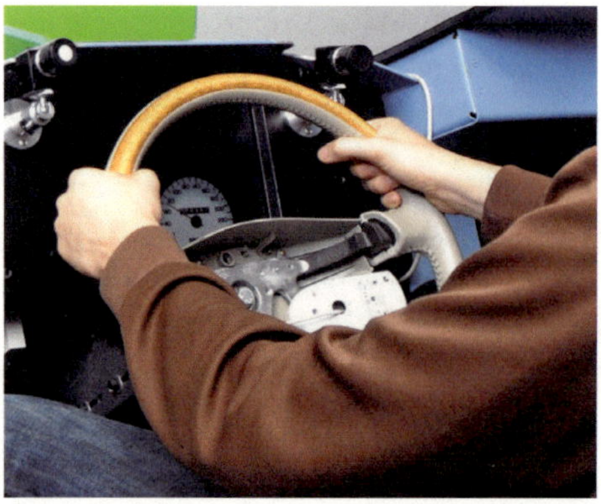

Fig. 3. A close-up of a subject holding the steering wheel, which could be perturbed or which could provide haptic guidance. The human reaction torque T_c and the resulting angular rotations X_c were measured.

During experiment 1, task-related information was shown by means of a Sanyo PLC-XU33 multimedia projector, projected on a screen in front of the subject at a distance of approximately 2.9 m from the eye-reference-point of the experiment subjects. The projector was positioned such that the centre of projection was aligned with the eye-reference-point. Refresh rate of the displayed image was 50 Hz. Graphical resolution of the projected image was 1280x1024 pixels at a screen width and height of 3.3x2.1 m^2.

3.2 Experiment 1: Neuromuscular Adaptability

The goal of the first experiment was to quantify the adaptability of the neuromuscular dynamics as a function of task and hand placement. Ten subjects (5 male, 5 female) participated in the first experiment. The subject's age was 26.4 (+/- 3.3) years. All subjects were recruited from the university student population. Participation was voluntary, no financial compensation was given.

Task instruction

Subjects were told they would experience torque perturbations on the steering wheel and were given three tasks to perform: resist the forces (or position task: PT), give way to the forces (or maintain force task: FT), and relax (RT). When resisting or giving way to forces, subjects received visual information of their task. During the 'resist force' - task a white, vertical line indicated the target position. A red, vertical line, starting in the middle of the screen indicated the current steering wheel position. The red, vertical line expanded upwards as a time-history of the measured wheel positions, so that subjects could monitor their performance. Performance is defined here as how well subjects could maintain the steering wheel position on the target position as indicated by the white line. For the 'give way' task, the goal was essentially to maintain zero force on the steering wheel, therefore the white, vertical line indicated zero force. The red, vertical line, showed a time-history of the measured wheel forces. For the relax task, no visual information was shown. Before the experiments, participants were told that for the force and position task, "...you will see a white line and a red column. In either task, the purpose is to maintain the red column on the while line to the best of your ability, while your steering wheel is disturbed." For the relax task they were told to "...do nothing, just leave your hands on the steering wheel, while it is being disturbed."

Hand positioning

The experiment was conducted for three hand positions on the steering wheel: both hands (BH), left hand only (LH) and right hand only (RH). When only one hand was used during the relax task, the steering wheel would have a bias angle to that side due to the weight of the arm turning the steering wheel somewhat. To prevent this, a bias torque of approximately ±0.2 Nm was added to the torque perturbation signal in these cases. This bias torque effectively put the steering wheel in the centre position with a passive arm holding it on either the left or right side.

Perturbation design

The torque perturbation was an unpredictable multi-sine signal, scaled such that for each task approximately similar steering wheel rotations were obtained in order to prevent effects of amplitude non-linearity (e.g., Stein & Kearney, 1995). The frequency content of the perturbation was designed according to the Reduced Power Method (Mugge et al., 2007). This method yields perturbations with full power at low frequencies (in this case 0.02 - 0.5 Hz) and only a small percentage of that power at higher frequencies (in this case up to 20 Hz). This is done to avoid the suppression of reflexive activity that occurs when exciting reflexes at frequencies beyond their bandwidth (van der Helm et al., 2002). The method effectively evokes low-frequent behaviour, while allowing the estimation of neuromuscular dynamics over a large bandwidth.

Experiment protocol

The nine different conditions (3 tasks, 3 hand positions) were each repeated four times. The positioning of the hands was randomized within the subjects. Between subjects the order of the task was also randomized. To prevent fatigue, the tasks were then alternated in this random order for each hand position and each repetition within each subject. Participants were trained for each task until satisfactory performance was. The total duration of the experiment was approximately 30 minutes.

Data Analysis

The following signals were logged at 100 Hz: steering wheel torque (T_c), steering wheel position (X_c), and torque disturbance (D). All repetitions were averaged in the time-domain. Subsequently, closed-loop system identification based on spectral densities (e.g., van der Helm et al., 2002) was done to calculate the dynamics of the human, of the steering wheel and of the combined physical interaction. They are all represented not as impedance, but as its mathematical inverse: the admittance, the causal relationship between input force and output position: admittance.

3.3 Experiment 2: Neuromuscular Adaptability for different Shared Control Impedance

The goal of the second experiment was to show how different neuromuscular settings (give way to forces, resist forces, relax) would influence shared control. A small group of three male subjects (mean age 30) participated in the experiment, for which no financial compensation was given.

Task instruction

Subjects were told they would experience torque feedback on the steering wheel from several shared control systems, some of them strong, some of them weak. This torque feedback would guide them to perform steering activity to make a fast lane change. Subjects were asked to hold the steering wheel with both hands (as shown in Figure 3) and to resist the torques, give way to them, or be relaxed in face of the forces.

Shared Control Design

The actuated steering wheel provided the subject with shared control, which was identical to the look-ahead based haptic guidance controller for curve negotiation used in previously published research (Mulder et al., 2008b). Essentially, the system guides drivers along an optimal path. The properties of the shared control could be tuned to yield desirable response, by means of two parameters: the force feedback gain and the stiffness feedback gain (Abbink et al., 2009). Through the force feedback gain, the strength of the feedback forces in response to look-ahead errors could be influenced (essentially determining the force F_{guide} from Figure 2). Stiffness feedback was an implementation of the idea to dynamically change impedance discussed in section 2.2. The additional stiffness acted around the optimal angle calculated by the look-ahead controller, and was designed to dynamically depend on the current lateral error with respect to the system's reference trajectory (the function *K(crit)* in Figure 2). Through the stiffness feedback gain, the gain on this lateral error could be increased. Note that because of the baseline steering wheel stiffness K_{sw}, there would always be some steering wheel impedance even if the stiffness feedback gain would be zero.

For this experiment, several settings were investigated, of which three will be presented here:

- the weakest shared controller (baseline force gain, no stiffness gains). The human has most authority in this situation – the driver easily overrides the haptic guidance controller in case there is disagreement on x_{opt};
- the medium shared controller (baseline force gain, double stiffness gain). The human and the haptic guidance controller have similar authority – the driver and controller present forces of similar magnitude to the interface;
- the strong shared controller (double force gain, double stiffness gain). The haptic guidance controller has most authority in this situation – the driver will have to use considerable force to override the haptic guidance controller in case there is disagreement on x_{opt}.

Note that although the shared control architecture is as proposed in this chapter, the gains were not based on neuromuscular measurements, but determined by trial-and-error. The purpose here was to show how different neuromuscular settings influence the functioning of different shared control systems.

Experiment protocol

Subjects were presented with a two-lane driving track on which the shared controller's reference trajectory would shift to the other lane and back, three times. The change in reference trajectory for the shared controller caused it to generate force feedback to follow that trajectory. The tracks were driven for the three shared control settings, and three different task instructions. The distance between changes in the reference trajectory was random, to prevent learning effects. The total duration of the experiment was approximately 10 minutes.

Data Analysis

The following signals were logged at 100 Hz: steering wheel torque (T_c), steering wheel position (X_c), and the lateral and longitudinal position of the car's centre of mass.

4. Experimental Results

4.1 Results for Experiment 1

Figure 4 shows the estimated admittances for a typical subject. These results were similar for all subjects. The squared coherence was generally high, indicating linear behaviour for the experimental conditions studied.

In the left column the solid lines denote the admittances estimated with both hands. There is a large difference in admittance at low frequencies. For example, subjects substantially reduced their admittance when resisting forces (position task, PT) compared to the relax task (RT). This indicates that, as expected, the steering wheel angles as a result of a external forces are much smaller when subjects try to resist those forces. It also shows that subjects can substantially increase their admittance when trying to give way. The wide range of admittances (FT more compliant than RT; PT behaviour much more stiff than RT) is consistent with previous experiments on the arms (Damveld et al., 2009) and the ankle joint (Abbink, 2006; Abbink 2007; Mugge et al., 2009).

Another result is that with both hands on the steering wheel, subjects could perform their task better (larger admittance during 'give way' tasks, and a smaller admittance during 'resist' tasks) than with only one hand. During the relax task, not much effect was found as a result of different hand placement.

In the middle column the estimated steering wheel dynamics are shown, which correspond to how the dynamics were set: that of a well-damped second-order system with eigen-frequency of 0.6 Hz. Naturally, the steering wheel dynamics are not affected by hand position or task instruction.

In the right column the total physical interaction dynamics was estimated, arising from both the human limbs and the steering wheel. It can be seen that the smallest admittance (i.e., the highest impedance) dominates the total physical response: during PT the total physical admittance is bounded by the driver, during FT the total physical admittance is bounded by the steering wheel stiffness.

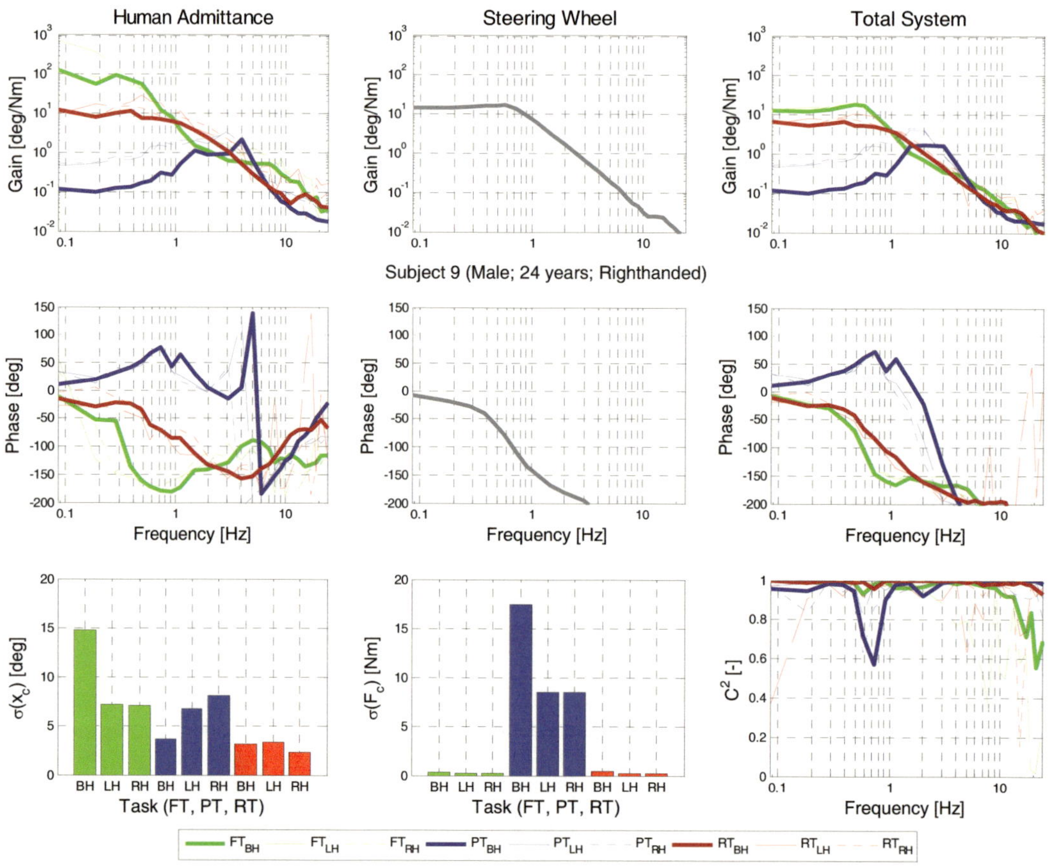

Fig. 4. Results of experiment 1: the estimated admittance for a typical subject, for three tasks (resist forces 'PT'; relax 'RT'; and give way to forces 'FT') and three hand positions: left hand only (LH - thin line), right hand only (RH - thin dashed line) and both hands (BH solid line). The top panels show the magnitude of the admittance, the middle panels the phase, and the bottom right panel the squared coherence. The lower left panel shows the standard deviations of the steering wheel angle, X_c. The lower middle panel shows the standard deviations of the steering wheel torques F_c. The left column shows the admittance of the human, the middle column that of the steering wheel, and the right column the combined physical interaction dynamics.

4.2 Results for Experiment 2

Figure 5 shows the results for a single lane change manoeuvre of a typical subject, guided by three different shared control systems: the lightest system (left column), the medium system (middle column) and the strong system (right column). The stronger the shared control, the stronger it guides the driver during relax and force tasks (give way) towards the optimal trajectory, but also, the more difficult it is to overrule the feedback forces and drive straight on (as can be seen from the forces f_c and position x_c).

Another interesting result is that by giving way (FT), the driver is always closer to the system's desired trajectory: the human is then cooperating with the system. The required forces to do so are small (in the same order of magnitude as during the relax task).

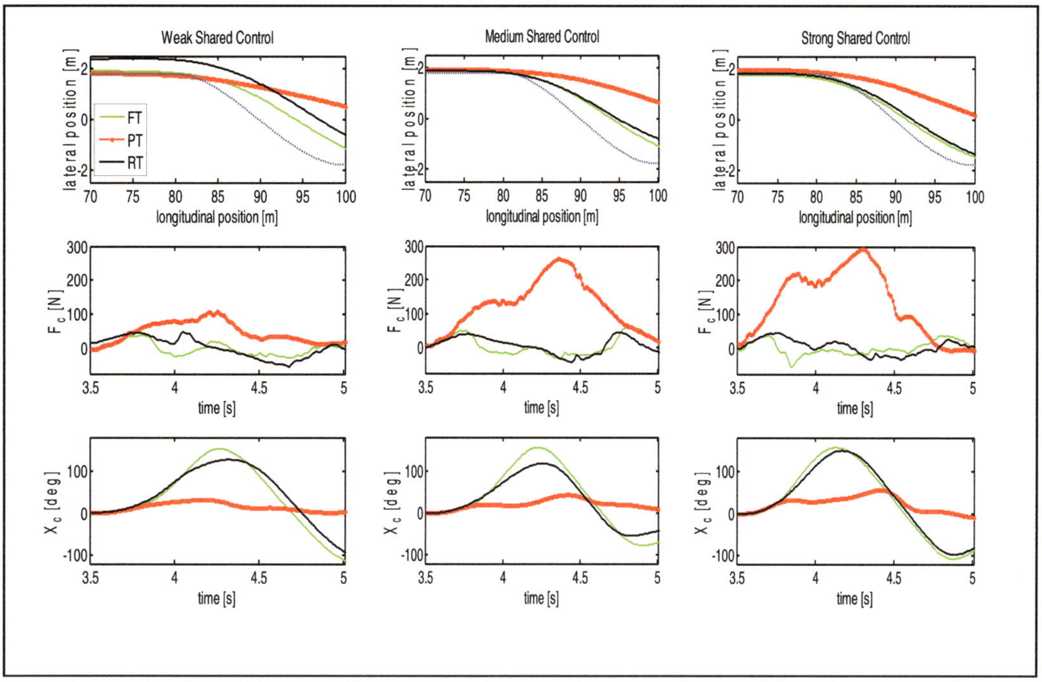

Fig. 5. Results of experiment 2: a single lane-change manoeuvre for a typical subject, to illustrate the influence of the strength of shared control and the neuromuscular dynamics on lane position (top), driver's force (middle) and steering wheel angle (bottom). The dashed line in the top row denotes the system's reference trajectory, to steer from the centre of one lane (1.8 m), to the centre of an adjacent lane (-1.8 m).

5. Discussion

The experiments showed that the possible adaptation range in human impedance control is extremely large when controlling a steering wheel: at low frequencies a factor of a 1000 could be distinguished between giving way to forces and resisting them. This adaptability confirms the underlying hypothesis of this chapter that it is difficult to design shared control forces if the neuromuscular impedance is not known. Even if the system's goals and controller completely match the human goals and control strategy, when trial-and-error tuning has tuned the forces to be optimal for a slightly 'resist forces' task (somewhere in between relaxed state and maximally resisting state) the feedback forces will be too large, and the human will have to resist them sometimes, or be satisfied with a different trajectory.

Moreover, the experimental results strengthen the evidence found in other studies (Abbink, 2006; Abbink, 2007), which suggest that minimizing force errors (i.e., giving way to external forces) is not only *possible*, but also *useful* when interacting with guidance forces from shared control systems. The second experiment - shared control for a lane-change - showed that also in that situation subjects could effectively give way to feedback forces. Consequently, appropriate steering actions could be made faster and with less effort, resulting in a trajectory that more closely matched the system's reference trajectory, without the need to increase feedback forces or control interface impedance.

The admittance results during relax tasks closely resembles those found in other studies (e.g., Pick & Cole, 2007), but that during 'resist force' tasks an even larger decrease in admittance was encountered for the subjects in the present study. This is probably caused by the different perturbation signals used. When using perturbations with full power up to 10 Hz, all reflexive activity will be suppressed, as has been shown in previous research (van der Helm et al., 2002; Mugge et al., 2007). The additional low-frequent stiffness found in the present study is likely the result of reflexive activity, although visual contributions may not be ruled out at low frequencies (below approximately 1 Hz).

The idea of scaling the impedance of the steering wheel (Abbink et al., 2009) has been shown in this study to be compatible with adaptations in neuromuscular impedance. The studied shared control system provides continuous support that can cause drivers to steer faster (when giving way to forces), and still be always overruled (when resisting forces). It was observed that at high authority levels of shared control the difference between giving way and relaxing became smaller. This corresponds to the results in experiment 1, which demonstrates that -according to the laws of mechanics - the strongest spring (highest impedance) dominates the dynamic behaviour of the combined physical interaction. In other words, at high authority levels of shared control the steering wheel became more stiff than the relaxed human impedance, reducing the influence of a more compliant human (during give way tasks) on the combined physical impedance.

Future Work

This chapter has provided arguments that it is beneficial to base shared control properties on neuromuscular analyses, as well as some experimental evidence. The designed shared control system with variable impedance should be tested more thoroughly then was done in experiment 2, with a larger subject group and with more in-depth analyses.

Even then, it is evident that more evidence is needed, in the form of a full design cycle for a novel shared control system based on the architecture presented in Figure 2. The design cycle should consist of in-depth modelling, shared control design, human-in-the-loop experiments, evaluation and model parameter estimation and validation. This will be the subject of further publications from the authors.

An important issue to address in future work is the extent to which the stationary measured neuromuscular response to perturbations during postural tasks corresponds to the actual impedance control during goal-directed movements of the steering wheel. To answer this question, two problems must be solved. First of all, unobtrusive estimations of admittance are needed while the human is engaged in a manual control task. Initial attempts during car-following (Abbink et al., 2006) and pitch control of an airplane (Damveld et al., 2009) are promising but require further investigation. Second, the time-variant nature of admittance needs to be quantified, for example through wavelets (e.g., Thompson et al., 2001).

Another interesting research spin-off would be to apply human motor-learning skills (Osu et al., 2002 ; Franklin et al. 2003) to the shared control system. If the system continuously feels resistance from the driver in certain curves, the system could learn that the driver cuts corners differently than the system and could, with time, update the reference trajectory or the internal model for the physical interaction (Goodrich & Quigley, 2004).

All such future research could shed more light on how humans control their movements and control forces when interacting with feedback forces and changing impedance of the control interface. This is expected to substantially assist in the design of shared control systems.

6. Conclusions

From a literature survey and the proposed novel shared control architecture, the following conclusions are drawn:

- two kinds of shared control systems can be recognized in literature
    - input-mixing shared control which changes the control input to the system
    - haptic shared control in which the support system and the human operator exchange forces on the control interface
- Haptic shared control offers the human the possibility of fast and intuitive communication about system's actions, as well as the possibility to respond through changes in neuromuscular impedance.
- Although haptic shared control systems have shown interesting benefits in a number of applications, several issues remain. Subjects have reported the feeling that one is not in complete control; large forces are needed to overrule the system
- Quantitative measurements of neuromuscular impedance can be used to understand the human response to forces, and can serve as a basis to design shared control forces. This step is expected to aid the design process of shared control systems and avoid the current trial-and-error tuning.
- Dynamically changing the impedance of the control interface is an interesting way to smoothly shift control authority, and provide more guidance only when needed. A larger impedance of the control interface communicates the criticality of a situation to the driver, and helps to attenuate control actions that the system deems undesirable.

From the experiments, the following conclusions can be drawn:

- Subjects could substantially adapt their neuromuscular impedance during a steering task. Compared to the relaxed state, they could increase their neuromuscular impedance (during 'resist force' tasks) or decrease it (during 'give way' tasks).
- In agreement with the rules of mechanics, the impedance of the combined physical interaction was shown to be dominated by the largest impedance
- A shared control support system to assist with lane changes was investigated for three different levels of control system authority. The larger the control interface impedance, the more closely the drivers matched the necessary steering angle to follow the desired trajectory.

Acknowledgements

Part of this work was supported by Nissan Motor Company, Ltd., and David Abbink is supported by the VENI Grant from NWO.

7. References

Abbink D.A. (2006). *Neuromuscular Analysis of Haptic Gas Pedal Feedback during Car Following.* Delft University Press, ISBN:978-90-8559-253-2 http://repository.tudelft.nl/file/447893/371671

Abbink DA (2007) Task instruction: the largest influence on Human Operator Control Dynamics. *Proceedings of World Haptics 2007,* pp. 206-211, Tsukuba, Japan, 22-24 March 2007.

Abbink, D.A & Mulder M. (2009). Exploring the dimensionalities of Haptic Feedback Support in Manual Control. *ASME Special Haptics Issue of JCSIE,* Vol. 9, No. 1, March 2009, pp 011006_1-9

Basdogan, C.; Kiraz, A.; Bukusoglu, I.; Varol, A. & Doğanay, S. (2007). Haptic Guidance for Improved Task Performance in Steering Microparticles with Optical Tweezers. *Optics Express,* Volume 15, No. 18, pp. 11616-11621.

Brandt, T.; Sattel, T. & Böhm, M. (2007). Combining Haptic Human-Machine Interaction with Predictive Path Planning for Lane-Keeping and Collision Avoidance Systems. *Proceedings of the IEEE Intelligent Vehicles Symposium,* Istanbul, Turkey, pp. 582-587.

Damveld, H.J.; Abbink, D.A.; Mulder, M.; Mulder, M.; van Paassen, M.M.; Van Der Helm, F.C.T. & Hosman, R.J.A.W. (2009). Measuring and Modeling the contribution of Neuromuscular Dynamics to Pitch Control Tasks. *In: Proceedings of the AIAA Conference,* August 2009, Chicago, USA

Doemges F. & Rack P.M.H. (1992b) Task-dependent changes in the response of human wrist joints to mechanical disturbance. *Journal of Physiology,* 447:575–585

Feldman, A.G.; Adamovich S.V.; Ostry, D.J. & Flanagan J.R. (1990) *In: Multiple Muscle Systems,* edited by Winters JM, Woo SL-Y. New York: Springer, 1990, ch. 43, p. 195–213.

Forsyth, B.A.C. & MacLean, K.E. (2006). Predictive Haptic Guidance: Intelligent User Assistance for the Control of Dynamic Tasks. *IEEE Transactions on Visualization and Computer Graphics,* Volume 12, No. 1, pp. 103-113.

Franklin, D.W.; Osu, R.; Burdet, E.; Kawato, M & Milner, T.E. (2003). Adaptation to stable and unstable dynamics achieved by combined impedance control and inverse dynamics model. *Journal of Neurophysiology* 90: 3270–3282

Goodrich, K.H.; Schutte, P. & Williams, R. (2008). Piloted Evaluation of the H-Mode, a Variable Autonomy Control System, in Motion-Based Simulation. *AIAA Conference,* August 2008, Hawaii pp.574-590

Goodrich, M.A. & Quigley, M. (2004) Learning Haptic Feedback for Guiding Driver Behavior. *Proceedings of the 2004 IEEE Conference on Systems, Man, and Cybernetics.* October 10-13, 2004, The Hague, The Netherlands.

Griffin, W.B.; Provancher, W.R. & Cutkosky M.R. (2005). Feedback Strategies for Telemanipulation with Shared Control of Object Handling Forces. *Presence,* 14(6): 720-731

Griffiths, P. & Gillespie R.B. (2005). Sharing Control Between Humans and Automation Using Haptic Interface: Primary and Secondary Task Performance Benefits. *Human Factors,* Vol.47, No. 3, Fall 2005, pp.574-590

Hammond P.H. (1956) The influence of prior instruction to the subject on an apparently involuntary neuro-muscular response. *Journal of Physiology* 132(1):17–18

Hogan, N. (1984). Adaptive Control of Mechanical Impedance by Coactivation of Antagonist Muscles. *IEEE Transactions on Automatic Control,* 29(8) (1984), pp. 681-690.

Jaeger R.; Gottlieb G. & Agarwal G. (1982) Myoelectric responses at flexors and extonsors of the human wrist to step torque perturbations. *Journal of Neurophysiology,* 48:388–402

Keen S.D., Cole D.J., (2006). Steering control using model predictive control and multiple internal models. *Proceedings of AVEC '06. The 8th International Symposium on Advanced Vehicle Control,* August 20-24, 2006, Taipei, Taiwan

Kragic, D.; Marayong, P.; Li, M.; Okamura, A.M. & Hager, G.D. (2005). Human-Machine Collaborative Systems for Microsurgical Applications. *International Journal of Robotics Research,* Volume 24, No. 9, pp. 731-741.

Lam, T.M.; Mulder M.; Van Paassen M.M.; Mulder J.A. & Van Der Helm, F.C.T. (2009). Force-Stiffness Feedback in Uninhabited Aerial Vehicle Teleoperation with Time Delay. *Journal of Guidance, Control and Dynamics,* Vol.32, No. 3, May-June 2009, pp.821-835

McRuer, D.T. & Jex, H.R. (1967) A review of quasi-linear pilot models. *IEEE Trans Human Factors Electron* 8(3):231–249

Mugge W.; Abbink D.A. & Van der Helm F.C.T. (2007). Reduced Power Method: how to evoke low-frequent behaviour while estimating high-bandwidth admittance. *Proceedings of the IEEE International Conference on Robotics and Rehabilitation,* Noordwijk, the Netherlands, June 2007

Mugge, W.; Abbink, D.A; Schouten, A.C.; Dewald, J.P.A. & Van der Helm, F.C.T. (2009). A rigorous model of reflex function indicates that position and force feedback are flexibly tuned to position and force tasks. *Experimental Brain Research,* Published online, August 2009

Mulder, M. (2007). *Haptic Gas Pedal Feedback for Active Car-Following Support.* Delft University Press, ISBN: 978-90-8559-266-2, http://repository.tudelft.nl/assets /uuid:008d10dc-3aa1-4b29-b445-579278543057/ae_mulder_20070130.pdf

Mulder, M.; Mulder, M.; van Paassen, M.M. & Abbink, D.A. (2008a). Haptic Gas Pedal Feedback. *Ergonomics,* Vol. 51, No. 11, pp.1710-1720.

Mulder, M.; Abbink, D.A. & Boer R. (2008b). The effect of Haptic Guidance on Curve Negotiation Behaviour of Young, Experienced Drivers, *Proceedings of IEEE SMC Conference,* pp. 804-809, Singapore, 12-15 Oct 2008

Osu, R.; Franklin, D. W.; Kato, H.; Gomi, H.; Domen, K.; Yoshioka, T. & Kawato, M. (2002). Short- and Long-Term Changes in Joint Co-Contraction Associated With Motor Learning as Revealed From Surface EMG. *Journal of Neurophysiology.,* 88, pp. 991–1004.

Osu, R., Kamimura, N., Iwasaki, H., Nakano, E., Harris, and C. M., Wada, Y. (2004). Optimal Impedance Control for Task Achievement in the Presence of Signal-Dependent Noise. *Journal of Neurophysiology* 92, pp. 1199–1215

Pick, A.J. & Cole, D.J. (2007). Dynamic properties of a driver's arms holding a steering wheel. *Proc. IMechE.* Vol. 221 Part D: J. Automobile Engineering, pp 1475-1486

Pick, A.J. & Cole, D.J. (2008). A Mathematical Model of Driver Steering Control Including Neuromuscular Dynamics. *Journal of Dynamic Systems, Measurement, and Control* MAY 2008, Vol. 130, pp. 031004 1-9

Pritchett, A.R. (2001). Reviewing the Roles of Cockpit Alerting Systems. *Human Factors in Aerospace Safety*, Vol. 1, No. 1, pp. 5-38

Rosenberg, L.B. (1993). Virtual Fixtures: Perceptual Tools for Telerobotic Manipulation. *Proceedings of the IEEE International Conference on Robotics and Automation*, pp. 76-82.

Sheridan, T.B. (2002). *Humans and Automation: System Design and Research Issues.* HFES Issues in Human Factors and Ergonomics Series, Volume 3, John Wiley, New York 2002, ISBN 0-471-23428-1

Stein R.B. & Kearney R.E. (1995) Nonlinear behavior of muscle reflexes at the human ankle joint. *Journal of Neurophysiology* 73(1):65–72

Switkes, J.P.; Rossetter E.J.; Coe I.A. & Gerdes J.C. (2006). Handwheel Force Feedback for Lanekeeping Assistance: Combined Dynamics and Stability. *Journal of Dynamic Systems, Measurement, and Control*, Volume 128, Issue 3, pp. 532-542.

Thompson, P.M.; Klyde, D.H. & Brenner M.J. (2001). Wavelet-based time-varying human operator models. *Proceedings of the AIAA Conference* August 6-9, Montreal, Canada

Toffin, D.; Reymond, G.; Kemeny, A. & Droulez, J. (2007). Role of steering wheel feedback on driver performance: driving simulator and modeling analysis. *Vehicle System Dynamics*, 45:4, 375 – 388

Van der Helm F.C.T.; Schouten, A.C.; De Vlugt, E. & Brouwn, G.G. (2002). Identification of intrinsic and reflexive components of human arm dynamics during postural control. *J Neurosci* 119: 1-14

Van Paassen, M.M. (1995). A Model of the Arm's Neuromuscular System for Manual Control. Proc. IFAC Analysis, Design and Evaluation of Man-Machine Systems, Cambridge, USA 1995.

Wolpert, D.M.; Miall, C. & Kawato, M. (1998). Internal models in the cerebellum. *Trends Cogn Sci* 2: 338–347

Factors Affecting the Perception-Based Compression of Haptic Data

Mehrdad Hosseini Zadeh
Kettering University
The United States of America

David Wang and Eric Kubica
The University of Waterloo
Canada

1. Introduction

The ability of technology to transmit multi-media content is very dependent on compression techniques since bandwidth affects how much information can be transmitted in a given amount of time. Researchers have investigated efficient lossy compression techniques for image compression (jpeg) (Miano J., 1999), audio compression (mp3) (Brandenburg K., 1999; Gersho A., 1994) and video compression (mpg) (Bhaskaran V., Konstantinides K., 1999) to facilitate the storage and transmission of audio and video.

Recently, haptics is becoming more important with its addition in various applications such as computer-aided design (CAD), tele-surgery, rehabilitation, robot-assisted surgery, and graphical user interfaces (GUI) to name a few. Haptic technology enables computer users to touch and/or manipulate virtual or remote objects in simulated environments or tele-operation systems. If haptic cues (e.g. touch sensations) are displayed in addition to visual and auditory cues, these VEs are called haptic-enabled virtual environments (HEVEs) (Srinivasan M. and Basgodan C., 1997).

If haptic data is to be stored, transmitted and reproduced, the efficient use of the available bandwidth and computational resources is a concern. Most lossy audio and visual compression techniques rely on the lack of sensitivity in humans to pick up detailed information in certain scenarios. Similarly, haptic perception-based lossy compression techniques utilize limitations in the sensitivity of human touch to create haptic models with much less detail and thus requiring less bandwidth for a given sensation. Essentially, perception-based approaches use the threshold or just noticeable difference (JND) of force perception to develop efficient compression techniques. Force JND is the minimum difference that we can notice between two forces: the base force and an increment/decrement of the base force (Gescheider G.A., 1997). The haptic data would be stored or sent over the network when the value of sampled force data was greater than the force threshold value. It is thus necessary to quantify the force threshold and to investigate the impact of important factors on the force threshold.

Most of the research in this field studied force perception with a human user in static interaction with a stationary rigid object (Hinterseer et al., 2005, 2006). It is equally important to

measure force JNDs when the user's hand and virtual objects are in motion (Zadeh et al., 2008). This chapter focuses on cases where the human user or the object are in relative motion. In addition, the effects of several factors, including user hand velocity, the base force intensity and the force increment or decrement on force perception are investigated.
This chapter is organized as follows. In Section 2, haptic compression techniques are addressed and perception-based compression techniques are reviewed. Section 3 reviews the sensory threshold of human force perception, Weber's law, several classical psychophysical methods, and previous work on the human haptic system. Section 4 presents an approach to incorporating velocity in the process of measuring the difference force threshold. First, the friction of haptic device is estimated to find the base force of force threshold. Then, an HEVE is constructed to study the effect of user's hand velocity on force perception. The experimental setup and procedure of experiments are described, and the results are presented and discussed. Section 5 studies the effects of the base force intensity and the force increment or decrement on the force threshold. The experimental setup and procedure of experiments are explained in detail, and the results are presented and discussed. Finally, Section 6 summarizes the findings and gives concluding remarks and directions on future research.

2. Haptic Compression Techniques

The haptic data compression techniques are divided into two main categories: statistical (Shahabi et al., 2002) and perception-based approaches (Hinterseer P. and Steinbach E., 2005). Statistical approaches mostly focus on the properties of the haptic signal. In contrast to the statistical approaches, perception-based approaches decrease the number of packets using a distortion metric based on the limitations of the human haptic system.
Ortega and Liu in Chapter 6 of *Touch in Virtual Environments* (McLaughlin et al., 2002) proposed a statistical method that employed similar approaches to those used in speech coding to analyze haptic data. They developed compression techniques that are more specific to the haptic data, including a low-delay coding scheme based on differential pulse code modulation (DPCM). They also presented an alternative coding approach that uses the knowledge of the underlying graphical model. Their findings show that they achieve a compression rate of a factor of 10 using the Low-Delay Predictive coding compression technique.
A variety of statistical methods were compared by Shahabi et al. (2002). They presented and evaluated alternative techniques for achieving efficient sampling and compression of haptic data such as the movement, rotation, and force associated with user-directed objects in a VE. They experimentally determined the benefits and limitations of various techniques in terms of the data storage, bandwidth and accuracy. Again, their study does not include perception-based approaches. However, they summarized the result of the statistical approaches that might be useful to compare with the perception-based ones.
Hinterseer et al. (2005) proposed a perception-based compression method to decrease the number of packets transmitted in a telepresence and teleaction system. They sent only haptic data over the network when the value of sampled sensor data is greater than a threshold value. The threshold value was determined in a psychophysical experiment. The results show a considerable reduction – of up to 90% in the packet rate and data rate – without any perceiveable effect on the fidelity and immersiveness of the telepresence system. Later, they extended their psychophysically motivated transmission method for multidimensional haptic data (Hinterseer P. and Steinbach E., 2006). They used an example of a three dimensional haptic interaction that haptic data are only generated and transmitted if the change in haptic variables exceeds

the JND of the human operator. Similar to their previous work, the approach reduces packet rates by up to 90% without impairing immersiveness.
Hinterseer et al. (2006) also presented a model-based prediction of haptic data signals that can be used as a haptic compression technique. This technique can be used to compress haptic data in Internet-based multimedia applications such as haptic-supported games and the haptic rendering of VEs. This method works on the basis of the psychophysical properties of human perception. A two-user tele-operation system was set up, including an operator side and a tele-operator side. A signal prediction model was used on both sides that enabled the users to send packets over the network if the current actual signal differs from the predicted signal by a force threshold. The method reduced the packet rate by up to 95% without impairing immersiveness. Later, Hinterseer et al. (2006) used fast Kalman filters on the input signals combined with model-based prediction of haptic signals.
Stability is one of the main issues in haptic systems. Instability might cause an undesirable feeling to the user and unrealistic interaction with the virtual environment. One of the most important approaches for designing a stable haptic display is the passivity-based (energy-based) approach. The extracted energy from the virtual environment can cause unrealistic feelings with severe destabilizing effects. Colgate J.E. and Brown J.M. (1994) have used a passivity-based model to design stable haptic displays. Kuschel et al. (2006) addressed the issue of stability in data compression algorithms that discard unnoticed data. They focused on guaranteed stability or passivity of a system that uses a lossy data reduction (LDR) algorithm. They proposed a classification scheme for a class of LDR algorithms and derived sufficient stability conditions.
Knowledge about the threshold of human force perception is essential in all reviewed perception-based compression techniques. It is thus necessary to investigate the impact of important factors on the force threshold, including the base force intensity, force increment/decrement, and velocity of the user's hand. However, the effects of these factors have not been addressed in the literature. This chapter studies a set of these factors when the user's hand is in motion.

3. Sensation, Perception and Psychophysics

In everyday life, we use our senses to interact with the environment. We can see, touch, smell, hear and taste the external world surrounding us through interactions that usually occur with an initial contact between an organism and its environment. Sensation mostly deals with the initial processes of detecting and encoding environmental energy during the interactions. Essentially, our sense organs convert the energy signals from the environment to bioelectric neural codes and send the codes to the brain (Schiffman, H.R., 2000). The cell receptors of the eye receive the light as environmental energy, transform it into bioelectric codes and then transmit the codes to the brain. Sensation not only deals with the study of the biological events such as the reaction of the eye cells to light energy, but also concerns the relation of sensory experiences to the functioning of sense organs.
In addition to sensations, psychological processes are also required to give meaning to the bioelectric neural codes. When we watch television, our eye initially detects a series of images. However, psychological processes enable us to perceive concepts from the images based on our past experiences, memory, or judgment. In other words, psychological processes present the visual events in a meaningful way. Perception deals with these psychological processes that are required to organize, interpret and give meaning to the output of sense organs. Thus,

the main objective of sensation and perception is to obtain accurate and reliable information about the environment (Schiffman, H.R., 2000).
Psychophysics refers to the methodology of studying perception. The methodologies from psychophysics are used to study perception (Gescheider G.A., 1997). Psychophysical methods enable us to establish a relation between certain features of environmental stimulation and sensory experiences. *Discrimination* is the most important perceptual problem that has been addressed in psychophysics. This problem involves the measurement of sensory thresholds, or the perceptual limits of the human sense organs (Brisben et al., 1999). In this study, the sensory thresholds of human force perception are measured in an HEVE.

3.1 Sensory Thresholds

The discrimination problem involves deciding whether two stimuli are identical or not. In order to find if there is any difference between the two stimuli, the smallest difference between two stimuli should be measured. The difference threshold or just noticeable difference (JND) is a measure of the minimum difference between two stimuli that is necessary in order for the difference to be reliably perceived. The first stimulus is called *base* stimulus, and the second stimulus is an increment/decrement of the base stimuli. The JND in the direction of stimuli increment is called the upper limen, and the JND in the direction of stimuli decrement is called the lower limen (Gescheider G.A., 1997). In discrimination experiments, the focus is mostly on the difference in the intensity of two stimuli. However, other dimensions of variation, such as frequency, intensity level, or adaptation time, have also been investigated (Gescheider G.A., 1997). Intensity is subjective quantity which can be triggered by different attributes of a stimulus. This study focus on the amplitude of force as force intensity.
In 1834, Weber studied the relationship between the difference thresholds or JNDs and the intensity levels of the base stimulus. He discovered that the JND increases significantly for very small intensities and decreases while the intensity of the base stimulus increases. For relatively large base stimuli, Weber found that the JND is a linear function of stimulus intensity. In other words, the difference threshold is always a constant fraction of the stimulus intensity for those base stimuli; this fraction is called Weber's fraction. This trend is observed by other researchers and is called the Weber trend (Gescheider G.A., 1997). The value of Weber's fraction is different for various senses.
The linear relationship is a valid law for all senses and sense organs. This relationship is called Weber's law, which can be represented as

$$\Delta\phi = c\phi \quad or \quad \Delta\phi/\phi = c, \tag{1}$$

where c is the constant Weber's fraction, $\Delta\phi$ is the change in the stimulus intensity that can just be noticeably different (JND), and ϕ is the starting intensity of the stimulus or base stimulus.

3.1.1 The Force Thresholds of the Human Haptic System

Srinivasan M. and Basgodan C. (1997) defined the human haptic system as the entire mechanical, sensory, motor and cognitive components of the body-brain system. Researchers have determined the force thresholds of the human haptic system in real world situations ((Jones L. A., 1989);Pang et al., 1991; Raj et al., 1985). Jones L. A. (1989), in a force matching experiment focused on a human elbow, found a JND ranging between 5% and 9% over a range of different base force values. Subjects were required to generate forces ranging from 15 to 85% of their maximum voluntary contraction (169-482 N). Pang et al. (1991) determined a JND that lies between 5% and 10% for pinching motions between finger and thumb with a constant resisting force. This JND was found to be relatively constant over a range of different base force values between 2.5 and 10 N. Raj et al. (1985) studied the ability of human subjects to discriminate between different magnitudes of weights. They found JNDs of 12%–13% for large base weights (80-200 g) lifted by the middle finger about the metacarpophalangeal (MCP) joint.

Allin et al. (2002) measured force JND in a VE. The goal was to use the force threshold to construct therapeutic force feedback distortions that stay below the threshold. The focus was on JND as applied to the index finger. The result was an average JND of approximately 10% over a number of subjects with a constant base force at 2.25 N. The conclusion was that the visual feedback distortions in a VE can be created to encourage the increment of force production by up to 10%, without a patient's awareness.

3.1.2 Force Thresholds and Motion

In the previous subsection, the reviewed studies have measured the force thresholds in the haptic display of stationary rigid objects, which interact with the operator's hand. However, motion is critical in many VR applications.

Very little research has considered the study of motion and perception in the haptic displays (Lederman et al. (1999); Jandura L. and Srinivasan M. A. (1994)). Lederman et al. (1999) investigated the effects of the speed of the relative motion on perceived roughness via a rigid probe. Several experiments were conducted based on the mode of touch, active or passive, and different ranges of velocities. It was realized that the effects are multiple and complex. The results show that increasing speed tended to render surfaces as smoother. It was also observed that the inter-element spacing for texture perception has a significant effect in addition to changes in the speed. In other words, perceived roughness decreases with increasing speed, up to the point where the probe tip is able to fall between the inter-element spaces, where the effect is reversed. This chapter also focuses on the effects of the relative velocity on the human haptic perception. However, the goal is to explore the limitations of the haptic perception in the haptic rendering of VEs.

Jandura L. and Srinivasan M. A. (1994) conducted torque discrimination experiments for a slow twisting motion. Subjects were asked to maintain a constant angular velocity, while a constant torque was applied on the subjects' hands. The results show that the JND for torque was 12.7% when the reference torque was 60 mN-m.

3.1.3 Psychophysical Methods for Measuring Thresholds

There are many methods to determine the absolute and difference thresholds. According to Gescheider (Gescheider G.A., 1997), methods of limits, constant stimuli, and adjustment are among the most well known methods for detecting absolute and difference thresholds. People are usually presented with the same stimuli on different occasions. However, they do not always respond in the same ways. The main reason for this is presumably that the neurosensory system allows a margin of error. Other sources of biases such as learning and adaptation, can also be a factor.

One of the best techniques for detecting sensory thresholds is the method of limits and it is not as time consuming as other methods. In this method, a subject is presented with a stimulus well above or below the expected threshold. On each trial, the subject indicates detection of the stimulus with a *yes* response, or non-detection with a *no*. The experimenter increments the stimulus on successive trials if the first stimulus presented is below the threshold, until the subject changes his response from *no* to *yes*. If the first stimulus is over threshold, the stimuli are gradually decremented in steps until the subject's response changes from *yes* to *no*.

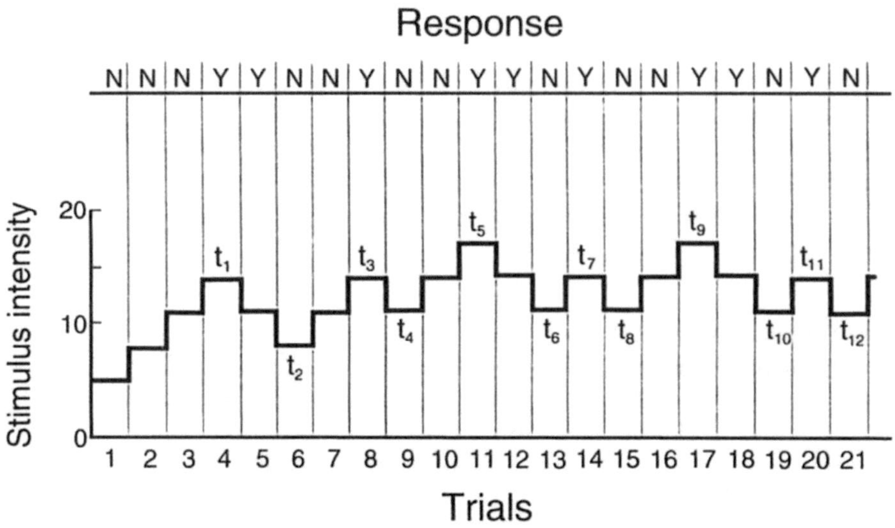

Fig. 1. Staircase method: *yes* (Y) or *no* (N) responses are shown in the top of figure. The transition points are indicated above and below of stairs Gescheider G.A. (1997).

A series is terminated immediately after the first change in response, and the transition point for that series is taken as the stimulus value halfway between the last two stimulus values. Several ascending and descending series can be conducted, and the absolute threshold is the average of the transition points over all of the series.

Another effective method is the *staircase method* which is a modification of method of limits for detecting absolute thresholds. It is very similar to the method of limits with the only difference being that each series does not terminate after a transition point, and the direction of the series is reversed. As shown in Figure 1, if the stimulus is being incremented, after the first *yes* response it will begin to be decremented, and vice versa.

The procedure is finished when a sufficient number of response transition points have been recorded. The result of averaging the transition points is the threshold. This method takes less time compared to other methods because only a few stimulus values that are far above or below threshold are presented. Although it is a very efficient method, its sources of biases are the same as the method of limits Gescheider G.A. (1997).

The Interweaving Staircase (IS) (Bernstein R. S., and Gravel J. S., 1990) method is a variation of the staircase method that is used to measure the JND in the direction of force increment and in the direction of force decrement. In the IS method, the experimenter starts by presenting a sequence of forces which is the base force plus the increment or decrement, then progressively increases or decreases in value. The subject responds with *yes* to increment or decrement or *no* to detecting changes in force value. When the subject's response changes from one or a series of the same response to the other response, as is the case of *yes, yes, yes* switching to *no*, the force value is recorded, and the direction of the force sequence is reversed from ascending to descending, or vice versa. These points are called transition points. The transition points are recorded and the JND value is the average value of the transition points.

The main advantage of the IS method is to reduce the possible biases compared to the original staircase method. In the IS method, a subject has to report one of the three possible responses, *increment, decrement,* or *no change.* Therefore, it is much more difficult for the subject to guess the response, and it is possible for the experimenter to check the response with the current direction of force whether ascending or descending.

4. The Effect of Velocity on Force Perception in HEVEs

This section reports the results of a pilot study that is conducted to investigate the relation between motion and human haptic perception. We study the effects of a user's hand velocity on force perception in an HEVE. The focus is on the determination of difference force threshold or JND by measuring the upper and lower limens of force JND. The force JND is obtained in the free motion condition of the PHANToM device when the device end-effector is grasped by a subject's hand. In free motion, there is no interaction with virtual objects, and no force feedback is applied on the subject's hand. The only force on the user's hand is a resistive force due to the backdrive friction of the device. Thus, this friction force is the base force for the force JND when no force feedback is applied. In the next section, Section 5, a full study is conducted to measure force JNDs for three base forces when force feedback is also applied on the subject's hand.

In two experiments, subjects are asked to report the just noticeable difference between the base force and an increment/decrement from it when they perceive the JND. The upper and lower limens of the force JND are quantified for three ranges of velocity: low (0.03 - 0.05 m/s), medium (0.12 - 0.15 m/s), and high (0.22 - 0.28 m/s).

The experiments are described in detail in Section 4.2. The upper and lower limens of force JND for the three ranges of velocity are presented in Section 4.3 and discussed in Section 4.4.

4.1 Hypothesis

4.1.1 H_1:

The force JND of human force perception increases when the velocity of user's hand increases in an HEVE.

4.2 Methods

This section describes the two conducted experiments, which use the same setup, task, and procedure. The direction of applied forces is the only difference between the two experiments. In the first experiment, the applied force is in the same direction of hand motion (aid force). Thus, the force partially cancels the friction, and decreases the resistive force. In the second experiment, the applied force is in opposition to the direction of the subject's hand motion (opposed force) and increases the resistive force.

4.2.1 Participants

There were eight right-handed participants who were between the ages of 27 and 34. All were regular computer users and students at the University of Waterloo. Participation was voluntary. The participants did not have any neurological illness or physical injury and had no more than trivial previous exposure to haptic interfaces. The experiment was conducted in accordance with the University of Waterloo ethical guidelines.

4.2.2 Apparatus

The PHANToM^{TM} Omni device was used in both experiments. This haptic device has been designed for a vast variety of applications, including medical, scientific and industrial. In general, some of the advantages of PHANToM device are their 3D force-feedback, the ability to operate in an office or desktop environment, compatibility with standard PCs and useful for a broad range of applications.

Omni devices have a relatively large workspace for desktop applications, suitable for a large range of hand motions, stiffnesses and motor forces to meet the specific requirements of this research project. Comparing to other haptic devices, this device is widely used in various applications because of its reasonable price. This device can generate maximum 3.3 N force, which is enough for the purpose of the experiments. The applied forces in the experiments in this study are less than 1 N. Another important characteristic of the device is the back-drive friction, which is reported as up to 0.26 N (*Sensable Technologies Inc.*). In Section 4.2.2.1, this friction and its variability are estimated for the part of work space that is used in the experiments. Essentially, the variability is important because we need to know the minimum detectable force output of the device.

The haptic device is connected to a personal computer through a Firewire interface card. The software has two processes, haptic and graphic, that are run on two 3GHz Pentium 4 computers running Windows XP. Force feedback is generated by the haptic process. The graphic process renders a 2D VE that is shown in Figure 2. The VE contains a colour ball and a colour bar. The colour ball represents the position of the device end effector (grasped by the subject's hand). The bar is stationary and has two green ends (targets). The center-to-center distance between the targets on the bar is 10.2 cm. As shown in Figure 3, a 17" LCD monitor, which is placed approximately 70 cm from the subject, is used to display the VE. The update rate of haptic (force) display is 1000 Hz.

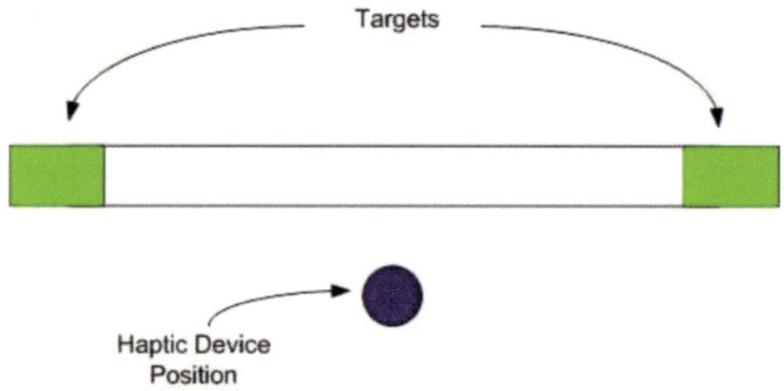

Fig. 2. The 2D VE that contains a 2D ball and a bar with two green target zones.

4.2.2.1 Estimation of the Device Friction

In the experiment, the base force is the resistive force due to the friction of the haptic device, which includes coulomb and viscous (damping) friction. Coulomb or dry friction is independent of velocity, however, viscous friction is proportional to the velocity of device end-effector (Berkelman, P. and Ji M., 2006), and is usually reported as a coefficient in Ns/m. Similar to coulomb friction, viscous friction is calculated in N when viscous damping coefficient is multiplied by velocity (m/s).

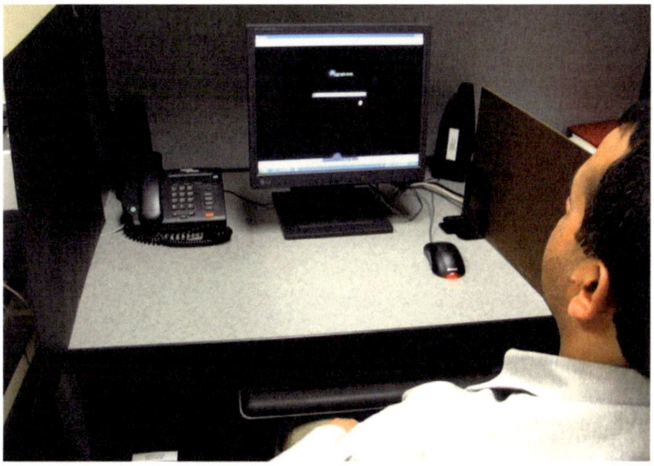

Fig. 3. The computer display shows the 2D VE.

The viscous frictions of PHANToM devices are very small because a cable-pulley transmission is used in these devices. Diolait et al. (2005) found that the coulomb friction is 0.038 N and the viscous friction coefficient is 0.005 N.s/m for PHANToM 1.0 haptic device. Thus, if the end-effector moves by 0.28 m/s, the viscous friction is 0.0014 N, which is negligible compared to the coulomb friction. Their measured friction is similar to the backdrive friction of the PHANToM 1.0, up to 0.04 N, as reported in the device specifications (*Sensable Technologies Inc.*).

The backdrive friction of the PHANToM Omni is reported up to 0.26 N, which is 6.5 times larger than the friction of PHANToM 1.0. Therefore, the Omni viscous friction is approximately 0.009 N if the end-effector of Omni moves by 0.28 m/s, which is the maximum velocity in the experiments. Thus, in all experiments, it is assumed that the resistive force is only due to the coulomb friction of the device, which is basically independent of velocity.

In addition, the preliminary experiments showed that the friction was variable within the workspace of the device. In other words, when we moved the device end-effector manually, we had to change the force intensity to maintain the motion with a constant velocity. Therefore, the friction and its variability were estimated within the part of workspace that was used in the experiments. The workspace was a 10.2 cm path, from -0.051 to 0.051 m on the x-axis of the device workspace.

In order to determine the friction, varying force profiles were applied to: a) move the end-effector from a static condition and b) keep an approximately constant velocity of the end-effector from the beginning to the end of the path. The applied force in b) should be equal to the friction if the force produces an equilibrium trajectory (the end-effector moves with a constant velocity on the whole path).

Initially, the end-effector was placed at a point (0.07 m on x-axis) before the beginning of the path. A relatively high intensity force was applied to the end-effector for 400 ms to move the end-effector toward the beginning of the path (0.051 m on x-axis). Finally, a weaker force was applied to the end-effector and this force was maintained until the device reached the end of the path.

Since the friction was variable, two frictions were estimated when the end-effector moved from right to left and left to right. To estimate the right to left friction, first, forces with different magnitudes were applied to find the force that could overcome the static friction. A 0.5 N force could initially move the end-effector, and overcome the static friction. Then, a weaker force of 0.26 N was applied to maintain a constant velocity (around 0.16 m/s). Figure 4 shows the trajectory of the end-effector when the force profile was applied. For the first 1000 ms, no force was applied, and then 0.5 N was applied for 400 ms followed by 0.26 N for 1600 ms.

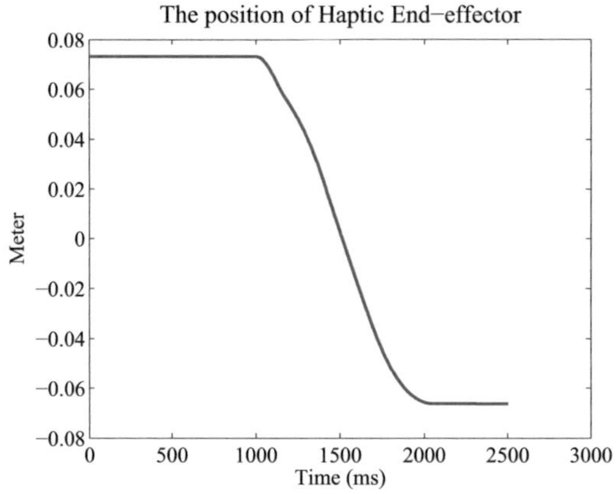

Fig. 4. The end-effector trajectory when no force was applied for 1000 ms, then a 0.5 N force was applied for 400 ms followed by a 0.26 N for 1600 ms.

To estimate the left to right friction, the force to overcome the static friction was 0.31 N, which was less than the applied force for the right to left. However, the force applied to maintain a constant velocity was slightly higher at 0.28 N.
Based on the results, the friction was 0.27 ± 0.01 N, which was the average of the two weaker forces for the right to left and left to right movements.
Other researchers ignored the friction force in their base force because the friction force is negligible compared to large base forces applied by the actuators such as 2.25 N in Allin's work, 2002. However, in this study, the small friction force should be taken into account because our base forces are small.

4.2.3 Design

In this pilot study, a mixed model design was used in the experiments (Reis & Judd, 2000). This model involves both a within-subject design as well as a between-subject design. In the mixed model design, several independent variables can vary within subjects and other variables can vary between subjects. The conducted experiments were devised to measure the force JNDs in a velocity-based scenario. The dependent variable was the force JND of human force perception. The independent variables were the velocity of subject's hand motion and the force increment/decrement. All participants experienced all three levels of the velocity because the main goal is to investigate the effect of the velocity. However, four subjects experienced the force increment or the force decrement since four subjects were enough to determine one limen of force JND. Participants were divided into two groups of four. One female and three male subjects were in each group. The first group participated in the experiment for the force increment and the second group participated for the force decrement. The order of the experiments and levels randomly assigned to the subjects.

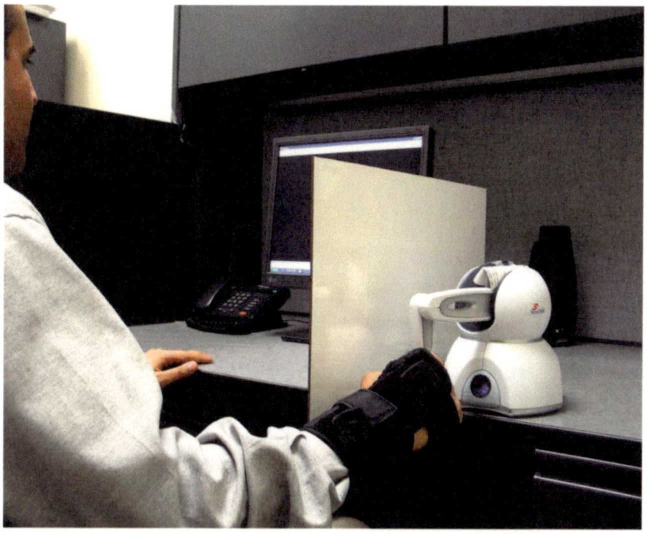

Fig. 5. The subject grasps the end-effector of the PHANToM^{TM} Omni and rotate his hand about his elbow.

4.2.4 Procedure

Each subject is seated on a chair facing a computer display and asked to place their right elbow on a side support. The wrist of the right hand is restrained with a wrist guard, as shown in Figure 5, so that wrist movements are locked to ensure that subjects just rotate their hands about their elbows. The subject grasps the end-effector of the haptic device.

During each experiment, the attention of the subject is directed to the display containing the 2D VE, as shown in Figure 2. The ball represents the device end-effector and moves when the subject moves the end-effector. The right arm and fingers of subjects are shielded from their own view with an opaque barrier to ensure subjects control their hands' movement via visual feedback from the display. The subject is asked to move his/her hand, back and forth, from left to right and then right to left, repeatedly. The subject is required to maintain the red ball between the green zones and not go beyond the zones.

Three ranges of reference velocity are selected based on two factors. First, the ability of subjects to carry out the experimental task at the velocity ranges. Second, having relatively large rooms among the ranges to study any potential significant difference of the force JNDs at the ranges. The selected ranges are low (0.03 - 0.05 m/s), medium (0.12 - 0.15 m/s), and high (0.22 - 0.28 m/s). To find the ranges at which subjects could complete the task, several subjects, other than the main eight subjects, carried out the task within various velocity ranges before starting the main experiments.

All subjects are required to maintain their hand velocity within the specified ranges in three different experiments. The colour of the ball in the display aids the subjects in maintaining the average value of their hands' velocity at the reference velocity. If the subject's velocity is within the range of reference velocity, the ball's colour is red. Otherwise its colour is yellow. Therefore, the subjects control their hands' velocity by observing the ball's colour. To ensure that subjects can control the velocity, they are given training before starting the main experiments.

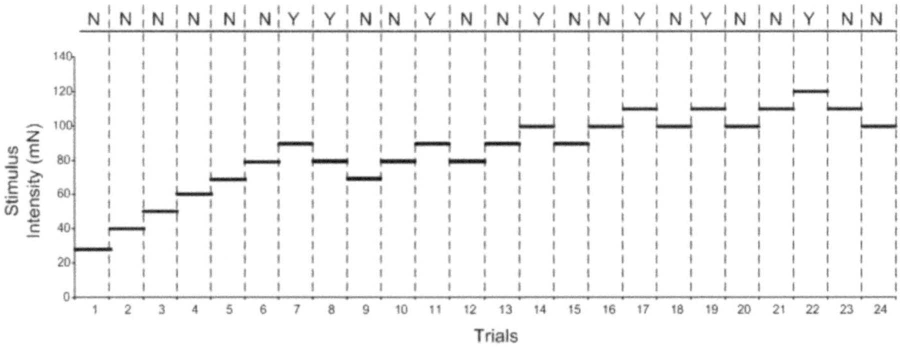

Fig. 6. The staircases of the applied forces. (*no*: N; *yes*: Y)

The average velocity is used because the subject stops at the end of the bar and moves towards the other side of the bar in the 2D VE, as shown Figure 2. If the velocity at each instant in time is used, then the ball's colour would turn to yellow at the end of the bar, and the subject might inadvertently apply extra force. This can distract the subject and affect the process of measuring the force JNDs. Thus, the mean velocity value is used as it does not change rapidly when the subject stops at the end of the bar, and the ball's colour does not turn to yellow.

The staircase method, which is explained in Section 3.1.3, is used to measure the force JNDs. In the middle of each trial, the experimenter applies a certain amount of either opposed or aid force to the subject's hand motion based on the staircase procedure. Each subject is asked to report any changes in the haptic sensations on their hand during each trial. Before applying the force, the experimenter ensures that each subject maintained the hand velocity within the reference range. The procedure is finished when 12 transition points are obtained. Therefore, the number of trials is variable. As a results, the duration of experiment is variable, and one experiment typically takes from 15 to 25 minutes. Twelve transition points are recorded and the force JND value is the average value of the transition points.

This procedure is repeated in three sessions for the three velocity ranges, low, medium, and high. Figure 6 shows the staircases of the force JND for one of the subjects in an experiment. Each subject is given training. The first session includes a familiarity phase and then the experiment is conducted for one of the velocity levels. In the second session, the subject does the same task with another velocity level. In the last session, the same task is done with the last velocity level.

The zero velocity is detected in the application of forces. The issue is encountered when the direction of motion frequently changes during a trial. For example, if the subject moves from left to right, the end-effector's velocity is positive. When the subject stops at the target and moves from right to left, the velocity's sign changes to negative, leading to a zero velocity at the targets. As a result, several sudden changes occur in the applied force, causing the device to switch discontinuously and jittering movement.

To overcome this problem, a model is developed using a narrow dead-zone as shown in Figure 7. In this model, if the velocity is within the velocity interval (dV), the applied force is set to zero by the dead-zone (dV). For these experiments, the $|dV|$ of 0.001 m/s is found to be sufficient to solve the problem. Our model is similar to the Karnopp (1985) model, which represents friction force at zero velocity.

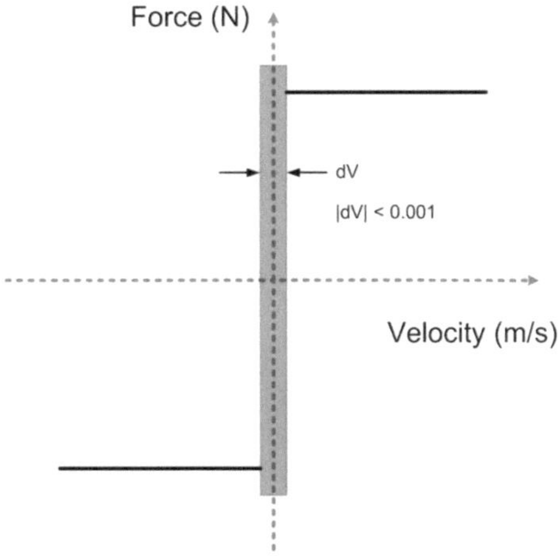

Fig. 7. The zero velocity detection model: no forces are applied on the subjects' hands when the velocity is within the interval dV.

4.3 Results

The average force JNDs across all subjects and for all levels of the velocity and force increment/decrement are shown in Table 1 and Figure 8. For example, the upper and lower limens of force JNDs are 18.91% (0.051 N) and 18.36% (0.049 N) when the subjects' hands are in the low velocity motion.

Rang of velocity (m/s)	Force Increment	Force Decrement	Average
Low (0.03-0.05)	18.91 ± 1.43	18.36 ± 0.9	18.63 ± 0.79
Medium (0.12-0.15)	27.08 ± 2.93	26.23 ± 2.85	26.66 ± 1.90
High (0.22-0.28)	36.19 ± 4.3	32.95 ± 3.00	34.57 ± 2.51
Average	27.39 ± 2.68	25.85 ± 2.21	

Table 1. The average force JNDs (%) of base friction force (0.27 N) and standard errors for all levels of the velocity and force increment/decrement across all subjects. The average JND of four subjects are included in each cell.

As shown in Figure 8, the average force JND values are in a range between 18.91% to 36.19% for force increment and 18.36% to 32.95% for force decrement, indicating that the force JNDs increase when the subject's hand velocity increases.

For the low velocity, the upper and lower limens are almost equal. However, the difference between the upper and lower limens slightly increases by increasing the velocity. The upper limen is 4% higher than the lower limen for high velocity.

To study the effect of the velocity and force increment/decrement, a two-way analysis of variance (ANOVA) is conducted. Statistical analysis is performed using a mixed (within and between-subject) analysis of variance (ANOVA) with $p<0.05$ as the rejection level.

The average of force JNDs are calculated for the three ranges of velocity across the two levels of force increment/decrement and shown in Figure 9. This figure also shows that the velocity

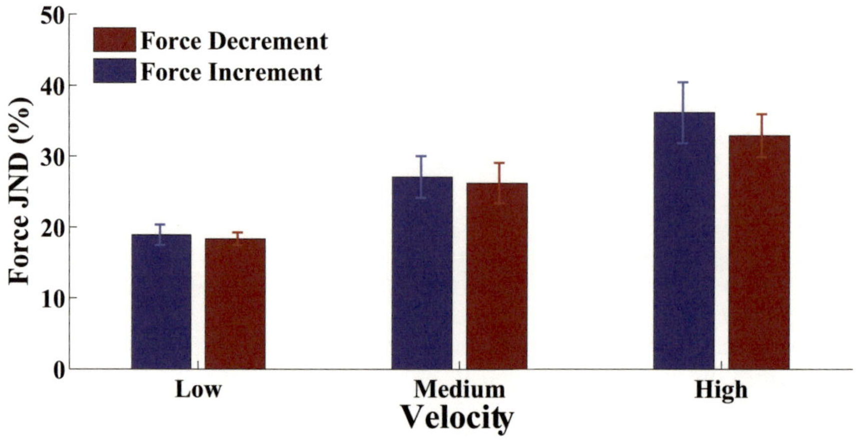

Fig. 8. The average of force JND across all subjects and standard errors for the three levels of velocities and the two levels of force increment/decrement. The results of ANOVA significantly supports the trend of increasing the force JND when the velocity increases, $p < 0.0001$.

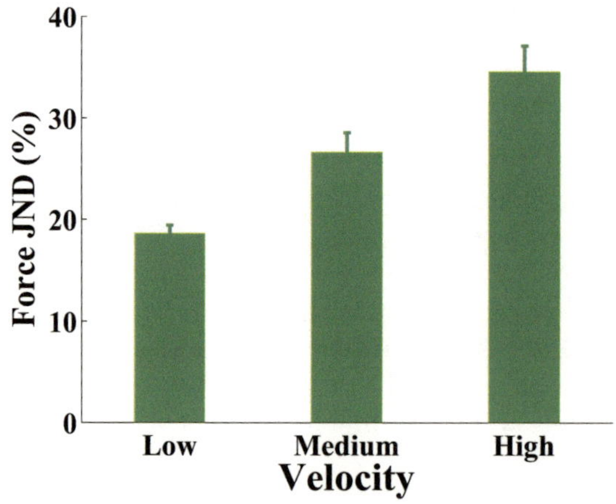

Fig. 9. The mean values and standard errors of force JND for the three ranges of velocity across the force increment and decrement.

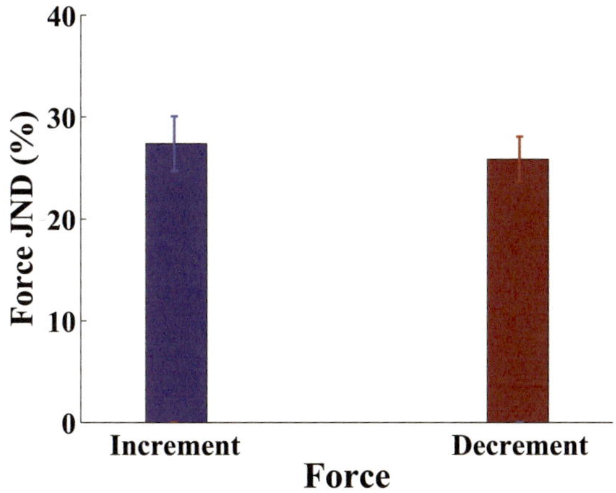

Fig. 10. The mean values and standard errors of force JND values across all ranges of velocity. The results of ANOVA also show no statistically significant difference between the force increment and decrement, $p = 0.6804$.

of the subject's hand has a significant effect on the force perception of the subject. For example, the force JND for high velocity is almost twice as large as the low velocity force JND with very small standard errors. The results of ANOVA significantly supports the trend of increasing the force JND when the velocity increases in Figures 8 and 9, $F(2, 12) = 56.75$ and $p < 0.0001$. The average of force JND were also calculated for the two levels of force increment and decrement across the three ranges of velocity and shown in Figure 10. As shown in the figure, the force increment and decrement are almost equal for all velocities, indicating that the upper and lower limens of force JNDs are somewhat symmetric. The results of ANOVA, $F(1, 6) = 0.19$ and $p = 0.6804$, also show no statistically significant difference between the force increment and decrement.

4.4 Discussion

An HEVE is constructed to study the effect of a user's hand velocity on force perception. An approach is presented to incorporate the velocity in the process of measuring the force perception threshold. The force JNDs are measured for three ranges of velocity. The trend of data, which is significantly supported by the results of an ANOVA, confirmed the hypothesis H_1, indicating that the force JND increases as the velocity of the user's hand increases in an HEVE.

The results also indicate that the upper and lower limens of force JND are almost equal for low and medium velocities, and the upper limen is slightly larger than the lower limen for high velocity motion. The results of an ANOVA also do not show any significant difference between the limens. In Section 5, the difference between limens will be investigated for smaller and larger base forces.

The results show that the measured force JNDs are larger than the JNDs measured by Pang et al., (1991) and Jones L. A. (1989), who determined the force JND in a range of 7%–10% for different muscle groups in hand and arm under various conditions. For example, Pang et al., (1991) found a JND that lies between 5% and 10% for pinching motions with a constant resisting force over base forces between 2.5 and 10 N.

Similarly, the force JNDs are higher than the JND measured in a VE by Allin et al., (2002), who found a 10% force JND on the index finger with a constant base force at 2.25 N. On the other hand, the low velocity JNDs are compareable to the JNDs obtained in a VE by Brewer et al., (2005) who found a 19.7% force JND for a 1.5 N base force. They also reported that their JND is larger than the JND in the literature, discussing several reasons such as the difference in the environment and tested joint, less subjects' training, and unfixed background dimensions. In this study, the small base force (0.27 N) can be the main reason that the JNDs are larger than the JNDs measured by Pang et al., (1991); Jones L. A. (1989); and Allin et al., (2002). The base force is much smaller than their base forces (1.5–10 N), and according to Weber's law, the JNDs for low base stimuli are larger than ones for high base stimuli. In the next section, Section 5, this difference will be investigated with different base forces to find if the higher JND in this section is due to a small base force.

5. The effect of force intensity on Force Perception in HEVEs

In this section, the force JNDs of the human haptic system are quantified and the effects of the base force intensity and the force increment/decrement on the force JND are investigated. An experiment is conducted for three levels of base force intensity. The Interweaving Staircase (IS) Bernstein R. S., and Gravel J. S. (1990) method is employed to measure the force JNDs. For the first level, 0.15 N force is applied in the same direction as the hand motion to partially cancel the backdrive friction of the haptic device (0.27 N). Therefore, the resulting resistive force on the subject's hand is 0.12 N, which is the first level of base force. This level is called the *low* base force.

For the second level, 0.15 N is applied in opposition to the direction of the hand motion. This force adds to the friction force, resulting in a 0.42 N resistive force on the subject's hand. This force is called the *medium* base force.

For the third level, 0.5 N is applied in opposition to the direction of subject's hand motion, resulting in 0.77 N force on the user's hand. This is called the *high* base force. Thus, the three resultant base forces are 0.12 N (low), 0.42 N (medium), and 0.77 N (high); two greater than the friction and one smaller.

The hypotheses are presented in the next subsection, and the experiment is described in detail in Section 5.2. The results are presented and discussed in Section 5.3.

5.1 Hypotheses

In Section 4, H_1, which is that the force JND increases when the velocity of user's hand increases, was tested. In this section, the following hypotheses are proposed and tested. These hypotheses are based on the results in the Section 4. H_2 is examined to investigate why the measured force JNDs in Section 4 were larger than the JNDs in the literature. H_3 is tested to find any significant difference between the upper and lower limens of force JND for a relatively high velocity motion and different base forces.

5.1.1 H_2:

Weber's law holds for force perception in an HEVE even when the user's hand is in motion. The force JND is larger for very small base force intensities and decreases as the base force intensity increases.

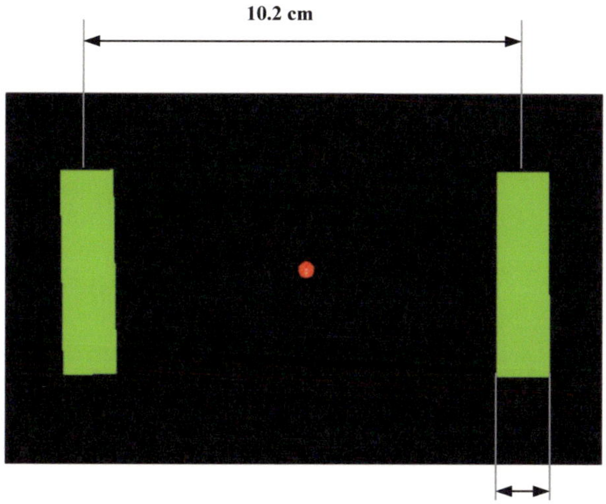

Fig. 11. The 2D virtual environment that contains a red 2D ball and two green rectangles.

5.1.2 H_3:

The upper and lower limens of force JND are not symmetric for all base forces when a subject's hand is in motion.

5.2 Methods

The experimental setup and procedure of the experiment are described. The intensity of the base force is the only difference between the three levels of the experiment.

5.2.1 Participants

There were 16 paid right-handed participants (eight females and eight males) between the ages of 22 and 33. All were regular computer users and students at the University of Waterloo, and had no neurological illness or physical injury that would impair hand function or force control ability. The experiment is conducted in accordance with the University of Waterloo ethical guidelines.

5.2.2 Apparatus

In this experiment, the same haptic device and monitor are used as in the previous section. A 2D VE is created and graphically rendered to users through the 17" LCD monitor. The VE is haptically rendered to subjects via the haptic device. As shown in Figure 11, the VE contains a 2D red ball and two green rectangles (targets). The center-to-center distance between the targets is 10.2 cm, and the width of the target is 1.3 cm in display coordinates and in the haptic device space. The ball represents the position of the end effector (grasped by the subject's hand). When the subject moves the end-effector, the ball moves on a horizontal line.

5.2.3 Design

A Repeated Measures (within subject) design Kuehl R. O. (2000) is employed in this experiment. Therefore, each subject is required to participate in all levels of the experiment plus a one-hour training session. The order of levels are randomly assigned to the subjects.

The base force intensity and the force increment/decrement are the independent variables. The base force intensity have three levels; low, medium, and high. The force increment/decrement factor have two levels based on the relative changes from the base force. At the half of trials in each base force level, the force increases from the base force, and at the other half, force decreases. The two levels of force increment/decrement are called increment and decrement.

5.2.4 Procedure

Similar to the experiments in Section 4, the subject is seated on a chair facing the monitor and asked to place their right elbow on a side support. The wrist of the right hand is restrained with a wrist guard, so that wrist movements are locked (to ensure that the subject just rotates his/her hand about his/her elbow). The subject grasps the device end-effector. Once the subject is seated comfortably, his/her right arm and fingers are shielded from his/her own view with an opaque barrier. Attention is directed to the monitor, which is placed approximately 70 cm from the subject.

As shown in Figure 12, each trial begins and ends with verbal commands (start and stop). Subjects start a task when they hear start from the experimenter. The task is explained later in *Task* subsection. Subjects stop and let go of the end-effector when they hear stop, and wait for 5-15 seconds before starting the next trial. During that time, no force is applied on the subject's hand, and the subject's hand is not in motion. Each trial has two intervals, and each interval lasts 15 seconds.

Figure 12 shows the first three trials of an experiment. In trial 1, the first force (F) is continuously applied on the subject's hand from the beginning of the trial until the end of the first interval. This force is 0.15 N in the same direction as the hand motion for low base level. The force vector is shown in Figure 13 as the aid force. The force is a 0.15 N for medium and a 0.5 N for high base levels. These forces are in opposition to the direction of the hand motion, and shown in Figure 13 as the opposed force. The relative direction of applied force to the hand motion does not change during an experiment.

At the beginning of the second interval, the second force is applied to the subject's hand. This force is either an increment or decrement from the first force. The trials with a force increment and decrement called *force increment* and *force decrement* trials, respectively. Each base force level of the experiment consists of 48 trials: 24 increment and 24 decrement trials. The order of trials was randomly chosen by the experimenter before starting the experiment.

The subjects are asked to detect changes in force value at the end of each trial. They respond with *yes* if they sense a force increment or a force decrement. They respond with *no* if they do not notice any changes. The trials with *no* and *yes* responses are called *unnoticed* and *noticed* trials, respectively. For instance, trial 1 is an unnoticed trial because the subject's response is No.

The force is increased/decreased by 0.02 N in the first trial of both force increment and decrement trials. The values of the force increment/decrement in next trials are determined based on the response of the subject in the current trial. Two variables are initialized by 0.02 N. One variable, which is called ΔF_{Inc}, saves the increment value for the next force increment trial, and the other one, ΔF_{Dec}, saves the force decrement value for the next force decrement trial. These variables would increase by 0.01 N if the response was No, and would decrease by 0.01 N if the response was *yes*. For example, ΔF_{Dec} value for trial 2 is 0.03 N (0.02 + 0.01) because the response is *no* in trial 1. Therefore, 0.15 N decreases by 0.03 N, and 0.12 N is applied at the second interval of trial 2. ΔF_{Dec} value would decrease by 0.01 if the response was *yes*.

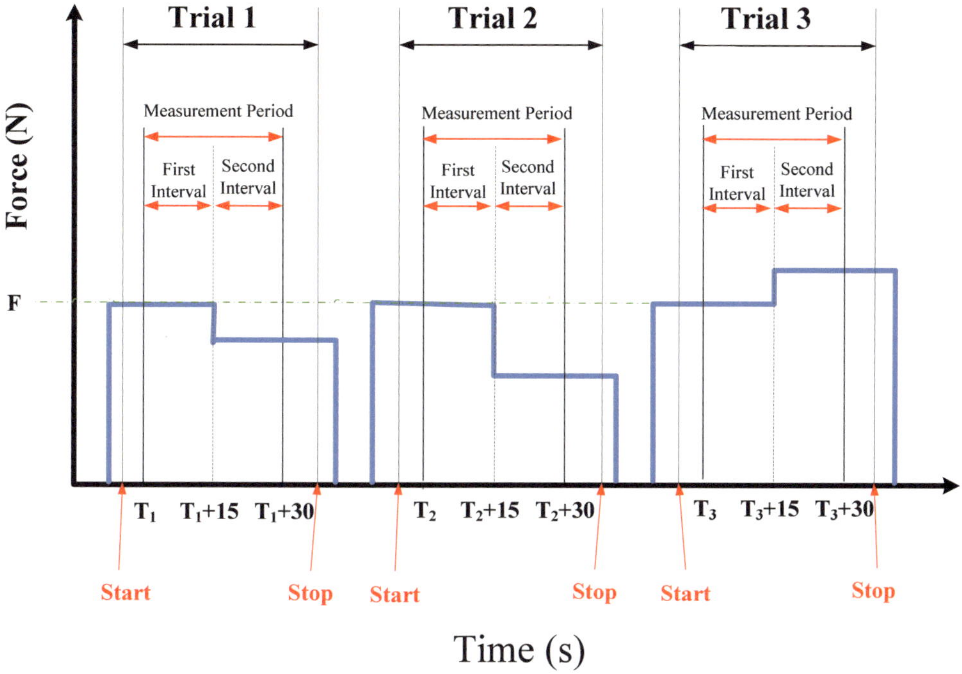

Fig. 12. The first three trials of an experiment(Times indicated are in seconds.)

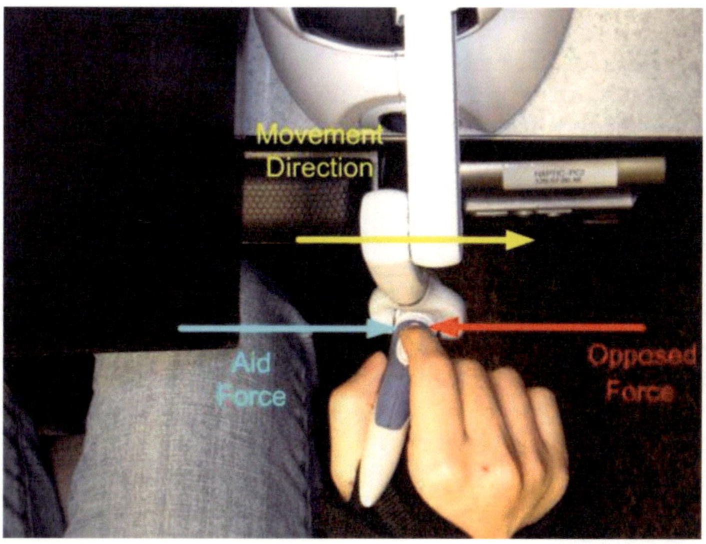

Fig. 13. The opposed and aid force vectors.

Base force Intensity	Force Inc./Dec.	Mean JND (%)	Standard Deviation	Standard Error
Low	Increment	64	22.36	5.59
Low	Decrement	43	17.47	4.37
Medium	Increment	15	6.93	1.73
Medium	Decrement	12	3.79	0.95
High	Increment	10	3.72	0.93
High	Decrement	11	3.76	0.94

Table 2. The average force thresholds (%), standard deviations, and standard errors for all levels of the base force and force increment/decrement.

The points at which the subject's response changes from *yes* to *no* or vice versa are called transition points. The direction of the force increasing/decreasing is reversed from increasing to decreasing, or vice versa at these points.
At the beginning of the experiment, the subject's responses might not be valid due to unfamiliarity with the type of force sensation. Thus, the first two transition points are neglected Cornsweet T. N. (1962). The force JND is the average values of the third transition point to the last one. To find the JND in %, this force value should be divided by the base force.

5.2.5 Task

The subject engages in a task similar to the Fitts' task (Fitts P.M., 1954). During each trial, subjects are asked to tap the two targets (green rectangles) by moving their hand to left and right. Each time the ball is within one of the targets, a hit is scored by subjects. An overshoot error occurs if they pass the target. An undershoot error happens if they did not reach the target. Subjects are asked to score as many hits as they can and carry out the task as rapidly as possible and as accurately as possible for a predetermined duration.
Unlike the Fitts' task, subjects are required to maintain their hand velocity within a specified range. The reference velocity range is set by the experimenter to 0.16-0.20 m/s based on the ability of a subject to carry out the task with an acceptable range of missing error (less than 15%). The missing error equals the sum of overshoots and undershoots divided by the total hits, overshoots, and undershoots. A training session is delivered to help subjects to get familiar with the task. It is required for subjects that carry out the task with less than 15% missing error at the end of training session and prior to the beginning of the experiment.
In this setup, the colour of the ball is also determined based on the hand's velocity and the reference velocity to help a subject to keep the hand's velocity within the range. If the subject's velocity is within the range, the ball's colour is red; otherwise its colour is yellow. The mean velocity value is monitored as it does not rapidly change when the subject stops at the target.
As shown in Figure 12, each trial has a measurement period, including two 15-second intervals (before and after force increment/decrement). The first interval is started when the experimenter ensures that the hand's velocity is within the reference range. The number of hits, overshoots, and undershoots are separately measured during each interval.

5.3 Results and Discussion

The average of JND values for all levels of the two factors are shown in Table 2 and Figure 14.

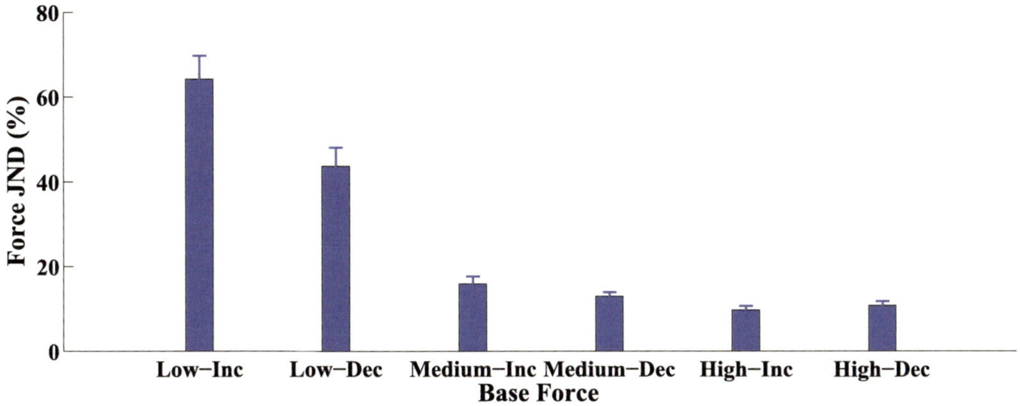

Fig. 14. The average and standard errors of force JND values for all subjects. (Inc = Force Increment, Dec = Force Decrement)

The result is analyzed using the repeated-measures (within subject) Analysis of Variance (ANOVA). The analysis is done at a significance level of 0.05.

As shown in Figure 14, there are several trends present in the data. One trend shows that the base force intensity has a major effect on the force JND. The force JND significantly decreases by increasing the base force intensity. The figure also shows a significant difference between the force increment and decrement of the low base force. The difference decreases for the medium and high base forces, indicating that there is an interaction between the base force intensity and force increment/decrement. The results of a two way ANOVA, $F(2, 30) = 12.28$ and $p < 0.0001$, also confirm the interaction between the base force intensity and force increment/decrement.

The results of a post-hoc Tukey test also confirm the large difference between the force increment and decrement of the low base force ($p < 0.0001$). This difference shows that the subjects notice the decrements of the low base force, Low−Dec, more easily than the increments, Low−Inc. This might be due to the fact that force is applied in the same direction of hand motion and the total resistive force is decreased on the subject's hand. This result rejects the null hypothesis in favour of H_3 hypothesis. In other words, the upper and lower limens of low base force JND are not symmetric.

The results in Figure 14 show a Weber trend, which is explained in Section 3.1. The force JND is noticeably large for the low base forces and decreases for the medium and high base forces. The results of the post-hoc test show a significant difference between the JNDs of the low base inc/dec and the medium or high base inc/dec ($p < 0.0001$). These results support the significant effect of the base force intensity on the force JND, rejecting the null hypothesis in favour of H_2 hypothesis.

In the previous section, Section 4, the force thresholds are determined with respect to a friction base force (0.27 N); however, that was for a different velocity range. To find the JNDs for the same velocity as the velocities implemented in this section, the JNDs for the friction are estimated based on a linear interpolation of JNDs for two ranges of velocities (0.12-0.15 and 0.22-0.28 m/s). The resulting force JNDs are 31.6% and 29.6% for the upper and lower limens of the friction base force. Figure 15 shows a Weber trend for the JNDs measured in the current and previous sections, confirming that the JNDs of small base forces are larger than high base

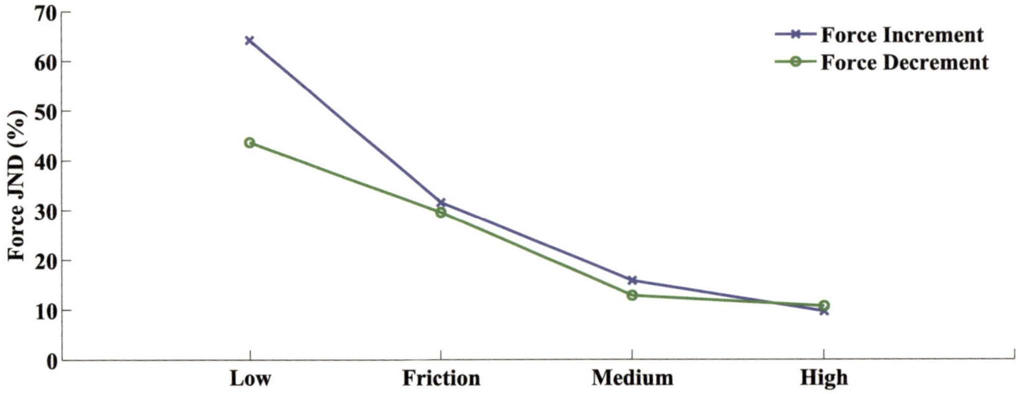

Fig. 15. The Weber's fraction for four base force intensities.

forces' JNDs. The JNDs for friction base forces are smaller than the low base force JNDs and greater than the medium base force JNDs.

Figure 15 does not show any significant difference between the force increment and decrement of the medium and high base forces. In other words, the upper and lower limens of JND are somewhat symmetric for medium and high base force intensities. The results of the post-hoc test also show no significant difference ($p = 0.9433$ for medium and $p = 0.9995$ for high).

The results show that, for applications that require motion within a constant velocity range, the JNDs are in the extremely small base force region of the Weber's fraction. For example, the low base force JNDs (62% and 38%) are comparable with the JNDs measured by Raj et al. (1985), who found that the human sensitivity is very low for small weights (20-60 g). Their results (JNDs ranging between 89% and 35%) indicate that as the base weights increases, JND decreases and remains relatively constant at weights above 200 g.

The standard errors (or standard deviations) of the low base force JNDs are greater than the JNDs of the medium and high base force. This indicates that the subjects are more confident in their reports about the medium and high base force JNDs.

The medium and high base force JNDs (around 13%) are very similar to the JNDs measured by Raj et al. (1985) who studied the ability of human subjects to discriminate between different magnitudes of weights. Their results show a JND of 12%–13% for relatively large base weights (80-200 g) lifted by the middle finger. The medium and high base force JNDs are also similar to the JNDs obtained by Jandura and Srinivasan (1994), who found 12.7% torque JND when the reference torque was 0.06 Nm.

The high base force JNDs (around 10%) are very similar to the JNDs measured by other researchers (Pang et al., (1991); Jones L. A. (1989); and Allin et al., (2002)). They found JNDs in a range of 7%–10% for different muscle groups in hand and arm under various conditions. (Jones L. A., 1989), in a force matching experiment about the elbow, found a JND ranging between 5% and 9% over a range of different base forces. Pang et al. (1991) found a 5% to 10% JND for pinching motions between the finger and thumb with a constant resisting force over base forces between 2.5 and 10 N. The high base force JNDs are almost the same as the JND measured in a VE by Allin et al. (2002) using the PHANToM^{TM} Omni device. They found a 10% force JND on the index finger with a constant base force at 2.25 N.

Our medium and high base force JNDs are much smaller than the JNDs obtained in a VE by Brewer et al. (2005) who found a 19.7% force JND (base force: 1.5 N) for the index finger of young subjects (ages 18–35) and a 31% force JND (base force: 2 N) for elderly subjects (ages 61–80). They confirmed that their JNDs are relatively high and discussed reasons why their JND is larger than the JND in the literature such as the difference in the environment and tested joint, less subjects' training, and unfixed background dimensions.

6. Conclusions and Future Directions

This study reports the results of experimental research designed to investigate the limitations of human force perception when the user's hand moves in a haptic-enabled virtual environment (HEVE). The thresholds of force perception are measured with respect to the factors such as the user's hand velocity, the base force, and force increment/decrement.

The results of this study have provided a basis for which the integration of the force JNDs in the presence of velocity can be used to transmit compressed haptic data unbeknown to the user. The threshold of human force perception plays a significant role in the development of these techniques. This study investigates the impact of important factors on the force threshold that affect these techniques when the user's hand is in motion. These factors include the base force intensity, force increment/decrement, and velocity of the user's hand.

The results show that force JNDs depend on the user's hand velocity, the base force and the force increment/decrement. Thus, these variables must be incorporated in an efficient haptic data compression algorithm when the user's hand is in motion. For example, if a user's hand is in a faster motion, fewer haptic details are required to be stored, calculated or transmitted.

The results indicate that haptic display developers cannot efficiently store or send the haptic data over the network when they are not aware of the previous applied force on the user's hand and if the forces increases or decreases. For example, the results and analysis of data in Section 5.3 show a Weber trend for the measured force JND, indicating that the force JND is significantly large for extremely small base forces and it decreases for the higher base forces.

The results indicate that the friction of haptic devices should be taken into account in the design of compression methods. In addition, the variability of friction is important. The variability of the OMNI device's friction did not largely affect the process of measuring the force threshold because it was very small. However, the variability of friction would be large and more complicated for many haptic devices and should be considered in developing a compression technique.

The human factors issues that are raised by the results of the experiments may guide future studies. For instance, based on the results, the effect of the base force on the JND of the human force perception is dependent on the force increment/decrement. This indicates that the interaction of these two factors should be taken into consideration in the design of haptic display of VEs. In addition, although the upper and lower limens of JND are almost symmetric for the medium and high base forces, they are not symmetric for the low base force. In other words, the user is not equally sensitive to the increment or decrement of applied forces for all base forces.

Time is critical in the development of compression techniques. Thus, time-efficient methods are essentials to measure the required force thresholds. Many psychophysical studies (Gescheider G.A. (1997)) have required long-term experiments to study human perception. For example in Pang et al., (1991) each experiment took hours with an average of 2048 trials for one experimental condition. In addition, the adaptation to force is also problematic in very long experimental sessions. In our study, each level of the experiment is completed within roughly a 50-minute session with 48 trials. The IS method takes less time compared to other methods because only a few stimuli values that are far above or below threshold are presented. As a result, a suitable compromise is found between the robust results and time to obtain specific data relevant to the development of perception-based compression methods.

7. References

Allin S., Matsuoka Y., and Klatzky R. L. (2002). Measuring Just Noticeable Differences for Haptic Force Feedback: Implications for Rehabilitation, *Symposium on Haptic Interfaces for Virtual Environment and Teleoperator Systems* pp. 299–302.

Berkelman, P. and Ji M. (2006). Effects of Friction Parameters on Completion Times for Sustained Planar Positioning Tasks with a Haptic Interface, *Proceedings of the 2006 IEEE/RSJ International Conference on Intelligent Robots and Systems* pp. 1115–1120. Beijing, China.

Bernstein R. S., and Gravel J. S. (1990). Method for determining hearing sensitivity in infants; The interweaving staircase procedure, *Journal of the American Academy of Audiology* **1**: 138–145.

Bhaskaran V., Konstantinides K. (1999). *Image and Video Compression Standards Algorithms and Architectures*, second edn, Kluwer Academic Publishers, USA.

Brandenburg K. (1999). MP3 and ACC explained, *Proceedings of the AES 17th International Conference on High Quality Audio Coding* . Florence, Italy.

Brewer B.R., Fagan M., Klatzky R.L. and Matsuoka Y. (2005). Perceptual limits for a robotic rehabilitation environment using visual feedback distortion, *Neural Systems and Rehabilitation Engineering, IEEE Transactions on [see also IEEE Trans. on Rehabilitation Engineering]* **13**(1): 1–11.

Brisben A. J., Hsiao S. S., and Johnson K. O. (1999). Detection of vibration transmitted through an object grasped in the hand, *Journal of Neurophysiology* **81**: 1548–1558.

Colgate J.E. and Brown J.M. (1994). Factors Affecting the Z-width of a Haptic Display, *Proceeding of the IEEE Int'l Conf. Robotics and Automation* pp. 3205–3210.

Cornsweet T. N. (1962). The Staircase-Method in Psychophysics, *The American Journal of Psychology* **75**(3): 485–491.

Diolaiti, N., Niemeyer, G., Barbagli, F., Salisbury, J.K., and Melchiorri, C. (2005). The effect of quantization and Coulomb friction on the stability of haptic rendering, *Proceedings of the First Joint Eurohaptics Conference and Symposium on Haptic Interfaces for Virtual Environment and Teleoperator Systems* pp. 237–246. 18-20 March.

Fitts P.M. (1954). The information capacity of the human motor system in controlling the amplitude of movement, *Journal of Experimental Psychology* **47**: 381–391.

Gersho A. (1994). Advances in speech and audio compression, *900-918* .

Gescheider G.A. (1997). *Psychophysics: The Fundamentals*, 3rd edn, Lawrence Erlbaum Associates.

Hinterseer P. and Steinbach E. (2005). Psychophysically Motivated Compression of Haptic Data, *In Proceedings of the Joint International COE/HAM - SFB453 Workshop on Human Adaptive Mechatronics and High Fidelity Telepresence* .

Hinterseer P. and Steinbach E. (2006). A Psychophysically Motivated Compression Approach for 3D Haptic Data, *In 14th Symposium on Haptic Interfaces for Virtual Environment and Teleoperator Systems* pp. p.35–41.

Hinterseer P., Steinbach E. and Chaudhuri S. (2006). Model-based Data Compression for 3D Virtual Haptic Teleinteraction, *IEEE International Conference on Consumer Electronics, ICCE 2006* .

Hinterseer P., Steinbach E., Chaudhuri S. (2006). Perception-Based Compression of haptic Data Streams Using Kalman Filters, *IEEE Intern. Conf. On Acoustics, Speech and Signal Processing* pp. pV–473–V–476.

Hinterseer P., Steinbach E., Hirche S., and Buss M. (2005). A novel, psychophysically motivated transmission approach for haptic data streams in telepresence and teleaction systems, *In Proceedings of the IEEE International Conference on Acoustics, Speech, and Signal Pro-cessing* pp. 1097–1100. Philadelphia, PA, USA.

Jandura L. and Srinivasan M. A. (1994). Experiments on Human Performance in Torque Discrimination and Control, *Proc. of the ASME Dynamic Systems and Control Division* **55-1**: 369–375.

Jones L. A. (1989). Matching forces: Constant errors and differential thresholds, *Perception* **18**(5): 681–687.

Karnopp D. (1985). Computer simulation of stick-slip friction in mechanical dynamic systems, *ASME Journal of dynamic Systems, Measurement and Control* **107**: 100–103.

Kuehl R. O. (2000). *Design of experiments : statistical principles of research design and analysis*, 2nd edn, Pacific Grove, CA ; London : Duxbury/Thomson Learning.

Kuschel M., Kremer P., Hirche S., and Buss M. (2006). Lossy data reduction methods for haptic telepresence systems, *Proceedings 2006 IEEE International Conference on Robotics and Automation ICRA 2006* . Las Vegas.

Lederman S.J., Klatzky R.L., Hamilton C.L. and Ramsay G.I. (1999). Perceiving roughness via a rigid probe: Psychophysical effects of exploration speed and mode of touch, *Haptics-e (Electronic Journal of Haptics Research)* **1(1)**: 1–20.

McLaughlin M.L., Joao P. Hespanha, and Gaurav S.S. (2002). *Touch in virtual environments: haptics and the design of interactive systems*, Prentice Hall.

Miano J. (1999). *Compressed Image File Formats: JPEG, PNG, GIF, XBM, BMP*, New York: ACM Press.

Pang X., Tan H.Z. and Durlach N. (1991). Manual discrimination of force using active finger motion, *Perception & Psychophysics* **49**(6): 531–540.

Raj D.V., Ingty K., and Devanandan M.S. (1985). Weight appreciation in the hand in normal subjects and in patients with leprous neuropathy, *Brain* **108**(1): 95–102.

Reis, H. & Judd, C. (2000). *Handbook of Research Methods in Social and Personality Psychology*, Cambridge University Press. ISBN 0521559030, 9780521559034.

Schiffman, H.R. (2000). *Sensation and perception : an integrated approach*, 5th edn, New York : Wiley.

Sensable Technologies Inc. (n.d.). http://www.sensable.com.

Shahabi C., Ortega A., and Kolahdouzan M.R. (2002). A Comparison of Different Haptic Compression Techniques, *Multimedia and Expo* .

Srinivasan M. and Basgodan C. (1997). Haptics in Virtual Environments: Taxonomy, Research Status, and Challenges, *Computers and Graphics* **21(4)**: 393–404.

Zadeh M.H., Wang D. and Kubica E. (2008). Perception-Based Lossy Haptic Compression Considerations for Velocity-Based Interactions, *Multimedia Systems Journal* **13**(4): 275–282.

Real-Time Support of Haptic Interaction by Means of Sampling-Based Path Planning

Michael Strolz and Martin Buss
Technische Universität München
Germany

1. Abstract

Haptic feedback enables the support of a human during the interaction with an environment. A variety of concepts have been developed to achieve an effective haptic support of the user in specific scenarios, e.g. *Virtual Fixtures*. However, most of these methods do not enable an adaptive support of the motion from a user within a (real or virtual) environment, which would be desirable in many situations. Especially when dynamical obstacles are involved or when the desired motion of the human is not known beforehand, an online computation of this support is essential, which should be based on a fast and effective determination of feasible motions.
In contrast to other methods, sampling-based path planning is applicable to arbitrary interaction scenarios and enables to find a solution if it exists at all. Thus, it seems to be ideally suited for a generic framework that is able to deal with various kinematics, as e.g. a virtual prototyping test bed for the haptic evaluation of mechanisms requires. At such a test bed, the path planner could directly be coupled to the haptic rendering of a virtual scene to assist a user in approaching a target.
This motivated the development of SamPP, a sampling-based path planning library with implementations of the most important algorithms. It can be used for nearly arbitrary rigid robots and environments. By performing numerous benchmarks, we prove the effectiveness and efficiency of SamPP. It is shown that a single-threaded version of the path planning can be used for real-time support of the haptic interaction at a novel actuated car door.
Furthermore, we enhance the path planning performance for unknown or dynamical environments significantly by the *OR-Parallelization* of different path planning queries. This *Generalized OR-Parallelization* is a novel concept that to the best knowledge of the authors has not been proposed beforehand. We show that for the case of dynamic environments the likelihood of a fast path planning result is higher with our approach. Thus, even in dynamic or unknown environments, a real-time support of haptic interaction can be achieved. Finally, we highlight four promising research directions to exploit the concept of Generalized OR-Parallelization:
1) Combination of PRMs and RRTs to achieve a synergy of the advantages of both concepts, 2) concurrent use of different parameter sets of path planning algorithms, 3) online adaptation of these parameter sets and 4) online adaptation of the types and numbers of parallel executed path planning programs.

2. Introduction

2.1 Support of Haptic Interaction

Haptic feedback enables the support of a human during the interaction with a virtual, shared, and/or remote environment. This is desirable for a broad range of applications, where the limited capabilities of humans should be improved or at least should not be detrimental. Examples include training of students and employees, manipulation of complex mechanisms, robotic surgery, and teleoperation in general (Esen, 2007).
A variety of concepts have been developed to achieve an effective haptic support of the user in specific scenarios. The most important one is the concept of *Virtual Fixtures*. Initially it has been proposed as a static, *rail-like* support to reduce the DOF of human motion (Rosenberg, 1993). Since then, a lot of extensions and variations of this concept have been developed, some of which even provide a dynamic, situation-dependent haptic support (Abott et al., 2003; Ammi & Ferreira, 2007; Davies et al., 1997; Kapoor et al., 2007; Lynch et al., 2002).
However, most of these methods do not enable an adaptive support of the interaction between a user and a haptic device. Rather, based on prior knowledge, they rely on a pre-computation of parts of the support method. One example is the offline determination of a desired path for surgical tools based on MRI data, where the desired start and goal configuration of the tools are known in advance (Li et al., 2007).

2.2 Path Planning

Especially when (real or virtual) environments with dynamical obstacles are involved or when the desired motion of the human is not known beforehand, an online computation of a collision-free path is essential. Path planning has been an active field in the past 15 years, and a variety of methods have been proposed.
A major drawback of many path planning algorithms is their lack of generality in terms of e.g. the existence of local minima. For instance, artificial potential fields which have been proposed for the assistance of haptic manipulation in the nano-scale (Varol et al., 2006) are prone to produce local minima in many handling scenarios.
With the recent introduction of sampling-based methods (Kavraki et al., 1996; LaValle et al., 1998), these limitations have been overcome, and high-dimensional path planning problems have been solved efficiently. Generally in sampling-based path planning, the geometry of both robot and workspace is considered based on discrete samples of the configuration of a robot. Various methodologies exist for the creation of these samples, which greatly influence the properties of the path planner depending on a given scenario. For the generated samples, a collision check is performed, often by openly available collision detection libraries as e.g. evaluated in (Strolz et al., 2008). The result is subsequently used by a path planning algorithm, which exclusively works in the configuration space (C-space) of the robot. To find a path for the robot, a local planner has to check whether two samples can be quasi-continuously connected without a collision.
Based on this, different strategies exist to find a path in the C-space: While *Single-Query* Planners as e.g. Rapidly-exploring Random Trees (RRT) (LaValle et al., 1998) create a path specifically for a given start and goal configuration, *Multi-Query Planners* as e.g. Probabilistic Roadmaps (PRM) (Kavraki et al., 1996) proceed in two steps: In the processing step, a number of samples is connected to form a *roadmap*. In the query step, the given start and goal configurations have to be connected to the roadmap. If this succeeds and if the

roadmap is connected, a solution surely exists and a suitable, optimized path can be found by a graph search. A comprehensive overview of the state of art in sampling-based path planning is given in (LaValle, 2006).

2.3 Performance Enhancement by Parallelized Sampling-Based Path Planning

It has been noted that some sampling-based path planning algorithms are (at least partially) *embarrassingly parallel* (Arnato & Dale, 1999). This means, that the path planning time can be drastically reduced by implementing the algorithm in a parallel manner and running it on suitable hardware. Impressive demonstrations of this are given in (Challou, 1995; Plaku, 2005), where a nearly linear speedup for an increasing number of processors has been reported.

Recently, it has been shown that another way of speeding up sampling-based path planning is to run a number of path planning queries in parallel on a suitable hardware (Klasing, 2009). It has been pointed out that with this *OR paradigm* the probability that none of the n queries finds a solution within a predefined time **t** is given by

$$1 - P_n(t) = (1 - P_1(t))^n \quad (1)$$

where P_1 denotes the probability that one query finds a solution within t (Challou, 1995). Obviously, this probability decreases rapidly with an increasing number of queries.

However, as noted in (Calisi, 2008), due to variations in the path planning environment there may be no single planner that will perform well in all possible situations. It is noted that "*an ideal motion planner would be a meta-planner using a suite of more specialized planners to cooperatively solve a motion planning problem. It would automatically apply the best-suited planner for each distinct region in the planning space and would produce regional solutions that could be composed to solve the overall motion planning instance.*" Furthermore, not only the choice of the algorithm itself but also its parameterization is a critical issue, because it drastically affects the performance of the path planning.

2.4 Contributions

Until the recent release of OpenRAVE (Diankov, 2008; OpenRAVE [Online]), there has been no easy-to-use, powerful generic path planning software. Thus, the sampling-based path planning library SamPP has been developed (Dömel, 2007) and subsequently improved, enhanced and evaluated. At first, we give an overview of SamPP and introduce the three most fundamental things about it: The representation of the robot and the environment, and the path planning algorithms. For the evaluation of SamPP, firstly it is successfully applied to a path planning scenario involving a robot with 10 DOF. Secondly, it is applied to different car door kinematics with 2 DOF, where it shows a superior performance (typical maximum path planning duration < 20 ms). Thirdly, the influence of the parameterization of the path planning algorithms is discussed and recommendations for the parameter tuning are given. A comparison with the state of the art, open-source sampling-based path planning libraries OpenRAVE and PP reveals that the performance of SamPP indeed is very high.

As explained in (Strolz et al., 2008), car doors with more than one DOF promise to improve the convenience of the access to cars. However, experiments on a Virtual Reality (VR) test

bed showed that users did not find the operation of car doors with several to be intuitive. We show that the single-threaded application of SamPP can be used for real-time support of the haptic interaction at such novel actuated car doors. The effectiveness of this haptic support with respect to user convenience is validated experimentally.
Furthermore, we enhance the path planning performance for unknown or dynamical environments significantly by an OR parallelization of ***different*** path planning algorithms. This is a novel concept that to the best knowledge of the authors has not been proposed beforehand. We prove that the likelihood of at least one fast path planning result is dramatically higher with our approached than with the parallel execution of several instances of a single path planner with a fixed parameter set. The reason is that the performance of a sampling-based path planner not only is subject to a stochastically process, but also depends greatly on the scenario at hand and the chosen parameters.

3. SamPP, a New Sampling-Based Path Planning Library

In this chapter, we introduce SamPP, a generic software library for Sampling-based Path Planning for rigid robots within arbitrary environments (Dömel, 2007). After describing the overall structure of the software and the representation of robot and environment, we present the implemented algorithms and an evaluation. Finally, we compare the performance to two recently released open source software libraries for sampling-based path planning, OpenRAVE (Diankov, 2008; OpenRAVE [Online]) and PP (PP [Online]).

3.1 Concept and Structure

SamPP has been intended to be part of a robotics control framework. Therefore, it was written in C++ (cross-platform) in an object-oriented manner as an API which is to be used in a client program. Using a specific parameter file which describes the path planning task at hand, a *SAMPP* object is instantiated there, and the path planning is executed.
A path planning task is fully defined by the following information:

- Description of the robot
- Description of the environment of the robot
- Start and goal configuration of the path

For solving the task, an algorithm and its parameterization have to be chosen. The algorithm needs a 3D representation of the path planning scenario to perform collision checking, which is built based on the description of robot and environment. Accordingly, we structured the software architecture in the following components:

1. ROBOT: Parametrized description of the kinematics and the 3D shape of the robot
2. ENVIRONMENT: Parametrized description of the 3D shape of all potential obstacles within the path planning scenario
3. WORLD_COLLISION and WORLD_VISUALIZATION: Structure representing the 3D scenario for the collision checking and the visualization engine
4. PLANNER: Selection and parametrization of the path planning algorithm
5. SAMPP: Path planning object based on previous five components

This way, a path planning query is performed by instatiating a SAMPP object, which will execute a path planning based on a chosen parameter set.

3.2 Representation of the Robot

The central consideration of sampling-based path planning is to find a collision free path for the robot in the configuration space (C-space) of the robot. The C-space depends on the specific kinematics of the robot, i.e. the number, the type and the limitations of its joints.
The motion of every rigid kinematics can be described by a combination of rotational and translational DOF. Even if a mechanism would exhibit different joints, e.g. a non-prismatic translational one, the position and orientation of all links could be expressed using additional *virtual* rotational and/or translational joints. This also holds for parallel links, where fewer overall DOF exist than the single joints would exhibit in sum.
To give a better understanding of the problems involved with creating a scheme for the representation of arbitrary robots, lets consider the robotic application of a car door with the two DOF ($\mathbf{q}_1$, $\mathbf{q}_2$) depicted in Figure 1. While the parts A and DOOR form an open tree-structured kinematic, due to the parallel mechanism the motion of the car door parts B and Z depend on ($\mathbf{q}_1$, $\mathbf{q}_2$). Thus, besides expressing rotational and translational DOFs and their limitations, we need to express the potential dependencies inherent to parallel mechanisms.

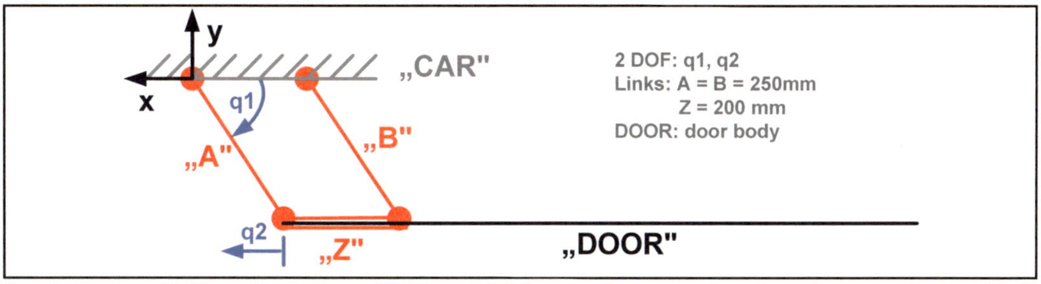

Fig. 1. Swing-Sliding Car Door (SSD) exhibiting both a rotational and a translation DOF, parallel links, and a closed kinematic chain.

By introducing dependent joints (dependent variables/dependent DOF), the problem of nonlinear and parallel kinematic configurations can be solved. For many real-world applications, a simple solution where the dependent joint configuration is calculated from the linear interpolation of predefined lookup table data is sufficient. This requires, that for every dependent joint a file has to be created that stores the lookup table.
A common way to represent kinematic chains is to use the Denavit-Hartenberg (DH) notation, where subsequently frames are created that describe a transformation from the base to the single links of the robot. This concept can be extended by introducing a parent for every frame, such that more than one child frame can be related to a frame. Thus, we build a tree structure, where each path represents a DH-like series of frames, which in combination with the dependent joints allows for representing parallel kinematics. This results in an intuitive tree-like robot description that can handle not only arbitrary open kinematic chains, but also kinematics with simple closed chains.
In robotics, it is often convenient to divide the configuration space in the configuration of the (usually) movable robot base on the one hand and the configuration of the joints of the manipulator on the other hand. The base configuration can generically be desribed by a transformation in respect to a world coordinate frame (maximum number of DOFs: 6). This equals a sequence of three translational and three rotational joints, all of which are

independent of each other. Thus, the base configuration can be expressed by a subset of the generic joint parameters.
Our generic definition of joint parameters is briefly described in the following:

- *ID*: Unique number of robot part (foundation of the overall kinematic tree)
- *PARENT*: *ID* of the predecessing robot part in the kinematic tree
- *REFJOINT*: [only if joint is of type dependent:] *ID* of reference joint
- *TYPE*: description of the DOF of the robot part
    - *RIGID*: the robot part represents no DOF
    - *TRANS*: translational DOF
    - *TRANS_CSTR*: constrained translational DOF
    - *TRANS_DPT*: no DOF, translational motion depends on *REFJOINT*
    - *ROT*: unconstrained rotational DOF
    - *ROT_CSTR*: constrained rotational DOF
    - *ROT_DPT*: no DOF, rotational motion depends on *REFJOINT*
- *MIN*: [only if joint is of type *_CSTR*:] minimum value of DOF
- *MAX*: [only if joint is of type *_CSTR*:] maximum value of DOF
- *DH_A*: Denavit-Hartenberg parameter (translation along x-axis)
- *DH_D*: Denavit-Hartenberg parameter (translation along z-axis)
- *DH_ALPHA*: Denavit-Hartenberg parameter (rotation around x-axis)
- *DH_THETA*: Denavit-Hartenberg parameter (rotation around z-axis)
- *WEIGHT*: weighting factor for this DOF

Accordingly, the base parameters are the subset without ID labels, joint type _DPT, and the Denavit-Hartenberg parameters.
Beside the kinematics, it is necessary to define parameters that take into account the influence of the single joints on the overall robot to ensure an efficient and effective path planning. The path planner needs to rate motions of the robot. A common measure for this is the change of the kinematic configuration of the robot, which results from the single joint displacements. In serial kinematic structures, a displacement of a joint near to the base usually has a significantly bigger impact on the displacement of the overall robot. This motivates to introduce a cost function that punishes big displacements, thereby allowing the path planner to work efficiently. Right now, we use a simple constant weighting WEIGHT of the individual joints to achieve this goal. The weighting has to be chosen heuristically based on the scenario at hand.
Furthermore, a discretization has to be defined for the single DOFs, because the path planning algorithm works in a discrete space, while the environment is continuous. The discretization $\mathbf{\Delta q}$ defines a lower bound which enables planning that can be considered quasi-continuously.
The distance of two states is calculated based on the simple L1 metric, thus all joint deviations are multiplied with their respective weight and summed, such that $\sum \mathbf{WEIGHT}(\mathbf{q}_k-\mathbf{q}_{k-1})$ results. If this sum is smaller than the threshold $\sum \mathbf{WEIGHT}(\mathbf{\Delta q})$ (minimum cost), no collision is considered to be feasible when moving from state k-1 to state k, and thus no collision check is performed. This means that, if the discretization is to coarse, the calculated path may not be collision-free. However, if the discretization is very fine, the efficiency of the path planning is significantly reduced. Thus, it is crucial to provide a parametrization that is appropriate for the example at hand.

For enabling collision checks and visualization, besides the kinematics a graphical 3D representation of the single robot parts is essential. Attention has to be paid to the handling of transformations and 3D data: The collision detection library and the visualization library may exhibit a different way to handle files and transformations.

3.3 Representation of the Environment

In contrast to the usually rigid and fixed robot kinematics, the environment may have to be altered during runtime because of moving obstacles. If obstacles are detected by sensors, they are often handled without semantic knowledge, i.e. shape primitives are used to describe a convex hull over their respective 3D geometry, compare e.g. (Strolz et al., 2008). Based on the assumption that only such shape primitives would be important in the modification of the environment during runtime, we defined data structures and accordingly transformation matrices for them. Thus, the environment objects can be altered, removed, or new ones can be inserted during runtime. Sometimes, it is more efficient to transform the objects rather than to create a new one.

3.4 Rapidly-exploring random Tree (RRT) Algorithms

Rapidly-exploring random Trees (RRTs, originally proposed in (LaValle, 1998)) are the most popular *Single Query* planning algorithms. A particularly successful modification is the bidirectional RRT: Instead of growing a tree from the start to the goal configuration, two trees are grown towards each other (Kuffner & LaValle, 2000).
There exist several expansion strategies for growing the tree. In the "classical" approach, the RRT is grown exactly one discretization step towards a sample. This can be extended by defining an upper bound for the expansion, e.g. five discretization steps. In contrast, the "visibility" approach iterates discretization steps towards the sample as long as the sample is not reached and no collision has been detected. We implemented these strategies, denoted as *RRT-cla* and *RRT-vis* in the following. Both algorithms require the start and the goal state as inputs. An optional parameter *timeout* enables to define a maximum duration for the path planning to quit the path planning for overly complex or even unsolvable problems. For an efficient handling of the search for nearest neighbors, we used kd-Trees and the open-source library ANN (Mount & Arya, 1997; ANN, [Online]).

3.5 Probabilistic Roadmap (PRM) Algorithms and their Parameterizations

PRM algorithms exhibit two phases: The processsing step, where the probabilistic roadmap is built, and the query step, which consists of connecting the start and the goal state to the roadmap and a consecutive search for the optimal path between them. Analogous to the RRT implementations, we implemented algorithms with "classical" and "visibility" expansion strategies: *PRM-cla* and *PRM-vis*.
The goal of building the map (*processing*) is to get a roadmap that provides a good coverage of the C-space. This can be heaviliy influenced by several parameters, which will be introduced in the following.
PrmMaxConnDist: Maximum distance between two states. This parameter defines to which extent the path planner behaves *classical* (low values, near resolution) or *visibility-based* (high values) while building the map.

As mentioned in the RRT section, the efficacy strongly depends on the environment at hand. Thus, with this parameter the path planning can be tuned for a class of scenarios. For instance, when rather dense environments have to be considered, a low value would be a good choice.
PrmInitialStates: Number of initial states which are randomly sampled before the algorithm tries to connect them. If all initial states are connected (or if the timeout condition is triggered), the building of the map is stopped.
The higher PrmInitialStates, the higher is the probability of a dense roadmap. In turn, this makes it more likely that the start and goal states can be connected with the roadmap in the query stage. However, a high number leads to a more complex roadmap which inhibits the path search. One way of finding a good setting can be to start with a rather low value. If it turns out that the start and/or goal state cannot be connected with the map, this number can adaptively be increased. Note that this functionality would have to be provided by the client program.
PrmMaxConnNumb: Maximum number of connections between a new collision free state and the roadmap. The higher this value, the better is the conjunction of the map, which tends to result in a smoother path and a longer path query.
In many applications, a value of up to 10 lead to good results.
PrmCleanMapRate: Rate of deletion of non-connected states. If a state is near an obstacle, it may be very difficult to connect it to the roadmap, which slows down the connection of the map. Therefore, the non-connected states are deleted with this rate. If this value is inappropriately low, it may be very difficult to build a map in a dense environment, because relevant states are deleted before being connected to the roadmap. Thus, this parameter be better only used if a relatively free C-space is assumed.
PrmMapRateExam: Rate of examination of the number of roadmaps. If the C-space is divided by obstacles such that not all states can be connected to one roadmap, some kind of timeout has to stop the attempt of the (infeasable) connection of the different roadmaps. This is done by examining the number of roadmaps at a constant rate. If the number did not change within one time interval, it is assumed that the different roadmaps can not be connected, and the proc. stage is terminated.
PrmMaxSampNumb: Maximum number of random samples. If this value is set, the proc. stage is terminated after this number of samples has been reached.
After the roadmap has been built, path planning *queries* can be executed. This involves firstly to connect the start and the goal state to the (same) roadmap. If this succeeded, one is sure that the states are connected, and a graph search as e.g. the famous A* algorithm can be performed to find the optimal path. Else, no path can be found, and an error is returned. Furthermore, a timeout results in an error, too.

4. Benchmark Results for SamPP

In the following, several benchmarks for SamPP are introduced and discussed. For all programs and scenarios, a PC with AMD Athlon(tm) 64 X2 Dual Core 5200+, 2 GB RAM and the operating system Linux Release 2.6.22-ipipe KDE 3.5.7 has been used. Only one of the two cores was used, and all programs were run 20 times.

In the results, **min** and **max** denote the minimum and maximum, and σ and **E** the standard deviation and expectation values of the path planning duration and the path length, respectively, of the 20 runs.

4.1 Application to a Robot with 10 DOF

Sampling-based path planning is superior to other path planning techniques especially if the number of DOF is high. To evaluate the efficiency of SamPP with respect to this, a scenario involving ViSHaRD10 (Ueberle et al., 2004) has been developed. ViSHaRD10 is a robot with 10 rotational DOF, as shown in Figure 2. Its special kinematic configuration does not allow a direct DH transformation from one joint to another for the joints 5, 8 and 9. Thus, for each of this joint two additional rigid joints have been used such that the robot kinematics could be described. As VRML model of these *pseudo joints*, very small cubes have been used, which are completely surrounded by neighboring joint models. Thus, they have neither influence on the path planning nor on the visualization.
The single joints of ViSHaRD10 are constrained by the wiring. We considered a restriction to **[-1.2 π 1.2π]** as appropriate to avoid damages, and applied this to every joint description. Furthermore, we had to find a suitable weighting for the joints. We did this for every single joint by using the maximum absolut worst-case displacement of all robot parts caused by a movement of this joint. These displacements were further used define the resolution for each joint.
The robot exhibits the highest versatility in the horizontal plane. Thus, a path planning scenario involving lots of motions in this plane was assumed to be most difficult, as it can constrain a high number of joints. For the evaluation, we used two scenarios.
Scenario 1 consisted of two narrow, parallel walls around the robot. The path planning task is to move the fully extended robot ($\mathbf{q}_{\{1..10\}} = \mathbf{0}$) to the opposite, fully stretched configuration ($\mathbf{q}_1 = \pi, \mathbf{q}_{\{2..10\}} = \mathbf{0}$).
Scenario 2 is an extension of scenario 1, where one additional short wall is placed exactly in the middle of the other two walls. It is shown in Figure 2 (r.). The start configuration is given by ($\mathbf{q}_1 = \pi, \mathbf{q}_2 = -\pi, \mathbf{q}_{\{3..10\}} = \mathbf{0}$), the goal configuration by ($\mathbf{q}_1 = -\pi, \mathbf{q}_2 = \pi, \mathbf{q}_{\{3..10\}} = \mathbf{0}$).

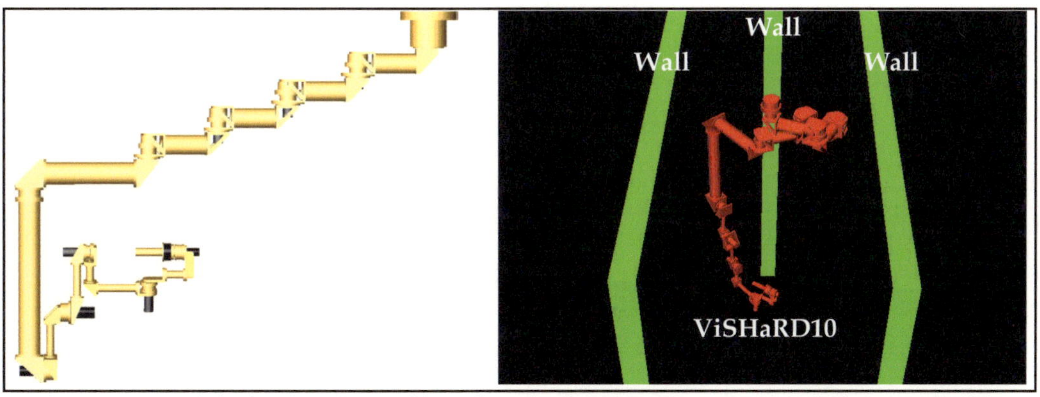

Fig. 2. VRML model of ViSHaRD10 (l.) and path planning scenario 2 with three walls (r.).

Due to the high number of dimensions, PRM algorithms are not appropriate for a fast single-shot query, because a good coverage of the C-space would require a very large number of states, such that the graph search on the roadmap would be much slower than a single query method. Thus, we only consider the two RRT algorithms *RRT-cla* and *RRT-vis* for these scenarios. The benchmark results are given in Table 1.

		Algorithm	min	max	σ	E
Scenario 1 (two walls)	Duration [s]	RRT-cla	0.471	6.435	1.475	2.618
		RRT-vis	0.086	1.309	0.422	0.387
	Path length [NORM]	RRT-cla	65.0	97.0	9.4	77.2
		RRT-vis	112.0	360.0	61.4	218.4
Scenario 2 (three walls)	Duration [s]	RRT-cla	2.099	7.438	1.127	3.537
		RRT-vis	3.026	43.079	11.659	17.125
	Path length [NORM]	RRT-cla	92.0	188.0	35.1	125.9
		RRT-vis	164.0	432.0	62.0	290.9

Table 1. Path planning benchmark results for the two ViSHaRD10 scenarios 1 and 2.

The environment of the first scenario with two walls is not very narrow in joint space. Therefore, *RRT-vis* outperforms *RRT-cla* in the duration measures by a factor of approximately 3 to 6. The differences in the normalized path lengths clearly exhibit that despite the postprocessing of the path the faster *RRT-vis* produced costs whose average was three times higher than the *RRT-cla*. This shows one dilemma of sampling-based path planning: By choosing an appropriate algorithm and by tuning parameters, a trade-off has to be found for the scenario at hand.

In the second scenario, the third wall leads to a very narrow area in the C-space. This limits the advantage of the *RRT-vis*, and consequently leads to a rather slow path planning when compared to *RRT-cla*. Again, the *RRT-vis* produces a much shorter path. For such an environment, the classic method is the best option.

Thus, by applying SamPP to a robot with 10 DOF, we have shown that the implementations *RRT-vis* and *RRT-cla* are able to plan a path in a relatively short time. In two complex scenarios, the *RRT-cla* exhibited a maximum planning time of 7.4 s. Furthermore, it found relatively short paths when compared to the visibility based method. This has also been visually observed when executing the planned path on the robot.

4.2 Preliminary Remarks on the Application to Different Scenarios with Car Doors

We apply SamPP to some car doors with 2 DOF and investigate the effect of different environments etc. As models for the car door a VRML file with 31728 polygons has been used, the obstacles were represented as approximated spheres with 400 polygons each.

The goal of the path planning is to provide a collision free path from a fully closed position to a given open position. The following methods are investigated:

- *RRT-vis*: visibility-based RRT implementation
- *RRT-cla*: classic RRT implementation
- *PRM-vis-P*: proc. stage of PRM-vis
- *PRM-vis-Q*: query stage of PRM-vis
- *PRM-cla-5P, PRM-cla-10P*: proc. stage of PRM-cla with 5/10 nearest neighbours
- *PRM-cla-5Q, PRM-cla-10Q*: query stage of PRM-cla with 5/10 nearest neighbours

4.3 Application to a Double-Four-Links Car Door (2 DOF)

In **scenario 3**, a car door with two serial links named Double-Four-Links Door is considered. Its kinematics is depicted in Figure 3 (r.). Though exhibiting four links and six joints, it only has two rotatory DOFs. Furthermore, due to the symmetry of the links, the door performs no rotation in world coordinates.

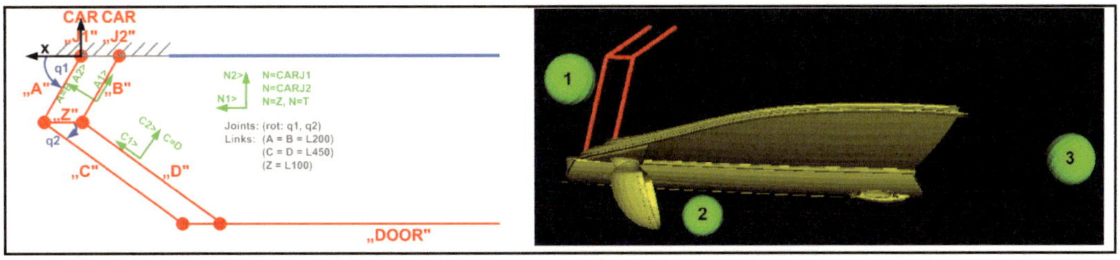

Fig. 3. Double-Four-Links Door (l.) within three obstacles (r.) (scenario 3).

We consider three different environments which consist of three spheres as is shown in Figure 3 (l.). The configuration space constrained by the environment is depicted in Figure 4 (m.). The C-space consists of 3 non-connected areas. As both the start and the goal state are located in area 2, a path can be found. Area 1 represents sphere 2 and, in combination with area 3, forms a narrow corridor. This surely is the bottleneck for the path-planning. If sphere 2 is varied only a little bit (**Δy=0.01m** nearer to the car, which has a length of **l=1.30m**), the corridor significantly narrows. In contrast, if sphere 2 is varied a little bit more (**Δy=0.10m** further away from the car), it is out of the workspace of the door and thus has no influence on the path-planning, see Figure 4 (l.). Area 2 is now a very large free space, and path planning should accordingly be very fast. This example illustrates how extremely small variations in the configuration of the obstacles can affect path planning.

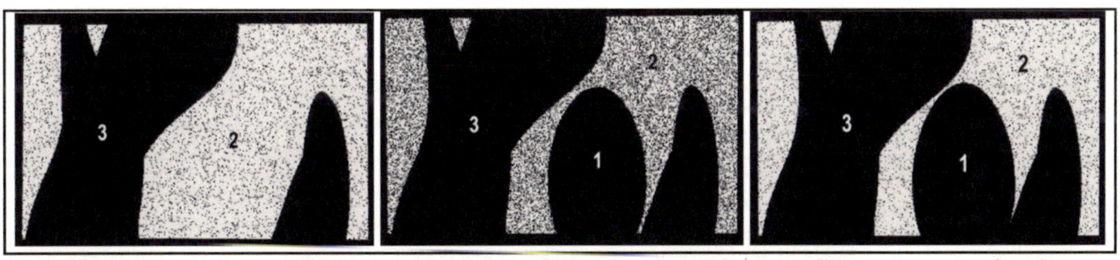

Fig. 4. Scenario 3: Broad (l.), narrow (m.) and very narrow (r.) configurations in the C-space given by slightly varying the position of obstacle 2 (see also Figure 3).

For all configurations of sphere 2 ("very narrow", "narrow", and "broad"), all path planning methods have been evaluated. The results are summarized in Table 2.
For configuration "very narrow", *RRT-cla* performs best. The PRM methods are considerably slower in the processing stage, but excel in the variations *PRM-cla-10Q* and *PRM-vis* in the query stage. If many queries are to be performed on such a kind of environment, PRM seem to be a good choice.
Interestingly, *PRM-cla-10* is faster then *PRM-cla-5* and *PRM-vis*. The reason for this must be that choosing 5 nearest neighbors leads to a roadmap which is too dense, while PRM-vis is to coarse. Thus, for every environment there is a range of connection length for which the

planning performs best. In this particular case, by chance we found a good balance, as both a higher and a lower value perform worse.
With respect to the length (cost) of the paths, there is no great difference between the planners for all three scenarios, see the example given in Table 2, scenario 3 "very narrow".
From the results for configuration "narrow", one can see that the RRT methods give a similar expectancy value, while exhibiting a significantly different variance. The reason is, that the *RRT-vis* sometimes "by chance" quickly finds a path through the narrow passage, but besides that works less efficient in such a kind of scenario. In contrast, from the PRM methods the *PRM-vis* performs best. This is due to the funnel-shaped C-space; if this was maze like, the results most likely would have been much worse.
While there has been a strong improvement in the time duration, the path lengths seem not to significantly differ from the ones of the "very narrow" ones.

		Algorithm	min	max	σ	E
Scenario 3 (broad)	Duration [ms]	RRT-cla	20	31	3	24
		RRT-vis	3	9	2	5
		PRM-cla-5P	22	48	8	35
		PRM-cla-5Q	7	17	3	11
		PRM-cla-10P	25	49	7	34
		PRM-cla-10Q	6	18	3	10
		PRM-vis-P	41	118	21	67
		PRM-vis-Q	4	13	2	6
Scenario 3 (narrow)	Duration [ms]	RRT-cla	33	49	4	38
		RRT-vis	13	102	21	35
		PRM-cla-5P	198	396	54	266
		PRM-cla-5Q	17	48	8	25
		PRM-cla-10P	117	160	31	231
		PRM-cla-10Q	7	15	3	22
		PRM-vis-P	86	187	26	120
		PRM-vis-Q	4	17	4	9
Scenario 3 (very narr.)	Duration [ms]	RRT-cla	31	66	8	44
		RRT-vis	21	375	95	115
		PRM-cla-5P	314	517	80	404
		PRM-cla-5Q	27	60	24	114
		PRM-cla-10P	240	382	40	275
		PRM-cla-10Q	14	38	6	23
		PRM-vis-P	374	548	102	448
		PRM-vis-Q	10	23	4	16
	Path length [NORM]	RRT-cla	39	42	0.9	40.5
		RRT-vis	39	46	2.0	41.1
		PRM-cla-5P	39	43	1.1	40.3
		PRM-cla-10P	39	43	1.1	40.5
		PRM-vis-P	39	42	0.8	40.3

Table 2. Path planning benchmark results for scenario 3 with variation of obstacle position.

4.4 Application to SCARA-like Car Door (2 DOF)

In scenario 4, SamPP has to be applied to the Two-Links Door which is depicted in Figure 5. The environment consists of four spheres. The main problem in doing this is to circumvent sphere 2 and to reach the state which is near the spheres 3 and 4. The C-space of this path planning problem is very narrow, as can be seen from Figure 5 (r.). In area 1 both the start and the goal configuration is contained, thus a valid path can be found. The representation of sphere 2 forms a long and narrow passage from the start state.

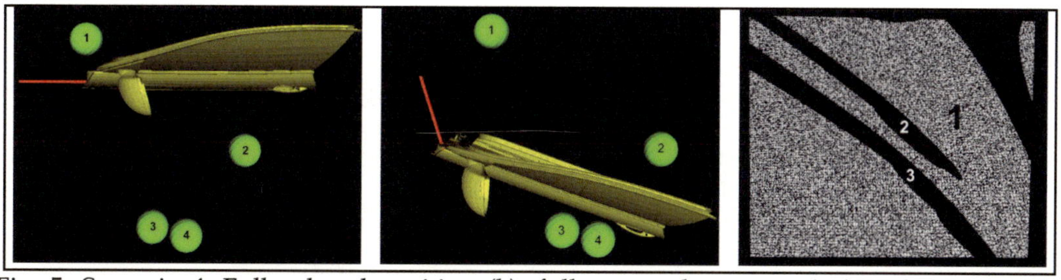

Fig. 5. Scenario 4: Fully closed position (l.), fully opened position (m.) and depiction of narrow passage in the C-space of the Two-Links Car Door.

		Algorithm	min	max	σ	E
Scenario 4 (very narr.)	Duration [ms]	RRT-cla	11	43	8	24
		RRT-vis	3	19	5	9
		PRM-cla-5P	75	168	23	103
		PRM-cla-5Q	6	17	3	11
		PRM-cla-10P	87	169	29	130
		PRM-cla-10Q	6	22	4	11
		PRM-vis-P	91	169	22	127
		PRM-vis-Q	4	19	4	9
	Path length [NORM]	RRT-cla	19	44	7.5	36.8
		RRT-vis	36	62	7.2	54.0
		PRM-cla-5P	39	47	2.2	42.3
		PRM-cla-10P	37	47	2.3	41.8
		PRM-vis-P	32	62	6.4	46.0

Table 3. Path planning benchmark results for scenario 4.

The RRT methods perform the path planning considerably faster than the PRM methods. The *RRT-vis* exhibits an expectation value of 9 ms, thereby even undercutting the expectation value of the PRM queries. If the corridor in the C-space would not have been straight but curved, the *PRM-cla* would have been better. All PRM methods require a maximum of more than 150 ms for building the map. This makes them not suited for real-time applications in scenarios like these.

The path lengths exhibit a significant variance for all methods, which is a hint that the path postprocessing performs very poor for scenarios like these. Thus, it might be beneficial to improve this algorithm.

4.5 Application to Car Doors with 2 DOF in the Presence of Many Obstacles

When interfacing the path planner with a sensor system (Strolz et al. 2009), a much higher number of primitive objects will be used to represent obstacles in the workspace of the door. This motivated to evaluate the influence of the number of obstacles on the path planner. We replaced the spheres of the environment (which represented vertical pillars) by 100 spheres each. This increase in the number of obstacles does barely affect the C-space.

From Table 4, it clearly can be seen that the RRT methods provide a much better performance than the PRMs for a single query. The reason is their reduce demand for collision checks: The PRMs suffer from the many collision queries that have to be performed when building the map. However, the maximum query time of the PRMs is significantly shorter than that of the *RRT-vis*. Thus, it is not possible to give a clear recommendation on whether to use PRMs or RRTs in a scenario with a high number of obstacles. In static scenarios, a combination might be a good choice: Two computers can be used, one running *PRM-vis*, the other *RRT-vis*. While the roadmap is built, only *RRT-vis* results are used for path planning. After that, as long as the environment does not change, both *RRT-vis* and a PRM-query a started simultaneously, and the faster result is used. For the evaluation scenarios, this would lead to a maximum time consumption for the "parallel query" of 68 ms, which might be fast enough to be used in an haptic assistance task.

		Algorithm	min	max	σ	E
Modified Scenario 3 (400 obst.)	Duration [ms]	RRT-vis	39	548	117	190
		PRM-vis-P	142	2084	382	1704
		PRM-vis-Q	16	66	11	41
Modified Scenario 4 (400 obst.)	Duration [ms]	RRT-vis	20	117	21	42
		PRM-vis-P	2497	2926	106	2643
		PRM-vis-Q	31	68	8	41

Table 4. Path planning benchmark results for modified scenarios 3 and 4 with 400 obstacles.

4.6 Short Performance Comparison to OpenRAVE

We wanted to find out whether our implementation of sampling-based path planning algorithms had a performance that is comparable to implementations of other researchers. Recently, the professional, open-source path planning library OpenRAVE (Diankov, 2008) has been released. Its RRT algorithms seemed to be suitable to benchmark our implementations of *RRT-cla* and *RRT-vis*.

At first, we installed OpenRAVE on the same Linux system that had been used for the evaluation of SamPP. We run the same scenarios which we described in the previous sections. The performance was really poor when compared to SamPP: All time measures were by approximately an order of magnitude worse than the ones for SamPP. For instance, the average time of the bidirectional RRT was 32.04 s (>> 0.39 s of our *RRT-vis*) for scenario 1 and 146 ms (>> 9 ms of our *RRT-vis*) for scenario 4. We could not explain this discrepancy, so we installed OpenRAVE on a virtual Linux system (Ubuntu) which was running on a Windows system (Windows XP, 2 GB RAM) and repeated the evaluation.

Despite the fact that the virtual Linux most likely increases the computational overhead, the results were much closer to the ones of SamPP. For instance, the average and minimum times of the bidirectional RRT was 2.45 s/0.53 s (> 0.39 s/0.09 s of our *RRT-vis*) for scenario 1 and 12 ms/5 ms (> 9 ms/3 ms of our *RRT-vis*) for scenario 4.

While these comparisons do not enable a fair overall judgement of the path planning performance (different system configuration, heavily dependence on specific scenario), they nonetheless lead to the following conclusions:

1. We were not able to identify the reason for the poor performance of OpenRAVE on the first system. Thus, we advice potential users of OpenRAVE or other complex path planning libraries to benchmark the software on different systems to minimize the risk of running it in a very suboptimal configuration.
2. SamPP is comparable to professional state-of-the-art implementations of samping-based path planning algorithms, as e.g. OpenRAVE or PP.

4.7 Remarks and Summary

We evaluated the performance of SamPP for executing path planning for a 10 DOF robot and for different 2 DOF car doors within an (in terms of the configuration space) very demanding environment. Due to the RRT and PRM algorithms, SamPP is able to solve a variety of path planning problems efficiently. For the case of 300 to 400 obstacles, nearly "worst-case" placed in the workspace of these car doors, we found typical mean values for the path planning time in the area of 50 ms for RRTs, 1500 ms for building a PRM and 30 ms for PRM queries. The evaluation results for scenarios 3 and 4 show that the performance of SamPP indeed is sufficient for the haptic real-time assistance of a human in various scenarios with 2 DOF. Independently of the planning algorithm, the path postprocessing seems to work quite well if there are no overly narrow passages in the C-space of the robot.
Note that the performance heavily depends on the environment at hand. The environments that we used for the evaluation often exhibited an uncluttered, rather free C-space. This promotes the visibility based methods. However, it has been shown that there is no "one size fits all" solution: depending on the environment at hand, variations of the parameter setting may decrease or increase the performance of the path planner.
Further, we observed that a comparison of the performance of PRM methods for fixed processing times showed that larger roadmap leads to longer query response time, and that a reduction of the number of initial states proved to give better results for our scenario. It is relatively hard to find an appropriate number of initial sample states for simple environments of the robot. The roadmap has to sufficiently cover the C-space to provide a very high probability that the start and the end goal can be connected to the map. A large and complex roadmap, in turn, cannot quickly be evaluated by a graph search algorithm. This problem cannot occur when using an RRT method, because the planner is focused on connecting a start configuration as efficiently as possible with the goal configuration, such that no "overly complex" connection structure results. For rather simple scenarios, the total planning time of *RRT-cla* is faster than a query on a roadmap. For such cases, it does make no sense to use PRMs at all.

5. Haptic User Support at a Virtual Car Door by Path Planning

5.1 System Description

In (Strolz et al., 2008), a system for the control of actuated car doors with arbitrary DOF has been introduced. This system should be augmented with an additional user support method given by an online path planning. An overview of the overall structure of the simulated system is given in Figure 6. The different modules are connected by UDP communication.

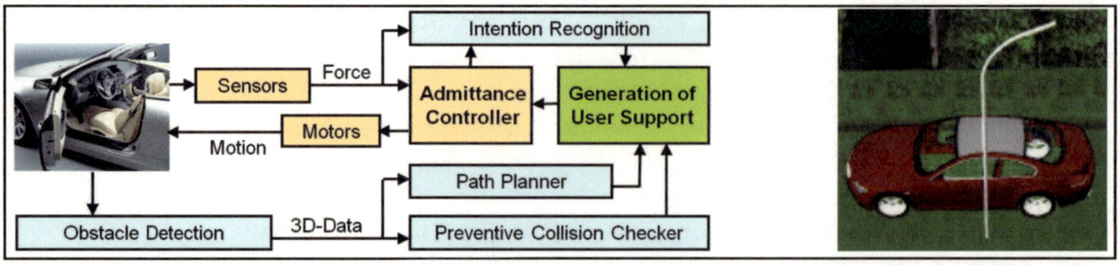

Fig. 6. Advanced car door control system with haptic user assistance by path planning, collision avoidance and intention recognition (l.) and its visual simulation (r.).

To achieve a precise path planning, a camera which monitors the workspace of the door and provides data about potential obstacles is simulated. The simulated data is continuously being sent to the path planning computer (in the form of primitive, convex shapes, e.g. spheres). Furthermore, the path planner continuously receives the start and goal configuration of the door from the door controller. For each new data packet, a path planning query trigger event occurs. As soon as the path planner finished a query and sent the collision-free path to the car door controller, it accepts such trigger events to restart path planning with the updated values.
In the car door controller, in the joint space a supportive force is calculated which points into the direction of the middle piece of the collision-free path. We chose an upper bound of 2 N for this bound, such that it predominantly does not change the motion of the mechanism itself, but rather gives motion cues to the user to achieve an intuitive interaction.

5.2 Experiment

To evaluate the effect of the haptic user assistance, an experimental user study has been conducted. We chose car door and obstacle configuration similar to scenario 4, see Figure 5. Our hypotheses were:

1. Users can handle the door easier and more intuitively if the door is actuated nad supportive forces are displayed to them.
2. The path planning support is helpful during the haptic interaction.

We designed the experiment such that different controller configurations were displayed, some of which included the path planning. By answering a questionaire, the participants should rate these configurations with respect to a reference scenario without path planning. The duration of the experiment was approximately 30 minutes, and 20 people (12 men; in average 26 years, 70 kg, 1.75 m) participated in it.

5.3 Results and Discussion

In Figure 7, some of the results are displayed. They show a predominant approval of the implemented car door control system with path planning. A T-test revealed that the rating of the two variations of the path planner assistance (with and without end positioning support) was significant on a 5% level ($F(0.95; 38) = 2.09$, $p = 0.017 < 0.05$) and ($F(0.95; 38) = 2.09$, $p = 0.0004 < 0.05$)). Thus, the path planner indeed brings a significant advantage to users when they handle a novel car door.

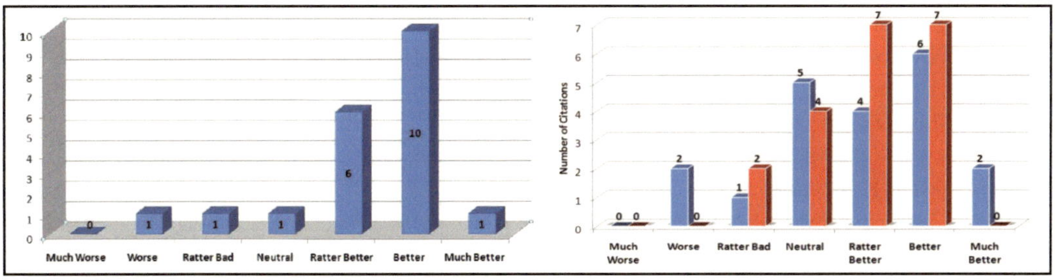

Fig. 7. Evaluation of the advanced car door control system: Comparison against reference scenario for the assistance in general (l.) and for two variations of the path planning assistance (r.) where the red bars represent an additional haptic support (Solhjoo, 2009).

6. Further Enhancement: Parallel Execution of Different Path Planners

6.1 Problem: There is no Best Algorithm

In the introduction and the evaluation section, it was highlighted that there is no overall best-performing path planning algorithm, because the kinematics of the robot and the structure of the environment have a huge impact on the level of difficulty of the path planning task. To clarify this, in Table 5 a composition of the fastest planners is given for slight modifications of scenario 3.

		Algorithm	min	max	σ	E
Scenario 3 (broad)	Duration [ms]	RRT-cla	20	31	3	24
		RRT-vis	3	9	2	5
		PRM-vis-P	41	118	21	67
		PRM-vis-Q	4	13	2	6
Scenario 3 (narrow)	Duration [ms]	RRT-cla	33	49	4	38
		RRT-vis	13	102	21	35
		PRM-vis-P	86	187	26	120
		PRM-vis-Q	4	17	4	9
Scenario 3 (very narr.)	Duration [ms]	RRT-cla	31	66	8	44
		RRT-vis	21	375	95	115
		PRM-vis-P	374	548	102	448
		PRM-vis-Q	10	23	4	16
Modified Scenario 3 (400 obst.)	Duration [ms]	RRT-vis	39	548	117	190
		PRM-vis-P	142	2084	382	1704
		PRM-vis-Q	16	66	11	41

Table 5. Composition of the fastest planners for modifications of scenario 3.

6.2 Solution: Parallelization of Different Algorithms (Generalized OR paradigm)

As already explained in the introduction, two research directions have been proposed in the past to speed up complex path planning problems:

1. Parallelization of subtasks of path planning algorithm:
   Decreasing the time consumption of specific path planning algorithms:
2. OR-parallelization of a specific path planning algorithm:
   Increasing likelihood of a fast result by executing several instances of one planner

We propose a promising third alternative:

3. OR-parallelization of different path planning algorithms:
   Increasing likelihood of a fast result by executing a number of instances of different planners and/or planner parametrizations

To prove this principle mathematically, we extend Equ. (1) (Challou, 1995) to the **Generalized OR paradigm**: Be $P_{1,2,..,k}(t)$ the probability that the different path planning programs 1, 2, ..., k do not find a collision-free path within the time t. Then, the probability that a path is found within t is

$$P(t) = 1 - P_{n+o+...+q}(t) = (1 - P_1(t))^n(1 - P_2(t))^o...(1 - P_k(t))^q \quad (2)$$

where n, o, ..., q denote the number of the parallel executed instances of the respective programs. The programs might be different in respect of the algorithm and/or the parametrization of the algorithm.

6.3 General remarks to the Generalized OR paradigm

The effect of this approach can be shown by the evolution of the probabilities of some random processes and their combinations. Several sequences of random numbers were generated based on an exponential distribution function. They are characterized by an exponential coefficient (8, 10, 9, 11 in our case) and a static time offset (0.30s, 0.15s, 0.25s, 0.18s) to represent the characteristics of different path planner evaluations.
Exemplary, in Figure 8 the probability of finding a collision-free path is depicted as a function of time and of number of programs. The arrow in the upper left axis indicates that for an increasing number of parallel path planning programs, the probability approaches a step function at time $t = t_{Offset} + t_{calc,\,min}$ which due to the probabilistical completness of sampling-based path planning would be achieved for an infinite number of simultaneously starting programms. The upper and lower axes show four different occurrences of path planning probability functions for 1 to 66 parallely running programms. In the middle axes, the combinations of 33 of the upper and 33 of the lower algorithms is depicted. Note that in both cases, a speedup with respect to the worse performing algorithm is achieved.

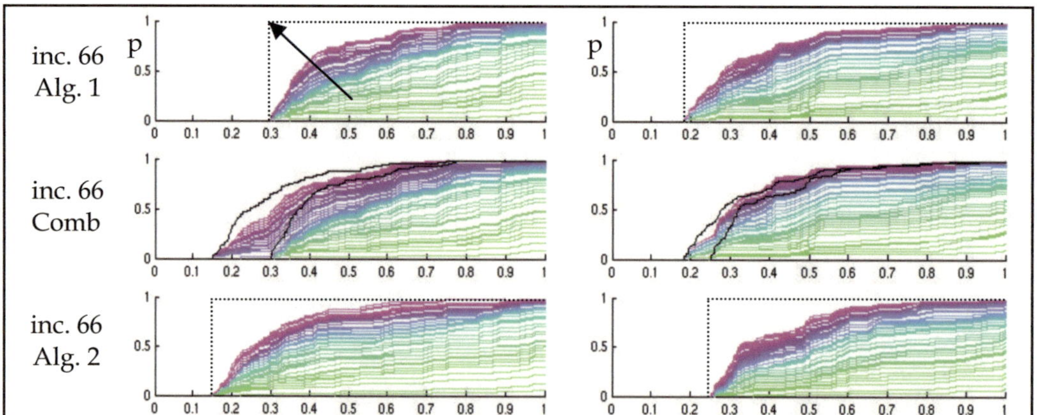

Fig. 8. Evolution of the probability of finding a collision-free path. The arrow indicates that for an increasing number of programs, the probability approaches a step function.

Based on Equ. (2), the general conclusion can be drawn that from an algorithmic point of view the performance of the overall sampling-based path planning will *always* increase if additional planners are started, because each planner contributes to the overall probability. In the following, we point out four advantages and research directions arising from this.

6.4 Potential Advantage 1: Synergy by combining PRMs and RRTs

Often, path planning queries can be faster calculated for existing PRMs than for single-shot RRTs. However, building the PRM requires a significant amount of time, which limits their application. The best option might be to build one ore more roadmaps while path planning queries are answered by other algorithms. Then, as long as the environment doesn't change significantly, the typically very efficient PRM queries can be performed. This way, both the advantages of PRMs and RRTs can be utilized. For the example given in Table 5, combinations of *RRT-cla, RRT-vis* and *PRM-vis* could drastically reduce the worst-case maximum duration of path planning both during and after building a PRM.

In Figure 9, the performance of the parallel execution of *RRT-cla* and *RRT-vis* is given for scenario 3. As had been expected from the results of Table 5, the *RRT-vis* was better in the broad configuration space and the RRT-cla in the very narrow one. Due to this combination, the poor performance of the *RRT-cla* in the very narrow case are barely noticable when compared to parallel executions of only *RRT-vis*. This underlines the increase of the reliability which is inherently achieved by the Generalized OR-parallelization.

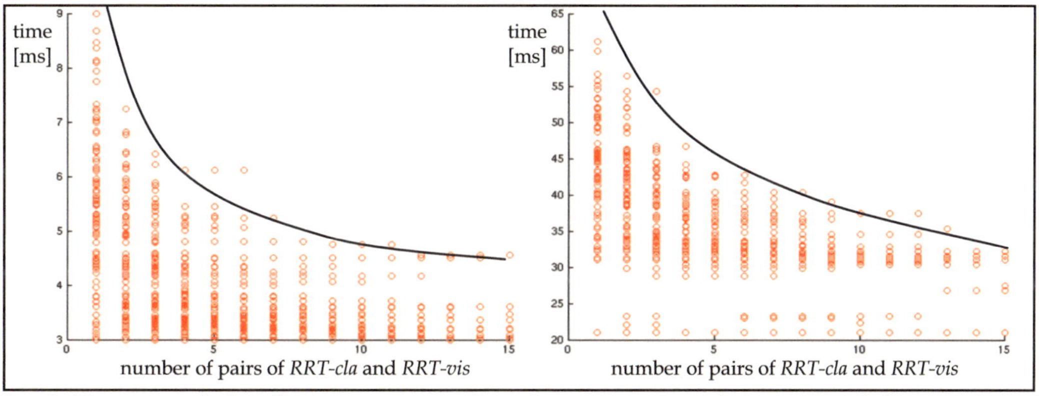

Fig. 9. Decrease of the shortest computation time per run with increase of the number of RRT-based path planner pairs for scenario 3 ("broad", l. and "very narrow", r.).

6.5 Potential Advantage 2: Utilization of Different Parameterizations of Algorithms

The choice of the parameters of an algorithm drastically influences its performance, see e.g. Section 3.6. One of the big problems with the parameterization is that due to the infinite combinations of robots and environments, most planners will perform badly for at least some "pathological" cases, where e.g. the C-space is extremely dense. However, the default parameter set of e.g. a PRM planner might not be designed for solving this particular case, but to perform well in the majority of the planning tasks. Using our approach, well-proven default and purpose-built parameter sets can be used for arbitrary scenarios.

6.6 Potential Advantage 3: Adaptive Parameterization of the Algorithms

Additionally to the utilization of different parameter sets for path planning algorithms, these parameters should be adapted online. In the previous sections, we pointed out that especially the performance of PRM planners relies on appropriate parameters such as the number of initial states or the desired density of the map. Based on PRM performance criteria such as query time and query success, these parameters can be adaptively balanced.

6.7 Potential Advantage 4: Advanced Adaptive OR-Parallelization Scheme

If there are enough processing resources that all relevant planning algorithms can be executed simultaneously, an advanced adaptive OR-parallelization can be realized: Based on the evolution of the path planning duration of the individual algorithms, the candidate(s) with the highest likelihood for fast path planning results is identified online and subsequently started more often than the other planners. Thus, based on the definition of specific criteria, an optimization of the OR-parallelization can be performed. This optimization should take into account the quality of the estimation of the path planning durations, e.g. it has to take care that sufficiently "non-optimal" algorithms are running.

7. Conclusion and Future Work

We have developed SamPP, a generic sampling-based path planning library and successfully applied to a variety of robots and environments. Due to the implementation of RRT and PRM algorithms, SamPP is able to solve low- as well as high-dimensional problems efficiently.

The ability to solve a high-dimensional path planning scenarios has been shown by the example of ViSHaRD10, a robot with 10 DOF.

Furthermore, we evaluated the performance of SamPP for executing path planning for different car doors with 2 DOF within an (in terms of free configuration space) very demanding environment. For the case of 300 to 400 obstacles, nearly "worst-case" placed in the workspace of these car doors, we found typical mean values for the path planning time in the area of 50 ms for RRTs, 1500 ms for building a PRM and 30 ms for PRM queries. The evaluation results show that the performance of SamPP indeed is sufficient for the haptic real-time assistance of a human in various scenarios with 2 DOF. Independently of the planning algorithm, the path postprocessing seems to work quite well if there are no overly narrow passages in the C-space of the robot.

Based on these results, we developed a "real-time" haptic support method and applied it to a virtual car door. An experimental user study revealed that the haptic support is appreciated by the users.

Furthermore, we enhanced the path planning performance for unknown or dynamical environments significantly by the *OR-Parallelization* of different path planning queries. This *Generalized OR-Parallelization* is a novel concept that to the best knowledge of the authors has not been proposed beforehand. We showed that for the case of dynamic environments the likelihood of a fast path planning result is higher with our approach.

Finally, we highlight four promising research directions to exploit the advantages of the concept of *Generalized OR-Parallelization*: 1) Combination of PRMs and RRTs to achieve synergy of the advantages of both concepts, 2) concurrent use of different parameter sets of path planning algorithms, 3) online adaptation of these parameter sets and 4) online adaptation of the types and numbers of parallel executed path planning programs.

Acknowledgement

This work has been supported by BMW Group in the framework of CAR@TUM.
First of all, the authors would like to thank Andreas Dömel for his valuable contributions during and after his Studienarbeit (Dömel, 2007). Furthermore, the authors would like to thank Klaas Klasing for his constant support and advice. Finally, the authors would like to thank Amir Solhjoo for his contributions in the user study (Solhjoo, 2009).

8. References

Abbott, J.J.; Hager, G.D. & Okamura, A.M. (2003). Steady-Hand Teleoperation with Virtual Fixtures. *Proceedings of the IEEE International Workshop on Robot and Human Interactive Communication*, Millbrae, California, USA, 2003.

Ammi M. & Ferreira, A. (2007). Robotic Assisted Micromanipulation System using Virtual Fixtures and Metaphors, *Proceedings of the IEEE International Conference on Robotics and Automation (ICRA)*, pp. 454-460, 2007.

ANN [Online]. *http://www.cs.umd.edu/~mount/ANN/*. Accessed on September 19th, 2009.

Arnato, N. & Dale, L. (1999). Probabilistic roadmap methods are embarrassingly parallel. *Proceedings of 1999 IEEE International Conference on Robotics and Automation*, 1999, pp. 688-694.

Calisi, D. (2008). Motion Planning, Reactive Methods, and Learning Techniques for Mobile Robot Navigation, *www.dis.uniroma1.it/~dottoratoii/db/relazioni/relaz_calisi_2.pdf* Accessed on September 19th, 2009.

Challou, D.; Boley, D.; Gini, M. & Kumar, V. (1995). A parallel formulation of informed randomized search for robot motion planning problems. *Proceedings of 1995 IEEE International Conference on Robotics and Automation*, 1995, pp. 709-714.

Davies, B.L.; Harris, S.J.; Lin, W.J.; Hibberd, R.D.; Middleton, R. & Cobb, J.C. (1997). Active compliance in robotic surgery--the use of force control as a dynamic constraint. *Proc Inst Mech Eng H.*, Vol 211, No. 4 (1997), pp. 285-292.

Diankov, R. and Kuffner, J.J. (2008). OpenRAVE: A Planning Architecture for Autonomous Robotics. *Technical Report CMU-RI-TR-08-34*, Robotics Institute, Carnegie Mellon University, Pittsburgh, USA, 2008.

Dömel, A. (2007). Entwicklung eines Pfadplaners für einen Virtual Reality-Versuchsstand. *Studienarbeit*, TU München.

Esen, H. (2007). Training in Virtual Environments via a Hybrid Dynamic Trainer Model. *PhD Thesis*, TU München, 2007.

Fischer, M.; Braun, S.C.; Hellenbrand, D.; Richter, C.; Sabbah, O.; Scharfenberger, C.; Strolz, M.; Kuhl, P. & Färber, G. (2008). Multidisciplinary Development of New Door and Seat Concepts as Part of an Ergonomic Ingress/Egress Support System. *FISITA 2008, World Automotive Congress*, Munich, 2008.

Kapoor, A.; Li, M. & Taylor, R.H. (2007). A Constrained Optimization Approach to Virtual Fixtures for Multi-Handed Tasks. *Proceedings of the 2007 IEEE International Conference on Robotics and Automation*, Orlando, Florida, May 2009.

Kavraki, L.; Svestka, P.; Latombe, J.-C. & Overmars, M. (1996). Probabilistic roadmaps for path planning in high-dimensional configuration spaces. *IEEE Transactions on Robotics and Automation*, Vol. 12, No. 4., pp. 566-580.

Klasing, K. (2009). Parallelized Sampling-based Path Planning for Tree-structured Rigid Robots, *Technical Report TR-LSR-2009-03-01-Klasing,* Institute of Automatic Control Engineering, TU München, 2009.

Kuffner, J.J. & LaValle, S.M. (2000). RRT-Connect: An Efficient Approach to Single-Query Path Planning. *Proceedings of 2000 IEEE International Conference on Robotics and Automation (ICRA 2000)*, Vol. 2, pp. 995-1001.

LaValle, S.M. (2006). *Planning Algorithms*. Cambridge University Press.

LaValle, S.M. (1998). Rapidly-exploring random trees: A new tool for path planning. *Technical Report TR 98-11*, Computer Science Dept., Iowa State University, Oct. 1998.

Li, M.;Ishii, M. & Taylor, R. H. (2007). Spatial Motion Constraints Using Virtual Fixtures Generated by Anatomy. *IEEE Transactions on Robotics*, Vol. 23, No. 1, pp 4-19.

Lynch, K.M.; Liu, C.; Rensen, A.S.; Kim, S.; Peshkin, M.; Tickel, T.; Hannon, D. & Shiels, K. (2002). Motion Guides for Assisted Manipulation. *International Journal of Robotics Research*, Vol. 21, No. 1 (2002), pp. 27-43.

OpenRAVE [Online]. *http://openrave.programmingvision.com/*. Accessed on September 19th, 2009.

Mount, D.M. & Arya, S. (1997). ANN: A Library for Approximate Nearest Neighbor Searching," *Proceedings of Center for Geometric Computing Second Ann. Fall Workshop Computational Geometry*, 1997.

Plaku, E.; Bekris, K.E.; Chen, B.Y.; Ladd, A.M. & Kavraki, L.E. (2005). Sampling-based roadmap of trees for parallel motion planning. *IEEE Transactions on Robotics*, Vol. 21, No. 4 (2005), pp. 597-608.

PP [Online]. *http://www.lsr.ei.tum.de/research/software/pp/*. Accessed on September 19th, 2009.

Rosenberg, L. (1993). Virtual fixtures: Perceptual tools for telerobotic manipulation. *Proceedings of IEEE Virtual Reality Annual International Symposium*, pp. 76–82, Sept. 1993.

Solhjoo, A. (2009). Further Development and Implementation of the Control of a Car Door with Two Actuated Degrees-of-Freedom. Master´s Thesis, TU München.

Strolz, M.; Mörtl, A.; Gräf, M. & Buss, M. (2009). Development, Control and Evaluation of an Actuated Car Door, *IEEE Transactions on Haptics*, Vol. 2, No. 3 (2009), pp. 170-180.

Strolz, M.; Mühlbauer, Q.; Scharfenberger, C.; Färber, G. & Buss, M. (2008). Towards a generic control system for actuated car doors with arbitrary degrees of freedom. *Proceedings of IEEE Intelligent Vehicles Symposium (IV 2008)*, pp. 391-397, Eindhoven, The Netherlands, June 2008.

Ueberle, M.; Mock, N. & Buss, M. (2004). ViSHaRD10, a novel hyper-redundant haptic interface. *Proceedings of the 12th International Symposium on Haptic Interfaces for Virtual Environment and Teleoperator Systems*, pp. 58-65, 2004.

Varol, A.; Gunev, I. & Basdogan, C. (2006). A Virtual Reality Toolkit for Path Planning and Manipulation at Nano-Scale. *Proceedings of the 14 th IEEE Symposium on Haptic Interfaces for Virtual Environments and Teleoperator Systems*, pp. 485-489, Washington D.C., USA, March 2006.

30

Sensory Properties in Fusion of Visual/Haptic Stimuli Using Mixed Reality

Itaru Kitahara, Morio Nakahara and Yuichi Ohta
University of Tsukuba
Japan

1. Introduction

This chapter introduces our experimental investigation about sensory properties in the fusion of visual/haptic stimuli by using Mixed-Reality (MR) technique. Especially, we focus on the discrepancy between the two stimuli.

When making a purchase from TV or online, we are sometimes disappointed by a product whose actual scale and material differ from our image, even though its appearance originally impressed us. This case indicates the use of integrated multiple sensory cues that include not only the visual but also the auditory and haptic to extract the properties of objects. However, the fusion of multiple sensory cues by interaction with each other has not been well examined. We introduce our developed system that can independently control the sensibility parameters of visual and haptic cues to study the effect of these cues on sensory properties.

MR techniques have been applied in factories to assist assembly, inspection and maintenance operations (Ohta & Tamura, 1999) (Wiedenmaier, et al, 2001) (Friedrich, 2002) (Fiorentino et al, 2002) (Nolle & Klinker, 2006). Recently, designing operations for industrial products are gathering attention as the next generation of MR applications (Navab, 2003) (Lee & Park, 2005) (Sandor et al, 2007). In ordinary designing operations, first, designers develop a broad plot of shape, appearance, and inner structure using a Computer Aided Design (CAD) system. After that, a mock-up, which is a dummy model of the designing product, is generated to examine such detailed information as a sense of touch and surface texture that is difficult to represent by CAD. However, generating a mock-up is very expensive, especially since it uses temporal resources. Thus, it is not practical to regenerate a mock-up whenever a design receives a minor change.

The display system shown in Figure 1 might create a new style of product design to reduce operation processes. For example, in ordinary product design, when a designer wants to evaluate different impressions caused by subtle changes of surface material, many similar preproduction samples must be generated that correspond to each change. However, design variations are usually limited because they are too expensive. On the other hand, using our proposed system, evaluation is possible by superimposing computer graphics (CG) textures of various appearances onto a design mock-up that solves not only cost problems but also the limitations of trial design variations.

To realize such a design support system, it is important to investigate how visual and haptic sensory sources are fused and affect each other.

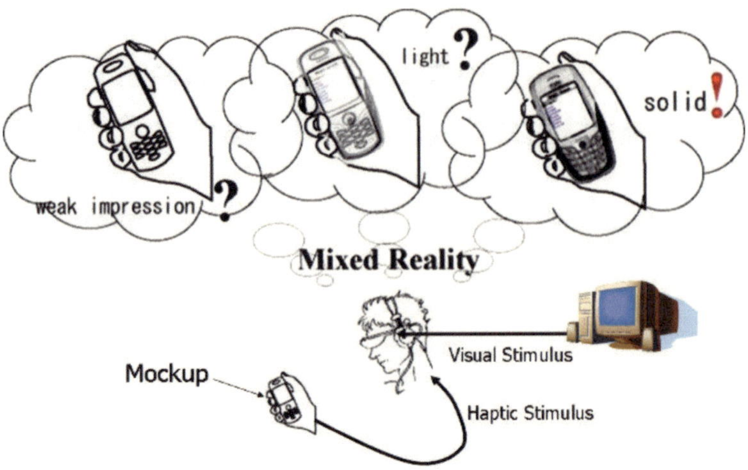

Fig. 1. Example of Designing Operation for Industrial Products by Using Mixed Reality. By using this system, evaluation is possible by superimposing computer graphics (CG) textures of various appearances onto a design mock-up that solves not only cost problems but also the limitations of trial design variations.

2. Fusion of Visual/Haptic Cues Using Mixed Reality

Visual cues seem to affect to estimate environmental properties. As a result, some research reports that haptic cues are affected by visual cues. Several studies have addressed this issue in the real world (Biocca et al, 2001) (Adams et al, 2001) (Rock & Harris, 1967) (Rock & Victor, 1964) (Lederman, & Abbott, 1981) (Hillis et al, 2002). In these researches, however, since subjects could not see an object, they had to imagine that they were grasping what they were looking at. The evaluating saturation is nowhere near the touching/holding operation in daily life, on the other hand, looking at and touching an object is important for evaluation. By focusing on such inconveniences, we developed a system that provides various impressions of an observed object by showing different visual information from the actual shape and material using an MR technique (Nakahara et al, 2007). Wang et al. also developed a MR system that fuses visual and haptic information (Wang et al, 2000). However, when the system developed, the quality of CG technology was not powerful to express subtle difference of appearance caused by changes of surface material. Then, the purpose of the investigation about sensory properties in fusion of visual/haptic stimuli is different from ours. Figure 2 shows an overview of our proposed system. A user perceives a tactile sensation by touching a real object. By displaying the object's appearance, the tactile sensation is merged with the visual sensation in the user's perception.

As a procedure to analyze sensory properties, we focus on two features of objects. One is the impression of texture that is intimately involved in the impression of products. The other is the sharpness of a cube's edge, which is strongly affected by both visual and haptic senses.

Below we introduce two experiments that evaluate the impression of texture and the sensation of sharpness by using our MR system.

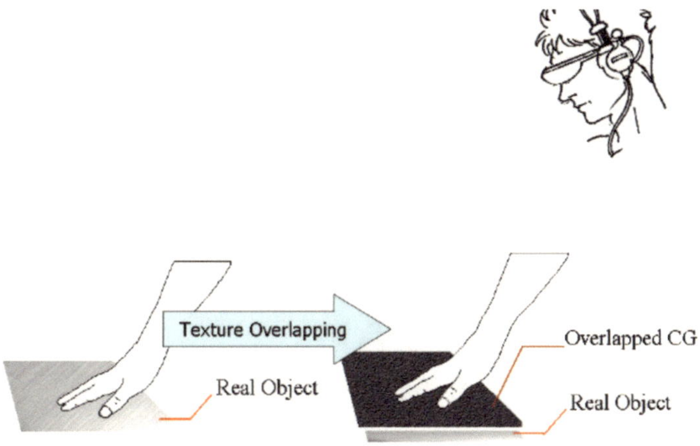

Fig. 2. Fusion of Visual/Haptic Cues Using Mixed Reality. A user perceives a tactile sensation by touching a real object. By displaying the object's appearance, the tactile sensation is merged with the visual sensation in the user's perception.

3. Subjective Evaluation of Texture Impression

We assume the impression of texture consists on two kinds: haptic and visual. Haptic texture is a stimulus given by the tactile sensation of touching an object, and visual texture is a stimulus given by its appearance. When touching glass material with closed eyes, we experience a tactile sensation that resembles the impres-sion of a "glass haptic texture." When looking at a glass material without touching, we experience a visual sensation that resembles an impression of a "glass visual texture." This section introduces our experimental evaluation that investigates whether it is possible to control the impression of a haptic texture by changing visual textures.

3.1 Experimental Environment

As shown in Figure 3, the experimental system can overlap various visual textures generated by computer graphics onto a real object. In this system, real objects are several plates made from different materials. We choose stone, cork, unglazed tile, steel, and wood as the materials of the plates. The stone has a rough surface, but it is not polished. When a subject strongly pushes the cork with a finger tip, its shape is deformed. The unglazed tile has a rough surface, but it is not cover coated. The surfaces of the steel and wood are smoothed by filing. An example of a subject's view is shown in Figure 4. An overlapping texture covers the entire real object.

Figure 5 shows an experimental scene. First, after we measure the temperature of a subject's hand, he/she puts on a thin latex glove. From pilot studies, we learned that haptic stimulus affects the texture impression more strongly than the visual stimulus. So we use a glove that deadens the haptic sensation to maintain balance.

Since humans can identify material by sensing inherent specific heat of each object, we maintained the temperature of the real objects at the temperature of a subject's hand by using a thermos-tatically-controlled electric carpet.
To maintain photometric consistency between real and virtual appearances, the system maps actual images captured by a high-end single-lens reflex camera at an identical position as a subject's viewpoint. We use a high-definition HMD that can display a 1280×1024 image to increase the evaluation reality as much as possible. If a subject's viewpoint differs from the viewpoints of other subjects, geometric and photometric inconsistencies are created between the visual cues. Subjects were instructed to fix their jaw at a prescribed position while they looked at a CG texture in the middle of an HMD, as shown in Figure 4.
These considerations described above allow evaluation of the impression of texture by only deriving visual and haptic stimuli.

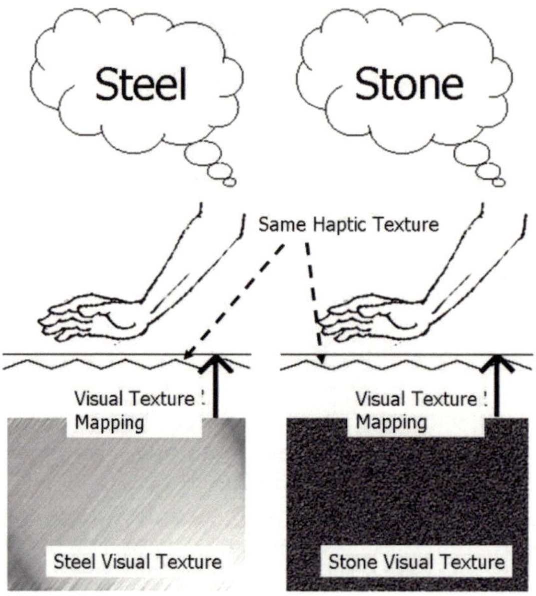

Fig. 3. Subjective Evaluation of Texture Impression. The experimental system can overlap various visual textures generated by computer graphics onto a real object.

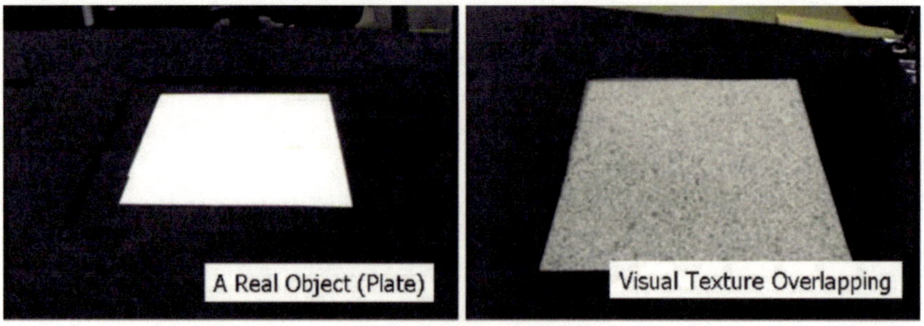

Fig. 4. Example of a Subject's View. An overlapping texture covers the entire real object.

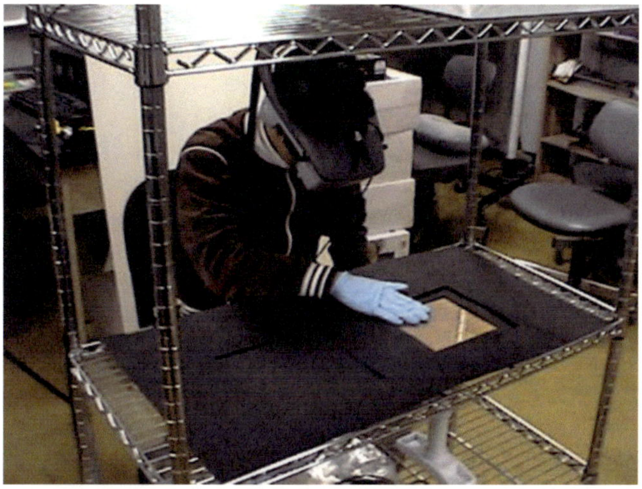

Fig. 5. An Experimental Scene of Evaluation. We use a glove that deadens the haptic sensation to maintain balance of haptic and visual stimuli.

3.2 Elimination of Occlusion by Image Matting

As shown in the picture on the left of Figure 6, when a subject moves a hand over a real object, the hand is occluded by the CG texture. As a result, subjects have difficulty feeling as they are actually touching a real object. We solve this problem by a skin color matting technique (Itoh et al, 2003) that utilizes a property that clusters the skin region in the chroma space. We defined a skin color model in chroma space in advance and segment the skin color region from captured images using the model. As shown in the picture on the right of Figure 6, generating an image is possible that does not spoil the appearance of the user's hand.

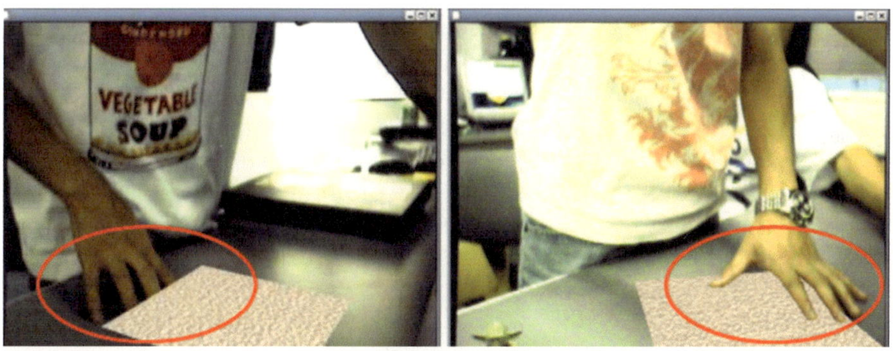

Fig. 6. Example of Occlusion: (Left) subject's finger region is occluded by CG; (Right) occlusion problem in finger region is solved.

3.3 Procedure of Subjective Evaluation

We evaluated the amount of mistaken sensations caused by the combinations of haptic and visual textures. Since each texture has five types of materials (stone, cork, unglazed tile, steel, and wood), there are 25 combinations. We analyzed texture impressions examining evaluation score which are answered by all subjects for all combinations. In all trials, subjects were permitted to take as much time as needed. The displayed textures are randomly chosen to control for order effects.

The subjective evaluations were conducted by ten male subjects in their 20s who were presented a randomly selected combination of haptic and virtual textures and then were answered whether their impressions matched the material they saw. A five-level rating scale was used. Scale 1 means "completely different impression from what I see." Scale 2 means a "different impression." Scale 3 means "No difference" Scale 4 means "almost identical impression what I see." Scale 5 means "completely identical." When the subject gives a high score with observing an MR object which has inconsistent visual and haptic texture, it shows that the visual cue has stronger influence than the haptic one for the impression of the object's texture.

3.4 Results and Discussion

Figure 7 shows the evaluation results. The horizontal axis represents the kinds of materials, and the vertical axis represents the mean evaluating rate for each material. The line with rhombus nodes indicates the result of displaying the visual texture of stone. The line with box nodes indicates the result of displaying the visual texture of cork. The line with triangle nodes indicates the result of displaying the visual texture of unglazed tile. The line with X nodes indicates the result of displaying the visual texture of steel. The line with asterisk nodes indicates the result of displaying the visual texture of unglazed wood.

When we used a cork plate as a real object, few subjects had a different impression from the real material when the visual texture is changed. Based on the questionnaire data, subjects identified the material by its surface softness. When we used a wood plate as a real object, some subjects commented that they could feel the surface softness. As a result, it was difficult to give an impression as if touching other materials.

Note that the evaluation rates of the haptic-stone/visual-steel and haptic-steel/visual-stone combinations are high, even though the haptic textures of their surfaces are quite different. In the questionnaire data, when touching a stone plate with a rough surface while looking at a visual texture of steel, one subject had the impression of touching a steel plate that was not well polished. On the other hand, when touching a steel-plate with a smooth surface while looking at the visual texture of stone, one subject had the impression of touching a well polished stone plate, such as granite or marble. From this result, we assume that if we already had some different impressions (e.g., smooth or rough) about touching materials from past experience, controlling the impression of the real object between the impressions is possible by changing the visual texture. The assumption can be assessed by comparing the rough surfaces of stone and unglazed tile. Because we rarely have impression that the surface of unglazed tile is smooth in daily life, when we use a smooth steel plate as a real object and overlap an unglazed tile texture onto the plate, few subjects had the impression that they were touching an unglazed tile.

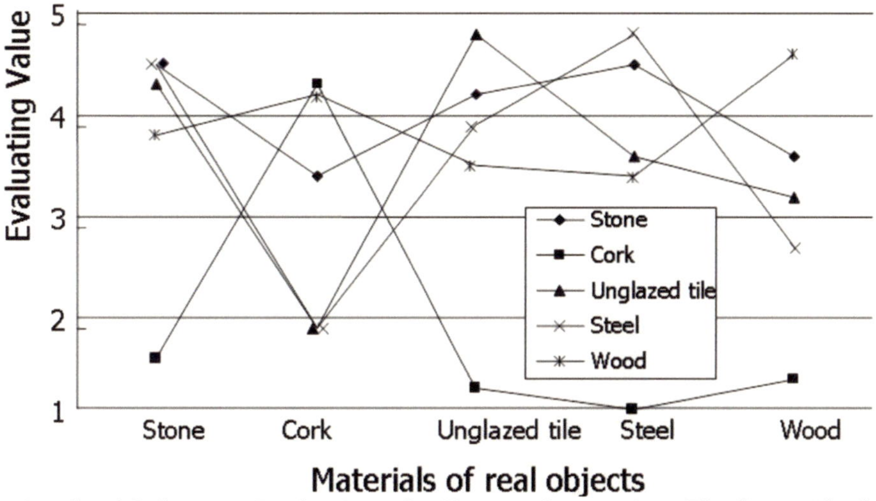

Fig. 7. A Result of Subjective Evaluations for Texture Impression. The line with rhombus nodes indicates the result of displaying the visual texture of stone. The line with box nodes indicates the result of cork texture. The line with triangle nodes indicates the result of unglazed tile texture. The line with X nodes indicates the result of steel texture. The line with asterisk nodes indicates the result of unglazed wood texture.

4. Subjective Evaluation of Sharpness

We conducted an experimental survey to investigate whether an edge is perceived sharper than its actual curvature (4 mm) by overlapping a sharper appearance (1 mm) on the surface. Figure 8 shows an overview of this experiment. In this experiment, we quantify the haptic stimulus by curvature radius of the edges of cubes.

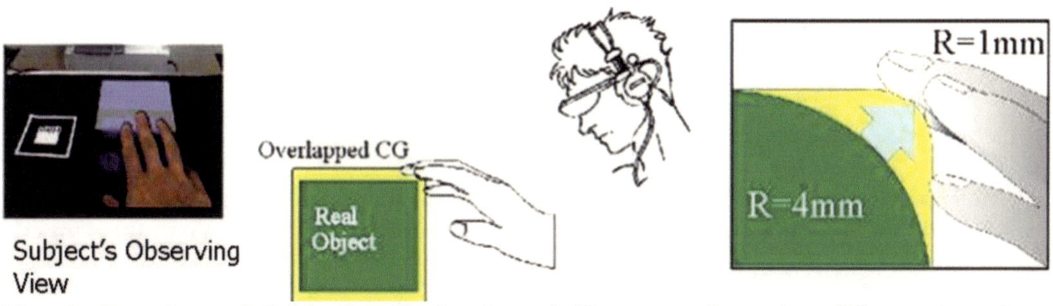

Fig. 8. Overview of Subjective Evaluation of Sharpness Sensation. We conducted an experimental survey to investigate whether an edge is perceived sharper than its actual curvature (4 mm) by overlapping a sharper appearance (1 mm) on the surface.

4.1 Experimental Environment

Figure 9 shows a picture of an experimental scene. The subject maintains his viewpoint while putting his jaw at a predefined position to preserve geometric and photometric consistency between the real and virtual information. As illustrated in Figure 10, the distance between the subject's viewpoint and a target object is about 30 cm and the tilt angle of the subject's line of sight is 45°.

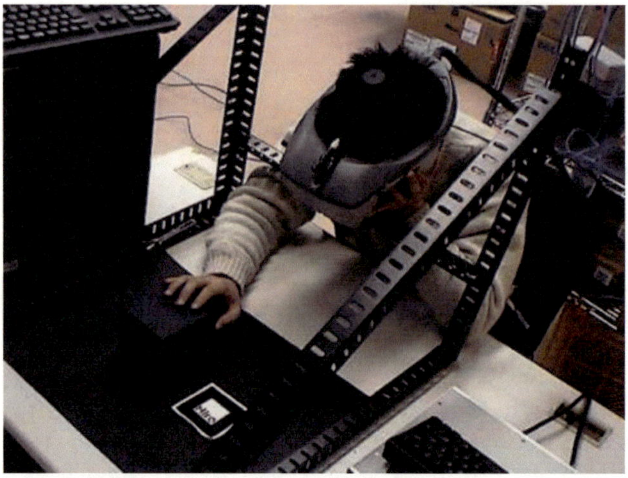

Fig. 9. Experimental of Subjective Evaluation of Sharpness. The subject maintains his viewpoint while putting his jaw at a predefined position to preserve geometric and photometric consistency between the real and virtual information.

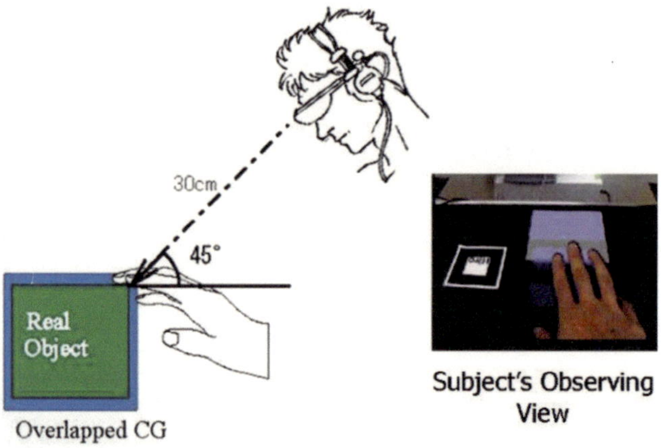

Fig. 10. Positional Relationship between a Real Object and a Subject. The distance between the subject's viewpoint and a target object is about 30 cm and the tilt angle of the subject's line of sight is 45°.

We prepared three cubes with 10 cm sides to control haptic stimuli. One cube has 12 edges of curvature radius from 0.0 to 1.1 mm, one has edges from 1.2 to 2.3 mm, and another has edges from 2.4 to 3.5 mm. A cube is shown in Figure 11. It is possible to generate various CG appearances of the cube by controlling the curvature radii of the CG edges.

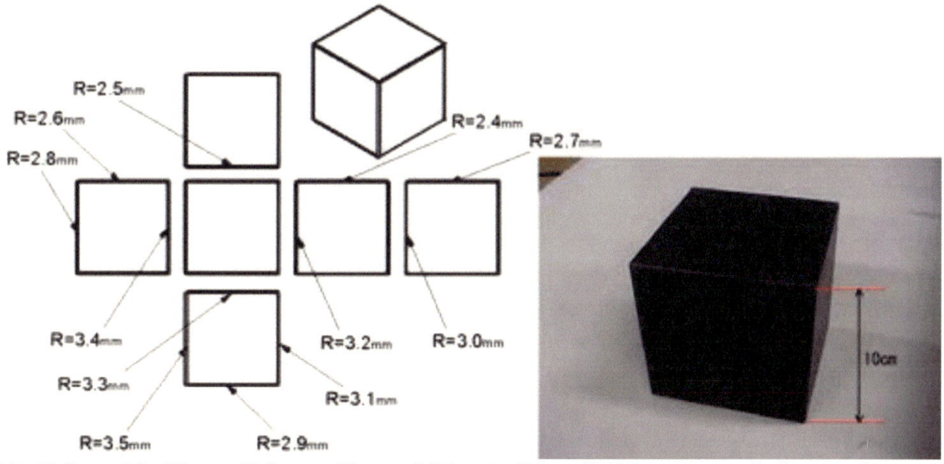

Fig. 11. Cube with 10 cm Sides to Control Haptic Stimuli. We prepared three cubes with 10 cm sides to control haptic stimuli. One cube has 12 edges of curvature radius from 0.0 to 1.1 mm, one has edges from 1.2 to 2.3 mm, and another has edges from 2.4 to 3.5 mm.

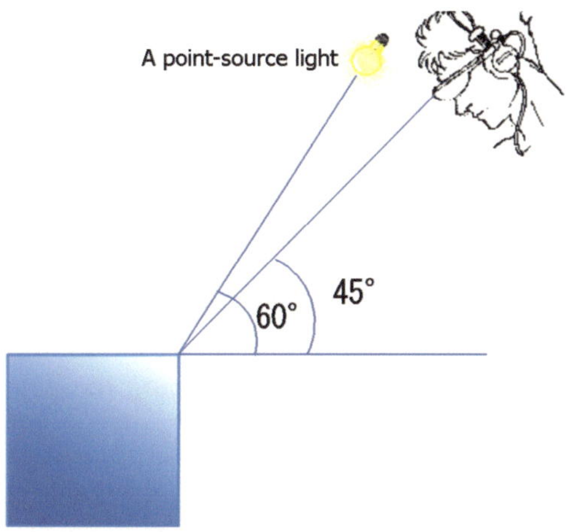

Fig. 12. Angle Between Horizontal Plane and Virtual Light is 60°. This angle is almost the same as the environment light of the expe-rimental room.

Twelve male subjects in their 20s evaluated sharpness sensations by touching a CG overlapped cube that contained a discrepancy between vision and haptic stimuli.
All subjects have visual acuity of nearsightedness over 1.0 to discriminate two lines with 0.14 mm interval which is generated by the sharpest edge in this research on an HMD.
A displayed virtual cube is illuminated by a point-source light. The angle between the horizontal plane and the light is 60°, as illustrated in Figure 12. This angle is almost the same as the environment light of the experimental room. By using ARToolKit (Kato & Billinghurst, 1999), the system overlaps the virtual cube onto a real cube. To prevent subjects from determining an edge's sharpness by referring to a cut plane of the edge, the system does not display the cut plane, as shown in Figure 13. To solve the CG appearance problem, which involves overlapping of the subject's hand in MR scenes, subject hands were extracted by using the same procedure described in Section 3.2.

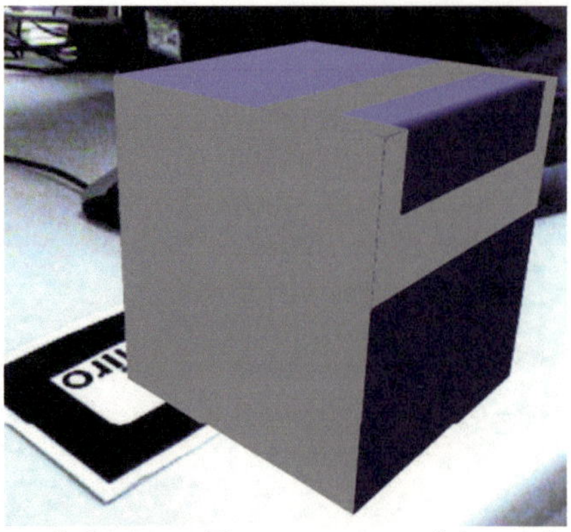

Fig. 13. Example of Displayed Image. To prevent subjects from determining an edge's sharpness by referring to a cut plane of the edge, the system does not display the cut plane.

4.2 Quantization of Curvature Radii Scale

In the matching process, it is better that each stimulus value can be clearly defined by subjects. In other words, when we used too roughly quantized stimuli in the evaluation, evaluation precision suffers. On the other hand, when we used too finely quantized stimuli, subjects cannot define the differences. Therefore we quantize the scale of the curvature radii as a unit to present to subjects.

Discrimination Threshold

As illustrated in Figure 14 physical stimulus differs from mental stimulus. We examined the discrimination thresholds of subjects by a psychology and statistics experiment. A discrimination threshold is the minimum distance at which subjects can define differences of stimuli. A method of limits detects a discrimination threshold by examining if a subject can detect differences between two different stimuli while changing the gap step by step. In this experiment, we examined a discrimination threshold (human's sensitivity) of sharpness by comparing reference stimulus R with standard stimulus R0. Reference stimulus R, which is the curvature radius of an edge, is changed at 0.1-mm intervals.

As illustrated in Figure 15 when a subject felt reference stimulus R was sharper than standard stimulus R0, he recorded "-". When a subject felt reference stimulus R was duller than standard stimulus R0, he recorded "+". When discrimination was difficult, he recorded "?". It is important to set an initial reference stimulus either large or small enough to easily define the difference between standard stimuli. We repeated the question-and-answer process until the subject recorded "?". A discrimination threshold is defined as a region within marked "?" by operating the process both upward and downward. We conducted evaluations with twelve male subjects in their 20s, all of whom have visual acuity of nearsightedness over 1.0.

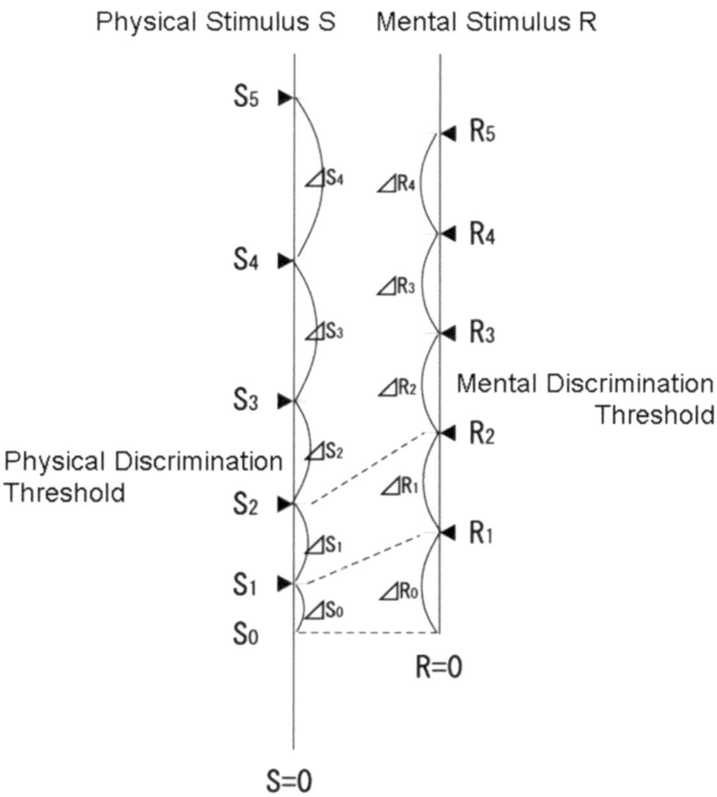

Fig. 14. Difference between physical and mental stimulus

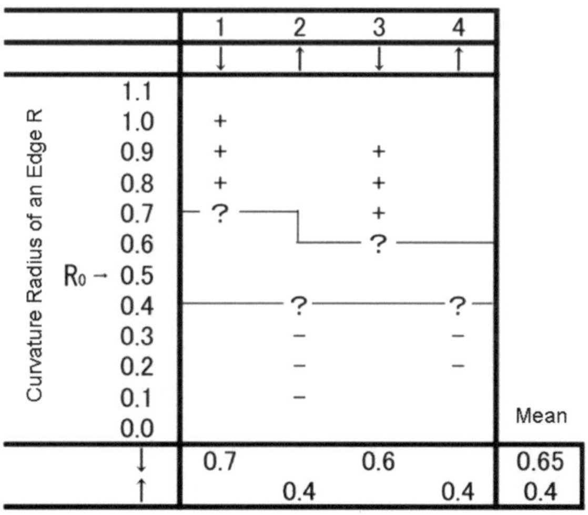

Fig. 15. Definition for Mental Discrimination Threshold.

Results

The estimated haptic and visual discrimination thresholds are shown in Tables 1 and 2. Visual discrimination thresholds are defined at 0.4-mm interval, but haptic discrimination thresholds are not. In order to investigate how visual/haptic stimuli interact with each other, common criteria are necessary. We define the common criteria as the minimum perceivable seven steps for both of visual/haptic discrimination thresholds, 0.2, 0.6, 1.0, 1.4, 1.8, 2.2, and 2.6 mm. Although, humans can discriminate differences less than 0.1 mm, due to the limitations of the accuracy processing machinery, it is not possible to estimate haptic discrimination thresholds less than 0.1 mm.

By considering different thresholds of visual and haptic information, we quantize the scale of the curvature radii into seven identical parts: 0.2, 0.6, 1.0, 1.4, 1.8, 2.2, and 2.6 mm.

Standard Stimulus (mm)	Discrimination Threshold (mm)	Standard Deviation
0.2	0.332	0.057
0.6	0.382	0.078
1.0	0.395	0.062
1.4	0.322	0.052
1.8	0.338	0.045

Table 1. Visual Discrimination Threshold

Standard Stimulus (mm)	Discrimination Threshold (mm)	Standard Deviation
0.0	0.000	0.000
0.1	0.000	0.000
0.2	0.130	0.053
0.4	0.270	0.078
0.7	0.238	0.049
1.0	0.237	0.069
1.3	0.300	0.063
1.6	0.418	0.095

Table 2. Haptic Discrimination Threshold

4.3 Procedure of Subjective Evaluation

First, as a reference of the matching process, subjects were presented a standard stimulus in three ways: only haptic, only visual, and both. When subjects are indicated to observe the object by using only haptic, subjects close the eyes, and then the experimenter leads their hand onto the object. When subjects are indicated to observe the object by only vision, subjects watch the object with putting their hands on the experimental table. When subjects are indicated to observe the object by using haptic and vision, subjects can watch and touch the object without any physical constraints.

After observing a standard stimulus, subjects are required to determine a corresponding stimulus by using only haptic, only vision, and both haptic and vision together. In all trials, subjects are permitted to take as much time as needed. The displayed stimuli for match-up are randomly chosen to control for order effects. When subjects require observing the next stimulus for match-up, the stimulus will be displayed after 15 seconds interval.

There are nine combinations of three displaying ways for standard stimulus and three displaying ways for mach-up stimuli. By executing multiple classification analysis to the result derived by the all combinations, we investigate whether human perception is affected by fusing visual and haptic cues.

If we conduct the experiment by using all perceivable seven steps for both of visual/haptic discrimination thresholds, huge amount of time and labor is needed. On the other hand, it is difficult to extract significant evidence to show that human perception is affected by fusing visual and haptic cues in the most of the trials, when the one stimulus is too week to affect the other stimulus. Thus, we conduct a preliminary experiment to choose combinations of visual and haptic stimuli that can easily introduce the influence caused by the fusion. As the result, a combination {visual: 2.2 mm / haptic 1.4 mm} is selected.

4.4 Result and Discussion

Results are illustrated in Figure 16 and Figure 17. The horizontal axis represents the types of matching procedures, and the vertical axis represents the mean evaluating value of the radii of edges. The line with rhombus nodes is the mean matching response when standard stimuli are presented only by haptic, the line with triangle nodes is only using vision, and the line with box nodes is using haptic and vision together.

In the first evaluation, subjects were given a 1.4 mm haptic curvature radius as a haptic stimulus and a 2.2 mm vision curvature radius as a visual stimulus. The result is shown in Figure 16.

When subjects received a standard stimulus as a 1.4 mm haptic curvature radius and determined a corresponding stimulus by only using haptic (the left rhombus node), they sensed it as 1.40±0.0 mm. On the other hand, when subjects received a standard stimulus as a 1.4 mm haptic curvature radius and a 2.2 mm vision one and determined a corresponding stimulus by only using haptic (the left box node), they sensed it as 1.64±0.2 mm by perceiving that the edge was blunter than the previous result. This result was derived by presenting a 2.2 mm vision stimulus as the standard stimulus.

When subjects received a standard stimulus as a 2.2 mm vision curvature radius and determined a corresponding stimulus by only using vision (the right triangle node), they sensed it as 2.20±0.0 mm. On the other hand, when subjects received a standard stimulus as a 1.4 mm haptic curvature radius and a 2.2 mm vision one and determined a corresponding stimulus by only using vision (the right box node), they sensed it as 2.12±0.4 mm by perceiving that the edge was sharper than the previous result. This result was derived by presenting a 1.4 mm haptic stimulus as the standard stimulus.

When subjects received a standard stimulus as a 1.4 mm haptic curvature radius and a 2.2 mm vision one and determined a corresponding stimulus by using both haptic and vision (the middle box node), they sensed it as 1.84±0.1 mm. This experiment shows that the haptic stimulus seems to be affected by visual stimulus when discrepancy exists between vision and haptic stimuli.

By applying the Student's t-test to our evaluation data, significance differences were found in effectiveness, caused by presenting a standard stimulus in three ways ($F(2.18) = 26.694$, $p<0.05$).

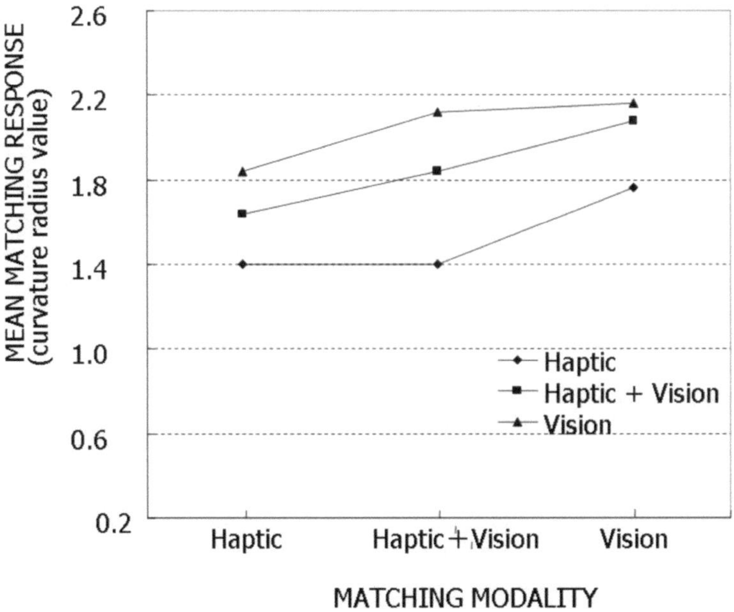

Fig. 16. Mean grit sizes selected as matches for visual/haptic, and visual/haptic standards; subjects touched an object with a 1.4 mm haptic curvature radius and a 2.2 mm vision one.

In the second evaluation, we switch the value of visual/haptic stimuli to control the order effect. Thus, a subject is given a 2.2 mm haptic curvature radius as a haptic stimulus and a 1.4 mm vision curvature radius as a visual stimulus. The result is shown in Figure 17.

When subjects received a standard stimulus as a 2.2 mm haptic curvature radius and determined a corresponding stimulus by only using haptic (the left rhombus node), they sensed it as 2.20±0.0 mm. On the other hand, when subjects received a standard stimulus as a 2.2 mm haptic curvature radius and a 1.4 mm vision one and determined a corresponding stimulus by only using haptic (the left box node), they sensed it as 2.16±0.2 mm by perceiving that the edge was sharper than the previous result. This result is derived by presenting a 1.4 mm vision stimulus as the standard stimulus.

When subjects received a standard stimulus as a 2.2 mm haptic curvature radius and a 1.4 mm vision one and determined a corresponding stimulus by using both haptic and vision (the middle box node), they sensed it as 2.04±0.2 mm. This experiment shows that the haptic stimulus seems to be affected by visual stimulus when discrepancy exists between vision and haptic stimuli.

By applying the Student's t-test to our evaluation data, significance differences were found in effectiveness, caused by presenting a standard stimulus in three ways, ($F(2.18)=36.394$, $p<0.05$).

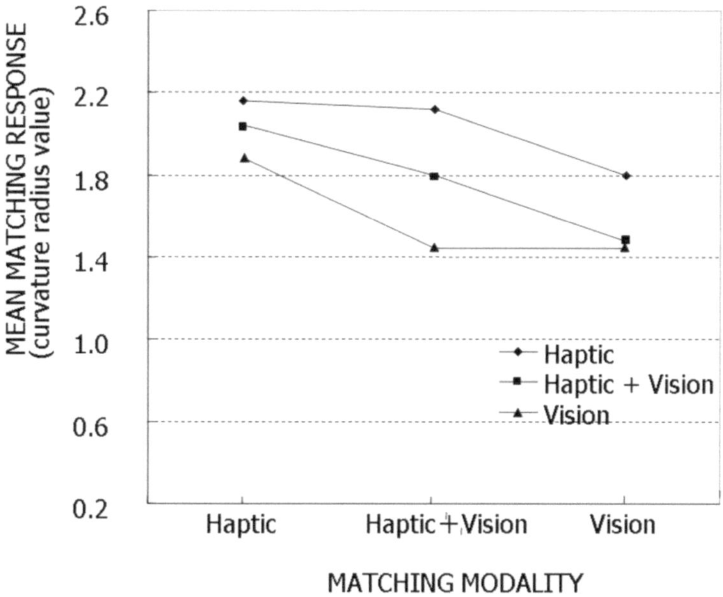

Fig. 17. Mean grit sizes selected as matches for visual/haptic, and visual/haptic standards; subjects touched an object with a 2.2 mm haptic curvature radius and a 1.4 mm vision one

These results of subjective evaluations for the sharpness of a cube's edge show that users perceive an edge to be controllable by presenting a duller or sharper CG edge.
We calculated the occupancy rate of haptic and vision stimuli for the evaluations by using the method introduced in Lederman's paper (Lederman & Abbott, 1981). Haptic and visual influences are calculated by the following equations:

$$\text{Haptic influence} = \frac{\text{Mean(Vision + Vision standard) - Mean(Vision standard)}}{\text{Mean(Vision standard) - Mean(Touch standard)}} \tag{1}$$

$$\text{Visual influence} = \frac{\text{Mean(Touch + Vision standard) - Mean(Touch standard)}}{\text{Mean(Vision standard) - Mean(Touch standard)}} \tag{2}$$

In these equations, Mean (Touch+Vision standard) is the mean evaluating value of the radius of an edge calculated from all subject evaluations that were presented standard haptic and vision stimuli. Mean (Vision standard) is the mean evaluating value of the radius of an edge calculated from all subject evaluations that were presented a standard vision stimulus. Mean (Touch standard) is the mean evaluating value of the radius of an edge calculated from all evaluations that were presented a standard haptic stimulus.
In the first evaluation, the occupancy rate of the vision stimulus is 57.1% and the haptic stimulus is 42.9%. In the second evaluation, the occupancy rate of the vision stimulus is 77.8% and the haptic stimulus is 22.2%. These results show that when a curvature radius becomes larger, the haptic sensation becomes duller. As a result, the occupancy rate of the vision stimulus increases.

6. Conclusion

This chapter introduced a system that can present visual/haptic sensory fusion using mixed reality. We investigated whether visual cues affect haptic cues. As a procedure to analyze sensory properties, we focused on two features of objects. One is the impression of texture that is intimately involved in the impression of products. The other is the sharpness of edge, which is strongly affected by both visual and haptic senses. From the result of the subjective evaluation on the impression of visual/haptic texture, we can derive an interesting assumption as follows; if we have learned from past experience that a material may sometimes have different haptic impressions (e.g., smooth and rough), we can control the haptic impression of a real object with the material by changing the visual texture overlaid on the object. Preliminary results of subjective evaluations on the sharpness of edge show that users perceive an edge to be duller or sharper than a real one when presented with an overlaid CG edge with a duller/sharper curvature.

7. References

Adams, WJ.; Banks, MS. & Van, Ee R. (2001). Adaptation to 3D distortions in human vision, *Nature Neuro-science*, Vol.4 (1063-1064)

Biocca, F.; Kim, J. & Choi, Y. (2001). Visual Touch in Virtual Environments: An Exploratory Study of Presence, Multimodal Interfaces, and Cross-Modal Sensory Illusions, *MIT Press, Presence*, Vol.10, No.3 (247-265), June

Fiorentino, M.; de Amicis, R.; Monno, G. & A. Stork. (2002). Spacedesign: a Mixed Reality Workspace for Aesthetic Industrial Design, *Proceedings. of International Symposium on Mixed and Augmented Reality (ISMAR02)*, (86-95)

Friedrich. W. (2002). ARVIKA-Augmented Reality for Development, Production and Service, *Proceedings. of International Symposium on Mixed and Augmented Reality (ISMAR02)*, (3-4)

Hillis, J. M.; Ernst, M. O.; Banks, M. S. & Landy, M. S. (2002). Combining Sensory Information: Mandatory Fusion Within, but Not Between, Senses, *Science*, Vol.298, (1627-1630)

Itoh, M.; Ozeki, M.; Nakamura, Y. & Ohta, Y. (2003). Simple and Robust Tracking of Hands and Objects for Video Indexing, *Proceedings. of IEEE Conference. on Multisensor Fusion and Integration for Intelligent Systems (MFI)*, (252-257)

Kato, H. & Billinghurst, M. (1999). Marker tracking and HMD calibration for a video-based augmented reality conferencing system. *Proceedings. of International Workshop on Augmented Reality (IWAR99)*, ACM, (85–94)

Lederman, S. J. & Abbott, S. G. (1981). Texture Perception: Studies of Intersensory Organization Using a Discrepancy Paradigm, and Visual Versus Tactual Psychophysics, *Journal of Experimental Psychology: Human Perception and Performance*, Vol.7, No. 4, (902-915)

Lee, W. & Park, J. (2005). Augmented Foam: a Tangible Augmented Reality for Product Design, *Proceedings of International Symposium on Mixed and Augmented Reality (ISMAR05)*, (106- 109)

Nakahara, M.; Kitahara, I. & Ohta, Y. (2007). ensory Property in Fusion of Visual/Haptic Cues by Using Mixed Reality, *Second Joint Conference, EuroHaptics Conference 2007 and Symposium on Haptic Interfaces for Virtual Environment and Teleoperator Systems (World Haptics 2007)*, (565-566)

Navab. N. (2003). Industrial Augmented Reality (IAR): Challenges in Design and Commercialization of Killer Apps, *Proc.eedings of International Symposium on Mixed and Augmented Reality (ISMAR03)*, (2-6)

Nolle, S. & Klinker. G. (2006). Augmented Reality as a Comparison Tool in Automotive Industry, *Proceedings. of International Symposium on Mixed and Augmented Reality (ISMAR06)*, (249-250)

Ohta、 Y. & Tamura, H. (1999). *Mixed Reality–Merging Real and Virtual Worlds-*, Ohmsha, Ltd.

Rock, I. & Harris, C. S. (1967). Vision and touch. *Scientific American*, Vol.216 (96-104), May

Rock, I. & Victor, J. (1964). Vision and touch: An experimentally created conflict between the two senses. *Science*, Vol.143 (594-596)

Sandor, C.; Uchiyama, S. & Yamamoto, H. (2007). Visuo-Haptic Systems: Half-Mirrors Considered Harmful, *Second Joint Conference, EuroHaptics Conference 2007 and Symposium on Haptic Interfaces for Virtual Environment and Teleoperator Systems (World Haptics 2007)*, (292-297)

Wang, Y & MacKenzie, C. L. (2000). The Role of Contextual Haptic and Visual Constraints on Object Manipulation in Virtual Environments, *Proceedings. of the SIGGCHI conference on Human factors in Computing Systems*, (532-539)

Wiedenmaicr, S. O.; Ochmc, L.; Schmidt, H. & Luczak, H. (2001). Augmented Reality (AR) for Assembly Processes - an Experimental Evaluation, *Proceedings. of IEEE and ACM International Symposium on Augmented Reality (ISAR2001)*, (185-186)

31

Expanding the Scope of Instant Messaging with Bidirectional Haptic Communication

Youngjae Kim and Minsoo Hahn
Korea Advanced Institute of Science and Technology
Korea, Republic of

1. Introduction

For the past five years, haptic interfaces have been applied to various commercial products. Most consumers are now familiar with the term *haptic*. Many among them use vibro-tactile feedback equipped touchscreen devices, although they may not have a clear understanding of what it is. According to the Google Trend result (http://www.google.com/trends/), Korean people type in and search for the keyword *haptic* more frequently than people in other countries. The traffic gaps between Korea and other countries are as follows.

Region	Traffic	std error		City	Traffic	std error
South Korea	1	0%		Seoul (South Korea)	1	0%
Vietnam	0.475	5%		Singapore (Singapore)	0.435	5%
Singapore	0.395	5%		Jakarta (Indonesia)	0.22	10%
Malaysia	0.25	5%		Ottawa (Canada)	0.21	10%
Philippines	0.23	5%		Bangkok (Thailand)	0.2	10%
Thailand	0.195	5%		Hong Kong (Hong Kong)	0.175	10%
Indonesia	0.18	10%		Delhi (India)	0.115	10%
Hong Kong	0.18	10%		Seattle (USA)	0.115	10%
Taiwan	0.145	5%		San Francisco (USA)	0.115	10%
India	0.14	5%		Los Angeles (USA)	0.11	10%

Table 1. Google Trend result on the keyword *haptic* (data acquired on Aug. 31, 2009)

In Table 1, the numbers in the Traffic column represent the relative values calculated upon the most dominant region (in this case, South Korea). As can be seen in Table 1, the search traffic of South Korea is twice higher than those of other countries such as Vietnam, Singapore, and the USA. It is mainly due to the marketing strategy of local cellular phone manufacturers that included the term *haptic* in their product names. The important point is not only that people are becoming familiar with the keyword, but also that many research and industry fields are starting to focus on haptic and its effects. For example, a car manufacturer may try to apply a haptic interface to the navigation controller, or a bank may introduce ATM's with a newly installed haptic feedback-equipped touchscreen. In short, haptic technology is making gradual changes in our daily lifestyle.

The initial goal of haptic technology is to facilitate the manipulation of devices. A vibro-tactile feedback enables a user to control a device more accurately and easily. For the next step, haptic aims to give intuitiveness to control target devices. This is mainly because, from a cognitive point of view, users expect a kind of reaction if he or she tries to command to the target.
Haptic technologies are widely employed in many areas these days, but in this chapter, we will focus on its communication usage only. As shown in many studies, haptic can be a type of daily messaging behaviours. Computer-mediated messaging technologies continue to evolve rapidly, and various types of messaging services are being marketed including short message services (SMS's) provided on a cellular phone, message-oriented networking services such as Twitter (Java et al. 2007), blogs with trackback and reply systems, and instant messenger applications that enable peer-to-peer communication in real-time. More innovative types of messaging will continue to emerge (Poupyrev, Nashida, and Okabe 2007). Regardless of the type of messaging, all services share a common goal of diversifying communications among people (Vilhjálmsson 2003). This study aims to improve messaging experiences more realistic by adding a framework for haptic interaction.
The term *haptic* means pertaining to the sense of touch, and thus haptic communication can be described as "communicating via touching". Bonanni had an insight into this concept and tried to implement it (Bonanni et al. 2006). He had studied the way to convey sensations from peer to peer. Rovers had introduced the vibro-tactile-pattern-embedded emoticon named HIM (A. F. Rovers and Van Essen 2004). His research method is quite similar to that proposed in this chapter. The vibro-tactile pattern is embedded into an emoticon so that users can feel more realistic sensations while engaged in instant messaging. VibeTonz (Immersion Corp 2007) is a commercialized vibro-tactile composer from Immersion. As a cellular phone with a touch screen or a conductive switch is being produced by a number of manufacturers these days, Immersion's VibeTonz technology is actively employed. VibeTonz can compose tactile output patterns along with a timeline. Although many researches led to touch-enabled emoticons (Chang et al. 2002; L. Rovers and Van Essen 2004; Aleven et al. 2006), most of these researches were limited to conveying vibro-tactile actuation. The component of touch and related sensations encompass not only tactile stimulus, but also temperature, sound, etc. For this reason, a framework to send and to receive the whole spectrum of haptic is strongly required. The objective of this research is to facilitate haptic communications among users and expand the scope of the computer-mediated conversation.
The bidirectional haptic means that a sensor and an actuator can be manipulated on a single framework. This is a simple concept, but most researches tend to focus on one side only. To achieve true haptic communication, a system providing both a sensor and an actuator within a single framework is needed. Brave introduced in-Touch (Brave and Dahley 1997) to synchronize each cylinder-like device. Two devices are connected and have both a sensor and an actuator in one single tangible object. When one user rolls one device, the motor in the other part starts to run. HAML (El-Far et al. 2006) is a haptic markup language which centers on the haptic description. This is a technical specification that tries to elevate to the MPEG standards. In this research, the Phantom device is mainly applied. HAMLET (Mohamad Eid et al. 2008) is a HAML-based authoring tool. Both HAMLET and this research aim to accomplish simplicity and efficiency in utilizing haptic for non-programmer developers and artists. However, our target users are rather general users than those of HAMLET, who uses the instant messenger as a daily communication tool. From the view of the description language, or the markup language, SensorML (Botts and Robin 2007) is one

of the specifications to describe a sensor. The object of this markup language is to provide the sensor information as detailed as possible including the manufacturer, hardware specifications, the data type to acquire a result, etc. It can be adopted into our work, but we concluded it is too verbose to apply this SensorML to our work.
In this study, TouchCon, a next-generation emoticon for haptic-embedded communication, is proposed. The architecture of the framework to represent haptic expressions in our daily messaging and chatting is also provided. In addition, included is the hardware specially designed for testing and the summary of user preference surveys with reference to the previous researches (Kim et al. 2009; Kim et al. 2009; Shin et al. 2007).

2. A Platform for Managing Haptic Communication

2.1 Overall Description

The proposed system enables a user to manipulate haptic interaction and to share it with others. To achieve this goal, we need to summarize the requirements of the system. The system needs to support haptic actuator control, sensor data acquisition, linkage with various applications, library management, etc. One important goal of this study is to resolve the haptic expression even when two devices are not identical.
For this reason, the haptic communication framework has been designed to achieve the flexibility and the scalability. The flexibility allows the framework to invite and to manipulate different devices. To support haptic-enabled hardwares, the framework must be capable of providing a standardized gateway. Thus, the architecture adopted here has a similar goal to the middleware system (Baldauf, Dustdar, and Rosenberg 2007) from the architectural point of view. The scalability means, the framework is extensible to adopt various sensors and actuators according to their descriptions. For that, the framework has to allow various protocols. Figure 1 shows the overall architecture of the platform.

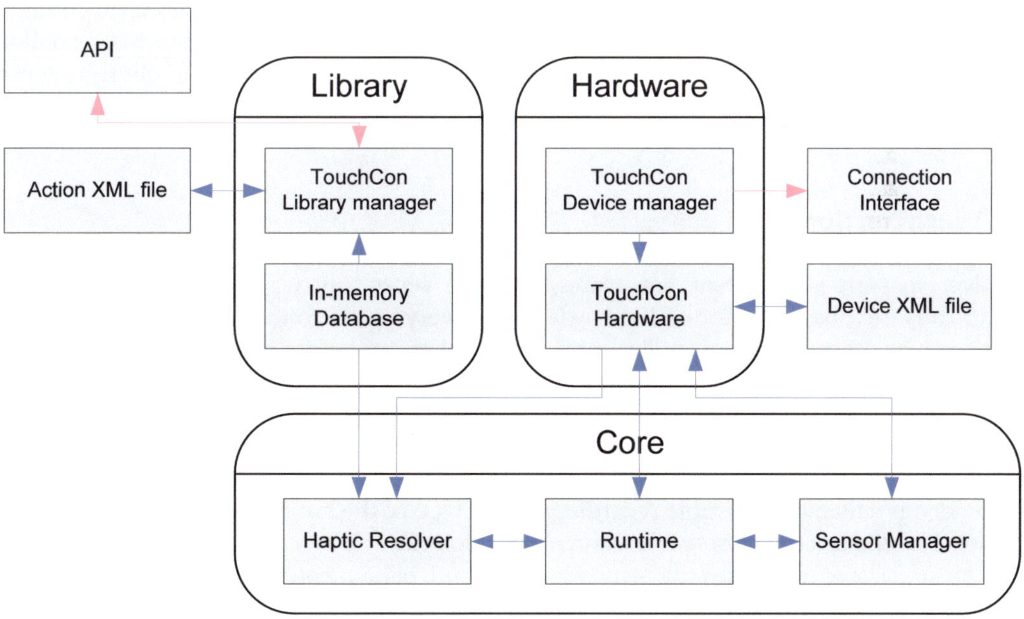

Fig. 1. Overall TouchCon architecture

The platform consists of three main parts; the core, the library, and the hardware. The core is a runtime to execute haptic interactions. The library handles haptic emoticons and their patterns, and the hardware deals with controllable hardwares. Before moving on to elaborate on each component, it must be explained that an *action* stands for a single motion of haptic.
Each module is described in Table 2.

Component Name	Description
TouchCon Core	Runtime of the framework
TouchCon Library	A list of TouchCons and a TouchCon, which is composed by a user or a haptic emoticon distributor
TouchCon Device	A hardware management of a TouchCon device (generally an actuator or a sensor)
Library XML file	An XML file which stores composed TouchCons
Device XML file	An XML file which stores hardware protocol specifications and acceptable commands
Connection Interface	Methods of communication through TouchCon hardware.

Table 2. Component description

To ensure the flexibility, we discriminate the library from the hardware at first. This allows for the framework to actuate similar haptic expressions with different hardware specifications. For example, there is only one red-coloured LED in the current hardware, the received TouchCon action could request to actuate the vibration motor. In this case, the resolver needs to interpret the TouchCon action into similar haptic expressions with current hardware specifications. In architectural point of view, if the hardware is directly coupled with the library and able to activate the identical hardware only, haptic expressions are limited to the hardware. To address this problem, the core runtime activates a function, i.e., the resolver, that interprets haptic expressions in accordance with hardware functionalities. The hardware monitors each available sensor and actuator so that the library acquires needed information to utilize them. For this reason, hardware management is relatively simpler than that of the library and the core in the framework.

2.2 TouchCon Core

The TouchCon Core consists of three components; the runtime to execute the library, the resolver to support different hardwares, and the sensor manager. The runtime module commands each haptic action to the hardware at every millisecond. In other words, a haptic action can be controlled in one millisecond. The runtime acts one of three behaviors with given TouchCon; activate user's hardware, transmit a TouchCon to a peer, or do nothing.
The *resolver* component modifies the input haptic action command when the hardware mismatch occurs. In other words, it compromises current hardware specifications and the input haptic expressions. Thanks to this resolver, the library can send TouchCon actions to the hardware as suitable as possible regardless of the type of the hardware attached to the user's device. The details of the resolver are given in Section 4.2.
The *sensor manager* processes the sensor input data. Unlike a general hardware management approach, the sensor management is done by the TouchCon Core. The reason why the sensor

is considered as the core component and not as the hardware one is that a sensor requires to process the acquired data. For example, the user can send a 'smile' haptic action as his/her laughing sound. Namely, the microphone can act as an input sensor to the framework and this is one of the useful scenarios in our work. In short, the input expression needs a decision to be described and sent as a TouchCon action format.

2.3 TouchCon Library

The TouchCon Library is a bundle of TouchCon actions. It can have one or more TouchCons according to the haptic expression. The library consists of three components; the TouchCon Library manager for organizing TouchCons, the in-memory database for storing temporary TouchCon actions, and the API (Application Programming Interface) for upper level applications. The TouchCon Library manager includes an XML parser to encode and to decode the given TouchCons with the TouchCon Library schema. Since all data handled in our work are designed to use the XML only, haptic contents can be authored with no length limitation. The specification of the schema and its example are given in the next section. The API allows external applications such as an instant messenger or the internet browser to communicate with the haptic framework. Unlike commonly used API approaches, our work is coupled with hardwares. For this reason, the API restricts to be invoked by one application only. If this restriction does not exist, the hardware might be collided by commands from multiple applications.

2.4 TouchCon Hardware

Since the scope of this study is not restricted to the vibro-tactile actuation, the hardware component can invite different protocols. Moreover, as haptic-enabled hardwares are being produced by various manufacturers, the framework should have a room to support them. If these future changes are not taken into consideration and thus only the limited haptic expressions can be executable, the results of this study may not be applicable in the near future. One of the possible solutions is to adopt an abstract layer above the hardware driver layer, and to simplify the hardware types and the commands. These approaches are used in Microsoft Windows HAL (Hardware Abstraction Layer) architecture and JINI home network one(Arnold et al. 1999; Russinovich and Solomon 2005). Once the hardware is attached to the framework, the abstract layer loads small description files and organizes available functionalities. In general, the hardware description files are located in the web or a local system. The advantage of this approach is to provide unified control points to other applications and to enable to invite various types of haptic-enabled hardwares.
Same approach is applied to our work. Once the device is connected and the description file, we call TouchCon Device XML, is loaded successfully, the TouchCon Device Manager expects the runtime to give some commands.

3. Haptic Description Language

We design two haptic description XML schemas in order to manage haptic commands and to activate haptic-enabled hardwares. Three factors must be taken into consideration to design schemas.

- Scalability: To include an abundance of haptic interactions and to support a combination of sensors and actuators, scalability must be considered in the system. This is the main reason why the XML format is adopted in this study.
- Flexibility: In this study, flexibility stands for adaptability. This means the schema can describe any form of the hardware interface. To incorporated with the framework, the developer must follow the suggested guidelines, but the developer's effort for the adaptation is minimized.
- Readability: According to Norman (Norman 2002), intuitiveness is an important factor in modern technology. From the view of consumer products, intuitiveness means easy-to-understand, easy-to-manipulate, and easy-to-use. Likewise, the schemas in this study have been carefully designed to be understood by general users as easy as possible. For example, the SensorML schemas that describe hardware specifications tend to be highly complicated because these formats are made to achieve more complex goals; to describe every kind of sensors in full details. Besides, our schemas require to describe the basic profile, the command list, and the data type only.

3.1 XML Schema for Haptic Device Description

As we introduced in Section 2.4, the objective of the device description is to incorporate various types of haptic-enabled hardwares together. To ensure the bidirectional haptic communication, both the sensor and the actuator must be described in a single schema. The method we use is to put the 'Output' attribute to each device description. The 'Output' attribute is allocated as a Boolean data type. If it sets to True, it indicates an actuator. Otherwise, it is a sensor. Even though the framework separates the sensor manager from the device manager (see Figure 1), the combination of sensors and hardwares in a schema is reasonable in the sense of *bidirectional haptic*. The details of the TouchCon device schema are summarized in Table 3. Note that the word 'TCon' is an abbreviation of TouchCon. As can be seen in this table, we designed it with less mandatory attributes.

Name	Attributes
TConDevices	(optional) Description: specifications or vendor information
TConDevice	(mandatory) Name: name of the controllable device Output: Boolean value for indicating sensor or actuator DataType: Property for protocol (optional) Description: information of the component
Property	(mandatory) Name: name to be displayed on the component Start: Start command End: End command

Table 3. Description on the haptic device schema

As can be seen in Table 3, we designed it with less mandatory attributes. Note that the word TCon is an abbreviation of TouchCon. The example using the schema is in Figure 2.

```xml
<?xml version="1.0" encoding="utf-8"?>
<TConDevices>
    <TConDevice Name="UpperLip" Output="True" Description="Mouth Upper Lip" DataType="String">
        <Property Name="Red" Start="U1AY" End="U1AN" />
        <Property Name="Green" Start="U2AY" End="U2AN" />
        <Property Name="Yellow" Start="U3AY" End="U3AN" />
        <Property Name="Blue" Start="U4AY" End="U4AN" />
        <Property Name="Purple" Start="U5AY" End="U5AN" />
        <Property Name="Cyan" Start="U6AY" End="U6AN" />
        <Property Name="White" Start="U7AY" End="U7AN" />
        <Property Name="Off" Start="U0AY" End="U0AN" />
    </TConDevice>
    <TConDevice Name="Pin" Output="True" Description="Pin" DataType="String">
        <Property Name="Left" Start="P1AY" End="P1AN" />
        <Property Name="Right" Start="P2AY" End="P2AN" />
        <Property Name="Both" Start="P3AY" End="P3AN" />
        <Property Name="Off" Start="P0AY" End="P0AN" />
    </TConDevice>
    <TConDevice Name="Heat" Output="True" Description="Heater" DataType="String">
        <Property Name="On" Start="H1AY" End="H1AN" />
        <Property Name="Off" Start="H0AY" End="H0AN" />
    </TConDevice>
</TConDevices>
```

Fig. 2. Example of the TouchCon device description

Figure 2 shows an example of the TouchCon Device XML schema. The root 'TConDevices' can contain multiple 'TConDevice' tags and one 'TConDevice' tag can contain multiple 'Property' tags. To understand the meaning of the example in Figure 2, we can see three actuators are involved in the framework; Upper Lip at line 3, Pin at line 13, and Heat at line 19. And also, we can identify that all three hardwares act as actuators from Output attributes. The values of each Start and End attributes inside the TConDevice tags are the unique commands for hardwares. These commands are totally dependent on the developer's hardwares. Currently, only ASCII strings are allowed to be used as commands.

3.2 XML Schema for Action Description

Unlike traditional text-based emoticons, the big changes in multimedia-enabled and haptic-embedded emoticons are able to deliver timeline-based actions. For example, a multimedia-enabled emoticon can play a small size animation with music. A haptic-embedded emoticon, the next generation of the emoticon, has additional features along with the timeline; a triggered hardware, its duration, and its property to be activated at each moment.

The TouchCon Action is a single element of hardware activation. And TouchCon Library is a bundle of actions. One action describes the device to be activated and its activation time. This is very similar to the music score. In other words, the TouchCon Library schema is the rule to write a score regarding haptic. Table 4 describes the schema of TouchCon Library and Action.

Name	Attributes
TCons	(optional) User: name of the author
TCon	(mandatory) Name: Name of the TouchCon action (optional) Image: small icon to display with the haptic action. Speed: running speed to be executed in the runtime component Description: information of the TouchCon.
Action	(mandatory) Device: Name of the device to be actuated StartTime: Start time in millisecond Duration: Duration time to play in millisecond (optional) Property: One of the device command

Table 4. Description on the haptic library schema

Figure 3 below shows an example of the TouchCon Library schemas in Table 4. According to Table 4, the library here has three levels of depth. We design the schema to have the minimum depth with many attributes, because the XML parser tends to slow down when the depth increases.

```
<?xml version="1.0" encoding="utf-8"?>
<TCons User="default">
    <TCon Name="Smile" Image="01.bmp" Speed="1" Description="">
        <Action Device="UpperLip" StartTime="0" Duration="30" Property="Purple" />
        <Action Device="LowerLip" StartTime="50" Duration="30" Property="Purple" />
        <Action Device="Vibrator" StartTime="100" Duration="50" Property="7_111111" />
    </TCon>
  <TCon Name="Kiss" Image="u_121.bmp" Speed="1" Description="">
    <Action Device="UpperLip" StartTime="0" Duration="50" Property="Red" />
    <Action Device="LowerLip" StartTime="50" Duration="30" Property="Purple" />
    <Action Device="Vibrator" StartTime="0" Duration="100" Property="3_111111" />
  </TCon>
</TCons>
```

Fig. 3. Example of the haptic device description

In contrast to the TouchCon Device schema, the TouchCon Library one is for users, not for developers. As we can see in Figure 3, one TouchCon Library (TCons) can contain one or more TouchCon Actions (TCon tags). And one TouchCon Action has a list of commands and times.

A single TouchCon Action can be represented as one haptic emoticon. Thus, it can be played on the user's hardware or sent to the peer's one.

3.3 TouchCon XML Parser

As all TouchCon-based data are handled and delivered in the XML format, the XML parser is installed in the framework. The TouchCon parser encodes and decodes TouchCon data;

the TouchCon Library, included actions, sensor specifications, and hardware descriptions. Once the TouchCon parser receives TouchCon Action data, it loads the data in the in-memory database in the FIFO manner. The in-memory database is an array-list so that it is expandable. There are pros and cons to make the in-memory data structure and the XML structure identical. Firstly, the pros; it has to be easy to convert, simple to understand for the user (or the developer), and easy to allocate for very large data. Now, the cons; it tends to cause memory abuse because of the unused TouchCon data, and it leads to the rather long processing time to be allocated into memory. Only two XML schemas were used in our framework, but the implemented TouchCon parser requires to interpret four types of XML data structures; TouchCon Library, TouchCon Action, TouchCon Device, and TouchCon sensor. One reason is that the Library is not just a bundle of actions, but additional information exists. And the other reason is the device and sensors are designed to share the same format for the realization of the bidirectional haptic concept (see Section 3.1), but from the view of the parser, they are not handled in the same way. In short, the two schemas are implemented to four structures.

4. Haptic Composer

This chapter introduces the Haptic Editor and the Haptic Resolver. Both aim to enhance the usefulness of the proposed framework. The Haptic Editor is a WYSIWYG editor with attached haptic hardwares. The Haptic Resolver is one of the modules in the TouchCon Core (see Figure 1), which negotiates haptic actuations when two corresponding peers use different hardwares.

4.1 Haptic Editor

The Haptic Editor is a timeline-based TouchCon editing tool. Today, many computer-savvy users are familiar with timeline-based multimedia editing tools such as Microsoft MovieMaker or Adobe Flash. Apart from the previous works (Aleven et al. 2006; Mohamad Eid et al. 2008), our Haptic Editor was designed in a WISIWIG manner. Basically, such a tool consists of two core parts; the horizontal part stands for time and the vertical part stands for elements. Timeline is labeled horizontally and elements are arranged vertically. Logically, the timeline and the involved elements are unlimited. Similar to common multimedia editing tools, our system is trigger-based one. Namely, each action is activated after the running time is passed at the designated moment.

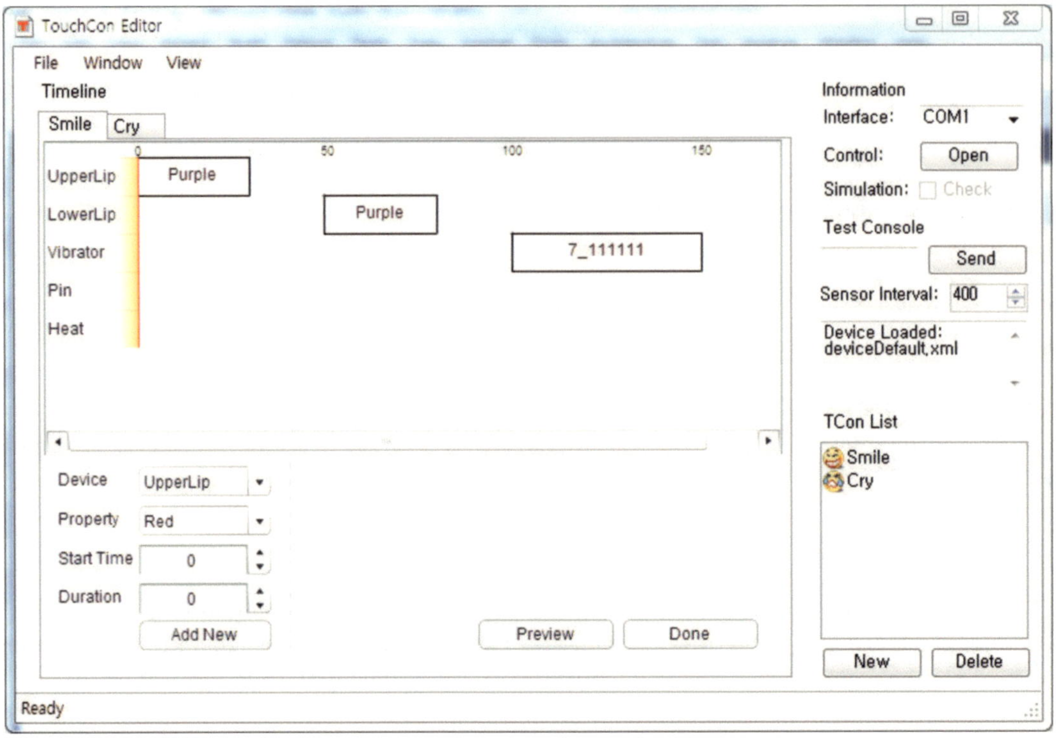

Fig. 4. Haptic Editor

Figure 4 shows a screenshot of the TouchCon Editor. This editor was designed to compose TouchCon Actions and to save them in the TouchCon Library file. The vertical layers indicate available (or controllable) haptic hardwares while the horizontal bars, durations of each action. The text label in the middle of the duration bar is for the property of the hardware. For example as in Figure 4, the label 'Red' indicates the light color of the LED.

The 'Preview' button at the bottom of the window executes (or plays) the current actions and activates the connected hardwares in order to test the composed results. When the user finishes making his/her own TouchCon Actions, the only thing to do is to click the 'Done' button to save the TouchCon haptic actions. Once the button is clicked, a popup window (save dialog) appears in order to incorporate a thumbnail image or additional descriptions.

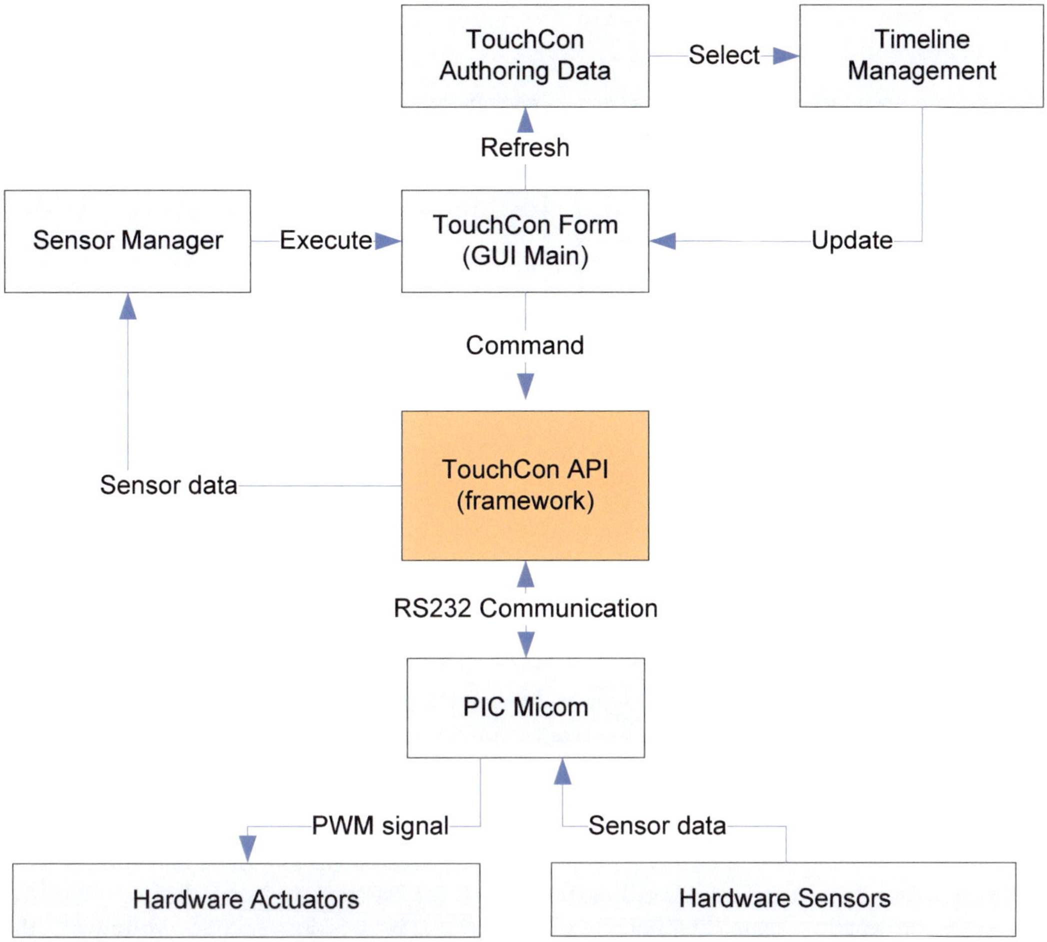

Fig. 5. Architecture of the Haptic Editor

Figure 5 illustrates how the Haptic Editor is constructed. The TouchCon framework communicates with a microcontroller through the RS232 serial port. The RS232 serial port can be replaced by the USB or the Bluetooth interface. The 'PIC Micom' stands for the Microchip® PIC microcontroller. We use an 8 bit microcontroller as the default, but the developer can use any type of microcontroller as far as the developer provides a proper TouchCon Device file.

As we can see in the middle (the orange-colored box), the Haptic Editor also uses the API of the TouchCon framework. The API allows the editor to create, append, remove, and arrange TouchCon Actions. The sensor is handled by the sensor manager. With the sensor data, the sensor manager executes one of three activities; activate user's hardwares, transmit a TouchCon to a peer, or do nothing. The decision along with the value from the sensor has to be defined in the TouchCon Action. Currently, the sensor-related implementation available in our work is only the rule-based decision. For instance, the 0-255 analog value (or 8 bit resolution) from a microcontroller can be categorized into three ranges and each range has its own activity. Generally, 0-30 is set to 'Do nothing' because such a low intensity value tends to be a noise.

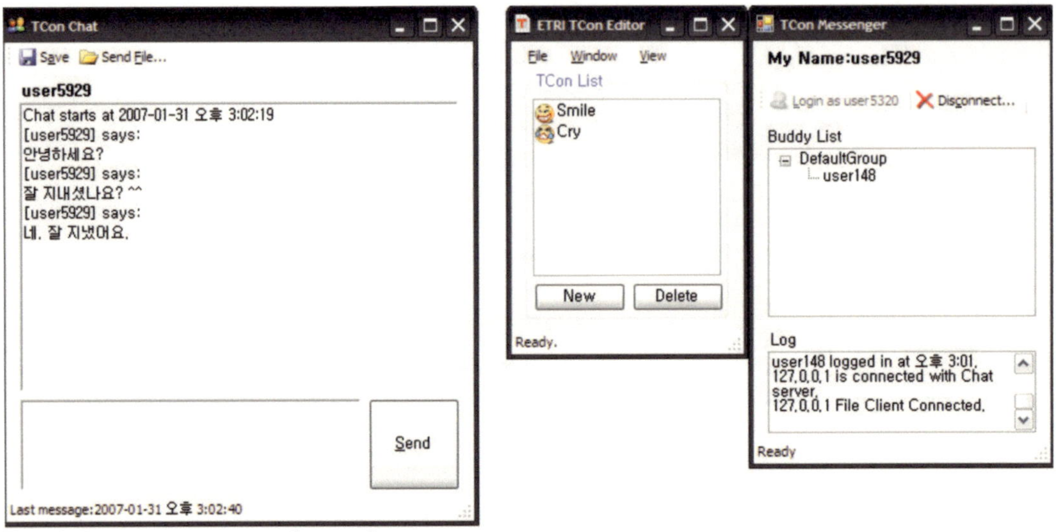

Fig. 6. Instant messenger for testing

A simple type of an instant messenger is implemented. This program is applied to the demonstration system and used for the evaluation and the survey. The demonstration and its result data are given in section 5.1. In Figure 6, three window-based programs are introduced. The left window is a chat window for the conversation among peers. Users can send text messages, graphical emoticons, or TouchCons. The middle window lists up the available TouchCons. This window is designed to be located nearby the chat window. The user can switch between TouchCon Editor and the list by clicking 'view' button. Namely, the user can easily create his/her own TouchCon while doing chat. Moreover, the messenger automatically adds new TouchCon to the list if the receiver does not have the TouchCon that the peer sends. Finally, the right window is a messenger server that shows available peers on the network. Entire programs are coded in C# language and run on the Windows XP operating system with the .Net Framework version 2.0.

4.2 Haptic Resolver

What happens if a peer sends TouchCons using a cellular phone and the other receives it with a laptop which cannot activate the received TouchCons? To solve this problem, the platform has to resolve this discrepancy and modifies the TouchCons from the sender to the acceptable and similar ones at the receiver.

Next is a simple example of the Haptic Resolver. At first, the magnitude of a TouchCon Action is analyzed. The three attributes to activate haptic actuators are the frequency, the amplitude, and the duration. Based on these, we can represent waveforms or the PWM (Pulse Width Modulation) signals accurately. We found that the waveform is very similar to sound signals. Thus, we utilize this metaphor to convert TouchCons or emoticons to haptic actuator signals through the resolver. Figure 7 shows an example of this conversion.

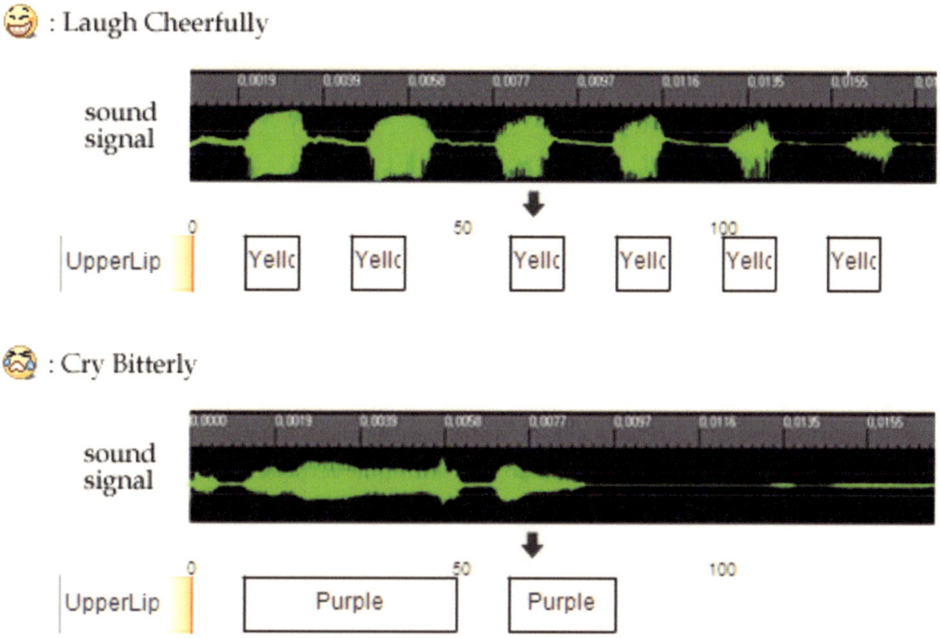

Fig. 7. Sound signals and vibration mapping patterns

The upper part of each box shows recorded sounds of different sensations. During the survey, subjects showed high preferences and high sensational sympathy for more than half of the haptic expressions when the sound mapping is applied. The preference survey results are described in Section 5.

5. Evaluation

To evaluate the proposed architecture, several hardware prototypes and software applications are implemented. This chapter introduces how such prototypes and applications work and how they can be utilized to expand the scope of human communications.

5.1 Implementation of Haptic Testbed for Instant Messenger Environment

A hardware testbed with various actuators and sensors is implemented. The testbed is designed for the instant messaging environment which is the main target of our system. Industrial designers joined the project and proposed the idea of the palm-rest-shaped silicon forms and a lip-shaped module to make a user feel more humane. The designer wants the user to touch and feel the hardwares like a small pet. For that, the hardwares were covered with the soft-feeling silicon material. In addition, we found that the silicon finish could prevent the user from being injured by embedded heater units.

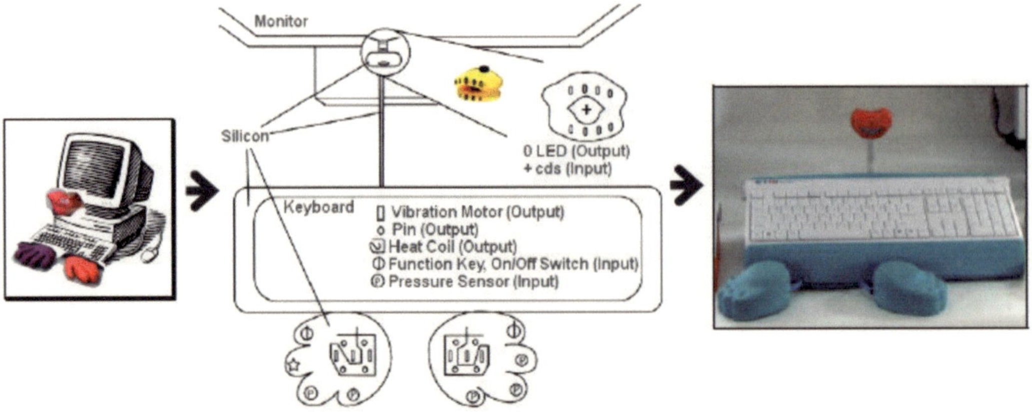

Fig. 8. Design and development process

Figure 8 describes hardware products and their embedded components. At first, a conceptual design was sketched. Then, sensors, actuators, and related circuits were placed in consideration of the hand positions on the products. Later, PCB boards are installed inside the specially designed foams.

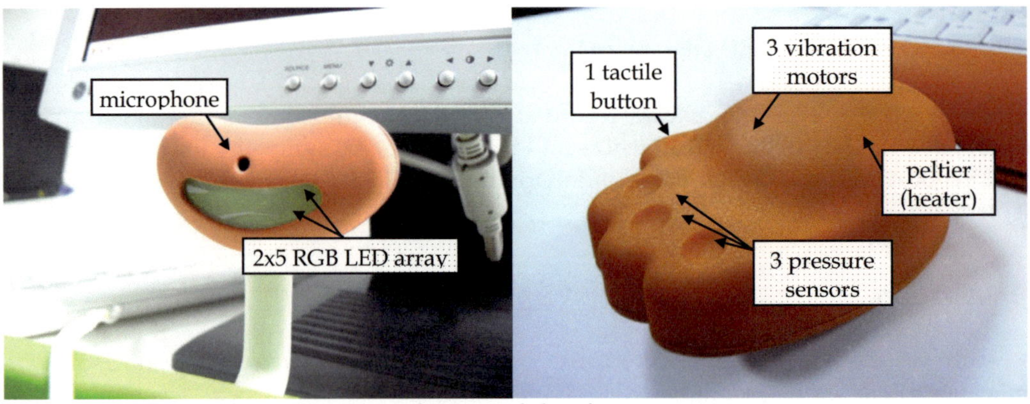

Fig. 9. Actuators and sensors inserted into each hardware part

As can be seen in Figure 9, one animal-foot-shaped palm-rest component has one tactile button, three pressure sensors, three vibration motors and one heater panel. The lip-shaped compartment has ten RGB-color LEDs and one microphone. The microphone can detect the user's touch. Each foot-shaped component is attached to the keyboard using a multiple-wire thick cable. This separated design allows the user to adjust the palm-rest position easily.

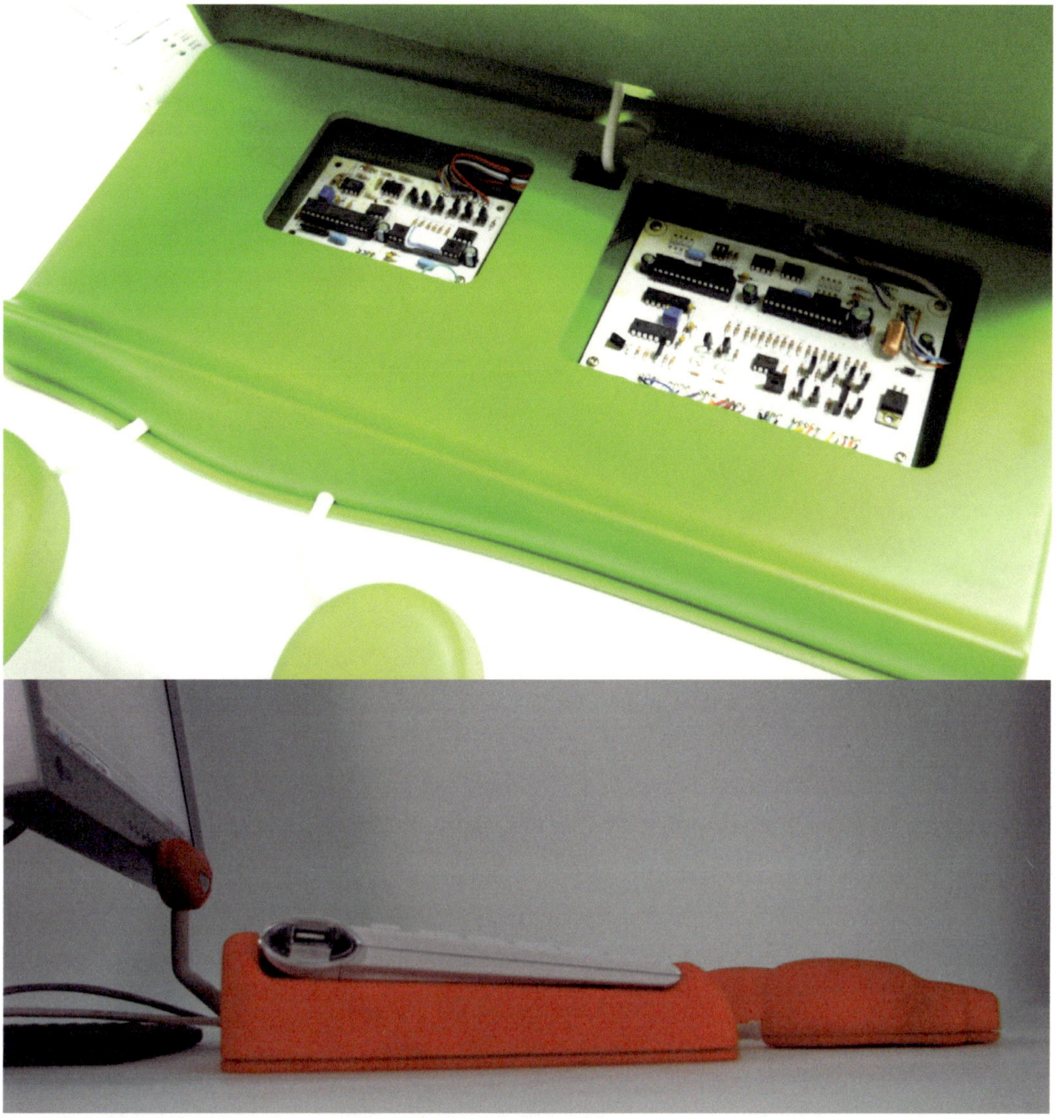

Fig. 10. Controller circuits underneath the keyboard base

Figure 10 shows the controller circuits underneath the keyboard. Thanks to the thin keyboard, i.e., the pentagraph-type keyboard, we can place circuits in the forms seamlessly without losing comfortable typing experiences. The two devices (above and below in Figure 10) are same devices except their color. The left circuit handles the lip-shaped component while the right circuit manages the animal-foot-shaped one. Both circuits use two microcontrollers in order to control the input and the output signal separately.

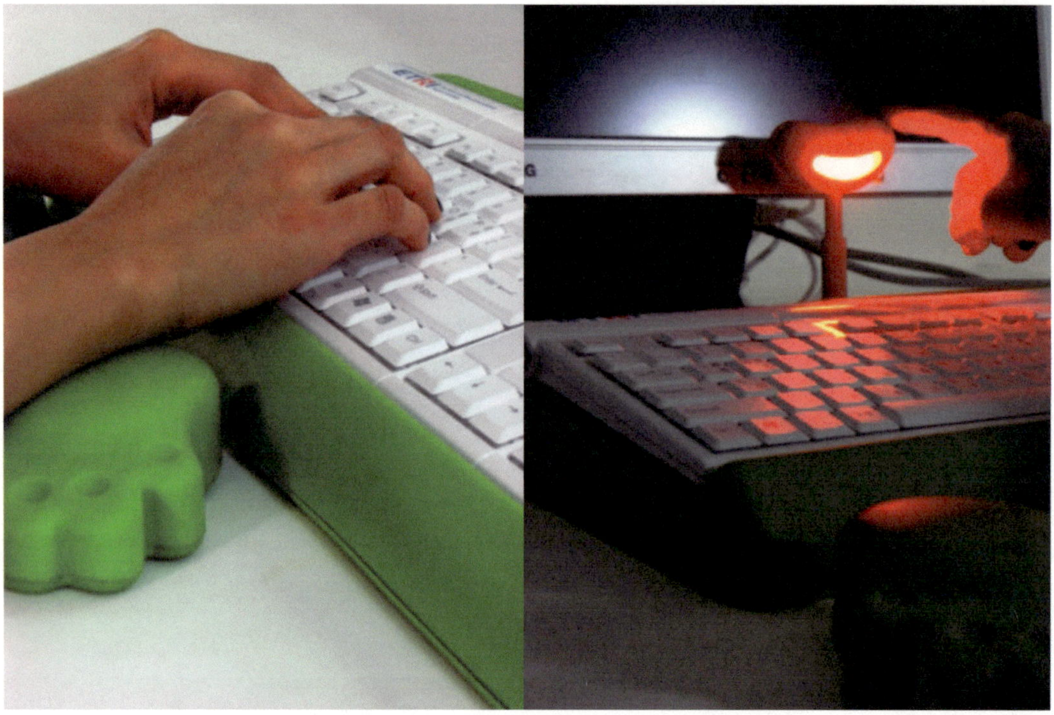

Fig. 11. Usage of prototype hardware

Figure 11 is an example of the hardware usage. The left picture shows how the user can feel the actuation of the vibration motor. The right picture illustrates how the light blinks when the user touches the lip-shaped component.

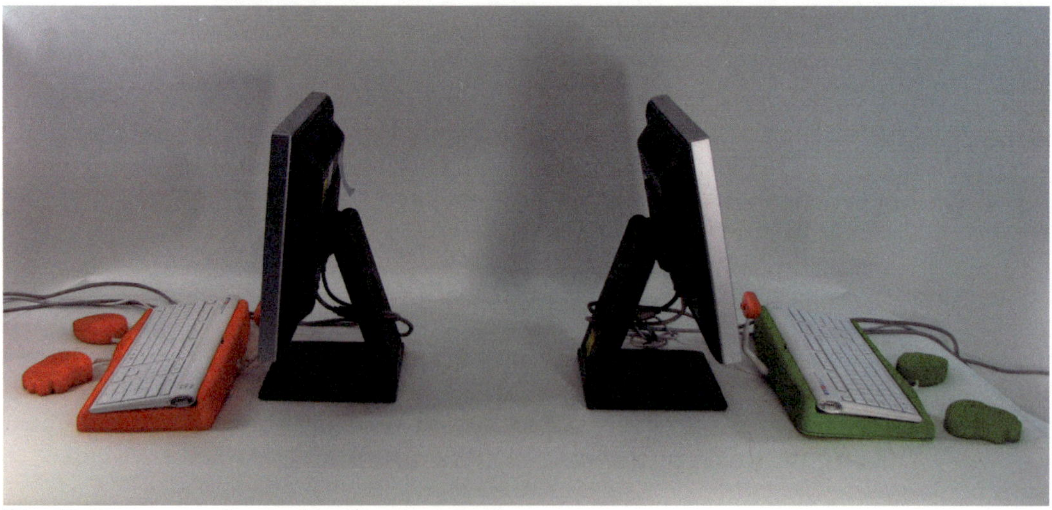

Fig. 12. Demonstration and evaluation setup

Figure 12 shows a pair of connected computers with our haptic testbed. Total three hardware sets in different colors (orange, green, and blue) were fabricated to survey the user preference. Two of them are used for the survey and the remaining one is for spare. The survey system was demonstrated at the Next Generation Computing Exhibition held in November, 2006, in Korea. During the exhibition, visitors were invited to experience our system and at the same time, the survey was also carried out.

5.2 User Test

The objective of the user test is to find out whether haptic expressions are sufficient to make users feel intended emotions. A total of 12 participants (six males and six females) were invited to evaluate TouchCons. Firstly, each TouchCons is presented to them, then they were asked to pick one best-matching emoticon from the list of six, that seemed to serve its purpose best. No prior information about the tactile or visual cues has been provided. Secondly, each participant was asked to evaluate the effectiveness of the TouchCons in representing different types of emotion. The average score was 1 point on a scale from -2 to 2 (five-point Likert scale). Figure 13 shows six selected emoticons and their haptic expressions while Figure 14 shows the two above-mentioned evaluation results.

Emotion Category	Emotion	TCON						
		Visual Expression	Tactile Expression					
			Vibrating Motor				Others	
			Voltage (min:0.1 ~ max:2.8)	Duration (ms)	Delay (ms)	Number of Times	Pin Actuator On/Off	Heat Display ON/OFF
Positive	Grin	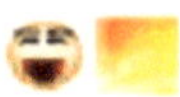	quick, light and regular vibration					
			1.9	100	100	5	off	off
Negative	Cry	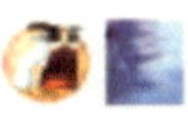	slow-moving vibration, hight -> weak -> mid -> weak stress					
			2.6 ->0.3 ->1.9->0.3	500->700 ->900->1100	0	1	off	off
	Anger	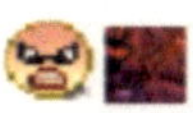	one of strong vibration + pin operation					
			2.6	200	0	1	on	off
Surprise	Surprise	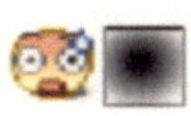	one vibration of thick and mid-stress					
			1.9->0.3	800->200	0	1	off	off
Winsome	Kiss	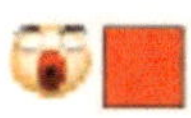	being strong gradually and continuously + Heat display operation					
			0.1->0.8 ->1.9->2.8	800->800 ->800->1500	0	1	off	on
State of Body	Sleepy	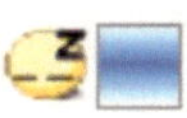	slow and regular vibration					
			0.3->1.9 ->0.3->1.9	1500	0	2	off	off

Fig. 13. Selected emoticons and haptic patterns

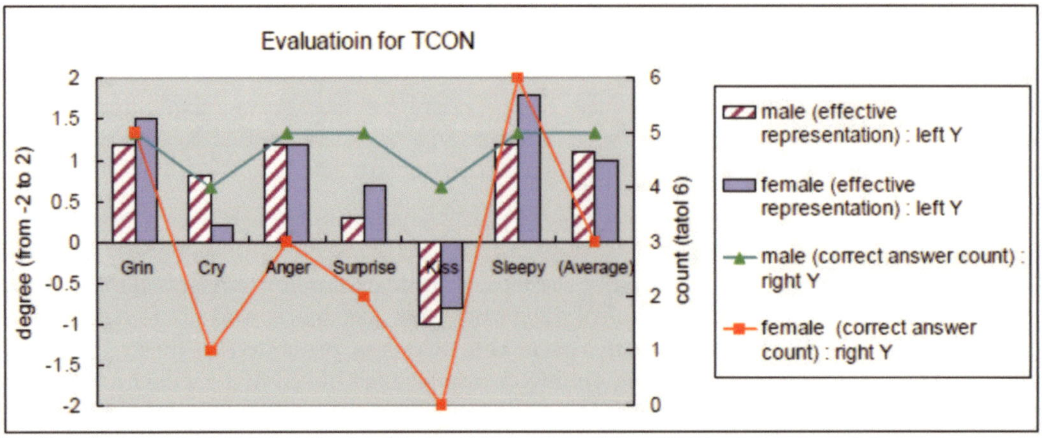

Fig. 14. Evaluation results for TouchCons

In Figure 14, the two lines indicate the first evaluation results (referenced on the right Y axis), and the bars indicate the second evaluation results (referenced on the left Y axis). The results show that the 'Kiss' TouchCon usually failed to give the sensation of kissing, but 'Sleepy' and 'Grinning' were rather successful. Note also that considerable differences exist between female and male users; the former tended to answer with the correct TouchCon less frequently and feel that the TouchCon patterns were less effective than the latter.
Although the TouchCon interface is more complex than that of text emoticons because users have to switch a window focus between the chat and the TouchCon list window, the average number of TouchCons used during each chat reached 14, while that of text emoticons was slightly higher than 17. Finally, a questionnaire survey was conducted after the free experience of the system. The questions included were how enjoyable, emotional, fresh, new, and absorbing the chatting experience was. Respondents were also asked how easy they thought it was to feel the tactile stimulus and how well the pattern chosen suited each type of emotion. Respondents gave the most positive responses on how fresh, new and enjoyable the chat felt (-2 is the most negative while +2 is the most positive). It was observed that males were more satisfied with the experience than females. Some more additional results can be found in our previous work (Shin et al. 2007; Jung 2008).

6. Conclusion

This work was conducted on the combination of two fields, i.e., haptic and social messaging. Haptic is one of the most attention-drawing fields and the biggest buzzwords among next-generation users. Haptic is being applied to conventional devices such as the cellular phone and even the door lock. Diverse forms of media such as blogs, social network services, and instant messengers are used to send and receive messages. That is mainly why we focus on the messaging experience, the most frequent communication of the device-mediated conversation.
We propose the integration of sensors and actuators in a single framework in order to make the usage be understood more easily. The specifications to manipulate hardwares require a very light burden to developers; they only need to know the command list which follows

the TouchCon Device schemas to cooperate their own haptic hardwares with our framework. In conclusion, the haptic communication system proposed in this study enables people to enjoy text messaging with haptic actions and can boost message-based communications among people.

7. References

Aleven, V., J. Sewall, B. M. McLaren, and K. R. Koedinger. 2006. Rapid authoring of intelligent tutors for real-world and experimental use. In *Advanced Learning Technologies, 2006. Sixth International Conference on*, 847-851.

Arnold, K., R. Scheifler, J. Waldo, B. O'Sullivan, and A. Wollrath. 1999. *Jini Specification*. Addison-Wesley Longman Publishing Co., Inc. Boston, MA, USA.

Baldauf, M., S. Dustdar, and F. Rosenberg. 2007. A survey on context-aware systems. *International Journal of Ad Hoc and Ubiquitous Computing* 2, no. 4: 263-277.

Bonanni, L., C. Vaucelle, J. Lieberman, and O. Zuckerman. 2006. TapTap: a haptic wearable for asynchronous distributed touch therapy. In *Conference on Human Factors in Computing Systems*, 580-585. ACM New York, NY, USA.

Botts, M., and A. Robin. 2007. Sensor model language (SensorML). *Open Geospatial Consortium Inc., OGC*: 07-000.

Brave, S., and A. Dahley. 1997. inTouch: a medium for haptic interpersonal communication. In *Conference on Human Factors in Computing Systems*, 363-364. ACM New York, NY, USA.

Chang, A., S. O'Modhrain, R. Jacob, E. Gunther, and H. Ishii. 2002. ComTouch: design of a vibrotactile communication device. In *Proceedings of the 4th conference on Designing interactive systems: processes, practices, methods, and techniques*, 312-320. ACM New York, NY, USA.

Eid, Mohamad, Sheldon Andrews, Atif Alamri, and Abdulmotaleb El Saddik. 2008. HAMLAT: A HAML-Based Authoring Tool for Haptic Application Development. In *Haptics: Perception, Devices and Scenarios*, 857-866. http://dx.doi.org/10.1007/978-3-540-69057-3_108.

El-Far, F. R., M. Eid, M. Orozco, and A. El Saddik. 2006. Haptic Applications Meta-Language. In *Tenth IEEE International Symposium on Distributed Simulation and Real-Time Applications, 2006. DS-RT'06*, 261-264.

Immersion Corp, A. 2007. HAPTICS: Improving the Mobile User Experience through Touch. http://www.immersion.com/docs/haptics_mobile-ue_nov07v1.pdf.

Java, A., X. Song, T. Finin, and B. Tseng. 2007. Why we twitter: understanding microblogging usage and communities. In *Proceedings of the 9th WebKDD and 1st SNA-KDD 2007 workshop on Web mining and social network analysis*, 56-65. ACM New York, NY, USA.

Jung, Chanhee. 2008. Design of Vibro-tactile Patterns for Emotional Expression in Online Environments. Thesis for the degree of Master, Information and Communications University. http://library.kaist.ac.kr/thesisicc/T0001759.pdf.

Kim, Y., Y. Kim, and M. Hahn. 2009. A context-adaptive haptic interaction and its application. In *Proceedings of the 3rd International Universal Communication Symposium*, 241-244. ACM.

Norman, Donald A. 2002. *The Design of Everyday Things*. Basic Books, ISBN 0-465-06710-7, Jackson, TN.

Poupyrev, I., T. Nashida, and M. Okabe. 2007. Actuation and tangible user interfaces: the Vaucanson duck, robots, and shape displays. In *Proceedings of the 1st international conference on Tangible and embedded interaction*, 212. ACM.

Rovers, A. F., and H. A. Van Essen. 2004. HIM: a framework for haptic instant messaging. In *Conference on Human Factors in Computing Systems*, 1313-1316. ACM New York, NY, USA.

Rovers, L., and H. A. Van Essen. 2004. Design and evaluation of hapticons for enriched instant messaging. In *Proceedings of EuroHaptics*, 4: Vol. 4.

Russinovich, M. E., and D. A. Solomon. 2005. *Microsoft Windows Internals, Microsoft Windows Server 2003, Windows XP, and Windows 2000*. Microsoft Press.

Shin, H., J. Lee, J. Park, Y. Kim, H. Oh, and T. Lee. 2007. A Tactile Emotional Interface for Instant Messenger Chat. *Lecture Notes in Computer Science* 4558: 166.

Vilhjálmsson, H. H. 2003. Avatar Augmented Online Conversation. Massachusetts Institute of Technology.

Youngjae Kim, Heesook Shin, and Minsoo Hahn. 2009. A bidirectional haptic communication framework and an authoring tool for an instant messenger. In *Advanced Communication Technology, 2009. ICACT 2009. 11th International Conference on*, 03:2050-2053. Vol. 03.

Realistic Haptics Interaction in Complex Virtual Environments

Hanqiu SUN
*Department of Computer Science & Engineering,
The Chinese University of Hong Kong,
Hong Kong*

Hui CHEN
*Shenzhen Institute of Advanced Integration Technology,
Chinese Academy of Sciences / The Chinese University of Hong Kong,
China*

1. Introduction

Simulating interactive behavior of objects such as soft tissues in surgical simulation or in control engine of VR applications has been extensively studied. Adding haptic information such as vibration, tactile array, force feedback simulation enhances the sense of presence in virtual environments. Recreating the realistic contact forces the user would perceive when interacting the virtual objects is in general difficult. Current haptic technology only effectively simulates interactive forces for simple cases, but rather limited when considering complex virtual scenes. Desirable properties in realistic haptics interaction include: the stable and smooth reflection forces at a high refreshing rate around 1KHz, and the smooth exhibition of object deformations and physical-realistic behaviors. Physically based haptic deformations and simulation are mostly computationally intensive and not suitable for interactive virtual-scene applications. Even so, integrating non-physical methods with haptic feedbacks is not natural, and cannot provide realistic physical simulation of deformable objects. VR applications strive to simulate real or imaginary scenes with which users can interact and perceive the realistic effects of their action in real time.

People investigate haptic interfaces to perform interactive tasks mainly in two aspects: to explore part of the environment and thus achieve tactile identification of objects, positions and orientations; to actively utilize force sensations to manipulate/deform objects in the touch-enabled immersive tasks. Researches on haptic display are currently focused on tool-object haptic interaction, during which the users feel and interact with the simulated environment through the tool of a given shape including the hand or fingers. The force feedbacks are generated based on the spring/damping linked to the dynamic haptic interface, but the proper values for those material properties are not always easy to derive from measured approaches. Touch-based surgical simulation is not only made to improve realism of virtual environments, but also to provide important diagnostic information through the sense of touch. Palpation is important to sense with hands during a physical examination, in which the doctor presses on the surface of the body to feel the organs or tissues underneath. We propose the novel body-based haptic interaction approach (Chen & Sun, 2006), which models the intrinsic properties of the tool and virtual objects during the touch-enabled palpation in medical simulation. During the virtual palpation force-sensing, the contact/frictional forces are evaluated based on Hertz's contact theory, and the press distribution with the contact is specified accordingly. Compliant contact models require surface geometry, material properties, and efficient interactive forces simulation. The non-linear viscoelastic behavior of typical tissues is mimicked using a volumetric tetrahedral mess-spring system, and high performance in computing the touch deformation is acquired to exhibit the typical human tissues in the real world.

More information channels have been provided recently to augment visual techniques with haptic methods, giving the modality for visualization and active data exploration. Most haptic devices utilize point interactions, resulting in a conflict between the low information bandwidth and further complication of data exploration. Unlike our sense of vision, haptic manipulation involves direct interaction with objects being explored, providing the most intuitive way of applying 3D manipulation in virtual scenes. Utilizing multi-resolution methods in haptic display provides a possibility to balance the conflict in the complex virtual scene. These combine the elegance of a recursive hierarchical spatial or geometric decomposition of the scene with the ability to provide simplified drawable representations for groups of related subobjects. We study the multi-resolution haptic interaction scheme of hybrid virtual models in the complex scene, in which the hierarchical imposter representations of surface/volume models are constructed. The optimal performance based on haptic-scene perceptual evaluation at run time is employed to meet both the visual and tangible interaction qualities, providing more information of objects transferred by detailed perceptions (spatial & physical) guided by the sense of touch.

2. Background

Users expected to manipulate the virtual worlds through the tool-based haptic interfaces in cyberspace as if in the real world. Many research efforts have been dedicated to this area (Salisbury et al., 2004), during which the users feel and interact with the simulated environment through the tool of a given shape including the hand or fingers. Most studies simplified the haptic tool-object interaction paradigm into multiple point contacts (Colgate et al., 1995), which provide a convenient simplification because the system needs only render forces resulting from contact between the tool's avatar and objects in the environment. The force feedbacks are generated based on the spring/damping linked to the dynamic haptic interface, and the proper values for those spring/damping constants are not always easy to derive from measured material properties. Lin and Manocha's groups worked on 6DOF haptic interactions (Gregory et al., 2000; Kim et al., 2002; Kim et al., 2003) that simulated the interaction between two 3D objects through convex decomposing of polygonal models to accelerate collision detection, and finally relayed a combination of penalty-based restoring forces of cluster contacts to the user.

Modeling of soft tissue deformation in tangible medical simulations is of great importance. The goal is to allow virtual tissues responding to user's manipulations in a physically realistic manner, as if possessing the true mechanical behavior of real tissues. Thus, tangible surgical simulators may become a safe and feasible alternative for enhancing traditional surgical training. Usually the complex surgical tools were modeled out of simple basic components with points and lines in medical simulation to achieve realistic and fast simulations. Basdogan et al. (Basdogan et al., 2001; Basdogan et al., 2004) have overviewed the research on distributed, collaborative haptic systems for laparoscopic surgery, where surgical tools of long, thin, straight probes and articulated tools for pulling, clamping, gripping, and cutting soft tissues were applied. Bielser et al. (Bielser et al., 1999; Bielser & Gross, 2000; Bielser & Gross, 2002) presented interactive open surgery scenarios applied with surgical hooks and scalpels.

Our sense of touch is spatially focused and has a far lower bandwidth in comparison with visual sense that has the largest bandwidth. Coupling interactive haptic rendering in complex virtual environment is important in tangbile scene navigation and exploration. Multi-resolution descriptions of the scene can provide a solution to the conflict between this low information bandwidth and the complexity of the virtual scene. El-Sana & Varshney (El-Sana & Varshney, 2000) introduced a Continuously-Adaptive Haptic rendering approach to reduce the complexity of the rendered dataset. Asghar et al. (Asghar et al., 2001) implemented multi-resolution descriptions of the scene in a haptic environment based on the affine median filter, providing users with view of varying resolution scene. Zhang et al. (Zhang et al., 2002) applied haptic rendering in different detail levels of soft object by subdividing the area of interest on a relatively coarse mesh model and evaluated the spring constants after haptic subdivision. Otaduy & Lin (Otaduy & Lin, 2003) provided a sensation preserving simplification algorithm based on multi-resolution hierarchies of object geometry for faster time-critical collision queries between polyhedral objects in haptic rendering.

Interactive rendering of complex virtual environments demands the desirable properties of tool-based haptic interaction, as the following:

- The interactive forces should reflect the characteristics between the touch tool and soft-tissue objects at an intuitive and stable way;
- The physical-realistic behaviours such as virtual palpation should be simulated smoothly in real-time;
- Multi-resolution tangible scheme should be established to maximize the perceptual information with larger force applied.

Here, the above properties realized in the recent researches are presented. In tangible simulation, the novel body-based haptic interaction approach that simulates the intrinsic properties of the tool and soft-tissue objects during the virtual palpation is presented. Further, the multi-resolution haptic interactive scheme of hybrid models is constructed to provide more detailed perceptions guided by our sense of touch in complex virtual scene.

3. Dynamic Tangible-active Palpation

Palpation is the essential diagnosis technique, commonly used in cancer diagnosis to find the size, consistency, texture, location, and tenderness of abnormal tissues. Currently, most simulated palpation forces were reduced to point-based interaction model with spring-damper linkage to simulate the contact between one or more fingertips and the virtual object. Some special haptics device was created and applied in breast palpation simulation.

The contact problem between two elastic solids that are pressed by the applied force was first solved by Hertz in 1882 (Landau & Lifshitz, 1986), under assumptions: the contact area is elliptical, each body is approximated by an elastic half-space loaded over an elliptical contact area, and the dimensions of the contact area must be small relative to the dimensions of each body. Hertz's theory yields stresses, deformations, and the shape of the interface formed at the two contacting bodies. These quantities depend on the elastic properties of the two bodies, the geometric shape at the contact, and the force used to push them together. Pawluk and Howe (Pawluk & Howe, 1999a; Pawluk & Howe, 1999b) investigated the dynamic force and distributed pressure response of the human finger-pad based on Hertz's theory, and developed a quasilinear viscoelastic model successfully explaining the observed measurements. Barbagli et al. (Barbagli et al., 2004) compared four physical models for rotational friction of soft finger contact and extended the god-object algorithm to simulate contact between one or more fingertips and a virtual object.

3.1 Haptic body-based palpation

Instead of point contact with mass only, we describe each contact as the body-based contact with elliptic paraboloid spheres, during the haptic tool-object interaction. Physical properties described by mass, volume, Poisson's Ratio and Young's Modulus with contacted objects are computed to reflect the intrinsic physical properties of the objects. Based on them, the contact/frictional palpation force-sensing between finger and virtual objects is simulated and the press distribution of the finger pad is specified accordingly. Hertz's contact theory based on solid bodies in contact is investigated to simulate the contact forces during the haptic tool-object interactions.

Basic force model

The virtual index finger is modelled as the single-layer sphere bodies bounding the surface of the forefinger in advance. Each sphere body $s_i(m_i, r_i, v_i, E_i)$ in the layer has four attributes: m_i is the mass of sphere body s_i, r_i is it's radius, v_i is the Poisson's Ratio and E_i is it's Young's Modulus (fundamental elastic constants reflecting the stiffness of the forefinger). In Figure 1, the left figure models show the simulation with one sphere attached to the finger tip, and the one simulated with 8-spheres to construct the volume of sphere bodies. The virtual index finger is modeled with a triangle-mesh surface object. The basic palpation force model between each sphere body and the object is constructed, shown in the righ part of Figure 1, as follows:

$$\vec{F} = \vec{F}_c + \vec{F}_\mu + \vec{F}_a \tag{1}$$

where $\vec{F}_c$ is the contact force between two solids based on Hertz's contact theory specified in equation (2); $\vec{F}_a$ is the ambient force in relation to the virtual finger, for example, the gravity $\vec{F}_g$ of the virtual finger and other compensation forces to balance the downward force of stylus tip of the haptic device; $\vec{F}_\mu$ is the frictional force caused by the roughness of the tissue surface in relation to the contact force and the gravity; and $\vec{F}$ is the integrated palpation force applied to the haptic interface.

When multi contacts are detected between the virtual index finger and the interacted tissue, each palpation force is evaluated using equation (1), and the final compound force is applied to the user through the haptic interface (Chen et al., 2007).

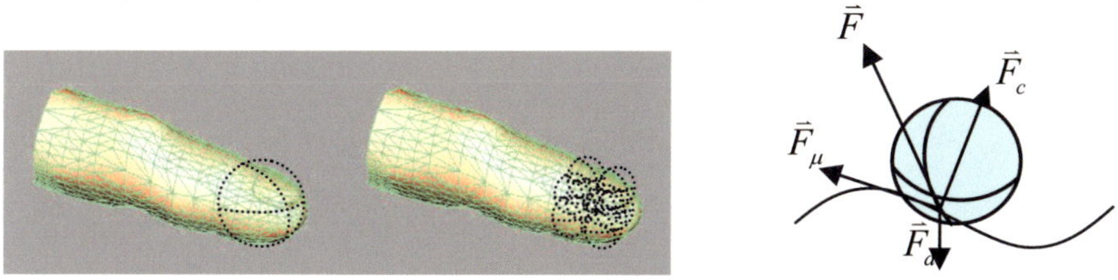

Fig. 1. Virtual finger simulation and body-based basic force model.

Palpation force-sensing
Hertz's contact theory yields stresses, deformation and the shape of the interface formed at two contacting bodies. These quantities depend on elastic properties, the object shape, the relative position of the two bodies at the point of contact and the force pushing them together. Although original Hertz contact load is based on the smooth (frictionless) contact, it can be developed to account for rough (frictional) surfaces. In virtual tangible palpation, the produced biomechanical behavior of the human tissues is evaluated. The virtual index finger is simulated with the properties of silicon rubber. The four typical human tissue categories, including skin, muscle, ligament, and bone, are simulated based on the physical properties specified. Figure 2 shows the tested environment of the virtual index finger and human tissue models, including the cuboid tetrahedral volume interacting via the virtual finger, the ligment, the cortical bone and the upper leg of human body respectively.

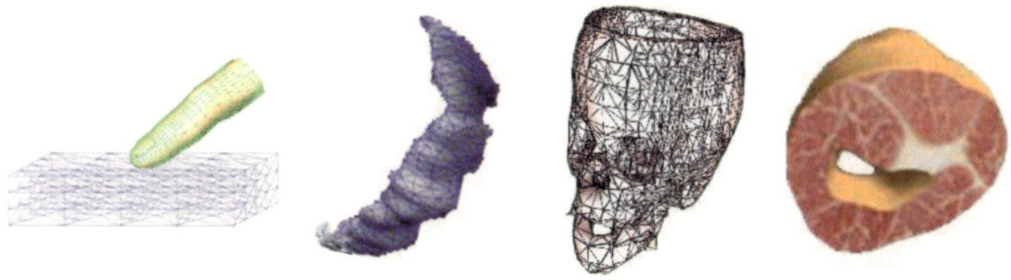

Fig. 2. Simulated human tissue models.

Normal contact force: Assuming $h << R$, and using the inverse of Hertz's contact theory based on solid bodies in contact, the contact force $\vec{F}_c$ exerted on the tool by the elastic deformation of the object is expressed below,

$$\vec{F}_c = h^{\frac{3}{2}} \frac{4}{3} \frac{1}{l_1 + l_2} \left(\frac{R_1 R_2}{R_1 + R_2} \right)^{\frac{1}{2}} \qquad l_1 = \frac{1 - v_1^2}{E_1} \qquad l_2 = \frac{1 - v_2^2}{E_2} \tag{2}$$

where h is the penetration depth between two contact bodies, v_i (i=1,2) is the Poisson's Ratio and E_i (i=1, 2) is the Young's Modulus that describe the elastic properties of two contact bodies respectively.

Pressure distribution: The distribution of the pressure over the contact area is given by the radius of the contact circle and the expression of the pressure, which is exerted on point ξ in the contact area. They are defined as follows:

$$a = \vec{F}_c^{\frac{1}{3}} \left(\frac{3}{4} (l_1 + l_2) \frac{R_1 R_2}{R_1 + R_2} \right)^{\frac{1}{3}} \qquad \vec{P}(\xi) = -\frac{3\vec{F}_c}{2\pi a^2} (1 - \frac{|\xi|}{a^2})^{\frac{1}{2}} \qquad \vec{P}_0 = -\frac{3\vec{F}_c}{2\pi a^2} \tag{3}$$

where ξ is measured from the center of the contact region, and a is the radius of the contact area. $\vec{P}_0$ specifies the contact pressure at the center of the contact area.

Firctional force: The frictional force on the contact area is determined by the contact force and the gravity force, as follows:

$$\begin{aligned} \vec{F}_{\mu g} &= \mu \vec{F}_g = \mu m g \qquad \vec{F}_{\mu c}(\xi) = \mu \vec{P}(\xi) \\ \vec{F}_{\mu c} &= \iint_{\xi < a} \vec{F}_{\mu c}(\xi) d\sigma \qquad \vec{F}_{\mu} = \vec{F}_{\mu g} + \vec{F}_{\mu c} \end{aligned} \tag{4}$$

where μ is the friction coefficient depending on the roughness of the object, $\vec{F}_{\mu g}$ is the frictional force in relation to the gravity of each body, $\vec{F}_{\mu c}$ is the frictional force caused by the contact force. $\vec{F}_{\mu c}(\xi)$ describes the frictional force of the unit area to the locally exerted pressure. The integration over the entire contact area is superposed to the final $\vec{F}_{\mu c}$. Finally $\vec{F}_{\mu}$ is the integrated dynamic frictional force between the virtual index finger and the tissue.

Figure 3 records the palpation force simulated between the virtual index finger and the touched tissues of bone/skin/ligment/muscle/upper leg. The force is depicted as a regression via a natural logarithm function. Here, the left graph shows the palpation force in relation to the indentation, and the right graph presents the force computed in relation to the local geometry of the contacted tissues. The simulated nonlinear force curves are similar to the typical load-deformation curves exhibited by corresponding human tissues.

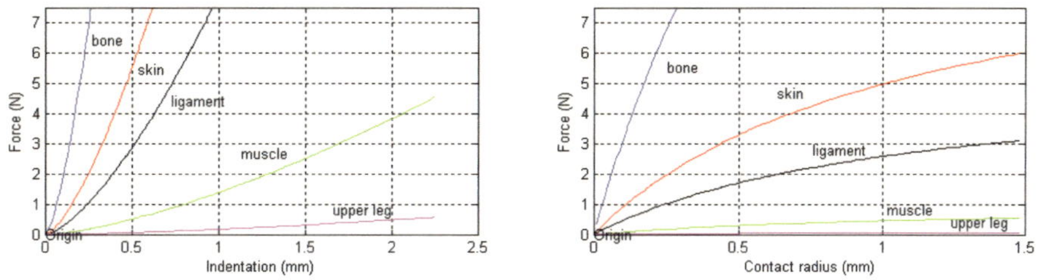

Fig. 3. Force evaluation between virtual finger and tissues.

3.2 Dynamic curvature estimation

An important step in our body-based haptic interaction model is constructing the equivalent sphere representing the shape of the object at the contact area dynamically. The mean curvature, describing insight to the degree of flatness of the surface, is applied to estimate the radius of sphere of the object at the contact area. Similar to normal vector voting (Page et al, 2001; Page et al., 2002) of curvature estimation on piecewise smooth surfaces, the mean curvature of contacted area is estimated dynamically during the haptic tool-object interaction.

Discrete approximation

Taubin (Taubin, 1995) showed that the symmetric matrix M_p at point p on a smooth surface,

$$M_p = \frac{1}{2\pi}\int_{-\pi}^{\pi} k_p(T_\theta)T_\theta T_\theta^t d\theta \qquad k_p^1 = 3m_p^1 - m_p^2 \qquad k_p^2 = 3m_p^2 - m_p^1 \tag{5}$$

has the equivalent eigenvectors to the principal directions $\{T_1, T_2\}$ and the eigenvalues $\{m_p^1, m_p^2\}$, where $\{m_p^1, m_p^2\}$ are related to the principal curvatures $\{k_p^1, k_p^2\}$ through a fixed homogenous linear transformation. As a result, the mean curvature can be acquired by $k_p = (k_p^1 + k_p^2)/2$. An approximation of the matrix on a discrete mesh is given by Taubin,

$$\widetilde{M}_p = \frac{1}{2\pi}\sum \omega_i k_i T_i T_i^t \tag{6}$$

where $\widetilde{M}_p$ denotes the approximation of M_p at vertex p through the combination of a finite set of directions T_i and curvatures $k_i \cdot \omega_i$ is a discrete weight version of the integration step and has the constraint $\sum \omega_i = 2\pi$. The two principal curvatures can be acquired by the eigen analysis of matrix $\widetilde{M}_p$.

Curvature estimation

The estimation of the mean curvature at the contact point p is transformed into the curvature voting of the vertices within q-rings' adjacent neighbourhood $Adj(p)$ shown in Figure 4 (where $Adj(p) = \{v \mid Dist(p,v) \le q\}$, $Dist(p,v)$ is the shortest path connecting point p with point v). All triangles within the neighborhood will vote to estimate the normal at the point, then the vertices within the same neighborhood will vote to estimate the curvature with the normal estimated. All voted normal N_i are collected through covariance matrix. The surface normal N_p at point p with surface patch saliency is evaluated as the corresponding eigenvector with the largest eigenvalue of matrix V_p. Each vertex $v_i \in Adj(p)$ has the curvature k_i, along the direction T_i with estimated normal N_p on point p,

$$k_i = \frac{\Delta \vartheta_i}{\Delta s_i}, \quad T_i = \frac{\vec{t_i}}{\|\vec{t_i}\|}, \quad \vec{t_i} = \overrightarrow{pv_i} - (N_p^t \overrightarrow{pv_i}) N_p \tag{7}$$

where $\Delta\vartheta_i$ is the change in the angle, and Δs_i is the shortest arc length fitting from v_i to p. And $\Delta\vartheta_i$ is obtained by the following,

$$\cos(\Delta\vartheta_i) = \frac{N_p^t \vec{n_i}}{\|\vec{n_i}\|} \quad \vec{n_i} = N_{vi} - (P_i^t N_{v_i}) P_i \quad P_i = N_p \times T_i \tag{8}$$

where N_{v_i} is the normal at vertex v_i, and $\vec{n_i}$ is its projection to the plane Π_v defined at point p with the normal N_p. Through collecting all voted curvatures, the discrete matrix $\tilde{M}_p$ in equation (6) is obtained. Thus two principle curvatures can be computed, and the sign of k_i is the same as the sign of $T_i^t \vec{n_i}$. The mean curvature radius $1/k_p$ is evaluated as the simulated radius in equation (2) at the contact area of the soft-tissue during virtual palpation.

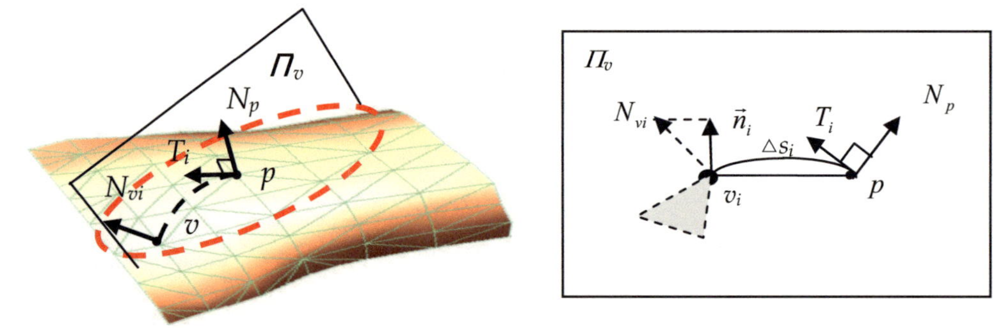

Fig. 4. Curvature voting from the vertices in neighborhood.

3.3 Soft tissue behavior simulation

The study of biomechanics shows that soft tissues are non-linear, time-dependent and history-dependent viscoelastic materials. It is difficult to precisely express the complex behavior of soft tissues in computer-generated organs. Here, human organs are simulated with viscoelastic behavior by volumetric tetrahedral mesh-spring systems with attention focused on small deformation restricted into a local area. It is convenient to extract multiple iso-surfaces among the different tissues. The tetrahedral element can support modeling of 3D organs with arbitrary shape.

The volumetric tetrahedral mass-spring system consists of mass points and connected springs along the edges. The Viogt rheological model is used to depict the time-dependent viscoelastic behavior of tissues. The linear springs obey the Hook's law, whereas the viscous dampers generate a resistance force proportional to the velocity. The dynamics of points are governed by the Newton's Second Law of motion. The nodal displacement of the ith point ($u_i \in R^3$) due to an external force F_i is given by the following,

$$m_i \ddot{u}_i + d_i \dot{u}_i + \sum_j \frac{\sigma_{ij}(|\vec{r}_{ij}| - l_{ij})}{|\vec{r}_{ij}|} \vec{r}_{ij} = F_i \tag{9}$$

where m_i is the mass of the point i, d_i is the damping constant of the same point, $\vec{r}_{ij}$ is the vector distance between point i and point j, l_{ij} is the rest length ,and σ_{ij} is the stiffness of the spring connecting two mass points. The right-hand term F_i is the sum of other external forces.

The motion equations for the entire system are assembled through concatenating the position vectors of the N individual mass points into a single $3N$-dimensional position vector U. Then the Lagrange's dynamics equation is satisfied,

$$M\ddot{U} + D\dot{U} + KU = F \tag{10}$$

where M, D and K are the $3N \times 3N$ mass, damping and stiffness matrices respectively. M and D are diagonal matrices and K is banded because it encodes spring forces which are functions of distances between neighboring mass points only. The vector F is a $3N$-dimensonal vector representing the total external forces acting on the mass control points. We can higly reduce the order of the dynamic computing by approximately fixing the vertices far from the acting forces.

In virtual palpations, the virtual index finger is modelled with a triangle mesh of 179 triangles, and the tested models are counted by the nodes and tetrahedrals (cube: 140/432; head: 456/1470; ligament: 601/1900; upper-leg: 728/2550). For dynamic finger-tissue collision detection, a ColDet 3D library is modified to detect multi contacts simultaneously. The working rate of this library is sufficient in considering the complexity of our experiments. The cost of force evaluation is mainly contributed by the curvature evaluation of the contacted tissues. Through restricting the deformation of the object within a local area, the refreshing rate of dynamic deformation during virtual palpation is fast. Our proposed dynamic tangible palpation model can guarantee a high refreshing rate of haptic interaction and meet the requirements of our visual update. Figure 5 illustrates the time-dependent viscoelastic mechanical properties of the simulated soft human tissues. In the left plot, the time step used is 0.01 to simulate the skin and the ligament tissues, and in the right plot, the time step used is 0.05 to simulate the muscle and a portion of the upper leg. The left part of the curve shows that the simulated creep is an increase in strain under constant stress; the right part of the curve shows that relaxation is a decrease in stress under constant strain. With higher elastic parameters in the simulated skin and ligament, the relaxation process is prolonged as it is more difficult to calm down to rest stage.

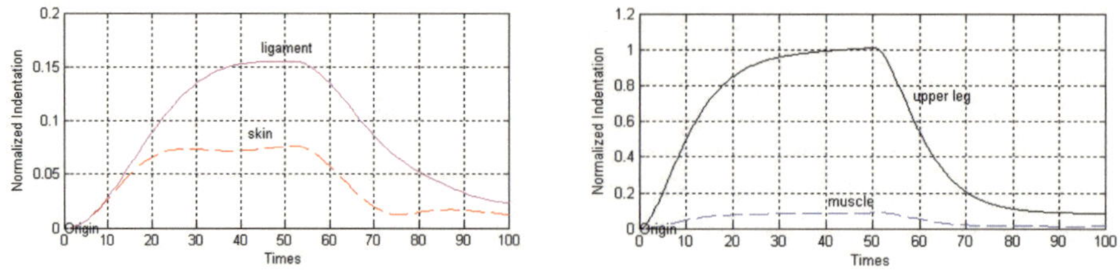

Fig. 5. Simulated soft-tissue palpation responses.

4. Multi-resolution Haptic Interactions

Developing a flexible multi-rsolution force evaluation scheme of tool-based haptic interactions within a complex virtual environment is of large demand. Compared with visual sense that has the largest bandwidth (Kokher, 1987), our sense of touch is spatially focused and has a far lower bandwidth. Thus, the rate at which information exchanged through touch is far less than that achieved through visual perception. Recent studies in haptic technologies provide more information channels that allow visual techniques to be augmented with haptic methods, giving an additional modality for visualization and active data exploration. Most haptic devices utilize point interactions, resulting in a conflict between the low information bandwidth and further complication of data exploration. Multi-resolution descriptions of hybrid models can provide a solution to the conflict between this low information bandwidth and the complexity of the virtual scene.

To effectively manage scene complexity, the recursive hierarchical descriptions are investigated with the ability to provide simplified drawable representations for groups of related subobjects. Shade et al. (Shade et al. ,1996) accelerated walkthroughs of complex environments with hierarchical image caching. Funkhouser and Sequin (Funkhouser & Sequin, 1993) noted that predictive level-of-detail selection could be used for active frame rate control. Mason and Blake (Mason & Blake, 1997) represented extensions of the predictive, but essentially non-hierarchical optimization approach to settle the optimization problem in hierarchical level-of-detail scene descriptions. Mason and Blake (Mason & Blake, 2001) further provided a graphical representation of the state spaces of hierarchical scene descriptions. Chen and Sun (Chen & Sun, 2004) established the body-based haptic interaction model in a unified multi-resolution framework.

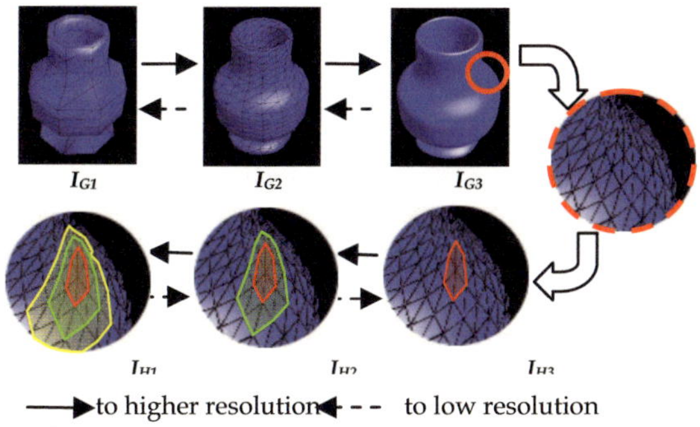

Fig. 6. Multi-resolution representations (graphics, haptics).

4.1 Multi-resolution tangible exploration

A detailed scene description of haptic interactions is complicated because it involves tracking continuously changing surfaces of the contacted objects being manipulated; evaluating the penetration depth that identifies the intersection volumes; resulting stress distribution in the materials. To simplify these complications, we employ the hierarchical description of hybrid models for both the visual display and haptic perception to balance the tangible-scene rendering requirements in interactive exploration.

Hierarchical Impostors

Hybrid virtual models, such as surfaces and volumes, are represented as multi-level information for both graphics display and haptic perception in our multi-resolution framework. Here, hierarchical imposters for graphics rendering and haptics perception have been constructed in advance, and selected to meet the real-time tangible-scene interactions. Hybrid objects in the virtual scene are rendered using different levels of graphics and haptics impostors. When the haptic input interacts and navigates the hybrid models, weight factors related with graphics impostors and haptics impostors are evaluated dynamically, to detect when and which of the objects should be traced up or down to a new level of displays. For instance, multi-resolution graphics imposters for triangle mesh surface data is obtained from Loop surfaces through subdivision (Sun et al., 2007), shown in upper rectangle pictures in Figure 6. Moreover, haptics imposters is derived from data model that represents the highest resolution, different curvature maps including mean curvature, Poisson's ratio and Young's modulus related with different parts or materials constructed with different adjacent neighborhood applied, shown in lower circle pictures in Figure 6.

The rendering of the interactive tangible scene is the optimal selection of graphics imposters and haptics imposters of the objects in the scene collectively. The pseudo code for controlling the force trigger logic with the haptic imposters is outlined in the following, thus the updated precision of tool-based haptic interface can lead to more or less detailed accuracy of interactive force perceptions.

```
HID := current displacement between haptic input and the object;
For each object that HID is in detecting area Do
Begin
   If HIP interacts with object Then
   Begin
         Evaluate the Force between HIP and object;
         If | Force | > Threshold_Fi Then
            Shift haptics impostor to a higher level;
            Load new haptic coefficients & parameters;
         Else
            Shift haptics impostor to a lower level;
            Load new haptic coefficients & parameters;
```

Tangible-scene interface

Haptic interactions in the virtual scene involve composing the hybrid objects, and exploring detailed graphics and haptics descriptive properties of the objects. Figure 7 is exampled system interface for hybrid tangible-scene exploration, during which two rendering servo loops, graphics and haptics, are involved. In the graphics rendering, object trees with selected graphics impostors are retrieved and taken into effect in each cycle. The cost for graphics display is the time for each cycle, which is reciprocal of graphics refreshing rate. In the haptics rendering, selected impostors are inserted into the haptic scene as touchable objects within the haptic-input influence range. Similar to graphics display, the cost of haptics is reciprocal of refreshing rate of the haptic system.

In our tangible-scene interface, the left side constructed a tree of control components, including virtual world, mouse control, display views, PHANToM haptic interaction, and navigation tools. Virtual world specifies the space and its center in the virtual scene. Mouse control traces the position and different actions (displacement, zoom, and rotate) related to each button. Display views setup the display attributes of the scene, including the display window, view point and direction, number of lights and location & property with each light. Haptic scene triggers the force feedback associated with the haptic interaction. PHANTOM specifies the coordinate of world, local movement and surface contacted point. Navigation tools specify the objects attached to the 6-DOF PHANToM input, which can be freely moved or rotated during the interactive haptic-scene navigation. Through the hybrid impostor hierarchy, different drawable representations and the haptic properties of virtual models such as stiffness, damping, and spring can be dynamically retrieved during the real-time haptic interactions.

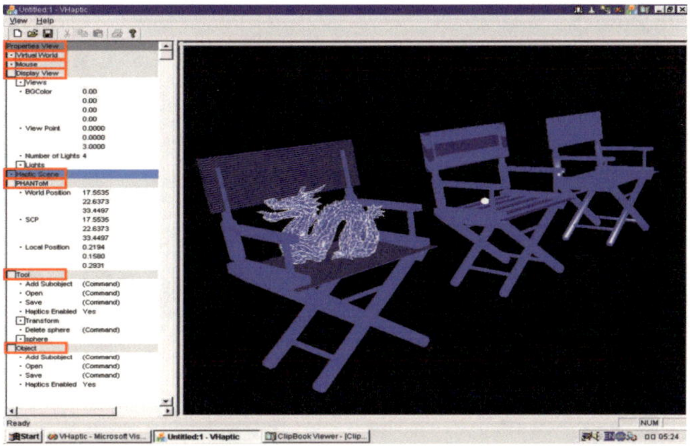

Fig. 7. Interactive haptic-tool interface.

4.2 Interactive scene evaluation

To convey the maximal perception qualities of the objects within the targeted tangible-scene cost, a heuristic value of each impostor computed in advance is defined as the benefit ratio of an object to its cost. The impostors of the objects are selected according to the descending order of their values until the targeted scene cost is met. If two impostors of the same object are both within the cost range, only one with the higher benefit is retained. When any selective update of impostor representations is triggered, the scene cost in graphics and haptics rendering is evaluated in order to meet the optimal performance and achieve the desired perception qualities of the haptic scene.

Two important scene criteria, cost and benefit of graphics and haptics impostors, have to be evaluated in interactive haptics exploration. The scene cost estimates time required to render the objects with different resolution in graphics/haptics processing, involving the coordinate transformations, collision detection, and evaluation of intersection point and normal. The upper limit of scene cost is reciprocal of rendering refreshing rate for graphics and haptics respectively. The benefit evaluates the contribution of impostors to model perception in the virtual environments. Ideally, it predicts the amount and accuracy of information conveyed to the user related with different rendering algorithm and object resolution. It is in general difficult to accurately model human perception and performance. In similarity, the size of perceptible area of an object after rendering is measured. Objects that appear larger to observer contribute more to vision, and the closer objects within the haptic-tool influence region contribute more touch-enabled details to haptics. An influenced area of the contacted force is computed as the constrained region to improve the working rate. During the haptic-scene interactions, our multi-resolution framework selects the imposters that are encapsulated for the optimal scene perfromance, acquiring both continuous graphics display and improved haptic perception qualities.

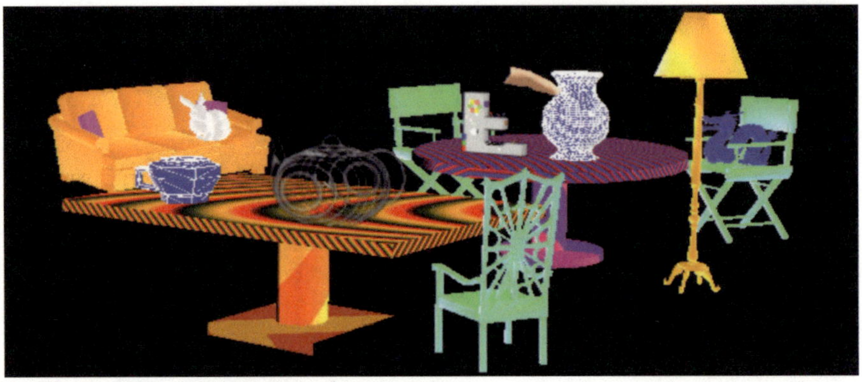

Fig. 8. Haptics-scene interactions and navigation.

The interactive haptic scene of hybrid models is constructed in Figure 8, with several surface datasets and volume objects placed on table, chair and sofa in the scene. During the haptic-tool interactions and navigation, different impostors of the hybrid objects are selected for the optimal graphics/haptics displays in real time. When haptic tool moves to and interacts with the kettle object, the most detailed kettle data on the table is exhibited in graphics and haptics rendering. The volume data of teapot in the middle of the table is shifted to a higher impostor level, within the influenced region of haptic input. Other objects such as F-shape and vase on the round table, dragon on the chair and bunny on the sofa remain in the same impostor representation, as far away from the haptic input. Figure 8 shows the impostor update of the hybrid tangible objects, while the haptic input passes teapot and interacts with vase on the round table within the influence region. The F-shape and vase in the scene go up to a higher impostor level, when closer to the moving haptic tool.

5. Conclusion

Most studies generally assumed that the contacts are point-based ones, and line/surface contacts are approximated by two or more point contacts. Based on the spring and damping linked to the dynamic haptic interface, the proper values for those dynamic parameters are not always easy to derive from measured material properties. Interactive rendering of complex virtual environments is important in scientific visualization and interactive scene navigation. Studies of haptic rendering of such complex-scene interaction for hybrid virtual models are scare. The focus of our work is to develop the novel body-based haptic interaction model that truly simulates the intrinsic physical properties of virtual objects interacting with the haptic tool. The contact forces are generated using our body-based force evaluation method based on Hert's contact theory. Physical properties of different object materials are computed to simulate the realistic touch perception between the body-based tools and interacting objects. We have applied the body-based interaction model in virtual palpation simulator, which is more suitable to enhance the touch sensation and exhibit the typical soft-tissue responsive behaviors. The non-linear viscoelastic behavior of human tissues is simulated via a volumetric tetrahedral mass-spring system, and high performance in computing is acquired by limiting the contact influence to reduce the order of dynamic systems. Further, we develop multi-resolution graphics/haptics rendering framework of tool-based haptic interactions and navigation in virtual environments. The hierarchical imposter representations of surface and volumetric models are constructed, and the optimal tangible-scene performance is evaluated at run-time to meet both the visual and haptic perceptual qualities.

In comparison with the other work studied haptic interaction in a special local area of the object (Asghar & Barner, 2001; Zhang et al., 2002), our proposed framework established a valuable attempt to integrate the multi-resolution haptic interactions and graphics rendering in complex virtual environments, providing more detailed perceptions (spatial and physical) guided by the sense of touch. Our future work will continue on investigating the constrained deformation of interested objects with the haptic interaction. We will work on more rigorous finite element model of soft-tissues behavior, and the interactive haptic interafce to effectively distinguish tissues by dynamic features, such as varying geometry shape, haptic textures, and touch-sensitive tenderness. The outmost of our goal is to incorporate more realistic haptic modes in tangible tasks, to realize more realistic real-world properties in the hybrid virtual environments.

6. References

Asghar, M. & Barner, K. (2001). Nonlinear multiresolution techni-ques with applications to scientific visualization in a haptic environment. *IEEE Transactions on Visualization and Computer Graphics*, Vol. 7, No. 1, page numbers (76–93), ISSN 1077-2626.

Barbagli, F.; Frisoli, A.; Salisbury, K. & Bergamasco M. (2004). Simulating human fingers: a Soft Finger Proxy Model and Algorithm, *In Proceedings of Haptic Interfaces for Virtual Environment and Teleoperator Systems (HAPTICS'04)*, pp. 9-17, ISBN 0-7695-2112-6, March 2004.

Basdogan, C.; Ho, C. & Srinivasan M.A. (2001). Virtual Environments for Medical Training: Graphical and Haptic Simulation of Laparoscopic Common Bile Duct Exploration. *IEEE transaction on mechatronics*, Vol. 6, No. 3, page numbers (269-285), ISSN 1083-4435.

Basdogan, C.; Rensselaer, S.; Kim, J.; Muniyandi, M.; Kim H. & Srinivasan M.A. (2004). Haptics in minimally invasive surgical simulation and training. *IEEE Computer Graphics and Applications*, Vol. 24, No. 2, page numbers (56- 64), ISSN 0272-1716.

Bielser, D.; Maiwald, V. A. & Gross M. H. (1999). Interactive Cuts through 3-Dimensional Soft Tissue. *Computer Graphics Forum (Eurographics '99)*, Vol. 18, No. 3, page numbers (31-38), ISSN 0167-7055.

Biesler, D. & Gross M. H. (2000). Interactive Simulation of Surgical Cuts, *Proceedings of Pacific Graphics*, pp. 116-125, Hong Kong, October 2000, IEEE Computer Society Press.

Bielser, D. & Gross M. H. (2002). Open surgery simulation. *Proc. of Medicine Meets Virtual Reality (MMVR 2002)*, pp. 57-62, Newport Beach, Ca, USA.

Chen, H. & Sun, H. (2004). Multi-resolution haptic interaction of hybrid virtual environments, *ACM Virtual Reality Software and Technology (VRST'2004)*, pp. 201-208, ISBN 1-58113-907-1, Hong Kong, China, November, 2004.

Chen, H. & Sun, H. (2006). Body-based haptic interaction model for touch-enabled virtual environments, *Presence: Teleoperators and Virtual Environments*, Vol. 15, No. 2, page numbers (186-203), ISSN 1054-7460.

Chen, H.; Wu, W.; Sun, H. & Heng. P.A. (2007). Dynamic Touch-enabled Virtual Palpation, *Journal of Computer Animation and Virtual Worlds*, Vol. 18, No. 4-5, page numbers (339-348), ISSN 1546-4261.

Colgate, J. E.; Stanley, M. C. & Brown, J. M. (1995). Issues in the haptic display of tool use. *1995 IEEE/RSJ International Conference on Intelligent Robots and Systems*, pp. 140-145, Pittsburgh, PA, ISBN 0-8186-7108-4, August, 1995.

El-Sana, J. & Varshney, A. (2000). Continuously-adaptive haptic rendering. *Virtual Environments 2000*, pp. 135-144.

Funkhouser, T. A. & Sequin, C. H. (1993). Adaptive display algorithm for interactive frame rates during visualization of complex virtual environments. *Proceedings of ACM Siggraph'93*, pp. 247–254, ISBN 0-201-58889-7.

Gregory, A.; Mascarenhas, A.; Ehmannl, S.; Lin, M. & Manocha, D. (2000). Six degree-of-freedom haptic display of polygonal models. *Proceedings of Visualization 2000*, pp. 139 -146, 549, ISBN 1-58113-309-X,Salt Lake City, Utah, USA, October, 2000.

Kim, Y.J.; Otaduy, M.A.; Lin, M.C. & Manocha, D. (2002). Six-degree-of-freedom haptic display using localized contact computations. *Proceedings of 10th Symposium on Haptic Interfaces for Virtual Environment and Teleoperator Systems (HAPTICS'02)*, pp. 209–216, ISBN 0-7695-1489-8, Orlando, FL, USA, 2002.

Kim, Y.J.; Otaduy, M.A.; Lin, M.C. & Manocha, D. (2003). Six-degree-of-freedom haptic display using incremental and localized computations. *Presence: Teleoperators and Virtual Environments*, Vol. 12, No. 3, page numbers (277-295), ISSN 1054-7460.

Kokher, K. J. (1987). The information capacity of the human fingertip. *IEEE transaction on Systems, Man, and Cybernetics*, Vol. 17, No. 1, page numbers (100–102), ISSN 0018-9472.

Landau, L. D. & Lifshitz, E. M. (1986). Theory of Elasticity. Vol.7 of Course of Theoretical Physics, page numbers (26-31), ISBN-13 978-0750626330, Pergamon Press.

Mason, A. & Blake, E. (1997). Automatic hierarchical level of detail optimization in computer animation. *Computer Graphics Forum*, Vol. 16, No. 3, page numbers (191–199), ISSN 0167-7055.

Mason, A. & Blake, E. (2001). A graphical representation of the state spaces of hierarchical level-of-detail scene descriptions. *IEEE Transactions on Visualization and Computer Graphics*, Vol. 7, No. 1, page numbers (70–75) , ISSN 1077-2626.

Otaduy, M. A. & Lin, M. C. (2003). Sensation preserving simplification for haptic rendering. *Proceedings of ACM Siggraph'03/ACM Transactions on Graphics*, Vol. 22, page numbers (543-553), ISSN 0730-0301.

Page, D. L.; Koschan, A.; Sun, Y.; Paik, J. & Abidi, M. (2001). Robust crease detection and curvature estimation of piecewise smooth surfaces from triangle mesh approximations using normal voting, *Proceedings of the International Conference on Computer Vision and Pattern Recognition*, Vol. I. pp. 162-167, Kauai, Hawaii.

Page, D.L.; Sun, Y.; Koschan, A.F.; Paik, J. & Abidi, M.A. (2002). Normal vector voting: crease detection and curvature estimation on large, noisy meshes. *Graphical Models*, Vol. 64, page numbers (199 – 229), ISSN 1524-0703.

Pawluk, D. & Howe, R. (1999a). Dynamic lumped element response of the human fingerpad. *Journal of Biomechanical Engineering*, Vol. 121, page numbers (178-183), ISSN 0148-0731.

Pawluk, D. & Howe, R. (1999b). Dynamic contact of the human fingerpad against a flat surface. *Journal of Biomechanical Engineering*, Vol. 121, page numbers (605-611) , ISSN 0148-0731.

Salisbury, K.; Conti, F. & Barbagli, F. (2004). Haptic rendering: introductory concepts. *IEEE Computer Graphics and Applications*, Vol. 24, No. 2, page numbers (24-32) , ISSN 0272-1716.

Shade, J.; Lischinski, D.; Salesin, D. H.; DeRose, T. & Snyder, J. (1996). Hierarchical image caching for accelerated walk-through of complete environments. *Proceedings of ACM Siggraph'96*, pp. 75–82, New Orleans, Louisiana, August, 1996.

Sun, H.; Wang, H.; Chen, H. & Qin, K.H. (2007). Touch-enabled Haptic Modeling of Deformable Multi-resolution Surfaces. *The Journal of Virtual Reality: Research, Development and Applications*, Vol. 11, page numbers (45-60), ISSN 1359-4338, Springer Verlag.

Taubin, G. (1995). Estimating the tensor of curvature of a surface from a polyhedral approximation. *Proceedings of the Fifth International Conference on Computer Vision*, pp. 902-907, ISBN 0-8186-7042-8, Cambridge, MA, USA, June 1995.

Zhang, J.; Payandeh, S. & Dill, J. (2002). Haptic subdivision: an approach to defining level-of-detail in haptic rendering. *Proceedings of 10th Symposium on Haptic Interfaces for Virtual Environment and Teleoperator Systems*, pp. 201–208, ISBN 0-7695-1489-8, Orlando, FL, USA, 2002.

33

Mapping Workspaces to Virtual Space in Work Using Heterogeneous Haptic Interface Devices

Ayano Tatematsu and Yutaka Ishibashi
Nagoya Institute of Technology
Japan

1. Introduction

In networked haptic environments, users can touch objects in a virtual space and feel the weight of the objects by manipulating haptic interface devices (Srinivasan & Basdogn, 1997). Thus, we can largely improve the efficiency of collaborative work such as remote surgery simulation and immerse ourselves in playing networked games.

On the other hand, a variety of haptic interface devices have been developed so far. The haptic interface devices have different specifications (e.g., the workspace size, position resolution, and exertable force) from each other. When we interconnect the devices over a network, the differences may cause some problems. There are a few papers addressing the problems (Hirose et al., 1998; Kameyama & Ishibashi, 2007; Fujimoto et al., 2008; Huang et al., 2008). In (Hirose et al., 1998), Hirose et al. develop basic software called Haptic Interface Platform (HIP), which does not depend on types of haptic interface devices. Then, they show that users do not notice meaningful differences in hardness in an experiment where the users recognize the hardness of an object although the users manipulate different types of haptic interface devices. In (Kameyama & Ishibashi, 2007), the authors clarify the influences of difference in workspace size between PHANToM Omni (Salisbury & Srinivasan, 1997) (just called Omni here) and PHANToM Desktop (Salisbury & Srinivasan, 1997) (called Desktop) for networked collaborative work and competitive work. They show that if the range of motion of a haptic interface device is not limited to a workspace which is smaller than the virtual space, there is no large influence of the difference on the efficiency of the collaborative work and the fairness of the competitive work. Otherwise, the efficiency of the collaborative work seriously deteriorates, and the fairness is damaged in the competitive work. In (Fujimoto et al., 2008), the authors handle collaborative work using Omni and SPIDAR-G AHS (Kim et al., 2003) (called SPIDAR). And they compare some methods of mapping workspaces to a virtual space. In (Huang et al., 2008), the authors treat collaborative work using Omni, Desktop, SPIDAR, and Falcon (Novint, 2007) when the size of a virtual space is small so that it is not necessary to map workspaces to the virtual space. However, the experiment with various haptic interface devices in the case where we need mapping (that is, the size of a virtual space is different from the size of each workspace) has not been performed.

In this chapter, we deal with collaborative work and competitive work using Omni, Desktop, SPIDAR, and Falcon. And we examine the influences of methods of mapping workspaces to a virtual space on the efficiency of the two types of work.
The rest of this chapter is organized as follows. Section 2 outlines the specifications of the haptic interface devices. Section 3 gives a brief description of the collaborative work and the competitive work. Section 4 explains system models of the two types of work. Section 5 describes methods of mapping. Section 6 explains the method of our experiment, and experimental results are presented in Section 7. Section 8 concludes the chapter.

2. Specifications of Haptic Interface Devices

When a user uses Omni or Desktop (see Figures 1(a) and (b)), the user manipulates the stylus of the device as if he/she had a pen. When he/she employs SPIDAR (see Figure 1(c)), he/she manipulates a globe (called the grip) hung with eight wires. In the case of Falcon (see Figure 1(d)), he/she manipulates a spherical grip connected with three arms. The workspace sizes of the devices are different from each other (see Table 1). In addition, the position resolution and exertable force of each device are different from those of the other devices.

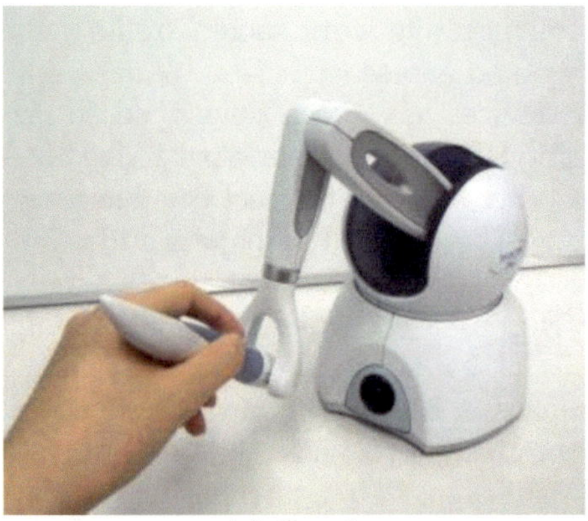

(a) Omni

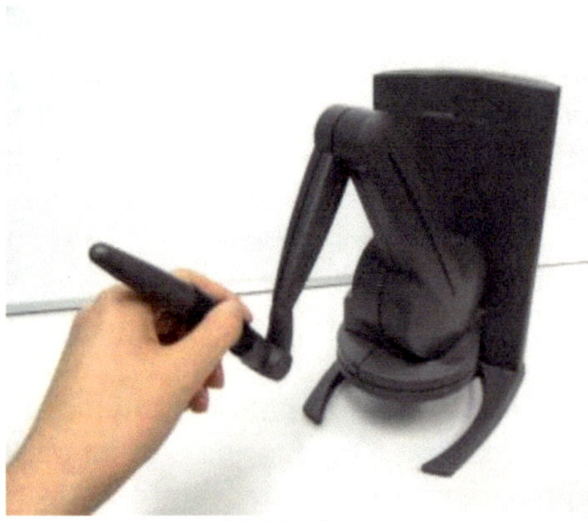

(b) Desktop

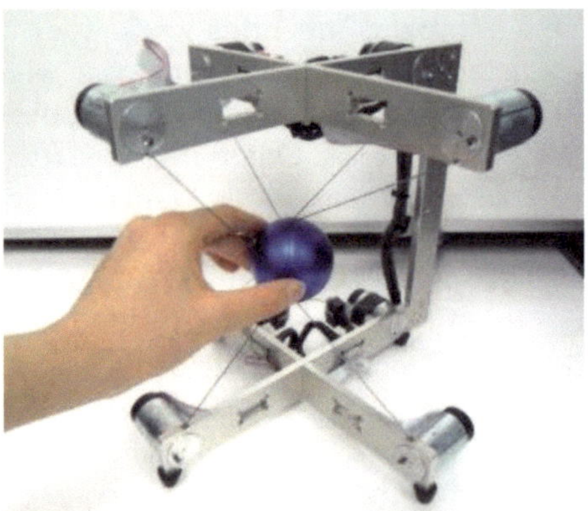

(c) SPIDAR

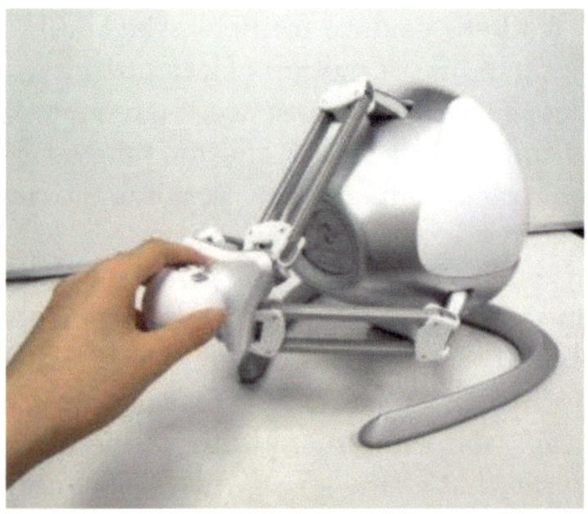

(d) Falcon

Fig. 1. Haptic interface devices

Device	Width [mm]	Height [mm]	Depth [mm]
Omni	160	120	70
Desktop	160	120	120
SPIDAR	200	120	200
Falcon	75	75	75

Table 1. Workspace sizes of haptic interface devices

3. Work Descriptions

We handle two types of work in which the difference in specifications excluding the workspace size among the four devices does not largely affect the efficiency of work.

3.1 Collaborative Work

Each of two users operates a haptic interface device, and the two users move a rigid cube (the length of each side is 30 mm, and the mass is 800 g) as an object collaboratively by holding the cube between the two cursors of the devices in a 3-D virtual space (width: 150 mm, height: 150 mm, depth: 140 mm. We will discuss the size of the virtual space in Section 5) surrounded by walls, a floor, and a ceiling (see Figure 2) (Fujimoto et al., 2008; Huang et al., 2008). The cursor of each haptic interface device moves in the virtual space when a user manipulates the stylus or grip of the device with his/her hand. The two users lift and move the cube collaboratively so that the cube contains a target (a sphere in Figure 2) which revolves along a circular orbit at a constant velocity. We do not carry out collision detection among the target, the orbit, and the cube or cursors.

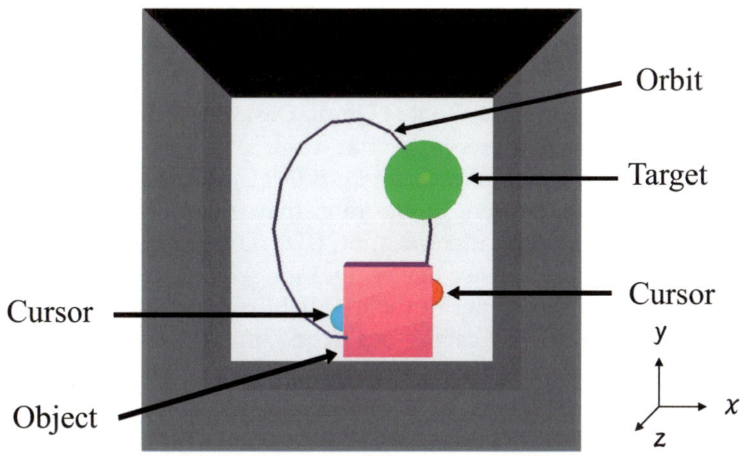

Fig. 2. Displayed image of virtual space in collaborative work

3.2 Competitive Work

Each of four players moves his/her object by lifting the object (the length of each side is 20 mm, and the mass is 750 g) from the bottom so that the object contains the target in a 3-D virtual space (width: 150 mm, height: 150 mm, depth: 140 mm. We will discuss the size of the virtual space in Section 5) as shown in Figure 3. If the distance between the center of the object and that of the target is less than 5 mm, we judge that the object contains the target.

When the target is contained by any of the four objects, it disappears and then appears at a randomly-selected position in the space. The four players compete on the number of eliminated targets with each other. The objects and target do not collide with each other, and the cursors do not collide with the target.

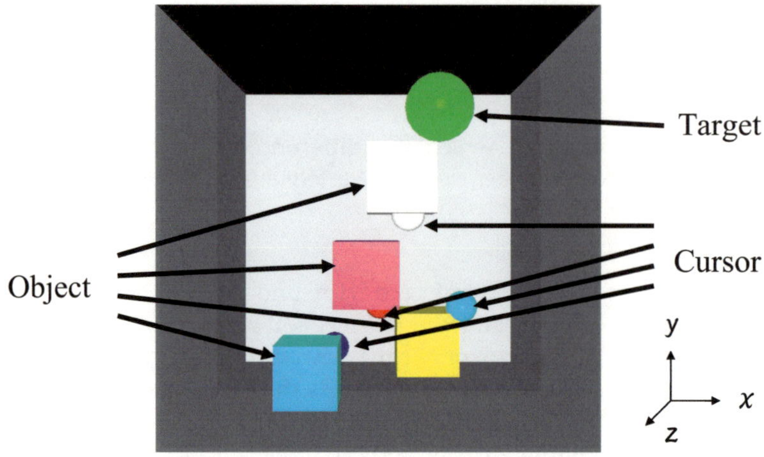

Fig. 3. Displayed image of virtual space in competitive work

4. System Models

4.1 Collaborative Work

A system model of the collaborative work is shown in Figure 4. The system model is based on a client-server model which consists of a single server and two clients (clients 1 and 2). As a haptic interface device, we employ Omni, Desktop, SPIDAR, or Falcon.

When the haptic interface device at a client is Omni, Desktop, or Falcon, the client performs haptic simulation by repeating the servo loop at a rate of 1 kHz (Novint, 2007; SensAble, 2004). And it inputs/outputs a stream of *media units* (*MUs*), each of which is the information unit for intra-stream synchronization, at the rate; that is, an MU is input/output every millisecond. Each MU contains the identification (ID) number of the client, the positional information of the cursor of the partner device, and the sequence number of the servo loop, which we use instead of the timestamp of the MU (Ishibashi et al., 2002). In the case where SPIDAR is used at a client, the client carries out haptic simulation at 1 kHz by using a timer and inputs/outputs a stream of MUs in the same way as that in the case where the other haptic interface devices are employed.

The server receives MUs from the two clients, and it calculates the position of the object based on the spring-damper model (SensAble, 2004). Then, it transmits the positional information of the object and cursor as an MU to the two clients.

When each client receives an MU, the client updates the position of the object after carrying out intra-stream synchronization control and calculates the reaction force applied to a user of the client. We employ Skipping (Ishibashi et al., 2002) for the intra-stream synchronization control at the clients. Skipping outputs MUs on receiving the MUs. When multiple MUs are received at the same time, however, only the latest MU is output and the others are discarded.

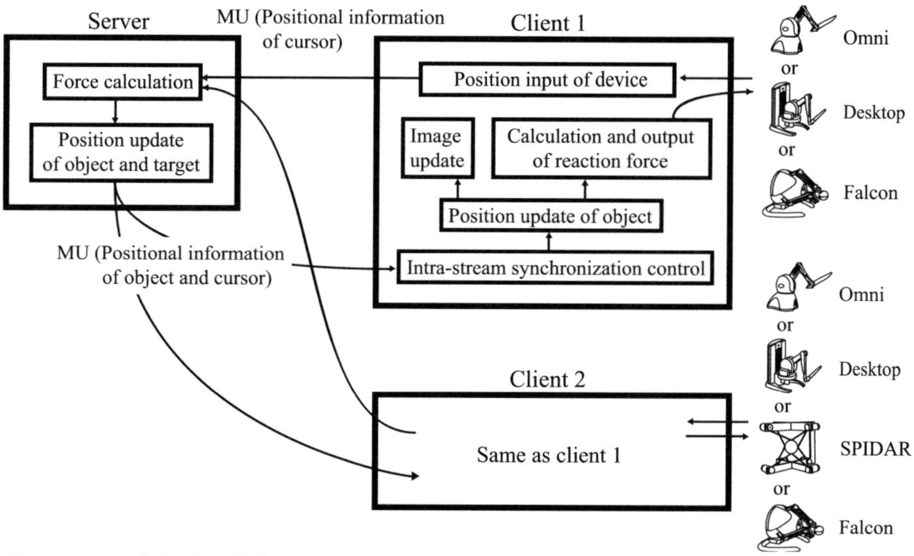

Fig. 4. System model of collaborative work

4.2 Competitive Work

Figure 5 shows a system model of the competitive work. The system model is similar to that of the collaborative work; that is, functions at the server and each client are almost the same as those of the collaborative work. The system model includes four clients (clients 1 through 4).

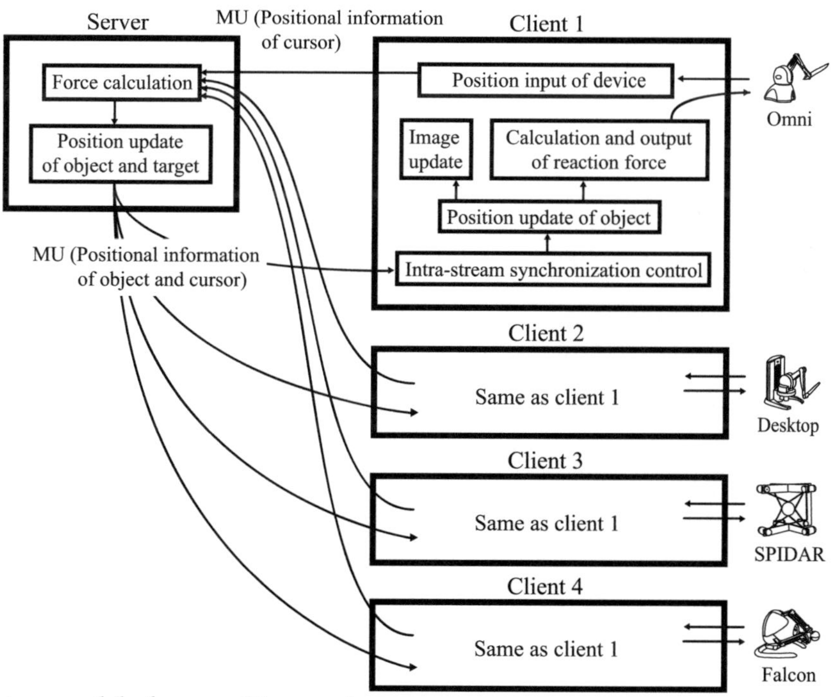

Fig. 5. System model of competitive work

5. Methods of Mapping

When the size of the virtual space is different from that of each workspace, there may exist domains that some of the haptic interface devices cannot reach in the virtual space. Therefore, it is necessary to map the workspace to the virtual space so that each device is able to work throughout the virtual space.

In this chapter, we deal with four cases in terms of the virtual space size. For explanation of the four cases, we define the *reference size* (width: 75.0 mm, height: 75.0 mm, depth: 70.0 mm) as the intersection of the four workspace sizes. In the first case, we set the virtual space size to half the reference size (width: 37.5 mm, height: 37.5 mm, depth: 35.0 mm). In the second case, the virtual space size is set to the reference size. In the third case, the virtual space size is set to one and a half times the reference size (width: 112.5 mm, height: 112.5 mm, depth: 105 mm). In the fourth case, the virtual space size is set to twice the reference size (width: 150 mm, height: 150 mm, depth: 140 mm). However, in the collaborative work, the first case is not treated since it was difficult to do the work due to the relation between the size of the object (see Section 3. The size of the object is constant independently of the size of the virtual space) and that of the virtual space.

This chapter handles the following two methods of mapping a workspace to the virtual space.

Method a: The workspace is uniformly mapped to the virtual space in the directions of the *x*-, *y*-, and *z*-axes (see Figure 6, which shows the shape of the workspace before and after mapping with Method a). In the case where the haptic interface device is Omni and the virtual space size is set to the reference size, for example, since the mapping ratio of the *z*-axis direction is one and the ratio is larger than those of the other axial directions, we also set the ratios of the other axial directions to one (see Tables 2, which show the mapping ratios in the two methods in the collaborative work in the case where the virtual space size is set to the reference size. We also show the mapping ratios in the collaborative work and competitive work in Tables 3 through 8).

Method b: The workspace is individually mapped to the virtual space in the direction of each axis so that the mapped workspace size corresponds to the virtual space size (see Figure 7, which shows the shape of the workspace before and after mapping with Method b).

In addition, we handled other two methods. In one method, the mapping ratio of each employed device is set to the largest mapping ratio among the employed devices in Method a. In the other method, mapping ratio of each employed device is set to the largest mapping ratio among the employed devices in Method b. However, experimental results of the two methods were worse than those of Method a.

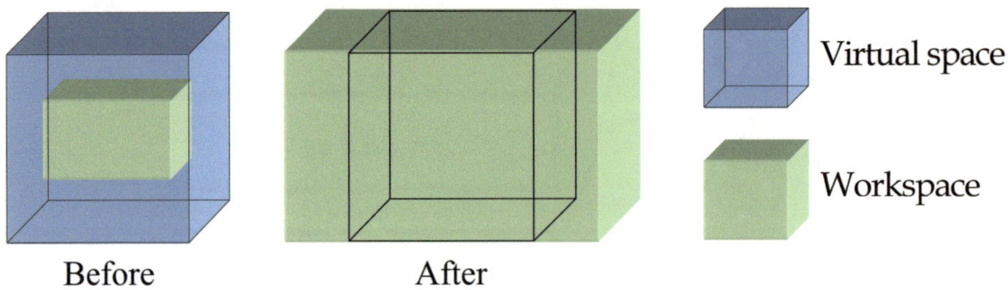

Fig. 6. Illustration of mapping with Method a

Method	Combination	Device	Ratio of x-axis	Ratio of y-axis	Ratio of z-axis
a	Omni-Omni	Omni	1.00	1.00	1.00
	Desktop-Desktop	Desktop	0.63	0.63	0.63
	Falcon-Falcon	Falcon	1.00	1.00	1.00
	Omni-Desktop	Omni	1.00	1.00	1.00
		Desktop	0.63	0.63	0.63
	Falcon-Omni	Falcon	1.00	1.00	1.00
		Omni	1.00	1.00	1.00
	Falcon-SPIDAR	Falcon	1.00	1.00	1.00
		SPIDAR	0.63	0.63	0.63
b	Omni-Omni	Omni	0.47	0.63	1.00
	Desktop-Desktop	Desktop	0.47	0.63	0.58
	Falcon-Falcon	Falcon	1.00	1.00	0.93
	Omni-Desktop	Omni	0.47	0.63	1.00
		Desktop	0.47	0.63	0.58
	Falcon-Omni	Falcon	1.00	1.00	0.93
		Omni	0.47	0.63	1.00
	Falcon-SPIDAR	Falcon	1.00	1.00	0.93
		SPIDAR	0.38	0.63	0.35

Table 2. Mapping ratios in two methods of mapping in collaborative work in case where virtual space size is set to reference size

Method	Combination	Device	Ratio of x-axis	Ratio of y-axis	Ratio of z-axis
a	Omni-Omni	Omni	1.50	1.50	1.50
	Desktop-Desktop	Desktop	0.94	0.94	0.94
	Falcon-Falcon	Falcon	1.50	1.50	1.50
	Omni-Desktop	Omni	1.50	1.50	1.50
		Desktop	0.94	0.94	0.94
	Falcon-Omni	Falcon	1.50	1.50	1.50
		Omni	1.50	1.50	1.50
	Falcon-SPIDAR	Falcon	1.50	1.50	1.50
		SPIDAR	0.94	0.94	0.94
b	Omni-Omni	Omni	0.70	0.94	1.50
	Desktop-Desktop	Desktop	0.70	0.94	0.88
	Falcon-Falcon	Falcon	1.50	1.50	1.40
	Omni-Desktop	Omni	0.70	0.94	1.50
		Desktop	0.70	0.94	0.88
	Falcon-Omni	Falcon	1.50	1.50	1.40
		Omni	0.70	0.94	1.50
	Falcon-SPIDAR	Falcon	1.50	1.50	1.40
		SPIDAR	0.56	0.94	0.53

Table 3. Mapping ratios in two methods of mapping in collaborative work in case where virtual space size is set to one and a half times reference size

Method	Combination	Device	Ratio of x-axis	Ratio of y-axis	Ratio of z-axis
a	Omni-Omni	Omni	2.00	2.00	2.00
	Desktop-Desktop	Desktop	1.25	1.25	1.25
	Falcon-Falcon	Falcon	2.00	2.00	2.00
	Omni-Desktop	Omni	2.00	2.00	2.00
		Desktop	1.25	1.25	1.25
	Falcon-Omni	Falcon	2.00	2.00	2.00
		Omni	2.00	2.00	2.00
	Falcon-SPIDAR	Falcon	2.00	2.00	2.00
		SPIDAR	1.25	1.25	1.25
b	Omni-Omni	Omni	0.94	1.25	2.00
	Desktop-Desktop	Desktop	0.94	1.25	1.17
	Falcon-Falcon	Falcon	2.00	2.00	1.87
	Omni-Desktop	Omni	0.94	1.25	2.00
		Desktop	0.94	1.25	1.17
	Falcon-Omni	Falcon	2.00	2.00	1.87
		Omni	0.94	1.25	2.00
	Falcon-SPIDAR	Falcon	2.00	2.00	1.87
		SPIDAR	0.75	1.25	0.70

Table 4. Mapping ratios in two methods of mapping in collaborative work

Method	Device	Ratio of x-axis	Ratio of y-axis	Ratio of z-axis
a	Omni	0.50	0.50	0.50
	Desktop	0.31	0.31	0.31
	SPIDAR	0.31	0.31	0.31
	Falcon	0.50	0.50	0.50
b	Omni	0.23	0.31	0.50
	Desktop	0.23	0.31	0.29
	SPIDAR	0.19	0.31	0.18
	Falcon	0.50	0.50	0.47

Table 5. Mapping ratios in two methods of mapping in competitive work in case where virtual space size is set to half reference size

Method	Device	Ratio of x-axis	Ratio of y-axis	Ratio of z-axis
a	Omni	1.00	1.00	1.00
	Desktop	0.63	0.63	0.63
	SPIDAR	0.63	0.63	0.63
	Falcon	1.00	1.00	1.00
b	Omni	0.47	0.63	1.00
	Desktop	0.47	0.63	0.58
	SPIDAR	0.38	0.63	0.35
	Falcon	1.00	1.00	0.93

Table 6. Mapping ratios in two methods of mapping in competitive work in case where virtual space size is set to reference size

Method	Device	Ratio of x-axis	Ratio of y-axis	Ratio of z-axis
a	Omni	1.50	1.50	1.50
	Desktop	0.94	0.94	0.94
	SPIDAR	0.94	0.94	0.94
	Falcon	1.50	1.50	1.50
b	Omni	0.70	0.94	1.50
	Desktop	0.70	0.94	0.88
	SPIDAR	0.56	0.94	0.53
	Falcon	1.50	1.50	1.40

Table 7. Mapping ratios in two methods of mapping in competitive work in case where virtual space size is set to one and a half times reference size

Method	Device	Ratio of x-axis	Ratio of y-axis	Ratio of z-axis
a	Omni	2.00	2.00	2.00
	Desktop	1.25	1.25	1.25
	SPIDAR	1.25	1.25	1.25
	Falcon	2.00	2.00	2.00
b	Omni	0.94	1.25	2.00
	Desktop	0.94	1.25	1.17
	SPIDAR	0.75	1.25	0.70
	Falcon	2.00	2.00	1.87

Table 8. Mapping ratios in two methods of mapping in competitive work in case where virtual space size is set to twice reference size

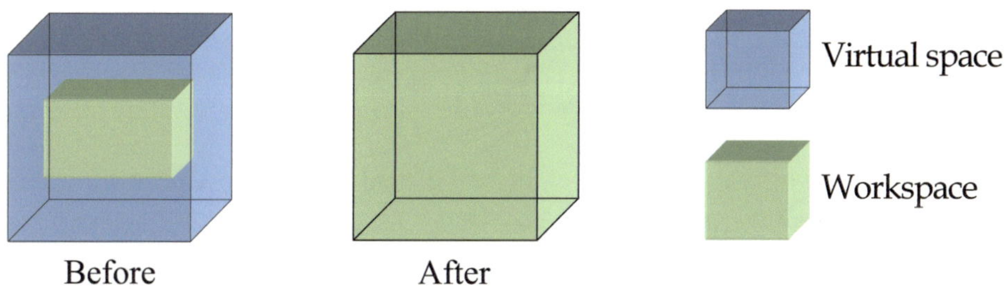

Fig. 7. Illustration of mapping with Method b

6. Method of Experiment

6.1 Experimental Systems

As shown in Figure 8, our experimental system in the collaborative work consists of a single server and two clients (clients 1 and 2). The server is connected to the two clients via an Ethernet switching hub (100 Mbps). In this chapter, we deal with the following six combinations as pairs of the devices: Omni-Omni, Desktop-Desktop, Falcon-Falcon, Omni-Desktop, Falcon-Omni, and Falcon-SPIDAR. These combinations are chosen from among pairs which have large differences in the efficiency of the work in (Huang et al., 2008).

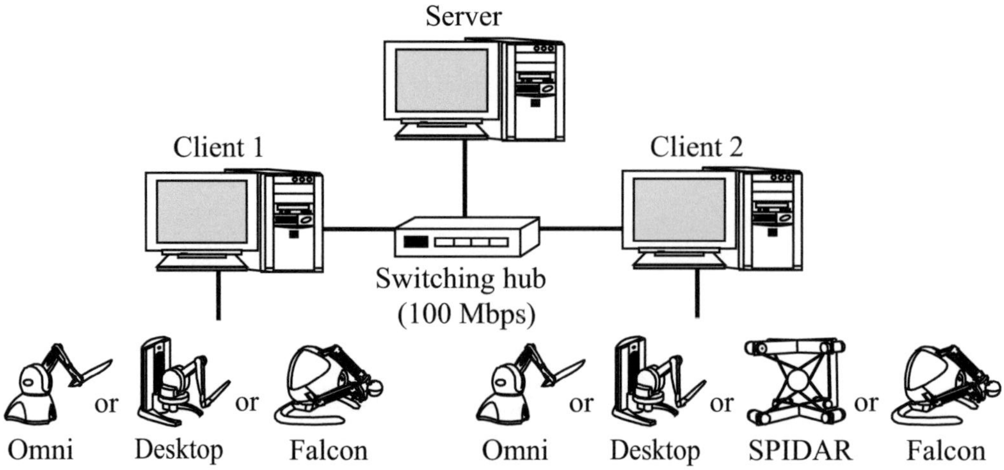

Fig. 8. Configuration of experimental system in collaborative work

Figure 9 shows our experimental system in the competitive work. The system consists of a single server and four clients (clients 1, 2, 3 and 4). The server is connected to the four clients via an Ethernet switching hub (100 Mbps). Clients 1 through 4 have Omni, Desktop, SPIDAR and Falcon, respectively.

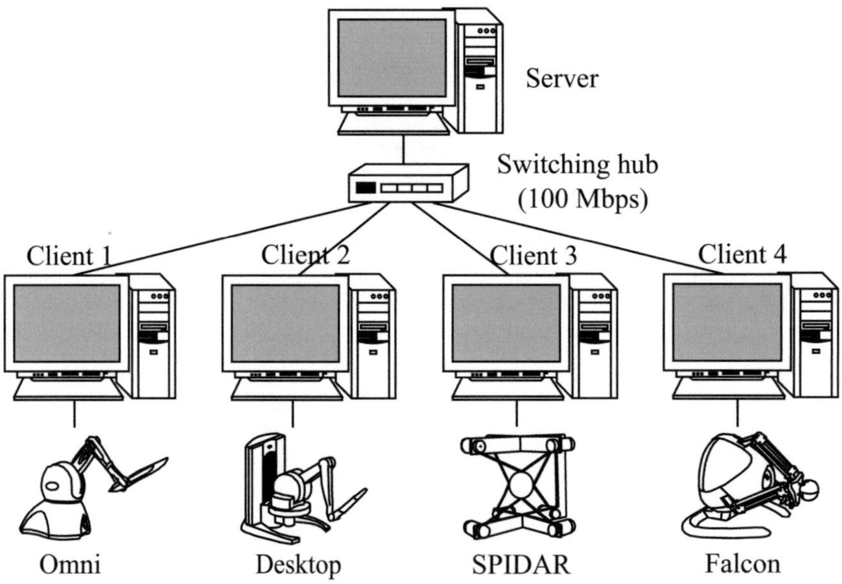

Fig. 9. Configuration of experimental system in competitive work

6.2 Performance Measure

As a performance measure, we employ the *average distance between cube and target* (Ishibashi et al., 2002) in the experiment on the collaborative work and the *average total number of eliminated targets* (Ishibashi & Kaneoka, 2006) in the experiment on the competitive work, which are QoS (Quality of Service) parameters. The average distance between cube and target is defined as the mean distance between the centers of them. This measure is related to the accuracy of the collaborative work. Small values of the average distance indicate that the cube follows the target precisely; this signifies that the efficiency of the work is high. The average total number of eliminated targets is closely related to the efficiency of the competitive work. Large values lead to high efficiency of the work.

In the collaborative work, two users operated haptic interface devices at clients 1 and 2. The experiment for each method was carried out 40 times. When the users operated different devices from each other, they exchanged the devices, and the experiment was done again. In the competitive work, four users operated devices at clients 1, 2, 3 and 4. The experiment for each method was also carried out 40 times. The users exchanged the devices every 10 times so that each user employed every device. The measurement time of each experimental run was 30 seconds in the two types of work.

7. Experimental Results

7.1 Collaborative Work

We show the average distance between cube and target for the two methods in Figures 10 through 12, where the virtual space size is set to the reference size, one and a half times the reference size, and twice the reference size, respectively. In the figures, we also display the 95 % confidence intervals.

In Figures 10 through 12, we see that as the size of the virtual space becomes larger, the average distance increases. From this, we can say that the larger the size of the virtual space, the more difficult the work.

From Figures 10 through 12, we also find that the average distance of Method a is smaller than that of Method b in all the combinations. The reason is as follows. In Method b, the movement distances of the cursor in the directions of the three axes are different from each other in the virtual space even if the movement distances of the stylus or grip in the directions of the three axes are the same in the workspace. Thus, the work with Method b is more difficult than that with Method a. In the case of Falcon-Falcon, the average distance of Method a is approximately equal to that of Method b. This is because the shape of the workspace of Falcon resembles that of the virtual space (the width, height, and depth of the workspace of Falcon are 75 mm, and those of the virtual space are 75 mm, 75 mm, and 70 mm, respectively, in the case where the virtual space size is set to the reference size).

From the above observations, we can conclude that Method a is more effective than Method b in the collaborative work.

7.2 Competitive Work

We show the average total number of eliminated targets for the two methods in Figures 13 through 16, where the virtual space size is set to half the reference size, the reference size, one and a half times the reference size, and twice the reference size, respectively. In the figures, we also display the 95 % confidence intervals.

In Figures 13 through 16, we see that as the size of the virtual space becomes larger, the average total number of eliminated targets decreases. From this, we can say that the larger the size of the virtual space, the more difficult the work.

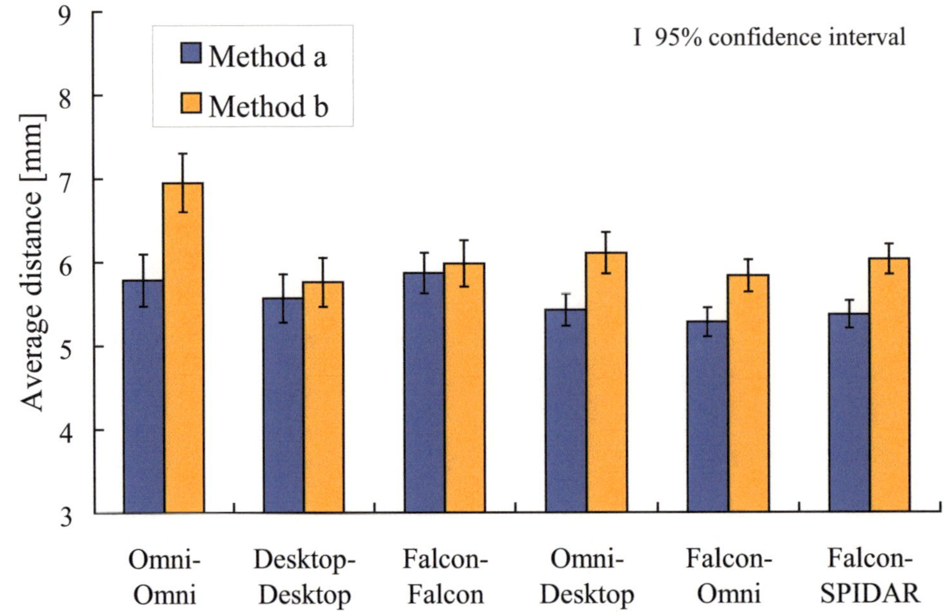

Fig. 10. Average distance between cube and target in case where virtual space size is set to reference size

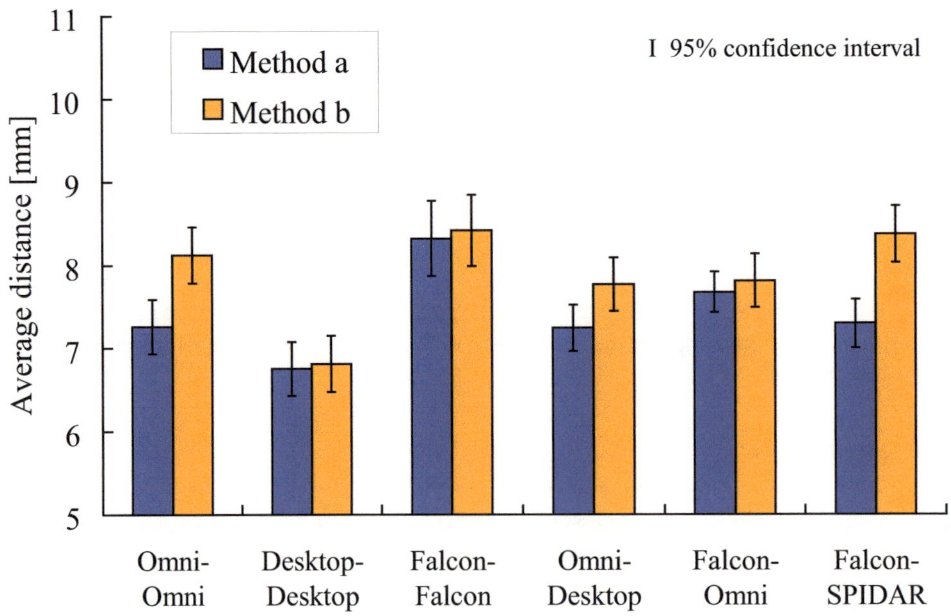

Fig. 11. Average distance between cube and target in case where virtual space size is set to one and a half times reference size

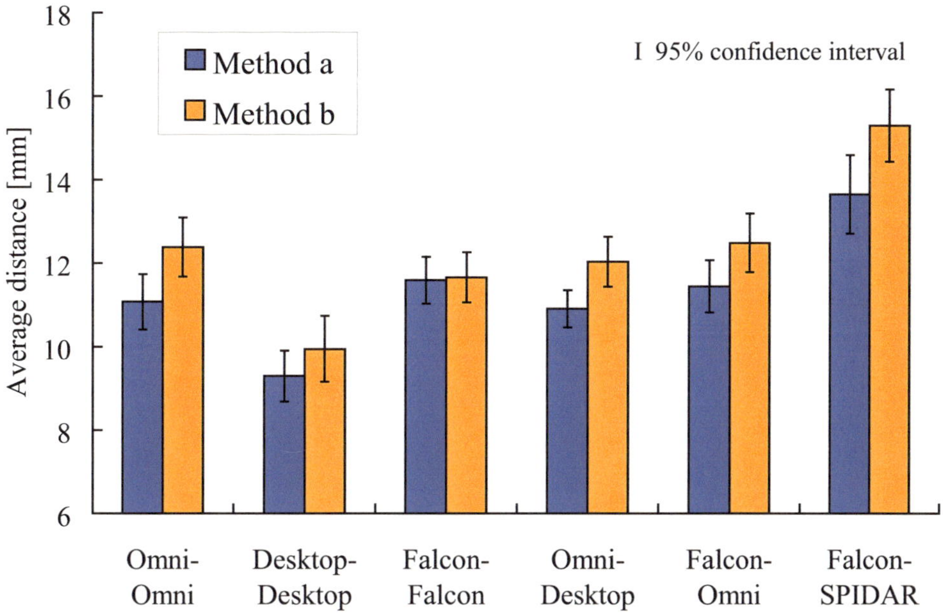

Fig. 12. Average distance between cube and target in case where virtual space size is set to twice reference size

From Figures 13, 14, and 16, we find that the average total number of eliminated targets of Method a is larger than that of Method b. The reason is similar to that in the case of the collaborative work. In Figure 15, the average total number of eliminated targets of Method b is somewhat larger than that of Method a. To clarify the reason, we examined the average number of eliminated targets at each haptic interface devices. As a result, the average number of eliminated targets of Omni with Method b was larger than that with Method a. This is because in the case of Omni, the mapping ratio of the x-axis with Method a is much larger than that with Method b owing to the shape of the workspace of Omni; therefore, it is easy to drop the cube in Method a.

From the above observations, we can roughly conclude that Method a is more effective than Method b in the competitive work.

8. Conclusion

This chapter dealt with collaborative work and competitive work using four kinds of haptic interface devices (Omni, Desktop, SPIDAR, and Falcon) when the size of a virtual space is different from the size of each workspace. We examined the influences of methods of mapping workspaces to the virtual space on the efficiency of work. As a result, we found that the efficiency of work is higher in the case where the workspace is uniformly mapped to the virtual space in the directions of the x-, y-, and z-axes than in the case where the workspace is individually mapped to the virtual space in the direction of each axis so that the mapped workspace size corresponds to the virtual space size.

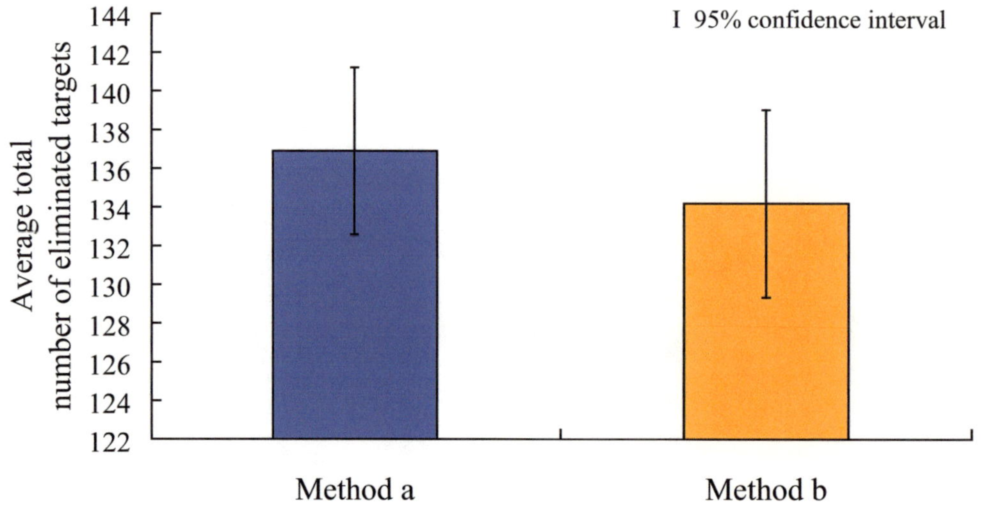

Fig. 13. Average total number of eliminated targets in case where virtual space size is set to half reference size

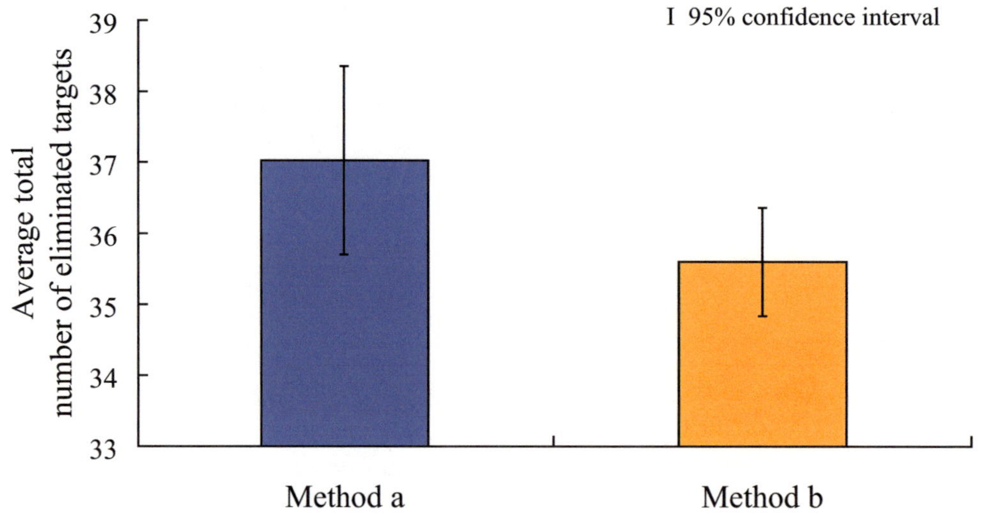

Fig. 14. Average total number of eliminated targets in case where virtual space size is set to reference size

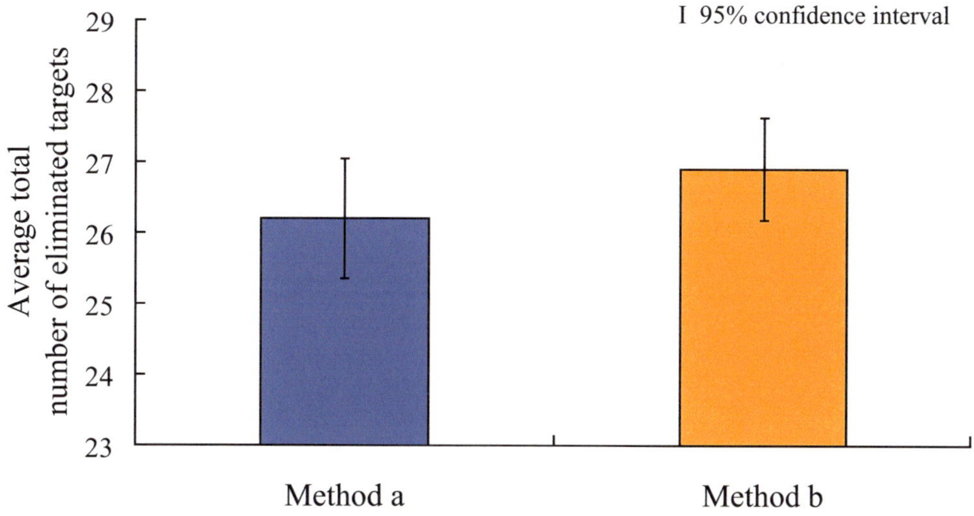

Fig. 15. Average total number of eliminated targets in case where virtual space size is set to one and a half times reference size

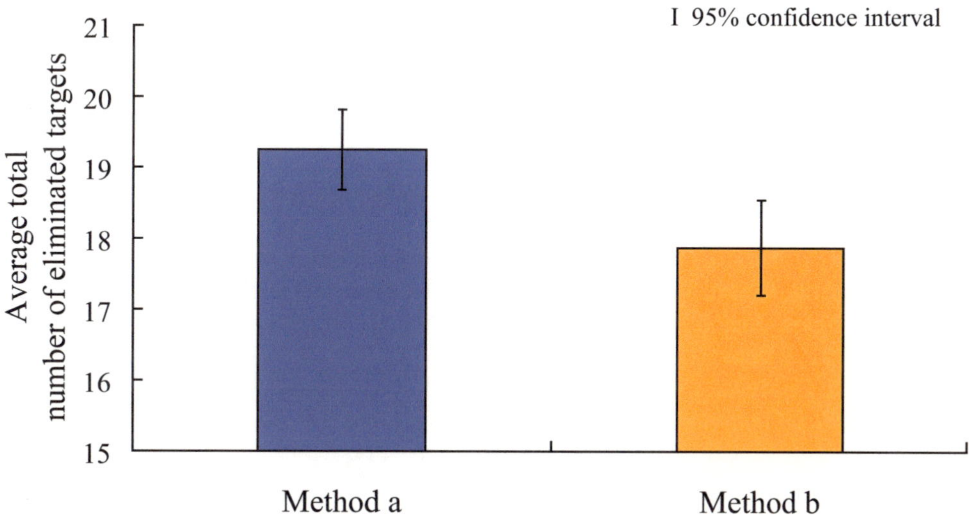

Fig. 16. Average total number of eliminated targets in case where virtual space size is set to twice reference size

As the next step of our research, we will handle other types of work and investigate the influences of network latency and packet loss.

Acknowledgments

The authors thank Prof. Shinji Sugawara and Prof. Norishige Fukushima of Nagoya Institute of Technology for their valuable comments.

9. References

Fujimoto, T.; Huang, P.; Ishibashi, Y. & Sugawara, S. (2008). Interconnection between different types of haptic interface devices: Absorption of difference in workspace size, *Proceedings of the 18th International Conference on Artificial Reality and Telexistence (ICAT'08)*, pp. 319-322

Hirose, M.; Iwata, H.; Ikei, Y.; Ogi, T.; Hirota, K.; Yano, H. & Kakehi, N. (1998). Development of haptic interface platform (HIP) (in Japanese). *TVRSJ*, Vol. 10, No. 3, pp. 111-119

Huang, P.; Fujimoto, T.; Ishibashi, Y. & Sugawara, S. (2008). Collaborative work between heterogeneous haptic interface devices: Influence of network latency, *Proceedings of the 18th International Conference on Artificial Reality and Telexistence (ICAT'08)*, pp. 293-296

Ishibashi, Y. & Kaneoka, H. (2006). Group synchronization for haptic media in a networked real-time game. *IEICE Trans. Commun., Special Section on Multimedia QoS Evaluation and Management Technologies*, Vol. E89-B, No. 2, pp. 313-319

Ishibashi, Y.; Tasaka, S. & Hasegawa, T. (2002). The virtual-time rendering algorithm for haptic media synchronization in networked virtual environments, *Proceedings of the 16th International Workshop on Communication Quality & Reliability (CQR'02)*, pp. 213-217

Kameyama, S. & Ishibashi, Y. (2007). Influences of difference in workspace size between haptic interface devices on networked collaborative and competitive work, *Proceedings of SPIE Optics East, Multimedia Systems and Applications X*, Vol. 6777, No. 30

Kim, S.; Berkley, J. J. & Sato, M. (2003). A novel seven degree of freedom haptic device for engineering design. *Virtual Reality*, Vol. 6, No. 4, pp. 217-228

Novint Technologies, Inc. (2007). Haptic Device Abstraction Layer programmer's guide, Version 1.1.9 Beta

Salisbury, J. K. & Srinivasan, M. A. (1997). Phantom-based haptic interaction with virtual object. *IEEE Computer Graphics and Applications*, Vol. 17, No. 5, pp. 6-10

SensAble Technologies, Inc. (2004). 3D Touch SDK OpenHaptics Toolkit programmer's guide, Version 1.0

Srinivasan, M. A. & Basdogn, C. (1997). Haptics in virtual environments: Taxonomy, research status, and challenges. *Computers and Graphics*, Vol. 21, No. 4, pp. 393-404

Collaborative Tele-Haptic Application and Its Experiments

Qonita M. Shahab, Maria N. Mayangsari and Yong-Moo Kwon
Korea Institute of Science & Technology, Korea

1. Introduction

Through haptic devices, users can feel partner's force each other in collaborative applications. The sharing of touch sensation makes network collaborations more efficiently achievable tasks compared to the applications in which only audiovisual information is used. In view of collaboration support, the haptic modality can provide very useful information to collaborators.

This chapter introduces collaborative manipulation of shared object through network. This system is designed for supporting collaborative interaction in virtual environment, so that people in different places can work on one object together concurrently through the network. Here, the haptic device is used for force-feedback to each user during the collaborative manipulation of shared object. Moreover, the object manipulation is occurred in physics-based virtual environment so the physics laws influence our collaborative manipulation algorithm. As a game-like application, users construct a virtual dollhouse together using virtual building blocks in virtual environment. While users move one shared-object (building block) to desired direction together, the haptic devices are used for applying each user's force and direction. The basic collaboration algorithm on shared object and its system implementation are described. The performance evaluations of the implemented system are provided under several conditions. The system performance comparison with the case of non-haptic device collaboration shows the effect of haptic device on collaborative object manipulation.

2. Collaborative manipulation of shared object

2.1 Overview

In recent years, there is an increasing use of Virtual Reality (VR) technology for the purpose of immersing human into Virtual Environment (VE). These are followed by the development of supporting hardware and software tools such as display and interaction hardware, physics-simulation library, for the sake of more realistic experience using more comfortable hardware.

Our focus of study is on real-time manipulating object by multiple users in Collaborative Virtual Environment (CVE). The object manipulation is occurred in physic-based virtual environment so the physic laws implemented in this environment influence our manipulation algorithm.

We build Virtual Dollhouse as our simulation application where user will construct a dollhouse together. In this dollhouse, collaborative users can also observe physics law while constructing a dollhouse together using existing building blocks, under gravity effects. While users collaborate to move one shared-object (block) to desired direction, the shared-object is manipulated, for example using velocity calculation. This calculation is used because current available physic-law library has not been provided for collaboration. The main problem that we address is how to manipulate **a** same object by two users and more, which means how we combine two or more attributes of each user to get one destination. We call this approach as shared-object manipulation approach.

This section presents the approach we use in study about the collaborative interaction in virtual environment so people in different places can work on one object together concurrently.

2.2 Related Work

In Collaborative Virtual Environment (CVE), multiple users can work together by interacting with the virtual objects in the VE. Several researches have been done on collaboration interaction techniques between users in CVE. (Margery, D., Arnaldi, B., Plouzeau, N. 1999) defined three levels of collaboration cases. Collaboration level 1 is where users can feel each other's presence in the VE, e.g. by representation of avatars such as performed by NICE Project (Johnson, A., Roussos, M., Leigh, J. 1998). Collaboration level 2 is where users can manipulate scene constraints individually. Collaboration level 3 is where users manipulate the same object together. Another classification of collaboration is by Wolff et al. (Wolff, R., Roberts, D.J., Otto, O. June 2004) where they divided collaboration on a same object into sequential and concurrent manipulations. The concurrent manipulation consists of manipulation of distinct and same object's attributes.

Collaboration on the same object has been focused by other research (Ruddle, R.A., Savage, J.C.D., Jones, D.M. Dec. 2002), where collaboration tasks are classified into symmetric and asymmetric manipulation of objects. Asymmetric manipulation is where users manipulate a virtual object by substantially different actions, while symmetric manipulation is where users should manipulate in exactly the same way for the object to react or move.

2.3 Our Research Issues

In this research, we built an application called Virtual Dollhouse. In Virtual Dollhouse, collaboration cases are identified as two types: 1) combined inputs handling or same attribute manipulation, and 2) independent inputs handling or distinct attribute manipulation. For the first case, we use a symmetric manipulation model where the option is using common component of users' actions in order to produce the object's reactions or movements. According to Wolff et al. (Wolff, R., Roberts, D.J., Otto, O. June 2004) where events traffic during object manipulations is studied, the manipulation on the same object's attribute generated the most events. Thus, we can focus our study on manipulation on the same object's attribute or manipulation where object's reaction depends on combined inputs from the collaborating users.

We address two research issues while studying manipulation on the same object's attribute. Based on the research by Basdogan et al. (Basdogan, C., Ho, C., Srinivasan, M.A., Slater, M. Dec. 2000), we address the first issue in our research: the effects of using haptics on a collaborative interaction. Based on the research by Roberts et al. (Roberts, D., Wolff, R., Otto, O. 2005), we address the second issue in our research: the possibilities of collaboration between users from different environments.

To address the first issue, we tested the Virtual Dollhouse application of different versions: without haptics functionality and with haptics functionality, to be compared. As suggested by Kim et al. (Kim, J., Kim, H., Tay, B.K., Muniyandi, M., Srinivasan, M.A., Jordan, J., Mortensen, J., Oliveira, M., Slater, M. 2004), we also test this comparison over the Internet, not just over LAN. To address the second issue, we test the Virtual Dollhouse application between user of non-immersive display and immersive display environments. We analyze the usefulness of immersive display environment as suggested by Otto et al. (Otto, O., Roberts, D., Wolff, R. June 2006), as they said that it holds the key for effective remote collaboration.

2.4 Taxonomy of Collaboration

The taxonomy, as shown in Figure 1, starts with a category of objects: manipulation of distinct objects and a same object. In many CVE applications (Johnson, A., Roussos, M., Leigh, J. 1998), users collaborate by manipulating the distinct objects. For manipulating the same object, sequential manipulation also exists in many CVE applications. For example, in a CVE scene, each user moves one object, and then they take turn in moving the other objects.

Concurrent manipulation of objects has been demonstrated in related work (Wolff, R., Roberts, D.J., Otto, O. June 2004) by moving a heavy object together. In concurrent manipulation of objects, users can manipulate in category of attributes: same attribute or distinct attributes.

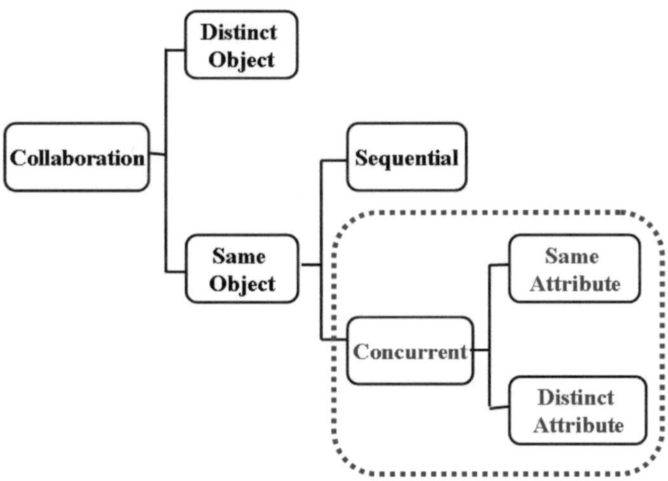

Fig. 1. Taxonomy of collaboration

2.5 Demo Scenario-Virtual Dollhouse

We construct Virtual Dollhouse application in order to demonstrate concurrent object manipulation. Concurrent manipulation is when more than one user wants to manipulate the object together, e.g. lifting a block together. The users are presented with several building blocks, a hammer, and several nails. In this application, two users have to work together to build a doll house.

The scenario for the first collaboration case is when two users want to move a building block together, so that both of them need to manipulate the "position" attribute of the block, as seen in Figure 2(a). We call this case as SOSA (Same Object Same Attribute). The scenario for the second collaboration case is when one user is holding a building block (keep the "position" attribute to be constant) and the other is fixing the block to another block (set the "set fixed" or "release from gravity" attribute to be true), as seen in Figure 2(b). We call this case as SODA (Same Object Different Attribute).

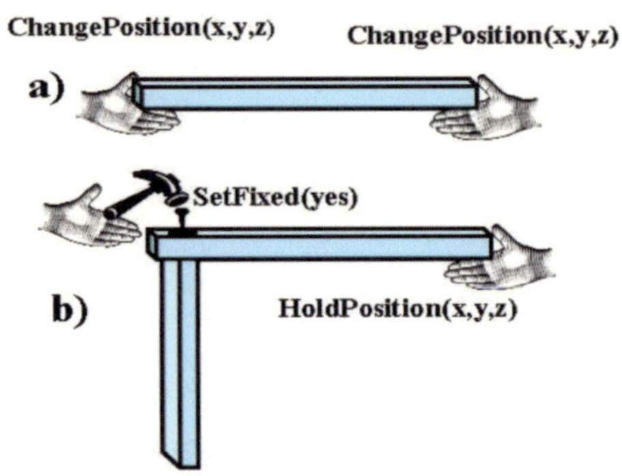

Fig. 2. (a) Same attribute, (b) Distinct attributes in Same Object manipulation

Figure 3 shows the demo content implementation of SOSA and SODA with blocks, hands, nail and hammer models.

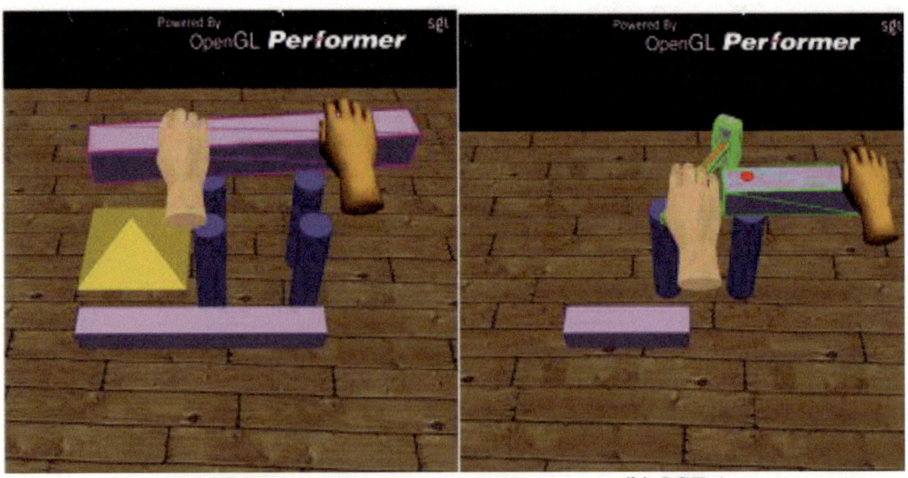

(a) SOSA (b) SODA

Fig. 3. Demo content implementation

2.6 Problem and Solution

Even though physics-simulation library has been provided, there is no library that can handle physical collaboration. For example, we need to calculate the force of object that pushed by two hands.

In our Virtual Dollhouse, user will try to lift the block and another user will also try to lift the same block and move it together to destination.

After the object reaches shared-selected or "shared-grabbed" status, the input values from two hands should be managed for the purpose of object manipulation. We created a vHand variable as a value of fixed distance between the grabbing hand and the object itself. This is useful for moving the object by following the hand's movement.

We encountered a problem of two hands that may have the same power from each of its user. For example, a user wants to move to the left, and the other wants to move to the right. Without specific management, the object manipulation may not be successful. Therefore, we decided that users can make an agreement prior to the collaboration, in order to configure (in XML), which user has the stronger hand (handPow) than the other. Therefore, the arbitration of two input values is as following (for x-coordinate movement case):

Diff = (handPos1-vHand1) - (handPos2-vHand2)

If abs(handPow2) > abs(handPow1)

Hand1.setPos(hand1.x-diff,hand1.y,hand1.z)

Else if abs(handPow1) > abs(handPow2)

Hand1.setPos(hand2.x+diff,hand2.y,hand2.z)

After managing the two hand inputs, the result of the input processing is released as the manipulation result.

Our application supports 6DOF (Degree Of Freedom) movement: X-Y-Z and Heading-Pitch-Roll, but due to capability of our input device, we did not consider Pitch and Roll as necessary to be implemented graphically.

X-Y-Z = (handPos1-vHand1 + handPos2-vHand2)/2

In Figure 4, the angle is the heading rotation (between X and Y coordinates). The tangent is calculated so that the angle in degree can be found.

tanA = (hand0.y-hand1.y)/(hand0.x-hand1.x)

heading = atan(tanA)*180/PI

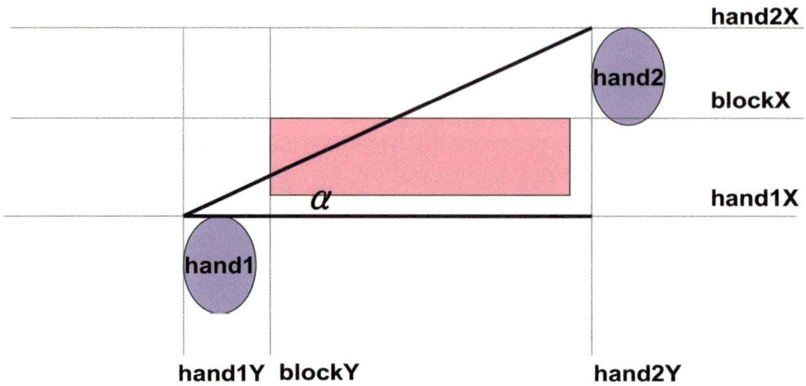

Fig. 4. Orientation of object based on hands positions

The final result of manipulation by two hands can be summarized by the new position and rotation as follows:

Object.setPos(X-Y-Z)

Object.setRot(initOri.x+heading, initOri.y, initOri.z)

Based on two user manipulation, three users manipulation can be calculated easily following the same algorithm. We have to choose which two hands against the other one hand (see Figure 5) based on hand velocity checking.

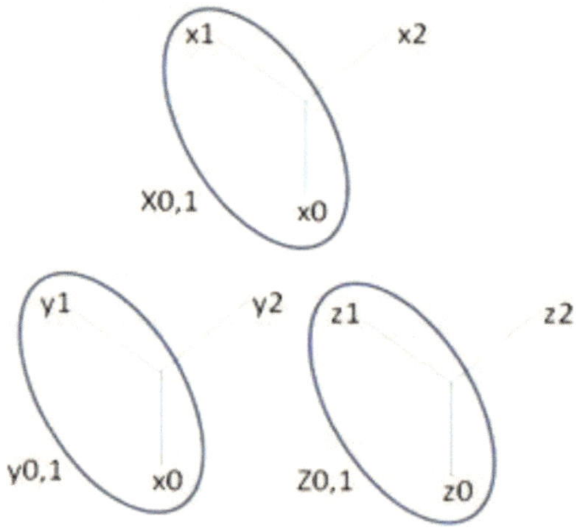

Fig. 5. Example of three users manipulation, Hand 0 and Hand 1 against Hand 2

After calculation, manipulation that made when three hands want to move an object together can be found below.

For each x, y, and z direction, check:

If abs(vel_hand0) >= abs(vel_hand1 + vel_hand 2)

Hand1 and hand2 follow hand0

Else if abs(vel_hand1) >= abs(vel_hand0 + vel_hand 2)

Hand0 and hand2 follow hand1

Else if abs(vel_hand2) >= abs(vel_hand0 + vel_hand 1)

Hand0 and hand1 follow hand2

2.7 Design of Implementation

(1) Virtual Dollhouse

We have built Virtual Dollhouse as our CVE. Our Virtual Dollhouse application is made based on OpenGL Performer (Silicon Graphics Inc. 2005) and programmed in C/C++ language in Microsoft Windows environment. VRPN server (Taylor, R. M., Hudson, T. C., Seeger, A., Weber, H., Juliano, J., Helser, A.T. 2001) is used to provide management of networked joysticks to work with the VR application. We use NAVER Library (Park, C., Ko, H.D., Kim, T. 2003), a middleware used for managing several VR tasks such as device and network connections, events management, specific modeling, shared state management, etc.
The physics engine in our implementation is an adaptation of AGEIA PhysX SDK (AGEIA: AGEIA PhysX SDK) to work with SGI OpenGL Performer's space and coordinate systems. This physics engine has a shared-state management so that two or more collaborating computers can have identical physics simulation states. Using this physics engine, object's velocity during interaction can be captured to be sent as force-feedbacks to the hands that are grabbing the objects.
The architecture of our implementation can be seen in Figure 7.

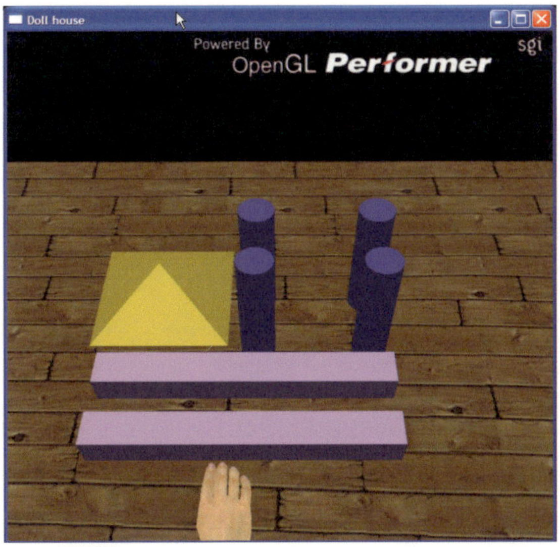

Fig. 6. Virtual Dollhouse as VCE

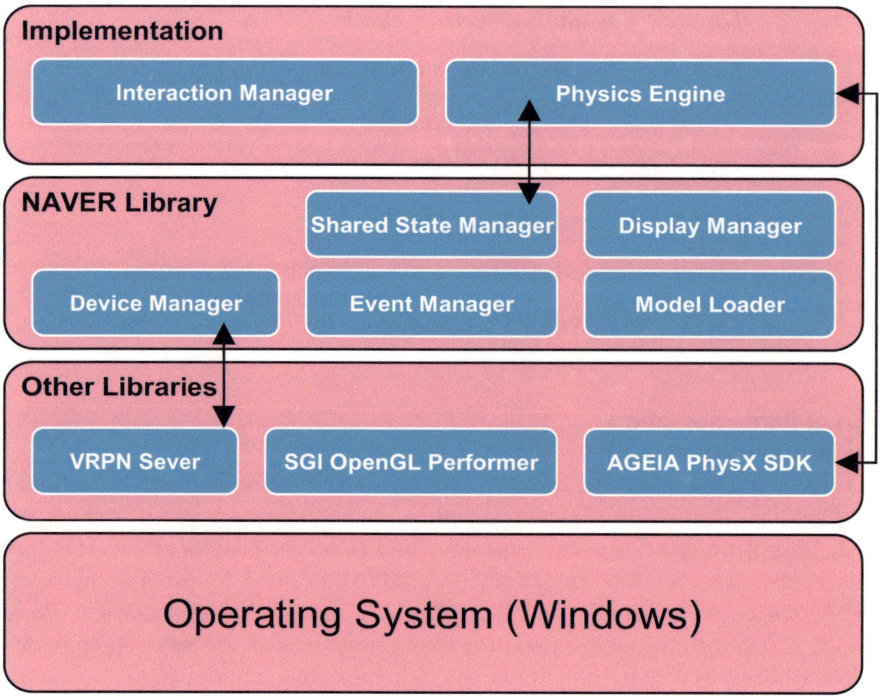

Fig. 7. System architecture of the implementation

To enable easy XML configuration, the application is implemented in a modular way into separate DLL (Windows' dynamic library) files. Using pfvViewer, a module loader from SGI OpenGL Performer, the dynamic libraries are executed to work together into one single VR application. All configurations of the modules are written in an XML file (with .pfv extension). The modules can accept parameters from what are written in the XML file, such as described in this figure below.

```
<id>physics</id>
<debug_key>d</debug_key>
<reset_key>s</reset_key>
<ground>nxground</ground>
<hammer>nxblock5</hammer>
<gravity_earth>0, 0,-9.81</gravity_earth>
<gravity_moon>0, 0,-1.62</gravity_moon>
<restitution>0.5</restitution>
<static_friction>0.5</static_friction>
<dynamic_friction>0.5</dynamic_friction>
```

Fig. 8. Configuration of physics simulation in XML file

(2) Three-Users Design and Implementation

Interaction status on the same object by three users is shared by showing several different states. These states are touched and selected by one, two, or three users. For user's graphical feedback purpose, these states are described by color yellow, cyan, green, magenta, red, and blue respectively (Figure 9).

- Object is touched by 1 hand (YELLOW)
- Object is touched by 2 hands (CYAN)
- Object is touched by 3 hands (RED)
- Object is grabbed by 1 hand (GREEN)
- Object is grabbed by 2 hands (MAGENTA)
- Object is grabbed by 3 hands (BLUE)
- Hand intersects with object (YELLOW)
- Hand grabs object (GREEN)

Fig. 9. Graphical feedback for three-users

Each user is represented by one hand avatar. We modify our previous algorithm in order to check all these "touch" and "select" status easier. We check object status instead of hand status that we used in our previous algorithm. "Select" status only can happen after "touch" status. In a frame, we will check the touching status for each object and define how many hand and which hand that touches the object. Still in the same looping of each object, we check the selecting status of that object and doing manipulation for that object based on how many hand selects that object.

We made our application fit with Joystick and SPIDAR (Sato, M. 2002) - WAND input. These devices will be used in our testing to give input to our simulation. BUTTON_PRESSED in the figure below represents the "selecting or grabbing" button from Joystick or WAND button.

```
Frame()
 for (each hand indexed ii)
     updateHand(ii);

 for (each object indexed jj) → based on each object
 {
     touched(jj) → check touching state
     for (each hand indexed ii) → then check all hands
     {
         if (hand is intersected) && (BUTTON_PRESSED [ii] == 0)
         {
             select_attach() → check grabbing state and attach each hand to object
             manipulateObj(jj); → move objects
         }
     } else {
         releaseObj(jj); → release objects
     }
     update physics simulation to interaction manager;
 }
 update hands movement to physics manager;
```

Fig. 10. Algorithm of the object and hand status

The algorithm for shared-object manipulation is extended from two user manipulation into three user manipulation. The calculation of movement for three users is made based on two users's manipulation. The different is we have to choose which two hands against the other one hand based on hand velocity checking.

2.8 Results

As result of our approach, we present the comparative study of two users and the simulation result of three users.

We have done comparative study for two users. Two users manipulate the same object together concurrently in: 1) PC and PC environment through LAN inside KIST and the Internet between KIST,Korea and Oita University, Japan through APII-Hyunhae-Genkai Network, 2) CAVE (Cruz-Neira, C., Sandin, D. J., DeFanti, T. A., Kenyon, R.V., Hart, J.C. 1992) and PC environment through LAN. The test also includes the comparative study between haptic (with force feedback) and non-haptic (no force feedback) device. We will use joystick as input device for PC environment. In the CAVE system, the input devices that used are SPIDAR for movement and WAND for object selecting/grabbing button.

Table 1 shows our experiment result. We test five times and calculate average time for completing the collaborative interaction.

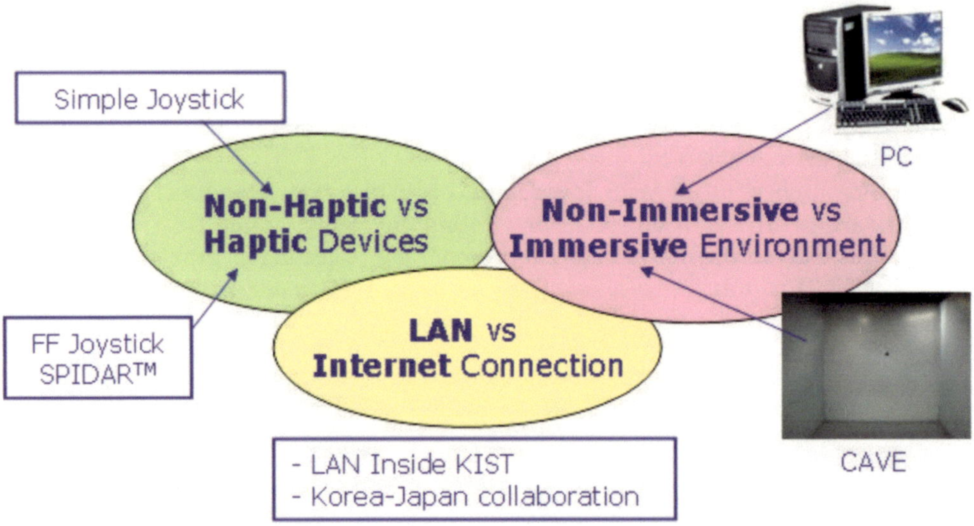

Fig. 11. Network Collaborative Interaction (NCI) Comparative Study

	PC-PC	PC-PC	CAVE-PC
	Non Force-Feedback	Force-Feedback	Force-Feedback
LAN Inside KIST	29.096s	21.344s	16.676 s
Internet (bw Korea and Japan)	43.55s	36.92s	-

Table 1. Comparison of network collaborative interaction in different immersion and different network environment

3. Summary

We have implemented an application for CVE based on VR systems and simulation of physics law. The system allows reconfiguration of the simulation elements so that users can see the effects of the different configurations. The network support enables users from different places to work together when interacting with the simulation, and see each other's simulation results.

From our series of testing of the application over different networks and environments, we can conclude that the use of haptics functionality (force-feedback device) is useful for users to feel each other's presence. It also helps collaboration to be performed more effectively (no time wasted). However, network delays caused problems on the haptics smoothness. In the future, we will update our algorithm by studying the possible solutions like indicated by Glencross et al. (Glencross, M., Jay, C., Feasel, J., Kohli, L., Whitton, M. 2007).

We also conclude that the use of tracker-type input device like SPIDAR is more intuitive for a task where users are faced with a set of objects to select and manipulate. From the display view of point, immersive display environment is more suitable for simulation of dealing with object manipulation that requires force and weight feeling, compared to non-immersive display environment such as PC.

Acknowledgment

This work was supported in part by KIST (Korea Institute of Science & Technology) through Development of Tangible Web Technology Project.

4. References

AGEIA: AGEIA PhysX SDK, http://www.ageia.com

Basdogan, C., Ho, C., Srinivasan, M.A., Slater, M. (Dec. 2000) An Experimental Study on the Role of Touch in Shared Virtual Environments. In: ACM Transactions on Computer Human Interaction, vol. 7, no. 4, pp. 443-460

Cruz-Neira, C., Sandin, D. J., DeFanti, T. A., Kenyon, R.V., Hart, J.C. (1992) The CAVE: audio visual experience automatic virtual environment. In: Communications of the ACM, vol. 35, issue 6, pp. 64-72

Glencross, M., Jay, C., Feasel, J., Kohli, L., Whitton, M. (2007) Effective Cooperative Haptic Interaction over the Internet. In: Proceedings of IEEE Virtual Reality Conference 2007. Charlotte

Johnson, A., Roussos, M., Leigh, J. (1998) The NICE Project: Learning Together in a Virtual World. In: IEEE Virtual Reality Annual International Symposium (VRAIS 98). Atlanta

Kim, J., Kim, H., Tay, B.K., Muniyandi, M., Srinivasan, M.A., Jordan, J., Mortensen, J., Oliveira, M., Slater, M. (2004) Transatlantic touch: A study of haptic collaboration over long distance. In: Presence: Teleoperator and Virtual Environments, vol. 13, no. 3, pp. 328-337

Margery, D., Arnaldi, B., Plouzeau, N. (1999) A General Framework for Cooperative Manipulation in Virtual Environments. In: 5th Eurographics Workshop on Virtual Environments. Vienna

Otto, O., Roberts, D., Wolff, R. (June 2006) A Review on Effective Closely-Coupled Collaboration using Immersive CVE's. In: Proceedings of ACM VRCIA. Hong Kong Roberts, D., Wolff, R., Otto, O. (2005) Supporting a Closely Coupled Task between a Distributed Team: Using Immersive Virtual Reality Technology. In: Computing and Informatics, vol. 24, no. 1

Park, C., Ko, H.D., Kim, T. (2003) NAVER: Networked and Augmented Virtual Environment aRchitecture; design and implementation of VR framework for Gyeongju VR Theater. In: Computers & Graphics, vol. 27, pp. 223-230

Ruddle, R.A., Savage, J.C.D., Jones, D.M. (Dec. 2002) Symmetric and Asymmetric Action Integration During Cooperative Object Manipulation in Virtual Environments. In: ACM Transactions on Computer-Human Interaction, vol. 9, no. 4

Sato, M. (2002) Development of string-based force display. In: Proceedings of the Eighth International Conference on Virtual Reality and Multimedia, Workshop 2. Gyeongju

Silicon Graphics Inc. (2005) , "OpenGL Performer," http://www.sgi.com/products/software/performer/

Taylor, R. M., Hudson, T. C., Seeger, A., Weber, H., Juliano, J., Helser, A.T. (2001) VRPN: A device-independent, network-transparent VR peripheral system. In: ACM International Symposium on Virtual Reality Software and Technology (VRST 2001). Berkeley

Wolff, R., Roberts, D.J., Otto, O. (June 2004) A Study of Event Traffic during the Shared Manipulation of Objects within a Collaborative Virtual Environment. In: Presence, vol. 13, no. 3, pp. 251-262

35

Using Haptic Technology to Improve Non-Contact Handling: the "Haptic Tweezer" Concept

Ewoud van West, Akio Yamamoto and Toshiro Higuchi
The University of Tokyo
Japan

1. Introduction

This chapter describes the concept named "Haptic Tweezer," which is in essence an object handling tool for contact-sensitive objects that are handled without any mechanical contact between the tool and the object, *with* the help of haptic technology. By combining haptic technology with conventional levitation systems, such as magnetic levitation and electrostatic levitation, intuitive and reliable non-contact object handling can be realized. This work has been previously published in journal and conference articles (van West, Yamamoto, Burns & Higuchi, 2007; van West, Yamamoto & Higuchi, 2007a;b) which form the basis of the information presented in this chapter.

Levitation techniques are very suitable for handling contact-sensitive objects because of the absence of mechanical contact between the levitator and the levitated object. Several negative effects such as contamination, contact damage, and stiction (Bhushan, 2003; Rollot et al., 1999) can be avoided by using these techniques. This can be vital for objects which are very sensitive to these problems such as silicon wafers, glass plates used in flat panel displays, sub-millimeter sized electronics, or coated sheet metal. The levitated object is held at a certain position from the levitation tool by actively controlling the levitation force. It compensates for gravitational, inertial, and disturbance forces, and the object appears to be suspended by an invisible spring. The advantages of levitation systems have led to the development of several non-contact manipulation systems.

While using non-contact handling techniques solves the problems related to the direct physical contact that exists in regular contact-based handling, it also introduces new difficulties as these systems behave differently from conventional contact-based handling techniques. Especially if the manipulation task has to be performed by a human operator, as is still often the case in R&D environments or highly specialized production companies, non-contact manipulation tasks can become very difficult to perform. The main reason for these problems is the fact that the stability of levitation systems against external disturbances is much lower than that of conventional handling tools such as grippers. Inertial forces and external forces can easily de-stabilize the levitation system if they exceed certain critical threshold values. In case of human operation, the motion induced by the human operator is in fact the largest source of disturbances. Especially in the tasks of picking up and placing, where the status of *non-levitated* changes to *levitated* and vice versa, large position errors can be induced by the downward motion. The air gap between the tool and the object can not be maintained as in

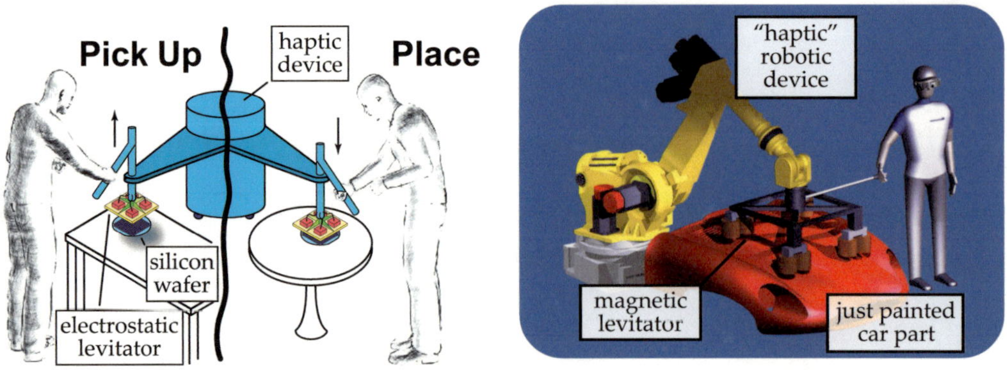

Fig. 1. A visual representation of the "Haptic Tweezer" concept. The human operator handles the non-contact levitator through the haptic device in order to augment in real-time the handling performance.

these tasks, the object is supported on one side by for example a table, while the levitator is moving down. If the motion is not stopped on time, contact between the levitator and object will occur, something which should be avoided at all cost in non-contact handling systems. In regular contact-based handling, the direct physical contact with the object directly transmits the reaction forces from the support which will stop the downward motion. The contact force also gives a tactile feedback signal on the grasping status *and* on whether or not the object is in mid-air or at a support. In levitation systems however, this direct contact force is missing and instead, the operator feels the reaction force of the levitation system which is far weaker and thus more difficult to sense. This means that the operator can easily continue his downward motion even though the object has already reached the correct position. This problem is even more eminent if the nominal levitation air gap between levitator and object is very small which is often the case in levitation systems. However, for the development of a practical non-contact handling tool, these challenges have to be overcome.

The main objective of this research is to develop a mechatronic non-contact handling tool that allows a human operator to perform simple manipulation tasks such as pick and place, in an easy and intuitive way. In order to realize that objective and overcome the challenges in terms of stability and robustness of such a human operated tool, a solution is sought in employing haptic technology to augment the human performance in real-time by active haptic feedback. This concept is named "Haptic Tweezer" and Fig. 1 shows some illustrations of the concept. The global idea is that haptic feedback compensates the disturbances coming from the human operator during manipulation tasks such as pick and place. By counteracting disturbances that would otherwise lead to instability (failure) of the levitation system, the haptic feedback will improve the performance of non-contact object manipulation. As the haptic feedback also restores in a sense the "feeling" of the levitated object, which was lost by the absence of physical contact, the task can be performed in an intuitive way.

The approach that is used for research on the "Haptic Tweezer" concept, has a strong experimental character. Several prototypes have been developed to investigate different aspects of the "Haptic Tweezer" concept. Two different levitation techniques have been used, magnetic levitation and electrostatic levitation, and control strategies based on both impedance control and admittance control were used in order to realize satisfactory results. The results have

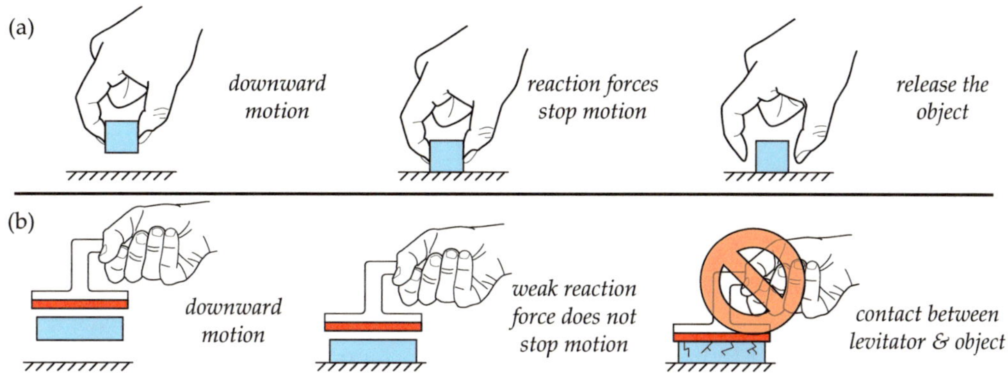

Fig. 2. Performing a placing task with (a) using direct physical contact, (b) using a non-contact levitation tool

shown that the haptic feedback has a significant beneficial contribution for handling objects without contact.

The general concept of the "Haptic Tweezer" concept will be further explained in the following section. A brief discussion on related research that uses haptic technology for real-time assisting applications is given in Section 3 and Section 4 will provide some basic background information on magnetic and electrostatic levitation systems. A first prototype that uses magnetic levitation and the impedance controlled haptic device PHANTOM Omni, is described in Section 5. Another prototype is described in Section 6, which uses electrostatic levitation and an in-house developed haptic device based on the admittance control strategy. The conclusions, describing the significance of the "Haptic Tweezer" concept, are given in the final section.

2. The "Haptic Tweezer" Concept

2.1 Basic concept

The concept of "Haptic Tweezer" uses the haptic device in a different configuration from most haptic applications. Typically, haptic devices are used in virtual reality applications or tele-operation systems to transmit tactile information, such that the operator can interact in a natural manner with the designated system. However, the output capabilities of the haptic device can also be used to modify, in real-time, the operators motion or force for other purposes. The human operator and the haptic device can perform a task collaboratively in which the haptic device can exert corrective actions to improve the performance of the task. This is precisely the objective of the "Haptic Tweezer" concept as the haptic device improves the task of non-contact handling by using haptic feedback to reduce the human disturbances to the levitated object.

The levitation systems used for non-contact handling have an independent stabilizing controller based on a position feedback loop. This same position information can be used as a measure of stability of the levitation system, i.e. large disturbances will induce large position errors in the levitation system. The largest levitation errors that are induced by the human operator will occur during the tasks of *picking up* and *placing*. This problem is graphically shown by Fig. 2, where a placing task is performed by using direct physical contact (a), as well as by using a non-contact levitation tool (b). In regular contact-based handling, the motion is

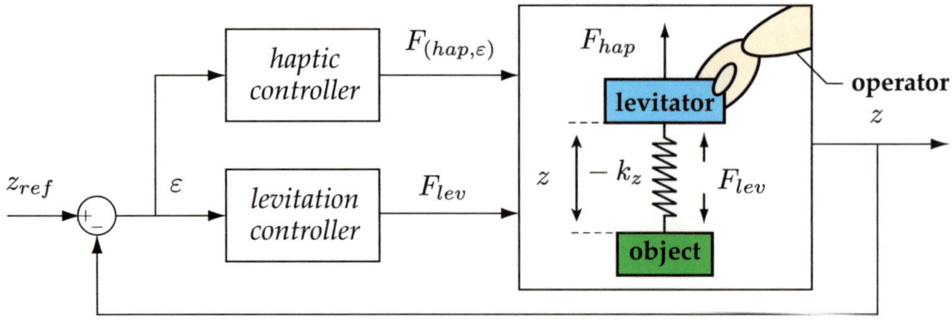

Fig. 3. Realization of an additional haptic force feedback loop

stopped by the reaction forces coming from the table, supporting the object. It also signals the operator that the correct location has been reached. In case of non-contact handling however, the downward motion is not stopped by the reaction forces from the levitation system as they are very weak. Furthermore, the human operator does not stop his motion as he can hardly "feel" the exact moment the object reaches the correct location. The induced position disturbance is too large for the levitation system and the air gap between levitator and object can not be maintained. The main focus of the "Haptic Tweezer" concept will lie in performance improvements for these pick and place tasks.

To compensate for the human disturbances, the haptic device will use the levitation position error to generate the haptic feedback to the operator. For example, if the human operator's downward motion reduces the air gap between the object and the levitation tool, the haptic device will generate a force to prevent this motion and thus avoid instability and damage. This is also shown in Fig. 3, where the haptic controller generates a feedback force $F_{hap,\varepsilon}$ based on the levitation position error ε. It is important to note that the haptic loop is an *addition* to the levitation controller that controls the force F_{lev} that stabilizes the leviation system. With the combination of the haptic controller *and* the levitation controller, a large induced position error will result in a reaction force from the levitation system (weak and hardly noticeable) and a force from the haptic device (strong) that counteract the position error. Furthermore, the haptic force sensation will naturally make the operator stop his downward motion as he can "feel" the status of the task he is performing. The haptic device allows the human operator to perform these pick and place tasks in a natural way and with improved performance as instabilities can be prevented.

2.2 Other contributing haptic effects

There are several other haptic effects that can further contribute to the "Haptic Tweezer" concept and a basic list of haptic effects comprising the "Haptic Tweezer" concept are described below and some are shown graphically in Fig. 4:

- Haptic feedback based on levitation position error (main)
- Damping force to restrict high accelerations
- Suppression of human hand vibration
- Virtual fixtures for guiding
- Gravity compensation of levitator and object

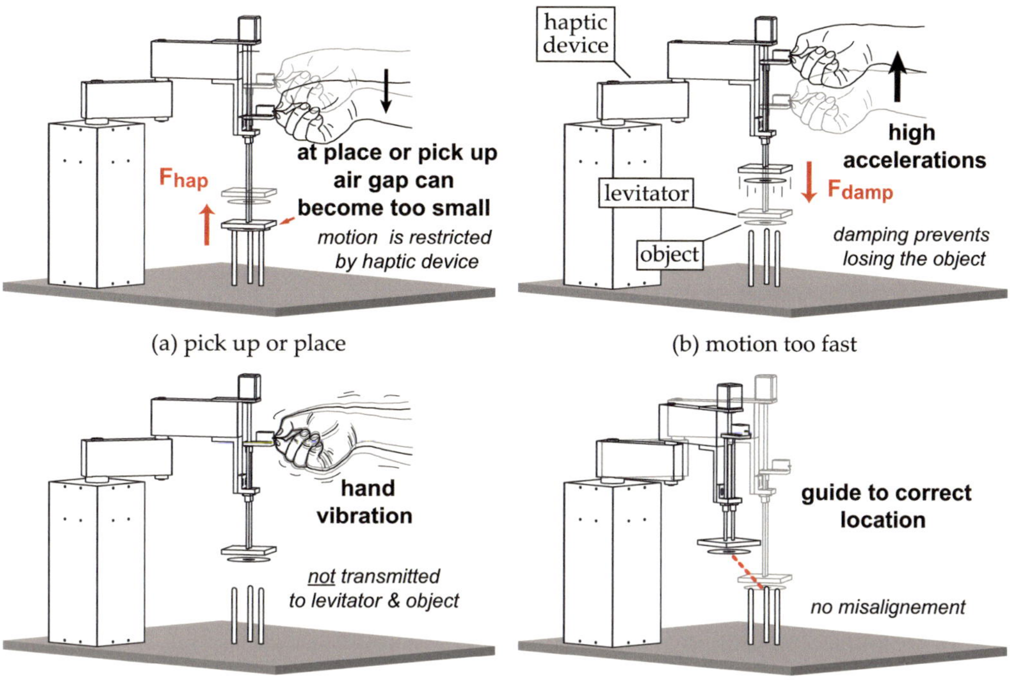

(a) pick up or place (b) motion too fast

(c) filter hand vibration (d) virtual fixtures (guiding)

Fig. 4. Several haptic effects that can contribute to the "Haptic Tweezer" concept

The effect of creating a virtual damping field will damp sudden accelerations that could be the result of wild motion and it will smoothen the resultant motion as shown in Fig. 4(b). The performance of precision handling can be further enhanced by filtering and suppressing the human natural hand vibrations as shown in Fig. 4(c). It can be realized through the mechanical structure of the haptic device and by filtering the operator's input. This idea is not unique to the "Haptic Tweezer" concept as other researchers have realized devices with the same objective and strategy, namely the Steady Hand Robot (Taylor et al., 1999). Virtual fixtures, shown in Fig. 4(d), can be used to guide the operator's motion and this technique is commonly used in various haptic applications. Lastly, the haptic device can assist in carrying the levitation system and object to reduce the task load of the operator. This list might be further extended with more effects at a later stage. However, the work presented in this chapter will mainly focus on the improvements that can be realized by the haptic feedback based on the levitation position error.

2.3 Various configurations & possible applications

The concept of "Haptic Tweezer" can be applied to various applications. In this section some configurations are described to give insight in where the "Haptic Tweezer" can be used. An overview is given in Table 1. However, this is just a selection of possible applications. The concept of "Haptic Tweezer" is general and can be applied to any situation which requires non-contact object handling and is therefore also not limited to only magnetic and electrostatic levitation systems.

In the first configuration, the "Haptic Tweezer" can be applied to handle very flat and thin fragile objects such as silicon wafers or the glass plates of Flat Panel Displays (FPD). Because of their large surface area, they can be levitated by electrostatic levitation which has the benefit that the levitation force is divided over the whole area and prevents bending (internal stress) of the flat objects.

The second configurations deals with precisely machined products which have to be moved without being contaminated. The tasks of picking up the object and placing it have to be performed with high accuracy which could be realized through the "Haptic Tweezer" concept.

In the third configuration, the "Haptic Tweezer" concept can be applied to handle objects in the (sub)-millimeter order. An example could be placing solder beads, which have to be aligned accurately for soldering of electronic chips. Or the assembly of minute parts, such as mechanical components like small gears and pins or assembly of electronic components on a printed circuit board.

In the last configuration, a piece of sheet metal that has been processed with a special coating (like paint) has to be transported without any contamination. This can be realized by magnetic levitation.

Application	Reason for non-contact handling	Levitation technique
1. Wafer / FPD glass plate handling	fragile	electrostatic
2. Precision placing	contamination	magnetic
3. Micro object handling	stiction	electrostatic / magnetic
4. Processed sheet metal	contamination	magnetic

Table 1. Several possible configurations / applications of "Haptic Tweezer"

3. Related research

The usage of haptic technology for real-time assisting applications, is a relatively new field within the haptic community that has an overlap with the field of Human-Machine Collaborative Systems (HMCS). The advantages of such a collaborative system are that the high precision and large endurance of robotic devices are combined with the intelligence and flexibility of a human operator. A system, in which a human operator and a robotic / haptic device work closely together, can realize results that would be not possible by only a robot or only a human operator. One field within the haptic community in which this development has taken place is the area of Computer Aided Surgery. The Steady Hand robots (Taylor et al., 1999), developed at the Johns Hopkins University (JHU), are a good example of such a class of assisting robotic tools. The key idea is that the tool the surgeon is holding, is kinematically connected to a mechanical device that provides high stiffness, high accuracy, and haptic feedback to the operator. The result is a smooth, tremor-free, precise positional control with capability of force scaling.

In the field of HMCS, the early collaborative robots, or *cobots* (Peshkin et al., 2001) are rather passive devices to support the human operator in terms of power (Hayashibara et al., 1997; Lee et al., 2000) that allows humans to perform heavier tasks for longer periods of time. An interesting development in this field which has brought the interaction even closer, is the development of wearable exoskeletons aiming to increase the human performance, with impressive results (Kazerooni, 1996; Kazerooni & Steger, 2006). In these systems, a close interaction between human and device is required and using haptic signals can facilitate this interaction as it allows more natural and comfortable operation. The fast processing of haptic signals by humans makes that haptic technology plays a key role for realizing systems that are intuitive to operate. Haptic signals can be used to present key information to an operator in for example augmented reality systems (Azuma et al., 2001; Azuma, 1997) to make the operator accept all the presented information more easily.

The possibilities are even larger as haptic devices can even transform sensory information, such as optical information, by presenting it haptically through the sense of touch. The Smart-Tool (Nojima et al., 2002) is a good example of such a system as it converts or "haptizes" information in real-time from an additional sensor into a haptic feedback. One example from their work shows the potential of such a system. The end-effector of the haptic device consists of the tool with an additional sensor, in this case, a surgical scalpel fitted with a reflectivity sensor. The objective will be to remove some unwanted tissue, for example a cancer growth, from a healthy organ, without damaging the healthy organ. For the experiment, the human tissue is replaced by a hard-boiled egg. A threshold in reflectivity is defined as a boundary between tissue that is safe to cut (egg white) and vital tissue (the egg yolk) that should be unharmed during a surgical cutting procedure. When the reflectivity sensor senses the egg yolk, a repulsive force is generated to compensate the operators cutting force. In such a way, the egg can be dissected without any effort from the operator. The strength lies in the ease with which such an operation can be performed and it shows the great potential of employing haptic technology. In addition, the usage of virtual fixtures (Rosenberg, 1993) can further enhance performance of some tasks as the operator's motion can be confined or guided, which increases performance of manipulation in for example medical tasks (Bettini et al., 2004; Lin et al., 2006).

4. Magnetic and Electrostatic Levitation

This section provides a brief introduction to the magnetic and electrostatic levitation systems used in this research. Both techniques have been researched by other researchers, so many literature is available on these subjects and this section is largely based on some of these works (Jin et al., 1994; 1995; Schweitzer et al., 1994).

4.1 Theoretical equations of motion

Magnetic and electrostatic levitation systems have similar characteristics as the generated attractive force is strong when the object is near the levitator, but gets quadratically weaker when the air gap increases. Therefore, according to Earnshaw's theorem (Earnshaw, 1842), active control is necessary for stable levitation. For a magnetic levitation system, as shown in Fig. 5 on the left side, the attractive electromagnetic force $\tilde{F}_{EM}$ is generated in a magnetic circuit that has a coil current $\tilde{i}$ and a permanent magnet. The force is given by

$$\tilde{F}_{EM} = \frac{A\mu_0 \left(\frac{B_r l_m}{\mu_0} + N\tilde{i} \right)^2}{(l_m + 2\tilde{z})^2}, \tag{1}$$

where A is the area of the magnetic flux path, μ_0 is the permeability constant, B_r is the remanent flux density of the permanent magnet, l_m is the length of the permanent magnet and N is the number of coil windings. For simplicity, the magnetic levitation is assumed to be quasi-static, and effects such as saturation, heat loss and leakage flux are ignored. Even though

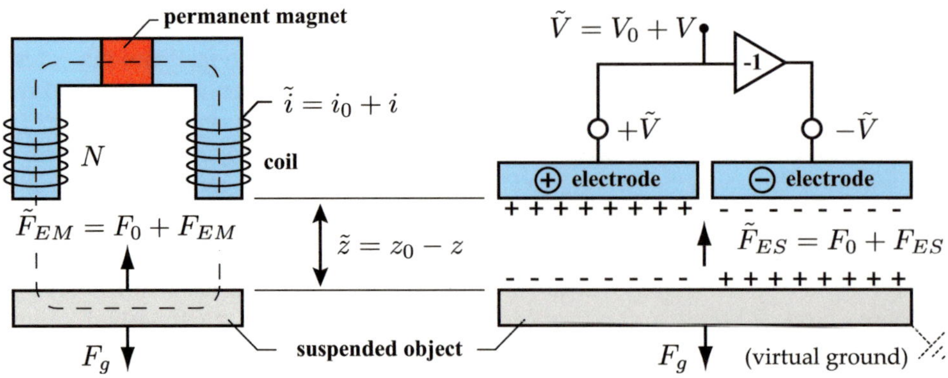

Fig. 5. Magnetic levitation system (left) and electrostatic levitation system (right). In magnetic levitation, the levitation force $\tilde{F}_{EM}$ is provided by a combination of a permanent magnet and an input current $\tilde{i}$. For electrostatic levitation, the levitation force $\tilde{F}_{ES}$ is generated by a high input voltage V applied to a pair of electrodes.

magnetic levitation can be realized without a permanent magnet, the permanent magnet reduces the required coil current since it provides a bias attractive force.

The electrostatic levitation system is shown in Fig. 5 on the right side; the attractive electrostatic force $\tilde{F}_{ES}$ is the result of an electric field that is generated by applying a high voltage $\tilde{V}$ to a pair of electrodes. The force is given by

$$\tilde{F}_{ES} = \frac{\varepsilon_0 A \tilde{V}^2}{2\tilde{z}^2}, \tag{2}$$

where A is the active area and ε_0 is the permittivity of air. By using a pair of positive and negative electrodes, the potential of the object can remain zero (virtual ground). For levitators controlling multiple n DOF, some of the electrodes can be combined, with a minimum of $n+1$ electrodes to control all DOF and maintain a zero potential of the object.

These levitation forces can be written in a more general form that holds for levitation systems where the levitation force $\tilde{F}(\tilde{u}, \tilde{z})$ is generated through input $\tilde{u}$ and also depends on the air gap $\tilde{z}$. Typically, the force equation is linearized around the operating point (u_e,z_e, and F_e) where the attractive force equals the gravitational force ($F_e = mg$). With deviations from the operating point as defined in the figure, the linearized force equation is

$$m\ddot{z} = k_u u + k_z z, \tag{3}$$

where m is the mass of the levitated object, k_u is the force-input factor, k_z is the force-displacement factor and

$$k_u = \frac{\delta \tilde{F}}{\delta u}(u_e, z_e), \quad k_z = \frac{\delta \tilde{F}}{\delta z}(u_e, z_e), \quad F_e = \tilde{F}(u_e, z_e). \tag{4}$$

The transfer function of this levitation system H_{SYS}, is derived from (3) in the Laplace conjugate domain, where each variable is capitalized and initial conditions are assumed to be zero:

$$H_{SYS} = \frac{Z(s)}{I(s)} = \frac{k_u}{ms^2 - k_z}. \tag{5}$$

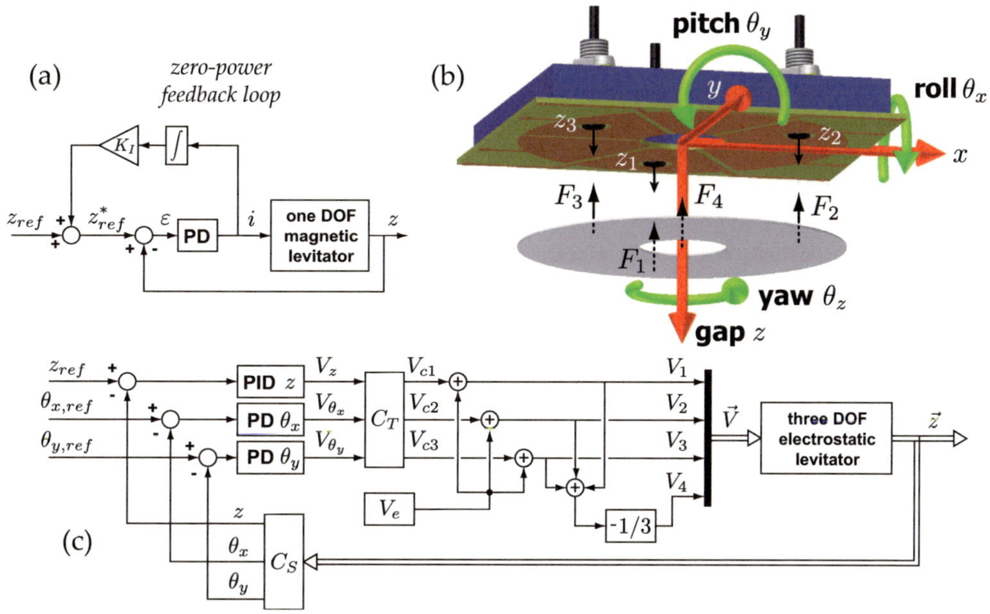

Fig. 6. (a) Zero-Power controller for magnetic levitation system. (b) Coordinate system for disk-shaped object used in electrostatic levitation. (c) Centralized controller for electrostatic levitation of a disk-shaped object.

It shows that the system behaves as an unstable mass-spring system because the spring stiffness is negative ($-k_z$). The following section will describe the stabilizing controller and how it influences the pick and place behavior.

4.2 Stabilizing levitation controller for one DOF

For a one DOF levitation system as (5), a simple Proportional-Derivative (PD)-controller is sufficient to realize stable levitation. The proportional gain will transform the negative spring constant to a positive value with stiffness $k = K_P \times K_u - k_z$. The derivative gain K_D will provide the necessary phase lead (damping) to the system such that there is enough phase-margin.

In addition to the PD-controller, an integral loop can be added to the system for further enhancing the controller performance. Such a loop can be a feedforward loop as in regular PID-control, or in a feedback loop, which is often lesser known. When the integral gain is a feedforward loop, the controller converges the steady state output to the reference *input* value to minimize the position or tracking error. However if the integral gain is in a feedback loop, the *output* of the controller is minimized. Such a controller is shown in Fig. 6(a) and is sometimes used in magnetic levitation systems to minimize power consumption under the name of Zero-Power controller (Morishita & Azukizawa, 1988). Power consumption can be minimal if the levitated object is in a position where the levitation force is almost completely provided by the permanent magnet. Current is still required to stabilize the system, but it can be virtually zero at steady state. If for example an additional load is added to the levitated object, the controller will bring the object to a new position, disregarding the original reference position input z_{ref}, closer to the levitator as the force from the magnet is stronger when the object is closer. It can be perceived as that the integral loop modifies the reference input to z^*_{ref}, which resembles a position in which the gravitational load is always balanced by the bias force of the levitation system (e.g. permanent magnet in magnetic levitation). The main benefit of Zero-Power controlled levitation systems and the reason why it is so suitable for non-contact transportation systems, is that the weight of the object can vary while still maintaining low power consumption for the manipulation task.

The integral gain loop in the levitation controller has another effect that is used in the *placing* task. The presence of such an integral loop allows to release the levitated objects automatically without any manual switching. This phenomena, which is described extensively in (van West et al., 2008), uses the integral controller wind up to reduce the holding force when a position error is temporarily forced to the levitated object. When, for example, the levitated object is brought to the desired location in the placing task, making contact at that location will reduce the air gap between levitator and object (the position error). For both Zero-Power and PID control, the result of this position error is that the controller will aim to increase the air gap by reducing the attractive force. The key point is that the integral gain will keep reducing the attractive force even if the position error is constant, due to the integral action. After some time, the attractive force has been reduced so much, that when the levitator moves away again and the position error changes sign, the object can not re-levitate the object and the placing has been realized automatically. Manually disabling the levitation force, on the other hand, would require precise timing as a release too early can drop the object, and a release too late can force the object to "stick" to the levitator. Automatic release will relief the operator in this regard and it contributes to perform the manipulation task intuitively. In the experimental results of the *placing* task, a more detailed description will be given using the experimental data.

For the *picking up* task however, having an integral gain in the levitation controller can be undesired for the same reason: integral controller wind up. If for example the picking up motion is too slow, the controller will increase the attractive force so much, that when the position is reached from which levitation is possible, the attractive force can be so large that instead of going to a stable position, it will "jump" and stick to the levitator. So in order to use the beneficial effects of the integral gain loop only when it is needed, it can be automatically switched on just after initial levitation (picking up) by a relay switch.

4.3 Multiple DOF levitation systems

While some objects can be levitated by actively controlling only one DOF, as will be shown in the first prototype of magnetic levitation of an iron ball, for most objects, multiple DOF have to be controlled for realizing stable levitation. For this purpose, multiple actuators and gap sensors have to be placed strategically around the object. However, it is not always necessary to control all six DOF with active control, as often a passive restoring force is present that naturally stabilizes some of the DOF. For levitating thin circular objects like an aluminium disk for example, it is natural to control only three DOF, namely the gap z, the roll θ_x, and the pitch θ_y, shown in Fig. 6(b). The lateral x- and y-direction are stabilized by a passive force that aligns the object with the levitator because in this position, the levitation field potential is the highest (Woo et al., 1995). As the side area is too small to place additional actuators, this force cannot be enhanced by means of control. Lastly, control of the yaw rotation θ_z is unnecessary due to the rotation symmetry of the object. As the actuators are all acting on the top surface of the object, the levitator can have the same form factor as the levitated object, which is very useful in the manipulation tasks of picking up and placing, where actuators on the side or bottom could be obstructive.

The controller structure for levitating an aluminium disk by electrostatic levitation is shown in Fig. 6(c) and it has a centralized control structure as each DOF is controlled by its own controller (Jin et al., 1995). The relative position of the disk is measured by three gap sensors, which are radially distributed around the z-axis at a radius R_s. Since these gap sensors will measure the distance z_i, $(i = 1,2,3)$ in local coordinates, they have to be transformed by a transformation matrix C_S to the correct DOF:

$$\begin{bmatrix} z \\ \theta_x \\ \theta_y \end{bmatrix} = \underbrace{\begin{bmatrix} 1/3 & 1/3 & 1/3 \\ \frac{-2}{3R_s} & \frac{1}{3R_s} & \frac{1}{3R_s} \\ 0 & \frac{-1}{\sqrt{3}R_s} & \frac{1}{\sqrt{3}R_s} \end{bmatrix}}_{C_S} \times \begin{bmatrix} z_1 \\ z_2 \\ z_3 \end{bmatrix}, \tag{6}$$

which assumes that tilting angles are small ($\sin(\theta) \approx \theta$). As the actuators have the same radial distribution as the gap sensors, the output from the controllers have to be transformed once again to generate the input signal for each actuator:

$$C_T = \begin{bmatrix} -1/3 & \frac{2}{3R_a} & 0 \\ -1/3 & \frac{-1}{3R_a} & \frac{1}{\sqrt{3}R_a} \\ -1/3 & \frac{-1}{3R_a} & \frac{-1}{\sqrt{3}R_a} \end{bmatrix}, \tag{7}$$

where R_a is the radius at which the actuating force occurs. By using C_T as the output transformation matrix, the proportional controller values of K_P will have the correct physical value of stiffness realized by control once they are multiplied with the force-input value of K_u.

In this case of electrostatic levitation, the positive electrodes are the controlling electrodes as they receive the output voltages of the controller V_i, $i = 1,2,3$. The negative electrodes receive a voltage that will simply maintain the total potential of the object at zero volt by setting $V_4 = -1/3 \sum V_i$, $i = 1,2,3$.

5. Prototype using magnetic levitation, PHANTOM Omni, and impedance control

The first prototype is realized to show how a combination of levitation system and haptic interface will perform. This prototype combines a magnetic levitation system with a commercially available haptic interface, the PHANTOM Omni (Sensable Technologies). This section describes the control strategy, the realized prototype, and the experiments that were performed to evaluate the overall performance.

5.1 Strategy for impedance controlled haptic devices

For the first prototype, the haptic device PHANTOM Omni has been used as it is commercially available at relatively low cost, and it can be easily equipped with a simple one DOF magnetic levitation system. The PHANTOM Omni is a haptic device based on the impedance control strategy, measuring the operator's position input and feeding back the haptic force (position in / force out). The implementation of the "Haptic Tweezer" concept for such a device is graphically shown in Fig. 7. The upper part shows the impedance structure of the haptic device with the position sensor measuring the human motion p, and the force actuator exerts the haptic feedback force F_{hap} based on a reference force F^*. One component of this reference force signal, F_v, comes from a virtual model that defines the haptic environment, and it

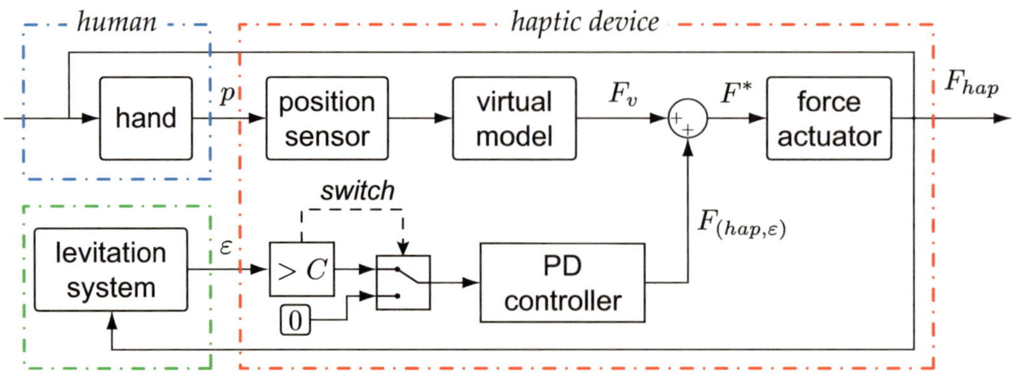

Fig. 7. Interaction between human, haptic device and the levitation based on the impedance control strategy

contains conventional parameters such as inertia and damping to realize comfortable motion. The additional haptic loop based on the levitation error ε is added to this virtual model such that a haptic force is generated as $F_{hap,\varepsilon}$ when the levitation error exceeds a certain threshold value C. The gain of this force can be regulated through a haptic PD-controller which acts like additional spring and damper elements for optimal results.

One drawback of using impedance controlled haptic devices, is that their performance in terms of output force and realizable stiffness is limited (van der Linde & Lammertse, 2003). This is a direct result of the design of these devices as they have to be lightweight and highly back-drivable to minimize their inertia and friction, which will always be felt by the operator. Such a limitation can be a problem if the levitation system is so sensitive that it requires larger force/stiffness values in order to compensate for the operators picking up or placing action. For the prototype discussed in this section, successful results could be obtained, but later on, another prototype will be described for which another type of haptic device had to be used.

5.2 Experimental setup

The magnetic levitation device consists of a hybrid electromechanical system and it is shown in Fig. 8, attached to the haptic device. The electromagnet has 530 windings in an E-core and a permanent magnet (type Nd-B-Fe, B_r = 1.2 T) is attached to the central leg. The air gap $\tilde{z}$ between the electromagnet and the object is sensed by an optical parallel beam linear sensor (Z4LB-S10V2, Omron). The absolute maximum coil current is limited at 1.2 A to prevent overheating of the coil. With this setup, only one DOF is actively controlled as the other two DOF are passively stable. The levitation controller is a Zero-Power controller as shown in Fig. 6(a) with the controller gains given in Table 2. Other parameters of the leviation setup are given in this table as well. Note that as mentioned earlier, a relay switch is implemented that automatically switches the integral feedback loop *off* for the *picking up* task.

The haptic controller, has a proportional gain K'_P on the air gap error and a gain K'_D on the differentiated air gap with values as shown in Table 2. Summed, a vertical upward force (z-direction) is generated at the stylus when an air gap is forced smaller, e.g. the object is placed on a surface. An extra stiffness is experienced by the operator, limiting the reduction of air gap. However, generating a haptic feedback force when there is a position error due to a larger air gap can give an undesirable effect. During the *picking up* task for instance, there

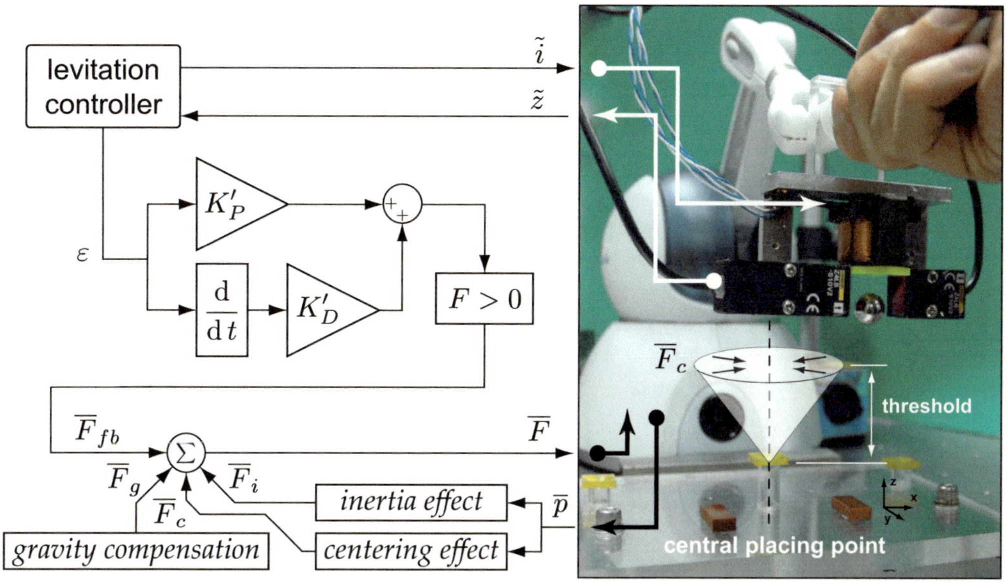

Fig. 8. Control structure for the prototype that uses magnetic levitation and the PHANTOM Omni to pick and place an iron ball, 12.7 mm in diameter

is a position error because the air gap between levitator and object is large. In this case, the haptic force would try to reduce the position error by moving the levitation device down to the object. As a result, the operator's motion is disturbed and he can no longer exert a controlled motion for the *picking up* task. Therefore, the haptic force can be limited to one direction only, namely the vertical upward direction and only when the position error is due to a smaller air gap. This is shown in Fig. 8 by the "$F > 0$"-block. The feedback force $\overline{F}_{fb}$ is further combined with a gravity compensating force $\overline{F}_g$ of 1.5 N to assist the user in carrying part of the weight of the levitation device (about 255 g) and artificial inertia ($\overline{F}_I$) is simulated to prevent sudden or rapid movements. The centering effect ($\overline{F}_c$) is used as a virtual fixture in the comparison experiment to guide the user to the correct pick and place location. It is further described in the comparison experiment, but also shown in Fig. 8. The total stiffness that is realized by the combination of magnetic levitation and haptic device is 452 N/m, which is roughly five times larger than the original stiffness realized by only the levitation controller. This is limited by the maximum force output of the haptic device and in fact a higher value of this stiffness is desired for this setup. As stronger haptic devices than the PHANTOM Omni are available, there is a potential to increase the performance here.

Another limitation of this prototype is the fact that the levitation device should be maintained level. This is necessary to keep stable levitation, but there is no mechanism present to achieve this. Thus, in this current setup, the operator has to maintain the horizontal position of the levitation device. It deviates from the concept that the tool should be natural and instinctive to use. Future prototypes should be designed to avoid this limitation.

5.3 Experimental results

To evaluate the additional performance of the haptic device to the levitation setup, three experiments based on a simple *pick and place* task were carried out. First, the details of the *picking up* task are presented followed by the details of the *placing* task. These tasks are then performed by a group of ten test subjects to evaluate the difference between the haptic effect *ON* and *OFF*. For this purpose, the iron ball has to be picked up and placed on a raised platform that has an absolute height of 63 mm.

Levitation		
Proportional gain	K_P	$2 \cdot 10^3$ A/m
Derivative gain	K_D	27.5 (A· s)/m
Integral gain	K_I	$1.2 \cdot 10^{-3}$ m/(A· s)
Force-current relation	k_u	$6.2 \cdot 10^{-2}$ N/A
Force-air gap relation	k_z	-32 N/m
MagLev stiffness	k_{MagLev}	92 N/m
Haptic Force		
Haptic proportional gain	K'_P	360 N/m
Haptic derivative gain	K'_D	210 (N· s)/m
Total Stiffness	k	452 N/m

Table 2. Control settings and other characteristics of PHANTOM-MagLev prototype

5.3.1 Picking up

Details of the *picking up* task are shown in Fig. 9. The moment the ball comes into the sensing range of the magnetic levitation, the control output is activated and the levitation system tries to get the ball to the reference air gap. When the air gap is reached from which levitation is possible, the ball will "jump" to the reference position with some overshoot after which it settles at the steady state position where controller current is zero. This overshoot and jump speed result in a repulsive force from the haptic interface at the stylus and the operator can feel that the ball is picked up through this force sensation. In this way, the object is picked up in a natural way by bringing the tool close to the object and because of the force sensation, the operator can feel the *picking up* is successful.

5.3.2 Placing

For the *placing* task, it is important to note that two effects will realize natural placing behavior. First of all the haptic interface will restrict the placing motion in such a way that the position error will remain within stable limits. Second, ZP-control allows for a natural release of the object due to the levitation controller wind up. Details of the *placing* task are shown in Fig. 10. The tool and object are moved down until the object makes contact with the surface (I). A forced reduction in the air gap leads to an upward force on the stylus (II) from the haptic device, which is experienced as an extra stiffness between the stylus and the object. Due to the behavior of the ZP-controller, the reduced air gap will increase the reference gap z^*_{ref} exponentially and the levitation system will try to bring the object to this larger air gap. The downward electromechanical force will increase (III) and so will the haptic upward force (IV). Due to the contact, the larger air gap cannot be realized until the operator retreats the tool from the object (V) and the air gap increases. As it takes time for z^*_{ref} to reduce, the reference gap is too large (levitation force is to weak) to re-levitate the ball (VI). The result is that the object will remain on the placing platform and placing is successful. In this way, both the ZP-controller and the haptic device contribute to a natural way of placing as the force sensation prevents

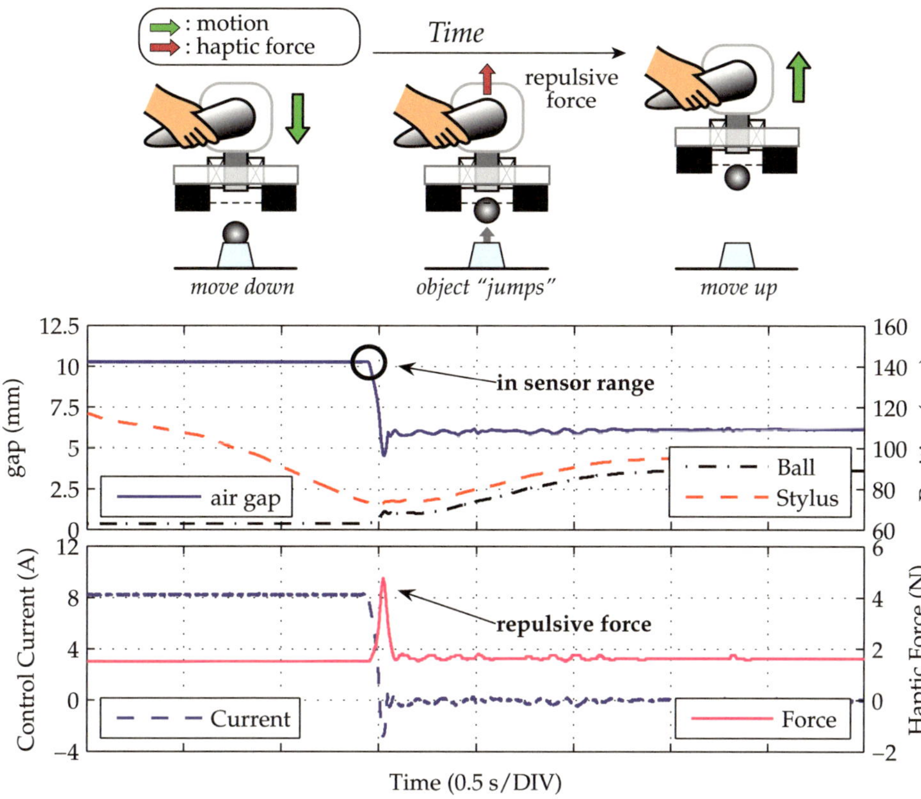

Fig. 9. Details of *picking up* with haptic assistance

instability and indicates when placing has been achieved. The placing sensation is natural and simple as there are no command or switch operations necessary to place the object. When the object makes contact at the desired location, further motion is prevented and the object will be automatically released.

5.3.3 Comparison experiment: approach

To evaluate the main effect of the haptic stiffness ($\overline{F}_{fb}$ in Fig. 8) on task performance, ten subjects (all male engineering students, age < 30 yr) with no experience on this device, performed a pick and place task. The only varying condition was the haptic stiffness either *ON* or *OFF*. As performance variables, the time for each task of *picking up* and *placing* is measured and failures are counted. Each subject had to perform 20 successful tasks while the number of attempts was not limited, but failures were recorded for later evaluation. Failures are classified as either "Stick", when the ball sticks to the levitation device, "Fell off", if the object was released but not on the desired location or as "Not Picked Up"/" Not Placed", when the attempt was made, but not successful without obvious failure.

The task duration is automatically measured as the difference in time when the operator moves the device passed a certain vertical height threshold, which is shown in Fig. 8. At this threshold, also the centering effect becomes active and a spring-like force related to the distance (in the horizontal XY-plane) to the central placing point will guide the operator to

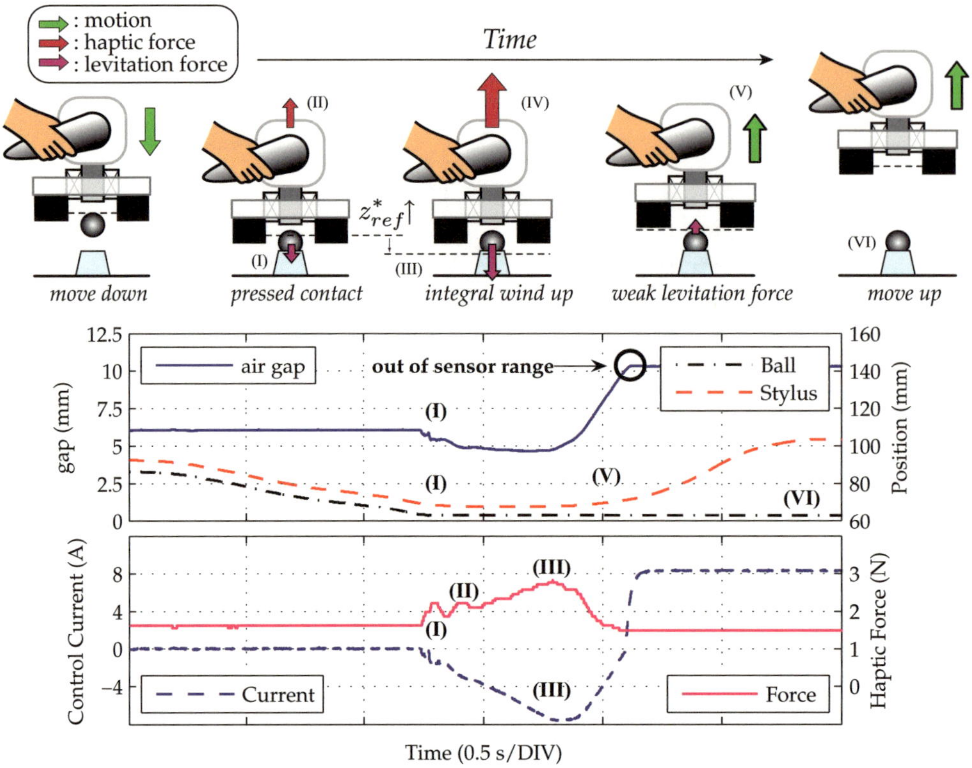

Fig. 10. Details of *placing* with haptic assistance

the right position. The spring stiffness of the centering effect is increased proportional to the vertical absolute position, giving a cone-shape vector field for constant centering forces.

Five subjects performed the task first with haptic stiffness *OFF*, followed by haptic stiffness *ON* (Group *OFF→ON*), but for the other half of the test subjects, the order was reversed (Group *ON→OFF*). All subjects were asked to perform the task in a natural way and they did not have any practicing time to get familiar with the setup, so they are considered as novice users. They also performed the same experiment at least a day later, with the only difference that they were given a 3 minute practicing time before each task, to enhance their skill and they are considered as experienced users. All experienced users performed the task in reversed order as when they were novice users.

With this approach, the performance can be evaluated under the effect of haptic stiffness. The average time of 20 *successful tasks* will give an indication on the handling speed, whereas the number of failures in the first 20 *attempts* can give insight on the frequency of failures. Also, the practicing effect can be analyzed by comparing the experienced group with the novice group. Any individual learning effect that might occur for the novice group within the 20 *successful tasks* is neglected as it can be considered equally distributed between the two groups.

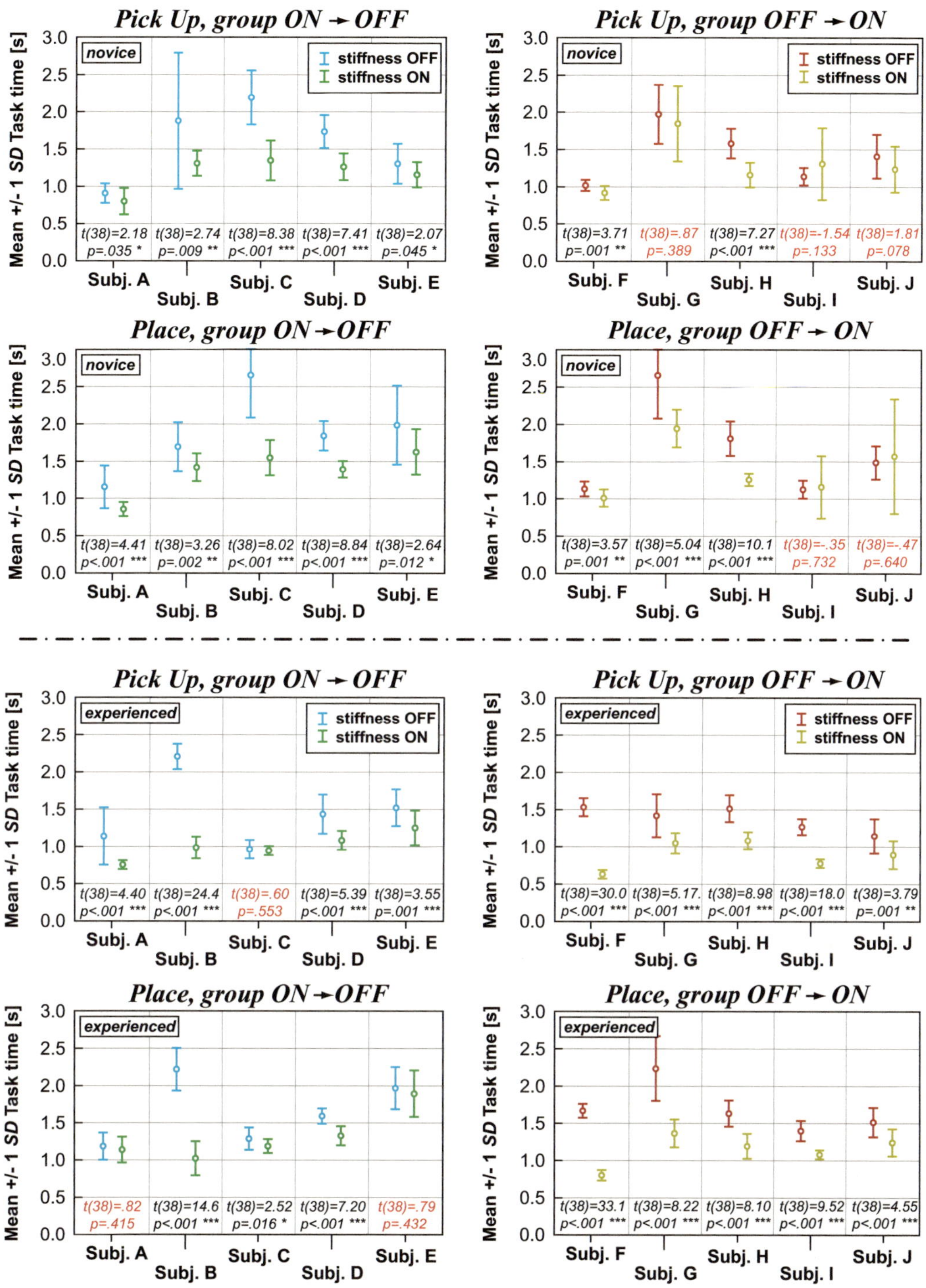

Fig. 11. Evaluation of *picking up* and *placing* by both novice operators (top four) and experienced operators (bottom four).

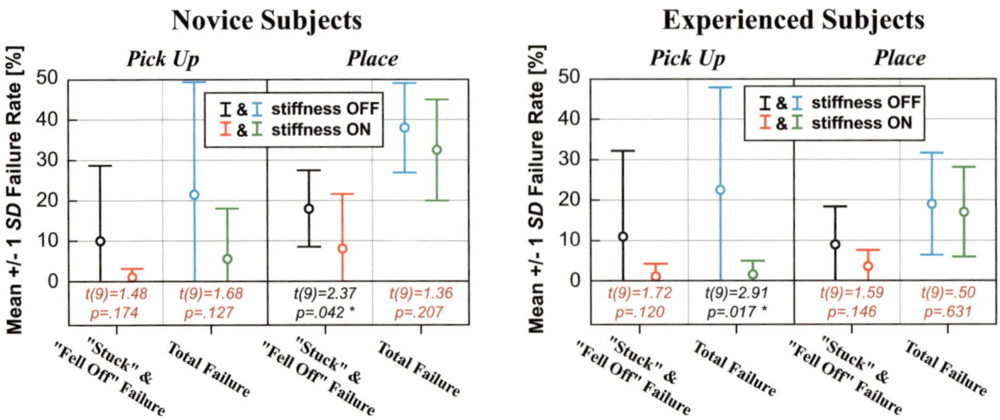

Fig. 12. Evaluation of the failure rates for both *picking up* and *placing*.

5.3.4 Comparison experiment: results

The average task time of 20 successful tasks is compared by an independent-samples T-test to verify if the task time is improved and the results are given in Fig. 11 for novice users (top four graphs) and for experienced users (bottom for graphs). A comparison of the failure rate of the first 20 *attempts* by a paired-samples T-test is provided in Fig. 12. Results, shown with an asterisk (*) have a p-value lower than the significance level $\alpha = 0.05$. Double asterisks (**) and triple asterisks (***) indicate significance levels of $\alpha = 0.01$ and $\alpha = 0.001$ respectively.

For novice users which performed the experiment in the order *OFF→ON*, the task time of both *picking up* and *placing* is significantly reduced with haptic stiffness *ON*, which could also be partly the result of a learning effect. For the novice users who performed the task in order *ON→OFF*, some improvements are not significant or even show deteriorated performance (e.g. Subj. I). Still the overall improvement is enough to support the positive effect of haptic stiffness. Moreover, the influence of the learning effect is further reduced by the practicing time given to each subject when they do the experiment again as an experienced user. The effect of haptic stiffness is more clear as all subjects performed significantly better in both tasks with few insignificant exceptions. The practicing effect improves the task time especially when the haptic stiffness is *ON* as can be seen in Table 3, where the average task times of all subjects are compared between the novice and experienced user by a paired-sampled T-test.

For the Failure analysis, a difference is made in strong failures such as "Stick" and "Fell Off", and weak failures as "Not Picked Up"/"Not Placed". In Fig. 12 both the weak failures and all failures (total) are shown for each case. Comparing the failure rates shows that in all cases there is a decrease of failure rate, which is however only significant in two cases.

At the *picking up* task, the failure rate is most clearly reduced for the experienced subjects as it is lower than 2%. It was observed that for some subjects the number of weak failures in the *placing* task did not reduce, but sometimes even increased. Due to the haptic stiffness, the operator can feel the contact as opposed to without the stiffness. This sensation caused in some cases the operator to move up more quickly than when the haptic stiffness was *OFF*. As a result, the contact time was not long enough to realize placing and the number of "Not placed"-failures increased.

Overall can be concluded that the effect of haptic stiffness has a positive contribution in the performance of non-contact object handling. However, the haptic stiffness was set the same

Condition	*M*	*SD*	*t(9)*	*p*
picking up, OFF, Novice	1.51	.43	.60	.566
picking up, OFF, Experienced	1.42	.34		
picking up, ON, Novice	1.24	.28	3.57	.006 **
picking up, ON, Experienced	.95	.19		
placing, OFF, Novice	1.75	.57	.49	.639
placing, OFF, Experienced	1.67	.36		
placing, ON, Novice	1.38	.32	1.71	.121
placing, ON, Experienced	1.23	.28		

Table 3. Practising effect by comparing Novice with Experienced

for all subjects, based on a general assumed placing motion. The experiments showed that an individual setting of the haptic stiffness is desired for this prototype as the placing motion varies per person and better individual results can be achieved. However, this is undesired for the final tool and improvements on the robustness for one optimum setting should be realized. In future work, the possibility to add other elements (e.g. a damper) to the spring or change its specific behavior to achieve this, should be studied.

With the reduction of task time and failures it is shown that it is more easy and instinctive to perform a pick and place task with haptic stiffness. Furthermore, with only a short time of practice, the performance increased and this indicates that the system has a degree of easiness to master.

6. Prototype using electrostatic levitation, SCARA-type haptic device, and admittance control

Another prototype has been developed for manipulating disk-shaped objects using electrostatic levitation. The haptic device used in this prototype is developed specific for this purpose but is still under development. This section describes the experimental setup and the results of the *picking up* and *placing* task.

6.1 Strategy for admittance controlled haptic devices

The limitations of impedance controlled haptic devices in terms of power and stiffness can give problems when the impedance controlled strategy of the "Haptic Tweezer" concept is applied to levitation systems which are very sensitive to disturbances, such as electrostatic levitation systems. For these systems, the levitation force is very weak and stable levitation is only possible at a very small air gap. Fig. 13 shows the difference in air gap between the magnetic levitation system used in the first prototype, and the electrostatic levitation system that will be described in this section. In order to apply the "Haptic Tweezer" concept also successfully to the electrostatic levitation systems, the requirements for the haptic device are higher. As the human operator's motion and force remain the same, the haptic device needs to be able to render a much higher stiffness for levitation systems with a small air gap.

By using an admittance controlled haptic device, these limitations can be overcome as an admittance controlled haptic device has the characteristics of being capable of rendering high

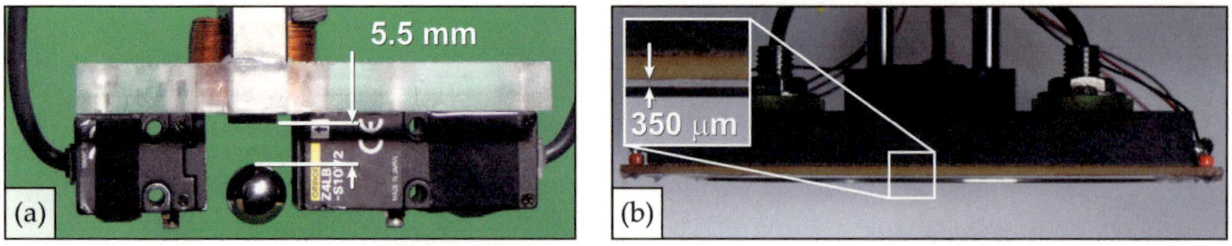

Fig. 13. Levitation system with different nominal air gap: (a) magnetic levitation of iron ball, (b) electrostatic levitation of aluminium disk

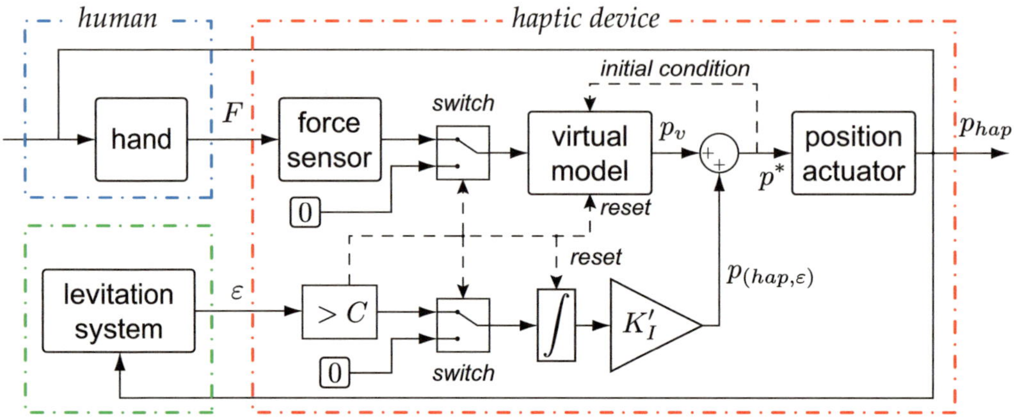

Fig. 14. Interaction between human, haptic device and electrostatic levitation

stiffness and outputting large forces. However, the strategy of admittance control is the inverse of impedance control as the haptic device measures the operator's force and gives a displacement based on the virtual model (force in, position out). This will require a modification on the implementation of the "Haptic Tweezer" concept.

Since the admittance control strategy is the inverse of admittance, the haptic contribution should also be inverted. Ideally that would mean that a force error is measured on the levitation system and a PI-controller adds a position signal to the virtual world output based on this force error. As in the levitation system itself, force is proportional to the air gap (in linearized case), this strategy should also work by substituting the levitation force error by the levitation position error. However, initial results were not satisfactory (unnatural feeling and damaging contact between object and levitator occurred) and the strategy for admittance controlled haptic devices had to be modified based on trial and error. Good results were achieved with the strategy as shown in Fig. 14.

The admittance control algorithm can be recognized in the upper part of the figure. The force from the operator is measured by a force sensor and this force is then sent to a virtual model. The virtual model calculates the position of the end-effector based on the effects acting on the object in the virtual model, such as damping, stiffness, and inertia. The position actuator gives the haptic position feedback p_{hap} that follows the reference position signal p^*.

The state of the electrostatic levitation system is indicated by levitation error ε. If the position error exceeds a certain threshold value C, it activates two switches that change the behavior of the total system. The first switch makes the input force to the virtual model zero, while the

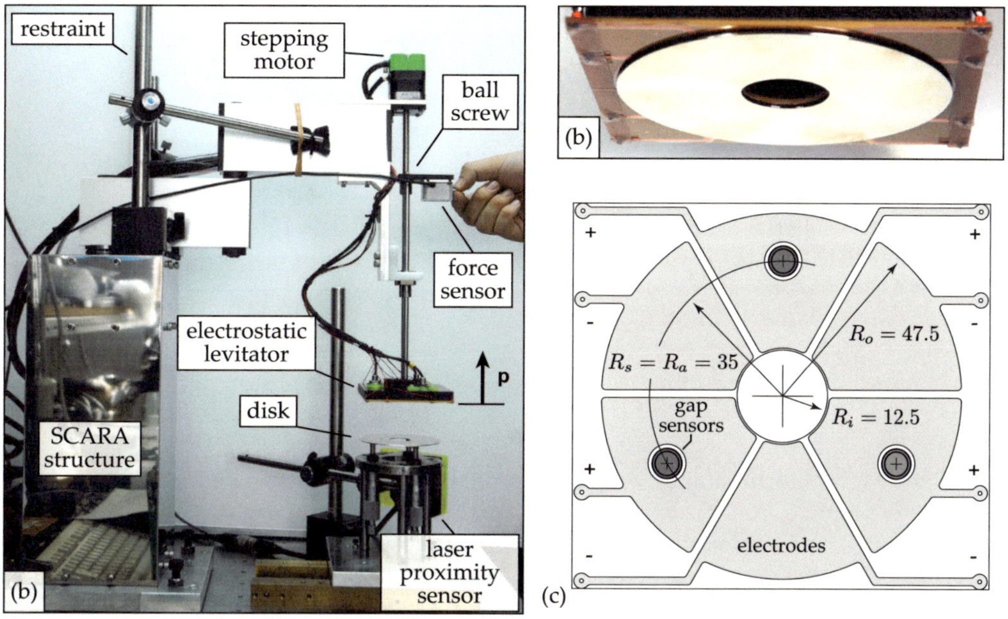

Fig. 15. (a) Prototype with electrostatic levitation and a SCARA-type haptic device. (b) The disk during stable levitation (air gap roughly 350 μm. (c) Details of the electrostatic levitator.

second switch allows the position error to pass through to an integrator. The threshold also sends a signal to the virtual model to reset any integrators inside the virtual model, and the results is a constant position output from the virtual model, which the operator experiences as he hitting a virtual wall. At the same time, the position error from the levitation system is integrated and added to the output of the virtual model as $p_{hap,\varepsilon}$. This minimizes the real levitation error ε as the end-effector with the electrostatic levitator moves up (positive p). When the error is again smaller than the threshold value C, the switches switch back to their previous value. To make sure that there are no discontinuities in the position signal that is sent to the position actuator, initial values for the virtual model are set at the moment of switching.

This strategy is further enhanced on two points to allow natural handling, which are not shown in Fig. 14 to avoid confusion. Firstly, the motion of the operator is automatically reduced when the levitator comes near the disk by using a high damping field, activated by a proximity sensor. Secondly, the switching criteria is extended to include the sign of force (positive/negative). That means that even if there is a levitation position error ($\varepsilon > C$), but there is a positive upwards force ($F > 0$), the position command p^*, will be entirely from the virtual model as the resulting motion will be upwards. This enhances the natural sensation to the operator.

6.2 Experimental setup

A general overview of the experimental setup is shown in Fig. 15, showing the complete prototype (a), the disk during stable levitation (b), and the details of the electrostatic levitator (c). An aluminium hard disk is used as the levitated object as it is freely available and reference literature is available (Jin et al., 1995). The haptic device is based on a SCARA-type robot (Padhy, 1992) and has three DOF, of which currently only one is actively controlled (vertical

Levitation		
Proportional gain z_c	K_{P,z_c}	$10 \cdot 10^6$ V/m
Integral gain z_c	K_{I,z_c}	$5 \cdot 10^6$ V/(m s)
Proportional gain θ_x, θ_y	$K_{P,\theta_x} = K_{P,\theta_y}$	$0.5 \cdot 10^6$ V/rad
Force-voltage relation	k_u	$2.8 \cdot 10^{-4}$ N/V
Force-air gap relation	k_z	-630 N/m
EstatLev stiffness	$k_{EstatLev}$	$2.2 \cdot 10^3$ N/m
Haptic Device		
Haptic integral gain	K'_I	10 s^{-1}
Mechanical stiffness	k	51 kN/m

Table 4. Control settings and other characteristics of electrostatic prototype

translation). More information on the development of this device can be found in (van West, Yamamoto & Higuchi, 2007b). For these experiments, the two rotational degrees of freedom are constraint to have only vertical motion. The input force is measured by a strain-gage load cell (Kyowa LVS-1KA, rated capacity: 10 N, force resolution: 50 mN) and the vertical displacement is generated by a direct motor drive ball screw (SiMB0802). The driving unit is a combination of a stepping motor with a ball screw directly connected to it, such that the need for a coupling is eliminated. As the lead screw is backlash-free, there is some friction in the mechanism. This friction however, will be eliminated by the admittance control loop up to the resolution of the force sensor. Furthermore, the position actuator is highly non-backdrivable, making it very suitable for admittance control.

The stepping motor is pulse-driven (max. 10 kHz) and the manufacturer guarantees no stepping out. Servo control is realized by feedback control on the pulses sent to the motor. The step resolution of the controlled system is set to 8 μm which fixes the maximum speed to 80 mm/s. As velocities in the virtual model can exceed this value, extra damping is automatically added to the virtual model when speed becomes larger than 75 mm/s.

A laser proximity sensor (Keyence LC2440) activates a high damping field when the distance between levitator and pick and place location becomes smaller than 2.5 mm by adding damping with a gradient of 50.000 Ns/m^2. For this experiment, the laser sensor has been mounted to the fixed world, but in the future it will be incorporated in the levitator to allow handling at any location. The nominal damping during normal moving is set to 4 Ns/m and the virtual mass is 1 kg. The haptic gain on the integral of the levitation error K'_I is 10 s^{-1}, set by trial and error.

The levitation air gaps are measured by three eddy-current displacement sensors (Keyence EX-800), which have a sensing range of 0 to 1 mm. The levitation system, virtual model and switching scheme are all integrated on the same digital signal processing (DSP) system, which is running at 20 kHz, with the controller settings as given in Table 4. Note that the Derivative gains (K_D) are zero as the air gap is so small that a natural damping exists and derivative gains are unnecessary. The reference gap is set to 350 μm and the bias voltage V_e is 920 V. The controller output is connected to four high voltage D.C. amplifiers (Trek 609C-6), which have an internal gain of 1000 and are limited on the control side to 1.6 kV in absolute value to prevent electric discharge.

6.3 Experimental results

The performance of this prototype is evaluated by performing a *picking up* and *placing* task. However, no comparison experiments are carried out as in fact it is nearly impossible for the human operator to hold the electrostatic levitator directly without losing the object, let alone performing a pick and place task. Performing the task with the haptic device, but *without* the haptic effect is too dangerous because of the high forces the haptic device can provide.

6.3.1 Picking up

Details of a typical *picking up* task are shown in Fig. 16(a). The force exerted by the operator on the haptic device (force sensor) is shown in the top. A negative force will result in a downwards motion until the disk is picked up and it is followed by a positive force to move levitator and disk upwards. The motion that is sent to the position actuator (p^*) is shown in the two middle plots. The change of speed, resulting from the high damping field is indicated in the graph. To show the influence of the haptic contribution, which is the integral of levitation error to position signal p^* at the switching moment, a zoomed plot of p^* is given together with the output from only the virtual model p_v. The difference between the two plots is the added integral of levitation error $p_{hap,\varepsilon}$. The levitation error itself is plotted in the lowest plot together with the threshold value, such that the switching moments can be easily recognized.

The *picking up* task can be described in four steps. First, the operator moves down by applying a downward force on the haptic device. Downward motion occurs and as soon as it comes in sensing range of the laser sensing, the damping field slows down the motion. Second, the disk comes in sensing range of the levitation gap sensors and will "jump" to the nominal levitation air gap of 350 μm (levitation error is zero). Due to the downward speed of the motion, almost directly after the levitating, the disk touches the support location again, creating a positive levitation error. The switch is activated and resultantly, the position p^* is upwards even though the operator's force is still a negative. This is experienced by the operator as touching a wall. Finally, a positive force from the operator will result in the upwards motion and picking up has been successful.

6.3.2 Placing

Details of a typical *placing* task are shown in Fig. 16(b), which follows the same structure as Fig. 16(a), with the operator's force on the top, the position signal in the middle, and the levitation error on the bottom. The force and motion profile are very similar to the *picking up* task. A negative force from the operator moves the levitated disk down and it is slowed down by the damping field upon detection by the laser sensor. The contact moment can be clearly seen by looking at the levitation error as well as the switching moments that prevent the air gap to become too small. Multiple switching moments can be observed as in fact the operator is still exerting a negative (downward) force. The positive force from the operator will move the electrostatic levitator up, while the disk remains at the support location and placing has been successful.

The actual release of the object is the result of the levitation controller wind up (not shown in the figure) due to the integral gain K_I as described earlier. The integrator reduces the attractive force as long as there is a positive levitation error. If this error persists for some time, the controller output is influenced in such a way, that even if the error is relieved, re-levitation is no longer possible (van West et al., 2008). With this strategy, placing becomes more easy as it is realized automatically.

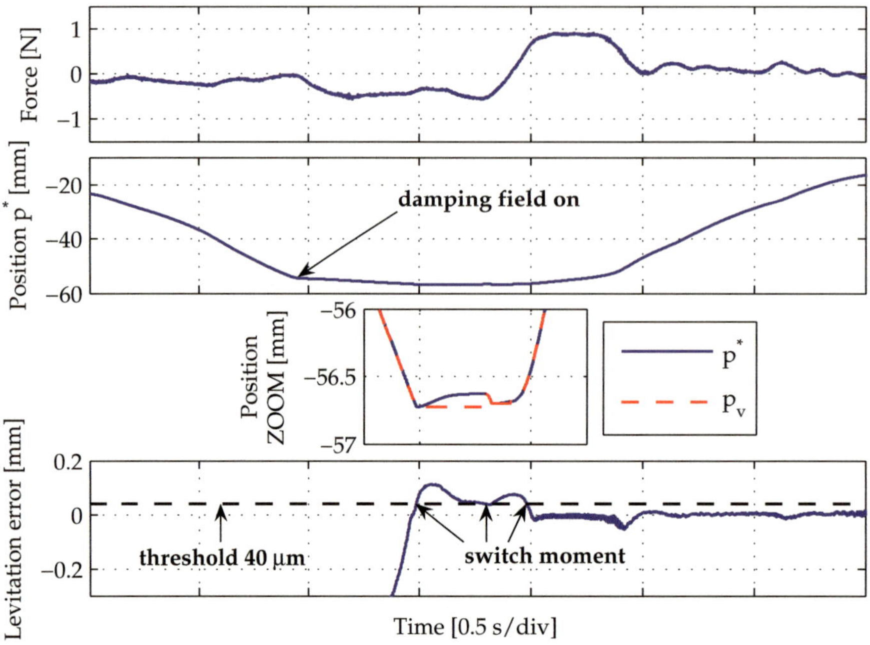

(a) Details of typical picking up

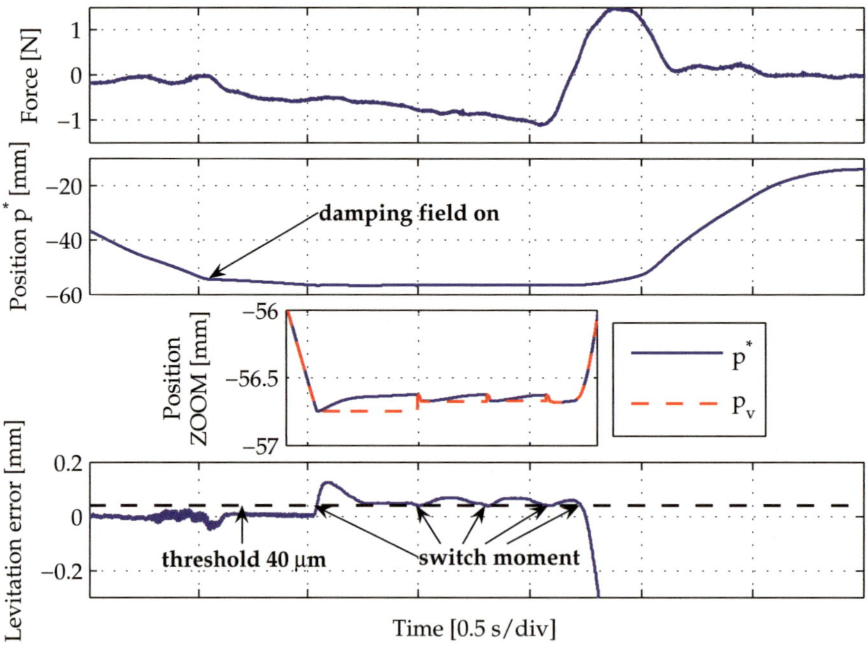

(b) Details of typical placing

Fig. 16. Manipulation using SCARA-type haptic device for electrostatic levitation handling

7. Conclusion

This research has proposed the concept of "Haptic Tweezer," which combines a haptic device with non-contact levitation techniques for intuitive and easy handling of contact-sensitive objects by a human operator. The levitation error of the levitated object is used as an input for the haptic device to minimize disturbances especially in the tasks of *picking up* and *placing*. The concept is evaluated by several prototypes of which two are described in this chapter, one using magnetic levitation and the haptic device PHANTOM Omni using an impedance controlled strategy, and a second prototype that uses electrostatic levitation and a SCRARA-type haptic device using the admittance control strategy. Experiments with the first prototype have showed that significant improvements can be realized through the haptic feedback technology. Not only the failure rates were reduced, but the manipulation time was faster indicating it is easier to perform the manipulation task with haptic assistance. The second prototype showed that the concept can also be successfully applied to handling objects with electrostatic levitation, which is more sensitive to disturbances than magnetic levitation and also has a much smaller levitation gap (350 μm). The haptic assistance makes it possible that a human operator can perform the tasks of *picking up* and *placing* of an aluminium disk which would not have been possible without any haptic assistance. Both cases demonstrate the potential of haptic assistance for real-time assisting in performing tasks like non-contact manipulation.

8. References

Azuma, R., Baillot, Y., Behringer, R., Feiner, S., Julier, S. & MacIntyre, B. (2001). Recent advances in augmented reality, *IEEE Computer Graphics and Applications* **21**(6): 34 – 47.

Azuma, R. T. (1997). A survey of augmented reality, *Presence: Teleoperators and Virtual Environments* **6**(4): 355–385.

Bettini, A., Marayong, P., Lang, S., Okamura, A. M. & Hager, G. D. (2004). Vision-assisted control for manipulation using virtual fixtures, *IEEE Transactions on Robotics* **20**(6): 953 – 966.

Bhushan, B. (2003). Adhesion and stiction: mechanisms, measurement techniques, and methods for reduction, *Journal of Vacuum Science & Technology B (Microelectronics and Nanometer Structures)* **21**(6): 2262 – 96.

Earnshaw, S. (1842). On the nature of the molecular forces which regulate the constitution of the luminiferous ether, *Trans. Camb. Phil. Soc.* **7**: 97–112.

Hayashibara, Y., Tanie, K., Arai, H. & Tokashiki, H. (1997). Development of power assist system with individual compensation ratios for gravity and dynamic load, *Proc. IEEE International Conference on Intelligent Robots and Systems IROS97*, pp. 640–646.

Jin, J., Higuchi, T. & Kanemoto, M. (1994). Electrostatic silicon wafer suspension, *Fourth International Symposium on Magnetic Bearings*, ETH Zurich, pp. 343 – 348.

Jin, J., Higuchi, T. & Kanemoto, M. (1995). Electrostatic levitator for hard disk media, *IEEE Transactions on Industrial Electronics* **42**(5): 467 – 73.

Kazerooni, H. (1996). The human power amplifier technology at the university of california, berkeley, *Robotics and Autonomous Systems* **19**(2): 179 – 187.

Kazerooni, H. & Steger, R. (2006). The berkeley lower extremity exoskeleton, *Journal of Dynamic Systems, Measurement and Control, Transactions of the ASME* **128**(1): 14 – 25.

Lee, H.-K., Takubo, T., Arai, H. & Tanie, K. (2000). Control of mobile manipulators for power assist systems, *Journal of Robotic Systems* **17**(9): 469 – 77.

Lin, H. C., Mills, K., Kazanzides, P., Hager, G. D., Marayong, P., Okamura, A. M. & Karam, R. (2006). Portability and applicability of virtual fixtures across medical and manufacturing tasks, *Proc. IEEE Int. Conf. Rob. Autom. ICRA06*, Orlando, Florida.

Morishita, M. & Azukizawa, T. (1988). Zero power control of electromagnetic levitation system, *Electrical Engineering in Japan* **108**(3): 111–120.

Nojima, T., Sekiguchi, D., Inami, M. & Tachi, S. (2002). The smarttool: A system for augmented reality of haptics, *Proc. Virtual Reality Annual International Symposium*, Orlando, FL, pp. 67 – 72.

Padhy, S. (1992). On the dynamics of scara robot, *Robotics and Autonomous Systems* **10**(1): 71 – 78.

Peshkin, M., Colgate, J., Wannasuphoprasit, W., Moore, C., Gillespie, R. & Akella, P. (2001). Cobot architecture, *IEEE Transactions on Robotics and Automation* **17**(4): 377 – 390.

Rollot, Y., Regnier, S. & Guinot, J.-C. (1999). Simulation of micro-manipulations: Adhesion forces and specific dynamic models, *International Journal of Adhesion and Adhesives* **19**(1): 35 – 48.

Rosenberg, L. B. (1993). Virtual fixtures: perceptual tools for telerobotic manipulation, *IEEE Virtual Reality Annual International Symposium*, Seattle, WA, USA, pp. 76 – 82.

Schweitzer, G., Bleuler, H. & Traxler, A. (1994). *Active Magnetic Bearings*, vdf Hochschulverlag AG an der ETH Zürich.

Taylor, R., Jensen, P., Whitcomb, L., Barnes, A., Kumar, R., Stoianovici, D., Gupta, P., Wang, Z., deJuan, E. & Kavoussi, L. (1999). a steady-hand robotic system for microsurgical augmentation, *International Journal of Robotics Research* **18**(12): 1201 – 1210.

van der Linde, R. & Lammertse, P. (2003). Hapticmaster - a generic force controlled robot for human interaction, *Industrial Robot* **30**(6): 515–24.

van West, E., Yamamoto, A., Burns, B. & Higuchi, T. (2007). Non-contact handling of hard-disk media by human operator using electrostatic levitation and haptic device, *Proceedings of the 2007 IEEE/RSJ International Conference on Intelligent Robots and Systems IROS'07*, San Diego, CA, USA, pp. 1106–11.

van West, E., Yamamoto, A. & Higuchi, T. (2007a). The concept of "haptic tweezer", a non-contact object handling system using levitation techniques and haptics, *Mechatronics* **17**(7): 345–356.

van West, E., Yamamoto, A. & Higuchi, T. (2007b). Development of scara-type haptic device for electrostatic non-contact handling system, *Journal of Advanced Mechanical Design, Systems, and Manufacturing* **2**(2): 180–190.

van West, E., Yamamoto, A. & Higuchi, T. (2008). Automatic object release in magnetic and electrostatic levitation systems, *Precision Engineering* **33**: 217–228.

Woo, S. J., Jeon, J. U., Higuchi, T. & Jin, J. (1995). Electrostatic force analysis of electrostatic levitation system, *Proceedings of the 34th SICE Annual Conference*, Hokkaido, Japan, pp. 1347–52.

36

Haptics and the Biometric Authentication Challenge

Andrea Kanneh and Ziad Sakr
University of Trinidad and Tobago, O'Meara Campus
Trinidad and Tobago

1. Introduction

There has been an increasing demand for on-line activities such as e-banking, e-learning and e-commerce. However, these on-line activities continue to be marred by evolving security challenges. On-line verification is now central to security discussions.

The use of biometrics for individual authentication has always existed. Physiological biometrics, which is based on physical features, is a widespread practice. Behavioural biometrics, however, is based on what we do in our day-to-day activities such as walking or signing our names. Current research trends have been focusing on behavioural biometrics as this type of authentication is less intrusive.

Haptics has come a long way since the first glove or robot hand. Haptics has played an immense role in virtual reality and real-time interactions. Although gaming, medical training and miniaturisation continue to prove the enrichments created by haptics technology, as haptic devices become more obtainable, this technology will not only serve to enhance the human-computer interface but also to enhance cyber security in the form of on-line biometric security.

Limited research has been done on the combination of haptics and biometrics. To date, dynamic on-line verification has been widely investigated using devices which do not provide the user with force feedback. Haptics technology allows the use of force feedback as an additional dimension. This key behavioural biometric measure can be extracted by the haptics device during any course of action. This research has significant implications for all areas of on-line verification, from financial applications to gaming. Future challenges include incorporating this technology seamlessly into our day to day devices and operations.

This chapter starts with a brief overview of security. This is followed by an introduction to key concepts associated with biometrics. Current on-line dynamic signature verification is then reviewed before the concept of the integration of haptics and biometrics is introduced. The chapter then explores the current published work in this area. The chapter concludes with a discussion on the current challenges of haptic and biometric authentication and predicts a possible path for the future.

2. Motivation

This chapter seeks to illustrate that the haptic force extracted from a user with a haptic device could be used for biometric authentication. It further shows that this form of authentication (using haptic forces) can potentially add to the accuracy of current on-line authentication.

3. The challenges of On-line Security

Security mechanisms exist to provide security services such as authentication, access control, data integrity, confidentiality and non repudiation and may include the mechanisms such as biometric authentication and/or security audit trails (Stallings, 2006).

On-line security is of particular importance especially for activities such as on-line banking or e-payments. Cyber attacks continue to increase and can take many forms. An example of this was the Banker Trojan which was created to copy passwords, credit card information and account numbers associated with on-line banking services from the user's PC.

In order for security mechanisms to work every link in the chain must work. This includes personal and/or resource passwords. People's habits or the security culture within organisations, such as sharing passwords or writing them down, or not logging off when they step away from the computer can break down most security systems. Often these habits are hard to monitor and prevent (Herath & Rao, 2009; Kraemera et al., 2009) yet in spite of this, text passwords remain popular as they are relatively easy to implement and still accepted by users. For the actual username–password method to be effective, it is essential that users generate and use (and remember) strong passwords that are resistant to guessing and cracking (Vu et al., 2007).

Biometric authentication cannot solve every problem with on-line security but it can be used to overcome some of these issues associated with passwords and system access. Biometric security can also provide a measure of continuous authentication when performing the actual transaction. The use of biometric security does not leave the user with something to remember or to write down. Dhamija and Dusseault (2008) suggest that users are more likely to accept a security system if it is simple to use.

4. Biometrics and Individual Authentication

4.1 Biometric Concepts

Biometrics is described as the science of recognizing an individual based on his or her physical or behavioural traits (Jain et al., 2006). Since a biometric is either a physical or behavioural characteristic of the user it is almost impossible to copy or steal. The use of biometrics as a security measure offers many benefits such as increasing individual user accountability or decreasing number of Personal Identification Numbers (PINs) and passwords per user. This in turn allows stronger security measures for remaining PINs and passwords.

Biometric security has existed since the beginning of man - recognising someone by face or voice. Fingerprint biometrics dates back to ancient China. A formal approach for commercial use dates back to the 1960s and 1970s as is the case with fingerprint scanning, which has been around since the late 1960s (Dunstone, 2001).

Biometrics authentication refers to both verification and/or identification. In verification the subject claims to be a specific person and a one-to-one comparison is done. Whereas, with identification the applicant's data is matched against all the information stored or the entire database to determine his/her identity. This is a one-to-many task.

There are many applications of biometrics for both security and confidentiality. These include law enforcement and forensics, access control, and preventing/detecting fraud in organisations, educational institutions and electronic resources. Biometric Encryption also exists. This is the process of using a characteristic of the body as a method to code/encrypt/decrypt data. This can be used in asymmetric encryption to generate the private key.

Jain et al. (2004) outlined some characteristics of efficient biometric systems:
(i) Universality — every person should have the characteristics.
(ii) Distinctiveness — no two persons should have the exact biometric characteristics.
(iii) Permanence — characteristics should be invariant with time.
(iv) Collectability —characteristics must be measurable quantitatively.
(v) Performance — the biometric system accuracy, speed, consistency and robustness should be acceptable
(vi) Acceptability — users must be willing to accept and use the system.
(vii) Circumvention —fooling the system should be difficult.

4.2 Biometric Techniques

There are two types of biometric techniques - physiological and behavioural. Physiological techniques are based physical characteristics. Examples include fingerprint recognition, iris recognition, face recognition, hand geometry (finger lengths, finger widths, palm width, etc.), blood vessel pattern in the hand, DNA, palm print (apart from hand geometry), body odour, ear shape and fingernail bed (apart from fingerprints).

Behavioural techniques are based on the things you do (a trained act or skill that the person unconsciously does as a behavioural pattern). Examples include voice recognition, keystroke recognition (distinctive rhythms in the timing between keystrokes for certain pairs of characters), signature recognition (handwriting or character shapes, timing and pressure of the signature process). Gait recognition or the pattern of walking or locomotion is also used as a biometric measure (Ortega-Garcia et al., 2004).

4.3 The Biometric Process

The Biometric Process has two stages - enrolment and authentication. Each user must first be enrolled in the system. Here the aim is to capture data from the biometric device which can identify the uniqueness of each subject as it is essential to establish a 'true' identity. The key features for each user are then extracted from this data and stored in a database. These features could be common for all users or customised, either by weights assigned to show the importance of the feature or by selecting different features, for each user. Usually before feature extraction/selection there is some form of pre-processing in which the data is made more manageable for extraction. Some form of normalisation or smoothing may be done at this stage. After the template is created for each user (during enrolment), a new sample is taken and compared to the template. This creates the genuine distance measure (Wayman, 2000). The average genuine distance for the whole sample population can be used as a common threshold or the threshold can be unique for each user.

During the authentication (identification and/or verification) process new samples taken from the subject are compared to the stored data and a match score is computed to determine the fit. The match score is compared to the threshold score and if it is greater that the threshold score this is not considered to be a fit. The general biometric process is shown in the figure below (Fig. 1.). This is them summarised in the table which follows (Table 1).

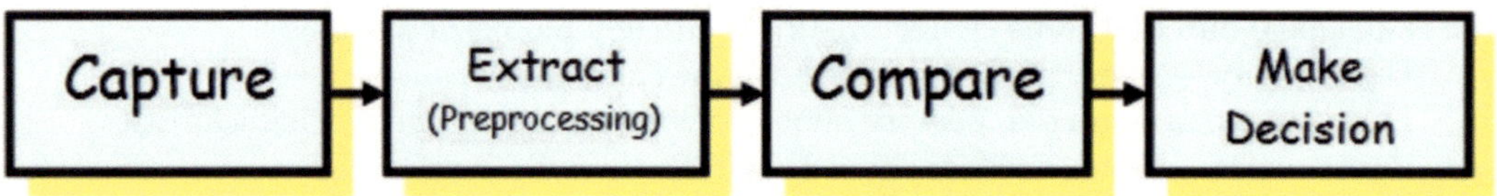

Fig. 1. The Biometric Process

Stage of Process	Activity
Capture	A physical or behavioural sample is captured by the system during enrolment. (Data Collection); this is influenced by the technical characteristics of the sensor, the actual measure and the way the measure is presented.
Extraction	Unique data is extracted from the sample and a template is created. Distinctive and repeatable features are selected. Feature templates are stored in the database.
Comparison/ Classification	The new sample is then compared with the existing templates. Distance Measures (DM) are calculated and compared to threshold(s). DM Never zero because of variability due to human, sensor, presentation , environment
Decision-making	The system then decides if the features extracted from the new sample are a match or a non-match based on the threshold match score.

Table 1. The Biometric Process explained

4.4 Some Challenges with Biometric Authentication

A biometric system cannot guarantee accuracy partly due to the variability in humans, the systems and the environment. Stress, general health, working and environmental conditions and time pressures all contribute to variable results (Roethenbaugh, 1997). Some of these factors are explained in Table. 2.

There are two main accuracy measures used: False Accept and False Reject. False Accept error occurs when an applicant, who should be rejected, is accepted. False Accept Rate (FAR) or Type II error rate is the percentage of applicants who should be rejected but are instead accepted. False Reject Rate (FRR) or Type I error rate is the percentage of legitimate users who are denied access or rejected. These two measures are also referred to as false match or false non-match rates respectively.

Since these are two different measures it is difficult to judge the performance of the system base on only one measure so both are usually plotted on a Receiving/Relative Operating Curve (ROC) (Martin et al., 2007; Wayman, 2000) which is a graph of FAR as a function of FRR (Gamboa and Fred, 2004). The equal error rate (EER) is defined as the value at which FAR and FRR are equal. This can be used as a single measure to evaluate the accuracy of the biometric system.

Factor affecting performance	Example
Environmental conditions	Extreme temperature and humidity can affect a system's performance
The age, gender, ethnic background and occupation of the user	Dirty hands from manual work can affect the performance of fingerprint systems
The beliefs, desires and intentions of the user	If a user does not wish to interact with the system, then performance will be affected. E.g. the user may deliberately control his/her typing speed
The physical make-up of the user	A user with no limbs cannot use hand or finger-based biometrics

Table 2. Factors affecting accuracy of biometric measurements

The UK Government Test Protocol for Biometric Devices (Mansfield et al., 2001) is a standard protocol which could be used for commercially available biometric devices. It suggests some time lapse between the collection of trials for template creation (to cater for the aging or learning process). Two common system errors are Failure to enrol and Failure to Acquire. Failure to enrol occurs when the system is unable to generate repeatable templates for a given user. This may be because the person is unable to present the required feature. Failure to acquire occurs when the system is unable to capture and/or extract quality information from an observation. This may be due to device/software malfunction, environmental concerns and human anomalies.

The following diagrams sums up some of the possible errors within each stage of the process.

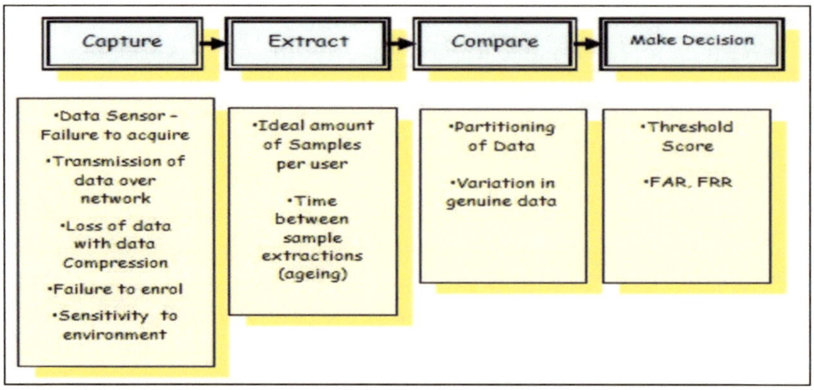

Fig. 2. Some possible errors within the Biometric Process

4.5. Multimodal Biometrics

A multimodal approach could be adopted to make a biometric system more secure. A layered or multimodal biometrics approach uses two or more independent systems or techniques to yield greater accuracy due to the statistical independence of the selected approaches. Therefore more than one identifier is used to compare the identity of the subject. This approach is also called multiple biometrics (Huang et al., 2008). Ortega-Garcia et al. (2004) refers to this as unimodal-fusion or monomodal-fusion.

5. Dynamic Signature Verification: a form of Biometric Authentication

Dynamic signature verification (DSV) can capture not only the shape of the image, as is done with static signature recognition, but also the space-time relationship created by the signature. Both static and dynamic signature verification are forms of biometric authentication.

Numerous studies have been done on dynamic signature verification - Plamondon (Plamondon & Srihari, 2000) and Jain (Jain et al., 2002) are just two of the popular names associated with these studies. Some of the work done on DSV follow.

In a study by Lee et al. (1996) individual feature sets as well as individual thresholds were used. The authors suggested that if time is an issue then a common feature set should be used. These features were captured using a graphics tablet (or digitising tablet, graphics pad, drawing tablet). Normalisation was done using factors such as total writing time (time-normalised features), total horizontal displacement, and total vertical displacement. Majority classifiers (implementing the majority decision rule) were used in the classification stage.

To decrease processing time a simple comparison was done before the classification stage - this took the form of 'prehard' and 'presoft' classifiers. This was done by comparing the absolute value of writing time of the signature being tested minus the average writing time. With the presoft classifier if this value was below a certain level (.2) the data did not need to be normalised before extraction. For the prehard classifier if this value was too high the data was instantly rejected. They were able to achieve 0% FRR and 7%FAR.

Penagos et al (1996) also used customised feature selection – the weight assigned to each feature was adjusted for each feature of each user. The common features selected were the starting location, size, and total duration of the signature. As in Lee et al. (1996) the threshold was also customised for each user. The customised thresholds were adjusted, if needed, until either their signatures were accepted repeatedly, or the maximum threshold value was reached. The experiment was conducted with the use of a digitizing tablet to extract features such as shape of signature, pressure (measured with the stylus), speed and acceleration. Normalisation was done on the time, position and acceleration values. They were able to achieve an 8% FRR and 0%FAR.

Plamondon & Srihari (2000) presented a survey paper on on-line and off-line handwriting recognition and verification. It suggested that at the time of this article (2000), even if verification was being researched for about three decades, the level of accuracy was still not high enough for situations needing high level of accuracy such as banking. The survey listed several techniques used for user verification, they include neural networks, probabilistic classifiers, minimal distance classifiers, nearest neighbour, dynamic programming, time warping, and threshold based classifier. One point highlighted was that before recognition noise is removed by a smoothing algorithm, signal filtering.

Jain et al. (2002) used writer-dependent threshold scores for the classification stage. For their experiment, like the ones above, a digitising tablet was used. The features were separated into Global (properties of the whole signature e.g. total writing time) and Local (properties that refer to a position within the signature e.g. pressure at a point). Prior to the feature selection stage a Gaussian filter was used to smooth the signatures. Number of individual strokes and absolute speed normalized by the average signing speed were some of the features used. Dynamic Time Warping was used to compare strings. The experiment yielded a FRR of 2.8% and a FAR or 1.6%.

Some studies focus on the best selection of the features, for example Lei & Govindaraju, (2005). In this paper they compared the discriminative power of the biometric features. Here the position features were normalised by dividing by the maximum height or maximum width. The authors compared the mean or average consistency for each feature, the standard deviation over subjects, and EER of selected features. The authors highlighted the fact that a high standard deviation implies that this feature may not discriminate itself among users. Low mean consistency implies that this feature varies among one user. The results showed that some features such as the speed, the coordinate sequence, and the angle were consistent and reliable.

In most studies the features were first normalised to make them easier to select and compare. Dimauro et al. (2004) suggested that the data should be first filtered then normalised in time-duration and size domain. Faundez-Zanuy (2005) stated that length normalisation was used because different repetitions of signature from a given person could have different durations.

Feature such as 2D position and speed were common features selected. McCabe et al. (2008) used other features such as aspect ratio (This is the ratio of the writing length to the writing height). Number of "pen-ups" (This indicates the number of times the pen is lifted while signing after the first contact with the tablet and excluding the final pen-lift). Top Heaviness (This is a measure of the proportion of the signature that lies above the vertical midpoint i.e., the ratio of point density at the top half of the signature versus the density at the bottom half), and Area (This is the actual area of the handwritten word). They used a neural network for user verification. The FAR was as low as 1.1% with a 2.2% FRR.

Recently Eoff and Hammond (2009) obtained accuracy of 97.5% and 83.5% for two and ten users respectively. The study was used to identify different user strokes on a shared (collaborative) surface. Here the authors used pen tilt, pressure and speed to classify users. A Tablet PC was used to capture the strokes of users.

Unlike the other studies discussed, C Hook et al. (2003) did not use the digitising tablet. They presented a study of a biometrical smart pen BiSP. In this study the pen itself was able to capture measures such as pressure and acceleration. This study took a multimodal approach - it also used fingerprint information as well as acoustic information for authentication. Results showed accuracy of up to 80% for user identification and 90% for user verification.

6. Haptic Devices and Biometrics

6.1 Haptics Force Feedback

Haptic, from the Greek αφή (Haphe) means pertaining to the sense of touch. Touch is different from sight and sound because with touch there is an exchange of energy between the user and the physical world: as the user pushes on an object, it pushes back on the user (Salisbury & Srinivasan, 1997).

Haptic interfaces allow a user to touch, feel, and manipulate three-dimensional objects in a virtual environment (Orozco et al., 2006).

Haptics not only refers to tactation (the distribution of pressure on the skin), it includes the study of movement and position, which is kinesthetics. Rendering techniques aim to provide reasonable feedback to users for instance the shape of the object, the texture of the surface and a sense of the force exerted by the user to achieve the task at hand (the mass of the object). Haptics applications can offer both spatial and temporal information.

The concept of the haptic force has been used in entertainment, training and education but, compared to these, haptics in security is relatively new. The haptic force can also be used to uniquely identify persons. The following diagram (Fig.3.) shows the force produced by two different subjects carrying out the same task. The individuals were provided with a surface which provided enough friction and softness to mimic a paper surface, and asked to write the same letter of the alphabet. As the number of users increase it is not as easy for the human eye to differentiate so this is why computer generated classification algorithms are applied.

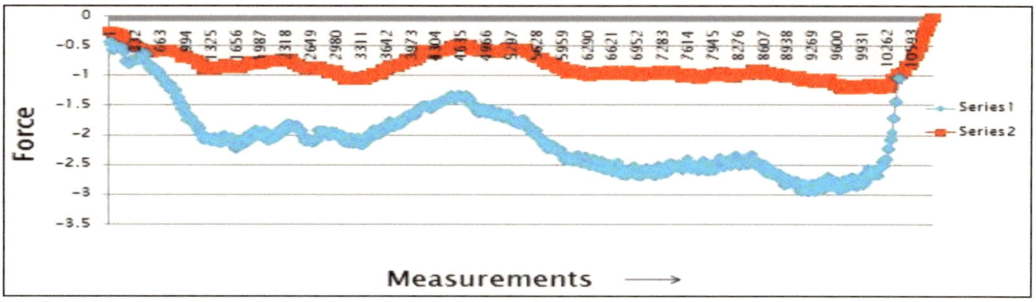

Fig. 3. Difference Force measurements produced by two users

While passwords and other access control provide some level of security, haptic devices can be used to supply behavioural biometrics such as force, position and angular orientation, which can provide ongoing/continuous security assessment while the user is using the system, thereby making haptics a good facilitator for (biometrics) signature recognition.

6.2 Haptics and Biometrics

A number of haptic devices exist, one of which is the PHANToM (The Personal Haptic Interface Mechanism) device (http://www.reachin.se/) which allows the user to feel virtual objects in a 3D space (Fig. 5).

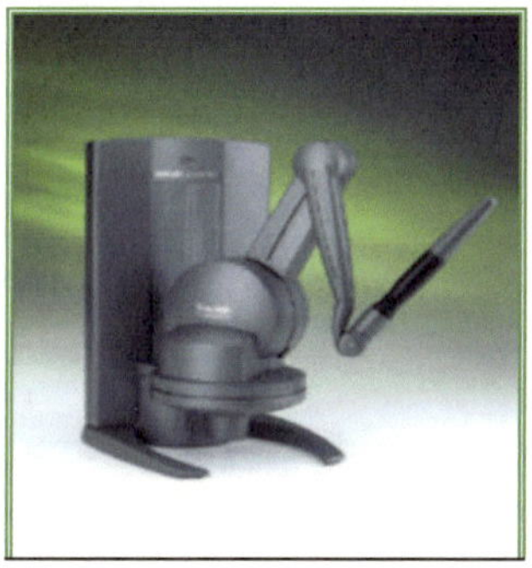

(a) The Phantom Desktop

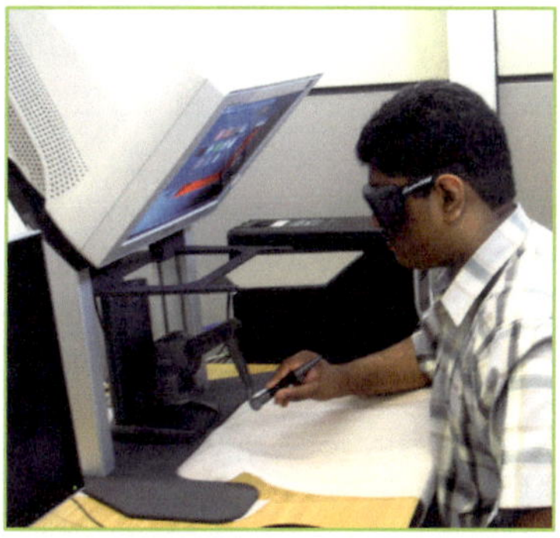

(b) The Reachin device form SensAble uses the Phantom Desktop as one of its components

Fig. 4. The Phantom Desktop and the Reachin Device

The PHANToM is part of the Reachin Desktop (Fig. 4b.). This device is able to extract and provide the same data as the digital tablets and more, such as force and torque, as well as the xyz (3D) coordinates all of which can fall under the heading of behavioural biometrics. Haptic devices can make biometric authentication (for access control) even more effective as the imposter using the device, to fool the system, can no longer just copy the visual output of the signature or activity, but now has to replicate the force produced by the user at a particular position, at the relative time (to the length of the signature) that that force was produced. Unlike the digitising tablet, haptic devices act like an output as well as input device. Even though the stylus tip of the digital tablets may sense pressure, they do not provide the force feedback to the user.

The following papers present several applications with haptics and biometrics. The work was done at the Distributed & Collaborative Virtual Environments Research Laboratory, University of Ottawa, Canada. Each application captured similar measurements such as force, time and momentum. The Reachin device was used in these studies. The general aim of these experiments was to explore the use of the Reachin haptic device to gain continuous authentication of the user based on the behavioural biometrics obtained from the interaction with the on screen application. Accuracy ranged from 80% (Orozco et al., 2005b) to 95.4% (Orozco et al., 2006a) with some initial findings showing the possibility of reaching accuracy as high as 98.4% (Orozco et al., 2006a). Classification algorithms comprised nearest neighbour, k-means, artificial neural networks and spectral analysis. Relative Entropy was used for feature selection. For the studies which follow the participants were given some time to familiarise themselves with the application.

The Virtual Phone experiment (Orozco et al., 2005a, 2005b) was conducted to analyse the unique characteristics of individual behaviour while using an everyday device (a virtual phone). 20 subjects were asked to dial the same code 10 times (Orozco et al., 2005b). Specific measures obtainable from the experiment include hand-finger positions, force applied to the keypad as well as time interval between pressing each key. The results of the experiment revealed that features such as force, velocity and keystroke duration were not as distinguishable as those related to the pen position. In this experiment they were able to attain about 20% FRR (Orozco et al., 2005b).

The Virtual Maze experiment (Orozco et al., 2006a, 2006b; El Saddik et al., 2007) aimed to identify the unique psychomotor (combined physical and mental) patterns of individuals participants based on their manipulation of haptic devices. In this case a virtual 2D maze on a 3D space was used. Data collected included xyz position, velocity, 3D force and torque from 39 subjects (Orozco et al., 2006a). Relative entropy was used for feature extraction, and comparison was done using Hidden Markov Models, Fast Fourier Transform spectral analysis and Dynamic Time Warping (Orozco et al., 2006b).

User dependent thresholds were also tested which improved the verification accuracy produce with a common threshold (Orozco et al., 2006a). The study also looked at the effect of introducing stress (Orozco et al., 2006a). This resulted in more variability and hence lower accuracy (66% FRR). The results of the paper showed that the haptic devices were more successful at verification than identification. They were able to attain 4.6%FRR with 16% FAR for verification (Orozco et al., 2006a).

The Virtual Cheque experiment (El Saddik et al., 2007) was created with the aim of removing any mental interference that could affect performance. Pen position, force exerted and velocity were extracted from the 16 subjects used. Relative entropy was first used to analyse the information content and signal processing was used to form the biometric profile. In classifier design a quantitative match score was calculated and used for the comparison and make decision stages. K-Means was used to cluster the features. It was found that Force data had the most information. The equal error rate fell between 6 % and 9% for the virtual cheque verification. Virtual signature verification was 8% FRR with 25% FAR. Some information was lost due to data compression which was used to reduce the storage requirement.

It is necessary to note that the authors concluded, based on their results, that these experiments (in this section) were more suitable for verification than identification (El Saddik et al., 2007). It was also observed that features such as speed became more consistent in the later trials than the initial ones as the participants became more comfortable with time (Orozco et al., 2005b; El Saddik et al., 2007).

Orozco et al. (2006c) also used a virtual grid. The user created a hapto-graphical password by navigating through the grid and selecting and connecting nodes on the grid, using a stylus. Features such as force, torque, angular orientation, and 3D position were selected. They also looked at pen-ups during the execution as was done in the study conducted by McCabe et al. (2008). Biometric classification was done with algorithms such as Nearest Neighbour and Artificial Neural Networks..

6.3 A Detailed description of a verification scheme

Our studies (Kanneh & Sakr., 2008a-d) presented a new algorithm for user verification. In our approach a fuzzy logic controller was used to mimic human reasoning in decision making. The user was instructed to trace a circle in particular direction. (Fig. 5.)

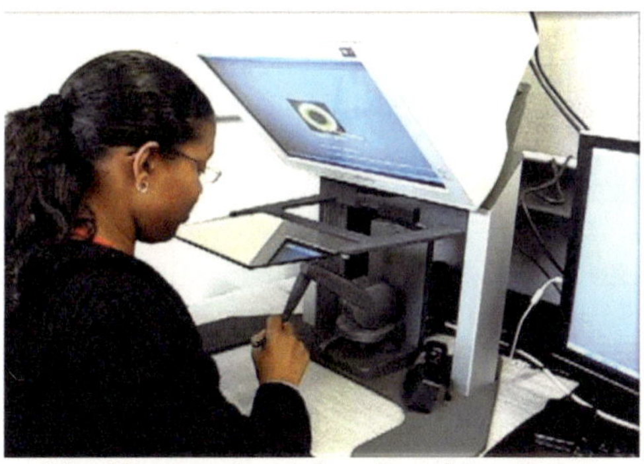

(a) User using the Reachin Device to trace the virtual circle

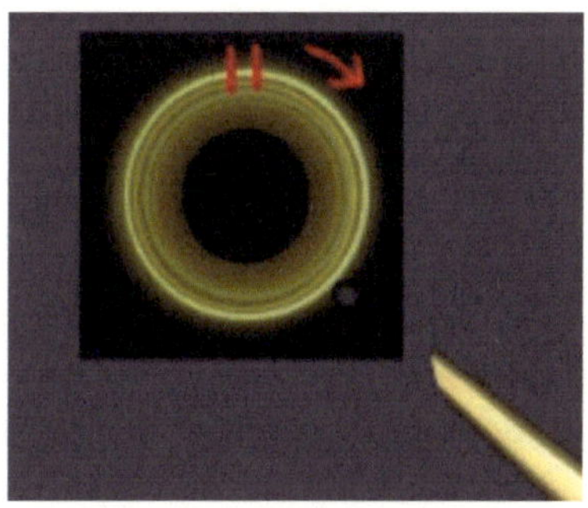

(b) The User Interface

Fig. 5. The Haptics and Biometrics Verification System

Limiting the direction was done to place some extra stress on the system to test just how effective the verification algorithm would be. In a real world application the user would be allowed to go in his/her preferred direction and this should improve the accuracy of verification even more. The Reachin Device and Application Programmer Interface (API) were used for this experiment. 9 participants were tested. These studies also introduced normalisation or standardisation of features based on their standard deviations. This process made each subject's data more distinguishable.

Principal Component Analysis was then used for feature selection. Seven features were chosen - force values at different positions, average size of the radius drawn, XYZ Distances and time. It was found that the XYZ distances provided the most information for this system. Based on the unique method of normalisation, as well as the use of the fuzzy logic templates for classification, the experiment yielded a verification accuracy of up to 96.25% with a 3.75% FRR and an 8.9% FAR (Kanneh & Sakr., 2008d).

The Reachin Haptic system used for these experiments (sections 6.2 and 6.3) exhibited the properties of a good biometric system outlined by Jain et al. (2004). The experiments showed that while some features were not distinguishable for every application such as force data with the virtual phone (Orozco et al., 2006c) the force data was key for the virtual cheque (El Saddik et al., 2007). This shows that there is no one recipe (group of algorithms) that could be applied to all experiments - the target application dictated the key features that could be used for classification.

7. Current Challenges with Haptics and Biometrics

Based on the current work discussed in sections 6.2 and 6.3 the concept of biometrics based on haptics is reasonable. The experiments all show that there is greater potential to be explored. As haptic devices become cheaper and more commonplace user acceptance of a new method of authentication will be more probable. There are some variability issues due to the users, system and environment which affect most biometric systems. In addition to this variability within the trials, handwriting can also change with time. Using soft algorithms such as fuzzy logic and neural networks reduces the effects of variability. Both neural networks and dynamic fuzzy logic can cope with the gradual change in handwriting.

Users also pointed out some Human-Computer Interaction (HCI)/ergonomics issues such as the difficulty, on first contact, to sense the distance to touch the virtual surface and the discomfort caused by not being able to rest down the hand when using the Rechin device (Kanneh & Sakr, 2008d) (see figures 4b and 5a). As the technology becomes more available some of these HCI issues would be resolved.

Coping with problem signers is another issue with biometric security (Penagos, 1996). These signers have very variable signatures making template creation (to yield good FAR and FRR) almost impossible. There is always the possibility of the failure to enrol and failure to acquire errors (Mansfield et al., 2001) where the user is not able to perform the action required by the system or produces features with insufficient quality to register. Fàbregas & Faundez-Zanuy, (2009) proposed a system to guide the user through the process which reduces this error and also identifies those individuals who cannot be enrolled.

With respect to haptic devices there is a key issue which needs to be addressed, that is interoperability across different operating systems and different versions of a device and device API. Haptic rendering is also still a work in progress as the haptic force sometimes becomes unstable under certain conditions.

Though biometrics presents a viable security measure there are some concerns specific to Biometrics. Standards are still being developed. Standards are essential for interoperability among vendors. Without standards biometrics is not cost beneficial to the potential user or the vendor. Another issue is that user data must be collected first to create the templates used for authentication. This becomes an issue for large-scale identification for example most terrorist are unknown. Security of the template database must also be addressed (Shan et al., 2008). When a typical password is compromised it can be changed. Unlike passwords, when a person's key feature (biometric) is copied, the template cannot be changed. This is referred to as the revocation problem (Panko, 2004).

According to Wayman (2000) and Mansfield et al. (2001) the sample size for biometric device evaluation should be large enough to represent the population and contain enough samples from each category of the population (from genuine individuals and impostors). In addition to this the test period should be close as possible to the actual period of the application's use. Both requirements increase the budget for testing and as a result, are usually not carried out.

There are other independent security issues which would not be solved with the use of a haptics device. Phishing and spam are just some of these issues. Shan et al. (2008) discuss various potential security threats to biometric systems, providing some food for thought when evaluating the storage and transfer of the unique biometric features in a biometric system. The authors seem to focus on this aspect as they appreciate the growing importance of e-commerce and the security of transactions.

8. Conclusion

The chapter shows that the potential for greater accuracy for on-line verification exists with the use of haptic devices by extracting data which is available from the digital tables in use as well as force data. Though experimental data using haptic devices are limited, the experiments covered showed that verification accuracy is very high- up to 96% (Kanneh & Sakr, 2008d). The potential exists for these results to be further improved with the use of customised threshold scores and customised feature selection (Lee et al., 1996; Penpgosl et al., 1996; Plamondon & Srihari, 2000).

Neural networks and other soft approaches can also be explored further with a view to increasing the authentication accuracy. There is a wealth of experiments with dynamic signature verification which could be altered by using a haptics device instead of the digital tablet.

It is worth noting that the haptics and biometrics experiments (sections 6.2 and 6.3) have been conducted in a controlled environment with engineering students as subjects. According to the target applications intended, the evaluation of the particular haptic device should again be done with the sample representative of the target population (Mansfield et al., 2001).

Haptics as a form of biometrics is a potential goldmine but it is still a work in progress. The accuracy of a biometric system can be further improved using a form of fusion with other independent biometric features or with the traditional password or smart card. These are multimodal approaches (discussed in section 4.5).

Haptics security need not only be applied to on-line activities. This concept of haptics and biometrics can be used within organisations for access to key areas. Both textual and graphical passwords could be supported with the use of haptic devices. Future research can explore the role of Haptics based biometric security in smart houses as ambient intelligence is gaining more and more interest.

Acknowledgements

Special thanks for the ongoing support of our families, as well as for the support of the staff and students of the University of Trinidad and Tobago and the Distributed & Collaborative Virtual Environments Research Laboratory, University of Ottawa.

9. References

Dhamija, R. & Dusseault, L. (2008) *The Seven Flaws of Identity Management: Usability and Security Challenges*. IEEE Security and Privacy, Vol. 6, No. 2, Mar./Apr. 2008, pp. 24-29, Institute of Electrical and Electronics Engineers (IEEE), USA

Dimauro, G., Impedovo, S., Lucchese, M.G., Modugno, R. & Pirlo, G. (2004). *Recent Advancements in Automatic Signature Verification*. Proceedings of the 9th International Workshop on Frontiers in Handwriting Recognition (IWFHR-9 2004), 0-7695-2187-8 Kokubunji, Tok, Oct. 2004, Institute of Electrical and Electronics Engineers (IEEE)

Dunstone, S. (2001). *Emerging Biometric Developments: Identifying The Missing Pieces For Industry*. Proceedings of Sixth International Symposium on Signal Processing and its Applications. vol.1. *pp*.351-354, 0-7803-6703-0, Kuala Lumpur, Malaysia, Institute of Electrical and Electronics Engineers (IEEE), USA

El Saddik, A., Orozco, M., Asfaw, Y., Shirmohammadi, S. & Adler, A (2007). A Novel Biometric System for Identification and Verification of Haptic Users. *IEEE Transactions on Instrumentation and Measurement*, Vol.56, No.3, (June 2007), (895-906), 0018-9456

Eoff, B.D. & Hammond, T. (2009). *Who Dotted That 'i'? : Context Free User Differentiation through Pressure and Tilt Pen Data*. Proceedings of Graphics Interface 2009, Vol. 324 pp. 149-156, 978-1-56881-470-4, Kelowna, British Columbia, Canada, 2009, Canadian Information Processing Society Toronto, Ont., Canada, Canada

Fàbregas, J. & Faundez-Zanuy, M. (2009). On-line signature verification system with failure to enrol management. *Science Direct Pattern Recognition Elsevier Ltd,* Vol.42 No.8, (September 2009), (2117-2126), 0031-3203

Faundez-Zanuy, M. (2005). Signature Recognition – State of the art. IEEE Aerospace and Electronic Systems Magazine, Vol. 20, Issue: 7, July 2005, pp: 28- 32, 0885-8985

Gamboa, H. and Fred, A. (2004). *A Behavioural Biometric System Based on Human Computer Interaction*. Proceedings of SPIE Vol. 5404, pp. 381-392, 2004.

Herath, T. & Rao, H.R. (2009). Encouraging Information Security Behaviors in Organizations: Role of Penalties, Pressures and Perceived Effectiveness. *Science Direct Decision Support Systems Elsevier Ltd, Vol.* 47, No. 2, (February 2009) (154–165), 0167-9236

Hook, C., Kempf, J. & Scharfenberg, G. (2003) .*New Pen Device for Biometrical 3D Pressure Analysis of Handwritten Characters, Words and Signatures*. Proceedings of the 2003 ACM SIGMM workshop on Biometrics methods and applications , pp: 38- 44, 1-58113-779-6, Berkley, California, 2003, ACM New York, NY, USA

Huang, Y., Ao, X., Li, Y & Wang, C. (2008). *Multiple Biometrics System based on DavinCi Platform*. Proceedings of 2008 International Symposium on Information Science and Engieering, Vol. 2, pp.88-92, 978-1-4244-2727-4, Shanghai, China, December 2008, Institute of Electrical and Electronics Engineers (IEEE), USA

Jain, A.K., Griess, F., & Connell, S. (2002). On-line Signature Verification. *Science Direct Pattern Recognition Elsevier Ltd.* Vol.35 (2002) (2002) 2963 - 2972

Jain, A. K., Ross, A. & Prabhakar, S. (2004), An introduction to biometric recognition. *IEEE Transactions on Circuits and Systems for Video Technology,* Vo1. 14, No. 1, (January 2004), (4–20), 1051-8215

Jain, A.K., Ross, A., & Pankanti, S. (2006) Biometrics: A Tool for Information Security. *IEEE Transactions on Information Forensics and Security,* Vol. 1, No. 2. (June 2006), (125-143), 1556-6013

Kanneh, A. & Sakr, Z. (2008a). *Intelligent Haptics Sensing and Biometric Security*. Proceedings of ROSE 2008 - IEEE International Workshop on Robotic and Sensors Environments, pp.102-107, 978-1-4244-2594-5, Ottawa - Canada, October 2008, Institute of Electrical and Electronics Engineers (IEEE), USA

Kanneh, A. & Sakr, Z. (2008b). Biometric User Verification Using Haptics and Fuzzy Logic. Proceeding of the 16th ACM international conference on Multimedia, pp. 937-940, 978-1-60558-303-7, Vancouver, British Columbia, Canada, October 2008, ACM New York, NY, USA

Kanneh, A. & Sakr, Z. (2008c). *Biometrics Security in a Virtual Environment.* Proceedings of 18th International Conference on Artificial Reality and Telexistence 2008, pp. 203-209, Keio University, Yokohama, Japan, December 2008.

Kanneh, A. & Sakr, Z. (2008d). *A Haptic and Fuzzy Logic controller for Biometric User Verification*. Proceedings of CERMA 2008 Electronics, Robotics, and Automotive Mechanics Conference, pp. 62-67, 978-0-7695-3320-9 , Cuernavaca, Morelos, Mexico. Sept./ Oct. 2008, IEEE Computer Society Washington, DC, USA

Kraemera, S., Carayonb, P. & Clemc, J. (2009). Human and organizational factors in computer and information security: Pathways to vulnerabilities. *Science Direct Computers and Security Elsevier Ltd.,* (April 2009) (1 - 1 2), doi:10.1016/ j.cose.2009.04.006

Lee, L., Berger, T. & Aviczer, E. (1996). Reliable On-Line Human Signature Verification Systems. *IEEE Transactions on Pattern Analysis and Machine Intelligence,* Vol. 18, No. 6, (JUNE 1996), (643 - 647), 0162-8828

Lei, H. & Govindaraju, V. (2005). A comparative study on the consistency of features in on-line signature verification. *Pattern Recognition Letters Elsevier Science Inc.* Vol.26 No.15 (November 2005), (2483–2489), 0167-8655

Mansfield, T., Kelly, G., Chandler, D. & Kane, J. (2001). *Biometric Product Testing.* Final Report. Issue 1. Centre for Mathematics and Scientific Computing, National Physical Laboratory, March 2001, doi: http://www.cesg.gov.uk/policy_technologies/biometrics/media/biometrictestreportpt1.pdf

Martin, A., Doddington, G., Kamm, T., Ordowski, M. & Przybocki, M. (2007). *The DET Curve in Assessment of Detection Task Performance.* National Institute of Standards and Technology and Department of Defense, USA. doi: http://www.itl.nist.gov/iad/mig//publications/storage_paper/det.pdf.

McCabe,A., Trevathan, J. & Read, W. (2008). Neural Network-based Handwritten Signature Verification. *Journal of Computers,* Vol. 8, No. 3, (2008), (9-22)

Orozco, M. & El Saddik, A. (2005a). *Recognizing and Quantifying Human Movement Patterns through Haptic-based Applications.* Proceedings of IEEE International Conference on Virtual Environments, Human-Computer Interfaces and Measurement Systems, pp-, 0-7803-9041-5, July 2005.

Orozco, M., Shakra, I. & El Saddik, A. (2005b). *Haptic: The New Biometrics-embedded Media to Recognizing and Quantifying Human Patterns.* Proceedings of the 13th annual ACM international conference on Multimedia, pp. 387 - 390, 1-59593-044-2, Hilton, Singapore, 2005, ACM New York, NY, USA

Orozco, M. Graydon, S. Shirmohammadi & A. El Saddik. (2006a). *Using Haptic Interfaces for User Verification in Virtual Environments.* Proceedings of IEEE International Conference on Virtual Environments, Human-Computer Interfaces and Measurement Systems, pp. 25 - 30, La Coruña - Spain, July 2006. Institute of Electrical and Electronics Engineers (IEEE), USA

Orozco, M., Asfaw, Y., Shirmohammadi, S., Adler, A.& El Saddik, A. (2006b) *Haptic-Based Biometrics: A Feasibility Study.* Proceedings of the Symposium on Haptic Interfaces for Virtual Environment and Teleoperator Systems, pp. 38, 1-4244-0226-3, 2006, IEEE Computer Society Washington, DC, USA

Orozco, M., Malek, B., Eid, M. & El Saddik, A. (2006c) *Haptic-Based Sensible Graphical Password.* Proceedings of Virtual Concept 2006, Playa Del Carmen, Mexico, Nov. / Dec. 2006, doi: http://www.discover.uottawa.ca/publications/files/VC2006Mauritz_V6.pdf

Orozco, M., Graydon, M., Shirmohammadi, S. & El Saddik, A. (2008). Experiments in Haptic-Based Authentication of Humans. *Springer Journal of Multimedia Tools and Applications,* Vol. 37, No. 1, (2008), (71-72), 1380-7501

Ortega-Garcia, J., Bigun, J., Reynolds, D & Gonzalez-Rodriguez. J. (2004). *Authentication gets Personal with Biometrics.* IEEE Signal Processing Magazine, Vol. 21, No. 2, pp. 50- 62, 1053-5888, March 2004.

Panko, R. (2004). *Corporate Computer and Network Security.* Pearson Higher Education. 0130384712, USA

Penagos, J.D., Prabhakaran, N. & Wunnava, S.V. (1996) *An Efficient Scheme for Dynamic Signature Verification.* Proceedings of the IEEE Southeastcon '96. 'Bringing Together Education, Science and Technology Department of Electrical & Computer Engineering, pp. 451-457, 0-7803-3088-9, Tampa, FL, USA, Apr 1996

Plamondon, R. & Srihari, S. N. (2000). On-line and off-line handwriting recognition: a comprehensive survey. *IEEE Transactions on Pattern Analysis and Machine Intelligence,* Vol. 22, No. 1, (January 2000), (63–84), 0162-8828

Roethenbaugh, G. (1997) *Biometrics Explained.* NCSA. Biometrics Editor 1997. Doi:http://www.incits.org/tc_home/m1htm/docs/m1050687.pdf

Salisbury, J.K. and Srinivasan, M. A. (1997). Phantom-Based Haptic Interaction with Virtual Objects. *IEEE Computer Graphics and Applications,* Vol.17, No. 5, (September 1997), (6 - 10), 0272-1716

Shan, A., Weiyin, R. & Shoulian, T. (2008). *Analysis and Reflection on the Security of Biometrics System.* Proceedings of IEEE 4th International Conference on Wireless Communications, Networking and Mobile Computing, 2008. WiCOM '08, pp. 1-5, 978-1-4244-2107-7, Dalian, Oct. 2008, Institute of Electrical and Electronics Engineers (IEEE), USA

Stallings, W. (2006) *Cryptography and Network Security,* Prentice Hall. 4/E . ISBN-10: 0-13-187316-4; ISBN-13: 978-0-13-187316-2, USA.

Vu, K-P. L., Proctorb, R., Bhargav-Spantzelb, A., Bik-Lam, T. , Cook, J, & Schultz,E. (2007). Improving Password Security and Memorability to Protect Personal and Organizational Information. *Science Direct International Journal of Human and Computer Studies Elsevier Ltd,* Vol. 65, No. 8, (April 2007), (744–757), 1071-5819

Wayman, J. 2000. *Technical Testing and Evaluation of Biometric Identification Devices.* Collected Works 1997-2000, August 2000 Version 1.2 National Biometric Test Centre, San Jose State University. doi: http://www.cse.msu.edu/~cse891/Sect601/textbook/17.pdf

Haptic virtual reality assembly – Moving towards Real Engineering Applications

T. Lim[§], J.M. Ritchie[§], R. Sung[§], Z. Kosmadoudi[§], Y. Liu[§] and A.G. Thin[‡]
[§]*Heriot-Watt University, School of Engineering and Physical Sciences, Scotland, UK.*
[‡]*Heriot-Watt University, School of Life Sciences, Scotland, UK.*

1. Introduction

The use of virtual reality (VR) in interactive design and manufacture has been researched extensively but its practical application in industry is still very much in its infancy. Indeed one would have expected that, after some 30 years of research, commercial applications of interactive design or manufacturing planning and analysis would be widespread throughout the product design domain. Similarly, investigations into virtual environments (VE) for assembly and disassembly tasks have been carried out for many years. Given the availability of moderately-priced high performance computing technology, many of these virtual manufacturing interfaces - which only stimulate the visual senses – have made actual physical contact during product development an increasingly rare occurrence.

"We're losing that tactile feel that we had before, and now we're trying to bring it back." Mike Levin, Vice President, Immersion Corporation (Immersion Corporation, 2008).

The first haptic device was developed and made commercial in the early 1990s (Salisbury et al., 1995). Today, haptics exists in many forms from electronic handheld devices to tele-operated robots. Yet outside of the research and engineering community, haptics remain a virtually unknown concept.

How will haptics and VR change the way we interact with the virtual world and how would it influence the way application developers and users (e.g. engineers, doctors, gamers, etc.) embrace the digital era? Already, entertainment and emerging online social networks have richly rendered 3D environments such as Second Life® (Linden Lab, 1999). What these environments lack though is the ability to navigate, manipulate and feedback 3D information kinaesthetically.

Virtual reality is a better understood concept with equally extensive research. However, one of the major but less well known advantages of VR technology pertains to data logging. For engineering purposes, logging the user provides rich data for downstream use to automatically generate designs or manufacturing instructions, analyse design and manufacturing tasks, map engineering processes and, tentatively, acquire expert knowledge (Ritchie et al, 2006). The authors feel that the benefits of VR in these areas have not been fully disseminated to the wider industrial community and - with the advent of cheaper PC-based VR solutions – perhaps a wider appreciation of the capabilities of this type of technology may encourage companies to adopt VR solutions for some of their product design processes. It is envisaged that the notion of unobtrusive logging can similarly be applied to other domains.

This chapter will describe applications of haptics in assembly demonstrating how user task logging can lead to the analysis of design and manufacturing tasks at a level of detail not previously possible; as well as giving usable engineering outputs. The study involves the use of a haptic feedback device (Phantom, Sensable Technologies, 1993) and a 3D system to analyse and compare this technology against real-world user performance. Through detailed logging of tasks in a haptic VR environment the study shows considerable potential in understanding how virtual tasks can be mapped onto their real world equivalent as well as showing how haptic process plans can be generated. The chapter also investigates methods to quantify how the provision of haptic feedback affects user performance, the enhancements from a physiological perspective and whether, through an association with game-based approaches, the working environment can be made more engaging. The chapter concludes with a view as to how the authors feel that the use of haptic VR systems in product design and manufacturing should evolve in order to enable the industrial adoption of this technology in the future.

2. Background

Various researchers have investigated sense of presence measurements simulation validity and human performance, in an effort to assess the effectiveness of force-feedback VR applications.

A classic example relates to peg-in-hole insertion operations. Insertion operations are an important aspect of assembly. Tight tolerances between both objects involved in the insertion, and associated positioning accuracies require some level of compliance, trajectory and force control. Ho and Boothroyd (1979) studied the intraposition of a peg into a hole and the circumposition of a part with a hole onto a peg. Their objective was to elicit chamfer designs that will minimise insertion times and, hence, overall assembly times. Rosenburg (1994) carried out an empirical study where participants were asked to execute a peg insertion task through a telepresence link with force-feedback. Five different haptic overlays were tested which included virtual surfaces, virtual damping fields, virtual snap-to-planes and snap-to-lines. The results indicated that human performance was significantly degraded when comparing telepresence manipulation to direct in-person manipulation. However, by introducing abstract haptic overlays into the telepresence link, operator performance could be restored closer to natural in-person capabilities. The use of 3D haptic overlays was also found to double manual performance in the standard peg-insertion task.

In the mid 1990s commercial force feedback interfaces appeared; such as the Phantom arm (Massie & Salisbury, 1994) which allows user interaction with virtual environments through a stylus. Gupta et al. (1997) investigated the benefits of multimodal simulation using VE technology for part handling and insertion compared to conventional table-based methods, as presented by Boothroyd et al. (2002). Their results showed that assembly task completion time increased in proportion to the complexity of the assembly operations required. However, the measured times were roughly double those required to carry out the operation in the real world. Although they employ two haptic arms their study was restricted to 2D simulations of the insertion operation. Significantly for the work reported in this paper the authors speculate that one of the contributory factors to task completion time was the lack of co-location.

For human computer interaction (HCI), Fitts' Law (Fitts, 1954) has generally been used as a quantitative means with which to measure the performance of human motor control of simple task. Fitts derived a quantitative predictor for the movement time needed for the successful completion of 2D targeting peg-in-hole-type tasks. There was, however, no consideration of shape at any stage.

Bayazit et al. (2000) reported that the lack of truly cooperative systems limits the use of haptic devices involving human operators and automatic motion planners. They presented a 'hybrid' system that uses both haptic and visual interfaces to enable a human operator and an automatic planner to cooperatively solve a motion planning query. By manipulating a virtual robot attached to the Phantom haptic device a sequence of paths were generated and fed to the planner. Haptic interaction comprised of tracking user motion, collision detection between haptic probe and virtual objects, computing reaction forces, and force rendering. An obstacle-based probabilistic roadmap method was used in conjunction with a C-Space toolkit to filter the haptically-generated paths and generate collision-free configurations for the robot.

Unger et al. (2001) described an experimental arrangement for comparing user performance during a real and virtual 3D peg-in-hole task. The task required inserting a square peg into a square hole via a 6 degree of freedom magnetic levitation haptic device and visual feedback. The goal was to understand human manipulation strategies. Their results indicate that haptic senses can discriminate between very fine forces and positions; however, it was found that overall task performance with real objects is best.

The sensory feedback capability of haptics lends itself naturally to tasks that require manual manipulation. Adams et al. (2001) conducted experiments to investigate the benefits of force feedback for VR training of assembly tasks. Three groups of participants received different levels of training (virtual with haptics, virtual without haptics, and no training) before assembling a model biplane in real world environment. Their results indicated that participants with haptic training performed significantly better than those without.

The Haptic Integrated Dis/Re-assembly Analysis (HIDRA) is a test bed application focused primarily on simulation of assembly procedures with force-feedback (Coutee et al., 2001). Their intention was to provide a development perspective relevant to haptically enabled simulations. The research efforts of Seth et al. (2005) fall into the similar assembly/disassembly category of analysis via visualisation with haptic force feedback. These reported examples are particularly useful for applications that provide tactile information regarding assemblability at the design stage. However, there is little evidence of data logged in order to output assembly instructions.

Similar to the vein of research here is the work by Gerovichev et al. (2002) on the evaluation of visual and haptic feedback for training needle insertion tasks in medicine. Promising results showed that the addition of force cues, along with real-time visual feedback, improved performance.

Yoshikawa et al. (2003) presented a methodology for observing human skill in a virtual space configured with haptic technology. A comparison between a real world square peg-in-hole task and a 2D simulation was performed. The virtual space incorporated dynamics and surface friction characteristics. Results indicated that stability of the haptic system can be improved with analogue circuitry so that human skills are better represented in the virtual environment. Bashir et al. (2004) developed a system to assess the influence equipment and its arrangement on the force, visual and augmented feedback and how this influences task completion times. Their experiment involved picking an object, placing it against a vertical surface and inserting it into a hole with a sliding motion. The effects of mass and clearance were not considered. Their results indicated 45% prolonged completion times with force feedback compared to real tasks.

Amirabdollahian et al. (2005) underlined the advantage of using assistive technologies to measure the effectiveness of a medical therapy regime. The peg-in-hole haptic assessment was the study of choice for quantifying upper limb skills. The set-up consists of a large virtual table with two identical cylindrical holes and a cylindrical peg that was to be repeatedly inserted by alternately moving between each of the holes with a Phantom device. Physical properties of the peg and hole such as diameter, peg weight and height, were taken into account. Position, velocity and reaction forces were logged at a sampling rate of 1000Hz. Inconclusive results were obtained but further clinical trials are being undertaken to investigate the usefulness of the haptic system as a means of assessing human performance, in particular arm skills and coordination.

Recent research points towards developing architectures for collaborative haptic virtual environments (CHVEs). The Collaborative Haptic Assembly Simulator (Iglesias et al., 2006) is one reported work that investigates assembly/disassembly simulation of mechanical components in a collaborative virtual environment. The system has the potential to manage large assemblies; unfortunately, they do not appear to have stored and managed the history of movements. A review on the application of haptics in nano robotics illustrates the advancement of VR and haptics (Ferreira & Mavroidis, 2006). However, only the exploratory influence and the associated sensory advantages of tactile feedback are reported.

There have been numerical studies evaluating the performance of haptic technologies in interaction with VR, the optimisation of the kinesthetic device design (Fritschi et al., 2008), as well as the human haptic perception (Bresciani et al., 2008). However there has been limited exploration into measuring the experience of haptic interaction. Haptic systems may provide force feedback and inherit the dynamics and movements of the tool they simulate but whether this provides the same feeling as it would had in reality needs further investigation. Comparing similar tasks in VR and real life based on the bio-mechanical reaction of the humans can lead to a scientifically more accurate and realistic haptic simulation (Kocherry et al., 2009).

While most of the published work on VR applications with force feedback shows the benefits of haptics, they do not discuss the automatic generation of qualitative information derived from assembly plans (syntax or semantics) developed within simulations in the virtual environment. Generally, haptics remains as a facilitator in guiding spatial exploration rather than as an output of task planning and in more general terms, manufacturing information. Extrapolating the cognitive procedures relating to assembly tasks (and even tacit exploration of the virtual components) during user interaction will provide information to better a product's design for manufacture and assembly (DFMA). User interactions captured through the haptic VR system provide a rich source of data that underlines knowledge, experience and intent. By analyzing this information optimizations can be made to procedural tasks and training strategies early in the development phase while making users aware of any faults.

The logging and reuse of associated information as an engineering task analysis tool within haptic VR environments is central to this work; indeed, the application of these methods is similar to a number of engineering task analysis applications covering both design and manufacturing assembly processes as well as early knowledge acquisition (Ritchie et al., 2006). Following a successful pilot study by Lim et al. (2006), while statistically inconclusive, it has shown that Design for Assembly (DFA) components had an impact on task completion time in the virtual environment. The initial study also exposed several inadequacies of the test bed, for example its functionality and ease of use, and aspects of human factors such as the associated cognitive and physiological perspective of how people perceive shapes in stereo and non-stereo modes. With this in mind the objective was to carry out the human factors' evaluation of a haptic assembly system via the use of a comparative assessment of virtual, virtual/haptic peg-in-hole assembly tasks against real world benchmarked equivalents. Further, measuring the physiological response using electromyography (EMG) can aid in the understanding of kinaesthetic responses between haptic VR and the real world tasks to potentially advance the state of the art and to achieve better and more accurate correspondence to reality for haptic based systems.

3. Motion Chronocyclegraphs

As advances in technology allow for more complex geometries to be manufactured, so too has the degree of complexities increased within component assembly. Therefore to automate assembly procedures it is useful to understand the cognitive insight of the human operator. A method that allows for such analysis is to track user-object interaction. The data obtained can then be plotted as a time-dependent profile describing motion together with position, orientation and velocity.

GROUP OF ACTIVITIES	NAME OF ACTIVITY	SYMBOL	COLOUR
1. EFFECTIVE OPERATION	USE		PURPLE
	ASSEMBLE		VIOLET
	DISASSEMBLE		LIGHT VIOLET
2. MANUAL OR VISUAL IDENTIFICATION	SEARCH		BLACK
	FIND		GREY
	SELECT		LIGHT GREY
	INSPECT		BURNT OCHRE
3. CONTROL ACTIVITY	GRASP		RED
	RELEASE LOAD		CARMINE RED
	HOLD		GOLD OCHRE
4. PRECISE MOVEMENTS	POSITION		BLUE
	PRE-POSITION		PALE BLUE
5. GENERAL MOVEMENT	TRANSPORT LOAD		GREEN
	TRANSPORT EMPTY		OLIVE GREEN
6. DELAY	PLAN		BROWN
	RESET FOR OVERCOMING FATIGUE		ORANGE
	UNAVOIDABLE DELAY		YELLOW
	AVOIDABLE DELAY		LEMON YELLOW

(a) Therblig Symbols

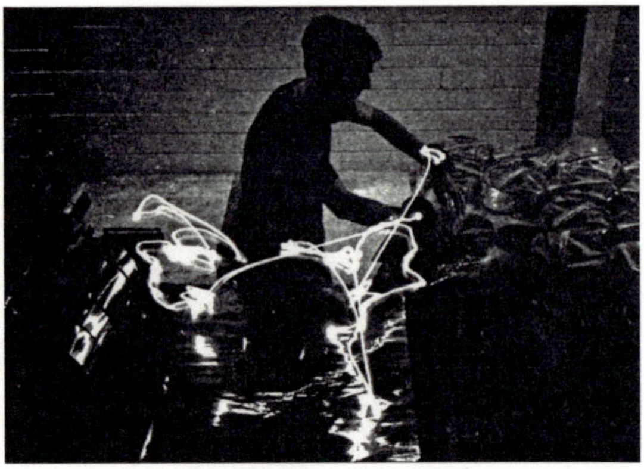

(b) Chronocyclegraph

Fig. 1. Gilbreth's Time and Motion Study (courtesy of Johnson & Ogilvie, 1972)

Therbligs are a set of symbols developed by Frank Gilbreth (Price, 1990; Johnson & Ogilvie, 1972) during the early 20th century to study assembly motions, where each symbol represented the mental and physical processes involved during an assembly task. Fig. 1(a) shows the 18 therblig units represent a set of fundamental motions required to perform a manual operation: Search; Find; Select; Grasp; Hold; Position; Assemble; Use; Disassemble; Inspect; Transport loaded; Transport unloaded; Pre-position for next operation; Release load Unavoidable delay; Avoidable delay; Plan; and Rest. As therbligs map onto each individual operation task, by analysing the therblig units associated with a process, unneeded movements can be eliminated to optimise and make efficient any task. For example, when numerous 'delay' therbligs associated with a particular assembly operation are evident then the efficiency for that specific task will have to be improved.

Gilbreth also devised chronocyclegraphs for motion studies (Price, 1990). The method involves attaching a light source to the hands of a person performing an assembly task. Using long-exposure photography of the whole assembly process, a result as seen in Fig. 1(b) is obtained. This result displays the path, known as the chronocyclegraph, that the user's hands have moved through during the assembly task and helps identify areas of inefficient movement by the user. By letting the light source flash at a known frequency, it can also help determine the velocity and acceleration of the hand movements.

Indeed, there is much to be gained from Gilbreth's seminal work on time and motion study. However, there is no literature that shows that these have been applied in any VR and/or haptic engineering environment.

4. Experimental methodology

Assembly is, classically, one of the most extensively studied manual processes in manufacturing. One strand of this work aims to quantify assemblies by analysis of the sequence of operations required to build a component. For example, Fig. 2 illustrates the relative time required for manual insertion of a peg into a hole for various geometries. Taking the insertion of a cylindrical peg into a round hole as its baseline time (i.e. 100%)

Haeusler (1981) reports a German study that estimated the relative times required to assemble different geometries. He estimated that the insertion of a round pegs into a chamfered hole took only 57% of the time required to complete the "nominal" case.

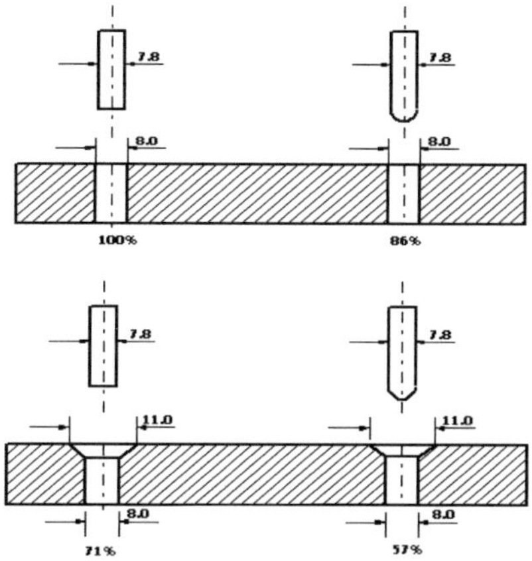

Fig. 2. Design for assembly (DFA). The diagram shows pegs and holes with varying feature shapes and relative assembly times (Haeusler, 1981).

DFA methodologies have quantified the relative times of real-world assembly tasks: grasping, acquisition, manipulation, and insertion. Could haptic assembly performance be benchmarked against previously quantified assembly times? This forms the rationale for the peg-in-hole assembly task in this study. The assembly process can be subdivided into three states; picking, placing and motion.

The peg-in-hole task requires inserting a peg into a block with a hole. Participants perform this both as a virtual 3D task where they are provided with different combinations of visual and force cues (through a haptic device) and the real world equivalent tasks.

The primary objective was to investigate simulator fidelity by comparing the time taken to carry out six different assembly tasks in a haptic VE with the following characteristics; rigid body dynamics, stereo display and haptic feedback, and so assess the relative impact of each technology on user cognitive and physiological performance. The peg-in-hole experiment was planned as a precursor to a more challenging assembly that involved a geared pump comprising five components.

4.1 Virtual task

Table 1 presents the experimental design for the virtual task. A binary label was used to indicate whether collision detection and stereovision was switched on (1) or off (0). There are six primary experimental steps, which are ordered such that tests are performed with/without collision detection (C/D) and with/without stereovision. The key feature of this experimentation was that the participants were totally unaware of any geometrical differences within components during this experimental programme.

Experiment ID	C/D	Stereo	Block Chamfer	Peg Chamfer	People x Reps
1	1	1	1	1	11 x 3
2	0	1	1	1	11 x 3
3	1	0	1	1	12 x 3
4	1	1	0	0	11 x 3
5	0	1	0	0	12 x 3
6	1	0	0	0	11 x 3

Table 1. Experimental design.

Allocation:
- Participants were randomly allocated to experiments 1, 2 or 3.
- Subsequently each was also randomly allocated to 4, 5, or 6.
- Each experiment had an equal number of participants.

Training:
- Each participant was given five minutes to briefly familiarise themselves with the virtual environment and haptic feedback.
- Shape manipulation requirements.
- Pick and place a peg into a hole using the haptic device.
- Applied force displacement with the picked object onto a stationary object to experience haptic feedback.

Instruction:
- Each participant was asked to move a peg from its starting position to the block and insert it.
- The process was repeated three times.
- Each participant was then asked to complete a questionnaire after the experiment.

Analysis:
- Log files recorded timestamps for the pickup of each peg until last release. This provided a task completion time (TCT) in seconds for each repetition.
- Log file names were uniquely defined for each participant.
- Perform error analysis.
- Video recording for each participant was taken to give more insight into both behaviour and errors.
- Statistical analysis was subsequently used to investigate the null hypothesis that: "The variability in performance between task pairs would be similar."

4.2 Real task

A similar number of participants were tasked to perform manual peg-in-hole insertions. Four different insertion routines were carried out in the following order:

1. Flat Peg/Flat hole (FPFH) – Insert flat end peg into a block with a chamferless hole.
2. Chamfered Peg/Flat Hole (CPFH) – Insert a peg with a 45° conical chamfered end into a block with a chamferless hole.
3. Chamfered Peg/Chamfer Hole (CPCH) - Insert peg with a 45° conical chamfered end into a block with a corresponding chamfered hole.
4. Flat Peg/Chamfer Hole (FPCH) - Insert flat end peg into a block with a 45° conical chamfered hole.

Each routine was repeated six times. The setup (Fig. 3) ensured that the distance between the peg and hole was fixed (at 40mm from the centre of the peg to the centre of the hole in the block) and that each participant was positioned according to their comfort of reach and eye level.

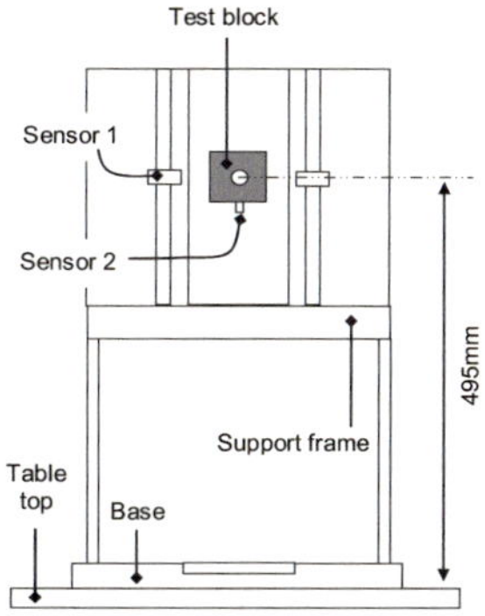

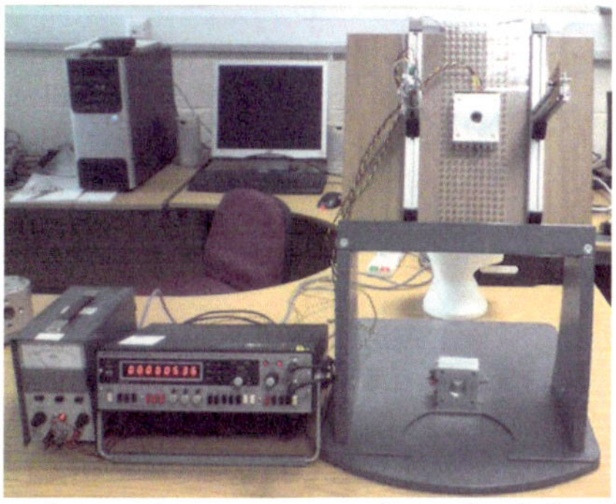

Fig. 3. Real world experimental setup. The schematic is presented on the left where sensor 1 and sensor 2 times peg insertion and retraction cycles.

Timings were taken only when the peg was displaced from its holder and stopped once the subject released upon a successful insertion. Fig. 4 details the dimensions for the block and peg used in the virtual world and for the real world experiment.

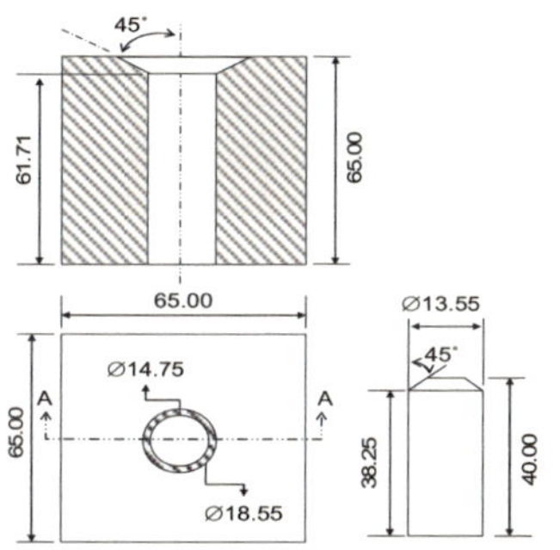

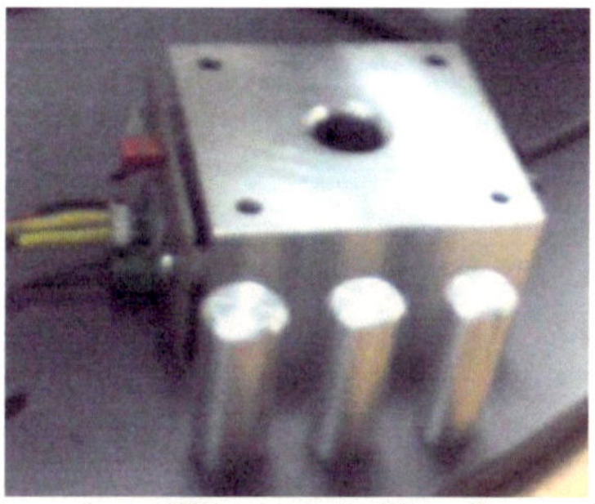

Fig. 4. Experimental block and peg (all dimensions in millimetres). The dimensional view on the left shows the peg and the block with its cross-sectional view along AA. The physical test block and pegs (diameters left to right - 14.85 mm, 14.48 mm and 13.54 mm) are shown on the right.

5. Implementation

The Haptic Assembly, Manufacturing and Machining System (HAMMS) was developed as a test bed to investigate and measure user interactions and response while performing various engineering tasks in a haptic VR environment. The hardware comprises a Phantom haptic device for interaction with the virtual environment, along with a pair of stereoscopic glasses (MacNaughton, 2008) for stereo viewing when required. The systems' hardware and architecture is presented in Fig. 5 and comprises the following components:

- Haptics Interface: Sensable Technologies OpenHaptics® Toolkit (Sensable Technologies, 1993), which provides device control for the Phantom Desktop and Omni, and supports polygonal objects, material properties, and force effects.
- Graphics Interface: The Visualization ToolKit (VTK, 1998) is used for rendering graphics, image processing, and visualization.
- Physics' Interface: AGEIA PhysX™ (AGEIA PhysX, 2008) technology provides the physics' engine that includes an integrated solver for fluids, particles, cloth and rigid bodies.

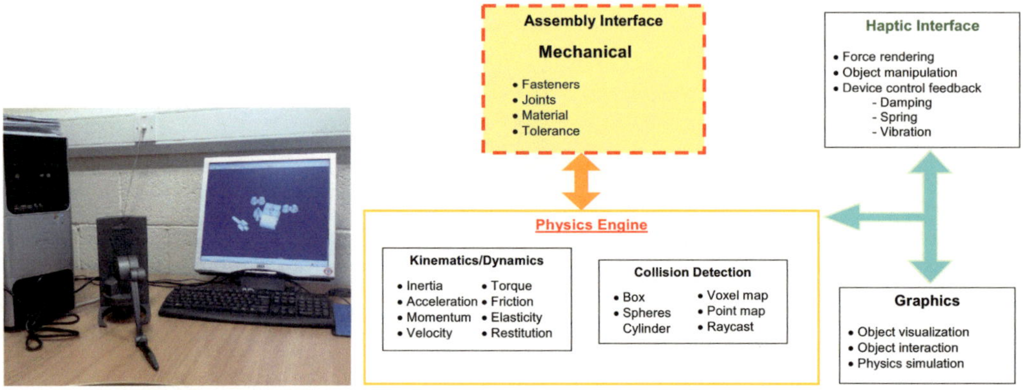

(a) Hardware (b) Architecture
Fig. 5. HAMMS hardware and dependencies.

Central to HAMMS is the physics' engine, which enables rigid body simulations in real time. State changes within the physics' environment update haptic rendering and vice versa. As haptic rendering relies on real time collision feedback from the physics engine, it is important that where possible convex hulls and/or primitive shapes are used to represent the objects in the physics' environment. The most important issue to address is the synchronization between the haptic and physics loops. Essentially, the physics loop runs at approximately 30-60 Hz while to create realistic sensations the haptic loop requires 1000 Hz. To avoid instabilities in force rendering, the input device and any rigid objects are uncoupled. Instead, the system uses the changing states in the physical simulation to influence the forces associated with the haptic rendering. The resulting events are then visualized through VTK.

HAMMS logs data for each virtual object in the scene including devices that are used for interaction. The basic logged data comprises position, orientation, time stamps, velocity and an object index (or identifying number). Fig. 6 illustrates the colour-coded therblig units adapted by HAMMS and its association to the logged data. By parsing through the logged data text files an assembly procedure can be automatically formulated.

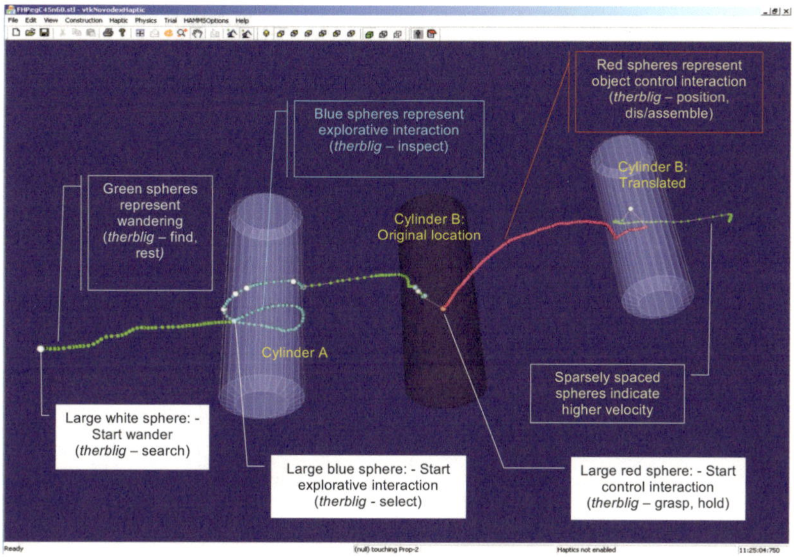

Fig. 6. HAMMS colour coded therbligs. Large spheres signify a start event while small spheres represent motion. Green indicates search, find or rest. Blue represents selection and inspection. Red identifies control events such as grasping, holding, translation, dis/assembly operations. Note: The shadowed cylinder in the middle shows the original position of the translated cylinder to the right.

To visualize the data stream, large spheres are used to signify the start of an event, while smaller contiguous spheres indicate the direction, speed, and location of exploration or controlled displacements. Velocity changes are indicated by the separation of the spheres, i.e. sparsely spaced spheres equate to higher velocity. The line joining all spheres is referred here as the motion-time-line (MTL).

6. Experimental Results and Analysis

A peg-in-hole experiment was performed to investigate how users responded to a simplistic assembly procedure in a haptic virtual environment. This experiment was designed as a precursor to a more challenging pump assembly. Two sets of experiments have been prepared: a real world set up and a virtual reality set up where the participant is given the impression of "forces" through a haptic device. The primary objective was to compare two different assembly tasks in a virtual environment with the following characteristics; rigid body dynamics, stereo display and haptic feedback, and so assess the relative impact of the technology against real world equivalent tasks and its influence on how a task is completed. As mentioned previously, the participants were not informed about chamfers being on the peg or hole.

6.1 Virtual vs. Real

A total of 34 participants were recruited for the virtual and real world peg-in-hole task. Each subject was randomly allocated to two experiments listed in Table 1 and the results charted in Fig. 7.

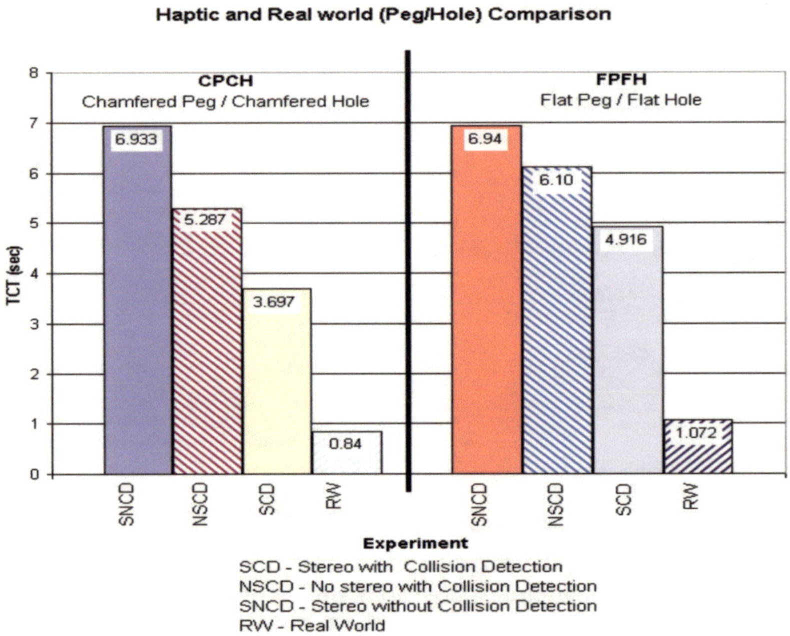

Fig. 7. Virtual and real world Peg-in-Hole task completion time (TCT) comparison. TCT for each experiment is indicated at the top of each column.

Chamfered Peg / Chamfered hole (CPCH): The results indicate the effects of augmented virtual environments through the use of force cues during an assembly task. Comparisons of stereo viewing show a gain of approximately 1.6 seconds on the overall task completion time (TCT). Where stereo is present but not collision detection, it was observed that participants took longer to align and insert the peg into the hole. This is reflected in the results (see SNCD in Fig. 7).

Flat Peg / Flat Hole (FPFH): This experiment also presents a similar trend to the CPCH experiment. Though less pronounced comparisons against stereo viewing again show a reduction (approximately 1.2 seconds) for TCT.

Interestingly, TCT for both SNCD experiments are nearly identical. This was due to subjects spending the majority of time aligning the peg in the hole. Since no force cues were present to indicate that the peg was in contact with the sides of the hole, the subjects relied heavily on visual perception.

Importantly, the virtual and real world experiments illustrate that shape is one predominant factor in reducing TCT. It appears that perception of size and shape, in addition to visual stimuli on haptic perception, has exposed the power of visual dominance over the other senses. It is also evident that manual manipulation of objects in virtual environments improves with haptic feedback.

Damping effects: In order to consider the haptic equipment's actual operational influence on performance, in a manner similar to that detected by Bashir et al. (2004), it was decided to investigate its inherent damping during operation. The architecture used for HAMMS meant that to approximate 'reality', phenomena such as gravity, restitution, material properties and friction were provided via a physics engine, which added an operational delay into the system. This adds further load to the system, and in the current development of HAMMS, generates a damped effect during object interaction (i.e. when using the haptic device to move an object). No motion damping effect is present while the user is touching virtual shapes; the haptic cursor response was instantaneous. Taking this into account, a series of displacement trials were carried out to establish a damping metric (Fig. 8).

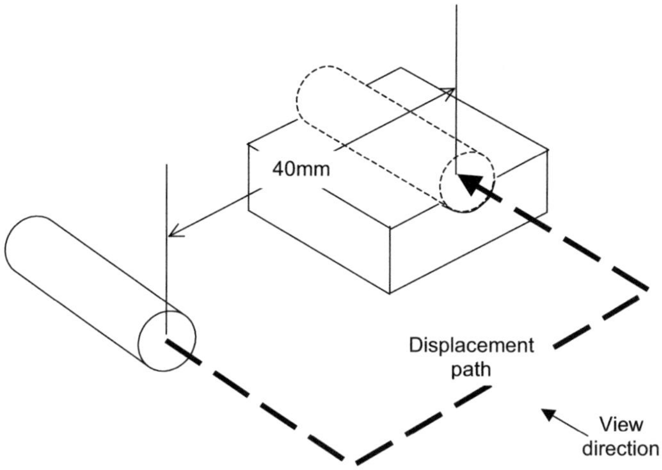

Fig. 8. Peg displacement test to determine haptic motion damping.

A total of 30 repetitions were executed and the average taken. The procedure involves picking up the peg, bringing it forward and placing it on a pedestal. The objects are reset automatically to their origins after each placement. The movements were carried out as quickly as possible. Each cursor path was recorded by logging cursor position and system time whenever a haptic device button message was processed by the operating system.

Fig. 9 presents the results after the effects of haptic damping (approximately 2 seconds) were removed from the original TCT. While the new figures are still a minimum of twice the real world experiment times, there is close correlation to real world assembly experience. This also supports the findings of Gupta et al. (1997) mentioned previously who measured times roughly double that in the real world. The results also show that the Haeusler factor (Haeusler, 1981) - 57% chamfered peg/hole to flat peg/hole - equates to 61% in the haptic domain and 78% in the real world. More improvements to the system on memory management and more efficient rigid body dynamic algorithms could potentially improve realism.

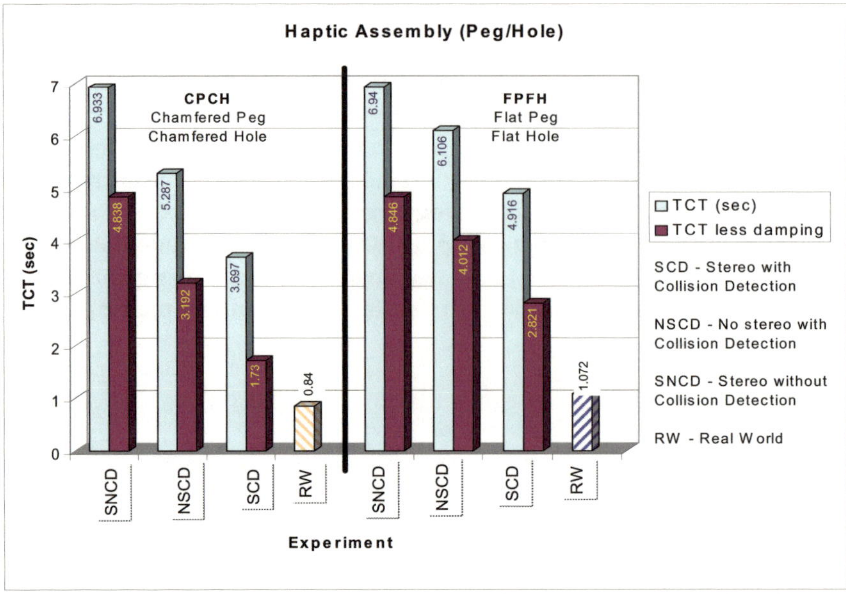

Fig. 9. Effect of virtual environment damping on task completion time (TCT). TCT for each experiment is indicated at the top of each column. The non-damping times have been superimposed to indicate the difference in TCT.

6.2 Physiological effects of haptic VR interface

Haptic displays provide users with the sense of touch and manipulation of objects. The haptic modality is a correlation of tactile and kinesthetic perception (Fritschi et al., 2008). In order for a user's grasp to be translated into free motion in the virtual mechanism, dynamic forces need to be calculated and returned to the user. An 'ideal' haptic device has a number of design criteria characterising its performance; dynamic properties, stiffness, output capability, workspace and extensibility (Ueberle et al., 2004).

In an effort to provide more intuitive interfaces, particularly for tasks involving exploration or manipulation of geometric entities, it is necessary to investigate users' sense of presence. It has been shown that users within virtual environments can exhibit parallax issues when exploring virtual geometric spaces although they would have easily understood a similar space in the real world (Baker et al., 1993; Robinson et al., 2007). Research in perceptual-motor coordination suggests why this effect might be occurring (Beal & Loomis, 1995). For example, physically walking through a complex environment allows a person to keep track of their position and where other key locations are with respect to their own position within that environment (Brooks, 1992). Similarly being able to physically touch and manipulate an object makes its shape and structure much more vivid than passively observing the same object (Burdea, 1996). Human visual sensors are spatially localised (Derrington et al., 2004); in contrast, haptic and kinaesthetic sensations are intrinsically three-dimensional. Thus studying how mechanical-VR interfaces can support human-scale workspaces, human-level dexterity, and haptic interaction while providing quantitative 3D precision becomes more compelling. The experiment here investigates the sense of motion or manipulation and the ability of users to interact mechanically with computational artefacts via haptic VR.

Fig. 10 shows the results of tactile feedback and how it has influenced the user's intent. Object control time-lines are represented by a series of red spheres. Blue spheres indicate that the user was exploring the shape (touching or finding a picking location). Green spheres indicate that the user was wandering (i.e. no interaction with virtual objects).

Fig. 10(b) clearly shows that without haptic feedback, tacit knowledge regarding the location of the peg as it passes through the hole is lacking, indicated by the sparsely separated object control lines (red spheres). However, when force cues are available, the user more accurately passes the peg through the hole, as shown in Fig. 10(c) and (d). The closely converging control lines indicate this as the peg enters the hole. Note also how the user has gained confidence about the environment (or workspace) when tactile information is available. Compared to the closely spaced red control spheres in Fig. 10(b), those shown in Fig. 10(c) and (d) are well separated, indicating that the user's motion and confidence has improved.

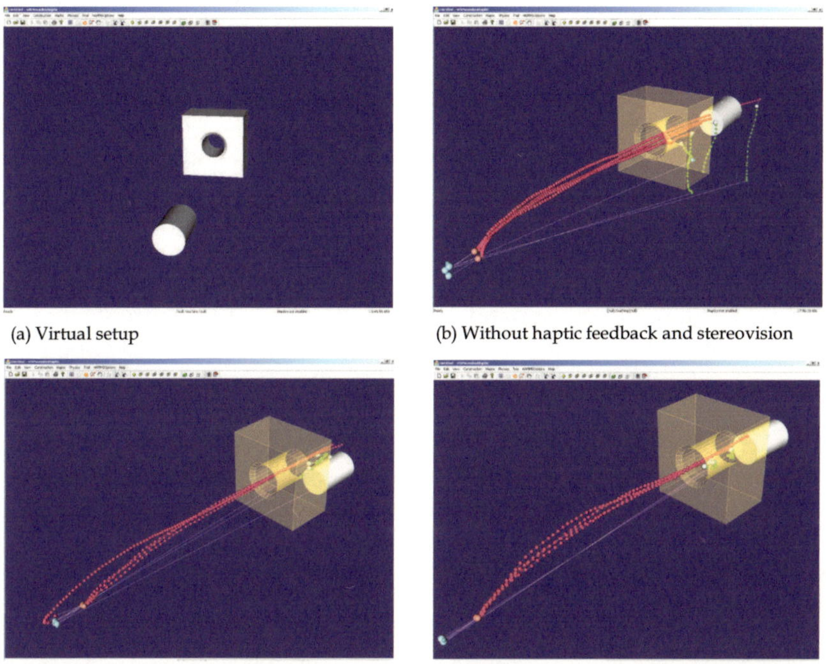

(a) Virtual setup

(b) Without haptic feedback and stereovision

(c) With haptic feedback, no stereovision

(d) With haptic feedback and stereovision

Fig. 10. Peg-in-hole motion chronocyclegraph. Frames b, c and d show four successive pick and place motions.

The vortex (twist) of the control lines indicates how the user is trying to orient the peg for a successful insertion. The amount of wavering in Fig. 10(b) compared to the precise motions attributed to augmented tactile information of the latter experiments clearly show the user has learnt to appreciate force cues to complete the task.

The effects of stereovision can clearly be observed in Fig. 10(d). The start (pick) event and the entry (insertion) event have been markedly improved as indicated by consistent picking and direction of motion. With stereovision the learning process is fast tracked, as there is better depth perception, reducing the guesswork during picking.

6.3 Haptic influence on motor control

The human body has a number of different sensory systems, namely somatic (touch-pressure, posture and movement, temperature, pain), vision, hearing, chemical (taste, smell) and vestibular (motion and position of head). VR by and large focuses on providing visual stimuli to the user whilst trying to avoid conflict with vestibular sensations that would result in dizziness or motion sickness in extreme cases. Haptic devices are used in conjunction with VR with intention of giving the user tactile feedback by providing touch and pressure stimuli to the digits and hands. However little is known about the nature of the user's experience from a kinaesthetic point of view.

Video games are rich multimedia environments that seek to provide engaging interactive experiences. Until relatively recently the predominant focus has been on the richness of the graphical game play environment. Whilst games developers and manufacturers have always being developing peripherals in order to provide more engaging ways to interact with games rather than the simple joystick, it is only in the last few years that so called "body-movement controlled video games" or "ExerGames" have become a commercial success. The Nintendo Wii console is worth considering in this context in that games for this console compensate for a relative lack of graphical computing power with varied and rich sound feedback and the physical interaction required to play games on the console. Research into player's experiences show that such an approach can facilitate an engaging experience without the highest possible degree of realism (Thin et al., 2009).

The term VR overtly implies an attempt to closely mimic reality. However, even in current systems, there is not a direct correspondence. The user of a VR environment can normally go beyond the confines of their human body in the equivalent real world and move through a virtual environment much more freely and easily, often at speed and defying gravitational and anatomical constraints. A shift in focus towards considering the nature of the user's interaction and experience opens up new avenues of development such that by augmenting or enhancing the VE, the user would experience something that is more intuitive and responsive to their needs and intentions. Examples of such augmentation would include "snap to" functionality, visual cues and guides, split screens presenting alternative views or specific details and proximity awareness through the use of sound (haptic feedback does not need to be confined to tactile sensations).

The nature of the interactive experience and how meaning is constructed by the user will in part depend on how "natural" or otherwise their experience of the VR system feels. This is not to say that a user cannot learn to use new systems and approaches and fit in to them but in order to gain widespread acceptance and adoption, it is desirable to try and fit within the range of a given user's existing experiences. Psychophysiological measurement techniques could potentially provide a way to evaluate how a user is sensing and responding to a given environment. Such techniques would be able to give measures of a user's intentions via electromyograhic activity of skeletal muscles (EMG), brain activity (electroencephalography, EEG) and eye movement tracking (electrooculography, EOG). Insight into a user's arousal and/or stress levels could also be gained (e.g. heart rate, temperature, blood pressures, galvanic skin response). Such physiological signals are likely to result in patterns of responses to different situations which are characteristics of certain subject responses, actions and also intentions.

A preliminary investigation was undertaken in order to assess the EMG response during both real world and virtual reality versions of the peg-in-hole task. Subjects sat in a seated position with the arm flexed and the elbow supported. EMG measurements were made of triceps and biceps activity whilst the movement of the arm was tracked using an electronic goniometer (Fig. 11). The signals were acquired using a specialised physiological recording system comprising a set of optically isolated analogue to digital converters under software control and sampled at 1 kHz. Data was stored and analysed using digital chart recording software. Subjects performed the peg-in-hole task for one minute and in that time performed 30 insertions and removals at a uniform rate. The real and virtual world tasks were performed in a randomised order. A screen shot from the physiological recording system is shown in Fig. 12.

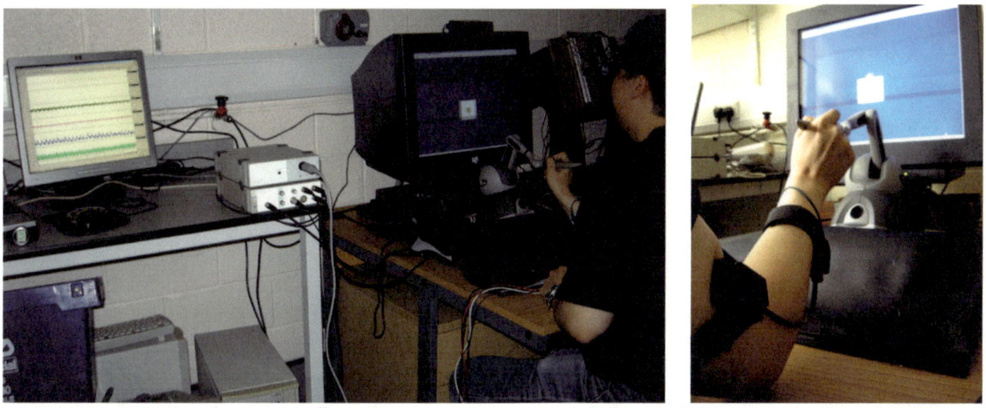

Fig. 11. Investigating haptic influence on motor control through biometric data logging. The experimental setup is shown on the left. The right image shows the goniometer attached to the subject's arm.

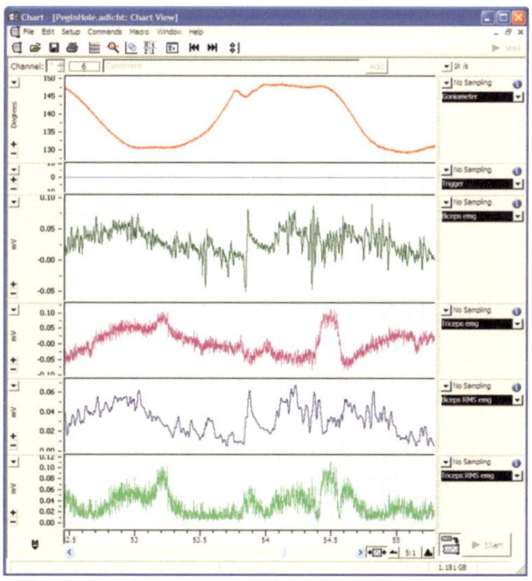

Fig. 12. Screenshot from Physiological recording system showing joint angle (goniometer), raw and RMS EMG signals from biceps and triceps muscles.

Representative EMG activity from the triceps muscle recordings performing the real and virtual peg-in-hole tasks are shown in Fig. 13. Whilst these EMG graphs are only preliminary data, there would appear to be differences between the two sets of traces, both in terms of the overall patterns of the traces and also in the degree of noise in the traces. The nature of haptic devices are such that it contains a certain degree of dampening of any movements by the user.

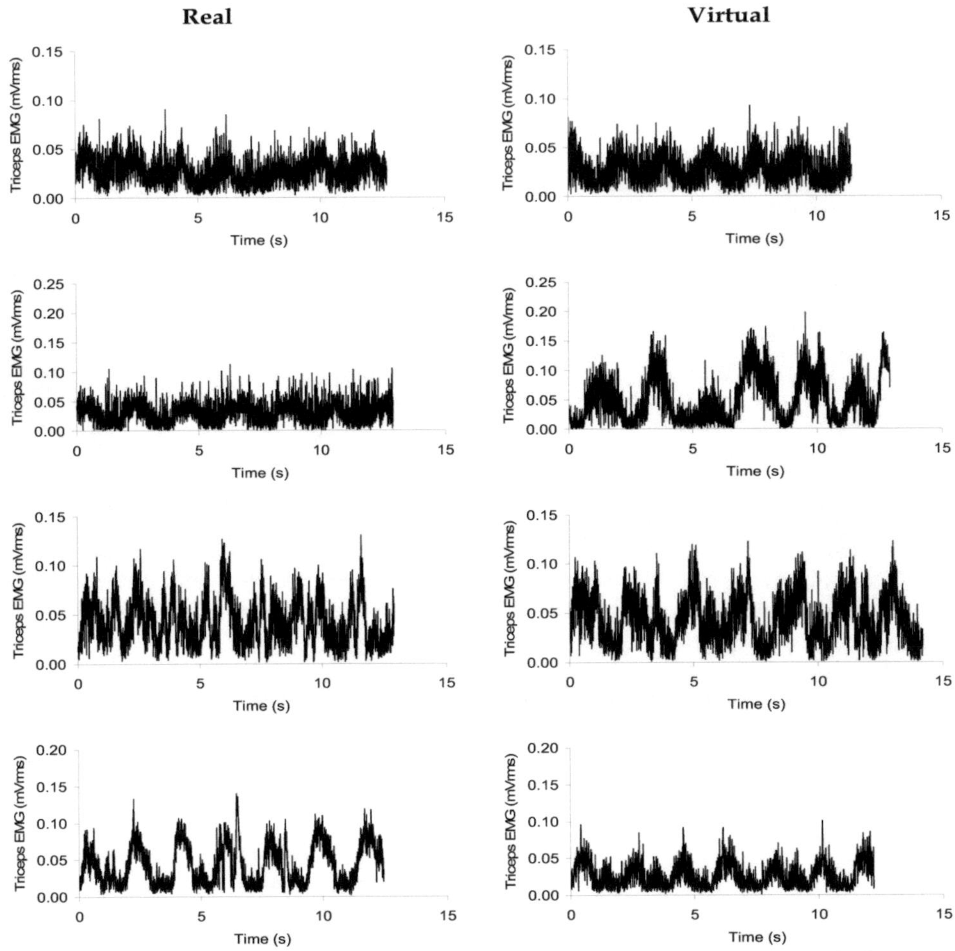

Fig. 13. Raw Triceps EMG traces for a sequence of 6 representative peg-in-hole insertions and removals for each subject. Real task traces are shown on left and virtual task traces on the right.

Human motor control is achieved through a combination of feed-forward and feed-back systems in combination with a central comparator. It has been suggested that noise in a physiological sensory system can enhance the flow of information by helping to aid discrimination (Schaefer et al., 2006). Theses preliminary results suggest that there may be an under-lying physiological difference in the nature of the real and virtual world peg-in-hole tasks that warrants further investigation. The use of psychophysiological techniques and approaches similar to those described above will help better understand the nature of users' experiences in VE and also provide insight into ways in which the environment may be augmented in order to provide more engaging experiences.

6.4 Effects of geometry

How much does a change in geometry affect assembly tasks when both visual and haptic information is available? It was decided to statistically investigate the cause and effect relationships between tasks by investigating those trials where only one parameter was changed. Due to the sample size a one-tail Student's t-test (Pearson & Kendall, 1970) was chosen at a 1% level. Table 2 presents a comparison of TCT (less damping) for two geometry pairs namely, CPCH and FPFH, under the effects of stereovision and collision detection feedback. Real world (RW) results for the corresponding virtual task are also shown.

Exp. ID	Geometry	World	Stereo	C\D	TCT (sec)	Std. Dev. TCT
1	Chamfered Peg Chamfered Hole (CPCH)	Virtual	1	0	4.838	2.853
2			0	1	3.192	1.864
3			1	1	1.73	1.481
4	Flat Peg Flat Hole (FPFH)		1	0	4.846	2.531
5			0	1	4.012	2.291
6			1	1	2.821	1.797
RW 1	CPCH	Real	1	1	0.84	0.144
RW 4	FPFH		1	1	1.072	0.251

Table 2. Comparison of geometry, stereovision and collision detection TCT (less damping). The highlighted rows indicate modal correspondence of virtual/real-world tasks.

The null hypothesis (H0) applied was: "The performance between task pairs will be the same." The alternative hypothesis (H1) was: "The factor changed in the experiment affected the outcome."

This test is designed for data that potentially alters under stereovision and/or collision feedback for CPCH or FPFH condition. The aim is to compare the amount of variability due to the predicted differences in scores between the two conditions as against the total variability in participants' scores. The predicted differences are calculated as a difference between the mean scores for the two groups. This difference between the means has to be compared against the total variance in all scores. If there were only random differences between the scores in the two conditions the variance due to the predicted differences would be relatively small in relation to the total variability in scores. The t-test results are shown in Table 3.

Pairs	Exp. ID	Geometry Comparison	World	Stereo	C\D	TCT (sec)	Std. Dev. TCT	T-Test
1	1 / 2	CPCH / CPCH	Virtual	1 / 1	1 / 0	1.73 / 4.838	1.482 / 2.853	1.22E-06
2	1 / 3	CPCH / CPCH	Virtual	1 / 0	1 / 1	1.73 / 3.192	1.482 / 3.192	5.89E-04
3	1 / 4	CPCH / FPFH	Virtual	1 / 1	1 / 1	1.73 / 2.821	1.482 / 1.797	9.15E-03
4	3 / 6	CPCH / FPFH	Virtual	0 / 0	1 / 1	3.192 / 4.012	1.482 / 2.291	0.11
5	4 / 5	FPFH / FPFH	Virtual	1 / 1	1 / 0	2.821 / 4.846	1.797 / 2.531	2.69E-04
6	4 / 6	FPFH / FPFH	Virtual	1 / 0	1 / 1	2.821 / 4.012	1.797 / 2.291	0.022
7	1 / 4	CPCH / FPFH	Real	1 / 1	1 / 1	0.84	0.144	1.77E-06
8	1 / 1	CPCH	Real / Virtual	1 / 1	1 / 1	0.575 / 1.73	0.107 / 1.482	1.74E-03
9	4 / 4	FPFH	Real / Virtual	1 / 1	1 / 1	0.979 / 2.821	0.191 / 1.797	3.41-E06

Table 3. t-test results (less damping) for the comparison between virtual and real TCT. CPCH - Chamfer on hole and peg. FPFH - no chamfers. Column 1 indicates the Pair number; Column 2 indicates the experimental pairing; Column 3 indicates the environment; Column 5 and 6 indicate whether stereovision and collision detection is in use - 1 (yes), 0 (no); Column 7 and 8 show each pairs' individual task completion time respectively; Column 9 presents the t-test results for each pair.

Pair 3 compares how differing geometries affect assembly performance. A highly significant difference between the two populations ($p<<0.01$) indicates that chamfers do make a significant difference over TCT reduction. Further, it clearly shows the benefit of stereovision when coupled with collision detection. Comparison of the real world experiments (Table 3, Pair 7) indicates that behaviour in the real world was the same regardless of peg/hole type ($p<<0.01$). Considering Table 3 results we can see that even though the peg (and similarly, the hole) chamfers are almost imperceptible, they have a significant influence on TCT. This further justifies the work by Unger (Unger et al., 2001) who showed that haptic senses can discriminate between very fine forces and positions and that real and virtual world placements strategies are essentially similar.

7. Assembly chronocyclegraphs – towards real world applications

Unlike the majority of reported work on assessing and generating assembly plans in a restricted manner, the pump assembly experiment was designed to be carried out with randomly placed components, rather than components whose final position was already known. This free-form type of assembly exercise is much closer to real-word assembly applications and novel in its application to assembly planning generation. Further, participants were not shown the actual assembly and had no prior knowledge of how each component fitted. Essentially, this test was about capturing a participant's perception and intent. The experiment was carried out in both the real and virtual environments to assess the haptic VR interface with a total of six participants.

The virtual and real components of a hydraulic gear pump are shown in Fig. 14. It comprises a pair of bushings, housing and a set of cogs. Each component is loaded into the scene and placed randomly. Participants were then instructed to assemble the components in their own time. This experiment was not about task completion time; rather, the objective is to gather information and understand how a human deduces the sequence of assembly and how they arrange the parts to fulfil their intent assisted by haptic feedback. Fig. 15 presents the chronocyclegraph results and associated therblig units of one such participant. The experiment was conducted with haptic feedback but without stereovision.

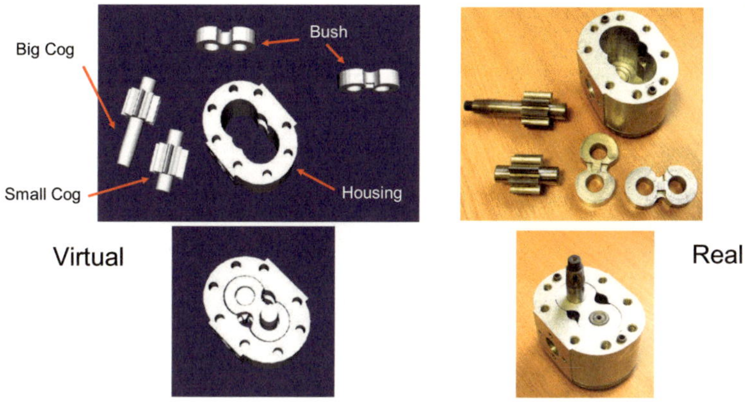

Fig. 14. Pump assembly. Virtual models on left, real on the right.

The MTL and therbligs (white and green spheres) showed in Fig. 15(a) depicts how the participant is navigating in the workspace. Sparsely separated green spheres and the few patches of compact spheres indicate that the participant has quickly identified the assembly sequence of the components. The blue spheres in Fig. 15(b) confirm the selection process through inspection (i.e. touching the object). From the results, it appears that during the assembly process of manipulation and insertion, participants were also preventing the object (the blue spheres directly above the highlighted cog in this example) from misalignment as it was being positioned. Fig. 15(c) shows the displacement of the components during assembly. From observation, the grasping and manipulation of the components consumed the most time. The vortices in the MTL clearly indicate that each component had to be reoriented for successful assembly.

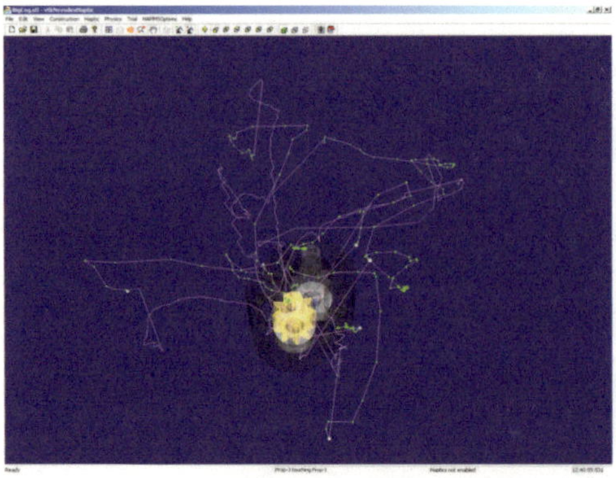

(a) Navigating and searching

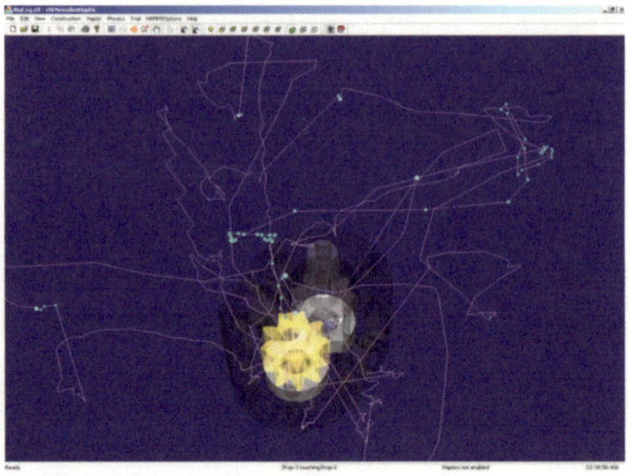

(b) Selection and inspection

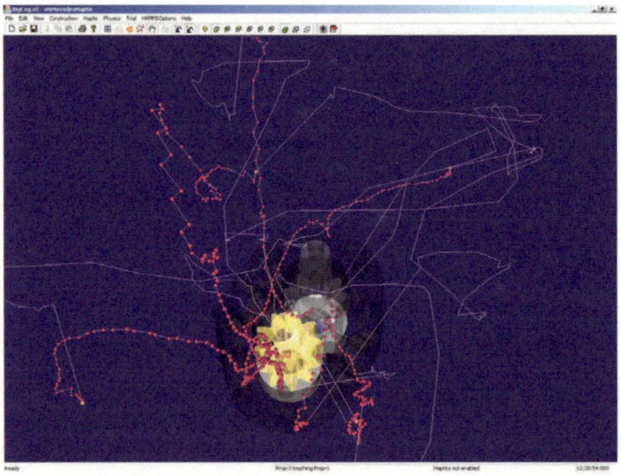

(c) Grasping and manipulating

Fig. 15. Chronocyclegraph analysis in HAMMS. The results indicate this participant has good shape perception and probably some knowledge on the functionality of each component. The MTL and therbligs show: (a) decisive navigation and (b) selection of parts, (c) the majority of time was spent on manipulating parts for assembly.

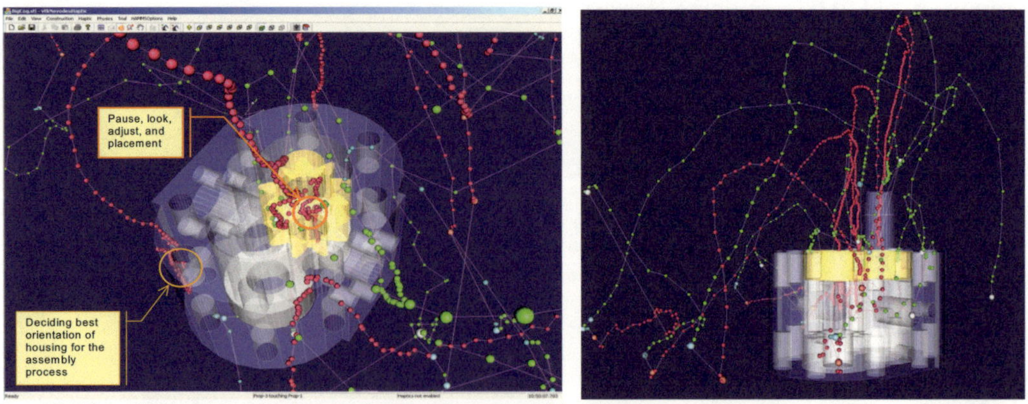

Fig. 16. Identifying through haptic interaction, possible decision making from MTL and therbligs.

Further insights to the process of selection can be observed in the MTL. For example, abrupt changes in direction during the search (green spheres) operation and selection (blue spheres) indicate that perhaps the initial approach was not suitable. When the participant pauses there is little positional and/or velocity change. This is reflected in the MTL as tight squiggles in the profile and/or along with very tightly packed spheres. This evidence is particularly visible as the participant brings an object close to its assembly point (Fig. 16). This form of output tantalizingly suggests that this approach can be used to detect manufacturing intent or confidence in decision making during the actual planning process; this will be further researched to see if there are ways in which decision-making processes and intent can be formalised automatically.

7.1 Generating assembly instructions

The logged data can be parsed to extract assembly instructions. Table 4 presents the assembly sequence of the pump component layout shown in Fig. 14(a). The prognosis of the MTL and its associated therbligs through visual analysis is liable to subjective interpretation. In order to ascertain its validity, the extrapolated information given in Table 1 can be use to crosscheck against the MTL.

HAMMS TRIAL ASSEMBLY PLAN

Op. Num.	W/Centre	Assembly Instruction	Tooling	Assembly Time Virtual (s)	Assembly Time Real (s)
10	Assy Station	Assemble Housing Pos(58.4883300,57.9209000,203.717230), Ori(-45.441740,-63.667560,-67.873010)	Hand assembly	6.961	3.0
20	Assy Station	Assemble Bushing Pos(-38.544190,22.1121600,42.7273800), Ori(55.8205900,-89.920540,89.9831100)	Hand assembly	14.672	12.0
30	Assy Station	Assemble Large Cog Pos(-45.852190,19.6320600,74.7069200), Ori(-24.664120,-86.972570,-89.210800)	Hand assembly	9.672	5.0
40	Assy Station	Assemble Small Cog Pos(-57.745910,20.6709500,98.0864500), Ori(-57.073800,-89.651550,-89.787970)	Hand assembly	12.719	6.0
50	Assy Station	Assemble Bushing Pos(43.4192370,75.5965990,157.523040), Ori(-55.059900,83.3759800,-95.860880)	Hand assembly	17.797	9.0

Table 4. Pump assembly plan automatically generated by extracting logged data. The total virtual time for the virtual assembly operation is 89.1 seconds while the real world 23.7 seconds. The positions and orientations shown correspond to the assembled unit.

Fig. 17 shows an overlay of assembly operations deduced from the logged data. This validity check is necessary in order to identify any discrepancies during the initial subjective interpretation of the MTL data. In this example, the bush associated with the assembly operation (Op Num 50) does not seem to be in the right place. Comparing to the bush's location in Fig. 14, the position of the bush when Op Num 50 begins is much farther away. The reason is that while manipulating the small cog (Op Num 40) there was a collision with the bush causing it to be displaced. Note that the position and orientation of each component in Table 4 correspond to the final assembled location.

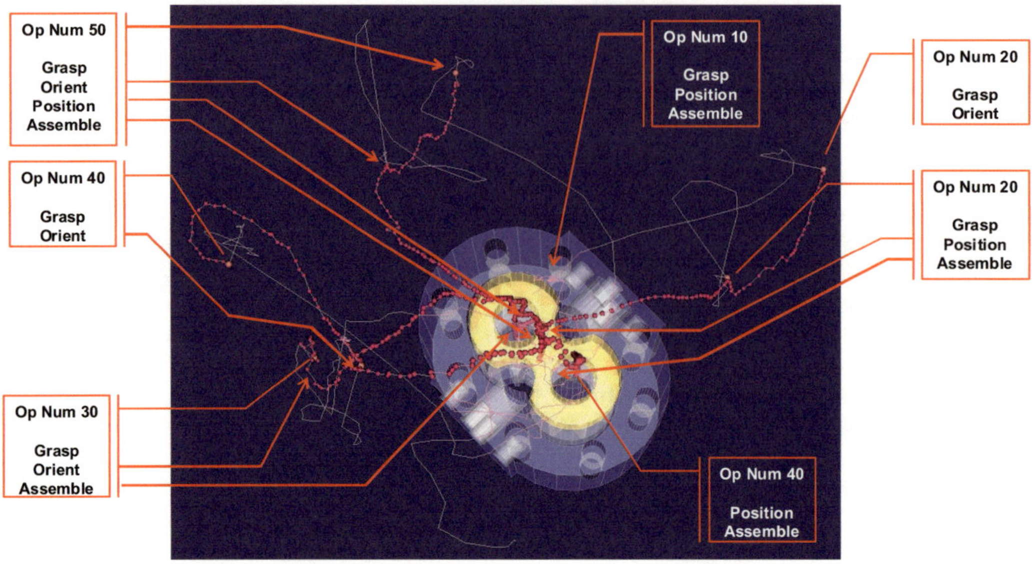

Fig. 17. Assembly operation crosscheck

As the experiment was designed without constraints or restrictions, participants were allowed to assemble the components in the manner they saw fit. Through observation and collected data, 90% of the assembly operations were sequenced in identical format as that described in Table 4. Only 2 participants assembled the small cog before the large cog. However, there was no change in timing trends with regards to aligning and inserting the cogs. The time required to fit the second cog once the first was install was always more (approximately 10 times) regardless of environment. The only notable difference was when 1 participant assembled the bushings and cogs first before slipping the housing over them. While the times recorded were much less for the cog/bush assembly, the participant spent the majority of time (40 seconds real world; 65 seconds virtual world) locating and aligning the housing such that it could be slipped into position.

8. Discussion

The overall objective of this work was to investigate the impact of a haptic VR environment on the user, its effectiveness and productivity for real engineering applications. In this context, the following observations support several important conclusions.

The experiments conducted have demonstrated that small shape change can affect assembly times in haptic VR environments; this is especially significant because the participants were unaware of any component shape changes. They have also shown that, in the case of chamfered features and flat features, the same relative reduction in TCT was recorded as the virtual technology used moves from stereo/no collision detection to stereo/full collision detection. In fact, with full stereo/haptics the best two computer-based performances were recorded for both chamfered and flat features.

The effect of chamfers can clearly be seen when compared against the non-chamfered results presented in Table 2. It can be seen that although the absolute assembly time in the stereo/haptic environment is significantly greater than that of the real world task, the relative difference between chamfered and flat peg insertion times, 61%, compare with published data surprisingly well (i.e. 57% as reported by Haeusler (Haeusler, 1981)).

The benefits of stereovision in virtual assembly environments are highlighted in Table 3 (Pair 4). In contrast to the real world, scalability is not an issue in virtual environments and subtle design alterations, even at micro level, can be simulated when augmented with haptic feedback.

The timings in Table 4 offers an important and interesting observation in that the virtual time gives the *planning time* when compared to actual planning experiments conducted in previous research (Sung et al, 2009).

The peg-in-hole tests have also highlighted several areas of the HAMMS system that needs to be improved. One such area is the damping effect caused by integrating various virtual engines. More efficient memory management and thread synchronization will be necessary to provide users with a better experience.

This work has also successfully used a haptic free-form assembly environment with which to generate assembly plans, associated times, chronocyclegraphs and therblig information. Also, it has been shown that by analyzing the chronocyclegraphs and interpreting user movements and interactions there is considerable potential for analyzing manufacturing methods and formalizing associated decision-making processes. Understanding and extracting the cognitive aspects in relation to particular tasks is not trivial. In the HAMMS environment, it requires dissecting the elements associated to human perception both in terms of visual cues and kinesthesia. It is envisaged that by logging user motion in the manner shown and outputting an interaction pattern over a task, the derived chronocyclegraph can be used to pinpoint areas of where and how decisions are made. HAMMS, as a test bed for investigating human factors, is still in its infancy and it is accepted that some areas, such as data collection methods and its visualization, can be improved. However, this early work indicated its potential as being much wider than simply validating assembly processes. The provision of auditory cues could also both further enhance a user's experience and provide clues on how the human sensory system synchronizes and process sound inputs with tacit and visual signals.

The assembly planning and knowledge capture mechanism presented here is simple and easily embedded in specific engineering processes, especially those that routinely handle important technical task, risk and safety issues. It is important to acquire engineering knowledge as it occurs while preserving the original format and intent. Collecting information in this manner is a more cost effective and robust approach than trying to create new documentation, or capture surviving documents years after key personnel have left the programme. The potential for this has been amply demonstrated in this work.

9. Conclusions

The subjective data on HAMMS system performance indicates that the intuitive nature of haptic VR for product interaction, which combine more than one of the senses in an engineering experience, bodes well for the future development of virtual engineering systems. Therefore, it can be concluded that emerging haptic technologies will be likely to result in the creation of natural and intuitive computer-based product engineering tools that allow a tactile experience through a combination of vision and touch.

The initiative to undertake preliminary investigation in order to assess the physiological response during both real world and virtual reality versions of assembly tasks is novel and has until now never been researched.

While haptic-VR technologies are beginning to find its way into mainstream industrial applications (Dominjon et al., 2007), from a usability and engagement standpoint there are still a number of issues to be addressed. Therefore the concept of employing a game-based approach is already being proposed as a way forwards to enhance engineering application (Louchart et al., 2009). Studies have shown that in a more relaxing game-like environment, users' strong desire to accomplish something produce better results. The nature of game playing is defined by the users' actions to reach an explicit goal, where one failure can provide the basis for a new attempt, or succeed and give acknowledgments and metrics of how well one has done. The goals, feedback and the mixture of failure and achievement provide a state of "flow" which encourages the process of learning (Björk, 2009). In healthcare there are many game-based rehabilitation applications (Dreifaldt & Lövquist, 2006) as well as surgical simulation training (Chan et al., 2009) to make the related process more rewarding, engaging and fun. There are a range of possibilities offered by gaming technologies. We believe that engineering application design can benefit from exploiting game-based approaches.

Haptics closes the gap in our current computer interfaces and has the potential to open up new possibilities. For engineers, blending haptics with recent advances such as in gaming, robotics and computer-numerical machine tools allows training for intricate procedures virtually, with increasingly accurate sensory feedback.

10. References

Adams, R.J.; Klowden, D. & Hannaford. B. (2001) Virtual Training for a Manual Assembly Task. *Haptics-e*, vol. 2, no. 2, pp.1-7. (http://www.haptics-e.org)

AGEIA PhysX (2008) Acquired by NVIDIA Corporation in 2008. Available: http://www.nvidia.com/object/physx_new.html.

Amirabdollahian, F.; Gomes, G.T. & Johnson, G.R. (2005) The Peg-in-Hole: A VR-Based Haptic Assessment for Quantifying Upper Limb Performance and Skills. *Proc. of the 9th IEEE Int'l Conf. On Rehabilitation Robotics*, pp. 422-425.

Bashir, A.B.; Bicker, R. & Taylor, P.M. (2004) An Investigation into Different Visual/Tactual Feedback Modes for a Virtual Object Manipulation Task. In: Proc. of the ACM SIGGRAPH Int'l Conf. on Virtual Reality Continuum and its Applications in Industry, pp. 359–362.

Bakker, N.H.; Werkhoven, P.J. & Passenier, P.O. (1993) The effects of proprioception and visual feedback on geographical orientation in virtual environments. *Presence: Teleoperators and Virtual Environments*, vol. 8, pp. 36–53.

Bayazit, O.B.; Song, G. & Amato, N.M. (2000) Enhancing Randomised Motion Planners: Exploring with Haptic Hints. *Proc. 2000 IEEE Int'l Conf. On Robotics & Automation*, San Francisco, pp. 529-536.

Beal, A.C. & Loomis, J.M. (1995) Absolute motion parallax weakly determines visual scale in real and virtual environments. *Proc. SPIE*, Bellingham, WA, vol. 2411, pp. 288–297.

Björk S. (2009) Gameplay Design as Didactic Design. *40th Annual Conference of International Simulation and Gaming Association*, Singapore 2009.

Boothroyd, G.; Dewhurst, P. & Knight, W. (2002) Product Design for Manufacture and Assembly. 2nd Edition. ISBN 0-8247-0584-X.

Bresciani1 J.P; Drewing P. & Ernst1 M.O. (2008) Human Haptic Perception and the Design of Haptic Enhanced Virtual Environments. *Springer Tracts in Advanced Robotics* volm 45, pp. 61-106.

Brooks, F.P. Jr. (1992) Walkthrough project: *Final technical report to National Science Foundation Computer and Information Science and Engineering*, Dept. Computer Science, Univ. North Carolina–Chapel Hill, TR92-026.

Burdea, G.C. (1996) Force and Touch Feedback for Virtual Reality. Wiley Interscience, New York. ISBN-10: 0471021415.

Chan W.Y; Ni D., Pang W.M., Qin J., Chui Y.P., Yu S.C.H. & Heng P.A. (2009) Make It Fun: an Educational game for Ultrasound Guided Needle Insertion Training. *40th Annual Conference of International Simulation and Gaming Association*, Singapore 2009.

Coutee, A.S.; McDermott, S.D. & Bras. B. (2001) A Haptic Assembly and Disassembly Simulation Environment and Associated Computational Load Optimization Techniques. *JOURNAL of Computing and Information Science and Engineering*, vol. 1, pp. 113-122.

Derrington, A.M.; Allen,H.A. & Delicato, L.S. (2004) Visual mechanisms of motion analysis and motion perception, Annu. Rev. Psychol., vol. 55, pp. 181–205.

Lövquist E. & Dreifaldt U. (2006) The design of a haptic exercise for post-stroke arm rehabilitation. *Proc. 6th Intl Conf. Disability, Virtual Reality & Assoc. Tech.*, Esbjerg, Denmark, 2006.

Dominjon L; Perret J & Lecuyer A; (2007) Novel devices and interaction techniques for human scale haptics, Springer-Verlag, pp. 257-266.

Ferrieira, A. & Mavroidis, C. (2006) Virtual Reality and Haptics for Nano Robotics: A Review Study. *IEEE Robotics and Automation Magazine*, Vol. 13, No. 2, pp. 78-92.

Fitts, P.M. (1954) The information capacity of human motor systems in controlling the amplitude of a movement. Journal of Experimental Psychology, vol. 47, 381-391.

Fritschi M; Esen H., Buss M, & Ernst M. (2008) Multi-modal VR Systems scale Haptics. *Springer Tracts in Advanced Robotics*, vol. 45, pp. 179-206.

Gerovichev, O.; Marayong, P. & Okamura, A.M. (2002) The effect of Visual and Haptic Feedback on Manual and Teleoperated Needle Insertion. *Proc. of the 5th Int'l Conf. on Medical Image Computing and Computer-Assisted Intervention-Part I*, vol. 2488, 147-154.

Gupta, R.; Whitney, D. & Zeltzer. D. (1997) Prototyping and Design for Assembly analysis using Multimodal virtual environments. *CAD*, vol. 29, no 8, pp.585-597.

Haeusler, J (1981) Design for Assembly - State-of-the-art. *Proc. of the 2nd Int'l Conf. on Assembly Automation*, Brighton, 109-128, ISBN 0903608162.
Ho, C. & Boothroyd, G. (1979) Design of chamfers for ease of assembly. *Proc. of the 7th Manuf Eng Trans*, North AME Metalwork Res. Conf., 345-354.
Iglesias, R.; Casado, S.; Gutierrez, T.; Garcia-Alonso, A.; Yap, K.M.; Yu, W. & Marshall, A. (2006) A Peer-to-peer Architecture for Collaborative Haptic Assembly. *Proc. of 10th IEEE Int'l Sym. On Distributed Simulation and Real-Time Applications (DS-RT'06)*, pp.25-34.
Immersion Corporation (2008), 801 Fox Lane, San Jose, California 95131 USA. (http://www.immersion.com/)
Johnson, S. & Ogilvie, G. (1972) Work Analysis. The Butterworth Group, London.
Kocherry J, Srimathveeravalli G, Chowriappa A.J., Kesavadas T. Shin G. (2009) Improving Haptic Experience through Biomechanical Measurements. *3rd Joint Eurohaptics Conference and Symposium on Haptic Interfaces for Virtual Environment and Teleoperator Systems*, USA, March, 2009, pp. 362-367.
Lim T., Dewar R., Calis M., Ritchie J.M., Corney J.R., Desmulliez M. (2006) A Structural Assessment of Haptic-based Assembly Processes. *1st International Virtual Manufacturing Workshop (VirMan'06)*, 26th March, Virginia, USA, 29.
Linden Lab (1999) Second Life® virtual world (http://secondlife.com/?v=1)
Louchart S; Lim T & Al-Sulaiman H.M; (2009) Why are video-games relevant test-beds for studying interactivity for Engineers? *40th Annual Conference of International Simulation and Gaming Association*, Singapore 2009.
MacNaughton, Inc. (2008) 1815 NW 169th Place, Suite 3060, Beaverton, OR 97006, USA. http://www.nuvision3d.com
Massie, T. & Salisbury, K. (1994) The PHANTom Haptic Interface: A Device for probing Virtual Objects. *ASME Winter Annual Meeting*, DSC-Vol. 55-1, pp.295-300.
Pearson, E.S. & Kendall, M.G. (1970) Gosset, William Sealy 1876-1937, *Studies in the History of Statistics and Probability*, Charles Griffin and Co., Volume I, pp. 355-404.
Price. B. (1990) Frank and Lillian Gilbreth and the Motion Study Controversy, 1907-1930. In: *A Mental Revolution: Scientific Management since Taylor*, Daniel Nelson, ed. The Ohio State University Press.
Ritchie, J.M.; Dewar, R.G.; Robinson, G.; Simmons, J.E.L. & Ng, F.M. (2006) The Role of Non-intrusive Operator Logging to Support the Analysis and Generation of Product Data using Immersive VR. *Journal of Virtual and Physical Prototyping*, V1, n2, pp. 117-134.
Robinson G.; Ritchie J.M.; Day P.N. & Dewar R.G. (2007) System design and user evaluation of CoStar: an immersive stereoscopic system for cable harness design, *Computer-Aided Design*, 39, pp. 245-257.
Rosenberg, L.B. (1994) Virtual haptic overlays enhance performance in telerpresence tasks. *Proc. SPIE Telemanipulator and Telepresence Technologies Symposium*, pp.99-108, Boston, October 31.
Salisbury, K.; Brock, D.; Massie, T.; Swarup, N. ; & Zilles, C. (1995). Haptic rendering: programming touch interaction with virtual objects. *In Proc. of the 1995 Symposium on interactive 3D Graphics*, Monterey, California, United States, April 09 - 12.

Schaefer, A.T.; Angelo, K.; Spors, H.; Margrie, T.W. (2006). Neuronal oscillations enhance stimulus discrimination by ensuring action potential precision. *PLoS Biol.*, 2006 Jun;4(6):e163.

SensAble Technologies (1993), Inc. 15 Constitution Way Woburn, MA 01801. (http://www.sensable.com/).

Seth, A.; Su, H-J & Vance, J. (2005) A desktop networked haptic VR interface for mechanical assembly. *Proc. of IMECE'05 ASME Int'l Mech. Eng. Congress and Exposition*, pp. 1-8, Nov. 5-11, Orlando, Florida.

Sung, R.C.W, Ritchie, J.M., Lim, T., Medellin, H. World Conference on Innovative VR 2009, WINVR09, February 25-26, 2009, Chalon-sur-Saone, France, Paper 713, ISBN 978-0-7918-3841-9.

Thin, A.G., Hansen, L. McEachen, D. Flow Experience and Mood States whilst Playing Body-Movement Controlled Video Games. Experience in Body-Movement Controlled Video Games. Manuscript under review.

Ueberle M; Mock N. & Buss M. (2004) VISHARD10, a Novel Hyper-Redundant Haptic Interface. *Proc. of the 12th Int'l Sym. on Haptic Interfaces for Virtual Environment and Teleoperator Systems (HAPTICS'04)*, 27-28 March 2004, pp. 58 - 65

Unger, B.J.; Nicoladis, A.; Berkelman, P.J.; Thompson, A.; Klatzky, R.L. & Hollis, R.L.. (2001) Comparison of 3-D Haptic Peg-in-Hole Tasks in Real and Virtual Environments. *Proc. of the IEEE/RSJ Int'l Conf. On Intelligent Robots and Systems*, pp.1751-1756.

VTK, The Visualization ToolKit. (1998) Kitware, Inc., 28 Corporate Drive, Suite 204, Clifton Park, New York 12065, USA. Available: http://www.kitware.com.

Yoshikawa, T.; Kawai, M. & Yoshimoto. K. (2003) Toward Observation of Human Assembly Skill Using Virtual Task Space. *Experimental Robotics VIII*, STAR 5, pp. 540-549.